DeMyer's

THE NEUROLOGIC EXAMINATION

Sixth Edition

Notice

DeMyer's
THE NEUROLOGIC EXAMINATION

A Programmed Text

Sixth Edition

José Biller, MD, FACP, FAAN, FAHA
Professor and Chairman
Department of Neurology
Loyola University Chicago
Stritch School of Medicine
Maywood, Illinois

Gregory Gruener, MD, MBA
Senior Associate Dean, Stritch School of Medicine
Director, Leischner Institute for Medical Education
Leischner Professor of Medical Education
Professor of Neurology, Associate Chairman
Maywood, Illinois

Paul W. Brazis, MD
Professor of Neurology
Mayo Medical School
Department of Neurology and Ophthalmology
Consultant in Neurology and Neuro-Ophthalmology
Mayo Clinic-Jacksonville
Jacksonville, Florida

Mc Graw Hill Medical

New York Chicago San Francisco Lisbon London Madrid Mexico City
Milan New Delhi San Juan Seoul Singapore Sydney Toronto

DeMyer's The Neurologic Examination: A Programmed Text, Sixth Edition

2 3 4 5 6 7 8 9 0 CTP/CTP 1 0 9 8 7 6 5 4 3 2

ISBN 978-0-07-170117-4
MHID 0-07-170117-6

This book was set in Berling by Glyph International.
The editors were Anne M. Sydor and Regina Y. Brown.
The production supervisor was Phil Galea.
Project management was provided by Rajni Pisharody, Glyph International.
The designer was Mary McKeon; the cover was designed by The Gazillion Group; cover image copyright © John W. Karapelou, CMI/Phototake.
China Printing & Translation Services, Ltd. was the printer and binder.

Library of Congress Cataloging-in-Publication Data

Biller, José, 1948- author.
Technique of the neurologic examination : a programmed text/Jose Biller, MD, FACP, FAAN, FAHA, Professor and Chairman, Department of Neurology, Loyola University Chicago, Stritch School of Medicine, Maywood, IL, Gregory Gruener, MD, MBA, Senior Associate Dean, Stritch School of Medicine, Director, Leischner Institute for Medical Education, Leischner Professor of Medical Education, Professor of Neurology, Associate Chairman, Maywood, IL, Paul W. Brazis, MD, Professor of Neurology, Mayo Medical School, Department of Neurology and Ophthalmology, Consultant in Neurology and Neuro-Ophthalmology, Mayo Clinic-Jacksonville, Jacksonville, FL.—Sixth Edition.
p. ; cm.
Neurologic examination
Includes bibliographical references and index.
ISBN-13: 978-0-07-170117-4 (pbk. : alk. paper)
ISBN-10: 0-07-170117-6 (pbk. : alk. paper) 1. Neurologic examination. I. Gruener, Gregory, author. II. Brazis, Paul W., author. III. DeMyer, William, 1924- Technique of the neurologic examination. IV. Title. V. Title: Neurologic examination.
[DNLM: 1. Neurologic Examination—methods—Programmed Instruction. WL 18.2]
RC348.D44 2011
616.8'0475—dc22

2010050656

International Edition: ISBN 978-0-07-176741-5; MHID 0-07-176741-X

...not for their elevated thoughts
Will their books be searched through but for
Some casual sentence, that allows conclusions...

—Bertolt Brecht

CONTENTS

PREFACE to the Sixth Edition

When it came to writing a preface, it was with some uncertainty whether we would compose a preface or a foreword for this edition of *DeMyer's The Neurologic Examination: A Programmed Text*. A preface is typically written by a book's author, while a foreword is an introductory essay by a different person that usually precedes it. The purpose of a preface is for the author to explain to the reader why the book was written or how it came into being while it typically ends with their acknowledgements to those who assisted in its conceptualization, development or who provided the author support through the endeavor. With that background it would seem that we are clearly the "different person" and should limit ourselves to a foreword, but we also have a tale to tell as to how we became involved at Dr. DeMyer's and his family's request.

One of us (JB) when Chairperson of the Department of Neurology at Indiana University School of Medicine not only knew but worked with and frequently collaborated with Dr. William E. DeMyer who was already a legend as a consummate and gifted educator blessed with insight, wisdom, and encyclopedic knowledge. His neuroanatomy course for the neurology residents was considered a highlight of their training and despite his encyclopedic and seemingly photographic memory he still reviewed and prepared before those sessions. This was never interpreted as a sign of uncertainty, but a demonstration of how deeply Dr. DeMyer felt about the importance of what he taught and respect for those he always felt privileged to teach. This book (and another he completed shortly before he died, *Taking the Clinical History; Oxford University Press,* 2009) emphasized his strong belief that the learner needed to be actively involved with their learning and the importance, if not the necessity, of self-observation and of course the need to practice.

It was always Dr. DeMyer's intent to revise and update this textbook, but as he became ill, he realized it may not be possible for him, but may be for others. He hoped to update his text, correct any errors, and improve the illustrations, but as to significant revisions, he did not feel they would be necessary. Those were the hopes he expressed to his family, his publishers and to us before he died on September 20th, 2008. Yet, for we who agreed to undertake this work there was some trepidation as to whether our task of updating or revision would maintain the voice of the author.

When Edith Grossman published her splendid translation of Miguel De Cervantes' *Don Quixote*[1] she expressed consternation ("fear") as to whether she would capture Cervantes' voice and expressed those concerns to Julian Ríos, the Spanish novelist. However, it was his "advice" to her which we took to heart and applied to the task Dr. DeMyer assigned to us.

> *... Cervantes, he said was our most modern writer, and what I had to do was to translate him the way I translated everyone else—that is, the contemporary authors whose works I have brought over into English. Julian's characterization was a revelation; it desacralized the project and*

[1]*Don Quixote* by Miguel De Cervantes. A new translation by Edith Grossman. Harper Perennial, 2005.

> *allowed me, finally to confront the text and find the voice in English. For me this is the essential challenge in translation: hearing,in the most profound way (I mean, to write) the text again in English...*

This 6th edition of the *DeMyer's The Neurologic Examination: A Programmed Text* has been retained in Dr. DeMyer's voice, but updated and refreshed where necessary (Bill would have accepted nothing less) and our publishers were of immense help in updating the formatting of the text and its illustrations. Presentation was always important to Dr. DeMyer and we all believe he would be happy with these changes. As we undertook this update what proved to be a pleasant surprise and source of satisfaction for us was that since the first edition in 1994, the text has essentially stood the test of time and fulfilled Dr. DeMyer's hoped for outcome in his preface to his fifth edition,

> *A masterful history and examination, conducted with competence and grace, leads to the physician's pleasure in discovery and to the patient's trust in the physician. No technologic procedure and computerized form can ever replace the mutual knowing process and bonding that occur during the clinical encounter. Mastery of the neurologic examination provides a giant step in achieving the clinical competence that fosters the maximum reward for you and the maximum benefit for your patients throughout your career.*

We are forever grateful to Dr. William E. DeMyer for his scholarship and professional competency that exemplified the very highest qualities of the physician, scientist, and teacher. It is our sincere wish that the readers of this textbook embrace Dr. DeMyer's hope for all of those who practice medicine and for the patients in our care; each encounter should always begin and end with our patients foremost in our mind. Oh, and by the way, this is our foreword.

José Biller, MD
Gregory Gruener, MD, MBA
Paul W. Brazis, MD

PREFACE to the First Edition

The purpose of this textbook is threefold: (1) to teach how to conduct a neurologic examination, (2) to review the anatomy and physiology for interpreting the examination, and (3) to show which laboratory tests help to clarify the clinical problem. This is not a differential diagnosis text or a systematic description of diseases.

Anyone who sets out to write a textbook should place the manuscript on one knee and a student on the other. When the student squirms, sighs, or gives a wrong answer, the author has erred. He should correct it right then, before the ink dries. That is the way I have written this text, on the basis of feedback from the students.

The peril of student-on-the-knee teaching is that, even though the student moves his lips, the words and voice remain the teacher's. To escape from ventriloquism, my text relies strongly on self-observation and induction. First, you learn to observe yourself, not as Narcissus, but as a sample of every man. Whenever possible, you study living flesh, its look, its feel, and its responses. Why study a textbook picture to learn the range of ocular movements when you can hold up a hand mirror? Why memorize the laws of diplopia if you can do a simple experiment on yourself whenever you need to refresh your memory? In the best tradition of science, these techniques supplant the printed word as the source of knowledge. The text becomes a way of extending your own perceptions, of looking at the world through the eyes of experience.

Because programmed instruction is the best way for the learner to judge whether learning has taken place, most of the text is programmed. The student is not abandoned to guess whether he has learned something; the program makes him prove that he has. Programming, if abused or overdone, becomes incredibly dull and unmercifully slow. The reader is required to inspect each grain of sand but should have been shown the whole shoreline at a glance. Some programs err by bristling with objectivity, causing one to ask, "Isn't there a human being around here somewhere? Didn't someone think this, decide it, maybe even guess at it a little?" For interludes, I use quotations, anecdotes, and poetry. I even stoop to mnemonics. Sometimes I cajole without pretending, as is customary in textbooks, that the pages have been purified, relieved of an author. I am very much here, poking my head out of a paragraph now and then or peering at you through an asterisk. When I see that you are weary from filling in blanks, I offer some whimsy. When you overflow with something to say, I ask for an essay answer. Sometimes you are invited to anticipate the text, to match wits against the problem without the spoon. At all times as you practice the neurologic examination, I stand at your elbow, guiding your moves and interpretations. You should be able to do an accomplished neurologic examination when you finish the book. And lastly, I include references. Only one reader in a hundred uses them? I am interested in him, too, in his precious curiosity.

These then are the secrets: a lot of self-observation, a lot of programming, some irony and humor, a few editorials, and occasionally a summarizing paragraph, like this one. And as the leaven, lest they vanish from medical education, reminders of the bittersweet flowers of the mind, of tenderness, of understanding and compassion, like this stanza from Yeats, because it is perhaps all that should preface a text like this, into which I have poured the best teaching that I can offer; yet the wish always exceeds the result, ah me, by far:

Had I the heavens' embroidered cloths,
Enwrought with gold and silver light,
The blue and the dim and the dark cloths
Of night and light and the half light,
I would spread the cloths under your feet;
But I, being poor, have only my dreams;
I have spread my dreams under your feet;
Tread softly because you tread on my dreams.

To the many colleagues who have shared their knowledge with me over the years, I am deeply grateful. I especially want to thank Dr. Alexander T. Ross, my own preceptor in clinical neurology, and many friends in the basic disciplines of neurology, Drs. Ralph Reitan, Charles Ferster, Sidney Ochs, Wolfgang Zeman, and Jans Muller. For their day-to-day help I thank my wife, Dr. Marian DeMyer, Dr. Mark Dyken, and the many medical students, interns, and residents who suffered through the stuttering phases of the programming. I also thank Miss Irene Baird, who meticulously, maternally made the drawings; Mrs. Faith Halstead, who typed and retyped the burgeoning manuscript; medical artist James Glore; and photographer Joseph Demma.

William E. DeMyer, MD

PREPARATION FOR THE TEXT

We assume that you know basic neuroanatomy and neurophysiology (but we review them anyway). The text teaches the necessary mental and manual skills for the neurologic examination (NE). Your teachers, then freed from teaching these skills by lecturing, can use precious class hours solely to examine patients (Pts). Then, if you can go directly after classes to the clinics and wards, you have the ideal situation for learning the NE.

At the outset, we find that students want to know just what constitutes an NE? Thus we start this text by outlining and demonstrating a full NE. Of course, you can't do the examination now, but you can use the outline in two ways: (1) refer back to it at the end of each chapter, to fit what you have learned into the total examination; (2) take it to the wards and clinics as a guide until you can wean yourself from it.

You must have on hand basic examining equipment (listed shortly) and some learning aids: colored pencils, a hand mirror, and for Chapter 4 a 2- to 3-in. foam rubber ball. Get all the items before starting.

Do the text in order. Skipping around invites confusion because each new step presumes mastery of the previous steps. Allow approximately one hour for each nine pages you want to study.

Because the text requires inspection of one's self and others, study in your own living quarters, preferably with a partner. **Do all tests and make all observations called for.** The ***doing*** results in active, permanent learning by developing your own powers of observation and manual skills. Most of your education to this point has consisted of memorizing lists or concepts compiled by someone else. Now you have to learn how to learn directly from the Pt through your own eyes, ears, and touch. That's what requires all of the ***doing*** and makes this text unique.

TABLE NE-1 • Abbreviations

AP	Anteroposterior
ARAS	Ascending reticular activating system
BE	Branchial efferent
BP	Blood pressure
C	Cervical
CAT	Computerized axial tomography
Cm	Centimeter
CNS	Central nervous system
Cps	Cycles per second
CrN	Cranial nerve
CrNs	Cranial nerves
CSF	Cerebrospinal fluid
EEG	Electroencephalogram
EMG	Electromyogram
Ex	Examiner
F	False
GSA	General somatic afferent
GSE	General somatic efferent
GVA	General visceral afferent
GVE	General visceral efferent
ICA	Internal carotid artery
L	Lateral, left, or lumbar
LMN	Lower motor neuron
LP	Lumbar puncture
MLF	Medial longitudinal fasciculus
Mm	Millimeters
MRA	Magnetic resonance angiography
MSR	Muscle stretch reflex
NE	Neurologic examination
O_2	Oxygen
OFC	Occipitofrontal circumference
Pt	Patient
R	Right
RBC	Red blood cells
RF	Reticular formation
S	Sacral
SA	Somatic afferent
SCA	Superior cerebellar artery
SCM	Sternocleidomastoid muscle
SSSS	Solely special sensory set (cranial nerves I, II, and VIII)
SVA	Special visceral afferent
T	True or thoracic
TNR	Tonic neck reflex
UMN	Upper motor neuron
V	Vertical
WBC	White blood cells

OUTLINE OF THE STANDARD NEUROLOGIC EXAMINATION

The text first outlines the NE of the conscious, responsive Pt and then of the unconscious Pt. Beginning with Chapter 1, the text then explains how to do each step.

I. INTRODUCTION

A. How the history guides the examination

The primary role of the examination becomes the testing of hypotheses derived from the history.

—**William Landau, MD**

1. You complete much of the NE during the history. Assess the Pt's word articulation, content of speech, and overall mental status. Inspect the facial features. Inspect the eye movements, blinking, and the relation of the palpebral fissures to the iris and look for en or exophthalmos. Inspect the degree of facial movement and expression and note any asymmetry. Observe how the Pt swallows saliva and breathes. Inspect the posture and look for tremors and involuntary movements.
2. Although you must do a minimum basic NE on every Pt, the history and preliminary observations focus attention on specific systems: motor or sensory systems, cranial nerves (CrNs), or cerebral functions. If the history suggests a spinal level lesion, successively test each dermatome for a sensory level and test the perianal region for loss or preservation of sacral sensation. If the history suggests a cerebral lesion, emphasize tests for memory, aphasia, apraxia, and agnosia.
3. Reproduce any circumstances, as discovered during the history, that trigger or aggravate symptoms:
   a. Dizziness when standing up: check for orthostatic hypotension.
   b. Episodic numbness and tingling in the extremities, syncope, or suspected epilepsy: Ask the Pt to hyperventilate for full 3 minutes.
   c. Weakness in climbing stairs: watch the Pt climb stairs.
   d. Trouble swallowing: give the Pt liquids and solids to swallow.
   e. Pathologic fatigability, particularly of CrN muscles: have the Pt make 100 repetitive eye movements and measure the width of the palpebral fissure at rest and following 1 minute of upward gaze.

B. How to ensure an orderly, complete examination

Younger practitioners are reported to be deficient in physical diagnosis. Unless you do an orderly NE, you will forget some part of it. Neurologists will complete the same tests, although the sequence may differ. Avoid using shortcuts. To remember the sequence we recommend, **lay out your instruments in the order of use.** Replace each instrument in your bag as you finish with it. When you have replaced every instrument, you will have done a complete examination. Lay out your instruments in this way:

Order	Instruments	Use
1.	Flexible steel measuring tape scored inmetric units	Measuring occipitofrontal and body circumferences, size of skin lesions, length of extremities, etc.
2.	Stethoscope	Auscultation over the neck vessels, eyes, and cranium for bruits
3.	Flashlight with rubber adapter	Pupillary reflexes, inspection of pharynx, and transillumination of the head of infants
4.	Transparent mm ruler	Measuring diameter of pupils and skin lesions
5.	Ophthalmoscope	Examining ocular media and fundi and skin surface for beads of sweat
6.	Tongue blades	Three per Pt: one for depressing tongue, one for eliciting a gag reflex, and one broken transversely for eliciting abdominal and plantar reflexes
7.	Opaque vial of coffee grounds*	Testing sense of smell
8.	Opaque vials of salt and sugar**	Testing taste
9.	Otoscope	Examining auditory canal and drum
10.	Tuning fork	Testing vibratory sensation and hearing (256 cps recommended) and temperature discrimination (see page 385)
11.	10 cc syringe	Caloric irrigation of the ear
12.	Cotton wisp	One end rolled for eliciting corneal reflex, the other loose for testing light touch
13.	Two stoppered tubes	Testing hot and cold discrimination
14.	Disposable straight pins	Testing pain sensation
15.	Reflex hammer	Eliciting muscle stretch reflexes and muscle percussion for myotonia
16.	Penny, nickel, dime, key, paper clip, and safety pin	Testing for astereognosis
17.	Blood pressure cuff	Routine blood pressure and orthostatic hypotension

*or standardized olfactory testing

**or standard taste test

II. MENTAL STATUS EXAMINATION

A. General behavior and appearance

Is the Pt normal, hyperactive, agitated, quiet, or immobile? Is the Pt neat or slovenly? Does the Pt dress in accordance with age, peers, sex, and background?

B. Stream of talk: does the Pt converse normally?

Is the speech rapid, incessant, under great pressure, or is it slow and lacking in inflection and spontaneity? Is the Pt tangential, discursive, or unable to reach the conversational goal?

C. Mood and affective responses

Is the Pt euphoric, agitated, inappropriately gay, giggling or silent, weeping, or angry? Does the Pt's mood appropriately reflect the topic of the conversation? Is the Pt emotionally labile, histrionic, expansive, or overtly depressed?

D. Content of thought

Does the Pt correctly perceive reality or have illusions, hallucinations, delusions, misinterpretations, and obsessions? Is the Pt preoccupied with bodily complaints, fears of cancer or heart disease, or other phobias? Does the Pt suffer delusions of persecution, surveillance, and control by malicious persons or forces?

E. Intellectual capacity

Is the Pt bright, average, dull, or obviously demented or mentally retarded?

F. Sensorium

1. Consciousness
2. Attention span
3. Orientation for time, place, and person
4. Memory, recent and remote
5. Calculation
6. Fund of information
7. Insight, judgment, and planning

III. SPEECH: DOES THE PT HAVE DYSPHONIA, DYSARTHRIA, DYSPROSODY, OR DYSPHASIA?

A. Dysphonia

Difficulty in producing voice sounds (phonating).

B. Dysarthria

Difficulty in articulating the individual sounds or the units (phonemes) of speech, the f's, r's, g's, vowels, consonants, labials (CrN VII), gutturals (CrN X), and linguals (CrN XII).

C. Dysprosody

Difficulty with the melody and rhythm of speech, the accent of syllables, the inflections, intonations, and pitch of the voice.

D. Dysphasia

Difficulty in expressing or understanding words as the symbols of communication.

IV. HEAD AND FACE

A. Inspect

1. What general impression does the Pt's face make? Do the features suggest a diagnostic syndrome? Any abnormalities in motility and emotional expression?
2. Inspect the head for shape and symmetry.
3. Inspect the hair of scalp, eyebrows, and beard.
4. Compare the palpebral fissures of the two eyes.
5. Inspect contours and proportions of nose, mouth, chin, and ears for malformations.

B. Palpate

For mature Pts, palpate the skull for lumps, depressions, or tenderness and palpate the temporal arteries. For infants, look for asymmetries palpate the fontanelles and sutures and record the occipitofrontal circumference.

C. Auscultate

For bruits over the neck vessels, eyes, temples, and mastoid processes.

D. Transilluminate

Attempt to transilluminate the skull of young infants.

V. CRANIAL NERVES

A. Optic group

CrNs II, III, IV, and VI

1. Inspect the widths of palpebral fissures, the interorbital distance, and the relation of lid margins to the limbus. Look for ptosis and en- or exophthalmos.
2. Visual functions: Test each eye separately for acuity (central fields) by newsprint or the Snellen chart and test peripheral fields by confrontation. Test for inattention to simultaneous visual stimuli, if a cerebral lesion is suspected.
3. Ocular motility: Test range of ocular movements and smoothness of pursuit as Pt's eyes follow your finger through all fields of gaze. During convergence, check for miosis. Do the cover-and-uncover test. Check for nystagmus and note any effects of eye movements on it.
4. Record size of pupils. Test pupillary light reflexes.
5. Do ophthalmoscopy. Record presence or absence of venous pulsations.

B. Branchiomotor group and tongue

Branchiomotor CrNs V, VII, IX, X, and XI and somatomotor CrN XII for the tongue

1. **CrN V:** Inspect the masseter and temporalis muscle bulk and palpate masseter muscles when the Pt bites.
2. **CrN VII:** Test forehead wrinkling, eyelid closure, mouth retraction, whistling or puffing out of cheeks, and wrinkling of skin over the neck (platysma action). Listen to labial articulations. Check for Chvostek's sign in selected cases.
3. **CrN IX and X:** Listen for phonation, articulation (labial, lingual, and palatal sounds) and check swallowing, gag reflex, and palatal elevation. Remember the gag reflex is often absent in healthy adults, and studies in stroke patients have not shown a consistent relation between an absent gag reflex and swallowing problems.
4. **CrN XI:** inspect sternocleidomastoid and trapezius contours and test strength of head movements and shoulder shrugging
5. **CrN XII:** lingual articulations, midline protrusion, lateral movements. Inspect for atrophy, and fasciculations.
6. If the history suggests pathologic fatigability, request 100 repetitive movements (eye blinks, etc.), and tests for diplopia by prolonged lateral gaze 7. Assess the rate, regularity, depth, and ease of respiration.

C. Special sensory group

CrNs I, VII, and VIII (CrN II already tested)

1. **Olfaction (CrN I):** Use aromatic, nonirritating substance, and test each nostril separately having the patients with eyes closed.
2. **Taste (CrN VII):** Use salt or sugar (test if CrN VII lesion is suspected).
3. **Hearing (CrN VIII):**
   a. Do otoscopy.
   b. Assess threshold and acuity by noting the Pt's ability to hear conversational speech and to hear a tuning fork, a watch tick, or finger rustling.
   c. If history or preceding tests suggest a hearing deficit, perform the air–bone conduction test of Rinne and the vertex lateralizing test of Weber.
   d. If the history suggests a cerebral lesion, test for auditory inattention to bilateral simultaneous stimuli and sound localization by using finger rustling.
   e. In infants, uncooperative, or unconscious Pts, try the auditopalpebral reflex as a crude screening test.

4. **Vestibular function (CrN VIII):** If the history indicates the need, test for the vestibulo-ocular reflex with the doll's eye maneuver or caloric irrigation and test for positional nystagmus.

D. Somatic sensation of the face

Test the sensation of the trigeminal area now to obviate returning to the face after examining the Pt's anogenital area and feet

1. Corneal reflex (CrN V–VII arc)
2. Light touch over the three divisions of CrN V
3. Temperature discrimination over the three divisions of CrN V
4. Pain perception over the three divisions of CrN V
5. Test buccal mucosal sensation in selected cases

VI. SOMATIC MOTOR SYSTEM

A. Inspection

1. Inspect the Pt's posture and general activity level and look for tremors or other involuntary movements.
2. Gait testing: free walking, toe and heel walking, tandem walking, deep knee bend; have a child hop on each foot, skip, and run.
3. Undress the Pt and assess the somatotype (the build or body Gestalt) but preserve modesty with drapes or underwear.
4. Observe the size and contour of the muscles. Look for atrophy, fasciculations, hypertrophy, asymmetries, and joint malalignments.
5. Search the entire skin surface for lesions, in particular neurocutaneous stigmata such as café-au-lait spots.

B. Palpate muscles

If on inspection they seem atrophic, or hypertrophic or the history suggests tenderness or spasms

C. Strength testing (Table 7-2)

1. **Shoulder girdle:** Try to press the arms down after the Pt abducts them to shoulder height. Look for scapular winging.
2. **Upper extremities:** Test biceps, triceps, wrist dorsiflexors, grip, and the strength of finger abduction and extension.
3. **Abdominal muscles:** Have the Pt do a sit up. Watch for umbilical migration.
4. **Lower extremities:** Test hip flexors, abductors and adductors, knee flexors, foot dorsiflexors, invertors, and evertors. (The previous deep knee bend tested the knee extensors, and toe walking tested the plantar flexors.)
5. Grade strength on a scale from 0 to 5 or describe as *paralysis* or *severe, moderate,* or *minimal weakness,* or *normal.* Record the pattern of any weakness such as proximal versus distal, right versus left, or upper extremity versus lower extremity.

D. Muscle tone and range of movements

Manipulate the joints to test for spasticity, clonus, rigidity or hypotonia, and range of movements.

E. Muscle stretch (deep) reflexes

Grade responses 0 to 4 (Table 7-3) and designate whether clonic. See Fig. NE-1.

1. Jaw jerk (CrN V afferent; CrN V efferent)
2. Biceps reflex (C5–6)
3. Brachioradialis reflex (C5-6)
4. Triceps reflex (C7–8)
5. Finger flexion reflex (C7–T1)
6. Quadriceps reflex (knee jerk; L2–4)
7. Medial Hamstrings reflex (L5–S1)
8. Triceps surae reflex (ankle jerk; S1–2)
9. Toe flexion reflex (S1–2)

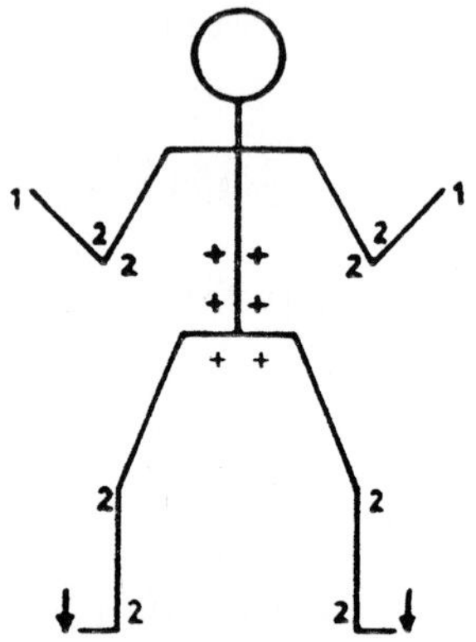

FIGURE NE-1. Stick figure for recording muscle stretch reflexes and abdominal, cremasteric, and plantar reflexes.

F. Percussion of muscle

Percuss the thenar eminence for percussion myotonia and test for a myotonic grip if the Pt has generalized muscular weakness.

G. Skin and muscle (superficial) reflexes

1. Abdominal skin and muscle reflexes (upper quadrants T8–9; lower quadrants T11–12) elicited by scraping the skin tangential to or toward the umbilicus. Look for umbilical migration (Beevor's sign) in Pts suspected of having thoracic spinal cord lesions.
2. Cremasteric reflex (afferent L1; efferent L2) elicited by scratching the skin of the medial thigh.
3. Anal pucker reflex (S4–5) and bulbocavernosus reflex (S3–S4) in Pts suspected of having sacral or cauda equina lesions.
4. Elicit the plantar reflex (Babinski's maneuver; afferent Sl; efferent L5–S1–2).

H. Cerebellar system (gait and hypotonia tested previously)

1. Finger-to-nose and rapid alternating hand movements
2. Heel-to-knee movement

I. Nerve root stretching tests

1. Do leg raising tests in Pts with low back or leg pain:
   a. The straight-knee leg raising test (Lasegue's sign)
   b. The bent-knee leg raising test (Kernig's sign)
2. In Pts with suspected meningeal irritation, test for nuchal rigidity and concomitant leg flexion (Brudzinski's sign) and do the leg raising tests.

VII. SOMATIC SENSORY SYSTEM

A. Superficial sensory modalities (include trigeminal area if not previously tested)

1. Light touch over hands, trunk, and feet
2. Temperature discrimination over hands, trunk, and feet
3. Pain perception over hands, trunk, and feet

B. Deep sensory modalities

1. Test vibration perception at fingers and toes
2. Test position sense of fingers and toes by using the fourth digits
3. Test for astereognosis
4. Do the directional scratch test
5. Romberg (swaying) test

C. Determine the distribution pattern of any sensory loss

Dermatomal, peripheral nerve(s), plexus, central pathway, or nonorganic.

VIII. CEREBRAL FUNCTIONS

A. Do a complete mental status examination, emphasizing tests of the sensorium (Section II of this outline).

B. Test higher level sensory functions, if the history or mental status examination suggests a cerebral lesion: test for graphagnosia, finger agnosia, poor two-point discrimination, right or left disorientation, topagnosia, and tactile, auditory, and visual inattention to bilateral simultaneous stimuli. Test for tactile inattention to simultaneous ipsilateral stimulation of face and hand and of foot and hand.

IX. CASE SUMMARY

A. Write a three-line summary of the pertinent positive historical and physical findings. (If you can't summarize it in three lines, you don't understand the problem.)

B. Write down a provisional clinical diagnosis and outline the differential diagnosis.

C. Make a list of the clinical problems.

D. Develop a sequential plan of management for

1. Diagnostic tests to differentiate the diagnostic possibilities
2. Therapy: state the therapeutic goals
3. Management of the emotional, educational, and socioeconomic problems that the illness causes the Pt
4. Identification of and prophylaxis for other persons now known as "at risk" because of the Pt's illness, if the illness is infectious, genetic, or environmentally induced

NEUROLOGIC EXAMINATION OF THE UNCONSCIOUS PATIENT

I. HISTORY

For the unknown Pt brought in off the street, two examiners are desirable, one for the emergency management of the Pt, and the other to obtain a history. Contact family, friends, police, the Pt's past physicians, or anyone who witnessed the events when the Pt lost consciousness. Ask about:

1. Possibility of head trauma.
2. A seizure disorder.
3. Insulin/diabetes mellitus, alcohol.
4. A recent change in mood, behavior, thinking, or neurologic condition.
5. Access to depressant medications or street drugs.
6. Allergies, insect bites, and other causes of anaphylactic shock.
7. Heart, liver, lung, or kidney disease.
8. Past hospitalizations for serious health problems.
9. Consider red herrings. Ask about any signs, such as abnormal pupils or strabismus, that may antedate the current episode of unconsciousness and confuse the diagnosis.

II. IMMEDIATE ABCDEE RITUAL FOR THE EXAMINATION OF THE COMATOSE PATIENT

On first approaching the comatose Pt, the examiner must follow a specific ritual, summarized by the **ABCDEE** mnemonic. This ritual detects any of the five **H's** that threaten the brain: Hypoxia, Hypotension, Hypoglycemia, Hyperthermia, and Herniation.

1. A and B = Airway and Breathing. Ensure that the Pt has an open airway and is breathing. Otherwise the brain, which requires a continuous supply of O_2 and glucose, will start to die within 5 minutes of total oxygen deprivation.
2. C = Circulation. The blood must circulate to deliver O_2 and glucose to the brain. Breathing and circulation must be restored within minutes.
3. D = Dextrose. The circulating blood must contain enough dextrose to nourish the brain.
4. EE = Examine the Eyes. Examination of pupillary size and reactions, the optic fundi, and the position and movement of the eyes spontaneously and in response to the vestibulo-ocular reflex reveals more about the neurologic status of the unconscious Pt than any other steps in the examination. Fixed pupils and fixed eyes indicate trouble.
5. Measure the body temperature.

III. PHYSICAL MANAGEMENT OF THE COMATOSE PATIENT

1. **Check respiration:** Observe the rate and rhythm of respiration. Note the Pt's color and verify air exchange by inspection, palpation, or auscultation. Look for suprasternal retraction and abdominal respiration. For inspiratory stridor, pull the mandible forward and reposition the Pt. For apnea, intubate and assist ventilation with an Ambu bag or ventilator and O_2 as needed. Note any odors such as alcohol. Before any neck maneuvers, stabilize the neck and spine, in case the Pt has had a neck injury.
2. **Check circulation:** Palpate and auscultate the precordium. If the Pt has no heartbeat, start cardiac resuscitation. Palpate the carotid and femoral pulses. Inspect for jugular vein distention and pedal edema. Take blood pressure.
   a. With hypotension, treat for shock. Secure an intravenous line and restore blood volume with normal saline or, Ringer's lactate, or whole blood or blood substitutes. See Section IV for processing of a blood sample.

b. With hypertension, consider a heart or brain attack (acute stroke) or hypertensive encephalopathy as the cause for the unconsciousness. Consider antihypertensive medication, but lower the blood pressure gradually over hours.

3. **Check blood sugar level:** Prick the Pt's finger for a glucose oxidase tape test (Dextrostix). Give 50 mL of 50% glucose intravenously stat for demonstrated or suspected hypoglycemia. Add 100 mg of thiamine daily if the Pt is suspected of being an alcoholic.
4. **Check the eyes:** Record the pupillary size in millimeters. Use a scale. Do not guess. Check the pupillary light reflex. With unilaterally or bilaterally dilated pupils that do not react to light, notify a neurosurgeon stat.
   a. Inspect for ptosis and spontaneous blinking and perform the eyelid release test and corneal reflex.
   b. Examine ocular alignment, position, and motility:
      i. Record alignment and the position of the eyes.
      ii. Record any spontaneous movements of the eyes.
      iii. Check the vestibulo-ocular reflex by the doll's eye test, unless a cervical injury is suspected. Otherwise, do caloric irrigation, if no ocular movements are elicited.
      iv. Do ophthalmoscopy. Record presence or absence of venous pulsations and the condition of the optic disc. Active venous pulsations virtually exclude increased intracranial pressure as the cause of unconsciousness.
   c. Test faciociliary and spinociliary reflexes.
   d. Remove contact lenses to preserve the corneas.
   e. Consider administering naloxone, if pinpoint pupils suggest opiate intoxication.
   f. Do not instill pupillo-active drugs.
5. **Record the Pt's temperature.**
6. **Inspect and palpate the Pt's head:** Look for localized edema or swelling from recent trauma. Look for blood behind the ear (Battle's sign) and around the eyes (raccoon eyes) and for blood or cerebrospinal fluid from the nose. Do an otologic examination to look for blood behind the eardrum, perforated tympanic membrane, or cerebrospinal fluid otorrhea.
7. **Test for nuchal rigidity:** Avoid neck manipulation, if a neck injury is suspected. In that case, obtain cervical spine films.
8. Inspect the Pt for persistent diagnostic postures, spontaneous movements, or patterned or repetitive movements:
   a. Note whether the Pt makes spontaneous and equal movements of the face and all four extremities or lies still in a flaccid or compliant, dumped-in-a-heap posture, indicating deep coma or flaccid quadriparesis.
   b. Look for a predominant posture:
      i. Persistent deviation of the eyes and head
      ii. Opisthotonus
      iii. Decerebrate (extensor) or decorticate (flexor) posturing
      iv. Clenched jaws or immobile neck or extremities, indicating tetanus
   c. Check specifically for hemiplegia by looking for paralysis of the lower part of the face on one side and of the ipsilateral extremities, as opposed to spontaneous or pain-induced movements on the opposite side.
      i. The affected muscles in acute hemiplegia are usually flaccid (hypotonic). Do the eyelid release test. Look for flaccidity of the cheek manifested by retraction on inspiration and puffing out during expiration. Inflict pain by supraorbital compression to check for unilateral absence of grimacing. Test muscle tone by passive manipulation of all extremities and do the wrist-, arm-, and leg-dropping tests.
      ii. Test the intact side of the hemiplegic Pt for **paratonia (gegenhalten).** Record the result of tonus testing *as normal, flaccid, spastic, rigid, paratonia,*

or flexibilitas cerea (waxy flexibility). Waxy flexibility occurs in catatonic schizophrenia and some organic encephalopathies.

d. Look for cyclic activities such as shivering, chewing movements, and tremors. Look for subtle manifestations of epilepsy such as eyelid fluttering, mouth twitching, myoclonic jerks, and finger or toe twitching.

9. **Strip the Pt completely:** Empty all of the Pt's pockets, purse, wallet, or belongings. Look for Identacards for diabetes or epilepsy, medications, suicide notes, or drug paraphernalia.
10. **Search the entire skin surface:** Look for needle marks indicating subcutaneous injections of insulin or intravenous injections, bruises, petechiae, entry wounds, and turgor. Roll the Pt over and check the back.
11. **Elicit the muscle stretch reflexes:** Begin with the glabellar tap to elicit the orbicularis oculi reflexes. Next, elicit the jaw jerk and work down through the customary stretch reflexes. Directly compare the reflexes on both sides of the body.
12. **Try to elicit Chvostek's sign:** Tap on the face at the point anterior to the ear and just below the zygomatic bone.
13. **Elicit the superficial reflexes:** Abdominal, cremasteric, and plantar reflexes.
14. **Attempt to elicit primitive reflexes:** Sucking, and lip-pursing reflexes, grasp reflexes, forced groping, and traction responses.
15. **Complete the physical examination:** Abdominal palpation and percussion. Percuss for a distended bladder.
16. **Initiate monitoring process and address Glasgow Coma Scale** (Sum totalling between 3 and 15): See Fig. 12-1
    a. Monitor pupillary size, equality and response to light, pulse, blood pressure, respiration, and temperature continuously or at regular frequent intervals. Consult a neurosurgeon about inserting an intracranial pressure monitor, if increased intracranial pressure is suspected.
    b. Record the Pt's level of consciousness by responses to voice, loud sound, light, and pain. Check the responses to pain inflicted by compression of the supraorbital notch and nail beds of all four extremities. Record the extremity response as *none, extension, flexion, appropriate brushing,* or *movement on command.*
    c. Proposed guideline for the neurologic examination in patients with altered levels of consciousness (Fleck and Biller, 2004, Table NE-2).

TABLE NE-2 · Guidelines for Neurologic Examination in Patients with Altered Levels of Consciousness

1. Mental Status
   a. Level of arousal
   b. Response to auditory stimuli (including voice)
   c. Response to visual stimuli
   d. Response to noxious stimuli applied both centrally and each limb
2. Cranial Nerves
   a. Response to visual threat
   b. Pupillary light reflex
   c. Oculocephalic (doll's eyes) reflex
   d. Vestibulo-ocular (caloric testing) reflex
   e. Corneal reflex
3. Motor Function
   a. Voluntary movements
   b. Reflex withdrawal
   c. Spontaneous and involuntary movements
   d. Tone (resistance to passive manipulation)
4. Reflexes
   a. Muscle stretch reflexes
   b. Plantar responses
5. Sensation (to noxious stimulation)

IV. LABORATORY TESTS FOR UNCONSCIOUS PATIENTS

1. Draw blood sample and anchor intravenous catheter or central line, as needed:
   a. Blood sugar (in addition to preliminary dextrose test tape)
   b. Complete blood cell count and hematocrit
   c. Blood urea nitrogen
   d. Arterial blood gases, pH, and osmolality
   e. Electrolytes (Na, K, Ca, and Cl)
   f. TSH
   g. Toxicology screen on blood and urine
   h. Typing and cross-matching
2. Place a vial of the Pt's serum in the refrigerator for later chemical or toxicologic testing, as indicated by new information.
3. Obtain urine specimen. Use an external bag or catheterize, if the Pt is in-continent or has a distended bladder. Freeze a sample of urine for later testing, as indicated by new information. Test the first specimen for:
   a. Specific gravity
   b. Sugar and ketones
   c. Protein
   d. Consider a toxicology screen
4. Insert a nasogastric tube or orogastric tube (if patient suspected of having a skull base fracture or nasal injury) and collect stomach contents in case the Pt has ingested poison or fails to improve and the diagnosis remains obscure. Save a sample of the aspirate for toxicology screening. However, inserting the tube may induce vomiting or gagging, thereby increasing the intrathoracic and the intracranial pressure.
5. Consider immediate computed tomography (CT) or MRI of the head.
6. Consider electroencephalographic monitoring, if a postictal state or status epilepticus is suspected.

V. MAKE A PROVISIONAL DIAGNOSIS

At the very least, assign the Pt to one of the five basic etiologic types of coma: *intracranial lesion, toxic-metabolic disorder, anoxia, ischemia,* or *mental illness.* See Fig. NE-2.

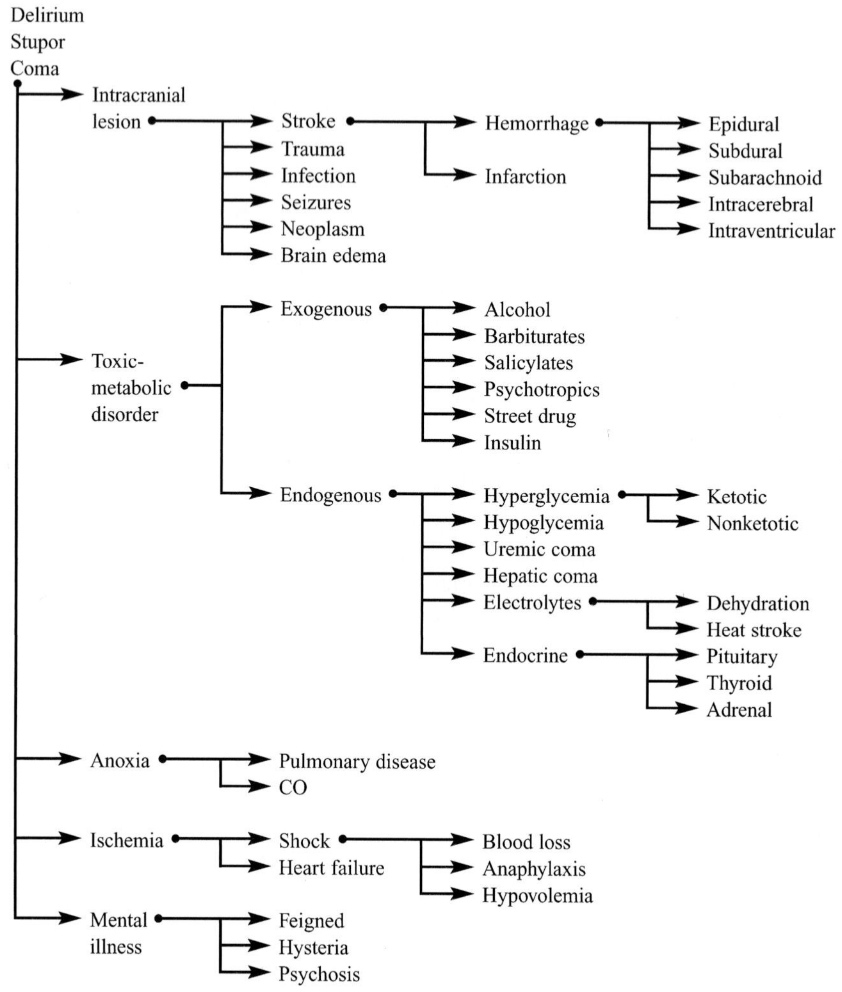

FIGURE NE-2. Categories for the differential diagnosis of the unconscious patient.

VI. SELECT THE SAFEST AND MOST CRITICAL TESTS TO CONFIRM OR REJECT YOUR PROVISIONAL DIAGNOSIS

Additional neurologic tests to consider are magnetic resonance imaging (MRI), lumbar puncture (LP), and angiography. In general, CT or MRI should precede the LP because the scan may disclose the diagnosis or impending brain herniation, making the tap unnecessary or dangerous. Obtain radiographs of the cervical spine, if trauma is suspected.

BIBLIOGRAPHY

Fleck JD, Biller J. Tips on the neurologic examination. Basic neurologic life support, James J. Corbett, Ed., BC Decker, Inc. 2004 236–257.

1 Examination of the Face and Head

Disease is of antiquity and nothing about it changes. It is we who change as we learn to recognize what was formerly imperceptible.

—Jean Martin Charcot (1825–1893)

I. INTRODUCTION TO THE NEUROLOGICAL EXAMINATION

A. Symptoms and signs of neurologic disease

Diseases that affect the nervous system manifest by *mental, motor,* or *sensory* symptoms and signs and by abnormal body contours (Fig. 1-1).

B. Steps in the neurologic examination

1. The neurologic examination (NE) consists of a series of simple, standardized steps. Each step focuses on a specific, readable end point. Most steps test a known neuroanatomic circuit. As end points, the examiner (Ex) selects:
   a. Simple behaviors, such as a pupil constricting to light or a finger flexing.
   b. Complex behaviors, such as walking, speaking, or writing.
   c. Specific body contours, such as head size or shape.
2. The Ex compares the result of each step with a "standard person" of like age, sex, and culture and judges each result as *normal, borderline,* or *abnormal.*
3. The steps use four types of operations: *inspections, questions, requests,* and *maneuvers.*
   a. **Inspections** disclose the patient's (Pt's) bodily contours and spontaneous and elicited behaviors.
   b. **Questions** determine the Pt's mental status and sensory perceptions.
   c. **Requests** or **commands** test the Pt's volitional responses.
   d. **Maneuvers** impose stimuli to elicit sensations and reflexes.

C. The NE as standardized assessment of designated behaviors

1. For the NE, we may define behavior as *any detectable change produced by neural activation of an effector.* The neural activation may arise voluntarily or reflexly.
2. Because only two types of effectors exist, namely *glands* and *muscles,* humans can produce behaviors by only two actions: by secreting something and by adjusting the length of their muscle fibers.
   a. By secreting we produce sweat, tears, saliva, mucus, hormones and digestive juices, and semen.

NEUROLOGIC SYMPTOMS AND SIGNS: Mental, Motor, and Sensory

MENTAL

- **Alterations of level of consciousness**
  - Lethargy/stupor/delirium/coma
  - Seizures/syncope/sleep disorders
  - Attention deficit
- **Cognitive dysfunctions**
  - Retardation/dementia
  - Amnesia, disorientation to time, person, and place
  - Illusions/hallucinations/delusions
  - Impaired insight, judgment and planning
  - Dyscalculia
  - Dysphasia/dyslexia/agnosia
- **Affective dysfunction**
  - Anxiety
  - Flat/emotional lability
  - Mania/depression
  - Phobias/obsessions
  - Episodic dyscontrol: rage and aggression

MOTOR

- **Somatomotor**
  - Fatigability/weakness/paralysis
  - Atrophy/hypertrophy of muscle/fasciculations/cramps/exercise intolerance
  - Hyperactivity
  - Hypo-/hyperkinesias: tremor, rigidity, dystonia, athetosis, chorea, tics
  - Spasticity/hypotonia
  - Dystaxia/dyspraxia
  - Dysphonia/dysarthria/dysphagia/dysprosody
  - Respiratory dysrhythmias: dyspnea/apnea/hyperventilation/cough/hiccoughing/sneezing
- **Visceromotor/homeostatic**
  - Cardiovascular: dysrhythmias/hypertension/hypotension
  - Vasomotor instability/flushing/Raynaud's phenomenon
  - Trophic skin/nail changes
  - Dyshidrosis: hyperhidrosis/anhidrosis
  - Bladder: dysuria/polyuria/oliguria/anuria/discoloration of urine
  - Bowel: anorexia/hyperphagia/vomiting/constipation/diarrhea
  - Sexual dysfunction: impotence/dyspareunia

SENSORY

- **Deficits of sensation**
  - Anesthesia/hypesthesia/numbness
  - Blindness/amaurosis/diplopia/scotomata/blurring
  - Deafness/hyperacusis
  - Anosmia/ageusia
- **Excessive sensation**
  - Pain: head, chest, abdomen, extremity, back, muscles, or joints
  - Neuralgia
  - Hyperesthias/tingling/tickling/itching
  - Nausea/cramping/bloating
  - Dizziness/vertigo
  - Tinnitus

FIGURE 1-1. Dendrogram summarizing neurologic symptoms and signs.

b. By adjusting the length of muscle fibers we can:
   i. Operate our skeletal levers to move ourselves and objects around.
   ii. Open and close or vibrate our apertures: vocal cords, eyelids, mouth, and other sphincters.
   iii. Move gases and liquids through our tubes (air, blood, secretions, food, feces, gametes, and urine).

c. All human behavior consists of secreting substances or changing the length of muscles' fibers. Whatever the behavior, it originates from nerve impulses traveling through neural circuits.

d. The definition of behavior excludes thinking per se, because the Ex cannot directly observe it. René Descartes (1596–1650) may have said, "I think therefore I am," but the Ex can gain access to the Pt's thoughts only if the Pt can display adaptive behavior, such as speaking, writing, or gesturing.

D. Corollaries of the definition of behavior

1. **All** behaviors and **all** thoughts depend on neuroanatomic circuits.
2. **Any** behavior conveys some information about the integrity of some neuroanatomic circuit. For example,
   a. Normal movements mean that the peripheral nerves are intact; that their endings are secreting adequate quantities of acetylcholine to the skeletal muscles; that the pyramidal and cerebellar pathways are intact; and that the substantia nigra is secreting adequate quantities of dopamine to the striatum.
   b. Normal movement means that a large amount of neural circuitry and a large volume of neural tissue are not the site of a lesion.
3. The concept of behavior and brain function as circuitry applies not only to the rational, conscious Pt but also to newborn infants, those in coma or a persistent vegetative state, and the diagnosis of brain death.
   a. If the brain is alive, not depressed by medication, toxins, or metabolic imbalance, and has the right temperature, the Ex can prove it is alive by using the NE to elicit some behavior.
   b. Conversely, the total absence of any behavior dependent on brain circuits proves that the brain is dead, if the requirements in **a**, above, are fulfilled.

E. The neural definition of behavior as applied to the success of the physician–patient relationship

And though I might be attracted or repelled (by the patient), the professional attitude which every physician must call on would steady me, dictate the terms on which I was to proceed.

—William Carlos Williams, M.D. (1883–1963)

We emphasize the stark biology of behavior not to deny the Pt's sentiency nor to dehumanize, but to create conditions that allow that sentiency to flow forth uninhibited by the physician's biases or censorship. Treating each Pt as a coequal organism consisting of neural circuits that operate a set of levers, apertures, tubes, and glands focuses on our elemental unity and limitations—the pathos of being human. "Because I was flesh and a breath that passeth away and cometh not again." By biological necessity, each of us originates, lives, and dies alike, and each of us exults and suffers alike. Ironically, in the necessity to recycle the food we eat, the water that quenches our thirst, and the air we breathe, as creatures sharing one biosphere, we continuously exchange with each other the very molecules that compose us. The oxygen atom cycling through me once cycled through you. If you regard all and every behavior objectively simply as clinical phenomena, as the product of neural circuits, operating glands, and adjusting the length of muscle fibers, you will react professionally, not socially in liking or disliking the Pt. You are not subject to the Pt's sorrows, seductions, and transgressions nor captive to your own reactions to the Pt's personality and life style. Free from fears of censure or entrapment, Pts can reveal their full sentiency and needs. Although you should achieve empathy, you must remain emotionally calm because you cannot think rationally when weeping over a Pt's illnesses, fuming about a Pt's behavior or faults, or feeling too attracted to the Pt. Perhaps this approach through elemental biology will work for you; if not, it may encourage you to find your own way to foster the professional humility and grace that enables Pts to fully reveal their personhood.

II. LOOKING AT EYES

You can see an awful lot just by looking.

—Attributed to Yogi Berra

If restricted to one part of the examination, choose inspection, the most efficient method of physical diagnosis. Inspection begins the moment you approach your Pt. Immediately you might notice pinpoint pupils and numerous needle scars over the antecubital veins. In two glances you suspect a drug addict. This is the diagnostic power of inspection. But wait a minute. Eye drops to treat glaucoma may have constricted the pupils, and repeated blood transfusions may have scarred the antecubital veins. The diagnostic value of signs emerges only after integration with a complete history and physical examination. No single diagnostic technique is sufficient.

After a lifetime of looking, you may consider yourself a keen observer. To test how well you have observed something, try to draw it. What you have seen well, you can draw well. Complete the requested drawings faithfully. They are tremendous tools.

Before starting this section, please get a hand mirror and a transparent millimeter ruler. Come on now; be fair. Give the tactics a chance.

A. Relation of the eyelid margins to the iris

1. An opening, the *palpebral fissure,* separates the upper and lower eyelid margins. See the vertical arrow in Fig. 1-2A.

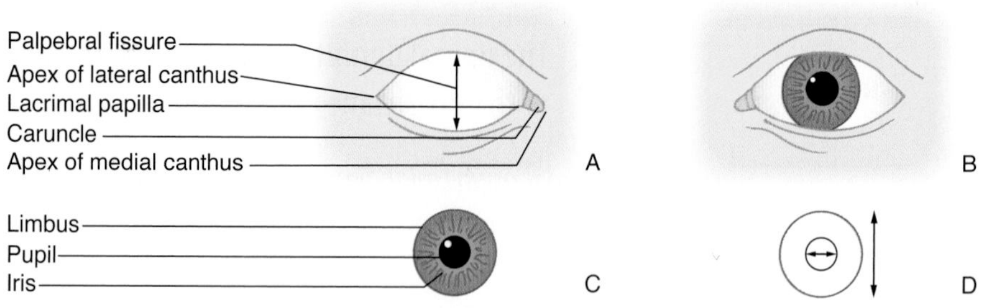

FIGURE 1-2. (A–D) Nomenclature of the external eye.

2. Observe your eyes in a hand mirror; in the space on the left side of this page, draw the exact contours of the margins of your upper and lower eyelids. Especially notice the configuration at the apices of the *medial* and *lateral canthi* (medial and lateral angles) of the palpebral fissure.
3. Compare your drawing with the one shown in Fig. 1-2A. Then look again into the mirror and identify the parts of your eye, as listed in Fig. 1-2A.
4. In Fig. 1-2A and in your mirror notice the *caruncle,* the tiny mound of meaty tissue that occupies the apex of the medial canthus.
5. In the mirror study the *iris,* the colored disc, surrounded by the white *sclera* (Fig. 1-2C). Is it uniform in color?

6. Next, in your mirror identify your *limbus* and *pupil*.
   a. The *external* circumference of the iris, at its junction with the white of the eye, forms the *limbus*.
   b. The *internal* circumference of the iris forms the *pupil*, the opening that admits light into the eye (horizontal arrow in Fig. 1-2D).
   c. The *cornea*, a transparent disc, covers the iris and pupil. The limbus also marks the external circumference of the cornea.
   d. Two types of abnormal corneal rings occur near the limbus. A golden-brown or brownish green corneal ring, the *Kayser-Fleischer* ring, formed by the deposition of copper in the Descemet membrane considered to be pathognomonic of Wilson hepatolenticular degeneration (may also be seen in other conditions such as aceruloplasminemia, primary biliary cirrhosis, Hardikar syndrome, and hypercupremia). A grayish-white ring, the *arcus senilis*, or arcus cornealis, is more prevalent with increasing age and is more frequently observed in men. A unilateral corneal arcus may be a diagnostic sign of carotid artery stenosis (absent on the side of the stenotic artery).

Note: Left of the vertical line is the answer column. Cover the answers with a card until you respond to the text. Then, after recording your response in the underlined blank, slide the card down to check your answer.

7. In your mirror study the relation of the upper and lower lid margins to the limbus and iris as you look straight ahead. Contrast where the margins of the upper and lower lids cross the iris. ____.

The upper lid partly covers the upper arc of the limbus, and the lower lid margin is virtually tangential to the limbus.

8. Set aside your mirror; from memory, draw the iris in the *left* eye of Fig. 1-3, showing the exact relation of the lid margins to the iris.

Check against Fig. 1-2B. If you erred, redraw the iris in the right eye shown in Fig. 1-3.

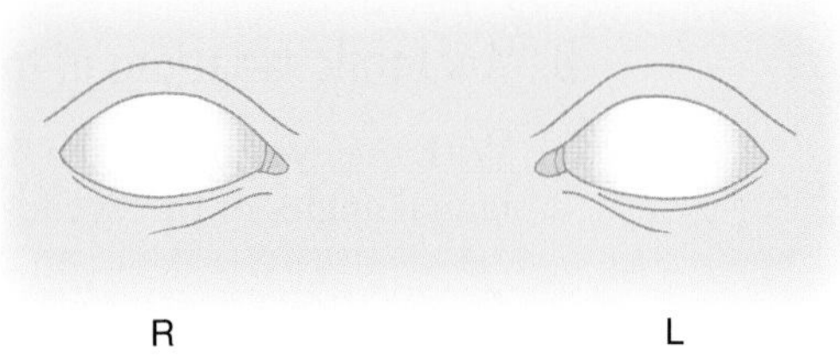

FIGURE 1-3. Blank for drawing the relation of the limbus, iris, and pupil to the lid margins when the patient looks straight ahead. L = left; R = right.

9. From memory, label the structures shown in Fig. 1-3 with the terms from Fig. 1-2, and check your results against Fig. 1-2.
10. Relation of limbus to canthi and caruncles when the eyes deviate.
    a. Look in your mirror and study another person to learn the relation of the limbus to the canthi and caruncles when the eyes turn as far as possible to the right or left. Remove eye glasses.
    b. With the eyes turned to one side as far as possible, how much scleral white shows between the limbus and the apex of the lateral canthus of the *abducted* eye? ____________________.

None or virtually none

    c. Although the lateral arc of the limbus reaches the apex of the lateral canthus, the medial arc cannot reach the apex of the medial canthus because the caruncle occupies it (Fig. 1-2A). Instead, the medial arc of the limbus reaches to, or nearly to, the lateral margin of the caruncle. Thus, with the eyes to one side, the limbus of the *abducted* eye reaches to, or nearly to, the apex (external angle); caruncle

__________ of the lateral canthus, and the limbus of the *adducted* eye reaches to, or nearly to, the lateral margin of the ______________.

11. In Fig. 1-4 draw the relation of the limbus, iris, and pupils to the lids when the Pt looks all of the way to the left.

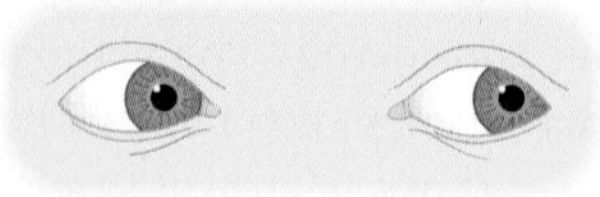

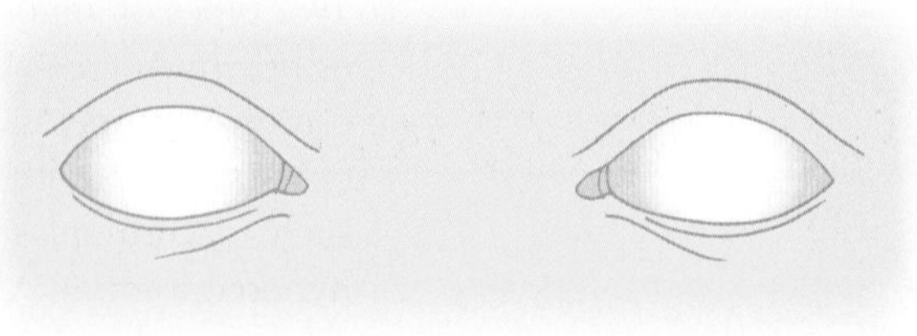

FIGURE 1-4. Blank for drawing the relation of the limbus, iris, and pupil to the lid margins when the patient looks to the left as far as possible.

12. A line drawn through the apex of the medial and lateral canthi of one eye defines the angle of the palpebral fissure (Fig. 1-5).

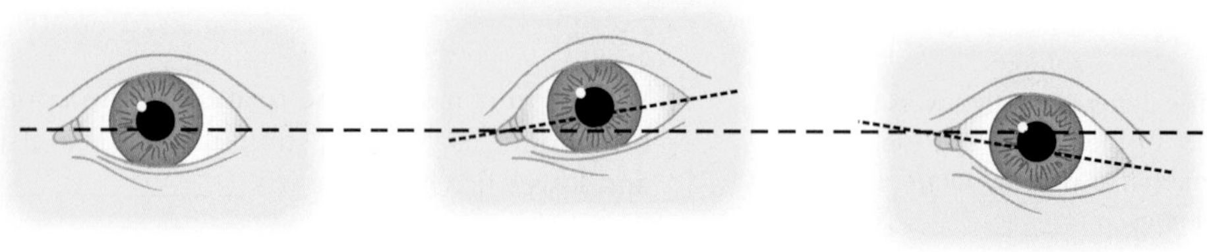

A Normal B Mongoloid slant C Antimongoloid slant

FIGURE 1-5. Left eye, showing angulations of the palpebral fissure.

B. Anatomic variations of the medial canthus

1. With the eyes at rest, the iris normally is nearly centered between the medial and lateral angles of the eyelids. See Fig. 1-6A.

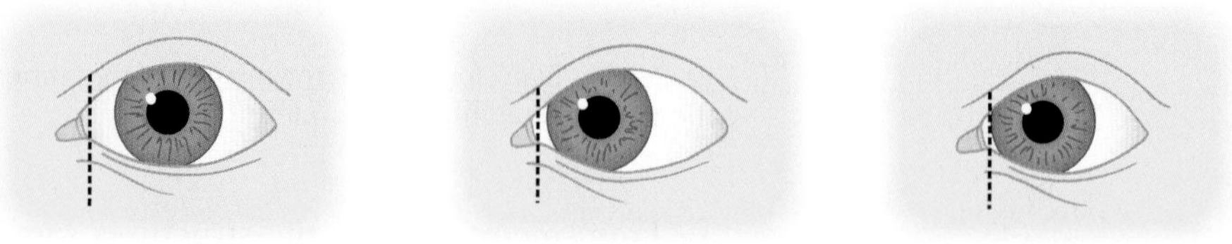

A Normal adult B Young child C Canthus dystopia

FIGURE 1-6. Left eye, showing variations in the relation of the medial canthus and lacrimal papilla (vertical line) to the corneal limbus. Note the decreasing distance between the caruncle and the medial margin of the limbus in (A), (B), and (C).

2. Look at an infant or young child and note that the medial canthus covers more of the conjunctiva than in adults. When the medial canthus is displaced laterally relative to the limbus, as in many young children, their eyes appear to deviate inward, although the eyes are perfectly straight, as in Fig. 1-6B.
3. Lateral displacement of the medial canthus, which moves the lacrimal punctum out toward the limbus, is termed *canthus dystopia* (*dys* = bad; *topos* = place; hence, badly placed canthus).

4. Sometimes a skinfold covers the medial canthus. Because the fold is *on* the canthus, it is called an *epicanthal fold*. In spaces A, B, and C in Figs. 1-7A to 1-7C, write down your diagnosis: *epicanthal fold*, *normal*, or *canthus dystopia*.

A ______________________

B ______________________

C ______________________

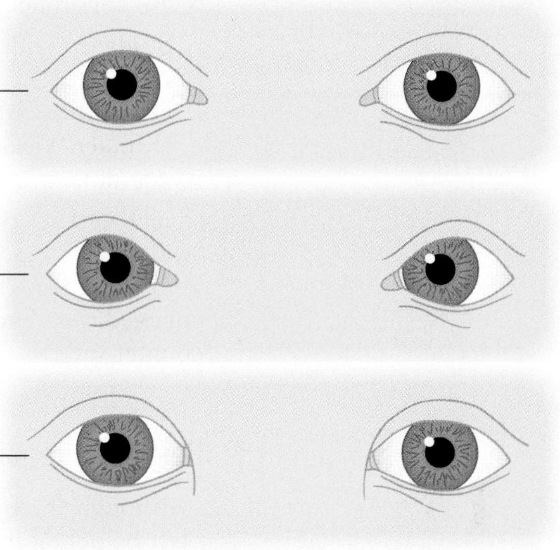

FIGURE 1-7. Write your diagnosis in blanks (A), (B), and (C).

C. Intercanthal and interorbital distances

1.9; 2.5

1. In Figs. 1-7A and 1-7B, measure the distance between the apices of the medial canthi in the normal eyes and those with canthus dystopia. The intercanthal distance of normal eyes is __________ cm and in canthus dystopia is __________ cm.
2. The measurement of 1.9 cm is the normal distance for a newborn. Measure your own intercanthal distance by holding up your ruler while looking in a mirror. It will be about 3 cm. See Jones (1997) for graphs of facial measurements.
3. Canthus dystopia or epicanthal folds cause the illusion of an increased distance between the eyes. The bone that forms the medial walls of the orbits sets the actual distance. This distance, the actual *interorbital distance*, can be measured only from skull radiographs, computed tomography (CT), or magnetic resonance imaging (MRI).
   a. If the medial orbital walls, and consequently the eyes, are set too far apart, the Pt has *orbital hypertelorism* (*hyper* = excessive; *tele* = far, as in *tele*phone).
   b. If the medial orbital walls and consequently the eyes are set too close together, the Pt has *orbital hypo*________________.

telorism

4. What canthal or lid anomalies could produce the illusion of hypertelorism, even with a short interorbital distance? ______________________________.

Epicanthal folds and canthus dystopia

5. What procedure would you order to decide whether a Pt has an abnormal interorbital distance? ______________________________________.

Skull radiographs, CT, or MRI

6. If the interorbital distance is too large, the Pt has __________ telorism; if too small, the Pt has __________ telorism.

hyper; hypo

7. Hypotelorism or hypertelorism increases the likelihood that the Pt has an abnormal brain (DeMyer, 1967, 1975, 1977).

D. Pupillary size

1. While holding up your millimeter ruler as you look in the mirror, measure and record the size of one pupil: ________ mm. Then measure it with the scale shown in Fig. 12-30 by holding it next to the Pt's eye.

2. Observe whether both pupils are exactly round and have the same diameter.
   a. Most people have exactly round, equal pupils, or isocoria (*iso* = equal; *cor* = pupil). The core is the center of something. The prefix *a-* or *an-* negates the term that follows. Thus, any congenital or acquired difference in pupillary size is called _________, which means *not equal pupils.*

anisocoria

   b. An abnormally small pupil is called *cormiosis,* or simply *miosis*.
   c. Study the width of your iris and its concentricity with the pupils. An eccentric pupil is called *corectopia* (core = center; ectopia = out of place). A form of corectopia with dorsomedially displaced pupils can occur in unconscious Pts (Kinnier Wilson pupil).
3. Pupils undergo an age-related change in size. The pupils of the newborn infant are small ("Gee, it's bright out here"). By adolescence, the pupils are their largest; the "wide-eyed," innocent look of the adolescent is a look once favored by women who used drops of atropine, or *bella donna* (= beautiful lady), to give them enlarged, sexy pupils. By old age, the pupils have become small, giving a flinty countenance.

E. Height of the palpebral fissure

1. Although the pupils normally are exactly equal, the height of the right and left palpebral fissures may differ slightly in normal persons, because of slight drooping of an eyelid. Pathologic drooping of the upper lid is called *ptosis*. Look in your mirror to see whether one of your lids droops more than the other.
2. Hold your mirror straight in front of your eyes and then move your mirror up and down but follow it only with your eyes while observing the surface area of your upper lid. In which direction do you see most of the surface area of the upper lid? ❒ Up/❒ Straight ahead/❒ Down

☑ Down

3. Notice in your mirror that, as the eyeballs rotate up and down, automatic adjustments keep the height of the palpebral fissure and the relation of the lid margins to the iris nearly the same. Such automatic adjustments are called *associated movements*. What would happen to vision if the eyelid margins did not adjust when the eyeballs rotated up or down? ______________________________ ______________.

The lid margins would cover the pupils and block vision when the person looked up.

4. Hyperthyroid Pts often show a sign called *lid lag*. As the eyeballs rotate down, the upper lid does not drop. You will see scleral white between the upper lid and the upper arc of the limbus.
5. Protrusion of an eyeball, called *exophthalmos* or *proptosis,* widens the palpebral fissure. A sunken eyeball, called *enophthalmos,* results in a narrow palpebral fissure.
6. Two conditions that reduce the height of the palpebral fissure are drooping of an eyelid, called ______________________, or a sunken eyeball, called ______________.

ptosis; enophthalmos

7. *Microphthalmia* means a pathologically small eyeball, and *macrophthalmia* mean a pathologically large eyeball. Correspondingly, the eyeball may have a *microcornea* or a *macrocornea*.
8. Write the correct diagnosis in Figs. 1-8A to 1-8F. Always compare the two eyes systematically: pupils, iris, and lids.
9. The foregoing ocular anomalies frequently occur in facial malformation syndromes. Measurement of the intercanthal, interpupillary, and interorbital distances aids in their diagnosis (Jones, 1997).
10. While inspecting the eyelids, note the rate of blinking. Infrequent blinking accompanies a number of conditions from hyperthyroidism to parkinsonism. The absence of blinking causes the eyes to have a "reptilian stare."

A. Ptosis and cormiosis on L (anisocoria)

B. Exophthalmia on R

C. Normal

D. Canthus dystopia

E. Macrocornea and pupillodilation (corectasia)

F. Miosis on L (anisocoria)

A ______________________

B ______________________

C ______________________

D ______________________

E ______________________

F ______________________

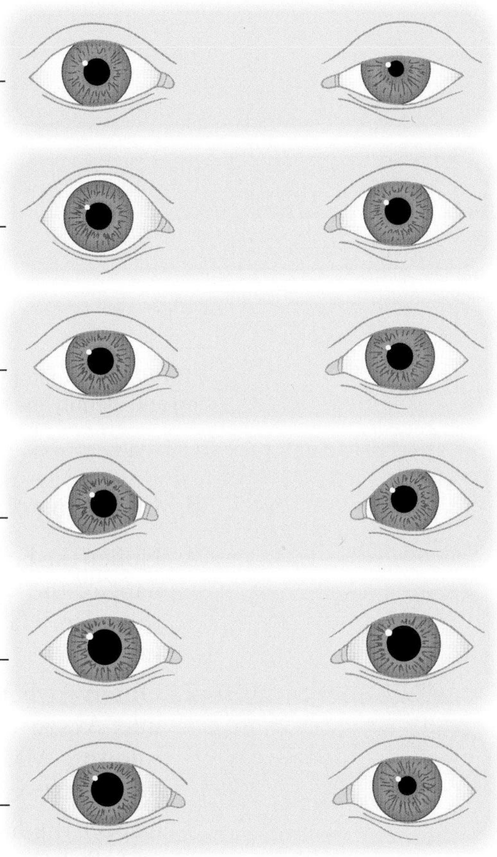

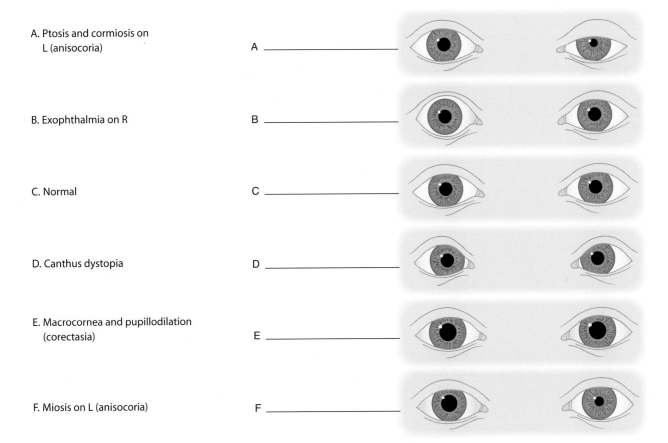

FIGURE 1-8. Write your diagnosis in blanks (A) to (F).

III. INSPECTION OF THE FACE, EARS, HAIR, AND SKIN

The human features and countenance, although composed of but some ten parts or little more, are so fashioned that among so many thousands of men there are no two in existence who cannot be distinguished from one another.

—Pliny the Elder (A.D. 23–79)

A. Inspection of the nose, mouth, chin, and ears

From abnormalities in the face alone, the perceptive Ex can diagnose literally hundreds of disorders, ranging from infectious diseases, such as leprosy, to endocrinopathies, mental, and neurologic disorders. After inspecting the entire face, start at the eyes and look systematically at the forehead, nose, mouth, chin, and ears.

1. **Nose:** Consider the bridge, the nostrils, and the relation of the nose to other facial proportions.
2. **Mouth:** Consider the vermillion border of the lips, the philtrum (the groove between the upper lip and the columella of the nose), median labial tubercle of the upper lip, and the line formed by lip closure. Do the lips make a horizontal closure line? Are the lips closed when the Pt's face is at rest? Does the mouth hang open, forming an inverted-U upper lip? Does the Pt have *micro*stomia or *macro*stomia?
3. **Chin:** Look for a small chin, *micro*gnathia, or a large protuberant chin, *macro*gnathia, as in pituitary gigantism (acromegaly).
4. **Ears:** Check for contour, shape, and asymmetry. Learn to draw a normal ear and label its parts as shown in Fig. 1-9.

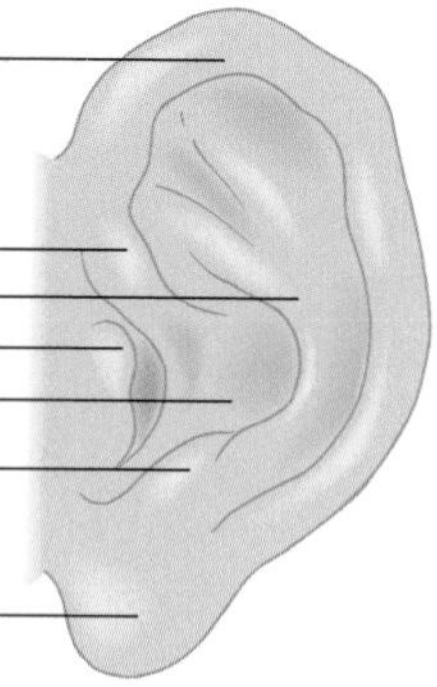

FIGURE 1-9. Anatomy of the normal ear, lateral view. Compare your own ear with that in the drawing and identify the parts.

B. Inspection of the hair of the scalp, eyebrows, and beard

1. Notice the border of the hairline. How does it relate to the forehead and to the nape of the neck? Is the hairline too high or too low? What is the texture of the scalp hair? Is the color nonuniform (poliosis). Is the hair absent in spots (alopecia)?
2. Observe whether the eyebrows are full, scanty, absent, or joined in the midline. Absence of the lateral part of the eyebrows is common in hypothyroidism. Midline union of the eyebrows (synophrys) occurs in some malformation syndromes.
3. Inspect the hair of the beard and face for its distribution and texture. Ask a male Pt how often he has to shave. Many disorders affect the distribution and texture of the hair: infections, congenital malformations, endocrine, and intersex syndromes. Use the Tanner Sexual Maturity Scale to describe secondary sexual characteristics.

C. Inspection of the skin of the face and general body surface

Various neurocutaneous stigmata are virtually pathognomonic of the underlying disease or correlate with neurologic deficits (Gomez, 1987; Hurko and Provost, 1999; Karabiber et al., 2002):

1. Multiple flat brown spots (café-au-lait spots): von Recklinghausen disease or neurofibromatosis (NF-1).
2. Irregular linear blotches of brown pigmentation of the infant's skin: incontinentia pigmenti.
3. Ash leaf-shaped white spots (naevus anemicus) and facial angiofibromas on the butterfly area and chin: tuberous sclerosis complex. Viewing the Pt in a dark room with a Wood's lamp (ultraviolet light of 360 nm) enhances discovery of the white spots.
4. Facial hemangiomas (Nevus flammeus) in the V1 distribution of the trigeminal nerve: Sturge-Weber syndrome (Bodensteiner and Roach, 1999).
5. Hypopigmented whorls: Hypomelanosis of Ito.
6. Hemangiomatous hypertrophy of one limb (most commonly the leg): Klippel-Trenaunay-Weber Syndrome.
7. Alcoholics have flushed skin when acutely intoxicated. Chronic alcoholics get spider nevi over the upper thorax, neck, and head, palmar erythema, multiple bruises, cigarette burns on the fingers, jaundice, gynecomastia, scaly, beriberi-like skin if malnourished, glossitis, and sparse chest, pubic, and axillary hair.

D. How to look at a face to diagnose malformation syndromes

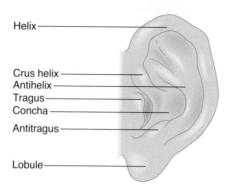

1. If the Pt's facial gestalt or some individual feature seems odd, the Pt may have a malformation syndrome, and it may affect the face and brain or other internal

organs. The face of such a Pt often predicts with some certainty the Pt's brain anomaly and intellectual potential, as in Down's syndrome and holoprosencephaly. Thus, in many instances, *the face predicts the defective brain* (DeMyer, 1975). Even if you cannot recite all of the possible facial malformations, by knowing the limits of normal, you can recognize the abnormal. The face is so important to humans that we have a special area of the cerebrum, the inferomedial temporo-occipital region, wired for facial recognition. (See prosopagnosia in Chapter 11.)

2. An understanding of facial embryology greatly expedites the diagnosis of malformation syndromes or other disorders affecting the face. The face derives from two morphogenetic sectors, the *frontonasal process sector* and the *branchial arch sector.*
   a. Figures 1-10 and 1-11 show these two sectors.

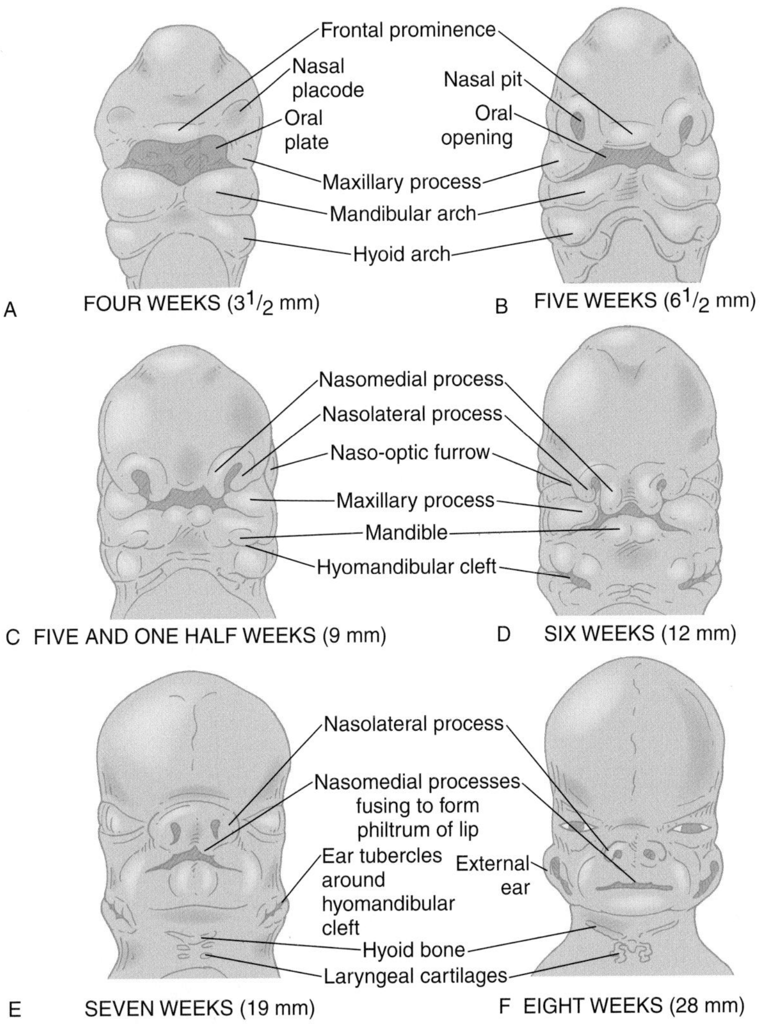

FIGURE 1-10. Embryogenesis of the face. Note the frontal prominence (frontonasal process) that forms the forehead and nose and the maxillary and mandibular processes that form the branchial arches.

   b. Notice in Figs. 1-10 and 1-11 that the embryonic frontonasal process (= frontal prominence) produces the *forehead, upper eyelids, nose,* and *medial third of the upper lip.*
   c. Notice that the branchial arch sectors produce:
      i. The *ears* (and the malleus, incus, and stapes of the inner ear).
      ii. The *maxillary* and *mandibular processes* and *lower eyelids, jaw,* and the *lateral thirds of the upper lip* and the entire *lower lip* and *chin.*

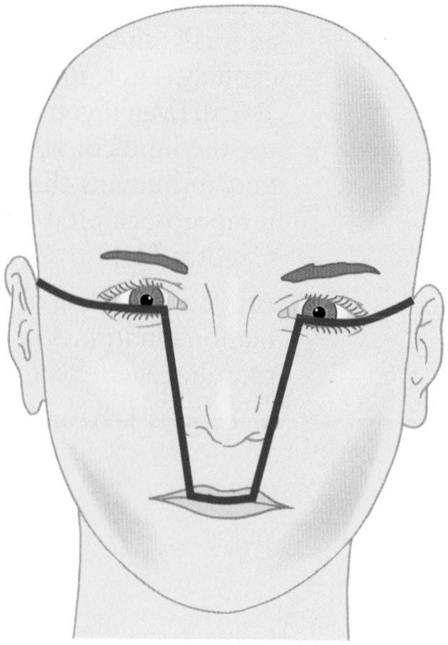

FIGURE 1-11. The heavy line divides the frontonasal sector of the face and the branchial arch sectors.

d. Notice that the frontonasal process produces the medial third of the upper lip and that the branchial arches produce the lateral thirds of the upper lip.

e. Notice the fusion sites between the medial third and the two lateral thirds of the upper lip. Failure of this fusion produces the common *lateral cleft lip* (harelip), whereas failure of development of the medial third of the lip produces a *median cleft lip*.

f. Defects of fusion between the processes of the branchial arches result in branchial cleft cysts in the neck.

3. A second method of localization of facial malformations involves dividing the face into three *transverse* sectors that cut across the morphogenetic sectors (Fig. 1-12).

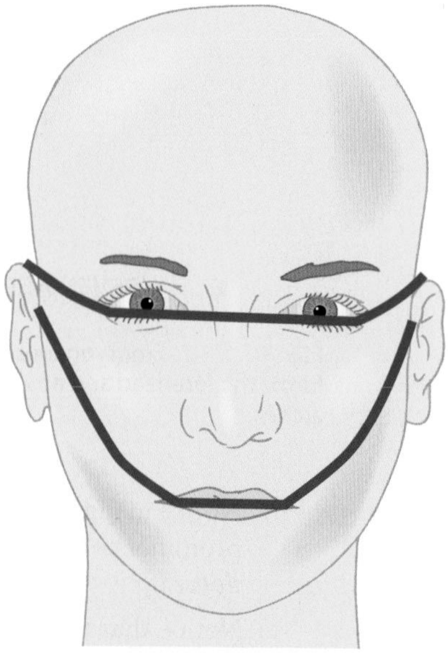

FIGURE 1-12. The lines divide the face transversely for descriptive purposes into upper, middle, and lower parts. Malformations may affect one, two, or all three parts.

4. Malformations may affect the frontonasal process only, resulting in orbital hypo- or hypertelorism or nasal malformations (DeMyer, 1967, 1975; Guion-Almeida et al., 1996); malformations may affect only the branchial arch section, resulting in lateral clefts of the lip and anomalies of the outer and middle ear and jaw; or malformations may affect derivatives of the frontonasal process and the branchial arch sector, resulting in a panfacial malformation syndrome that affects the entire face.
5. **Procedure for facial analysis**
   a. First observe the Pt's facial gestalt.
   b. Then systematically divide the face into parts for individual inspection. Start at the hair and forehead and work down to the chin.
   c. Imagine the face as a pair of eyes. Are they too close together or too far apart? Are the pupils unequal? Simply ask and answer such questions as you inspect the Pt's forehead, nose, mouth, chin, and ears.
6. Decide whether the Pt has a *pan*facial anomaly, such as Down's syndrome, or whether the malformation localizes mainly or exclusively to a *sector* of the face, based on its morphogenesis.
7. Finally, having identified the anomalies, consult a syndrome compendium to make the diagnosis (Bysse, 1990; Canepa et al., 2001; Gorlin et al., 2001; Jones, 1997; Winter and Baraitser, 2001).

E. A test panel for facial diagnosis

To test your acumen in facial diagnosis, study each Pt in Figs. 1-13A to 1-13L from the hairline down and record any abnormalities. Then check your findings in frame F. Grade yourself on the "honor system."

F. Descriptions of patients in montage of Fig. 1-13

1. Figure 1-13A shows an infant with rounded face, slight mongoloid obliquity of the palpebral fissures, open mouth, inverted-U-shaped upper lip, short upper extremities. The frog-legged position of the lower extremities reflects hypotonia: Down's syndrome, trisomy 21.
2. Figure 1-13B shows an infant with high forehead (abnormal upper sector as shown in Fig. 1-12), large head, antimongoloid obliquity of the palpebral

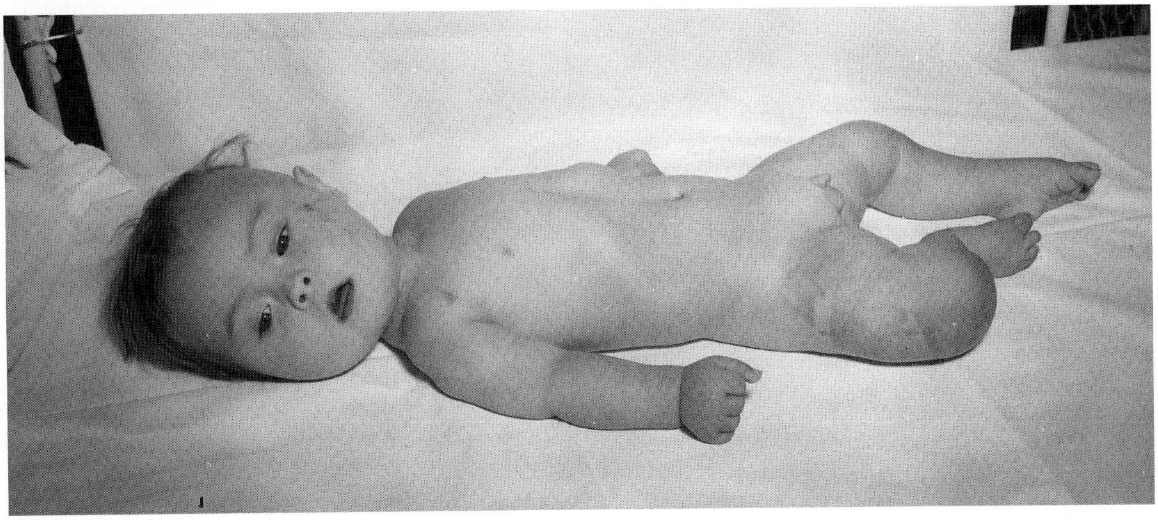

A

FIGURE 1-13. Montage of facial and skin abnormalities detected by inspection. See (F) after you have described the Pts yourself. Figures 1-13E and 1-13F show the same Pt.

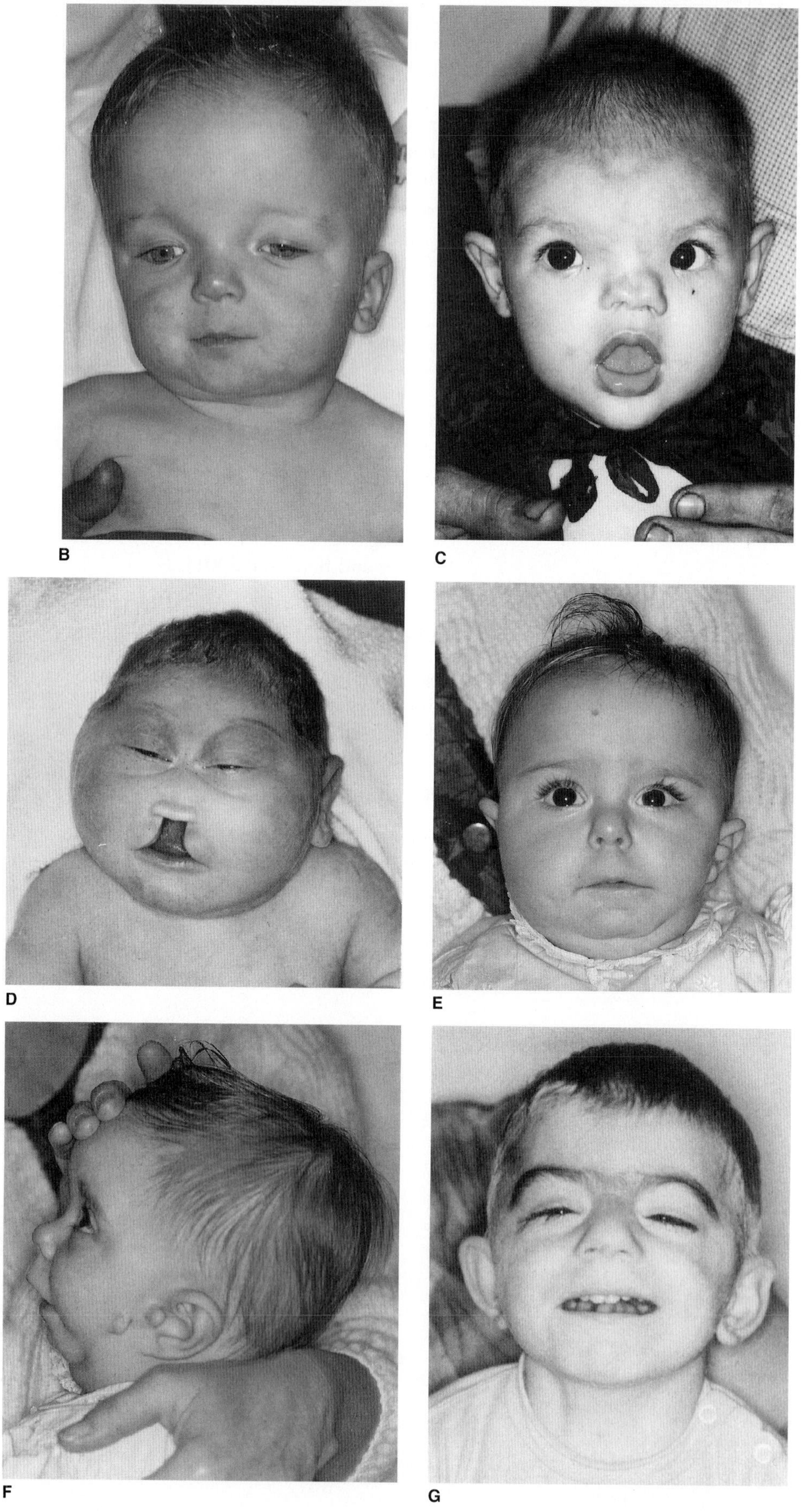

FIGURE 1-13. (Continued)

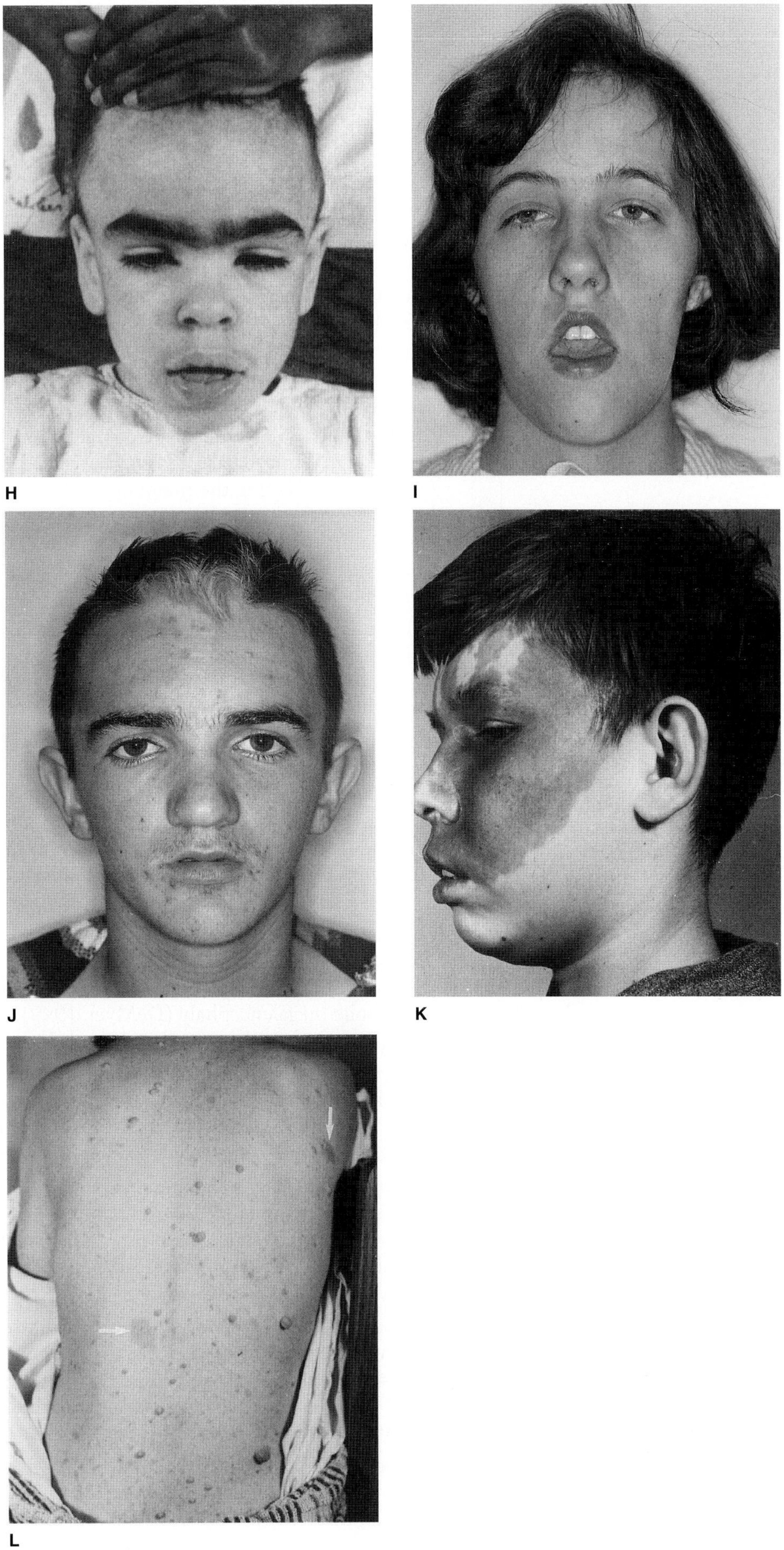

FIGURE 1-13. (Continued)

fissures, and orbital hypertelorism. Radiographic examination disclosed agenesis of the corpus callosum. The infant was mildly mentally retarded.

3. Figure 1-13C shows a boy with "widow's peak" hairline (midline V-shaped extension of hair pointing downward), hypertelorism plus canthus dystopia plus epicanthal folds, flat nasal bridge with slight median groove, and broad philtrum: median cleft face syndrome (DeMyer, 1967, 1975), also called frontonasal dysplasia. Such patients generally are mentally normal.
4. Figure 1-13D shows a newborn infant with microcephaly, orbital hypotelorism, flat nasal bridge, and median cleft of the upper lip. The apparent ptosis is caused by some lid edema and the fact that the infant has its eyes turned somewhat downward. The facial malformation is restricted to the frontonasal process sector (Figs. 1-10 and 1-11). This face is pathognomonic for holoprosencephaly, a brain malformation of the type shown in Fig. 1-24. Such Pts are severely retarded (DeMyer, 1975).
5. Figure 1-13E shows an infant girl showing normal hairline and forehead. On the left side notice the small palpebral fissure, hypoplastic zygoma and mandible, downward displaced ear, and slight macrostomia: unilateral first branchial arch syndrome (affecting the mandible and maxilla, from the first branchial arch). The frontonasal process sector of the face is normal. Notice the symmetrical corneal light reflections, indicating intact ocular muscles, which derive from somites, not from branchial arches. A small pigmented nevus is present on the right side of the forehead.
6. Figure 1-13F shows the lateral view of patient shown in Fig. 1-13E. Notice the malformed tragus and extra tag of tissue and the hypoplastic left mandible (hypoplasia of the first branchial arch). The rest of the ear, from the second branchial arch, is well-formed.
7. Figure 1-13G shows a boy with midline eyebrows (synophrys), small midfacial segment (the middle of the three horizontal sectors of the face; Fig. 1-12), little or no philtrum, mild micrognathia, and mental retardation: Cornelia de Lange's syndrome. The patient also had a lumbar hair patch and hypoplasia of the radius and thumb, typical of this syndrome. The apparent ptosis was caused by squinting from the bright light used for photography.
8. Figure 1-13H shows a boy with megalocephaly and high forehead, coarse facial features, midline eyebrows, slight hypertelorism, concave nasal bridge, very broad philtrum with thick lips, and an open mouth (from thickened tongue): Hurler's syndrome, mucopolysaccharidosis. The megalocephaly is secondary to metabolic megalencephaly (DeMyer, 1999).
9. Figure 1-13I shows a young woman with very slight ptosis on the right, bilateral temporal and masseter muscle atrophy (hollowing of the temples and posterior cheeks giving a so-called "hatchet face" appearance), expressionless face, and sagging jaw with inverted-U-shaped upper lip: myotonic dystrophy. Males have frontal baldness.
10. Figure 10-13J shows a young man with white forelock, slight synophrys, slight hypertelorism, and heterochromia of the iris. Notice especially the medial part of the iris of the left eye. He was mildly deaf. All of these features are diagnostic of Waardenburg's syndrome, type II. Type I patients have dystopia canthorum. He also has incidental acne.
11. Figure 1-13K shows a boy with port wine stain, affecting the maxillary division of the trigeminal nerve (see Fig. 10-2) and, to a lesser extent, the ophthalmic division: Sturge-Weber syndrome of angiomatosis (Bodensteiner and Roach, 1999). The patient had epileptic seizures due to meningeal and cortical involvement by the angiomatosis.

13. Figure 1-13L shows the back of boy with multiple neurofibromas and café-au-lait spots (arrows): neurofibromatosis, type I. This disorder, like Sturge-Weber syndrome, belongs to the neurocutaneous syndromes, a group of congenital diseases that affect the brain and skin.

BIBLIOGRAPHY · Inspection of the Eyes, Face, Hair, and Skin

Norms for Ocular and Facial Measurements

Farkas LG. *Anthropometry of the Head and Face in Medicine.* Amsterdam, Elsevier/North Holland, 1981.

Jones KL. *Smith's Recognizable Patterns of Human Malformation*, 5th ed. Philadelphia, W.B. Saunders, 1997.

Craniofacial Anomalies

Bodensteiner J, Roach ES, eds. *Sturge-Weber Syndrome.* Mt. Freedom, Sturge-Weber Foundation, 1999.

Bysse ML, ed. *Birth Defects Encyclopedia*. Cambridge, Massachusetts, Blackwell Scientific Publications, 1990.

Canepa G, Maroteaux P, Pietrogrande V, eds. *Dysmorphic Syndromes and Constitutional Diseases of the Skeleton*. Padova, Piccin Nuova Libraria, 2001.

DeMyer W. The median cleft face syndrome: differential diagnosis of cranium bifidum, hypertelorism, and median cleft nose, lip, and palate. *Neurology* 1967;17:961–971.

DeMyer W. Median facial malformations and their implications for brain malformations. *Birth Defects* 1975;11:155–181.

DeMyer W. Orbital hypertelorism. In: Vinken PJ, Bruyn GW, eds. *Handbook of Clinical Neurology, Vol. 30*. Amsterdam, North-Holland Publishing Company, 1977, Chap. 9, pp. 235–255.

Gomez M, ed. *Neurocutaneous Diseases. A Practical Approach*. Boston, Butterworths, 1987.

Gorlin RJ, Cohen MM, Hennekam RCM, eds. *Syndromes of the Head and Neck*, 4th ed. New York, Oxford University Press, 2001.

Guion-Almeida ML, Richieri-Costa A, Saavedra D, et al. Frontonasal dysplasia: analysis of 21 cases and literature review. *Int J Oral Maxillofac Surg* 1996;25:91–97.

Hurko O, Provost TT. Neurology and the skin. *J Neurol Neurosurg Psychiatry* 1999;66: 417–430.

Jones KL. *Smith's Recognizable Patterns of Human Malformation*, 5th ed. Philadelphia, W.B. Saunders, 1997.

Karabiber H, Sasmaz S, Turanh G, et al. Prevalence of hypopigmented maculae and caféau-lait spots in idiopathic epileptic and healthy children. *J Child Neurol* 2002;17:57–59.

Stricher M, Van Der Meulen J, Raphael B, Mazzola R, eds. *Craniofacial Malformations.* Edinburgh, Churchill Livingstone, 1990.

Winter EM, Baraitser M. *London Dysmorphology Database and Photolibrary*, 3rd ed. Oxford, Oxford Electronic Publishing, 2001.

IV. PALPATION OF THE HEAD, AUSCULTATION, AND THE NEUROVASCULAR EXAMINATION

A. Palpation of the head

1. The laying on of hands, an ancient habit of healers, serves at once as a source of information to the physician and of comfort to the Pt. After inspection, grasp the Pt's head between your fingertips (or your own head in lieu of a Pt) and, using fairly firm pressure, search for soft spots, lumps, depressions, and areas of tenderness. Palpate your own frontal and parietal eminences. Which region is the widest, the frontal or parietal? By feeling along the midline and then out laterally, locate the depression, the site of the coronal suture, between the frontal and parietal eminences. Feel in the midline posteriorly, where the nape of the neck meets the skull, for the skull bump called the *external occipital protuberance*.
2. Section VI describes the palpation of the sutures and fontanels of the infant calvaria.

B. The neurovascular examination

Patients suspected of cerebrovascular disease require a thorough neurovascular examination involving *palpation* and *auscultation* of the head and arteries and *blood pressure* measurements (Roach et al., 2010). Check for asymmetry of the right- and left-side arteries.

1. **Palpation of arteries**
   a. **Temporal arteries:** Lay your index finger lightly, just in front of your tragus, and follow the pulsating temporal artery as far distally as possible. Note any prominence, nodularity, or tenderness of the artery.
   b. **Subclavian arteries:** Lightly place your fingertips 2 to 3 cm across the proximal part of the clavicle, just lateral to the origin of the sternocleidomastoid muscle. Try this in thin-skinned, lightly muscled individuals to learn how to locate the artery.
   c. **Remaining arteries:** Palpate the radial, femoral, and dorsalis pedis arteries. If you suspect occlusive disease of the carotid artery, avoid palpating it.
2. **Auscultation of the head and neck for bruits**
   a. A bruit is but an indication of non-laminar flow and can have many causes. Aneurysms, arteriovenous malformations or fistulae, and occlusive vascular disease may cause bruits over the carotid arteries or head (Sandock et al., 1982; Roach et al., 2010). Normal infants and children to age 5 years often have benign bruits over the head. A continuous venous hum is generally innocuous. Sometimes normal adults have benign bruits over the carotid arteries, but a strong, localized bruit, over the carotid bifurcation increases the likelihood of a cerebral infarction but not necessarily in the arterial territory corresponding to the bruit (Howard et al., 1989). Particularly if the Pt has hypertension, diabetes, or coronary artery disease. Cervical bruits may also be due to flow augmentation due to contralateral carotid artery stenosis, external carotid artery pathology, arterial kinks, sounds transmitted from a more proximal source, turbulent flow due to anemia, hemodialysis, or hyperthyroidism.

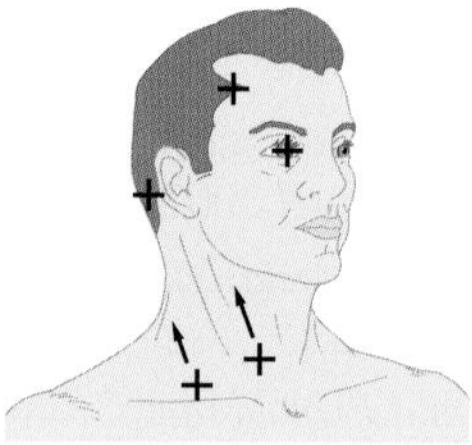

   b. Pathologic bruits become audible over the carotids after approximately 50% stenosis. The loudness may increase as the stenosis increases. At approximately 90% stenosis, the most ominous bruit appears, which has a soft, high-pitched sound that continues throughout systole into diastole. At 95% or greater stenosis, the bruit disappears.
   c. To survey for bruits of the neck vessels, gently place a rubber-edged stethoscope bell at various sites along the carotid and vertebral arteries (Fig. 1-14A) and over the supraclavicular fossa for the subclavian artery. If you suspect

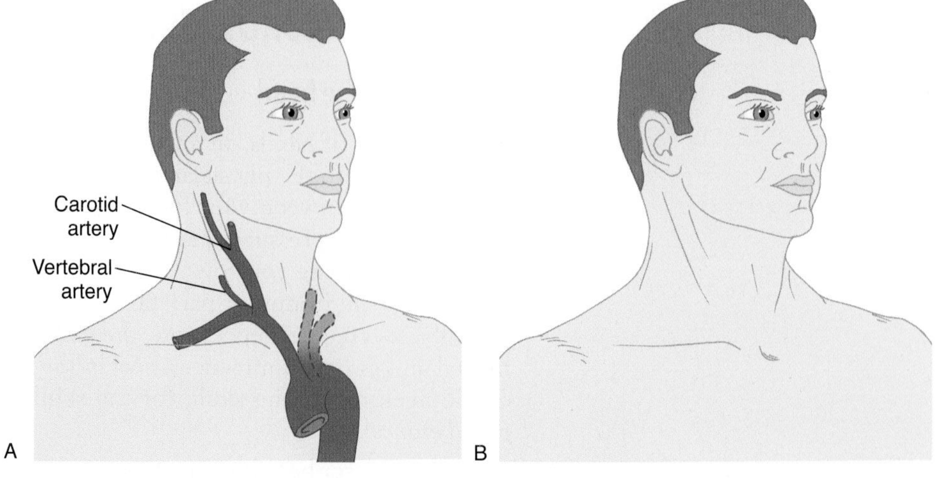

FIGURE 1-14. Auscultation of the neck vessels for bruits. (A) Phantom view of carotid and vertebral arteries in the neck. (B) Blank to mark sites of auscultation for bruits.

occlusive arterial disease, avoid compressing the carotid artery. Carotid bruits ordinarily are heard along the anterior edge of the sternocleidomastoid muscle, and vertebral artery bruits are heard along the posterior edge. Listen carefully at the carotid bifurcation, below the angle of the mandible.

d. Then place the bell over the mastoid processes, frontal and parietal regions, and over each eye after the Pt gently closes and then relaxes the eyelid. The bell will keep the lid closed, protecting the cornea. Place the bell of the stethoscope over your own eye and listen to the sound as you tense and relax your eyelids.

e. In Fig. 1-14B, draw lines showing where to place the stethoscope bell to listen for carotid or vertebral artery bruits and then mark X's at the other sites to place the bell to listen for a cranial bruit.

f. Using your stethoscope, listen to what (I hope) is the silence over your own head. Can you hear heart or breath sounds when you auscultate your carotid arteries? ______________________.

g. When you place the bell over the eye, after the Pt has closed the eye, what do you have to ask the Pt to do to eliminate muscle noise? ________________.

Relax the eyelid. The light pressure of the bell will keep the lid closed to protect the cornea.

h. In summary, you will hear intracranial bruits best with the bell of the stethoscope over the eyes, carotid artery bruits over the bifurcation, and subclavian bruits over the supraclavicular fossa.

i. Further investigation of a bruit may require duplex ultrasonography, magnetic resonance angiography, computed tomography angiography, or catheter cerebral angiography.

3. **Blood pressure measurement in patients suspected of cerebrovascular disease**

   a. Measure the blood pressure in both arms. A consistent difference of more than 10 to 20 mmHg between the two arms suggests proximal occlusive disease, usually of one of the subclavian arteries. See Chapter 12, for blood pressure measurement in suspected orthostatic hypotension.

   b. Measure the blood pressure of the femoral arteries and palpate the pulse. Hypertension in the arms and a reduced pulse and blood pressure in the femoral artery suggest coarctation of the aorta.

BIBLIOGRAPHY · Palpation of the Head, Auscultation, and the Neurovascular Examination

Howard VJ, Howard G, Harpold GJ, et al. Correlation of carotid bruits and carotid atherosclerosis detected by B-mode real-time ultrasonography. *Stroke* 1989;20:1331–1335.

Roach ES, Bettermann K, Biller J. *Toole's Cerebrovascular Disorders*, 6th ed. Cambridge, Cambridge Press, 2010.

Sandock BA, Whisnant JP, Furlan AJ, Mickell JL. Carotid artery bruits: prevalence survey and differential diagnosis. *Mayo Clin Proc* 1982;57:227–230.

C. Percussion

1. Percussion or compression over the frontal and maxillary sinuses and mastoid processes may disclose tenderness when these cavities are infected, but the percussion noted from the skull itself has little diagnostic value.
2. To test for the pain of sinusitis, have the sitting Pt lean forward with the trunk on the legs and head down, and then have the Pt perform a Valsalva maneuver. The increased venous pressure acting on the already swollen mucosa increases sinus pain, which will then have a pounding character corresponding to the pulse.
3. Try transillumination of the frontal and maxillary sinuses.
4. To further check for sinusitis and mastoiditis, obtain plain skull films, CT, or MRI to look for mucosal thickening, an air-fluid level, or opacification.

V. TRANSILLUMINATION OF THE INFANT'S HEAD

A. Purpose

Transillumination of an infant's head may disclose excessive amounts of extra and intracranial fluid and may indicate the need for CT or MRI of the brain (Fig. 1-15).

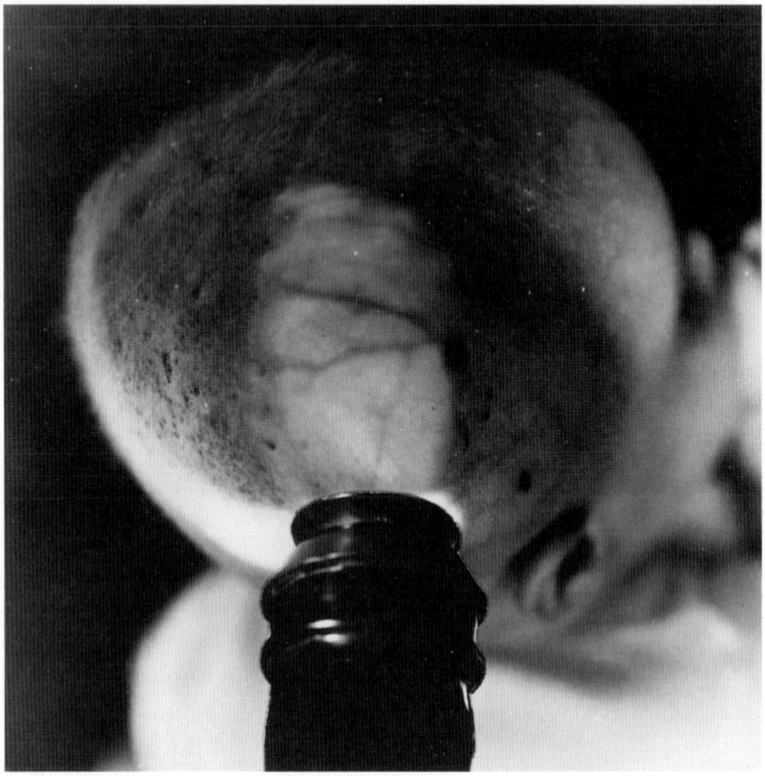

FIGURE 1-15. Localized transillumination of the parietal region. A parietal craniotomy was done to relieve combined intracerebral and subdural hematoma caused by a head injury. Clear fluid then accumulated between the dura and cerebrum (subdural hygroma) and gradually bulged through the surgical defect in the parietal bone. Observe the scalp vessels coursing over the bulge.

B. Technique

Take the infant into a completely dark closet and allow several minutes for your eyes to adapt to the darkness. Place an ordinary flashlight fitted with a rubber adaptor against the infant's head and move it over the entire calvarium, including the posterior fossa (Rabe, 1967; Sjögren and Engsner, 1972).

C. Results

Normally, a small halo of light, smaller than 1 cm in diameter, appears around the adaptor margin. Four conditions may enlarge the halo or even cause the entire head to light up.

1. Edema of the scalp, caused by birth injury or infiltration of intravenous fluid (Fig. 1-16A).
2. Increased fluid in the subdural space (subdural hygroma) or in the subarachnoid space (Fig. 1-16B).
3. Increased fluid within the brain because of thinning by hydrocephalic stretching, destruction, atrophy, or hypoplasia (Figs. 1-16C and 1-16D).
4. Premature infants with huge fontanels and very thin cranial bones.

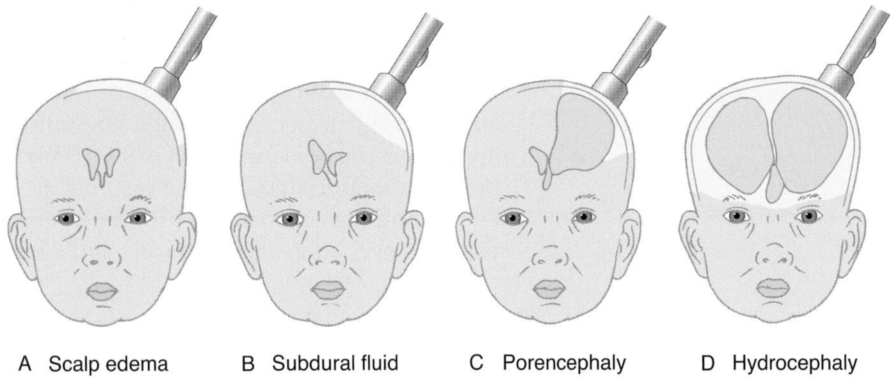

FIGURE 1-16. Head transillumination with lesions at different sites.

D. Systematic analysis of the causes for cranial transillumination

First consider whether the fluid that transilluminates is *out*side or *in*side the calvarium. If outside, the fluid must be in the scalp or subgaleal space.

1. **Detection of scalp edema by the pitting test:** Bruising and infiltration of fluid given through a scalp vein most commonly cause scalp edema. The *pitting test* discloses it: Press the ball of your finger firmly against the scalp in the area of transillumination. Continue pressing until your fingertip directly feels the bone. After removal of your finger, a pit remains.
2. **Detection of subgaleal fluid:** Subgaleal fluid elevates the scalp from the calvarium. The bone can be felt by *ballottement*. Finger pressure readily discloses the distance between the scalp and skull, but the scalp does not pit (unless it is also edematous).
3. **Location of fluid inside the skull**
   a. Fluid inside the skull occupies the subdural or subarachnoid spaces or is intracerebral. If intracerebral, the fluid occupies the ventricles or a cyst (Figs. 1-16C and 1-16D).
   b. Acutely after a head injury, epidural blood is too opaque to transilluminate. Exact localization of intracranial fluid often requires imaging (Chapter 13). Sometimes subdural fluid is diagnosed by inserting a needle through the lateral angle of the anterior fontanel or a burr hole, if the fontanels have closed.
4. To prove that you can systematically analyze transillumination, place your hand on top of your head and recite the possible extracranial and intracranial locations of the fluid. Then complete Table 1-1.

TABLE 1-1 • Tests for Locating Excess Fluid When the Head Transilluminates

Location of fluid	Test procedure to verify

Scalp; Fingertip pressure for pitting edema
Subgaleal space; Fingertip ballottement for elevation of scalp
Subdural space; Radiographic imaging or taps
Within the brain; Radiographic imaging

a. In the absence of the cerebellum or in the presence of a large cyst, the posterior fossa (inferior occipital region) transilluminates. Thus, for a thorough examination, move the flashlight over the entire cranium.
b. Transillumination has little value in Pts older than 18 months. The thicker, well-ossified skull will not transmit light. Transillumination in an older Pt

outside the calvarium, in the scalp or subgaleal space

would usually mean that the fluid was located ________________________.

5. By adding transillumination to the NE, which consists of inspection, palpation, auscultation, and occipitofrontal circumference (OFC) measurement, you will appreciate Harvey Cushing's (1869–1939) remark that we have increasing numbers of laboratory tests, "... the vast majority of which are but supplementary to, and as nothing compared with, the careful study of the Pt by a keen observer using his eyes and ears and fingers and a few simple aids."

BIBLIOGRAPHY · Transillumination of the Infant's Head

Rabe E. Skull transillumination in infants. *Gen Pract* 1967;36:78–88.

Sjögren I, Engsner G. Transillumination of the skull in infants and children. *Acta Paediatr Scand* 1972;61:426–428.

VI. THE BONES AND SUTURES OF THE CRANIUM

A. Origin of the skull bones

The cranial bones arise in cephalic mesoderm by two different histogenetic sequences. The *endochondral bone* of the cranial base develops from preformed cartilage. The *membranous bone* of the cranial vault and facial skeleton develops directly from osteoid.

Mnemonic: Learn the four endochondral bones of the cranial base in Fig. 1-17. Then you can easily remember the membranous origin of all of the other skull bones.

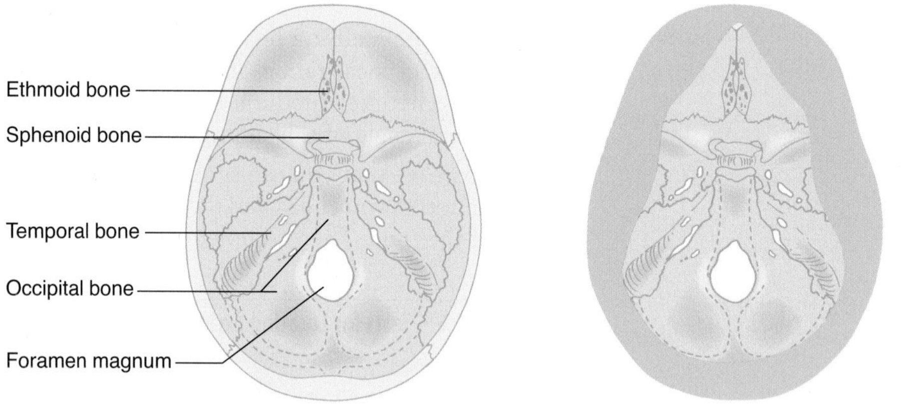

FIGURE 1-17. Interior view of skull base on the left. The right side shows only the endochondral bones.

B. Functional arthrology of the cranium

1. When a cavity separates the two bones at a joint, the joint is a *diarthrosis*. Connective tissue forms a capsule around the joint space and its cavity. If connective tissue also occupies the space between the bones, leaving no joint cavity, the joint is a *synarthrosis*.
2. The temporomandibular joints and joints of the ear ossicles are *diarthroses*. All other skull joints are *synarthroses*.
3. During morphogenesis, *cartilaginous* connective tissue united the joints of the endochondral bones at the cranial base. Such synarthroses are called *synchondroses*. Similarly, *fibrous* connective tissue united the membranous bones

of the cranial vault and of the face to each other and to endochondral bones. Those synarthroses where the large, flat bones of the cranium contact each other are *sutures*.

sutures; synchondroses

4. Wherever membranous bones contact each other or endochondral bones, the joints are called ________________, but wherever endochondral bones contact other endochondral bones, the joints are called ________________.
5. In fetuses, the fibrous connective tissue at the sutures is broad and somewhat pliant. Where the fibrous connective tissue forms large, nonossified membranes between the margins of some skull bones, the sites are called *fontanels*. Learn the *sutures, fontanels,* and *bones* in Fig. 1-18.

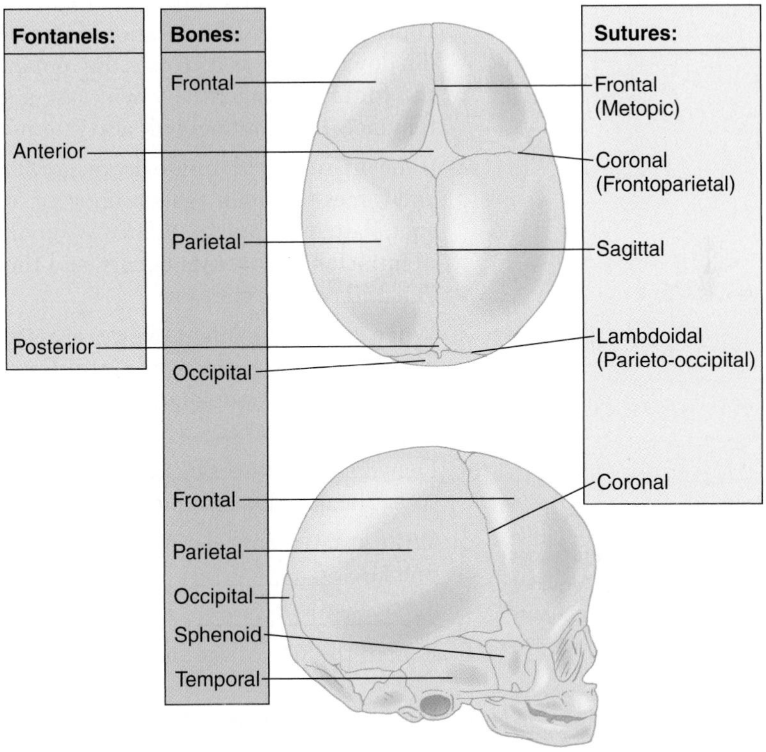

FIGURE 1-18. Fontanels, bones, and sutures of the infant cranium. Top: superior view of cranium. Bottom: lateral view of cranium.

frontal and parietal

6. The bones that border the largest fontanel, the *anterior*, are the ____________ bones.

C. Pliancy of the synarthroses in the infant's cranium

☑ fontanels

1. A fontanel is a sheet of fibrous connective tissue that bridges the gaps at the intersections of the sutures in the neonatal skull. Later the fontanels ossify. The sheet of connective tissue at the fontanels allows an up and down, diaphragm-like action, whereas the narrower connective tissue strip at the sutures permits only a limited, hinging action. Thus the infant skull is most pliant at the ❑ sutures/ ❑ fontanels.

fontanels, sutures, synchondroses

2. The cartilage uniting the synchondroses of the cranial base is less pliant than fibrous connective tissue. Rank the three skull synarthroses, the *synchondroses, fontanels*, and *sutures*, in order from most to least pliant: ________________, ________________, and ________________.
3. During morphogenesis and birth, the cranium serves the contradictory functions of *plasticity* and *rigidity*. The plasticity of the cranium permits expansion and deformation, whereas the rigidity of the bones protects the brain during passage

through the birth canal. The suture margins may overlap one another, thus damaging the brain by compression or by rupturing veins and venous sinuses.

4. The relative rigidity of the synchondroses prevents buckling of the skull base against the brainstem during birth, which would imperil the passenger even more than deformation of the calvarium.

D. Response of the anterior fontanel to changes in intracranial pressure

1. To the palpating finger, the anterior fontanel is pliant, as every mother knows because she calls it the "soft spot." Physicians often mistakenly describe the normal anterior fontanel as "flat." The normal anterior fontanelle in fact will be slightly *concave*, if you support the infant upright when it is not struggling or crying, because gravity causes the brain to sag away from the calvarium. As you run your finger across the anterior fontanel from one side to the other, the finger will dip down a little as it crosses the fontanel. In addition, a beam of light that crosses the fontanel tangentially will cast a shadow on the concavity of the normal fontanel. The fontanel will also pulsate.

2. If the infant is held upside down, gravity distends the intracranial veins with blood and forces the brain against the roof of the skull. The anterior fontanel, the soft spot, flattens or bulges slightly. When the infant is held upright, the opposite shift in intracranial contents occurs, and the fontanel assumes its normal ❐ concave/❐ flat/❐ convex contour.

☑ concave

3. When crying, the infant expires against a partly closed glottis. Contraction of the expiratory muscles increases intrathoracic pressure. The venous system transmits the pressure intracranially. As the intracranial pressure increases, the anterior fontanel ❐ becomes sunken/❐ bulges/❐ does not change.

☑ bulges

4. Dehydration reduces blood and tissue volume, thereby reducing intracranial pressure. The anterior fontanel ❐ sinks more/❐ bulges more/❐ does not change.

☑ sinks more

5. Write a statement relating the contour of the anterior fontanel to the intracranial pressure. ______________________________.
______________________________.

Increased intracranial pressure causes a bulging (convex) anterior fontanel, whereas low intracranial pressure causes a more sunken (more concave) fontanel.

6. Record the size of the fontanel in the infant's medical record.

E. Mechanism of normal enlargement of the cranium

1. During the gentle expansion of the fetal and infant brain, bone progressively deposits along the suture margins, keeping them from separating. The most important growth occurs along the *sagittal*, *coronal*, and *lambdoidal* sutures. Study Fig. 1-19.

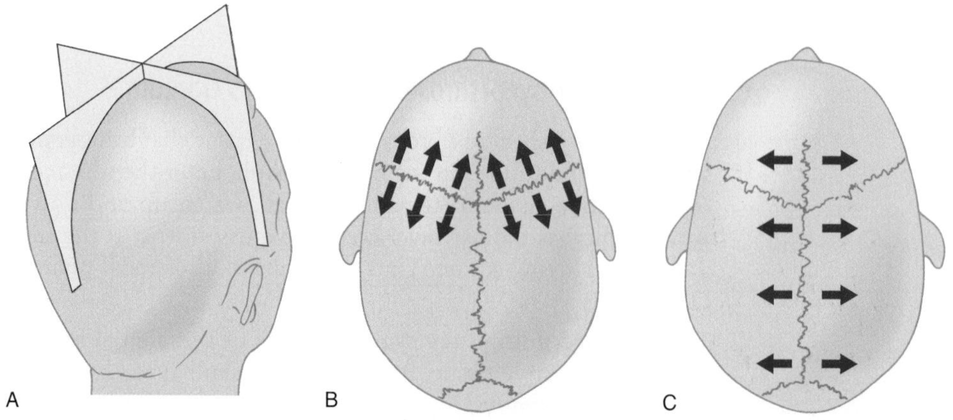

FIGURE 1-19. The sagittal and coronal sutures and the direction of head enlargement from their growth zones. (A) Schematic projection of the planes of the sagittal and coronal sutures. (B) Growth along the coronal suture increases the anteroposterior diameter of the head. (C) Growth along the sagittal suture increases the lateral diameter of the head.

☑ anteroposterior

2. Bone deposition along the *coronal* suture increases the head diameter that is perpendicular to it, i.e., the ☐ anteroposterior/☐ lateral diameter.

lateral

3. Bone deposition along the *sagittal* suture increases the head diameter that is perpendicular to it, i.e., the ________________ diameter.

anteroposterior

4. Bone deposition along the parieto-occipital (lambdoidal) suture would increase the ________________ diameter of the calvarium.

perpendicular

5. As a general rule, we can state that growth along a suture margin increases the head diameter that is ________________ to the plane of the suture.

Brachycephaly

6. Study the head shapes of your classmates. Some will have unusually short and wide heads, others will have long and thin heads. Both groups will have heads with approximately the same circumference. Therefore, a head that is relatively small in one diameter will, in compensation, enlarge in the opposite diameter. Anthropologists designate short-headedness as *brachycephaly* (*brachy* = short) and long-headedness as *dolichocephaly* (*dolicho* = long). Which head type would have the greatest lateral diameter? ________________

sagittal; coronal

7. In *brachycephaly*, growth from the ________________ suture proceeds rapidly relative to that from the ________________ suture.

coronal; sagittal

8. In *dolichocephaly*, growth from the ________________ suture proceeds rapidly relative to that from the ________________ suture.

F. Closure of the sutures and fontanels

1. With maturation, the cranium becomes increasingly rigid because the synchondroses, sutures, and fontanels progressively unite and finally ossify completely. Before the synarthroses ossify, we say they are "open." Afterward, they are "closed." The time of closure of the various sutures by ossification varies considerably (Table 1-2).

TABLE 1-2 • Time of Ossification of Some Cranial Synarthroses

Synarthrosis	Time ossification completed
Frontal (metopic) suture	2 y
Coronal suture	30 y
Basilar synchondroses	2–20 y
Anterior fontanel	1.5 y (range, 3–27 mo)
Posterior fontanel	Birth to 2 mo

☑ sutures of the cranial vault

2. The anterior fontanel usually closes by 18 months (normal range, 4 to 27 months). If increased intracranial pressure occurs *before* closure, the anterior fontanel reflects it first by bulging. Suppose increased intracranial pressure began *after* that time. Which synarthrosis would yield next to the pressure, the ☐ synchondroses of the cranial base or ☐ the sutures of the cranial vault?

Increases

3. Palpation will disclose wide separation, or "splitting," of the sutures. Otherwise, skull radiographs or CT are essential. If the sutures split, what happens to the head size? ________________.

4 to 6 years

4. Although suture closure by ossification continues into adulthood, functional closure by dense connective tissue occurs much earlier. By 10 to 12 years of age, the sutures have adhered so firmly, although not ossified, that they no longer yield to increased intracranial pressure. If a 16-year-old girl has a big head and split sutures, as shown by a skull radiograph, what is the minimum time she could have had increased intracranial pressure? ________________.

Bulging anterior fontanel, split sutures (as shown by palpation or radiography), and increased head size.

5. List three physical signs of pathologically increased intracranial pressure in a young infant.____ ________________.

VII. MISSHAPEN HEADS: CRANIOSYNOSTOSES, DEFORMATIONAL (POSITIONAL) MOLDING, AND CONGENITAL DEFORMITIES

A. The craniosynostoses

1. In the craniosynostoses, one or more sutures and fontanels do not form or, if formed, ossify and close prematurely, resulting in a misshapen head. The excessive bone growth along the suture lines causes palpable ridges.

Decreases head and brain size

2. If the major sutures close in the fetus or young infant during the brain's growth phase, how would it affect head size and brain size? ________________.

Increases

3. In the absence of sutures and fontanels, what would happen to the intracranial pressure? ________________.
4. To treat craniosynostoses, surgeons create artificial sutures by removal of strips of bone from the calvarium. The Ex must recognize craniosynostosis in young infants, because early treatment produces the best cosmetic results and prevents subsequent complications: increased intracranial pressure, brain damage from restricted brain expansion, and blindness from optic nerve compression (Shillito and Matson, 1968).
5. Diagnostic terms for abnormal head shapes caused by craniosynostosis:
   a. The terms *dolichocephaly* and *brachycephaly* describe normal variations in the length or width of the skull. The sutures are basically normal. Clinicians use special terms to differentiate the abnormal head shapes caused by craniosynostosis from normal variations. (The terms here follow Ford's usage [1973], but you will find many synonyms and some discrepancies across investigators).

coronal (or coronal/lambdoidal)

   b. The pathologic condition of *short*-headedness from craniosynostosis is *acrobrachycephaly* (Fig. 1-20A). The closed suture is the ________________ suture.

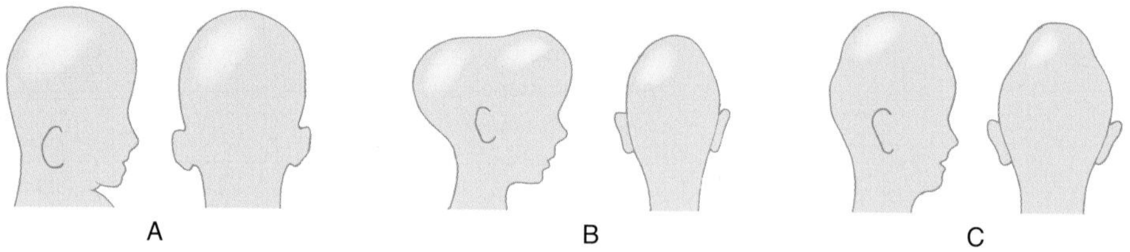

FIGURE 1-20. Silhouettes of abnormal head caused by craniosynostosis. (A) Acrobrachycephaly, (B) Scaphocephaly, (C) Oxycephaly.

sagittal

   c. In acrobrachycephaly, the head becomes too wide because it expands perpendicular to the less affected suture, the ________________ suture.

sagittal

   d. The pathologic condition of *long*-headedness from craniosynostosis is called *scaphocephaly* (*scapho* = skiff or boat). The head resembles an inverted boat (Fig. 1-20B). The closed suture is the ________________ suture.

coronal

   e. In scaphocephaly, the head becomes long because it expands perpendicular to the less affected suture, the ________________ suture.

All major sutures, the coronal/lambdoidal and sagittal, are closed.

   f. The pathologic head shape shown in Fig. 1-20C is called *oxycephaly* (*oxy* = keen or sharp). The lateral and anteroposterior diameters are reduced. What does this head shape imply about the cranial sutures? ________________.
   g. Complete Table 1-3.

TABLE 1-3 • Comparison of Terms for Head Shapes

Skull shape	Term for extreme variation of normal skull	Pathologic term for craniosynostosis
Skull too short and wide		
Skull too long		
Skull too short and narrow	None	

Brachycephaly; acrobrachycephaly
Dolichocephaly; scaphocephaly
Oxycephaly

h. Would acrobrachycephaly, scaphocephaly, or oxycephaly most likely cause microcephaly and increased intracranial pressure? Explain. ____.

Oxycephaly. Neither major suture allows skull expansion, thus limiting head size and brain growth in lateral and anteroposterior diameters.

6. The increased intracranial pressure in craniosynostosis causes the weakest part of the calvarium to yield. Because it cannot expand at the sutures or fontanels, the thin orbital plates bulge downward, causing the eyes to protrude. The general term for eyeball protrusion is ______________.

exophthalmia (exophthalmos or proptosis)

7. Clinical detection of craniosynostosis
   a. Clinical recognition of craniosynostosis requires *inspection* of the infant's head shape and *palpation* along the sites of the major sutures. The finger will detect absence of the sutures and fontanels and replacement by a bony ridge along the suture lines.
   b. Skull radiographs or CT confirms the bony overgrowth and absence of the sutures (CT directly shows bone, whereas MRI does not).
8. A 2-month-old baby with a short head would raise the suspicion of a deficiency of growth from the ______________ suture.

coronal (or coronal/lambdoidal)

9. How would you determine whether the child has brachycephaly, a normal variant, or craniosynostosis of the coronal suture, i.e., acrobrachycephaly? ____.

Palpate for a bony ridge along the suture lines and order skull radiographs or a CT scan. Also, when the Pt has a borderline head size or shape or an unusual face, always check the somatotype of parents and siblings.

10. Complete Table 1-4 to fix the diagnostic terms for head shapes firmly in mind.

TABLE 1-4 • Terms for Abnormal Head Shapes

——— cephaly	Too short a skull because of a lack of coronal suture
——— cephaly	Too long a skull because of a lack of sagittal suture
——— cephaly	Too long a skull without craniosynostosis
——— cephaly	Short, narrow skull because of craniosynostosis
——— cephaly	Short skull without craniosynostosis

Acrobrachycephaly
Scaphocephaly
Dolichocephaly
Oxycephaly
Brachycephaly

11. Craniosynostosis of various types occurs in numerous syndromes, many with congenital malformations of the brain and extremities. See Ashwal (1999) and Cohen (1986).

BIBLIOGRAPHY · Craniosynostosis

Ashwal S. congenital structural defects. In: Swaiman KE, Ashwal S, eds. *Pediatric Neurology. Principles & Practice*, 3d ed. St. Louis, Mosby, 1999, Chap. 17, pp. 234–300.

Cohen MM, ed. *Craniosynostosis: Diagnosis, Evaluation, and Management*. New York, Raven Press, 1986.

Ford F. *Diseases of the Nervous System in Infancy, Childhood and Adolescence*, 6th ed. Springfield, Charles C. Thomas, 1973.

Shillito J Jr, Matson D. Craniosynostosis: a review of 519 surgical patients. *Pediatrics* 1968;41:829–853.

B. The asymmetrical head: plagiocephaly and deformational molding of the cranium

1. Intrinsic diseases such as craniosynostosis, rickets, and syphilis alter head shape, as does extrinsic pressure. Striking examples of molding of the cranium and the feet by extrinsic pressure occurred in certain societies that sought to beautify girls by tightly bandaging the head and feet during infancy.
2. If an infant has an abnormal position in utero or if a neurologic deficit, such as hemiplegia or hemianopia, causes it to recline on one part of its head after birth, the head deforms to become flat on the "down" side.
3. If the young infant reclines too much on its back, the occiput becomes symmetrically flattened (DeMyer, 2002). The prolonged sleeping position of infants on their backs to avoid sudden infant death syndrome has caused a distinct increase in deformational or positional occipital flattening (Huang et al., 1996; Marshall et al., 1997; Mulliken, 1999). The brachycephaly is usually mild, more or less symmetrical, and self-correcting as the infant learns to sit up and spends less time on its back. The long periods that premature infants spend on the sides of their heads causes a deformational long-headedness, a dolichocephaly, that also tends to self-correction.
4. If the infant reclines on one parieto-occipital region, it flattens, and the head becomes skewed or asymmetrical. When the head molding, prenatally or postnatally, produces head asymmetry, the condition is called *plagiocephaly*. Extracranial lesions that may accompany plagiocephaly are torticollis and vertebral malformations. Sometimes no cause for skull asymmetry can be identified.
5. Although usually bilateral, craniosynostosis may obliterate the sutures only on one side of the head. The affected hemicranium is small, causing an asymmetrical calvarium and face. Some investigators prefer to limit the term *plagiocephaly* to the deformity caused by craniosynostosis.
6. Plagiocephaly affects the whole base of the skull and often causes a tilt of the base. With deformational plagiocephaly, the unilaterally flattened occiput displaces or rotates the ipsilateral ear and cheek *forward* (Fig. 1-21A).
7. With the much rarer craniosynostotic plagiocephaly, which may occur from unilateral lambdoidal synostosis, the restricted hemicranium fails to expand, and the ear and cheek ipsilateral to the flattening are displaced *backward* relative to the normal forward growth on the opposite side (Fig. 1-21B).
8. Use the "two-forefingers" test to determine the degree of rotation of the skull base: look down on top of the infant's head and insert your forefingers lightly into the external end of each ear canal. Normally the fingers should align exactly. In plagiocephaly, the degree of offset of the fingers reflects the degree of rotation of the calvarial base.
9. Because torticollis may accompany the plagiocephaly, palpate the sternocleidomastoid muscle for a hematoma or fibrotic tightening.
10. Plagiocephaly from lambdoidal synostosis may warrant surgical correction, whereas the much commoner deformational plagiocephaly usually responds to positioning and application of a molding helmet (Marshall et al., 1997; Mullikan et al., 1999).
11. In any event, an abnormal size or shape of the skull raises the question of an abnormal brain (Miller and Clarren, 2000), often requiring further investigation by MRI or CT. Computed tomography can depict the skull and sutures in three dimensions.

C. Misshapen heads in neonates, other than plagiocephaly

1. The most common conditions are molding of the head during birth and consequent scalp edema, frank caput succedaneum, subgaleal hematoma, and cephalohematoma, all from birth trauma, and meningocele or meningoencephalocele, which are malformations. In the conditions caused by birth trauma, the scalp has closed in the midline.
2. *Meningoceles* or *meningoencephaloceles* are saclike protrusions in the midline and may occur from the occipital region to the forehead. They resemble a "topknot."

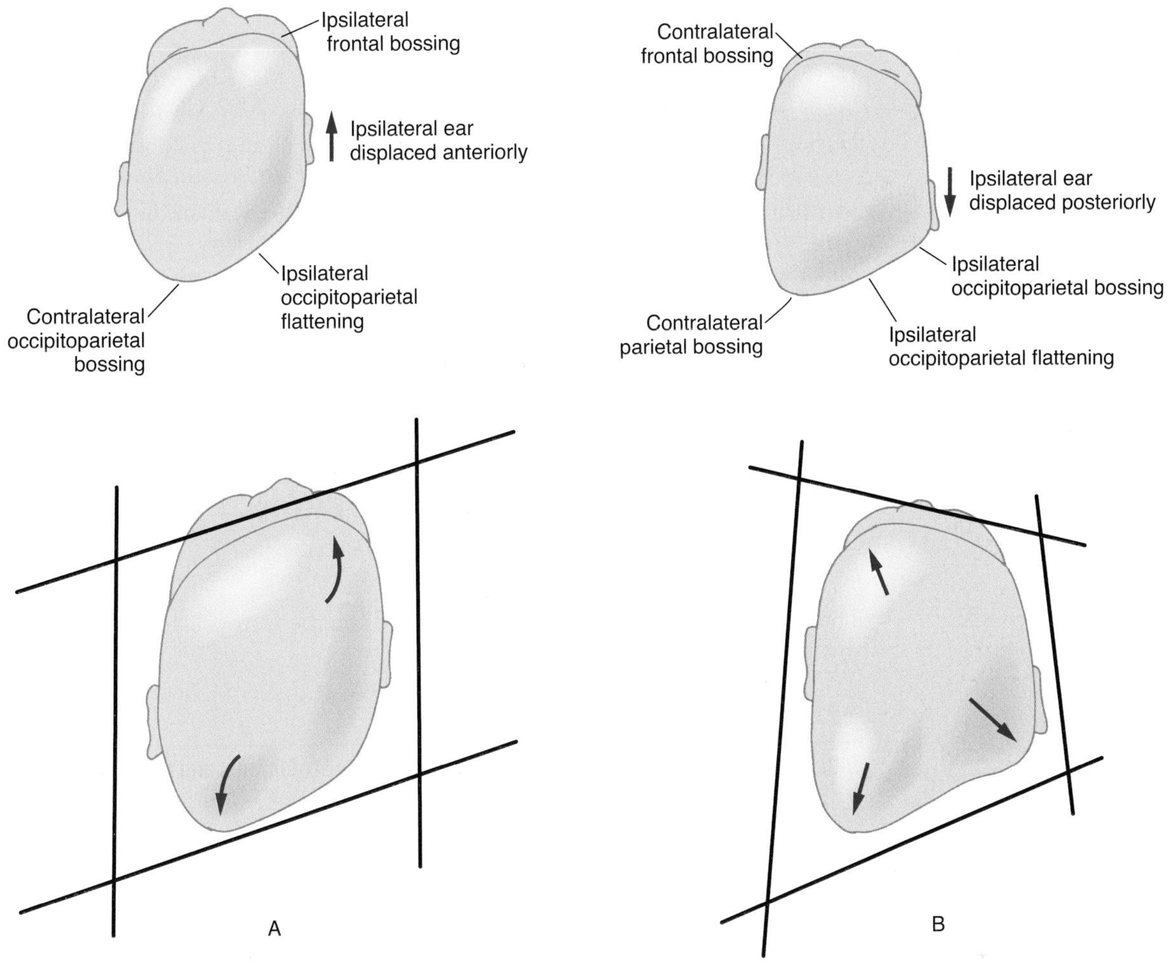

FIGURE 1-21. Top view of plagiocephaly. (A) The two left drawings show simple deformational or positional molding of the head and its effect on the prominence of the occiput and cheek. The sutures are open on both sides. (B) The two right drawings show the effect of unilateral craniosynostosis in restricting head growth on the right side. Notice the difference in the forward positioning of the forehead and cheeks between (A) and (B). (Reproduced with permission from Marshall D, Fenner GC, Wolfe A, et al. Abnormal head shape in infants. *Int Pediatr* 1997;12:172–177.)

Meningoceles generally transilluminate, whereas meningoencephaloceles generally do not.

3. In *scalp edema* or in the frankly hemorrhagic scalp edema called *caput succedaneum*, the infant has a scalp swelling that alters the head contour smoothly, usually symmetrically, and at the vertex (Volpe, 2001). Scalp edema, whether from injury or infiltration of intravenous fluid, transilluminates readily, but the greater the hemorrhage, the more opaque the lesion.
4. In *subgaleal hemorrhage*, the blood occupies a space between the external periosteum and the galea aponeurotica of the scalp. It does not transilluminate. It may cause significant blood loss.
5. In *cephalohematoma*, blood dissects the external periosteum away from one of the large, flat calvarial bones, usually the parietal. The lesion thus causes a localized bulge, limited by suture lines. The adherence of the periosteum at the sutures arrests the spread of the lesion to adjacent bones. A unilateral parietal hematoma is limited *medially* by the *sagittal* suture, *frontally* by the *coronal* suture, and *posteriorly* by the *parieto-occipital* (*lambdoidal*) suture. The underlying bone sometimes has a fracture.
6. By palpation, scalp edema pits, subgaleal hematoma is fluctuant or allows ballottement, and a cephalohematoma is very firm. None of these extracranial lesions pulsate, whereas meningoceles or any other lesion connected to the intracranial space do. Final diagnosis of the lesion and its consequences for the brain may require imaging by ultrasound, CT, or MRI.

BIBLIOGRAPHY · Misshapen Heads

DeMyer W. Small, large or abnormally shaped heads. In: Maria BL, ed. *Current Management in Child Neurology*, 2nd ed. Hamilton, BC Decker Inc., 2002, Chap. 49, pp. 299–304.

Huang M, Gruss J, Mouradian WE, et al. The differential diagnosis of posterior plagiocephaly: true lambdoid synostosis versus positional molding. *Plast Reconstr Surg* 1996;98:765–774.

Marshall, D, Fenner GC, Wolfe A, et al. Abnormal head shape in infants. *Int Pediatr* 1997;12:172–177.

Miller RI, Clarren SK. Long-term developmental outcomes in patients with deformational plagiocephaly. *Pediatrics* 2000;105:e26.

Mulliken JB, Woude DL, Vander DL, et al. Analysis of posterior plagiocephaly: deformational versus synostotic. *Plast Reconstr Surg* 1999;103:371–380.

Volpe JJ. *Neurology of the Newborn*, 4th ed. Philadelphia, W.B. Saunders, 2001.

VIII. THE SIZE OF THE HEAD AND BRAIN

A. Determinants of head size

The head size of any given individual depends on the factors listed in Table 1-5. Learn this table.

TABLE 1-5 · Determinants of Occipitofrontal Circumference of Infants and Children

Age
Genetic background
Sex
Family somatotype
Volume of intracranial contents
Brain size
Amount of fluid in the ventricles and meningeal spaces
Volume of blood in the intracranial vessels
Space-occupying lesions
Ability of calvarium to expand (open or closed sutures)
Thickness of the calvarial bones, scalp, and hair

B. Measuring the head size: the occipitofrontal circumference (OFC)

1. The two most important measurements of the newborn infant are its birth weight in relation to gestational age and its OFC (Raymond and Holmes, 1994; Roche et al., 1987; Sher and Brown, 1975; Sheth et al., 1995; Volpe 2001). Record every infant's OFC at every examination (DeMyer, 1999, 2002). Place a tape measure around the maximum OFC, from the *external occipital protuberance (inion)* to the *glabella*. Figures 1-22A to 1-22D show the normal values, which differ by age and sex.
2. **Mnemonic for the infant's OFC:** The average full-term newborn weighs approximately **3500 g.** The birth OFC is approximately **35 cm.** The OFC increases, on average, about 1 cm per month, making the average OFC at 1 year about 47 to 48 cm.
3. An OFC beyond +2 standard deviations from the mean always raises suspicion of an abnormal brain, particularly with normal body weight, chest circumference, length, and body proportions. Measure the OFCs of parents and siblings to make allowance for normal variations of somatotype (DeMyer, 1999; Weaver and Christian, 1980).
4. Too large a head is called *macro*cephaly (*megalocephaly*), and one that is too small is called *micro*cephaly (Opitz and Holt, 1990). An infant's head may be too large or too small at birth, or the head may become abnormal in size later on. To best recognize an abnormal trend in head size as the infant develops, plot successive OFC measurements on a chart (Fig. 1-23). In Fig. 1-23, trend line A represents an abnormally enlarging head, and trend line B represents a lagging head size.

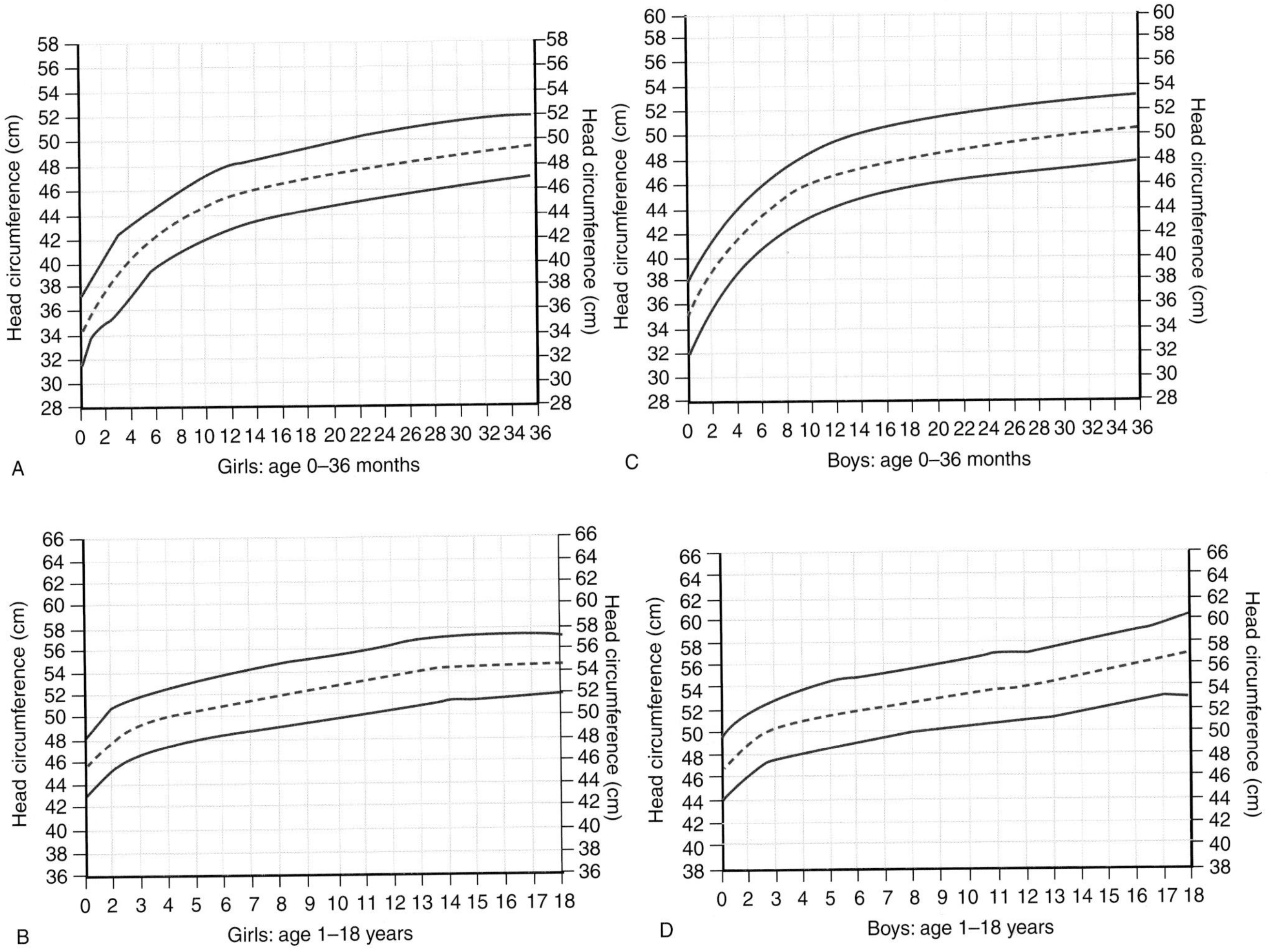

FIGURE 1-22. Growth curve for the occipitofrontal circumference. The areas shown for males and females include 2 standard deviations above and below the mean. Ninety-five percent of normal children fall within these limits.

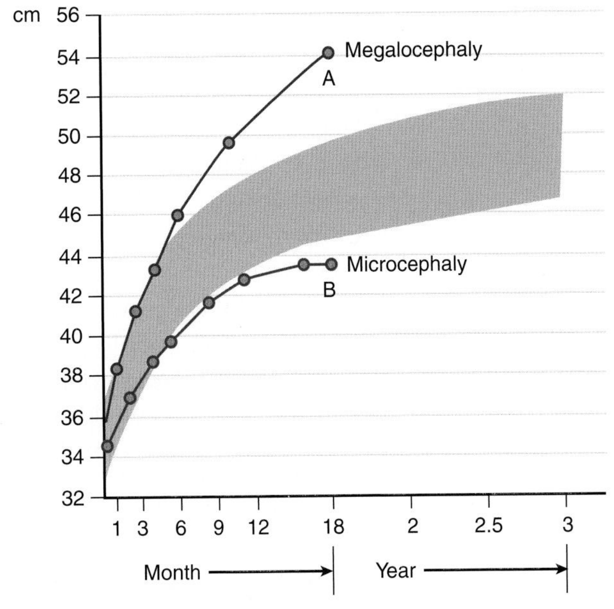

FIGURE 1-23. Successive plots of abnormal head sizes. The shaded area represents ±2SD from the mean.

BIBLIOGRAPHY · Measuring the Head Size

DeMyer W. Microcephaly, micrencephaly, megalocephaly and megalencephaly. In: Swaiman K, Ashwal S, eds. *Pediatric Neurology,* 3rd ed. St. Louis, Mosby, 1999, Chap. 18, pp. 301–311.

DeMyer W. Small, large and abnormally shaped heads. In: Maria BL, ed. *Current Management in Child Neurology,* 2nd ed. Hamilton, BC Decker, 2002, Chap. 49, pp. 299–304.

Opitz JM, Holt MC. Microcephaly: general considerations and aids to nosology. *J Craniofac Genet Dev Biol* 1990;10:175–204.

Raymond GV, Holmes LB. Head circumference standards in neonates. *J Child Neurol* 1994;9:63–66.

Roche AF, Mukherjee D, Guo S, et al. Head circumference reference data: birth to 18 years. *Pediatrics* 1987;79:706–712.

Sher PK, Brown SB. A longitudinal study of head growth in pre-term infants. II: differentiation between "catch-up" head growth and early infantile hydrocephalus. *Dev Med Child Neurol* 1975;17:711–718.

Sheth RD, Mullett MD, Bodensteiner JB, et al. Longitudinal head growth in developmentally normal preterm infants. *Arch Pediatr Adolesc Med* 1995;149:1358–1361.

Volpe JJ. *Neurology of the Newborn,* 4th ed. Philadelphia, W.B. Saunders, 2001.

Weaver D, Christian J. Familial variation of head size and adjustment for parental head circumference. *J Pediatr* 1980;96:990–994.

C. Relation of head size to brain size

1. The technical term for the head is *cephalon* and that for the brain is *encephalon*. If the brain or encephalon is too small and weighs too little, the condition is called *micrencephaly*. If the brain is too large and weighs too much, it is called ________________.

megalencephaly or macrencephaly

2. Of necessity, a Pt with microcephaly has ❒ megalencephaly/❒ micrencephaly/ ❒ a normal brain size.

☑ micrencephaly

3. Of necessity, a Pt with megalencephaly must have megalocephaly, but a Pt with megalocephaly does not necessarily have megalencephaly. *Megalocephaly* is simply a statistical description of head size, not a diagnosis or a synonym for megalencephaly. In megalocephaly, the brain may be normal in weight, too large, or too small. In fact, Pts with little or no cerebrum (hydranencephaly) may have *microcephaly, normocephaly*, or *megalocephaly*. Thus, the encephalon may be much smaller than suggested by the OFC. When the brain fails to fill the cranium, fluid occupies the extra space. Study Fig. 1-24.
4. Select the correct statement about head size and brain size:
   a. The OFC and brain weight have a strict, linear correlation in normal and pathologic conditions.
   b. Even though the OFC and brain weight generally correlate, the OFC predicts the maximum weight the brain may have, but not the minimum.
   c. Even though the OFC and brain weight generally correlate, the OFC predicts the minimum weight the brain may have, but not the maximum.
   d. None of these answers apply.

☑ b

5. The relation of head size to intelligence is complex. As the OFC approaches and exceeds ±2 standard deviations from the mean, the likelihood of an abnormal brain increases. Some evidence suggests that a head size slightly larger than average correlates with increased intelligence and protects against dementia (Tisserand et al., 2002), but children with neurofibromatosis, muscular dystrophy, and autism have heads larger than average and yet have below-average IQs.

D. Head size, brain size, and hydrocephalus

1. Whenever the volume of cerebrospinal fluid (CSF) is significantly increased, the condition is called *hydrocephaly* (= *hydrocephalus*), irrespective of brain size or

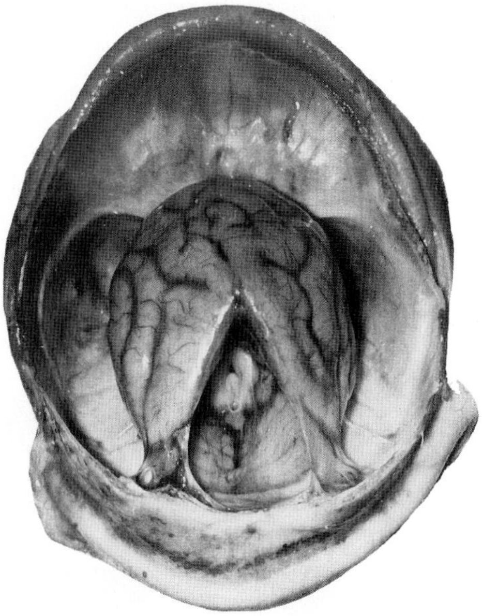

FIGURE 1-24. Postmortem photograph of a micrencephalon in a microcephalic skull. When this patient died at the age of 4 months, the occipitofrontal circumference was only 32 cm (normal, 41 cm). Despite the tiny head, the disproportionately small brain failed to fill the intracranial space. [Reprinted with permission from DeMyer W, White P. EEG in holoprosencephaly (arrhinencephaly). *Arch Neurol* 1964;11:507–520.]

CSF

head size, irrespective of the location of the CSF, whether within the ventricles or subarachnoid space, and irrespective of the intracranial pressure. Thus, the one condition necessary to justify the term *hydrocephaly* is an excessive volume of ________________ within the intracranial cavity.

2. The Pt shown in Fig. 1-24 happened to have *microcephaly* and *micrencephaly*. The disproportionately small brain left a large fluid-filled space. Thus, this Pt had hydrocephaly, microcephaly, and micrencephaly.
3. Hydrocephaly has a second meaning, a triad of *increased volume of* CSF, *increased intracranial pressure,* and usually *increased head size*. If the excessive CSF is under pressure in the ventricles, the cerebral wall thins, the ventricles dilate, and the head size increases, if the sutures have not closed (Fig. 1-25).
4. With an undersized brain, as from atrophy, hypoplasia, or destructive lesions, the excessive CSF may merely fill in the unoccupied space (nature abhors a vacuum). In this condition, called *hydrocephalus ex vacuo*, the intracranial pressure is normal. Does the term *hydrocephaly* apply correctly? ❒ Yes/❒ No. Explain. ____.

☑ Yes. The first definition, the purely quantitative one, applies even though the Pt does not have increased intracranial pressure

5. Thus far, the terms *micro-*, *megalo-*, and *hydro-* have been used quantitatively to mean too much or too little of something. Thus, they are descriptive terms, like gigantism or dwarfism, not diagnoses. An abnormal head size usually requires radiographic visualization of the size and shape of the brain and its ventricles and subarachnoid spaces. Visualization techniques include ultrasound in fetuses and very young infants and CT or MRI (see Chapter 13).

E. Causes of megalocephaly

1. One of five conditions usually causes megalocephaly. Be able to recite these. See DeMyer (1999) for a full list of differential diagnoses for megalocephaly (Fig. 1-26).
2. An unfortunate, all too common cause of a bulging fontanel and an enlarged head is a battered or shaken infant who has a subdural hematoma and brain edema and who most likely has had seizures. The caretakers provide an implausible

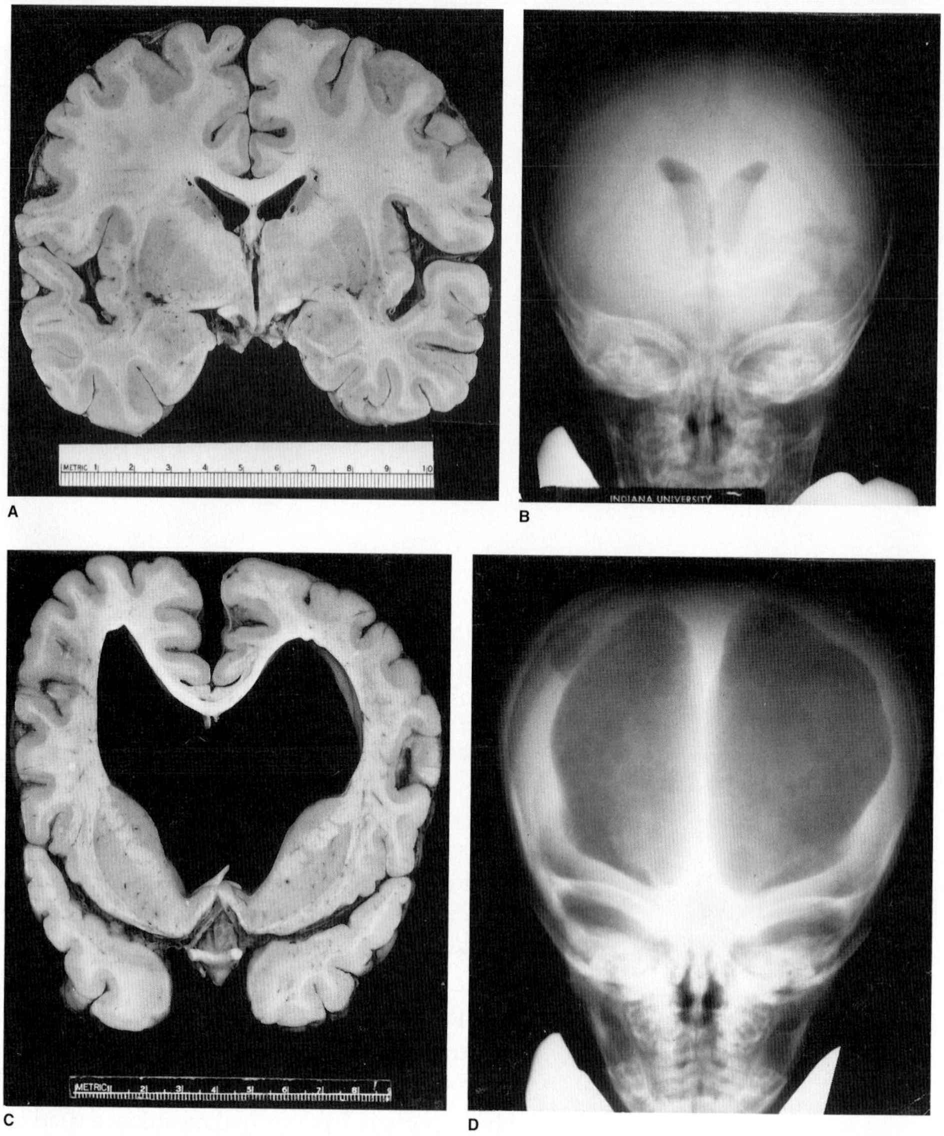

FIGURE 1-25. Coronal sections of the brain. (A) Normal brain showing configuration of the anterior horns of the lateral ventricles. (B) Normal anterior horns as shown by radiography (in this case, pneumoencephalography). (C) Dilated anterior horns in a patient with obstructive hydrocephalus. (D) Radiograph of dilated anterior horns in a patient with obstructive hydrocephalus.

history: "He rolled off of the couch" or "He crawled out of the crib"—remarkable feats for a 3-month-old infant. The NE shows an obtunded infant with multiple bruises involving the scalp, ear, or remainder of the body, a bulging fontanel, split sutures, retinal hemorrhages, and often fractures of the skull, ribs, or long bones. The lesions are of various ages, indicating repeated assaults. The shaken rather than the battered baby may lack the skin signs and multiple fractures but has the brain lesions.

F. Review of steps in the NE of a patient with megalocephaly or microcephaly (DeMyer, 1999)

1. In infants, palpate the fontanelle and sutures and attempt to transilluminate the cranium.
2. Compare the somatotype and OFC of the Pt with those of siblings and parents. Does the Pt match or differ from the family pattern?
3. Obtain MRIs if the history or examination discloses slow development. Note that

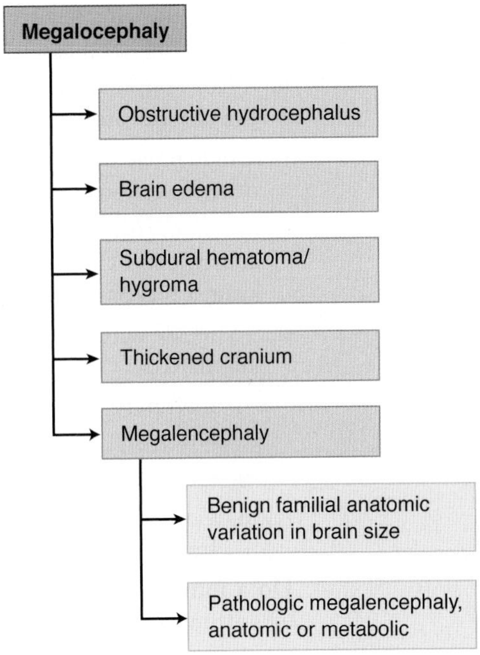

FIGURE 1-26. The five most common causes for megalocephaly.

MRI is almost always superior to CT in diagnosing intracranial lesions, except in a few acute emergencies when intracranial bleeding is suspected. Use CT to show the cranial bones, the sutures, and calcified intracranial lesions (Alper et al., 1999; Barkovich, 2000).

BIBLIOGRAPHY · Abnormalities of Head Size and Brain Size

Alper G, Ekinci G, Yilmaz Y, et al. Magnetic resonance imaging characteristics of benign macrocephaly in children. *J Child Neurol* 1999;14:678–682.

Barkovich AJ. *Pediatric Neuroimaging*, 3rd ed. Philadelphia, Lippincott Williams & Wilkins, 2000.

DeMyer W. Microcephaly, micrencephaly, megalocephaly and megalencephaly. In Swaiman K, Ashwal S, eds. *Pediatric Neurology*, 3rd ed. St. Louis, Mosby, 1999, Chap. 18, pp. 301–311.

DeMyer W. Small, large or abnormally shaped heads. In Maria BL, ed. *Current Management in Child Neurology*, 2nd ed. Hamilton, BC Decker, 2002, Chap. 49, pp. 299–304.

Tisserand DJ, Bosma H, Van Boxtel MPJ, et al. Head size and cognitive ability in non-demented older adults are related. *Neurology* 2002;56:969–971.

IX. THE GENERAL RULES FOR THE NEUROLOGIC EXAMINATION

Having learned some of the steps of the NE, you can now appreciate the general, operational, analytic, and attitudinal rules that determine success or failure.

A. Operational rules for the neurologic examination

1. **Follow the prescribed technique for each step of the NE.**
2. **Systematize the NE:** The actual order is less important than the fact that you follow an order:
   a. **Anatomic order:** Work from top to bottom (rostrocaudal order).
   b. **Functional order:** Test for mental, motor, and sensory dysfunctions in packages; the Standard NE (see Introduction) follows this rule.

3. **Quantify the NE:** Measure the measurable and grade or scale the rest. **Numbers comprise the language of science.**
   a. Record pupillary size, OFC, limb circumference, weight, etc., when relevant to the clinical problem.
   b. Grade muscular strength from 0 to 5, muscle stretch reflexes from 0 to 4+, or other functions as minimally, mildly, moderately, or severely abnormal.
   c. Match or titrate the Pt's functions against your own whenever possible: visual acuity, extent of visual fields, sensory thresholds, and strength (biceps pull against biceps pull).
   d. To decide whether a body part deviates from normal, compare it against three standards:
      i. Compare each part with the established norm for a person of like age and sex.
      ii. Compare each part with its mate on the opposite side.
      iii. Compare the Pt with the family members. Does the Pt match or deviate from the genetic traits of the family?
4. **Do a minimum screening NE on every Pt (Chapter 15):** You must examine everything pertinent to the clinical problem, but you cannot and need not do every conceivable test on every Pt. You can extend or reduce the Standard NE to adapt to the clinical problem. The Pt with acute pain radiating down a leg requires a considerably different NE from that for the unconscious Pt. The Pt's age, mental status, the symptoms that require investigation, and the diseases suspected require intelligent adaptation of the Standard NE.
   a. Gather in the gestalt of the Pt: Appraise the total impact of the Pt's personality, facial appearance, and somatotype. Then inspect the Pt part by part.
   b. Inspect every square centimeter of skin and mucous membrane.
   c. Look into every opening.
   d. Feel every part.
   e. Listen over the chest, abdomen, head, and blood vessels.
   f. Smell every odor.

B. Analytic rules for the NE

1. **Record all end-point results objectively:** Record what actually occurred during each operation of the NE, not an interpretation.

Interpretation: The Pt withdrew his leg from pain.
Observation: Pinprick elicited leg flexion.

Notice how the second statement records the operation performed (pinprick) and the behavioral result (leg flexion). A brain-dead Pt with an intact spinal cord or a paraplegic might reflexly withdraw the leg but could not have "felt pain."

2. **Think circuitry:** After recording the findings objectively, interpret their pathophysiologic implications and convert to technical terminology, e.g., the observed weakness and hyperreflexia on one side becomes hemiplegia from pyramidal tract interruption. The interpretation locates the lesion in the circuits of the nervous system. Thus far, Chapter 1 has not introduced circuitry, but subsequent chapters will discuss it extensively.
   a. As corollaries of the definition of behavior on page 1, we can state that:
      i. **All** behavior depends on neuroanatomic circuitry.
      ii. **Every** behavior, spontaneous or induced, that the Pt can or cannot produce conveys valuable information as to the integrity of the underlying circuits.

b. By "thinking through" the circuits responsible for each end action tested, the Ex plugs into and can determine which circuits of the nervous system are intact or impaired, e.g.:

   i. If the pupil constricts to light, the circuit from the retina to the midbrain and back to the pupilloconstrictor muscle is intact. If the pupil does not react, a lesion, anatomic or pharmacologic, blocks the circuit at some point.

   ii. If the large toe flexes in response to plantar stimulation, the pyramidal tract and the afferent and efferent nerve fibers of the foot are intact; if the toe extends (Babinski sign), the pyramidal tract is interrupted. Thus, blockage of certain circuits may alter the effector actions in characteristic ways.

3. **Localize the lesion:** Postulate an anatomic site where the lesion has interrupted a nerve, pathway, or circuit.

   a. Because the clinical signs of lesions at different levels of a circuit vary, the NE discloses which level the lesion has interrupted.

   b. For a weak or paralyzed Pt, the NE localizes the lesion to the pyramidal tract, ventral motoneuron, nerve root, peripheral nerve, neuromyal junction, or the muscle itself.

   c. For a blind Pt, the NE localizes the lesion to the retina, optic nerve, chiasm or optic tract, the geniculocalcarine tract, or the calcarine (visual) cortex itself.

   d. By knowing the anatomic conjunctions of the various neural circuits, the Ex can localize the lesion to a specific anatomic site. A VI cranial nerve palsy and a contralateral hemiplegia localize the lesion to the basis pontis, near the pontomedullary junction, at the conjunction of the VI cranial nerve and the pyramidal tract.

4. **Propose an etiologic diagnosis**: For example craniosynostosis is the cause of the Pt's abnormal head shape. By integrating the history, anatomic localization, pathophysiology, and the probability of various diseases, the Ex achieves a presumptive etiologic diagnosis, which in turn determines any required laboratory workup to reach a final etiologic diagnosis. The final etiologic diagnosis sets the prognosis and therapy.

5. This catechism summarizes the analytic process applied to every Pt:

   a. Is there a lesion?

   b. Where is the lesion?

   c. What is the lesion or disease present?

   d. How do I confirm the diagnosis?

   e. What is the therapeutic and preventive management?

C. Attitudinal and ethical rules for success in the NE

First and foremost, the success of the NE depends on the Ex's mindset and ability to react nonjudgmentally.

1. **React professionally:** Accept every Pt with equal humility and grace, whether the Pt is a murderer, pedophile, grossly retarded, or a genius and whether the Pt has a hangnail or acquired immunodeficiency syndrome. Accept all of the Pt's behavior objectively as clinical phenomena, as the activation of glands and muscles by nerve impulses shuttling through neuroanatomic circuits. **You cannot complete a competent, analytical evaluation while plagued with emotions of attraction or repulsion or while making moral judgments about the Pt's lifestyle and worthiness.**

2. **Communicate with the Pt during the examination**

   a. Proper communication ensures full Pt cooperation and confidence. Reassure the Pt that a particular test will not hurt, or prepare the Pt if the test causes discomfort.

b. Remember that everyone has doubts about how they will measure up under scrutiny and whether the physician will discover something dreadful. During the NE, you may want to comment briefly on your findings: "Your blood pressure is OK." "Your eyes check out normal." Patients will appreciate the communication, but avoid extensive discussions. Wait until the end of the examination for that.

i. For the anxious but neurologically normal Pt, the recital of normal findings will provide some assurance.

ii. For the neurologically impaired Pt, the recital of abnormal findings assures the Pt of your care and concern. When you summarize your conclusions at the end of the examination, the Pt will understand the evidence for your conclusions and will more readily accept the correct management.

3. **Expect the abnormal:** Expect that every observation, question, request, or maneuver will disclose an abnormality. The trained mind discovers what it is trained to discover. Look for abnormalities, anomalies, asymmetries, malalignments, and dysfunctions. The expectation of normality inevitably results in loss of vigilance and a sloppy or incomplete examination (Fowkes, 1986). If you expect that the eardrums or rectum will be normal, you won't examine them carefully, if at all.

4. **Enjoy each NE**

a. Convert parts of the NE into a friendly contest or game.

i. **Visual fields:** Ask the Pt, "Let's find out whether you can see out as far to the side as I can."

ii. **Strength testing:** "Don't let me win."

iii. **Sensory testing:** "Let's see how light a touch you can feel."

b. Such challenges elicit the Pt's interest and best performance and maintain your own interest. Then both you and the Pt will enjoy the NE. If you do something 20 times a day for the rest of your career, you may as well learn how to enjoy it.

c. The NE gives you the privilege of entering and sorting through the Pt's neural circuits to discover the way lesions alter mental, motor, and sensory functions. If you remain curious, inquisitive, and take pride in your knowledge, technique, and competence, the whole process of the NE and its derivative conclusions becomes immensely gratifying or downright fun. Viewed this way, each NE becomes an opportunity for enjoyment. That is what I want this text to offer you: the skill to do a competent, enjoyable NE.

BIBLIOGRAPHY

Fowkes FGR. Diagnostic vigilance. *Lancet* 1986;1:493–494.

D. Review of the initial examination of the head and face

To ensure mastery you need to review and rehearse these general principles and the techniques of this chapter. Although you may prefer to call it practicing, behavioral psychologists would say that they want you to emit the terminal behavior of the learning sequence. By terminal behavior, the psychologist means that you should produce those recitations and performances that provide evidence to you and anyone watching that you have learned what you should have. First, review the Learning Objectives for Section VIII, page 48. Then, with a partner, practice the "terminal behavior" outlined in Section IV, A to E, of the Standard NE (see Introduction).

Learning Objectives for Chapter 1

The Learning Objectives match the order of the text. Follow along in the text to check the correctness of your responses.

I. INTRODUCTION TO THE NEUROLOGICAL EXAMINATION

1. The end point of each operation of the NE is the observation of some bodily contour or some spontaneous or elicited behavior. Define behavior as applied to the NE.
2. State the two general types of effectors through which humans express behavior.
3. Discuss how viewing all Pts as biological co-organisms who share identical needs and life processes may aid the physician in responding nonjudgmentally to each Pt. If this approach does not seem effective for you, discuss this subject with others to learn their methods of avoiding emotional entanglements.

II. LOOKING AT THE EYES

A. Relation of the eyelid margins to the iris

1. Make a drawing of the eye, label the following structures, and point them out on another person or yourself in your mirror: medial and lateral canthi, corneal limbus, iris, pupil, caruncle, and lacrimal papilla (Fig. 1-2).
2. Make a drawing that shows the relation of the limbus to the upper and lower eyelid margins when the Pt looks straight ahead (Fig. 1-3).
3. Make a drawing that shows the relation of the limbus to the canthi and caruncle when the Pt holds the eyes as far as possible to the side (Fig. 1-4).
4. Describe and name the abnormal angulations of the palpebral fissures (Fig. 1-5).

B. Anatomic variations of the medial canthus

1. Draw or describe an epicanthal fold.
2. Contrast canthus dystopia and an epicanthal fold (Figs. 1-6 and 1-7).

C. Intercanthal and interorbital distances

1. Define these eye abnormalities: canthus dystopia, epicanthal folds, hypertelorism, and hypotelorism ptosis, enophthalmia and exophthalmia, anophthalmia, microphthalmia, and macrophthalmia (Figs. 1-7 and 1-8).
2. Name two anomalies of the medial part of the eyelid that may falsely indicate hypertelorism.
3. Name the diagnostic procedure necessary to establish true bony ocular hypertelorism and hypotelorism.

D. Pupillary size

1. What is the size of the normal pupil in millimeters in ordinary light?
2. Define isocoria, anisocoria, miosis (cormiosis), corectasia, and corectopia.
3. Describe two types of rings that appear in the cornea near the limbus and state their clinical implications.
4. Describe the normal variations in the size of the pupil from term birth to old age.

E. Height of the palpebral fissure

1. Define ptosis of the eyelid.
2. Describe the sign called "lid lag" as seen in hyperthyroidism.
3. Describe the effect of exophthalmia and enophthalmia on the height of the palpebral fissure.

Learning Objectives for Chapter 1

III. INSPECTION OF THE FACE, EARS, HAIR, AND SKIN

1. Name in order the parts of the face that the Ex must systematically inspect.
2. Draw and label the parts of the external ear (Fig. 1-9).
3. Name two abnormalities of the eyebrows and their clinical implications.
4. Name three types of congenital skin lesions or spots and the diagnostic implications for neurologic disease.
5. Describe the parts of the face that derive embryologically from the frontonasal process and the branchial arch sectors (Figs. 1-10 and 1-11).
6. Describe the three horizontal subdivisions of the face useful for describing facial malformations (Fig. 1-12).
7. Restudy the Pts shown in Fig. 1-13, write down the abnormalities, and check with the caption of each figure.

IV. PALPATION OF THE HEAD, AUSCULTATION, AND THE NEUROVASCULAR EXAMINATION

1. Describe the normal bumps and depressions felt on palpation of the calvarium.
2. Demonstrate how to palpate the superficial temporal arteries.
3. Describe and demonstrate auscultation of the neck and head for bruits (Fig. 1-14).
4. Describe the type of carotid bruit that indicates a significantly occluded carotid artery and an increased risk of stroke in adults.
5. Describe the sites to percuss or compress the head for tenderness when sinusitis or mastoiditis are suspected.

V. TRANSILLUMINATION OF THE INFANT'S HEAD

1. Describe the conditions for proper transillumination.
2. State the size of the normal halo around the flashlight during transillumination of the head.
3. Describe how to differentiate scalp edema from subgaleal fluid.
4. Place your hand on top of your head and describe the sites of fluid in order from superficial to deep that may transilluminate (Fig. 1-16).
5. State the age range for the usefulness of transillumination.

VI. THE BONES AND SUTURES OF THE CRANIUM

1. State the difference in the histogenetic origin of the bones of the skull base and the flat bones of the calvarium.
2. Name the endochondral bones of the skull base (Fig. 1-17).
3. Distinguish between a *synarthrosis* and a *diarthrosis* and state which cranial joints are diarthroses.
4. Recite the fontanels, bones, and sutures of the calvarium (Fig. 1-18).
5. Name the bones that border the anterior fontanel (Fig. 1-18).
6. Rank the calvarial synarthroses (synchondroses, fontanelles, and sutures) in order of pliancy.
7. Describe the contour of the normal fontanel in a neonate or young infant and describe two techniques for demonstrating the normal (or abnormal) contour.
8. Describe the proper conditions for examining the contour of the anterior fontanel of an infant and explain why you would not attempt to judge the contour of the fontanelle when the infant is struggling or crying.
9. Describe the process that keeps the sutures from separating during normal brain growth.

Learning Objectives for Chapter 1

10. State the rule that relates head shape to the plane of the sutures (Fig. 1-19).
11. Explain the meaning of "closure of the sutures" and describe when functional closure of the sutures occurs.
12. State the average time for closure of the anterior fontanel and the range.
13. List three physical findings on examination of the head of an infant that indicate increased intracranial pressure.

VII. MISSHAPEN HEADS: CRANIOSYNOSTOSES, DEFORMATIONAL (POSITIONAL) MOLDING, AND CONGENITAL DEFORMITIES

1. Define craniosynostosis.
2. Describe the adverse effects of craniosynostosis on the nervous system.
3. Contrast the terms *brachycephaly* and *dolichocephaly* with *acrobrachycephaly* and *scaphocephaly.*
4. Describe the state of the sutures in oxycephaly.
5. Describe the effects of craniosynostosis on the orbits and eyes.
6. Describe the findings on physical examination that lead to the diagnosis of craniosynostosis.
7. Describe two causes for plagiocephaly and describe how they affect the prominence of the cheek and occiput (Fig. 1-21).
8. What is the radiographic procedure of choice to investigate craniosynostosis?
9. Describe the location of caput succedaneum.
10. Describe the unique feature of a cephalohematoma that distinguishes it from a caput or subgaleal hemorrhage.

VIII. THE SIZE OF THE HEAD AND BRAIN

1. Describe the factors that determine head size.
2. Draw the normal curve for the increase in the OFC after birth and show trend lines indicating evolving macrocephaly (megalocephaly) and evolving microcephaly (Fig. 1-23).
3. Recite the mnemonic for remembering the mean head size at birth and at age 1 year.
4. Distinguish among megalocephaly (macrocephaly), hydrocephaly, and megalencephaly (macrencephaly).
5. Discuss the use and limitations of the OFC in predicting the actual size and weight of the brain (Fig. 1-24).
6. State the two definitions of hydrocephaly. (Hint: Without increased pressure and with increased pressure)
7. Name five general categories of causes for megalocephaly (macrocephaly; Fig. 1-26).
8. Describe the physical findings and complications that identify a battered infant.

Learning Objectives for Chapter 1

IX. THE GENERAL RULES FOR THE NEUROLOGIC EXAMINATION

1. Describe some techniques or principles that ensure a systematic orderly NE.
2. Describe several measurements or scales useful in recording the NE.
3. Describe the types of comparisons made to determine whether any particular finding on the NE is normal or abnormal.
4. Explain the utility of the "thinking circuitry" or why that term is the neurologist's watchword.
5. Recite the five-question catechism that summarizes the analytic process applied to every Pt. (Hint: It starts with, "Is there a . . . ?")
6. Explain why the physician replaces the usual social and emotional reactions with a professional reaction.
7. Discuss whether to approach each operation of the NE with the attitude that the finding will be normal or abnormal.
8. As the overall Learning Objectives of Chapter 1 describe and demonstrate how to examine the face and head by inspection, palpation, percussion, transillumination, and auscultation.

2 A Brief Review of Clinical Neuroanatomy

But chieflye the anatomye
Ye oughte to understande:
If ye will cure well anye thinge,
That ye doe take in hande.

—John Halle (1529–1566)

I. GROSS SUBDIVISIONS OF THE NEURAXIS

To interpret the neurologic examination (NE), you must have a firm grasp of basic neuroanatomy. If you just groaned, let us distinguish two types of neuroanatomy: *tongue tip* neuroanatomy is used on the spot in the clinic, and *fingertip* neuroanatomy is researched as the need arises. This chapter clearly separates the two.

A. Two main parts of the nervous system

The nervous system consists of the *central nervous system* and the *peripheral nervous system*.

1. The *central nervous system* (= CNS = neuraxis) consists of the *brain* and *spinal cord*. See Fig. 2-1.
2. The *peripheral nervous system* (PNS) consists of:
   a. *Cranial nerves* (CrNs) and their *ganglia*
   b. *Spinal nerves* and their *ganglia* and *plexuses*
   c. *Autonomic nerves* and their *ganglia*, *plexuses*, and *nerves*
3. To cleanly separate the PNS from the CNS, simply snip all cranial and spinal nerves at their attachment sites to the brain and spinal cord.

B. Cutting the neuraxis into its gross subdivisions

1. **To separate the brain from the spinal cord:** Locate the foramen magnum shown in Fig. 2-1 and sweep a scalpel transversely across the neuraxis at the level of the foramen magnum. The plane of that cut defines the *medullocervical junction*.
   a. The *brain* is *rostral* to the cut.
   b. The *spinal cord* is *caudal* to the cut.
2. **Definition of the brain:** The whole brain consists of the *brainstem*, *cerebellum*, *diencephalon*, and the *cerebral hemispheres*. Identify them in Fig. 2-1.

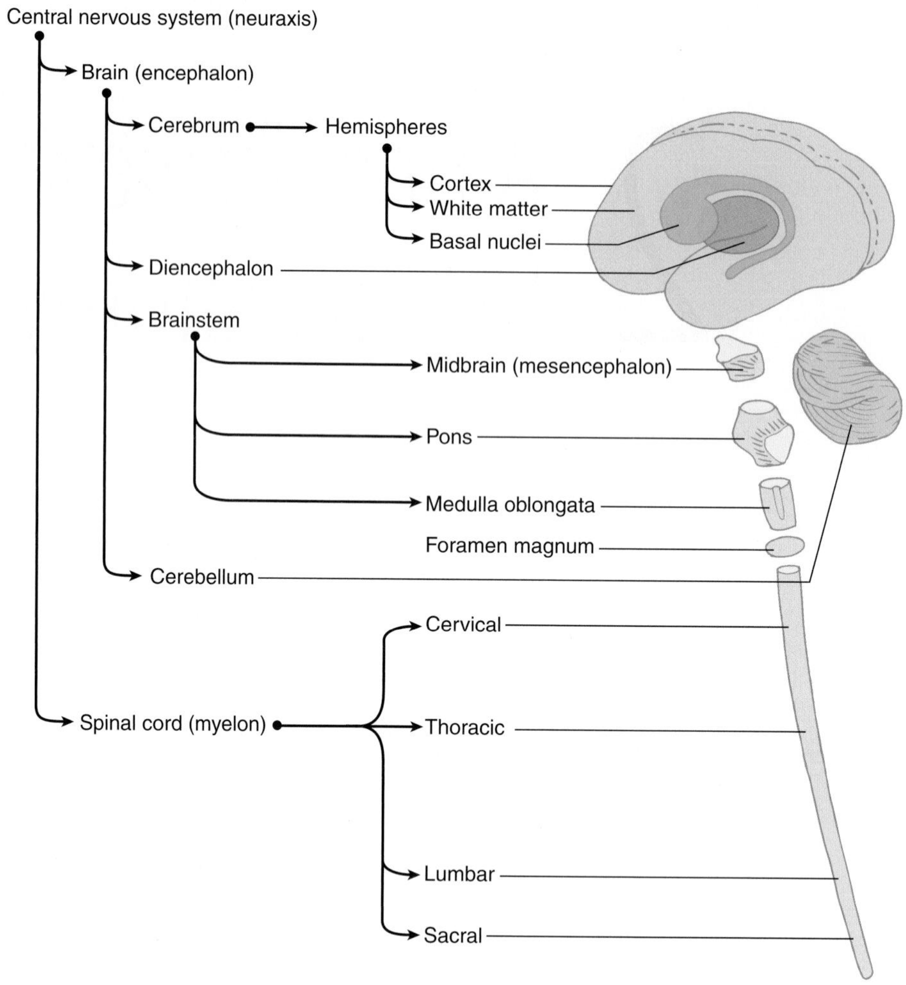

FIGURE 2-1. Lateral view of the neuraxis (central nervous system), showing its gross subdivisions.

3. **To separate the brainstem from the rest of the brain, make the following cuts:**
   a. Transect the neuraxis just as the midbrain (= mesencephalon) emerges from the base of the cerebrum (Fig. 2-1). (Technically the plane of transection runs from the postmammillary sulcus to the posterior commissure.) The *rostral* cut surface of the *midbrain* abuts on the *caudal* cut surface of the *diencephalon* (Fig. 2-1).
   b. Then, to separate the *cerebellum* from the brainstem, slice through the cerebellar peduncles that attach it to the pons (Figs. 2-1 and 8-3). The *brainstem* remains.
   c. To separate the brainstem into its three parts, the *midbrain, pons,* and *medulla,* make transverse cuts at the *midbrain-pontine junction* and at the *pontomedullary junction* (Figs. 2-1 and 2-20).
   d. The *diencephalon* and *cerebrum* remain.
4. **To separate the diencephalon from the cerebrum, core it out with a wire loop:** The basal ganglia and deep cerebral white matter surround the diencephalon. To detach these structures from the cerebrum, insert a wire loop from the base of the cerebrum, where the diencephalon presents as the hypothalamus with its mammillary bodies, infundibulum, and optic chiasm (Fig. 2-20). After coring out the diencephalon, the *cerebrum* remains.
5. **Definition of the cerebrum:** The cerebrum consists of two cerebral hemispheres. Sections of each hemisphere show that the cerebrum consists of:
   a. *Cortex,* a surface coating of alternating layers of neuronal perikarya and neuronal process (Fig. 13-10).

b. *Deep white matter,* consisting of nerve fibers (Fig. 13-10).

c. *Basal ganglia (basal nuclei),* comprises the corpus striatum [caudate nucleus and putamen], globus pallidus, nucleus accumbens, substantia nigra, and subthalamic nucleus, consisting of masses of neurons.

d. *Lateral ventricles,* consisting of cavities filled with spinal fluid (Figs. 13-1 and 13-10).

6. **Learn to reproduce** Fig. 2-1. It is core knowledge.

C. Fissures and sulci of the cerebrum

The cerebral surface displays two types of crevices: *fissures* and *sulci.*

1. Landmark *fissures* include:

   a. The *interhemispheric* (longitudinal) *fissure* that separates the two cerebral hemispheres (Fig. 13-7).

   b. The *Sylvian* or *lateral fissure.* Its *anterior* part separates the temporal from the frontal lobe, and its *posterior* part separates the temporal from the parietal lobe (Fig. 2-2A).

2. Landmark *sulci* include:

   a. The *central sulcus* that separates the frontal and parietal lobes laterally (Fig. 2-2A).

   b. The *parieto-occipital sulcus* that separates the parietal and occipital lobes medially (Fig. 2-2B).

   c. The *calcarine sulcus* that divides the occipital lobe into superior and inferior halves (Fig. 2-2B).

D. Boundaries of the cerebral lobes

1. Each hemisphere has four major lobes, *frontal, parietal, temporal,* and *occipital,* so named because anatomists had already given these names to the overlying bones of the skull.

2. Some lobar boundaries are natural landmarks, others are arbitrary lines. Learn to draw Figs. 2-2A and 2-2B. Then test yourself with frames 3 to 12.

3. The plane of the central sulcus divides the *posterior* margin of the ________________ lobe from the *anterior* margin of the ________________ lobe.

frontal; parietal

4. Notice in Fig. 2-2A that the hemisphere forms a U-shape around the Sylvian fissure, with the frontal and parietal lobes above the fissure and the temporal below. The Sylvian fissure extends *anteriorly* and *posteriorly* to the plane of the central sulcus (Fig. 2-2A). The *anterior* part of the Sylvian fissure divides the ________________ lobe above from the ________________ lobe below.

frontal; temporal

5. The *posterior* part of the Sylvian fissure divides the ________________ lobe above from the ________________ below.

parietal; temporal

6. Laterally, the occipital lobe abuts superiorly and anteriorly on the ________________ lobe and inferiorly and anteriorly on the ________________ lobe.

parietal; temporal

7. Laterally, the line that divides the occipital lobe from the parietal and temporal lobes extends from the ________________ notch to the ________________ notch.

superior preoccipital; inferior preoccipital

8. Taking the midpoint of the line connecting the preoccipital notches, how do you divide the parietal from the temporal lobe? ________________.

Draw a perpendicular line until it meets the Sylvian fissure

9. Medially, the occipital lobe is divided from the parietal lobe by a natural boundary, the ________________ sulcus.

parieto-occipital

10. Describe how to divide the occipital from the temporal lobes on the medial aspect of the hemisphere. ________________.

Draw a line to connect the inferior preoccipital notch to the junction of the calcarine and parieto-occipital fissures (Fig. 2-2C)

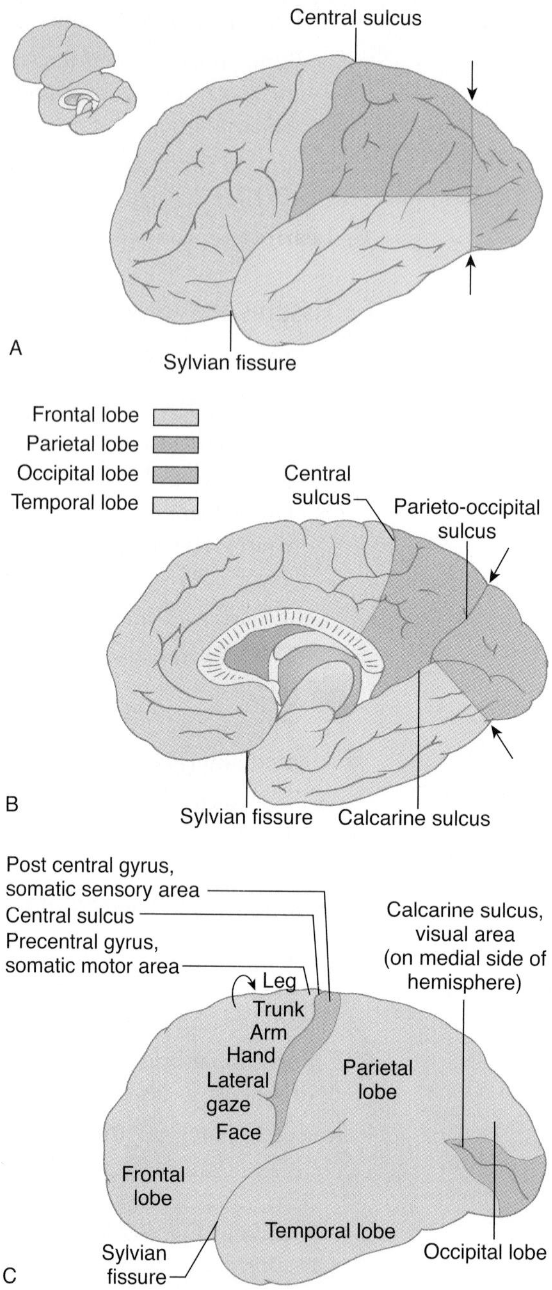

FIGURE 2-2. Lobes of the cerebrum. (A) Lateral view of the left cerebral hemisphere. (B) Medial view of the right cerebral hemisphere. Upper arrow: superior preoccipital notch; Lower arrow: inferior preoccipital notch. (C) Lateral view of the left cerebral hemisphere showing the location of somatomotor, somatosensory, visual, and auditory regions. The leg area of the sensorimotor cortex extends onto the medial aspect of the hemisphere.

parietal

11. **Mnemonic:** By knowing all the boundaries of just one lobe, you can fairly well define the boundaries of all four major lobes. The keystone lobe is the ________________ lobe.

12. Draw medial and lateral views of the cerebrum and demarcate and label the major fissures, sulci, and lobes. Compare your drawing with Figs.2-2A and 2-2B.

E. The olfactory and limbic lobes

1. Previous neuroanatomists have recognized an olfactory lobe, consisting of the olfactory bulbs and tracts and their immediate cortex. See the olfactory lobe (in black) shown in Fig. 2-3. This lobe contains original neural tissue that unites the

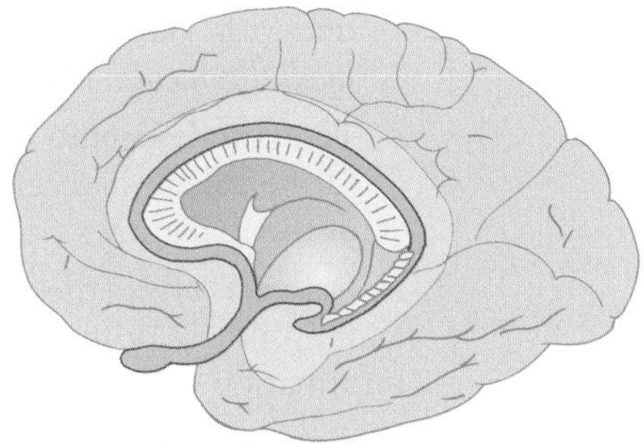

FIGURE 2-3. Medial view of the left cerebral hemisphere showing the limbic lobe (entire light blue ring) and the olfactory lobe (entire yellow ring inside limbic lobe and the olfactory bulb and tract extending anteriorly and inferiorly from the ring.

hemispheres across the midline, forming the median stalk from which the two hemispheres expand outward.

2. From the medial parts of the four traditional lobes, Paul Broca (1824–1880) separated another lobe, the ***limbic lobe*** (Fig. 2-3).
3. Notice in Fig. 2-3 that the limbic lobe (stippled) forms a concentric ring around the inner ring formed by the olfactory lobe (in black). The general term for such an anatomic junction, as of the cornea with the sclera, is *limbus,* hence the term *limbic lobe.*

Ring mnemonic for all cerebral lobes: The parietal lobe is the keystone lobe. If you understand the U- or C-shape of the cerebral hemisphere around the Sylvian fissure and can draw the boundaries of the parietal lobe, you will know the boundaries of the frontal, parietal, occipital, and temporal lobes. The limbic lobe, or limbic ring, attaches the four lobes to the hemispheric hilus. The olfactory lobe comprises the hilus. The olfactory bulbs extend forward from the ring of the olfactory lobe (Fig. 2-3).

F. Functional localization in the cerebral cortex

Various areas of the cortex serve different functions. The cortex contains *somatomotor areas, sensory receptive areas, association areas,* and *limbic areas.*

1. Somatomotor cortex
   a. The primary *somatomotor cortex* occupies the *precentral gyrus,* located just in front of the central sulcus (Fig. 2-2C). Secondary and supplementary motor areas exist also.
   b. The somatomotor cortex originates (gives rise to) the pyramidal tract, the pathway that mediates volitional movements. Pyramidal tract axons also arise in the postcentral gyrus (Russell and DeMyer, 1961).
2. **Sensory receptive cortex:** *somatosensory, auditory,* and *visual.*
   a. The *somatosensory* receptive cortex occupies the *postcentral gyrus,* just behind the central sulcus (Fig. 2-2C).
      i. It receives the somatosensory pathways from the thalamus (diencephalon). This cortex receives the general somatosensory pathways that result in conscious appreciation: touch, pain, temperature, and the discriminative senses, such as position sense and stereognosis.
      ii. The somatomotor and somatosensory cortices represent the body parts upside down (Fig. 2-2C).
   b. The *auditory receptive cortex* consists of transverse temporal gyri in the hidden part of the temporal lobe that forms the floor of the Sylvian fissure, buried

under the parietal lobe (Fig. 2-2C). It receives the auditory pathway from the *medial geniculate body* of the thalamus.

c. The *visual receptive cortex* occupies the superior and inferior banks of the calcarine sulcus. It receives the visual pathway from the *lateral* geniculate body of the thalamus.

3. *Association cortex* (the blank cortex in Fig. 2-2C) receives and sends pathways to and from these primary receptive sensory cortices, associating the primary sensory information with its meaning and with motor responses.
4. *Limbic cortex* mediates emotions and their expression in autonomic and endocrine activities and overall behavior. Phylogenetically, the limbic lobe is derived from the olfactory system, with which it retains close anatomic connections, including the amygdala, hippocampal formation, temporal lobe, and hypothalamus (Gloor, 1997).
   a. Hippocampal, thalamic, and limbic circuits also mediate recent memory. Diseases such as herpes simplex encephalitis and other limbic encephalopathies (paraneoplastic, antibody mediated, etc.) that attack the temporal lobe impair emotional expression and recent memory, as do diffuse cerebral diseases.
   b. The rabies virus strongly attacks the hippocampus. The patient (Pt) suffers hydrophobia in association with the throat spasms of the disease.
   c. Deep midline neoplasms, such as gliomas of the septum pellucidum, hippocampus-fornix, corpus callosum, and adjacent limbic lobe, also frequently cause changes in emotionality and loss of recent memory.

BIBLIOGRAPHY · Gross Subdivisions of the Neuraxis

DeMyer W. *Neuroanatomy*, 2nd ed. Baltimore, Williams and Wilkins, 1998.

Duvernoy HM. *The Human Brain Stem and Cerebellum. Surface, Structure, Vascularization, and Three-Dimensional Section Anatomy with MRI.* New York, Springer-Verlag, 1995.

Duvernoy HM. *The Human Brain. Surface, Three-Dimensional and MRI.* New York, Springer-Verlag, 1991.

Gloor P. *The Temporal Lobe and Limbic System.* New York, Oxford University Press, 1997.

II. THE NEURON AND THE NEURON DOCTRINE

A. Definition of a neuron

Neurons are the parenchymal cells of the nervous system. Each neuron consists of a *nucleus* (karyon), a *cell body* (perikaryon), and one or more *branches.*

1. Most neurons typically display two types of branches, *dendrites* and *axons* (Fig. 2-4).
   a. Dendrites convey nerve impulses *toward* the perikaryon.
   b. Axons convey nerve impulses *away* from the perikaryon.
2. Some branches of some neurons (amacrine neurons) defy simplistic classification as axons and dendrites.

B. Function of neurons

1. The basic function of neurons is communication. When stimulated, neurons produce nerve impulses that communicate with other neurons, or effector cells (gland cells or muscle cells), to activate or inhibit them.
2. The nerve impulse can be electronically recorded and measured as an *action potential.* The action potential, a wave of electrical depolarization, propagates along the surface of the neuronal membrane to end feet at the axonal tips. The end feet form *synapses* on a dendrite, perikaryon, or an axon of one or more neurons, or on an effector cell. A synapse consists of:
   a. A *presynaptic membrane* provided by an axonal end foot
   b. A synaptic cleft
   c. A *postsynaptic membrane* of a neuron or effector cell

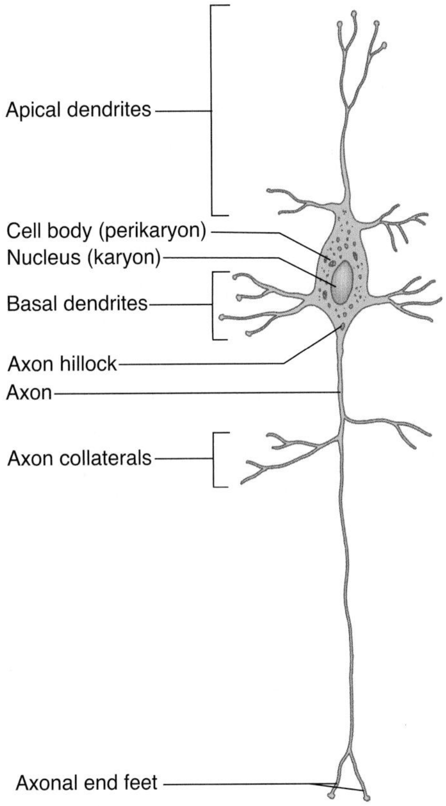

FIGURE 2-4. Typical components of a multipolar neuron. (Reproduced with permission from DeMyer W. *Neuroanatomy,* 2nd ed. Baltimore, Williams & Wilkins, 1998.)

3. The branching of dendrites increases the surface area of any given neuron to receive larger numbers of synapses. The branching of axons increases the number of synapses a given neuron can disperse to subsequent neurons or effector cells.
4. At a synapse, the axonal tip or end foot releases a chemical called a *neurotransmitter.* The neurotransmitter crosses the synaptic cleft to attach to receptor sites on the postsynaptic membrane that alters its electrical polarization.
   a. *Excitatory* neurotransmitters *depolarize* the postsynaptic cell, thereby promoting impulse generation.
   b. *Inhibitory* transmitters *hyperpolarize* the postsynaptic cell, thereby opposing impulse generation.
5. The simplest communication loop, called a *reflex arc,* involves an *afferent* neuron that responds to a stimulus, one central synapse that fires an *efferent* neuron that then activates an *effector.*
6. A synapse acts as a one-way valve. At a synapse impulses flow from the incoming axon to the next neuron. In Fig. 2-5, the flow of impulses is ❒XWY/❒WXY/❒YXW.

☑ WXY

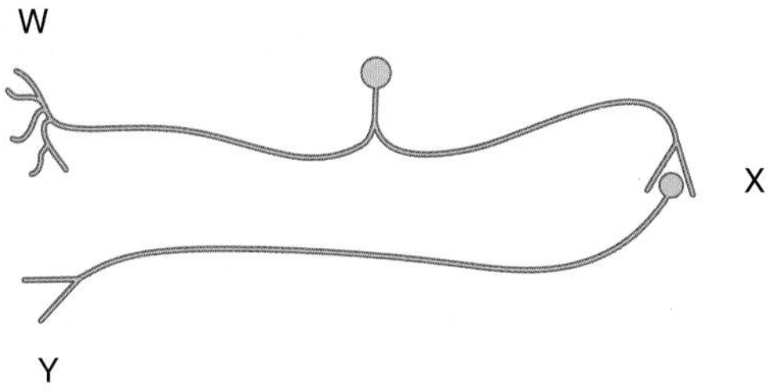

FIGURE 2-5. Conventional representation of a synapse at X. A receptor is any sensory nerve ending (W). Y is any motor synapse on a secretory cell or a muscle fiber.

C. The six tenets of the neuron doctrine

The doctrine asserts that the neuron is the *anatomic, functional, directional, genetic, pathologic,* and *regenerative* unit of the nervous system (Shepherd, 1991).

1. Each neuron is an *anatomic* unit. A continuous surface membrane separates each neuron from all other cells.
2. Each neuron is a *functional* unit. The neuron is the smallest unit capable of receiving, generating, and transmitting nerve impulses.
3. Each neuron is a *directional* unit. In general, a neuron in a circuit conducts impulses in only one direction, from dendrite to axonal tip (amacrine cells excepted).
4. Each neuron is a *genetic* unit. Each neuroblast develops by mitosis from a primitive precursor cell; neuroblasts then differentiate into populations of specific neurons that differ in structure, biochemistry, and connections.
5. Each neuron is a *pathologic* unit:
   a. Any part of a neuron separated from its perikaryon dies, although the rest of the cell may live. If the perikaryon itself dies, all branches die.
   b. Although neurons live or die as individuals, they exist as populations or species. Because of genetic differences in biochemistry and structure, the various species of neurons differ in susceptibility to disease. A pathogen such as a genetic defect, virus, or toxin may affect only one susceptible neuronal species, whereas neighboring species survive. If the pathogen affects retinal neurons, the Pt becomes blind; if it affects auditory neurons, the Pt becomes deaf.
   c. This differential susceptibility leads to an almost endless number of genetic or toxic diseases that cause systematized degeneration of specific types of neurons.
6. Each neuron is a *regenerative* unit. Most mature neurons cannot multiply, but some can regenerate axons.
   a. After transection of an axon, the distal part, severed from its perikaryon dies, a process called *Wallerian degeneration*.
   b. The surviving neuronal perikaryon of a peripheral axon may regenerate its severed axon. Peripheral nerves therefore can effectively and functionally regenerate, but effective axonal regeneration of severed major tracts of CNS axons in humans apparently does not occur. The promotion of axonal and neuronal regeneration ranks as one of the most important areas of research (Mehler and Kessler, 1999; Ochs, 1977; Tuszynski and Kordower, 1998).
7. **Review Section II C until you can recite the six tenets of the neuron doctrine.**

BIBLIOGRAPHY · Neuron Doctrine, Degeneration, and Regeneration

Mehler MF, Kessler JA. Progenitor cell biology. Implications for neural regeneration. *Arch Neurol* 1999;56:780–784.

Ochs S. The early history of nerve regeneration beginning with Cruikshank's observations in 1776. *Med Hist* 1977;21:261–274.

Shepherd GM. *Foundation of the Neuron Doctrine.* New York, Oxford University Press, 1991.

Tuszynski MH, Kordower J, eds. *CNS Regeneration.* Orlando, Academic Press, 1998.

III. THE SPINAL CORD, SOMITES, AND SPINAL NERVES

How to get to the clinic through the muck and slime of phylogenesis and a little help from set theory.

A. Somites and the segmental level of the neuraxis

1. During ontogeny and phylogeny, paired tissue masses, *somites,* develop along each side of the neuraxis, up to the midbrain level (Fig. 2-6A).

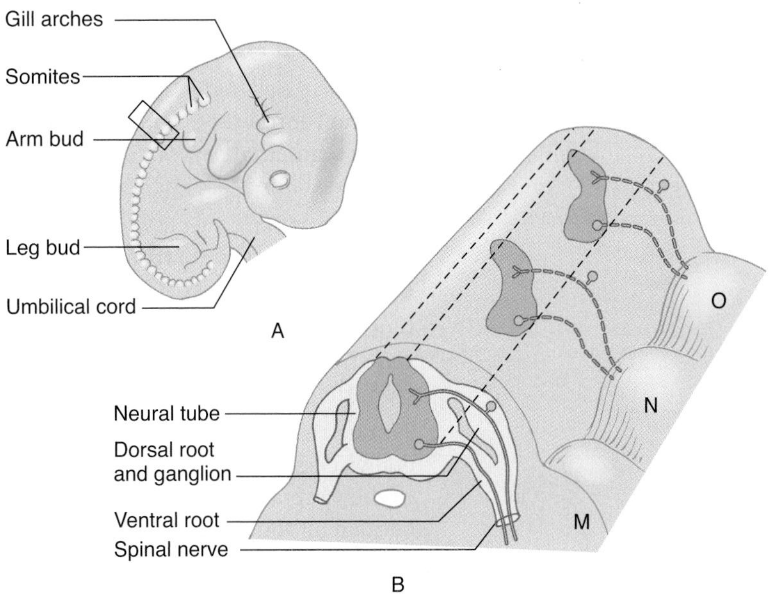

FIGURE 2-6. Somites in a 5-week-old human embryo. (A) Serial arrangement of the somites lateral to the neuraxis. (B) Enlargement of neuraxis and somites blocked off in A. Notice that each somite (M, N, and O) receives one nerve (created by the union of one dorsal root and one ventral root).

2. The spinal cord and brainstem, the parts of the neuraxis that send nerves to the somites or segments, constitute the *somite* or *segmental level* of the nervous system. The rostralmost nerve to a somite, CrN III, attaches to the midbrain. It is also the rostralmost motor CrN.
3. The diencephalon and cerebrum are the *suprasegmental levels* of the neuraxis.
4. The primitive cells of each somite differentiate into a *dermatome, myotome,* and *sclerotome.* The dermatome spreads out under the epidermis to form the dermis, the myotome differentiates into muscle, and the sclerotome becomes bone. These tissues form the extremities and parietes, or wall, of the body.

B. Spinal nerves and the theory of nerve components

1. Each pair of somites receives a pair of spinal nerves and a pair of spinal arteries. Autonomic branches of the spinal nerves innervate the underlying viscera. The spinal cord innervates approximately 30 pairs of somites through 30 pairs of spinal nerves: 8 cervical, 12 thoracic, 5 lumbar, and 5 sacral.
2. A *dorsal* root and a *ventral* root unite to form each spinal nerve (Figs. 2-6 and 2-7).

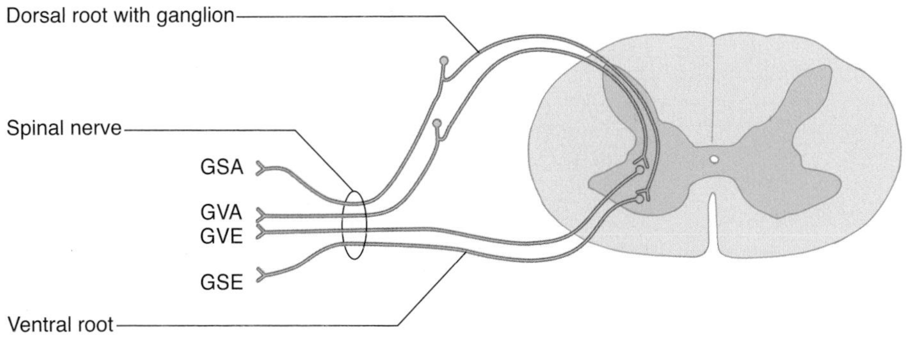

FIGURE 2-7. Cross section of spinal cord showing the typical four functional types of axons in a spinal nerve. GSA = general somatic afferent; GSE = general somatic efferent; GVA = general visceral afferent; GVE = general visceral efferent.

3. The *theory of nerve components* states that the nerve roots and peripheral nerves convey afferent and efferent axons of specific functional types.
   a. The *law of Bell and Magendie* states that the dorsal roots convey *sensory* axons and the ventral roots convey *motor* axons. The internal plan of the gray matter of the segmental nervous system reflects this sensorimotor dichotomy because the dorsal horns are mainly sensory and the ventral are mainly motor.
   b. Notice that *perikarya* in *dorsal root ganglia* provide the axons of the somatosensory afferents (GSAs) from the dermatome, myotome, and sclerotome and viscerosensory afferents (GVAs) from the viscera (Fig. 2-7).
   c. Notice that *perikarya* in the *ventral horns* of the spinal gray matter provide somatic efferent (GSE) axons. GSE axons innervate the striated muscle derived from the myotomes.
   d. Notice that *perikarya* in the *intermediolateral horn* (Fig. 2-12A) provide general visceral efferent (GVE) axons to innervate glands and the smooth muscle of the viscera (via a synapse in an outlying ganglion). Virtually all spinal nerves contain all four components: **GSA, GVA, GVE,** and **GSE.**
4. Figure 2-7 shows that the GSA or GVA axons can synapse *monosynaptically* on their respective GSE or GVE motor neurons. Read all circuit diagrams by tracing along the course of the nerve impulses. In Fig. 2-7, start at a receptor ending, e.g., the GSA receptor. Trace the impulse centrally past the dorsal root ganglion to the motoneuron. Excitation of the motoneuron then causes contraction of the skeletal muscle fibers innervated by the GSE axon.
5. Draw and label a cross section of the spinal cord showing the dorsal and ventral horns and roots and their functional nerve components. By means of arrows, indicate the course of impulse flow, beginning at a receptor and ending at an effector. Check your drawing against Fig. 2-7.

C. Three functional types of neurons: afferent (sensory), efferent (motor), and internuncial

1. The perikaryon of all *afferent neurons,* except for the retina, occupy dorsal root ganglia of the spinal nerves or their counterpart ganglia on the CrNs, including the trigeminal ganglion, cochlear, and vestibular ganglia, genicu-late ganglion, olfactory ganglion, and, by analogy, the retina.

Rule for the origin of afferent systems: All afferent systems, including smell but not vision, originate in nodules of neurons called *sensory ganglia,* located outside the CNS on a CrN or spinal nerve.

   a. **Dispersion of afferent axons:** The proximal branches of the perikarya in dorsal root ganglia enter the CNS. After entering the CNS, the afferent axons may synapse (Fig. 2-8):
      i. At the level of entry
      ii. After ascending or descending
      iii. After decussating
   b. The afferent axon may synapse on efferent neurons monosynaptically (Fig. 2-7) or on one or more internuncial neurons (Fig. 2-8). The number of internuncials between afferent axons and efferent neurons varies from none to countless.
2. **Efferent neurons** (= motoneurons = lower motoneurons)
   a. Consist of *somatic* and *autonomic lower motoneurons* (LMNs). The brainstem also contains a group of *branchial efferent* (BE) *lower motoneurons.*
   b. The perikarya of these LMNs is always within the CNS, but their axons exit into the PNS to reach their effectors.

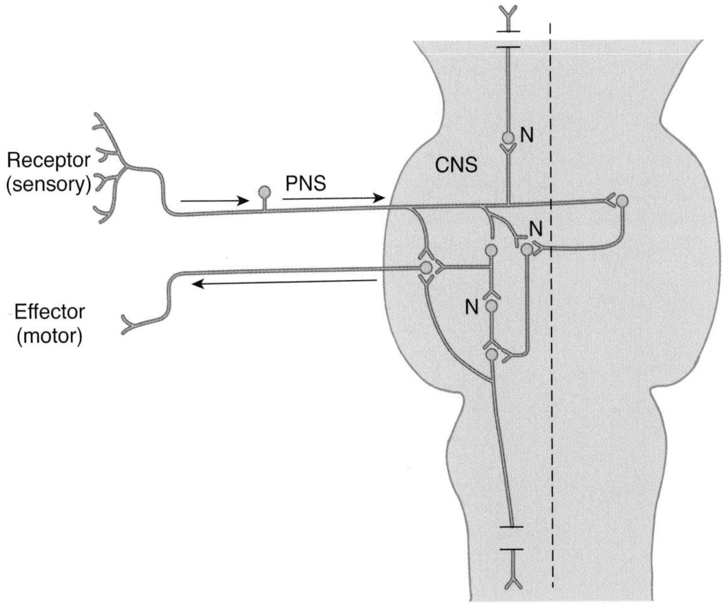

FIGURE 2-8. Polysynaptic reflex arc consisting of a **primary sensory neuron** in a dorsal root ganglion, any number of **internuncial neurons** in the CNS, and a **motoneuron** that innervates an effector. Contrast with the monosynaptic arc shown in Fig. 2-7. CNS = central nervous system; N = neuron; PNS = peripheral nervous system.

3. The *internuncial* or *intercalary neurons* interpose themselves between the afferent and efferent pools (Fig. 2-8).
   a. Because internuncials remain entirely within the CNS and do not enter peripheral nerves, the theory of nerve components excludes them.
   b. Internuncial neurons comprise the vast majority of all CNS neurons. They provide polysynaptic circuits of greater complexity and plasticity than do the direct monosynaptic reflex arcs that can produce only simple muscular twitches (Figs. 2-8 and 7-4).

D. Somite migrations and the law of original innervation

1. The phylogenetic specializations leading to limb and head development obscure the simple serial arrangement of the somites. The proximal portions of the dermatomes attenuate as they extend into the limbs. They are stretched so thin that C4 abuts on T2 in the final state of the dermatomes (Figs. 2-9 and 2-10).
2. Notice that dermatome C7 extends to the middle finger and divides dermatomes C5 and C6 from C8 through T1. C7 then can be regarded as the "axis" of symmetry of the brachial plexus (DeMyer, 1998). Learn this fact and the following mnemonic. The information is valuable at the bedside.

Mnemonic for dermatomal distributions (Fig. 2-10):

1. C2 abuts on the trigeminal nerve at the interaural line, a "hood" distribution. C1 does not have a sensory branch.
2. C3 and C4 cover the shoulders in a "cape" distribution, where a cape would rest. Therefore, remember that C2, C3, and C4 have a "hooded cape" distribution.
3. C5 through T1: Remember the C7 mnemonic. March down the superior aspect of the arm for C5 and C6 to C7. Then march back up the inferior aspect from C7 to C8, T1, and T2.
4. T4: the nipple level.
5. T10: the umbilicus
6. L1: the groin.
7. L5: the large toe (L = large toe).
8. S1: the small toe (S = small toe).

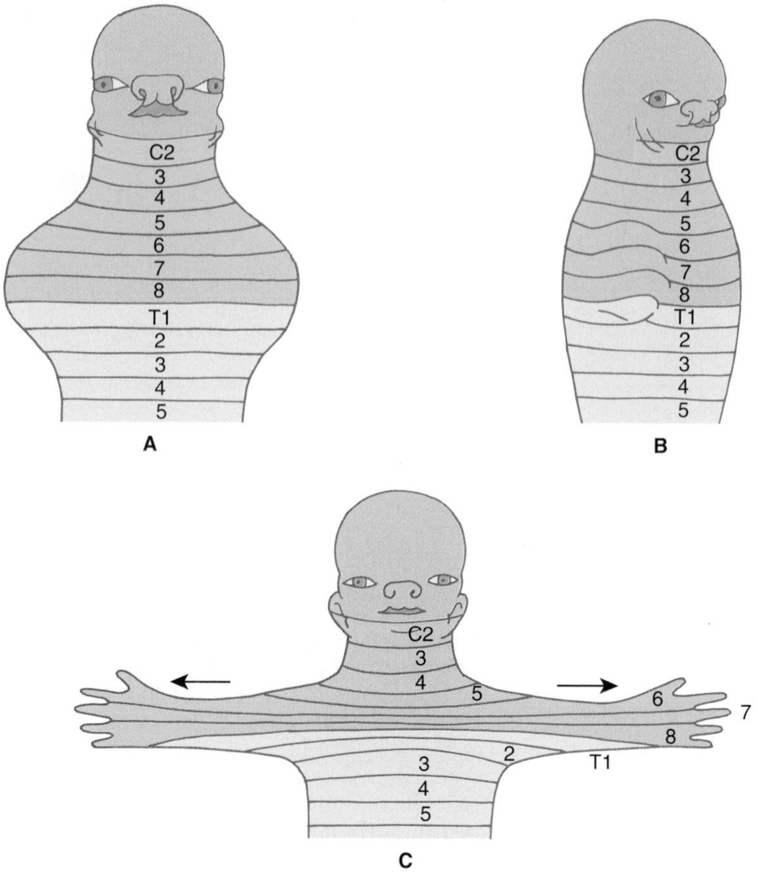

FIGURE 2-9. Dermatomal dislocations caused by development of the limbs. Notice that C2 is the first of the cervical dermatomes. Cranial nerve V innervates facial sensation. See Fig. 2-10.

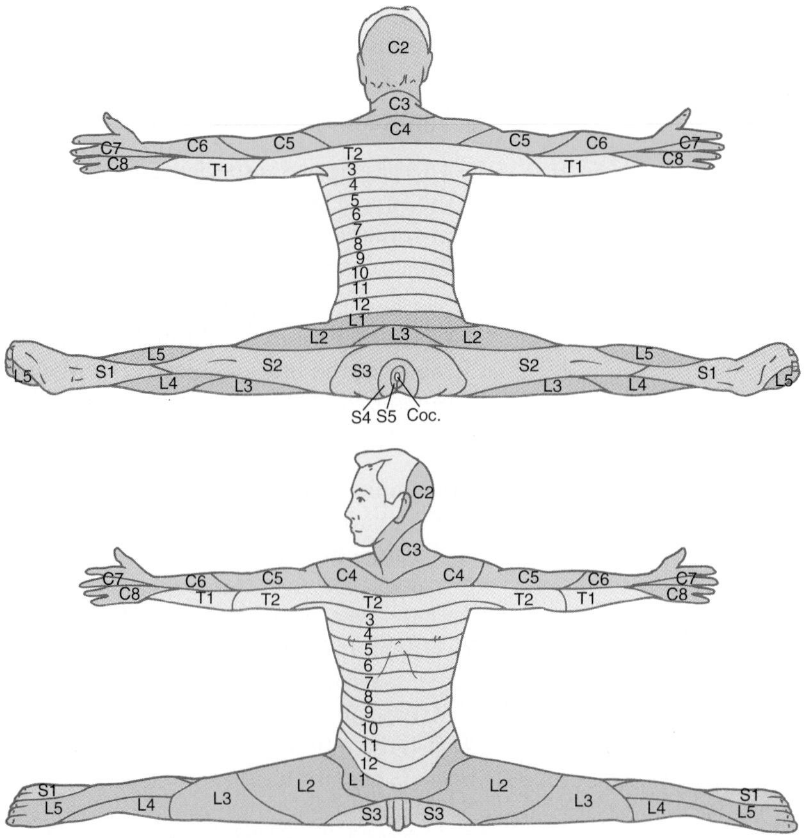

FIGURE 2-10. Sensory innervation areas by dermatomes. The numbers correspond to the spinal cord level of the dermatomes. C = cervical; L = lumbar; S = sacral; T = thoracic. (Reproduced with permission from Haymaker W, Woodhall B. *Peripheral Nerve Injuries,* 2nd ed. Philadelphia, W.B. Saunders, 1962.)

3. The myotomes and sclerotomes also migrate. For example, the myotomes of cervical somites 3, 4, and 5 combine to produce the diaphragm. They migrate to the level of T12 and drag their somite nerves, united as the *phrenic nerves*, along with them from the cervical region. Many of the extremity muscles also contain contributions from more than one myotome. Table 2-1 lists the segmental innervations of the skeletal muscles, and Table 2-2 lists the segmental levels of some clinically important reflexes. Use these tables for reference, as needed.

TABLE 2-1 · Segmental Innervation of Muscles

Action tested	Roots	Nerves	Muscles
Cranial			
Closure of eyes, pursing of lips, exposure of teeth	Cranial VII	Facial	Orbicularis oculi, orbicularis oris, etc.
Elevation of eyelids, movement of eyes	Cranial III, IV, V	Oculomotor, trochlear, abducens	Extraocular
Closing and opening of jaw	Cranial V	Motor trigeminal	Masseters, pterygoids
Protrusion of tongue	Cranial XII	Hypoglossal	Lingual
Phonation and swallowing	Cranial IX, X	Glossopharyngeal, vagus	Palatal, laryngeal, and pharyngeal
Elevation of shoulders, anteroflexion, and turning of head	Cranial XI	Spinal accessory	Trapezius, sternocleido mastoid
Brachial			
Adduction of extended arm	C5, C6	Brachial plexus	Pectoralis major
Fixation of scapula	C5, C6, C7	Brachial plexus	Serratus anterior
Initiation of abduction of arm	C5, C6	Brachial plexus	Supraspinatus
External rotation of flexed arm	C5, C6	Brachial plexus	Infraspinatus
Abduction and elevation of arm up to 90 degrees	C5, C6	Axillary nerve	Deltoid
Flexion of supinated forearm	C5, C6	Musculocutaneous	Deltoid
Extension of forearm	C6, C7, C8	Radial	Triceps
Extension (radial) of wrist	C6	Radial	Extensor carpi radialis longus
Flexion of semipronated arm	C5, C6	Radial	Brachioradialis
Adduction of flexed arm	C6, C7, C8	Brachial plexus	Latissimus dorsi
Supination of forearm	C6, C7	Posterior interosseous	Supinator
Extension of proximal phalanges	C7, C8	Posterior interosseous	Extensor digitorum
Extension of wrist (ulnar side)	C7, C8	Posterior interosseous	Extensor carpi ulnaris
Extension of proximal phalanx of index finger	C7, C8	Posterior interosseous	Extensor indicis
Abduction of thumb	C8	Posterior interosseous	Abductor pollicis brevis
Extension of thumb	C7, C8	Posterior interosseous	Extensor pollicis longus and brevis
Pronation of forearm	C6, C7	Median nerve	Pronator teres
Radial flexion of wrist	C6, C7	Median nerve	Flexor carpi radialis
Flexion of middle phalanges	C7, C8, Tl	Median nerve	Flexor digitorum superficialis
Flexion of proximal phalanx of thumb	C8, T1	Median nerve	Flexor pollicis brevis
Opposition of thumb against fifth finger	C8, T1	Median nerve	Opponens pollicis
Extension of middle phalanges of index and middle fingers	C8, T1	Median nerve	First, second lumbricals
Flexion of terminal phalanx of thumb	C8, T1	Anterior interosseous nerve	Flexor pollicis longus
Flexion of terminal phalanx of second and third fingers	C8, T1	Anterior interosseous nerve	Flexor digitorum profundus
Flexion of distal phalanges of ring and little fingers	C7, C8	Ulnar	Flexor digitorum profundus
Adduction and opposition of fifth finger	C8, T1	Ulnar	Hypothenar
Extension of middle phalanges of ring and little fingers	C8, T1	Ulnar	Third and fourth lumbricals

(*Continued*)

TABLE 2-1 · Segmental Innervation of Muscles (Continued)

Action tested	Roots	Nerves	Muscles
Adduction of thumb against second finger	C8, T1	Ulnar	Adductor pollicis
Flexion of proximal phalanx of thumb	C8, T1	Ulnar	Flexor pollicis brevis
Abduction and adduction of fingers	C8, T1	Ulnar	Interossei
Crural			
Hip flexion from semiflexed position	L1, L2, L3	Femoral	Iliopsoas
Hip flexion from externally rotated position	L2, L3	Femoral	Sartorius
Extension of knee	L2, L3, L4	Femoral	Quadriceps femoris
Adduction of thigh	L2, L3, L4	Obturator	Adductor longus, magnus brevis
Abduction and int. rotation of thigh	L4, L5, SI	Superior gluteal	Gluteus medius
Extension of thigh	L5, SI, S2	Inferior gluteal	Gluteus maximus
Flexion of knee	L5, SI, S2	Sciatic	Biceps femoris, semitendinosus, semimembranosus
Dorsiflexion of foot (medial)	L4, L5	Peroneal (deep)	Anterior tibial
Dorsiflexion of toes (proximal) and distal phalanges)	L5, SI	Peroneal (deep)	Extensor digitorum longus and brevis
Dorsiflexion of great toe	L5, SI	Peroneal (deep)	Extensor hallucis longus
Eversion of foot	L5, SI	Peroneal (superficial)	Peroneus longus and brevis
Plantar flexion of foot	S1, S2	Tibial	Gastrocnemius, soleus
Inversion of foot	L4, L5	Tibial	Tibialis posterior
Flexion of toes (distal phalanges)	L5, SI, S2	Tibial	Flexor digitorum longus
Flexion of toes (middle phalanges)	S1, S2	Tibial	Flexor digitorum brevis
Flexion of great toe (proximal phalanx)	S1, S2	Tibial	Flexor hallucis brevis
Flexion of great toe (distal phalanx)	L5, SI, S2	Tibial	Flexor hallucis longus
Contraction of anal sphincter	S2, S3, S4	Pudendal	Perineal muscles

SOURCE: Reprinted with permission from Adams RA, Victor M. *Principles of Neurology,* 4th ed. New York, McGraw-Hill, 1989.

4. **The law of original innervation: Wherever a somite derivative migrates, it retains its original somite nerve.** Even when a muscle or bone receives contributions from several somites, each spinal nerve continues to innervate only the tissue that derived directly from its original somite. Only the thoracicoabdominal wall retains the nerves, muscles, ribs, and intercostal vessels in their primordial somite sequences, without migrating, because no limbs develop (Fig. 2-10).
5. **Plexuses versus peripheral nerve distributions**
   a. To reach their original somites, the axons of the spinal nerves may detour in the *cervical, brachial,* and *lumbosacral plexuses* to share peripheral nerves to the limbs.
   b. No plexuses develop in the thoracicoabdominal region because of the lack of limbs.
   c. The peripheral nerves *distal* to the plexuses have dorsal and ventral root axons from more than one spinal cord segment. **A lesion in or distal to a plexus causes deficits that exceed the innervation field of one somite.**
   d. By mapping the patterns of sensory or motor loss and comparing them with those shown in Figs. 2-10 and 2-11, the examiner (Ex) can decide whether the Pt suffers from a *dorsal root (dermatomal), plexus,* or a *peripheral nerve* lesion.

TABLE 2-2 · Segmental Innervation of Spinal Reflexes

Deep (muscle stretch) reflexes	Superficial reflexes	Methods of elicitation	Normal results	Segment(s) traversed
Biceps		Tap biceps tendon	Flexion of the forearm at the elbow	C5 to C6
Triceps		Tap triceps tendon	Extension of the forearm at the elbow	C6 to C7
Brachioradial		Tap styloid process of the radius, with forearm held in semipronation	Flexion of the forearm at the elbow	C5 to C6
Finger flexion		Flick palmar surface of the tip of the finger	Flexion of the fingers	C7 to Tl
Abdominal muscle stretch reflexes		Tap lowermost rib, tap finger placed on rectus abdominis or tap symphysis pubis	Contraction of the abdominal wall or, when the symphysis is tapped, adduction of the legs	T8 to T12
	Abdominal skin-muscle reflexes	Stroke skin of the upper and lower abdominal quadrants	Contraction of the abdominal muscles and retraction of the umbilicus to the stimulated side	T8 to T12
	Cremasteric	Stroke skin of the upper and inner thigh	Upward movement of the testicle	Ll to L2
Adductor		Tap medial condyle of the tibia	Adduction of the leg	L2 to L4
Quadriceps		Tap tendon of the quadriceps femoris	Extension of the lower leg	L2 to L4
Triceps surae		Tap Achilles tendon	Plantar flexion of the foot	L5 to S2
	Plantar	Stroke sole of the foot	Plantar flexion of the toes	S1 to S2
	Anal	Prick skin of the perianal region	Constriction of the anal sphincter—"anal wink"	S4 to Co1
	Bulbocavernous	Prick skin of the glans penis	Contraction of the bulbocavernosus muscle and constrictor urethrae	S3 to S4

E. Segmental composition and motor distribution of the major peripheral nerves from the spinal plexuses

Note: Study Sections E-1 to E-3 but learn only the principal movements served by the major peripheral nerves. This material is not programmed, but you need to know it.

1. **Motor distribution of the cervical plexus:** Roots C1 to C4.
   a. This plexus innervates:
      i. The neck muscles that turn the head and open the jaw
      ii. The trapezius muscle in conjunction with CrN XI
      iii. The diaphragm
   b. The phrenic nerve is the single most important nerve in the body because it innervates the diaphragm. It arises from C3 through C5. C4 usually supplies most of its axons. The nerve may be *pre* fixed (C2–C4) or *post* fixed (C4–C6).
2. **Motor distribution of the extremity nerves of the brachial plexus (roots C5 to T1):** This plexus innervates a number of proximal muscles of the shoulder girdle and issues five major terminal nerves for the arms, as follows:
   a. The axillary or *circumflex nerve* (C5–C6) is the *elevator* nerve of the arm because it innervates the deltoid muscle.
   b. The *musculocutaneous nerve* (C5–C7) is the *flexor* nerve of the arm. It flexes the brachium on the shoulder and the forearm on the brachium. The only arm flexor muscle not innervated by the musculocutaneous nerve is the brachioradialis muscle, which is innervated anomalously by the radial nerve, an extensor nerve.
   c. The *radial nerve* (C5–C8) is the *extensor* nerve of the arm (elbow, wrist, and fingers), but it does not extend the distal phalanges. It also supplies the brachioradialis, which flexes the elbow.

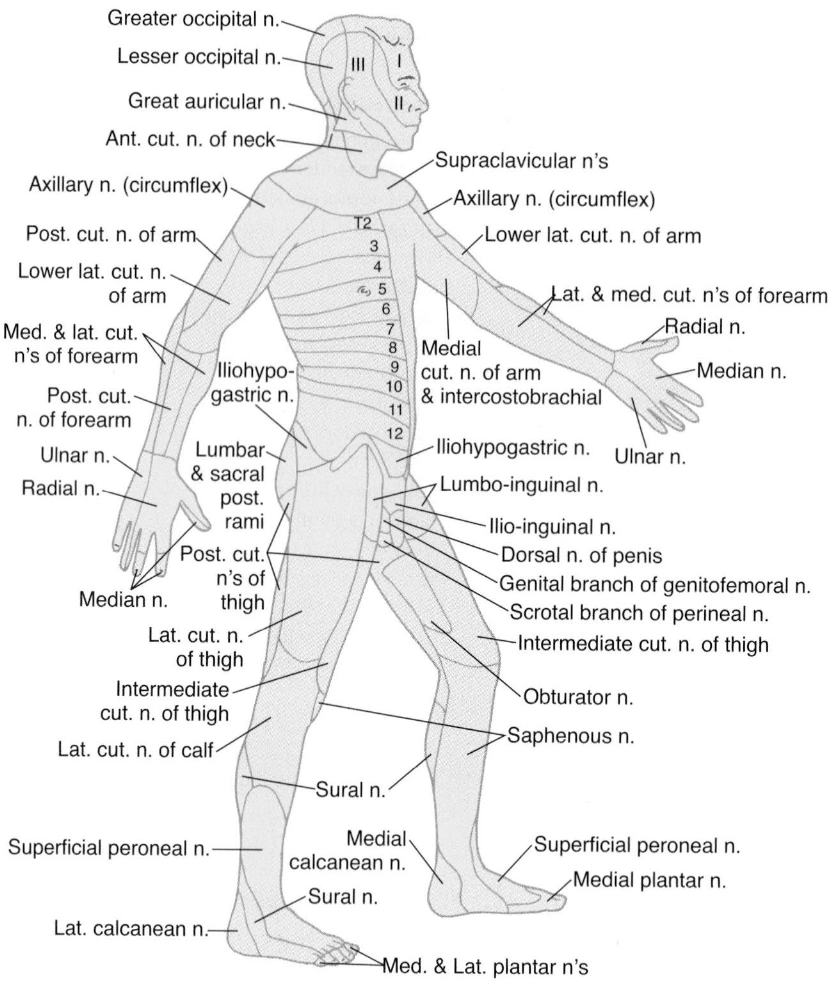

FIGURE 2-11. Sensory innervation areas by peripheral nerves. Peripheral nerves may contain axons from one or more somite nerves. By using Figs. 2-10 and 2-11, the clinician can determine whether the patient's sensory loss matches a dermatomal or peripheral nerve distribution. n. = nerve. (Reproduced with permission from Haymaker W, Woodhall B. *Peripheral Nerve Injuries,* Philadelphia, W.B. Saunders, 1945)

d. **Recap:** Can you name the elevator nerve of the arm, the flexor nerve of the elbow, and the extensor nerve of the elbow, wrist, and fingers?

e. The *median nerve* (C6–C8) is a *flexor* nerve of the wrist. It innervates the long forearm muscles that flex the wrist and the fingers, and inner-vates five intrinsic hand muscles. See the LLOAF/2 mnemonic below.

f. The *ulnar nerve* (C7 and C8) is a *flexor* nerve of the fingers

   i. In the forearm, the ulnar nerve innervates the flexor carpi ulnaris exclusively and, with the median nerve, innervates long flexors of the wrist.

   ii. In the hand, the ulnar nerve innervates all interossei, lumbricals to digits 4 and 5, and the adductor pollicis.

3. **The muscles acting on the digits of the hand**

   a. The lumbrical muscles, innervated by median and ulnar nerves, *flex* the proximal phalanges and *extend* the distal phalanges.

   b. The interossei, innervated by the ulnar nerve, flex the proximal phalanges, extend the distal phalanges, and waggle the fingers laterally (adduct and abduct the fingers).

   c. The thumb action tests the three motor nerves that control the digits:

      i. **Radial:** *extension* of the thumb

      ii. **Median:** *abduction* of the thumb and opposition of the thumb to the little finger

iii. **Ulnar:** *adduction* of the thumb

iv. **Median and ulnar:** flexor brevis of the thumb

v. Chapter 7 describes clinical testing of these actions

4. **Here is a mnemonic summary, if you care to learn it.**

Mnemonic for the motor innervation of the major brachial plexus nerves (formed by the union of ventral rami of spinal nerves C5–T1):

Axillary (circumflex) C5–C6: arm elevation (deltoid).

Musculocutaneous C5–C7: flexor nerve of the shoulder and elbow (except for the brachioradialis muscle, which is innervated by the radial nerve).

Radial C5–C8: extensor nerve of the elbow, wrists, and fingers, except the distal phalanges, which are extended by the intrinsic hand muscles.

Median C5–T1: flexors of the wrist; five intrinsic muscles of the hand: three thenar and lateral two lumbrical muscles. **LLOAF/2 (mnemonic within a mnemonic):** LL = Lateral two Lumbricals, O = Opponens pollicis, A = Abductor pollicis brevis, F = half of the Flexor pollicis brevis.

Ulnar C7–T8–T1: flexor carpi ulnaris and all intrinsic muscles of the hand except for the opponens pollicis, abductor pollicis brevis, and half of the flexor pollicis brevis; ulnar intrinsics (the interossei, medial two lumbricals) flex metacarpophalangeal joints of fingers.

Mnemonic within a mnemonic: The action of the thumb tests three of the long motor nerves of the brachial plexus:

Extension: radial nerve.

Opposition to little finger: median nerve.

Abduction: median nerve.

Adduction: ulnar nerve

5. **Motor distribution of the lumbosacral plexus (formed from the ventral rami of spinal nerves L1–S4):** This plexus provides proximal branches to the glutei and hip abductors and adductors. The major terminal nerves to the extremities are

   a. The *femoral nerve* (L2–L4): the *extensor* nerve of the knee.

   b. The *obturator nerve* (L2–L4): the *adductor* nerve of the thigh.

   c. The *sciatic nerve* (L4–S3): the *flexor* nerve of the knee and the *flexor* and *extensor* nerves of the foot and toes and the invertors and evertors of the foot. The largest of the peripheral nerves, the sciatic can be regarded as consisting of three nerves:

      i. The *hamstring* nerve that branches to the knee flexors

      ii. The *tibial* nerve that branches to the posterior muscles of the calf

      iii. The *common peroneal* nerve that branches to the anterior muscles

   d. After giving off hamstring branches, the sciatic nerve divides in the popliteal space into the *tibial* and *peroneal nerves:*

      i. The *tibial nerve* (L4–S3) innervates the *plantar flexors* of the foot and toes and the muscle that *inverts* the foot when the foot plantar flexes.

      ii. The *peroneal nerve* (L4–S1) innervates the *dorsiflexors* of the ankle and toes and the muscle that *everts* the foot when the foot dorsiflexes.

   e. The *pudendal nerve* (S2–4), a somatic nerve, innervates the urogenital diaphragm, voluntary bowel and bladder sphincters, and sexual sensation.

   f. The *pelvic splanchnic nerve* (nervi erigentes), a visceral nerve, innervates the bladder and internal sphincters and is the vasomotor for erection of the penis and clitoris.

F. The axonal pathways in the spinal cord

1. Learn the nomenclature and location of the pathways of the spinal cord depicted in Figs. 2-12A to 2-12C. Figure 2-12 contains the essential information for bedside examination of a Pt with a spinal cord lesion.

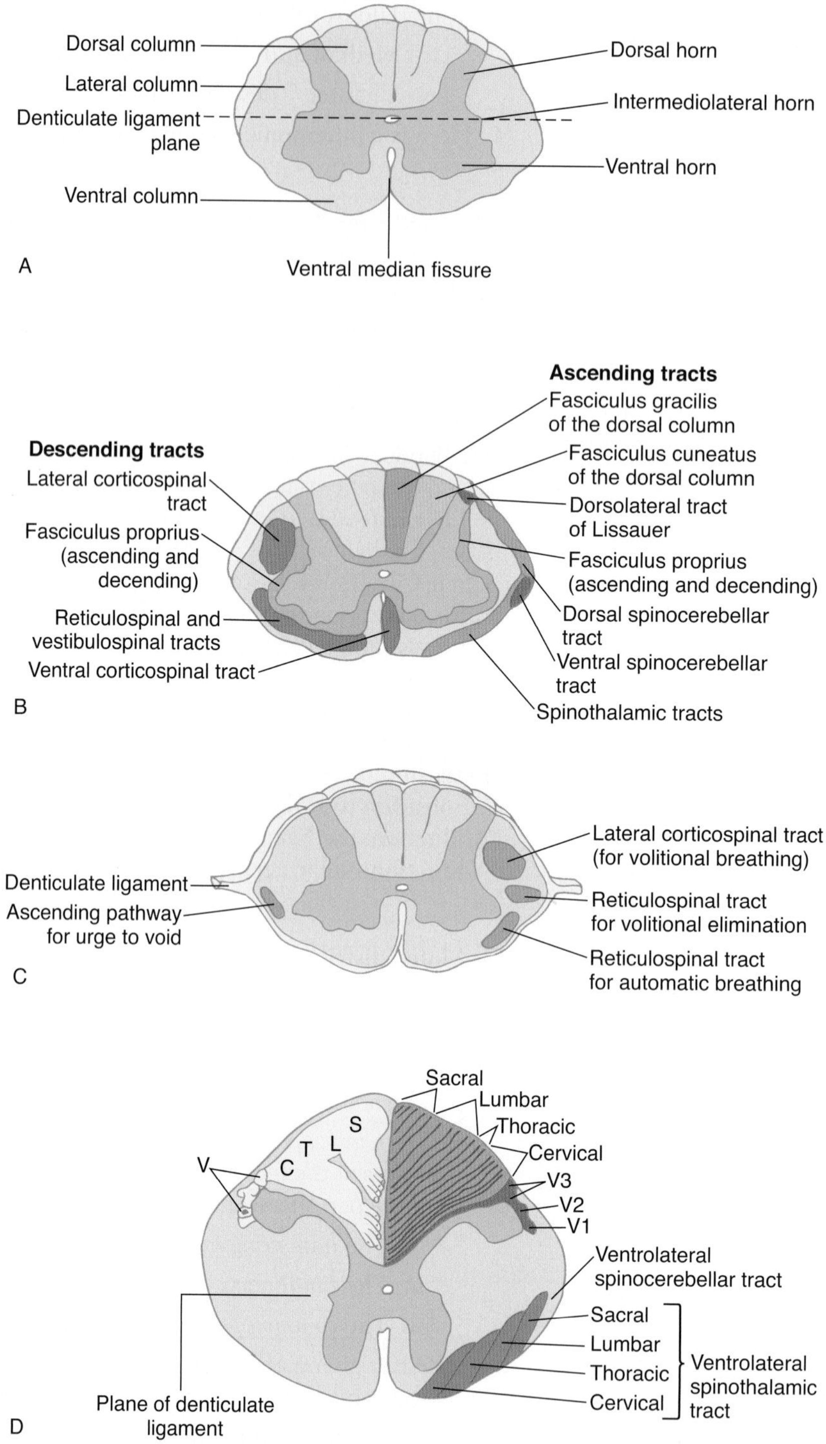

FIGURE 2-12. Cross sections of the spinal cord. (A) Nomenclature for regions of the spinal cord. Note the plane of the denticulate ligament that divides the cord into dorsal and ventral halves. (B) Location of the major descending and ascending tracts of the white matter. (C) Location of the pathways for visceral functions and breathing. (D) Topographic lamination of axons in the dorsal columns and the lateral spinothalamic tract for pain and temperature. (Reprinted with permission from DeMyer W. *Neuroanatomy*, 2nd ed. Baltimore, Williams & Wilkins, 1998.)

Mnemonic for the cross-sectional anatomy of the spinal cord: Divide the spinal cord into **dorsal** and **ventral** halves by a line from one denticulate ligament across to the other (Fig. 2-12A). The sensory nuclei of the gray matter, the lateral corticospinal tract, the dorsal spinocerebellar tract, and the white matter of the dorsal columns are **dorsal** to the denticulate plane. **Everything else that has clinically testable functions is at that plane or ventral to it.**

2. The pathways of the spinal cord arise from neurons in the dorsal root ganglia *outside* the CNS or from neurons *inside* the CNS. The axons of the *fasciculi gracilis* and *cuneatus* and of the *dorsolateral tract of Lissauer* arise from primary sensory neurons outside the CNS, in the dorsal root ganglia. All other tracts arise from neuronal perikarya within the CNS.
3. The primary axons that form the *fasciculi gracilis* and *cuneatus* travel up the dorsal columns of the cord to synapse on secondary neurons at the cervicomedullary junction (see Fig. 2-28). The secondary axons then decussate to form the *medial lemniscus,* which synapses on somatosensory nuclei of the thalamus that relay to the somatosensory cortex. This pathway mediates the so-called *deep sensory modalities* of position sense, vibration, stereognosis, pressure, two-point discrimination, and direction of movement.
4. The dorsolateral tract consists of primary axons from the dorsal root ganglia that synapse at the level of entry or after traveling up or down the cord only one or two segments. These primary axons synapse ipsilaterally in the spinal gray matter on secondary neurons whose axons decussate and ascend in the ventrolateral columns as *spinothalamic tracts.* These axons mediate pain and temperature (see Figs. 2-12 and 2-28).
5. The other spinothalamic tract component mediates touch. The primary axons of this pathway synapse in the dorsal horn and cross and ascend in the ventrolateral columns of the cord with the pain and temperature pathway (Fig. 2-28).

IV. ANATOMIC ORGANIZATION OF THE BRAINSTEM

A. For clinical neurology you must know:

1. The three *longitudinal* and three *transverse* subdivisions of the brainstem
2. The location of the major tracts on cross section of the brainstem and their decussations
3. The name and number of the CrNs and their composition
4. The location of the CrN nuclei
5. The point where each CrN attaches to the neuraxis and exits from the skull

B. Three transverse and three longitudinal subdivisions of the brainstem

1. The three *transverse* subdivisions of the brainstem, the *mesencephalon, pons,* and *medulla* (Fig. 2-1), consist of three continuous *longitudinal* layers, *tectum, tegmentum,* and *basis* (Fig. 2-13).
2. The *tectum* (= roof, the roof of the brainstem) consists of the quadrigeminal plate that roofs the midbrain aqueduct and the anterior and posterior medullary vela that roof the fourth ventricle of the pons and medulla.
3. The *tegmentum* (= covering, the covering of the basis) separates the tectum from the basis. It consists of tracts and vitally important neurons grouped into various nuclei.
4. The *basis* (= the bottom, the bottom layer of the brainstem).
   a. The basis mesencephali, basis pontis, and basis medullae (the medullary pyramids) convey the longitudinally coursing corticofugal motor pathways, consisting of the *pyramidal* tract and the *corticopontine* tracts.
   b. In addition, the basis of the pons contains nuclei that swell it enormously. These nuclei receive the corticopontine tracts and relay them to the cerebellum. This pathway comprises the large belly of the basis pontis (Figs. 2-1, 2-16, and 2-17).

C. Cross-sectional organization of the brainstem

Learn Fig. 2-14, which shows the plan for the arrangement of gray and white matter along the length of the brainstem. Figures 2-15 to 2-18 show the regional variations, for reference.

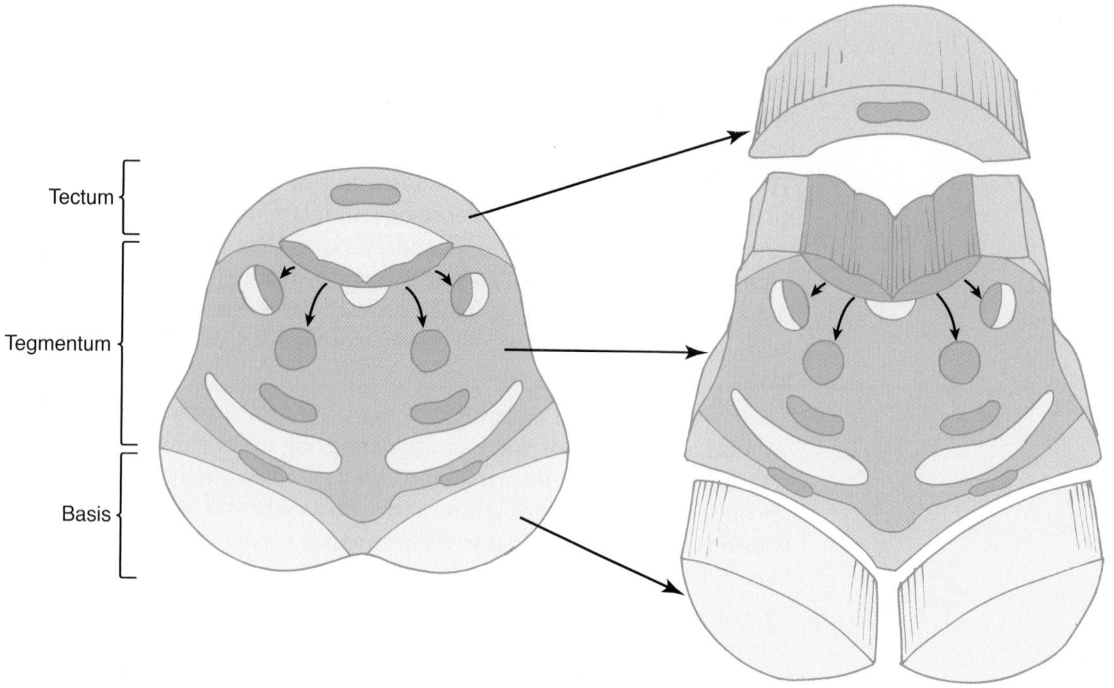

FIGURE 2-13. Exploded view of a generalized cross section of the brainstem to show the three longitudinal subdivisions: tectum, tegmentum, and basis.

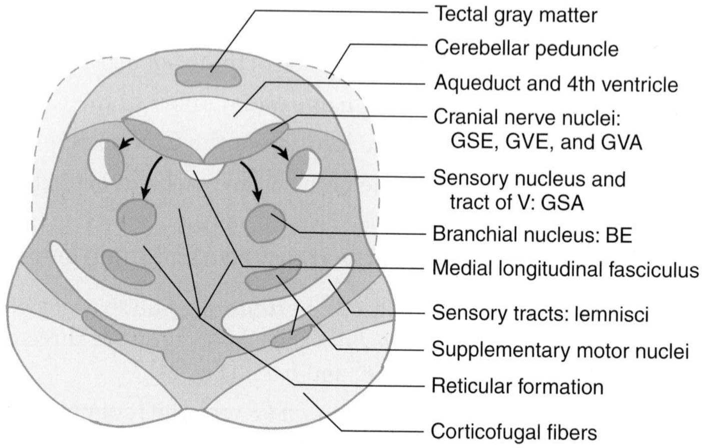

FIGURE 2-14. Generalized cross section of the brainstem. Nuclei are stippled with random dots, the reticular formation is stippled with lattice dots, and the white matter is white. Learn this figure. BE = branchial efferent; GSA = general somatic afferent; GSE = general somatic efferent; GVA general visceral afferent; GVE = general visceral efferent.

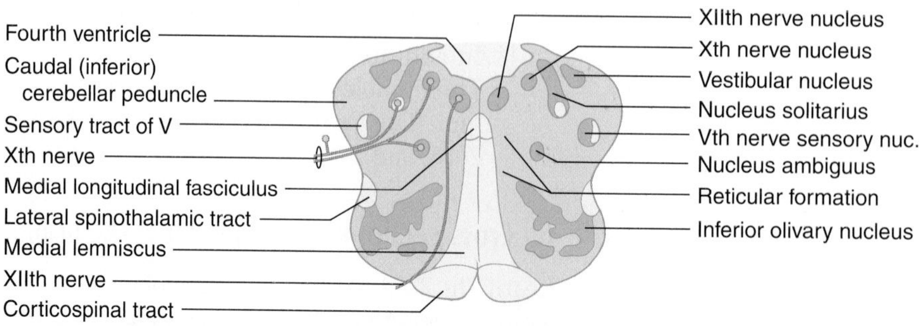

FIGURE 2-15. Transverse section of the medulla oblongata.

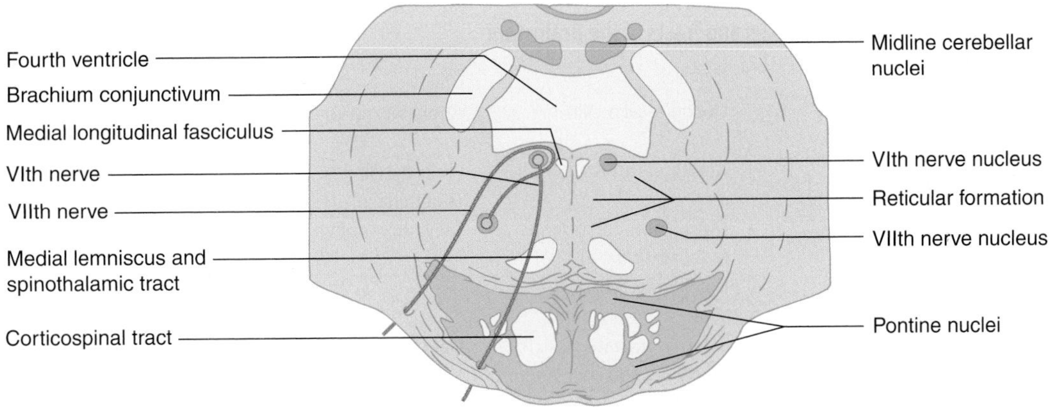

FIGURE 2-16. Transverse section of the pons at the level of the VIIth nerve (caudal).

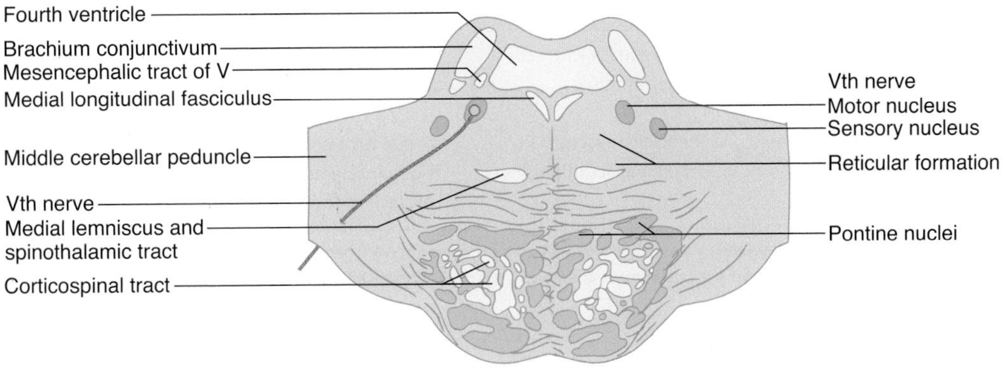

FIGURE 2-17. Transverse section of the pons at the level of the Vth nerve (rostral).

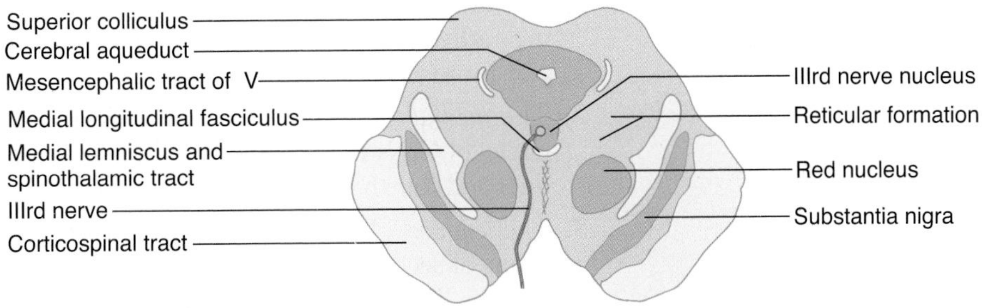

FIGURE 2-18. Transverse section of the mesencephalon (midbrain) at the level of the IIIrd nerve.

D. The tegmental gray matter consists of *CrN nuclei, supplementary motor nuclei,* and *reticular formation*

1. The *CrN nuclei* are scattered along the tegmentum, toward its dorsal half. The BE nuclei are ventrolateral to the GSE nuclei (Fig. 2-14).
2. *Supplementary motor nuclei* occupy the ventral half of the tegmentum, or the basis in the special case of the pons.
   a. The *midbrain* contains the substantia nigra and red nucleus (Fig. 2-18 and Table 2-3).
   b. The *basis pontis* contains the pontine nuclei (Figs. 2-16 and 2-17 and Table 2-3).
   c. The *medulla* contains the inferior olivary nuclei (Fig. 2-15).
3. The *reticular formation* is a mixture of neuronal perikarya, axons, and dendrites that fills in the tegmental space not occupied by nuclei or tracts (Table 2-3 and Figs. 2-14 to 2-18). Many regions mediate motor functions.

TABLE 2-3 · Summary of Cranial Nerve Nuclei and Tracts of the Brainstem

Structure	Upper cervical cord	Medulla	Pons	Mesencephalon
GSE nucleus	Ventral motoneurons	Hypoglossal n. (XII)	Abducens n. (VI)	Oculomotor n. (III) Trochlear n. (IV)
BE nucleus	Spinal accessory n.	Ambiguus n. (IX, X)	Facial n. (VII) Trigeminal n. (V)	—
GVE nucleus	—	Dorsal motor n. of vagus	Salivatory n. of VII	Pupilloconstrictor n. (III)
GVA nucleus	—	N. solitarius (IX, X)	—	—
SVA nucleus (taste)	—	N. solitarius (VII, IX, X)	—	—
GSA nucleus	Dorsal column n.	External cuneate n.	Main sensory n. of V	Mesencephalic n. of V
SSA nuclei	—	Vestibular and cochlear n. (VIII)		
Supplemental motor nuclei	—	Reticular formation Inferior olivary n.	Reticular formation N. of basis pontis	Reticular formation Substantia nigra, red n.
Tracts	Corticospinal, MLF Spinocerebellar tracts Spinal root of V	Corticobulbar Corticospinal, MLF Caudal cerebellar peduncle Spinal root of V	Corticobulbar Corticospinal, MLF Middle cerebellar peduncle Descending root of V	Corticobulbar Corticospinal, MLF Rostral cerebellar peduncle Ascending root of V
Lemnisci	Spinal lemniscus (spinothalamic tracts) Beginning of trigeminal lemniscus	Spinal lemniscus Medial lemniscus Trigeminal lemniscus	Spinal lemniscus Medial lemniscus Trigeminal lemniscus Lateral lemniscus	Spinal lemniscus Medial lemniscus Trigeminal lemniscus Lateral lemniscus

ABBREVIATIONS: BE = branchial efferent; GSA = general somatic afferent; GSE = general somatic efferent; GVA = general visceral afferent; GVE = general visceral efferent; MLF = medial longitudinal fasciculus; n. = nucleus or nuclei; SSA = special somatic afferent; SVA = special visceral afferent.

E. The brainstem white matter (Figs. 2-14 to 2-18 and Table 2-3)

1. The brainstem transmits many short, medium, and long ascending and descending pathways. Many arise in or course to the reticular formation and supplementary motor nuclei.
2. The *medial longitudinal fasciculus* interconnects the vestibular nuclei with the nuclei of CrNs III, IV, and VI and the spinal cord. It runs just ventral to the aqueduct and fourth ventricle (Figs. 2-14 to 2-18 and 5-1).
3. The *lemnisci* (Table 2-3 and Figs. 2-14 to 2-18 and 2-28), by definition, convey axons of secondary sensory neurons that terminate in a somatosensory thalamic nucleus. The thalamic nucleus then relays to the respective sensory areas of the cerebral cortex.
4. Long descending *corticofugal motor tracts,* consisting of the *pyramidal* and *corticopontine tracts,* run in the basis.
5. The *cerebellar pathways,* consisting of afferent and efferent tracts, course along the lateral and dorsal aspects of the pons, where they form *cerebellar peduncles* that attach the cerebellum to the pons (Fig. 8-3).

F. Review exercise for the composition of the brainstem

1. Trace the perimeter shown in Fig. 2-14 two times on scrap paper. From memory draw in and label the white matter. Compare your drawing with Fig. 2-14.
2. On the second figure, draw in and label the gray matter and compare with Fig. 2-14.
3. From memory, draw the perimeter of the generalized brainstem cross section and insert and label the white and gray matter. Match your drawing against Fig. 2-14.

G. Functional significance of the additional neurons and tracts of the brainstem

1. The additional brainstem circuitry expands the internuncial neuronal pool beyond that available in the spinal cord gray matter. Like the spinal nuclei, the CrN nuclei mediate monosynaptic reflexes, but the additional neurons in the reticular formation, supplementary motor nuclei, quadrigeminal plate, and cerebellum provide polysynaptic circuitry for complicated brainstem reflexes controlling posture, eye and body movements, breathing, feeding, and homeostasis.
2. The vestibular nuclei and cerebellum add additional internuncial sensory circuits for the brainstem. The cochlear nuclei and superior olivary nuclei of the auditory pathway similarly add their circuitries.

V. ANATOMIC REVIEW OF THE 12 PAIRS OF CRANIAL NERVES

So the present classification of the cranial nerves into 12 numbered pairs was devised by a German medical student (Samuel Soemmering, 1755–1830) nearly two centuries ago. Its basis is the holes in the floor of the skull through which nerves extend out from the cranial cavity to organs as diverse as the eyes and the bowels. Only in part does it sort the nerves according to their function or ultimate distribution. Although rather arbitrary and awkward, it seems likely to be with us for some time.

—C. Wilbur Rucker

A. Number and name of the cranial nerves

1. By definition, a CrN is any major nerve trunk that traverses one of the major foramina in the base of the skull. Learn Table 2-4.

TABLE 2-4 · **Exit Foramina for the Cranial Nerves in the Base of the Skull**

Anterior fossa	I	Perforations in cribriform plate
Middle Fossa	II	Optic foramen
	III, IV, VI, and ophthalmic division of V	Superior orbital fissure
	Maxillary division of V	Foramen rotundum
	Mandibular division of V	Foramen ovale
Posterior Fossa	VII and VIII	Internal auditory meatus
	IX, X, and XI	Jugular foramen
	XII	Hypoglossal foramen

2. The CrN *number* corresponds to the rostrocaudal sequence in which the nerve exits the base of the skull (except XI). The number very nearly duplicates the rostrocaudal sequence by which the CrNs attach to the brain (Fig. 2-20).
3. The CrN *name* conveys at least something about the components, function, or distribution of the nerve. Learn Table 2-5.

B. Functional summary of the cranial nerves

Learn Table 2-6. It lists the function of each CrN in the fewest words. It is the ultimate simplification. You need Tables 2-4 to 2-6 at your tongue tip.

TABLE 2-5 · **Relation of Cranial Nerve Name to Anatomy or Function**

Cranial Nerve		
Number	Name	Functional or anatomic significance of name
I	Olfactory	It smells.
II	Optic	It sees.
III	Oculomotor	Its muscles move the eyeball.
IV	Trochlear	Its muscle moves the eyeball after running through a trochlea.
V	Trigeminal	It has three large sensory branches to the face.
VI	Abducens	It abducts the eye.
VII	Facial	It moves the muscles of all facial orifices.
VIII	Vestibulocochlear	It equilibrates, hears.
IX	Glossopharyngeal	It supplies taste fibers to the tongue and activates the pharynx during swallowing.
X	Vagus	It is a vagrant, wandering from the pharynx to the splenic flexure of the colon.
XI	Spinal accessory	It arises from neuronal cell bodies in the cervical spinal cord, runs into the skull, out again, and conveys accessory fibers to the vagus.
XII	Hypoglossal	It runs under the tongue.

TABLE 2-6 · **Function of the Cranial Nerves**

Number	Function
I	Smells
II	Sees
III, IV, and VI	Move eyes; III constricts pupil
V	Chews and feels the front of the head
VII	Moves the face, tears, snots, tastes, salivates
VIII	Hears, equilibratesh
IX	Tastes, salivates, swallows, monitors carotid body and sinus
X	Tastes, swallows, lifts palate, phonates, afferent and parasympathetic efferent to thoracicoabdominal viscera
XI	Turns head, shrugs shoulders
XII	Moves tongue

C. Special functional components of the cranial nerves

Some CrNs retain the four general nerve components present at spinal levels (GSE, GVE, GVA, and GSA; Fig. 2-7), but three special functions, one motor and two sensory, are added, making seven possible components.

1. Special motor nuclei, *special BE nuclei*, innervate the skeletal muscle derived from the gill arches.
2. *Special visceral afferent* (SVA) *axons* for *taste* and *special somatic afferent* (SSA) *axons* for *auditory* and *vestibular* functions require special nuclei and pathways. Any given CrN may contain one or more but never all of the seven possible components (Table 2-7).

D. Mnemonic classification of cranial nerves into three sets: *solely special sensory set, somatic set,* and *branchial set*

1. From phylogenetic and embryologic data and the theory of nerve components, we can segregate the 12 pairs of CrNs into three sets:
   a. A solely special sensory set (SSSS)
   b. A somite (somatic) set
   c. A branchial set

TABLE 2-7 · Functional Types of Axons in the Spinal Nerves and in the Three Sets of Cranial Nerves

	Functional Type of Axon						
	GSE	BE	GVE	GVA	SVA	GSA	SSA
Spinal nerves	+		+	+		+	
Cranial nerves							
1. Solely special sensory set							
I					+		
II							+
VIII							+
2. Somatomotor set							
III	+		+			+*	
IV	+					+*	
VI	+					+*	
XII	+					+*	
3. Branchial set							
V		+				+	
VII		+	+	+	+	+	
IX		+	+	+	+	+	
X		+	+	+	+	+	
XI		+				+*	

*Cranial nerve V may mediate the GSA component by anastomosing with the somite nerves.

ABBREVIATIONS: BE = branchial efferent; GSA = general somatic efferent; GSE = general somatic efferent; GVA = general visceral afferent; GVE = general visceral efferent; SSA = special somatic afferent; SVA = special visceral afferent.

2. The *SSSS* contains *three* CrNs: I (smell), II (vision), and VIII (hearing and equilibrium). These nerves convey no motor fibers to effectors. Three other CrNs, VII, IX, and X, mediate the one other special sense, taste.
3. The *somite set* (= somatic set) contains *four* CrNs: III, IV, VI, and XII. Because these nerves innervate cranial somite derivatives (eye and tongue muscles), they are direct homologs of the spinal nerves. All belong to the GSE category.
4. The *branchial set* contains *five* CrNs, V, VII, IX, X, and XI, that serially innervate the derivatives of the branchial (gill) arches (Fig. 2-19). Because the branchial arches develop only in the head region, only CrNs contain BE axons.

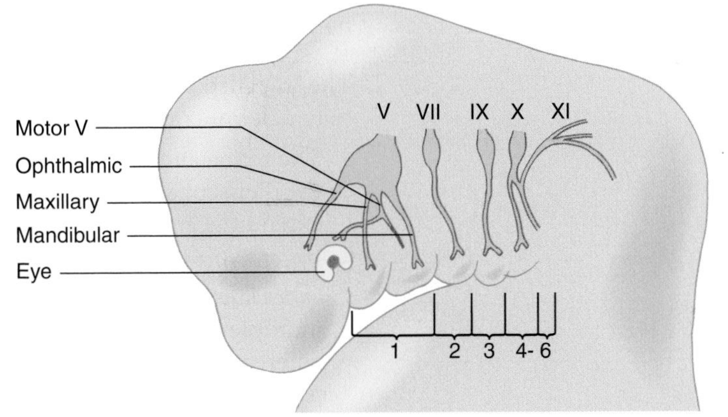

FIGURE 2-19. Six-week-old human embryo showing the innervation of the branchial arches (arabic numerals) by the branchial set of cranial nerves (roman numerals). The first arch (1) divides into two processes, the maxillary and the mandibular.

E. The SSSS of cranial nerves I, II, and VIII

1. *CrN I*, the olfactory nerve, consists of axonal filaments from perikarya located in the olfactory ganglia in the nasal mucosa (Fig. 9-1).
   a. This olfactory ganglion corresponds to the dorsal root ganglion of a spinal nerve.
   b. The olfactory axons penetrate the cribriform plate to synapse on the olfactory bulb. See the olfactory bulb in Fig. 2-20.

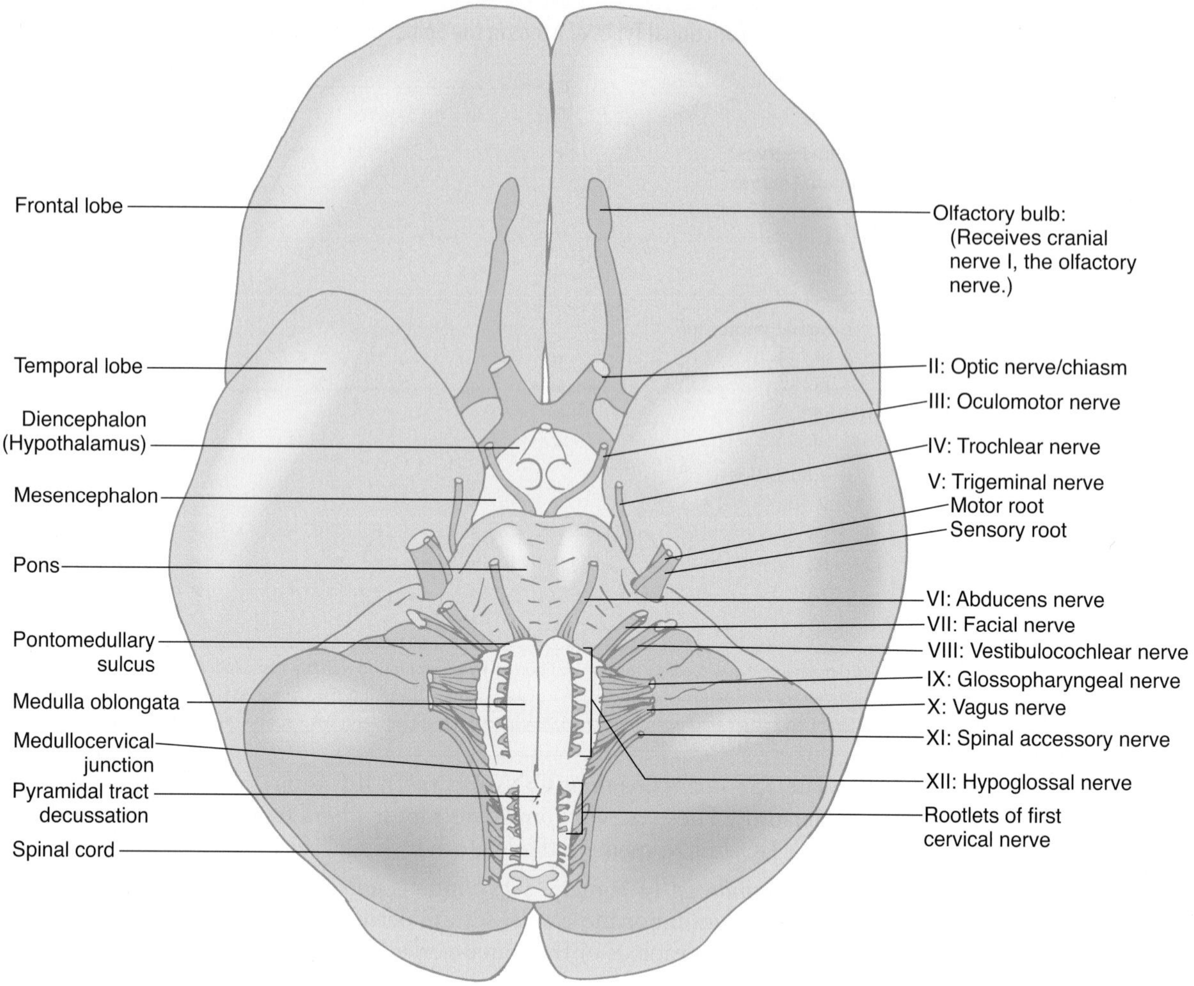

FIGURE 2-20. Ventral aspect of the brain showing where the cranial nerves attach. The origin of cranial nerve IV, which attaches to the dorsal surface of the mesencephalon, does not appear in this view.

2. The so-called *CrN II*, the optic nerve, is neither developmentally nor histologically a peripheral nerve.
   a. The retina and optic stalks develop as evaginations from the hypothalamus of the diencephalon (Fig. 2-22). The retinas, at the distal end of the optic stalks, extend the actual wall of the neuraxis out to the body surface to detect light.
   b. Proximally, the two optic stalks remain attached to the hypothalamus as the *optic chiasm* (Figs. 2-20 and 2-26). Demyelinating diseases of the CNS, such as multiple sclerosis, that affect oligodendroglial myelin, attack the optic nerves, whereas a different set of diseases attack the Schwann cell myelin of true peripheral nerves.
3. *CrN VIII*, the vestibulocochlear nerve, conveys afferents from the cochlear apparatus for detecting sound and the vestibular apparatus for detecting motion and the pull of gravity. Of the three special sensory CrNs, only VIII has typical peripheral nerve histology.

F. The somite set of cranial nerves: III, IV, VI, and XII

1. Fate of the rostralmost cranial somites and their nerves
   a. Of the dozen somites that arise at the brainstem level, only a few survive the travail of evolution. The cranial dermatomes retrogress, but some myotomes remain. The first cervical dermatome (C1) usually also disappears. Hence, the rostralmost dermatome is at the level of C _______________.

C2. Review Fig. 2-10 if you missed this answer

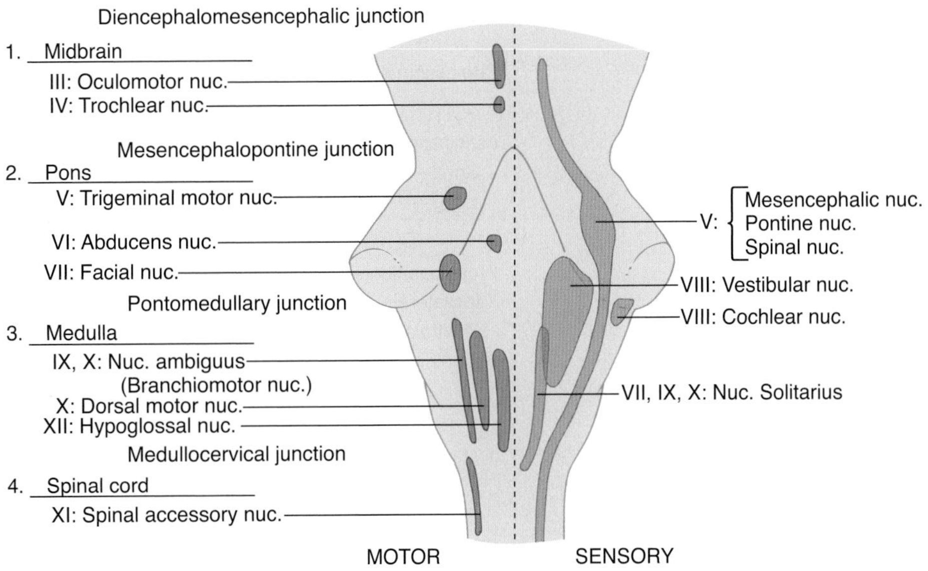

FIGURE 2-21. Phantom dorsal view of the cranial nerve nuclei in the brainstem and the rostral portion of the cervical cord, motor nuclei are on the left, and sensory nuclei are on the right.

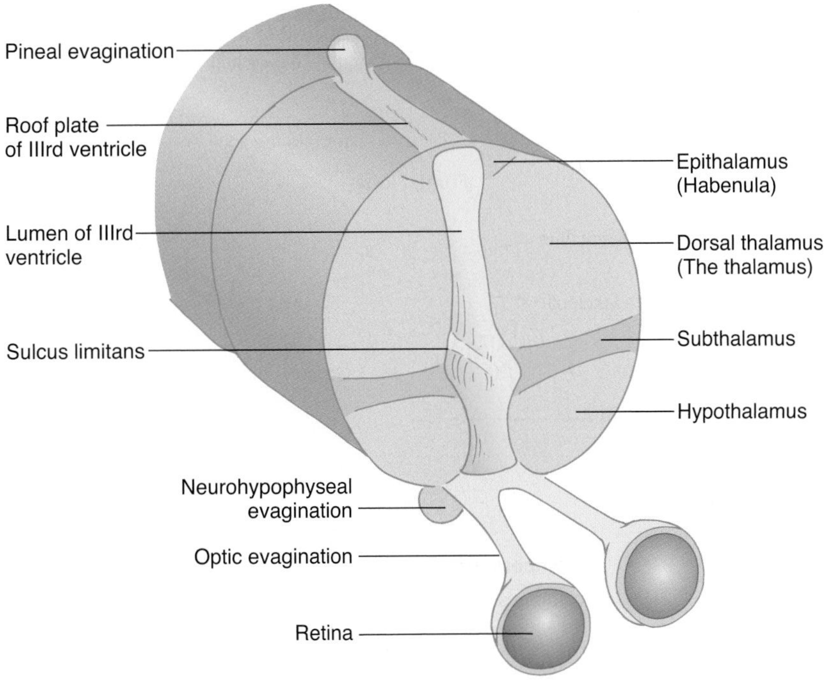

FIGURE 2-22. Transverse (coronal) section of the embryonic diencephalon, showing its four nuclear zones bordering the third ventricle. (1) Epithalamus. (2) Thalamus dorsalis. (3) Thalamus ventralis (subthalamus). (4) Hypothalamus.

III; IV; VI. (If you had trouble recalling, sort through the CrNs one by one, from I to XII. See Table 2-5.)

b. Of the rostral myotomes, three survive, wondrously transformed into the ocular muscles. The law of original innervation requires these three myotomes to retain their three original nerves. The numbers of the three somite CrNs that innervate the eye muscles are _____, _______, and _______.

☑ GSE

c. To supply skeletal muscle derived from somites, these nerves must have a ❒ GVA/❒ GSE/❒ GVE component.

d. We will assume that any nerve supplying GSE fibers to a skeletal muscle also returns proprioceptive (GSA) fibers from it. Because these nerves lack individual dorsal root ganglia, their proprioceptive afferents presumably come from anastomotic branches from a collective ganglion that is on CrN V, the trigeminal (= Gasserian) ganglion.

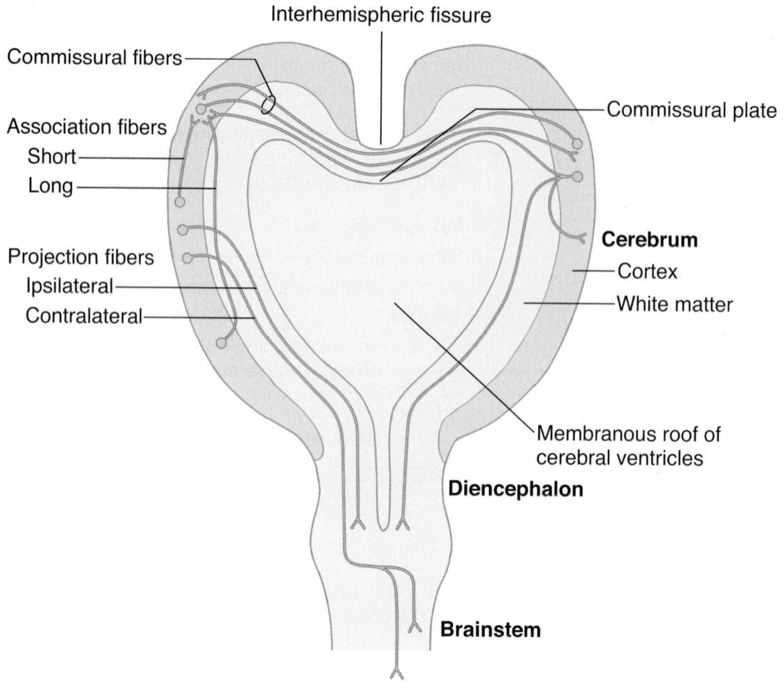

FIGURE 2-23. Horizontal section of embryonic brain showing the course of the association, commissural, and projection fibers. (Reproduced with permission from DeMyer W. *Neuroanatomy,* 2nd ed. Baltimore, Williams and Wilkins, 1998.)

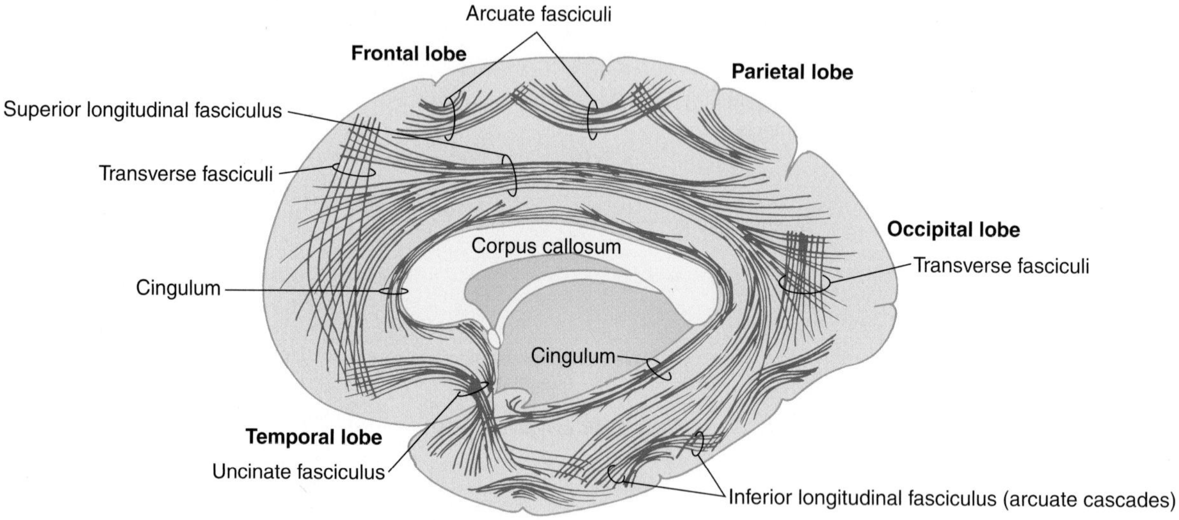

FIGURE 2-24. Sagittal section of mature cerebrum showing the projection pathways (for reference).

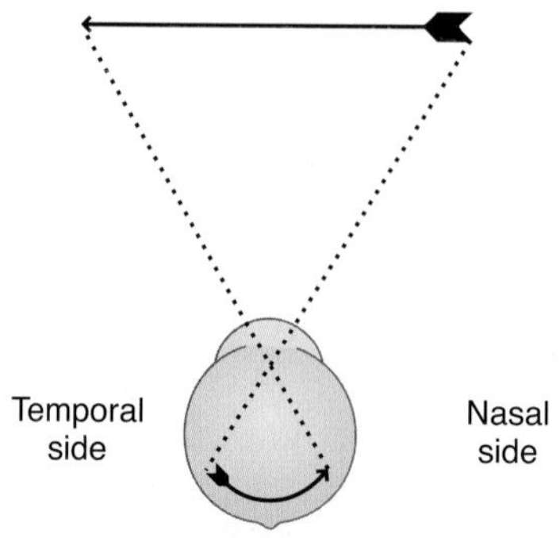

FIGURE 2-25. Diagram showing the reversal of the retinal image of an object.

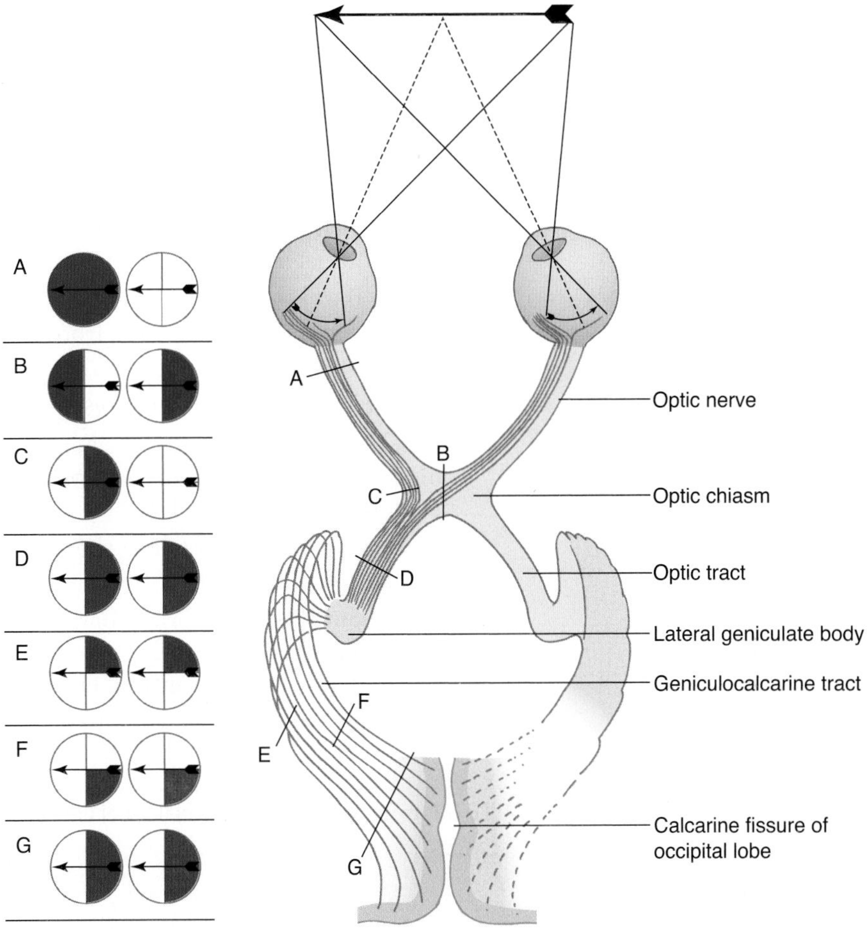

FIGURE 2-26. Diagram showing the topographic projection of the visual field on the calcarine cortex of the occipital lobe in higher animals with binocular stereoscopic vision. The small scale of the drawing precludes showing the synapse of the retinogeniculate axons at the lateral geniculate body. A to F indicate lesion sites and the corresponding defects produced in the visual field.

e. Of the somite CrNs, only III conveys GVE axons from the brainstem (Table 2-7). These GVE axons innervate the *pupilloconstrictor muscle,* which adjusts pupillary size, and the *ciliary muscle,* which adjusts lens thickness. No GVA fibers return to the neuraxis in any somite nerve.

2. **Fate of the middle and caudal cranial somites:** The *middle* cranial somites disappear, as do their nerves. The *caudal* cranial somites donate their myotomes to the tongue and their sclerotomes to the base of the skull, but their dermatomes disappear. Although CrN XII runs to the tongue muscles as a single trunk, it conveys axons from several somites. Because it does not innervate any visceral organs or special senses, XII has only two components, ❐ GSE/❐ GVE/❐ GVA/❐ GSA.

☑ GSE and ☑ GSA

3. The disappearance of many of the middle group of somites accounts for the absence of the somite nuclei between CrNs XII and VI and between VI and IV. Notice this discontinuity in Fig. 2-21.

4. Review Table 2-7 and then complete Table 2-8 to summarize the components of the somatic set of CrNs.

	III	IV	VI	XII
GSA	+	+	+	+
GVA				
GVE	+			
GSE	+	+	+	+

TABLE 2-8 · Nerve Components of the Somite Cranial Nerves

	III	IV	VI	XII
GSA				
GVA				
GVE				
GSE				

G. The branchial set of cranial nerves ..."or human face divine"

1. To the poet Milton, it was the human face divine, created in final form, by a deity and passed along from generation to generation without a history. But to the biologist, William Gregory (1929), the face evolved gradually from the branchial arches and frontonasal process (Fig. 1-10). He stated "that the real ancestral face belonged not to a precreated man but to a poor mud-sucking protochordate of pre-Silurian times; that when in some far-off dismal swamp a putrid prize was snatched by scaly forms, their facial masks already bore our eyes and nose and mouth."
2. In creating the cheeks, jaws, and ears, the branchial arches usurped the retrogressive cranial somites. Thus the face, from fish to man, recapitulates the phylogeny of the branchial arches.
3. The branchial arches remarkably resemble somites in fundamental plan.
   a. Thus, branchial arches are paired and arranged serially, and each pair receives only one pair of nerves and only one pair of arteries. See Fig. 2-19 and compare it directly with Fig. 1-10.
   b. The branchial arches produce the dermis, muscles, and bones of the cheeks, jaws, and ears (Fig. 1-10).
   c. Throughout their transformations, the branchial arch derivatives retain their original branchial nerve. Chapter 6 on clinical testing diagrams the individual CrNs. For now learn the introductory descriptions in Tables 2-5 to 2-7.
4. Complete Table 2-9 to review the branchial CrNs.

V	trigeminal
VII	facial
IX	glossopharyngeal
X	vagus
XI	spinal accessory

For functions see Table 2-6

TABLE 2-9 · Summary of the Branchial Set of Cranial Nerves

Arch number	Nerve number	Name	General function
1			
2			
3			
4			
5–6			

5. Complete Table 2-10 to review the three sets of CrNs.

Somatic: III, IV, VI, XIII
Branchial: V, VII, IX, X, XI
Solely special sensory: I, II, VIII
For functions check Table 2-6

TABLE 2-10 · Summary of the Nerves in Each of the Three Sets of Cranial Nerves

Name of set	Characterized by	Nerves in set
1.	(1 per body segment)	
2.	(1 per gill arch)	
3.	(no motor axons)	

H. Mnemonic for the attachment sites of the cranial nerves to the brain

1. Learn now, once and for all, that CrNs VI, VII, and VIII (a *somite*, a *branchial*, and a *special sensory* nerve) attach, in *ventrodorsal* order, at the *pontomedullary sulcus.* See Fig. 2-20.
2. By knowing this one fact and the unique attachment sites of the olfactory and optic nerves, you can fairly well deduce where all other CrNs attach:
   a. All CrNs with numbers *less* than VI must attach *rostrally* to the pontomedullary sulcus.
   b. CrNs III to V must attach *caudally* to CrN II and *rostral to* the pontomedullary sulcus (Fig. 2-20).
   c. All CrNs with numbers *greater than* VIII must attach *caudally* to the pontomedullary sulcus.

3. In Fig. 2-20, learn the labels on the two sides and color each set of CrNs with a different color. Then do the test frames 4 to 14.

I
4. The only CrN with an extracranial ganglion synapsing directly on a bulb that evaginates from the base of the cerebrum is number ______.

II
5. The stalk of a diencephalic evagination forms CrN ______.

VII; pontomedullary
6. The only SSSS CrN with true peripheral nerve histology is CrN ______. It attaches to the brainstem at the ______________________________ sulcus.

III; ☑ mesencephalon
7. The rostralmost somite nerve and the rostralmost motor CrN is ______. It attaches to the ❐ diencephalon/❐ mesencephalon/❐ pons.

III; IV
8. The unique exit site of CrN IV from the tectum (dorsum) of the mesencephalon does not appear in Fig. 2-20. No other CrN attaches dorsally. The two CrNs attached to the mesencephalon are ______ and ______.

V
9. The CrN that attaches to the lateral sides of the bulging belly of the pons is ______.

VI; VII; VIII
10. Three CrNs attach at the pontomedullary sulcus in ventrodorsal order, ______, ______, and ______.

IX; X; XII
11. Three additional CrNs attach to the medulla: ______, ______, and, ______.

XI
12. The *only* CrN attaching to the spinal cord is ______.

Note: CrN XI qualifies as a CrN because although it enters the posterior fossa through the foramen magnum, it then exits through the jugular foramen, thus meeting the definition of a CrN (Section V A-1).

13. In Fig. 2-20, notice that CrNs III, VI, and XII and the first cervical nerves that are phylogenetically homologous, attach in a *parasagittal line* along the brainstem. To remember this fact, draw a colored line in Fig. 2-20 from the attachment sites of CrN III through VI, and XII and the rootlets of the first cervical nerve.

☑ lateral to (Fig. 2-20)
14. The branchial set (CrNs V, VII, IX, X, and XI) then attach ❐ lateral to/❐ medial to/❐ in line with the somatic set.

15. Draw Fig. 2-20 from memory.

I. Location of the cranial nerve nuclei

Note: In Fig. 2-21 connect the motor CrN nuclei of the somite and branchial sets of CrN motor nuclei with different colored lines. Use the same color for the somite set as you used in Fig. 2-20.

Next complete frames 1 to 11. In thinking out the answers, sort through the CrNs one by one, from I to XII, for each question.

III and IV
1. The CrN nuclei limited to the mesencephalon are ______________.

V, VI, and VII
2. The CrN motor nuclei limited to the pons are for CrNs ______________.

cochlear; vestibular
3. The two CrN sensory nuclei that straddle the pontomedullary junction and serve CrN VIII are the ______________ and ______________ nuclei.

IX, X, and XII
4. The CrN motor nuclei limited to the medulla are for CrNs ______________.

solitarius; IX and X
5. The sensory nucleus limited solitarily to the medulla is called the nucleus ______________. It serves the visceral sensory functions of the medullary branchial nerves numbered ______________.

V
6. The one CrN nucleus extending from the spinal cord to the mesencephalon belongs to CrN _________.

V (sensory); XI (motor)

7. The two CrN nuclei found in the rostral part of the cervical cord are (sensory) _______ and (motor) _______.

I; II

8. The only CrNs attaching to the brain rostral to the mesencephalon are _______ and _______.
9. In column 1 of Table 2-11, list in rostrocaudal sequence, the numbers of the branchial CrNs. Then complete the rest of Table 2-11.

V	(trigeminal), pons
VII	(facial) pons
IX	(ambiguus) medulla
X	(ambiguus) medulla
XI	(spinal accessory) spinal cord

TABLE 2-11 · Number, Name, and Location of Branchial Efferent Nuclei (Rostrocaudal Order)

Number of cranial nerve	Name of branchial motor nucleus	Anatomic subdivision of neuraxis containing the nucleus

The somatic nuclei (GSE) are all paramedian, that is, adjacent to the median or midsagittal plane, and the nerves attach in a paramedian line along the brainstem. The branchial nuclei (BE) align more laterally and their nerves attach more laterally. (The actual location of the branchial nuclei with respect to the somatic nuclei is ventrolateral. See Figs. 2-14 to 2-18 and 2-21.)

10. Describe how the sites of the nuclei and sites of brainstem attachment of the somatic set of CrNs (GSE) are located with respect to the midsagittal plane. Then describe how the branchial set of CrNs (BE) are located with respect to the somite CrNs.____
____
______________________________________.
11. Draw Fig. 2-21 from memory to ensure that you know the locations of the CrN nuclei.

J. An "elimination" mnemonic for learning the distribution of the branchial nerves: V, VII, IX, X, and XI

1. First, eliminate V and XI.
   a. CrNs V and XI are relatively simple in composition and distribution.
      i. Both are sensorimotor nerves and have only BE and GSA components (Table 2-1).
      ii. Neither nerve conveys special senses or GVE (autonomic axons) to glands or smooth muscle (Table 2-7).
   b. CrN V has a huge GSA component for facial skin and related mucous membranes and cavities (Fig. 10-2). It conveys BE axons to the chewing muscles (Fig. 6-1) and returns proprioceptive, GSA fibers, from them.

Mnemonic for CrN V: CrN V feels the face and chews (Fig. 6-1).

   c. CrN XI conveys BE axons to the sternocleidomastoid and trapezius muscles that turn the head and shrug the shoulders. CrN XI returns only a small contingent of proprioceptive (GSA) axons. It closely resembles the somite set.
2. Common plan of branchial CrNs VII, IX, and X.

Note: With CrNs V and XI eliminated, three complicated CrNs, VII, IX, and X, remain. They all convey the same components and adhere to a common plan but pursue radically different peripheral courses. Compare with Tables 2-7 and 2-12.

a. All three CrNs, VII, IX and X, convey BE axons to striated muscle derived from a gill arch.

b. All three convey GVE (preganglionic parasympathetic) axons to a peripheral ganglion located in or near one of the large exocrine glands of the head or to glands in mucous membranes or viscera.

i. *CrN VII* sends GVE axons to the *lacrimal glands* and to the *mucous glands* of the nasal mucosa via the sphenopalatine ganglia (Figs. 6-5 and 6-6) and to the *submandibular* and *sublingual* glands via the submandibular ganglia.

TABLE 2-12 · Nerve Components of Cranial Nerves VII, IX, and X and Their Peripheral Distributions

Nerve	Branchiomotor (BE)	Visceromotor (VE) (all parasympathetic)	VA	Taste (SVA)	SA
VII	To all muscles of the face and facial orifices and to the stapedius muscle	To lacrimal, submandibular, and sublingual glands: all large exocrine glands of head except the parotid; to the nasal mucosa	From posterior nasopharynx and soft palate	From anterior two-thirds of the tongue	Cutaneous twig to ear
IX	To the pharyngeal plexus for swallowing	Parotid gland and pharyngeal mucosa	Soft palate and upper pharynx, carotid body and sinus	From the posterior third of the tongue	Cutaneous twig to ear
X	To the pharyngeal plexus and laryngeal muscles (via the accessory branch of XI)	To glands of the pharyngeal and laryngeal mucosa and to the glands and smooth muscle of thoracicoabdominal viscera; inhibitory axons to the heart	Pharynx and larynx and thoracicoabdominal viscera	From the region of the epiglottis	Cutaneous twig to ear

ABBREVIATIONS: BE = branchial efferent; SA = somatic afferent; SVA = special visceral afferent; VA = visceral afferent; VE = visceral efferent.

ii. *CrN IX* sends GVE axons to the parotid gland via the otic ganglion and to the glands of the pharyngeal mucosa (Fig. 6-9).

iii. *CrN X* sends GVE axons to the glands of the pharyngeal and laryngeal mucosa and to the smooth muscle and glands of the thoracicoabdominal viscera, as far as the splenic flexure of the colon (Fig. 6-10).

c. All three CrNs, VII, IX and X, convey GVA fibers from the palatopharyngeal mucosa. The Xth nerve also carries afferents from the thoracicoabdominal viscera (Fig. 6-10).

d. All three convey SVA fibers for taste: *CrN VII* from the anterior two-thirds of the tongue, *IX* from the posterior third, and *X* from the palatal orifice: rostrocaudal sequence.

e. All three convey GSA fibers from the skin of the external auditory canal but no auditory or vestibular fibers. The ear twigs from these nerves underscore the complex origin of the ear from several branchial arches. The skin area of CrN V on the face and the skin twigs of VII, IX, and X demonstrate retention of the dermis of the branchial arches.

3. CrNs IX and X differ from VII in innervating palatal and pharyngeal muscles during swallowing, the carotid sinus and carotid body, and the larynx for phonation. CrN X, the vagrant nerve, is unique in wandering through the thoracicoabdominal viscera to the splenic flexure.

BE, GVE, GVA, GSA, and SVA (Tables 2-7 and 2-12)

4. **List the five nerve components of VII, IX, and X.____________________.**

5. **Special features of CrN VII:**

a. By eliminating the GSA cutaneous twig to the ear and the GVA palatopharyngeal sensory innervation as clinically insignificant, we can reduce CrN VII to its BE, GVE, and SVA components, its clinically important components

(Figs. 6-4 and 6-5). Read the quotation from Bell, page 231. Realize that, through this nerve, we wink, smile, frown, cry, taste, salivate, and produce mucus in the nose. This leads to a mnemonic:

Mnemonic for remembering the functions of CrN VII: CrN VII *tears, snots, tastes, salivates,* and *moves the face.* It innervates all facial movements (except for eyelid elevation by CrN III) and mandibular movements by CrN V (Figs. 6-5 and 6-6).

b. CrN VII travels through the parotid gland but does not innervate it (Fig. 6-5). CrN IX innervates the parotid gland.

VI. THE RETICULAR FORMATION

A. Anatomic definition of the reticular formation

1. The reticular formation (RF) consists of tegmental neurons more or less loosely arranged into nuclear groups connected by countless, multisynaptic, internuncial circuits.
2. The RF extends through the tegmentum from the *rostral* end of the spinal cord into the *caudal* end of the diencephalon. RF fills the tegmental space not occupied by CrN nuclei, supplementary motor nuclei, or tracts in transit.
3. The RF receives collaterals from sensory, motor, and autonomic pathways that traverse the brainstem and returns pathways to every part of the CNS.

B. Functions of the reticular formation

1. The RF mediates functions as diverse a breathing and consciousness. A midpontine transection divides the RF into *rostral* and *caudal* halves that somewhat separate its major functions.
2. The *rostral*, or pontomesencephalic, half of the RF sends ascending pathways to the thalamus and cerebral cortex. This *ascending reticular activating system* mediates consciousness and the waking state. Chapter 12 discusses the neuroanatomy of consciousness.
3. The *caudal*, or pontomedullary, half of the RF mediates various vital reflexes related to breathing, feeding, homeostasis, control of the blood pressure and pulse, alimentation and elimination, and control of posture and eye movements.
   a. Destruction of the caudal half of the RF does not impair consciousness, if respiration and blood pressure are artificially maintained.
   b. The caudal part of the RF, through CrNs V, VII, IX, X, and XII, controls the oronasopharyngeal conduits for feeding, breathing, and vocalizing.
      i. *Feeding-related actions* include sucking, chewing, salivating, and swallowing.
      ii. *Breathing-related actions* include phonation, sneezing, coughing, sighing, and hiccoughing. To phonate and articulate speech and yet maintain the blood CO_2 and O_2 levels requires coordination of facial, oropharyngeal, laryngeal, diaphragmatic, intercostal, and abdominal muscles.
      iii. Sensory receptors innervated via CrNs IX and X and neurons located directly in the medullary RF itself control breathing and blood gases. Chapter 6 discusses the neuroanatomy of breathing.
   c. The caudal pontomedullary RF likewise mediates autonomic reflexes of the thoracicoabdominal viscera that control blood pressure, pulse, bronchial diameter, gastrointestinal motility, and elimination.
4. The pontine RF is necessary for sleep regulation. Lesions of the pontine tegmentum abolish rapid eye movement sleep and greatly reduce the amount of nonrapid eye movement sleep.

VII. THE DIENCEPHALON

A. The four nuclear subdivisions of the diencephalon: nuclear zones consist of the *epithalamus, thalamus dorsalis, thalamus ventralis (subthalamus),* and *hypothalamus*. These structures form the roof, walls and floor of the third ventricle (Figs. 2-22 and 13-10B)

B. The epithalamus consists of the *pineal body, habenula,* and membranous *roof* plate of the third ventricle (Fig. 2-22)

C. The thalamus (thalamus dorsalis)

1. To know the brain, you must know the thalamus. The thalamus consists of diverse nuclei that modulate all *mental, motor,* and *sensory* functions, including cognition, memory, speech, and affective experience.
2. The thalamus receives ascending sensory pathways (except for smell); ascending motor impulses from the RF, cerebellum, and basal motor nuclei; the ascending reticular activating system; and limbic pathways.
3. Thalamocortical and corticothalamic feedback circuits link the thalamic nuclei with motor, sensory, association, and limbic areas of the cerebral cortex. Almost everything that enters or exits the cortex must submit to thalamic modulation. As a corollary, thalamic lesions can impair the mental, motor, and sensory functions of the cortex, causing, for example, dementia, loss of memory, dysphasia, and various sensory and motor deficits.
4. The thalamus contains five groups of nuclei:
    a. *Sensory nuclei* receive the optic tract and the medial, lateral, spinal, and trigeminal lemnisci and relay to the respective sensory areas of the cerebral cortex (Table 2-13). Only smell lacks a direct thalamic relay nucleus.

TABLE 2-13 · Origin of the Lemnisci, Thalamic Relay Nucleus, and Cortical Projection from the Thalamus

Lemniscus and origin	Thalamic relay nucleus	Cortical area of projection
Spinal, spinal gray matter	n. ventralis posterior (lateralis)	Somesthetic cortex of the postcentral gyms
Medial, n. gracilis and cuneatus	n. ventralis posterior (lateralis)	Somesthetic cortex of the postcentral gyms
Trigeminal, spinal n. of CrN V	n. ventralis posterior (medialis)	Somesthetic cortex of the postcentral gyms
Lateral, cochlear n.	Medial geniculate body	Auditory receptive area, transverse gyri of temporal lobe
Optic tract, retina	Lateral geniculate body	Visual receptive area, calcarine cortex of occipital lobe

ABBREVIATION: n. = nucleus.

Thalamic sensory relay mnemonic: All sensory pathways known to reach consciousness relay to the cerebral cortex through a specific thalamic sensory nucleus, except for smell.

b. *Somatomotor nuclei* relay impulses from the cerebellum, RF, and basal motor nuclei to the motor cortex. These connections modulate the output of the motor cortex through the pyramidal tract.

c. *Midline* and *intralaminar nuclei* relay ascending reticular activating impulses to the cortex at large, mediating alerting responses and consciousness.

d. *Association nuclei* mediate cognition by relaying to the association cortex of the frontal, parietal, temporal, and occipital lobes (Figs. 2-2C and 2-3). Association cortex does not directly receive sensory pathways or originate axons for the pyramidal tract.

e. *Limbic nuclei* interconnect with the limbic lobe.

D. The *subthalamus* (thalamus ventralis) consists of the subthalamic nucleus of Luys and the zona incerta that belong to the basal motor nuclei (Fig. 2-32)

E. The *hypothalamus* controls homeostatic and autonomic functions and emotional expression in close collaboration with the limbic lobe, hippocampus, amygdala, periaqueductal gray matter, and pituitary gland

VIII. CONNECTIONS AND WHITE MATTER OF THE CEREBRUM

A. Ontogeny of cortical connections

1. The cerebral pathways are best understood from their ontogeny. An axon growing from its cortical perikaryon might form three possible types of pathways: *association*, *commissural*, and *projection*.
   a. **Association pathways:** An outgrowing axon may connect with an *ipsilateral* cortical neuron to *associate* the functions of the two neurons (Fig. 2-23).
      i. Numerous long and short association pathways course through the cerebral white matter to connect the various cortical areas of one hemisphere.
      ii. The longest such association fibers extend rectilinearly or in sweeping arcs through the white matter to connect frontal, occipital, and temporal lobes and the areas in between (Fig. 2-24).
   b. **Commissural pathways:** An outgrowing axon that crosses the midline to end in a mirror image site on the opposite side is, by definition, a *commissural fiber.* The largest number of commissural fibers runs through the corpus callosum (Figs. 13-10A and 13-10B). Smaller commissures exist at all levels of the neuraxis.
   c. **Projection pathways:** An outgrowing cortical axon may end *ipsilaterally* or *contralaterally* on an infracortical *internuncial* or an *efferent* neuron (Fig. 2-23). Such an axon *projects* the cortical influence down to the next neuron in line.
      i. Axons that cross the midline to end on non-mirror image sites are called *decussations,* to distinguish them from commissures.
      ii. Like commissures, decussations occur at all levels of the neuraxis.
      iii. The term *projection* applies generically for efferent connections at any level, not just cortical projections.

associational; commissural; projectional

2. In summary, outgrowing cortical axons establish pathways of three types: ______________, ______________, and ______________.

Commissures connect mirror image points of the cortical or nuclear gray matter of the two sides of the CNS, whereas decussations connect non-mirror image sites.

3. A given axon may collateralize to form all three types of connections: associational, commissural and projectional. See right side of Fig. 2-23.
4. What is the essential difference between commissures and decussations? ____ ______________________________.

B. Review of the pathways in the cerebral white matter

1. *Association pathways,* long and short, connect ipsilateral cortical areas.
2. *Commissural pathways* connect mirror image cortical areas of the two cerebral hemispheres.

3. Cortical *projection pathways* connect the cortex with ipsilateral or contralateral infracortical neurons. Major cortical projections include *corticostriatal, corticothalamic, pyramidal* (corticobulbar and corticospinal), and *corticopontine pathways.*
4. *Thalamocortical pathways* connect the various thalamic nuclei to various cortical areas.
5. Most of the incoming and outgoing cortical pathways, including the massive corticothalamic and thalamocortical circuits, fan out from or funnel down through the internal capsule (Fig. 13-10). See the geniculocalcarine tract in Figs. 3-4 to 3-6 for an example of a fan.
6. Lesions of the white matter disconnect various cortical areas from each other and from the thalamus, resulting in *cerebral disconnection syndromes* of dementia, dysphasia, dyspraxia, amnesia, spatial neglect, and alterations of affect, consciousness, and cognition.

IX. THE CONTRALATERALITY OF THE SENSORY PATHWAYS: THE DECUSSATIONS IN THE NEURAXIS AND THE LAW OF CONTRALATERALITY OF CEREBRAL SENSORIMOTOR PATHWAYS

A. The contralateral representation of the visual fields

1. To localize lesions that interrupt the long CNS pathways, you must know where they decussate. A lesion *rostral* to a decussation causes *contralateral* deficits, whereas a lesion *caudal* to a decussation causes *ipsilateral* deficits.
2. To explain decussations we had best start, surprisingly, with viewing an arrow in space.
   a. The physical properties of light and the physical optics of the eye (the pinhole camera effect of the pupil) form an inverted, real image on the retina (Figs. 2-25 and 2-26).
   b. Each site on the retinal image corresponds to a site on the arrow, but each half of the retina represents the *opposite* half of the visual field (Fig. 2-26).
   c. The mind then creates a mental image that projects or interprets an image that falls on one half of the retina as coming from the opposite side, i.e., from the location of the real object.
3. From these facts comes an intriguing theory that, phylogenetically, the wiring diagram of the visual system depends on:
   a. The physical properties of light.
   b. The physical optics of the eye.
   c. The necessity to unite the halves of visual space so that the mind can scan the entire visual field in continuity (Santiago Ramon y Cajal).
4. Because mammals have a cerebral cortex, the pathway from the retina runs to the lateral geniculate body (a thalamic nucleus) and from it via the geniculocalcarine tract to the calcarine cortex of the occipital lobe (Fig. 2-26). This pathway conveys the image of each right or left half of the visual field in uninterrupted fashion because of the compensatory semidecussation of axons at the optic chiasm (Fig. 2-26). **The crucial fact is that each hemisphere mediates the visual field from the contralateral half of space.**
5. **Inversion of the sensorimotor homunculus in the paracentral region**
   a. The retinal image is reversed not only *laterally* but also *vertically* (Fig. 2-27). Thus, the *lower* half of the retina receives the *top* half of the visual field and projects it to the calcarine cortex in topographic order (Fig. 2-27).
   b. This inversion of the vertical arrow may account for the inverted homunculus of motor and sensory representation in the pre- and postcentral gyri (Fig. 2-27), because then the mind has only to make one inversion to make the retinal input correspond to external reality.

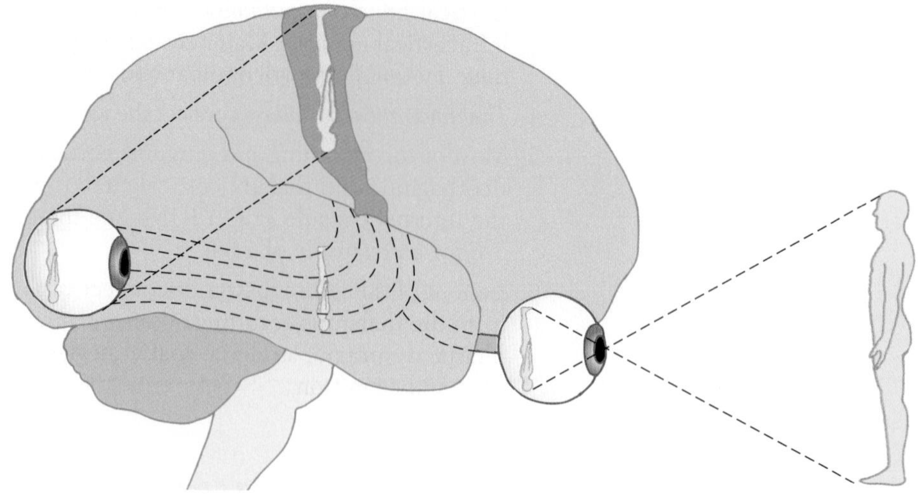

FIGURE 2-27. Diagram showing the inversion of the visual field on the retina and the subsequent inverted representation of the visual field in the calcarine visual cortex and the sensorimotor cortex of the paracentral region.

BIBLIOGRAPHY · Contralateral Representation of the Visual Fields

Ramon y Cajal S. *Recollections of My Life, vol. VIII*. Horne Craige E, trans. Philadelphia: Memoirs of the American Philosophical Society, 1937.

Rucker CW. The concept of a semidecussation of the optic nerves. *Arch Ophthal* 1958;59:159–171.

B. The contralaterality of the somatosensory pathways

1. The cerebral hemisphere that receives its visual information from the contralateral half of space also receives the somatosensory information from the contralateral half of the body. Then the association area of that hemisphere can readily integrate the visual stimuli and proprioceptive and tactile stimuli from the contralateral limbs.
2. **The primary, secondary, and tertiary neuron plan of the somatosensory pathways:** Start tracing a somatosensory pathway at the receptor ending from its *primary neuron* in a dorsal root ganglion (Fig. 2-28).
   a. The *peripheral* branch of a dorsal root neuron receives a stimulus representing the *superficial* modalities of touch, pain, or temperature or the *deep* modalities of form, texture, vibration, position sense, direction of movement, stereognosis, and barognosis.
   b. The *central* branch synapses on a secondary neuron in the spinal cord gray matter. The axon of the secondary neuron then decussates and ascends to the thalamus as a lemniscus. **The critical factor in tracing a sensory pathway is the level of the secondary neuron because the decussation occurs at that level.**
      i. The *primary axons* for the *deep sensory modalities* enter the spinal cord white matter and ascend through the *ipsilateral* dorsal column to synapse on the nuclei gracilis and cuneatus located at the cervicomedullary junction (Figs. 2-28 and 10-14). The axons from the secondary neurons in these nuclei then decussate at that level (as the internal arcuate decussation). The axons turn rostrally in the *contralateral* half of the brainstem, where they ascend as the medial lemniscus to the thalamus.
      ii. The primary axons for the *superficial modalities of pain and temperature* synapse on their secondary neurons at or near the level of entry of each dorsal root into the CNS. The axons of the secondary neurons then decussate and

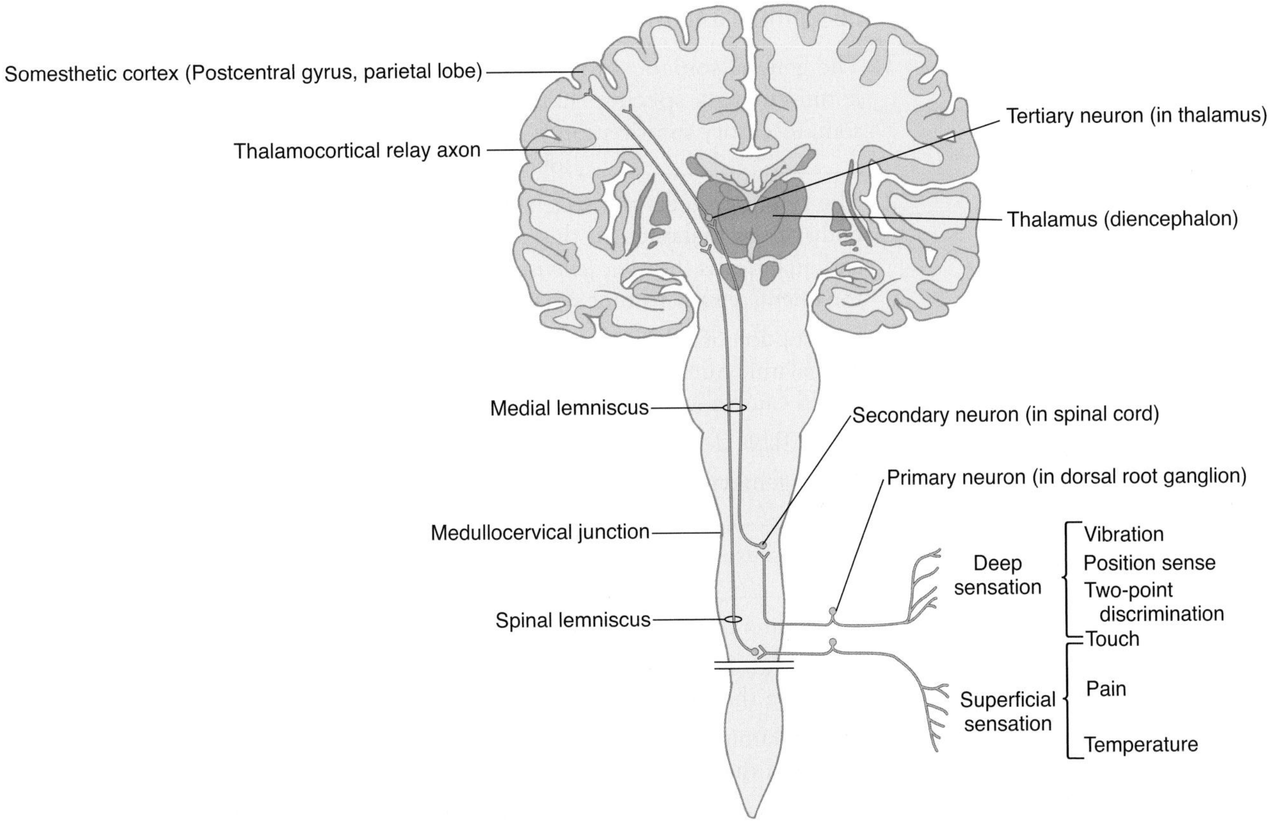

FIGURE 2-28. Decussation of the somatosensory pathways. The pathway for deep sensation decussates at one level, the cervicomedullary junction. The pathway for pain and temperature synapses at or near the level of entry of the primary axon up and down the cord. The impulses that mediate light touch travel in both pathways.

turn rostrally in the *contralateral* ventrolateral quadrant of the spinal cord white matter. This pathway of second-order neurons is called the *spinal lemniscus* to designate that it ends in the thalamus (Figs. 2-28 and 10-6).

c. The *superficial modality of touch* is mediated by dorsal and ventral column pathways. The ventral column component comprises part of the spinal lemniscus (Fig. 2-28).

The law of the level of decussation of the somatosensory pathways: The general somatosensory pathways decussate at the level of the nucleus for the perikarya of the second-order neurons. The law holds for the spinothalamic, spinocerebellar, touch, pain and temperature, and dorsal column pathways.

3. The *third-order neuron* of the somatosensory pathways resides in a sensory relay nucleus of the thalamus. The thalamic neurons relay to the ipsilateral somatosensory cortex in the postcentral gyrus of the parietal lobe (Fig. 2-28). Association fibers then connect the visual and somatosensory areas with other association cortices.
4. The pathways of two special senses, smell and hearing, are partial exceptions to the contralaterality law. Their stimuli, odors and sounds as distinct from light, go around corners and over obstructions. Contrary to other sensory pathways, the ascending pathways for hearing contain about an equal number of decussated and undecussated axons (Fig. 9-7). Thus, **a unilateral CNS lesion does not ordinarily cause a strongly lateralized hearing loss.**

C. The lemnisci and the role of the thalamus in sensation

postcentral; parietal

1. The general somatic and special sensations, except for smell, relay through a lemniscus to a specific thalamic nucleus. The thalamus then relays general somatosensory information (GSA) to the ____________ gyrus of the ____________ lobe.
2. The retina projects the special sense of vision (SSA) to the lateral geniculate body of the thalamus. In this sense, the optic tract is an analog of the lemnisci and qualifies as the *optic lemniscus.* Another SSA sense, hearing, projects through the *lateral lemniscus* that synapses in the medial geniculate body.

☑ contralaterally

3. Interruption of a decussated somatosensory (GSA) pathway through a lemniscus, its thalamic nucleus, or the pathway up to and including the post-central gyrus would cause a loss of sensation ❒ bilaterally/❒ ipsilaterally/❒ contralaterally.
4. Learn Table 2-13 and then do test frames C-5 to C-10.

trigeminal

5. The trigeminal sensory nuclei for facial sensation send axons to the thalamus via the ____________ lemniscus.

medial (or medial and spinal lemnisci)

6. Somatosensory impulses from the remainder of the body run to the thalamus via the ____________ lemniscus.

lateral

7. The auditory pathway runs to the thalamus via the ____________ lemniscus.

☑ secondary
crossed

8. In general, lemnisci contain axons from ❒ primary/❒ secondary/❒ tertiary perikarya that have ____________ the midline.

lateral geniculate; medial geniculate

9. The thalamic sensory relay nucleus for *vision* is the ____________ body and that for *hearing* the ____________ body.

dorsal root ganglion; thalamic

10. The perikarya of the primary neurons of a somatosensory pathway occupy ____________, whereas the tertiary neurons occupy a ____________ nucleus.

D. Union of the lemnisci in the brainstem

1. The lemnisci unite in the brainstem to travel as one to the thalamus.
   a. The medial lemniscus proper originates in the dorsal column nuclei (nuclei gracilis and cuneatus) of the medullocervical junction (Fig. 2-28).
   b. As the *medial* lemniscus travels rostrally into the pons, the *spinal* and *trigeminal lemnisci* merge with it. The name *medial lemniscus* still applies even though its composition differs along the brainstem. In the rostral pons, the *lateral lemniscus* merges along the dorsolateral edge of the medial lemniscus.
2. The domain of the lemnisci on transverse section of the brainstem.
   a. No long pathway runs along the *tectum*, but a cerebellar pathway cuts through it.
   b. Only corticofugal tracts run through the basis.
   c. Thus *all* lemnisci run through the tegmentum. Trace the medial lemniscus through the tegmentum in Figs. 2-15 to 2-18.

E. Sensation as the basis of movement

1. In reaching out to pick up an object, you have to locate it and guide the action of your muscles to it. The brain can guide movement by immediate or remembered information from the visual and somatosensory systems. By decussations, these systems bring the sensory information from one side to the *contralateral* cerebral hemisphere.
2. The hemisphere that receives the sensory information from the contralateral half of space also contains the motor cortex that directs the volitional movements of the contralateral extremities, via the pyramidal tract.

X. THE CONTRALATERALITY OF THE PATHWAY FOR VOLITIONAL MOVEMENTS: THE PYRAMIDAL TRACT

It would seem, therefore, that we may look upon the pyramidal system as an internuncial, a common pathway by which the sensory system initiates and continuously directs, in willed movements, the activities of the nervous motor mechanisms. This sensory afflux is a condition of willed movements, and unless we consider both in association we cannot hope to see the purpose of either.

—F. M. R. Walshe

A. Function of the pyramidal tract

1. The pyramidal tract mediates willed movements. It begins in the motor cortex, located in the precentral and, to a lesser extent, the postcentral gyri.
2. The pyramidal tract projects through the deep white matter of the cerebrum to synapse on internuncial or efferent neurons in the brainstem and spinal cord. It consists of two components, *corticobulbar* and *corticospinal* (Fig. 2-29).

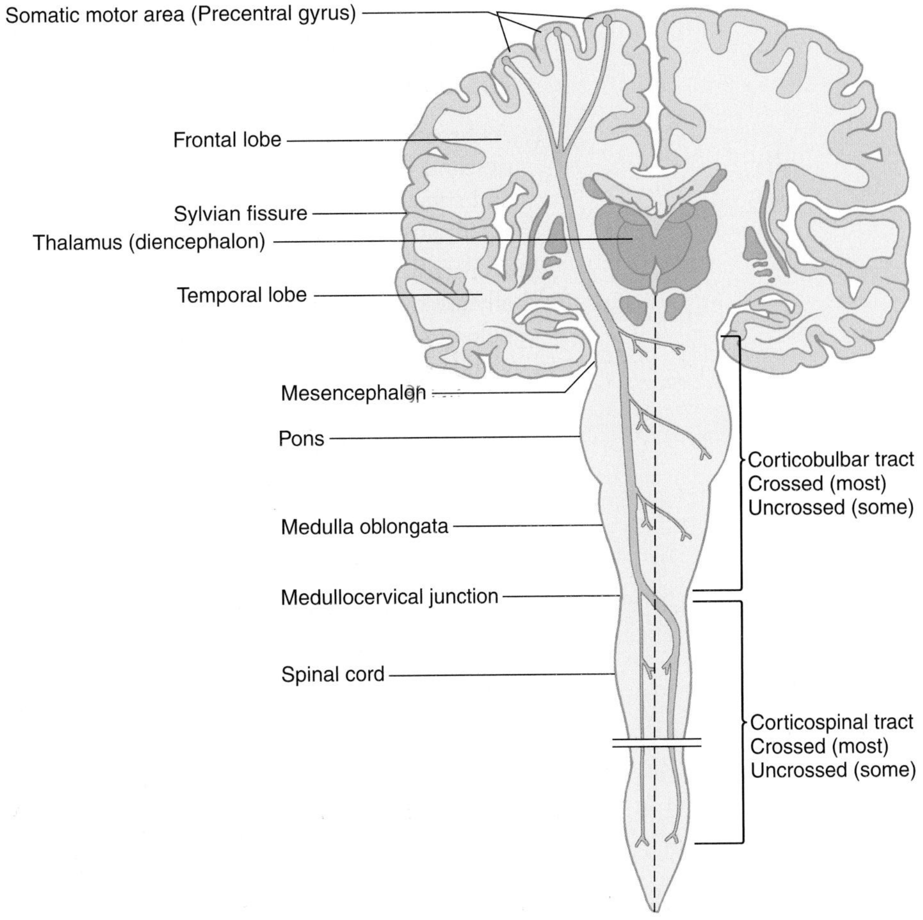

FIGURE 2-29. Coronal section of the neuraxis showing the corticobulbar and corticospinal components of the pyramidal tract pathway from the cerebral motor cortex to the brainstem and spinal cord.

a. The *corticobulbar* component decussates at various levels to synapse on brainstem neurons (Fig. 2-29). Figure 5-1 shows one of the most important corticobulbar tract decussations, in the pathway for volitional conjugate horizontal gaze. Preview it at this time by tracing through it, starting from the cortex.

b. The *corticospinal* component mostly decussates at the cervicomedullary junction, where the dorsal column sensory pathways also decussate (Fig. 2-29). A variable number of corticospinal axons descend ipsilaterally in the spinal cord.

B. Paresis and paralysis after pyramidal tract interruption

1. Interruption of the pyramidal tract in the cerebrum or brainstem paralyzes most volitional movement on the *contralateral* side of the body. Complete or nearly complete paralysis on one side is called *hemiparalysis* or, more commonly, *hemiplegia*. Incomplete paralysis on one side is called *hemiparesis.*
2. Interruption of a pyramidal tract *rostral* to its decussation causes hemiplegia ❒ ipsilateral/❒ contralateral to the lesion.
3. Interruption of a pyramidal tract just *caudal* to its decussation causes hemiplegia ❒ ipsilateral/❒ contralateral to the lesion.
4. Pyramidal tract interruption in the cerebrum affects both components of the pyramidal tract, the cortico_________________ and cortico___________.
5. Pyramidal tract interruption *caudal* to its decussation affects only the cortico _________________ tract.

Answers (margin): ☑ contralateral; ☑ ipsilateral; bulbar; spinal; spinal

C. The pyramidal tract and the concept of upper motor neurons and lower motor neurons

1. As broadly defined, upper motoneurons (UMNs) include all motor tracts that descend from the brain to the lower motor neurons (LMNs) in the brainstem and spinal cord, i.e., the pyramidal, rubrospinal, tectospinal, reticulospinal, and vestibulospinal tracts. No UMN axons leave the neuraxis.
2. As narrowly defined, UMNs indicate only the pyramidal tracts. Clinicians generally use this definition. All other motor pathways, basal motor and cerebellar, etc., belong to the *extrapyramidal system.*
3. LMNs are the motoneurons in the brainstem or ventral horns of the spinal cord that send their axons into the PNS. The somatomotor LMNs, branchial and somatic, activate skeletal muscles. The visceromotor (autonomic) LMNs activate smooth muscles and glands.

D. UMN (pyramidal tract) versus LMN paralysis

1. The hallmark of pyramidal tract interruption is paresis, or paralysis of volitional movements of the parts, not the individual muscles. Volitional movements, even if ostensibly simple, usually involve more than one muscle. If you flex your finger, pucker your lips, or lift your arm, more than one muscle springs into action. Movements, then, are compounded of the actions of several muscles.
2. The hallmark of LMN, or motor nerve, interruption is paralysis of only the individual muscle supplied. This type of paralysis is called *LMN paralysis* to differentiate it from UMN paralysis.
3. If the patient has paresis or paralysis of one muscle or a restricted set of muscles, with normal movements otherwise, the lesion involves the ❒ UMNs/ ❒ LMNs.
4. If the patient has paresis or paralysis of movements of one side of the body, sparing the other side, the lesion most likely affects the ❒ UMNs/❒ LMNs.

Answers (margin): ☑ LMNs; ☑ UMNs

☑ movements; ☑ muscles

a. Taking some poetic license, we may summarize this conclusion by saying that UMN lesions paralyze ❐ movements/❐ muscles, whereas LMN lesions paralyze ❐ movements/❐ muscles.

b. Despite this general rule, very tiny lesions of the motor cortex can, in rare instances, paralyze restricted movements of the fingers (Kim et al., 2002).

XI. LATERALITY OF CLINICAL SIGNS OF CEREBELLAR LESIONS

A. The cerebellum and the motor cortex

1. The sensory system, the cerebellum, basal motor nuclei, thalamic somatomotor nuclei, and motor cortex function by *modulating* each other.
   a. To *modulate* means to control the *force, velocity, distance, amplitude,* and *trajectory* of volitional movements and the required *sequence of activation* of the muscles.
   b. The pyramidal tract transmits the final modulation of the motor cortex to the muscles during volitional activation. The pathways of the various components of the motor system decussate in accordance with the law of cerebral contralaterality.
2. The clinical effect of dysmodulation differs depending on whether the lesion affects the cerebellum, sensory pathways, thalamus, or the basal motor nuclei.
   a. Lesions of the cerebellum or its pathways result in uncoordinated contractions of the muscles during volitional activation. Such uncoordinated movements are called *cerebellar ataxia* (Chapter 8). The Pt also displays a tremor during volitional movements but not at rest.
   b. The affected parts are very floppy and hypotonic. Drunkenness serves as a prime example of all of the cerebellar signs.
3. *Afferents* to the cerebellum come from:
   a. Olivary nuclei of the medulla.
   b. Sensory systems, in particular the proprioceptive system (spinocerebellar tracts and vestibular system).
   c. The cerebro-cerebello-cerebral circuit. Trace this pathway in Fig. 2-30.
4. *Efferents* that convey cerebellar modulation to the motor cortex run from the cerebellar dentate nucleus to the somatomotor nuclei of the thalamus that relay to the cerebral motor cortex. Trace the dentato-thalamo-cortical pathway in Fig. 2-30. Notice the decussation of this pathway in the caudal midbrain (Fig. 2-30).
5. Next trace the pyramidal tract down through its decussation (Fig. 2-30). Thus, the cerebellar circuit requires *three* decussations to finally reach and modulate the LMNs.
   a. The cortico-ponto-cerebellar pathway decussates in the ________________.
   b. The dentato-thalamic pathway decussates in the ______________________.
   c. The *corticobulbar* components of the pyramidal tract decussate at levels along the brainstem, whereas the *corticospinal* component decussates at the ______________________ junction level.

basis pontis

caudal midbrain

medullocervical

B. Laterality of cerebellar signs

1. The cerebellar pathway, with its two decussations (Fig. 2-30) and the third, pyramidal decussation, explains a clinical aphorism: Cerebral hemisphere lesions cause *contralateral* motor signs, but cerebellar hemisphere lesions cause *ipsilateral* motor signs.

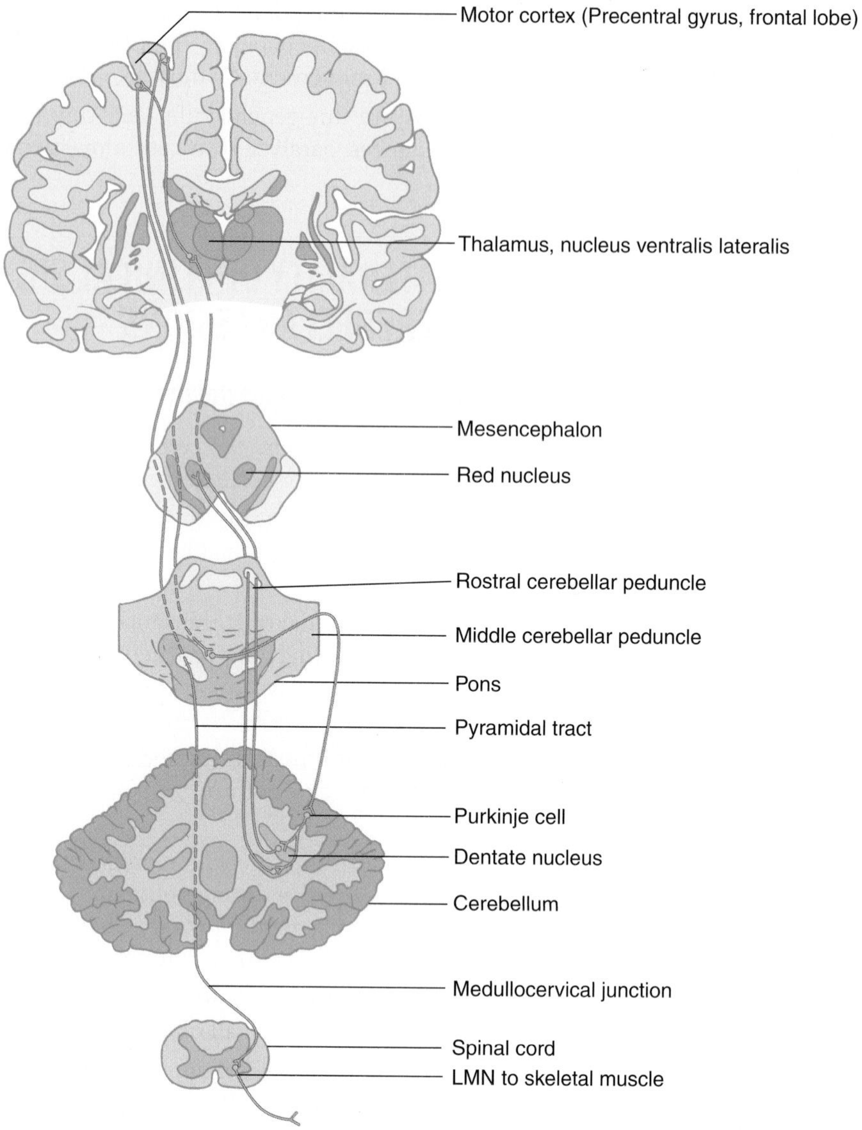

FIGURE 2-30. Diagram of the cerebro-cerebello-cerebral circuit. The circuit from one cerebral motor area to a cerebellar hemisphere and back crosses the midline twice. Thus, one cerebellar hemisphere coordinates the muscular contractions projected by the pyramidal tract of the opposite cerebral motor cortex. Because it decussates, the pyramidal tract then produces coordinated movements on the side of the body *ipsilateral* to the cerebellar hemisphere.

☑ **ipsilateral;** ☑ **contralateral.** Examine Fig. 2-30 if you don't understand the answer.

2. A lesion of the one cerebellar hemisphere would cause ❐ ipsilateral/❐ contralateral ataxia, whereas a lesion of the dentatothalamic tract rostral to its decussation in the midbrain would cause ❐ ipsilateral/❐ contralateral ataxia.

XII. LATERALTY OF CLINICAL SIGNS OF LESIONS OF THE BASAL MOTOR NUCLEI

A. Definitions

1. Refer to Fig. 2-31 and learn the subdivisions of the corpus striatum.
2. Originally the corpus striatum belonged to a group of nuclei called the *basal ganglia*, which also included the claustrum and amygdala. Now the amygdala is classified with the limbic system, and the function of the claustrum remains uncertain.

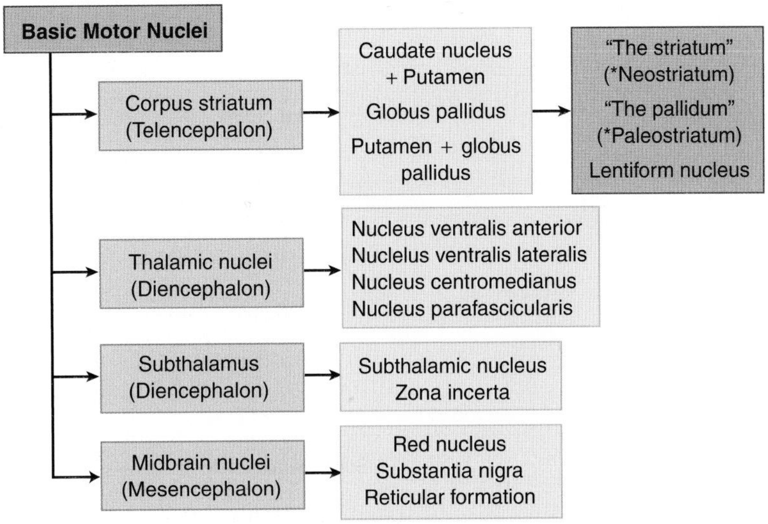

FIGURE 2-31. Dendrogram showing the components of the basal motor nuclei (extrapyramidal system) and their locations in the central nervous system. * Obsolete terms.

3. The basal motor nuclei, situated in proximity at the base of the brain, modulate somatomotor activity by means of numerous feedback circuits that ultimately relay through the thalamus to the motor cortex.
4. Taken together, the basal motor nuclei constitute the *extrapyramidal system* (Fig. 2-31).
5. **Clinical signs of lesions of the basal motor nuclei**
   a. Muscular rigidity.
   b. Bradykinesia (difficulty in initiating and slowness in executing voluntary movements).
   c. Hyperkinesias (involuntary movements) consisting of
      i. Tremor, frequently of a part at rest.
      ii. Patterned involuntary movements called *chorea*, *athetosis*, and *dystonia*. The type and distribution of the movements depend on the nuclei or pathways interrupted (Chapter 7).

B. Connections of the basal motor nuclei and laterality of clinical signs

1. The basal motor nuclei project to the motor cortex through the ipsilateral somatomotor nuclei of the thalamus (Fig. 2-32).
2. Thus, a *unilateral* lesion of the basal motor connections results in motor signs expressed *contralaterally* through dysmodulation of the motor cortex and the crossing of the pyramidal tract (Fig. 2-32).
3. The evidence that basal motor nuclei pathways operate by modulating the output of the cerebral motor cortex comes from the fact that involuntary movements, such as chorea, disappear contralaterally after destruction of the motor cortex or the pyramidal tract. Of course, contralateral voluntary movements also disappear. Similarly, ataxia cannot appear without the voluntary movement mediated by the pyramidal tract. **We come to the heretical conclusion that pyramidal tract interruption paralyzes voluntary and involuntary movements.** This statement applies to the effects of acquired lesions in previously normal brains. Infants born with no pyramidal tracts do make movements, which must come from extrapyramidal sources.
4. A key difference between basal motor nuclei signs and cerebellar signs is that ataxia appears only during voluntary movements, whereas involuntary movements

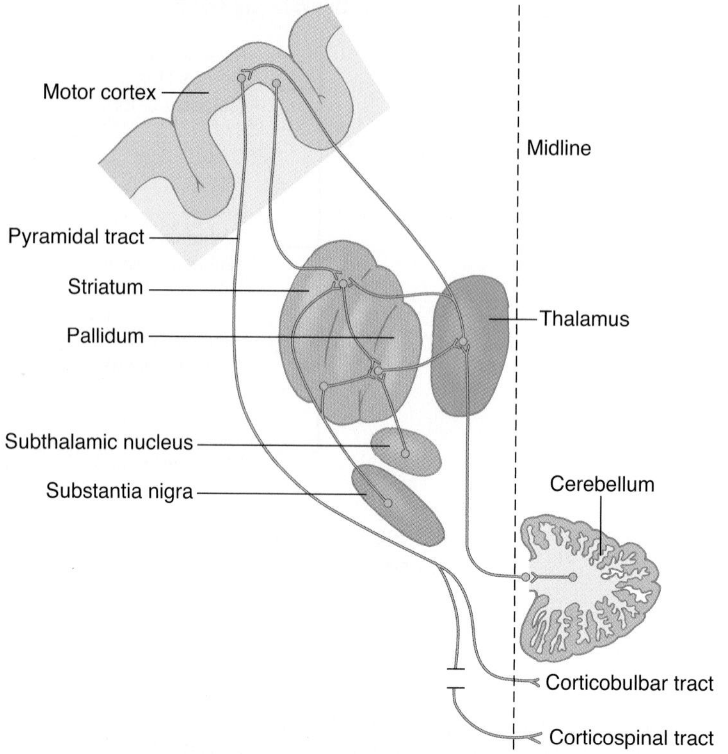

FIGURE 2-32. Diagram for conceptualizing the maze of basal motor circuits that feedback through the thalamus into the ipsilateral cerebral motor cortex. The decussation of the pyramidal tract then projects the influence of the basal motor nuclei modulation of the motor cortex to the contralateral side.

may be superimposed on muscles at rest or superimposed on voluntary actions. Almost all abnormal involuntary movements caused by lesions in the basal motor nuclei disappear during sleep.

5. Review the summary of the clinical syndromes of motor systems lesions in Table 2-14.

TABLE 2-14 · Brief Summary of Clinical Syndromes of Lesions at Various Levels of the Motor System

Level of motor system affected	Clinical signs
Lower motoneurons	Paralysis of individual muscles
Pyramidal tract (upper motoneurons)	Paralysis of movements in monoplegic, hemiplegic, paraplegic, or quadriplegic distributions
Basal motor nuclei	Rigidity Bradykinesia Postural instability Involuntary movements Tremor at rest Patterned hyperkinesias Dystonia, athetosis, and chorea Signs may be unilateral or bilateral
Cerebellum	Ataxia/hypotonia/tremor during movement Signs may be unilateral or bilateral

XIII. SUMMARY OF DECUSSATIONS AND CONTRALATERALITY

Learn Table 2-15.

TABLE 2-15 · Summary of the Clinically Important Sensorimotor Decussations of the Central Nervous System

Pathway	Site of decussation
Optic decussation	Optic chiasm (Fig. 2-26)
Somatic sensory decussations	
Pain and temperature	Near or at levels of entry of the dorsal root axon (Fig. 2-28)
Light touch	Two routes: near or at levels of entry and the cervi comedullary junction (Fig. 2-28)
Vibration and position sense (deep modalities)	Cervicomedullary junction (Fig. 2-28)
Descending reticulospinal tract for breathing	Cervicomedullary junction at the obex, dorsal to other decussations (Fig. 6-17)
Pyramidal tract	
Corticobulbar component	Various sites along the brainstem (Fig. 2-29)
Corticospinal component	Cervicomedullary junction (Fig. 2-29)
Horizontal eye movement pathway	
Corticobulbar component	Decussates broadly from the midbrain level to the rostral pons (Fig. 5-1)
Medial longitudinal fasciculus component	Decussates near the VI nerve level to make the medial rectus act equal to the lateral rectus, thus fulfilling Hering's law (Fig. 5-1)
Cerebro-ponto-cerebello-thalamo-cerebral pathway	Decussates at the pons on the way down from the motor cortex and the midbrain on the way back up to the thalamus and motor cortex (Fig. 2-30)

XIV. REVIEW OF THE LAW OF CONTRALATERAL HEMISPHERIC SENSORY AND MOTOR CONNECTIONS

1. **The contralaterality law applies to the decussations of all long sensory and motor pathways:** One cerebral hemisphere receives most of its somatosensory and visual sensory information from the contralateral side of the body or the contralateral half of space and in turn controls the motor activity of the contralateral side of the body (Louis, 1994).
2. Using a colored pencil, superimpose the pyramidal pathway of Fig. 2-29 onto Fig. 2-28. Then mentally trace a nerve impulse from a somatic sensory receptor to the cerebral cortex and back to the motoneurons via the pyramidal tract while noting the decussations.
3. Table 2-15 summarizes the clinical correlates of lesions at various sites in the motor system.

BIBLIOGRAPHY · Contralaterality

Kim JS, Chung JP, Sang Ha. Isolated weakness of index finger due to small cortical infarction. *Neurology* 2002;58:985–986.

Louis ED. Contralateral control: evolving concepts of the brain-body relationship. *Neurology* 1994;44:2398–2400.

Learning Objectives for Chapter 2

I. GROSS SUBDIVISIONS OF THE NEURAXIS

1. Make a lateral-view diagram showing the major subdivisions of the central nervous system (neuraxis; Fig. 2-1).
2. Define *brain, cerebrum,* and *brainstem* (Fig. 2-1).
3. Name, in rostrocaudal order, the three transverse subdivisions of the brainstem (Fig. 2-1).
4. Describe how to separate the brainstem from the cerebrum and spinal cord.
5. Name the four levels of the spinal cord in rostrocaudal sequence (Fig. 2-1).
6. On lateral and medial drawings of the cerebrum, label and describe the boundaries of the four traditional lobes of the cerebrum (Fig. 2-2).
7. On a medial drawing of a cerebral hemisphere, shade the olfactory lobe and the limbic lobe of Broca (Fig. 2-3).
8. Describe and draw the location of the somatosensory, auditory, visual, and motor cortices.
9. State, in principle, the functional significance of the association cortex.
10. State, in principle, the functional significance of the limbic lobe.

II. THE NEURON AND THE NEURON DOCTRINE

1. Draw and label a typical neuron (Fig. 2-4).
2. Define a synapse and explain how it functions.
3. Explain the six tenets of the neuron doctrine summarized by the statement that the neuron is the anatomic, functional, directional, genetic, pathologic, and regenerative unit of the nervous system.
4. Explain why so many genetic, toxic, and viral diseases cause degeneration of only one specific group of neurons but spare other neuronal groups.
5. Describe the difference in regeneration of central versus peripheral axons.

III. THE SPINAL CORD, SOMITES, AND SPINAL NERVES

1. Define a somite and describe the types of tissue derived from it.
2. Define the segmental and suprasegmental parts of the CNS.
3. State the law of Bell and Magendie with respect to the dorsal and ventral roots.
4. Draw a cross section of the spinal cord showing the composition of a spinal nerve. Label the functional types of axons (nerve components) in the dorsal and ventral roots of the typical spinal nerve (Fig. 2-7).
5. Describe the location of the perikarya of the three functional types of neurons, afferent (primary sensory), internuncial, and efferent (motor neurons), and the relation of their axons to the CNS and PNS.
6. Explain, in principle, the functional importance of internuncial neurons (Fig. 2-8).
7. Explain why dermatome C4 abuts on T2 (Figs. 2-9 and 2-10).
8. Recite the mnemonic for remembering the distribution of the dermatomes.
9. Explain why the diaphragm receives its innervation from cervical segments 3, 4, and 5 (the law of retained original innervation).
10. Explain why the distribution of the dermatomes and peripheral nerves differs in the extremities but conforms in the thoracic region (Figs. 2-9, 2-10, and 2-11).
11. Describe, in principle, the movements (e.g., flexion of the elbow) mediated by the major terminal peripheral nerves of the spinal plexuses: circumflex, musculocutaneous, radial, ulnar, median, femoral, obturator, sciatic, tibial, peroneal, pudendal, and pelvic splanchnic.

Learning Objectives for Chapter 2

12. Recite the LLOAF/2 mnemonic for the motor distribution of the median nerve.
13. Describe how to test the integrity of the motor functions of the radial, ulnar, and median nerves in a Pt whose entire forearm and hand are encased in a case, except for the thumb, which is free to move.
14. Draw a cross section of the spinal cord to show the location of the clinically important tracts (Fig. 2-12).
15. Contrast the difference in the location of the secondary neuron of the somatosensory pathways that run through the dorsal and ventral columns.

IV. ANATOMIC ORGANIZATION OF THE BRAINSTEM

1. Name, in rostrocaudal order, the three transverse subdivisions of the brainstem (Fig. 2-1).
2. Name, in dorsoventral order, the three longitudinal plates or subdivisions of the brainstem (Fig. 2-13).
3. Draw a generalized cross section of the brainstem and label the clinically important regions of gray and white matter (Fig. 2-14 and Table 2-3).
4. Name the large supplementary motor nuclei in the ventral part of the midbrain tegmentum, basis pontis, and the ventral part of the medullary tegmentum.
5. Describe the location of the major tracts of clinical significance seen on cross section of the medulla, pons, and midbrain.
6. Explain, in principle and by giving examples, why the brainstem has more elaborate pools of internuncial neurons (reticular formation) than the spinal cord.

V. ANATOMIC REVIEW OF THE 12 PAIRS OF CRANIAL NERVES

1. Define a CrN.
2. Give the number, name, and foramen of exit of the CrNs (Tables 2-4 and 2-5).
3. Describe, in the fewest possible words, the function of each CrN (Table 2-6).
4. Divide the CrNs into three functional sets and list the number of the CrNs belonging to each set (Table 2-7).
5. Describe the embryologic origin of the olfactory and optic bulbs.
6. Explain why demyelinating diseases of the CNS would attack the optic nerve but not the other two special sensory nerves, I and VIII.
7. Make a table of the nerve components of the somite set of CrNs (Table 2-8).
8. Describe, in principle, the fate of the rostral, intermediate, and caudal cranial somites.
9. Describe which part of the face derives from branchial arches.
10. Describe the fundamental morphologic similarities of branchial arches and somites.
11. Name, in ventrodorsal sequence, the CrNs that attach to the pontomedullary sulcus. Explain why knowledge of this one fact helps you to remember where all of the remaining CrNs attach.
12. Draw a ventral view of the brain to show where the CrNs attach (Fig. 2-20).
13. Draw a dorsal phantom view of the brainstem showing the locations of the motor and sensory CrN nuclei. Draw the motor nuclei on one side and the sensory nuclei on the other (Fig. 2-21).
14. Describe, in principle, the similarities in the peripheral distribution of CrNs VII, IX, and X (Table 2-12).
15. Describe how the peripheral distribution of the CrNs relates in more or less rostrocaudal sequence to the rostrocaudal sequence of the nuclei of VII, IX, and X in the brainstem (Table 2-12).

Learning Objectives for Chapter 2

16. Make a table of the nerve components of the 12 CrNs (Table 2-7).
17. Recite the mnemonic for remembering the functions of CrN VII.

VI. THE RETICULAR FORMATION

1. Give an anatomic definition of the RF.
2. State, in principle, the major functional differences between the rostral (pontomesencephalic) and caudal (pontomedullary) parts of the RF.

VII. THE DIENCEPHALON

1. State, in dorsoventral order, the four nuclear zones that comprise the diencephalon (Fig. 2-22).
2. Describe, in principle, the projections of the thalamus (thalamus dorsalis) to the cerebral cortex.
3. Describe, in principle, the five functional nuclear subdivisions of the thalamus.
4. State the system to which the subthalamus belongs.
5. State, in principle, the role of the hypothalamus.

VIII. CONNECTIONS AND WHITE MATTER OF THE CEREBRUM

1. Name the three types of pathways taken by axons of cortical neurons.
2. Distinguish between commissures and decussations.

IX. THE CONTRALATERALITY OF THE SENSORY PATHWAYS

1. Draw the visual pathway from the retina to the cerebral cortex in the human brain (Fig. 2-26).
2. Draw the pathway for pain and temperature sensation from the periphery to the cerebral cortex (Fig. 2-28).
3. Give a plausible explanation for the inverted representation of the body topography in the sensorimotor cortex.
4. Draw the pathways for superficial and deep sensation from the periphery to the cerebral cortex (Fig. 2-28).
5. Describe the two pathways for touch from the periphery to the cerebral cortex (Fig. 2-28).
6. Explain the significance of knowing the location of the second-order neuron in a somatosensory pathway.
7. Recite the lemnisci and their origins and terminations, naming the nucleus and its cortical projection area (Table 2-13).
8. Describe the differences in the composition of the medial lemniscus at its origin at the medullocervical junction and in its course through the rostral part of the brainstem.
9. Locate the lemniscal crescent on cross sections of the brainstem (Figs. 2-14 to 2-18).
10. Discuss the importance of sensation for movement.

X. THE CONTRALATERALITY OF THE PATHWAY FOR VOLITIONAL MOVEMENTS: THE PYRAMIDAL TRACT

1. State the two components of the pyramidal tract and draw the pyramidal pathway from its origin to its termination (Fig. 2-29).
2. Explain the difference in the laterality of paralysis from interruption of the pyramidal tract in the brain as contrasted to the spinal cord.
3. Define UMNs and LMNs.
4. Contrast the effect of UMN and LMN lesions on movements and muscles.

Learning Objectives for Chapter 2

XI. LATERALITY OF CLINICAL SIGNS OF CEREBELLAR LESIONS

1. Discuss the meaning of modulation of movements by the cerebellum, basal motor nuclei, thalamus, and somatosensory systems.
2. Describe, in principle, the afferent and efferent connections of the cerebellum.
3. Diagram the circuit that explains the laterality of signs due to a lesion of the right cerebellar hemisphere (Fig. 2-30).

XII. LATERALITY OF CLINICAL SIGNS OF LESIONS OF THE BASAL MOTOR NUCLEI

1. Recite the subdivisions of the corpus striatum (Fig. 2-31).
2. List the additional basal motor nuclei of the extrapyramidal system (Fig. 2-31).
3. Recite the motor deficits caused by lesions of the basal motor nuclei (Table 2-15).
4. Diagram, in principle, the circuit that explains the laterality of choreiform movements of the left extremities secondary to a lesion of the right caudate-putamen (Fig. 2-32).
5. Explain the effect of an interruption of the pyramidal tract on voluntary and involuntary movements.
6. Recite, in principle, the major clinical signs that are caused by lesions of the LMNs, UMNs (pyramidal), cerebellum, and basal motor nuclei (extrapyramidal system; Table 2-15).

XIII. SUMMARY OF DECUSSATIONS AND CONTRALATERALITY

1. Cover the right column of Table 2-15 and work down the left column, reciting the sites of the decussations.

3 Examination of Vision

Seasons return; but not to me returns Day, or the sweet approach of even or morn, Or sight of vernal bloom or Summer's rose, Or flocks, or herds, or human face divine.

—John Milton (On His Own Blindness, at Age 43)

I. ANATOMY OF THE EYEBALL

Learn to draw Fig. 3-1 sight unseen.

II. DUAL ORGANIZATION IN THE OPTIC SYSTEM

A. Two cranial nerves, II and V, convey afferents from the eye to the brain

1. The *optic nerve, cranial nerve* (CrN) *II,* conveys the afferent axons for two functions, the special sense of vision and pupilloconstriction.
2. The *trigeminal nerve,* CrN *V,* conveys the afferents for general sensation:
   a. Ocular pain
   b. Tearing reflex
   c. Corneal reflex
   d. Proprioception from the extraocular muscles

B. Two motor systems, *peripheral* and *central,* innervate the intra- and extraocular muscles

1. *Peripheral* ocular motor nerves consist of CrNs III, IV, and VI and the carotid sympathetic nerve.
2. *Central* ocular motor systems control the peripheral movements. The central systems find, fixate, focus/align on, and follow visual targets. CrNs III, IV, and VI innervate the extraocular muscles for these actions.

C. Two images, a real *retinal image* and a *mental* or *visual image,* made by the mind

1. **Start with an arrow as the visual target** (Fig. 3-2).
   a. Each retina receives an inverted *real* or *actual image,* due to the physical optics of the eye.
   b. Neurophysiologic processing then converts this real retinal image into an abstraction called a *visual image.*
2. **Projection of the visual image by the mind**
   a. As Fig. 3-2 shows, the light rays that form the *nasal* half of the retinal image come from the ❐ temporal/❐ nasal half of the object viewed.

☑ temporal

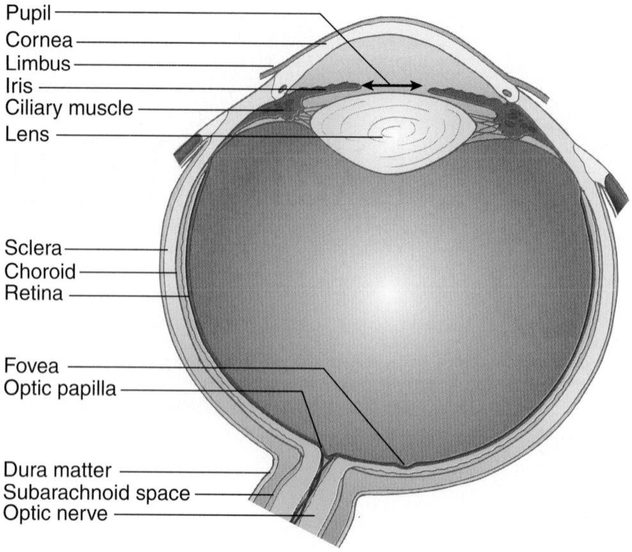

FIGURE 3-1. Horizontal section of the right eye, seen from above.

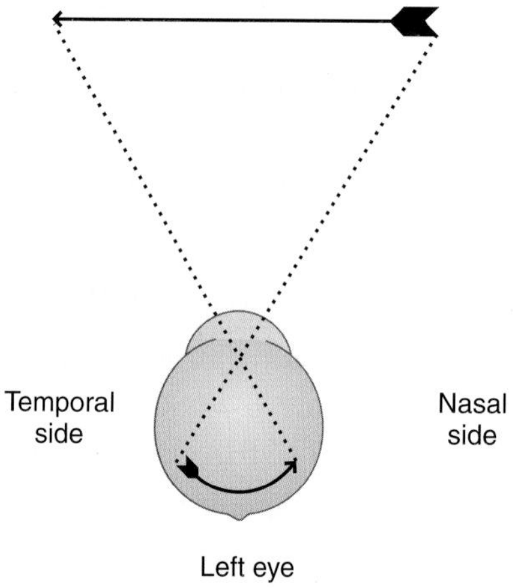

FIGURE 3-2. Retinal image formed during monocular fixation with the left eye.

☑ nasal

b. By a process of learning, we associate the point of retinal stimulation with the reverse half of space. Hence, if light rays fall on the *temporal* half of the retina, the mind perceives the object as located in the ❒ temporal/❒ nasal half of space.

lower

c. If the image of an object falls on the *nasal* side of the retina, we would reach for the object in the *temporal* half of space. Similarly, if the image falls on the *upper* half of the retina, we would reach for the object in the ____________ half of space.

opposite or reverse

d. Thus the **law of projection of the visual image** states that the mind projects the visual image derived from one half of the retina to the ____________ half of space.

e. This particular law exemplifies a general law of sensation: **The mind projects afferent impulses to their usual site of origin in all sensory systems.** If an electrode stimulated your right auditory nerve, you would experience a sound as if it came from the right side of space. If you bump your ulnar nerve at the elbow, you would feel a shock down your forearm into your little finger, even when no afferent impulses arose from the finger itself. In each case, we say that, when afferent impulses reach the brain, the mind projects or refers them to their usual site of origin.

D. Two areas of the retina: *central* and *peripheral* areas

1. The retina consists of a *central circular macula* and a *peripheral zone* that concentrically surrounds the macula (Fig. 3-3).

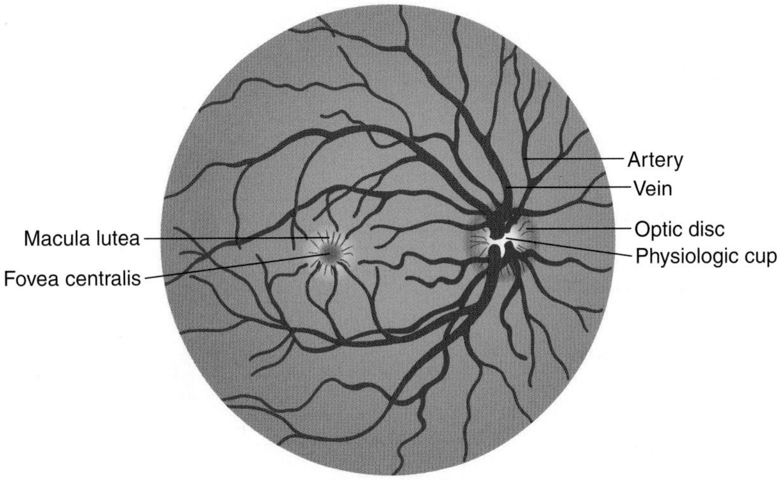

FIGURE 3-3. Drawing of the fundus of the right eye.

2. **The retina has two types of receptors:**
   a. *Cones* in the macula
   b. *Rods* in the periphery
3. **The retina provides two fields of vision, central and peripheral. Each field has two functions:**
   a. The *cone* receptors of the macula mediate the two functions of the central field of vision:
      i. Visual acuity
      ii. Color vision

Mnemonic of the C's for the function of the Cones: The Cones, located Centrally in the maCula, mediate visual aCuity, and Color vision.

   b. In the *periphery* of the retina, concentrically surrounding the macula, *rod* receptors mediate the two functions of the peripheral field of vision:
      i. Night vision
      ii. Motion detection
4. **Neuronal layers of the retina**
   a. Light initiates afferent impulses for vision and pupilloconstriction by exciting the rod and cone receptors of the retina.
   b. The *unipolar* rod and cone neurons synapse on the *bipolar* neurons of the adjacent layer of the retina.
   c. The *bipolar* neurons synapse on *multipolar* neurons of the ganglion cell layer. The axons from the multipolar neurons converge on the *optic disc* in a special pattern, pierce the *lamina cribrosa* of the sclera, and form the *optic nerve* that emerges from the back of the eyeball and joins the *optic chiasm*.

E. Dual pathways in the optic nerve

The optic nerve runs from the retina posteriorly through the optic chiasm where it divides into two *optic tracts*. Each optic tract contains two sets of axons.

1. One set of axons comes from the *ipsilateral, temporal half* of the retina (Fig. 3-4).

A. Complete blindness, L eye

B. Complete bitemporal hemianopia

C. Complete nasal hemianopia, L eye

D. Complete R homonymous hemianopia

E. Complete R superior homonymous quadrantanopia

F. Complete R inferior homonymous quadrantanopia

G. Complete R homonymous hemianopia

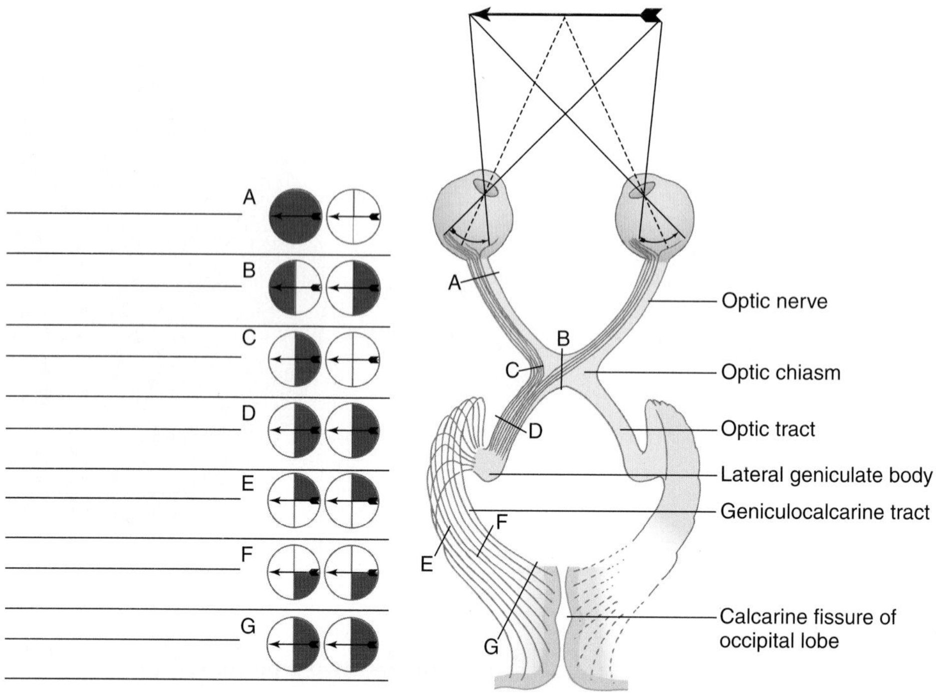

FIGURE 3-4. The visual pathway from the retinal images to the calcarine cortex of the occipital lobe, as seen from above. The letters on the left indicate lesion sites and the visual field defects they would cause.

2. A second set of axons comes from the *contralateral, nasal half* of the retina. These two groups of axons unite the right and left visual half fields from each eye.

F. Dual pathways branch from the optic tract

The optic tract conveys *visual* and *nonvisual* axons posteriorly from the chiasm.

1. The *nonvisual axons* of the optic tract go to the *pretectum* of the midbrain and to the *hypothalamus*.
   a. The *retinopretectal tract* synapses in the *pretectum* and midbrain for pupilloconstriction to light (Fig. 4-30).
   b. The *retinohypothalamic tract* synapses on the paraventricular nucleus and mediates the diurnal cycle of sleep and wakefulness.
2. The *visual axons* in the optic tract, the *retinogeniculate* tract, synapse on the lateral geniculate body of the thalamus (Fig. 3-4).
   a. The *geniculocalcarine tract* then synapses on the primary visual (calcarine) cortex (Figs. 3-4 to 3-6).
   b. The association cortex surrounding the calcarine cortex then interprets the significance and meaning of the visual image.

G. Dual banks of the calcarine cortex

1. The primary visual cortex forms dual, *upper* and *lower,* banks along the calcarine fissure on the medial surface of the occipital lobe (area 17 of Brodmann; Figs. 2-2, 3-4, and 3-5A).
2. The macula is represented toward the occipital pole of area 17. The remaining retina is topographically represented forward (Fig. 3-5B).

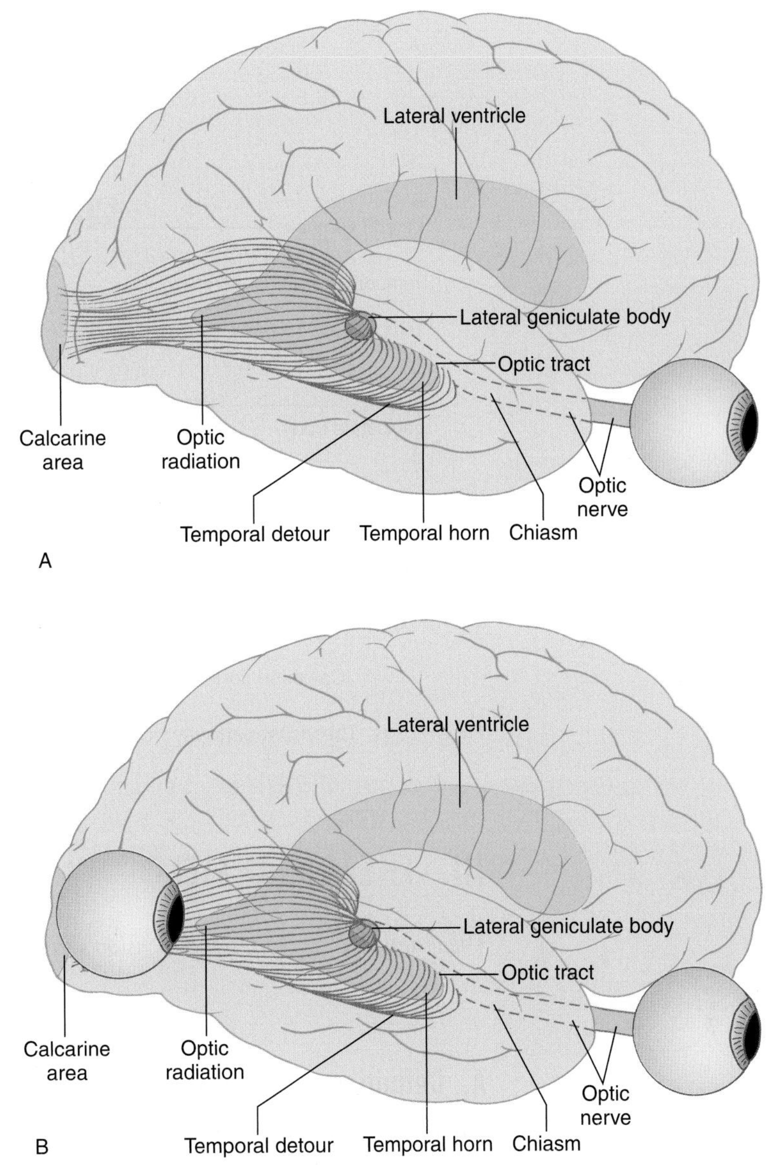

FIGURE 3-5. (A) The visual pathway from the retina to the calcarine area, as seen from the right side. (Reproduced with permission from Cushing H. The field defects produced by temporal lobe lesions. *Trans Am Neurol Assoc* 1921;47:374–423.) (B) The visual pathway from retina to the calcarine area, as seen from the side with a hemisectioned eyeball moved back to cap the occipital pole of the cerebrum.

Mnemonic for the representation of the macula and upper and lower halves of the retina on the calcarine cortex: Make a sagittal hemisection of an eyeball and place the hemisection on the occipital pole, as in Fig. 3-5B. The actual macula of the eyeball then rests on the occipital pole, which receives the projection from the macula. The rest of the visual cortex represents the successively more forward sectors of the retina. The upper half of the retina rests on the upper bank of the calcarine cortex, and the lower half rests on the lower bank of the calcarine fissure.

H. Review of the visual pathway

Think through the afferent pathway for vision until you know it. First of all, notice in Fig. 3-4 that, when both eyes focus on the arrow, the real images fall on corresponding parts of the retina. Then proceed through the retinal rods and cones; bipolar layer; multipolar layer, optic nerve, optic chiasm; optic tract; geniculate body synapse; and geniculocalcarine tract to the primary visual cortex around the calcarine fissure.

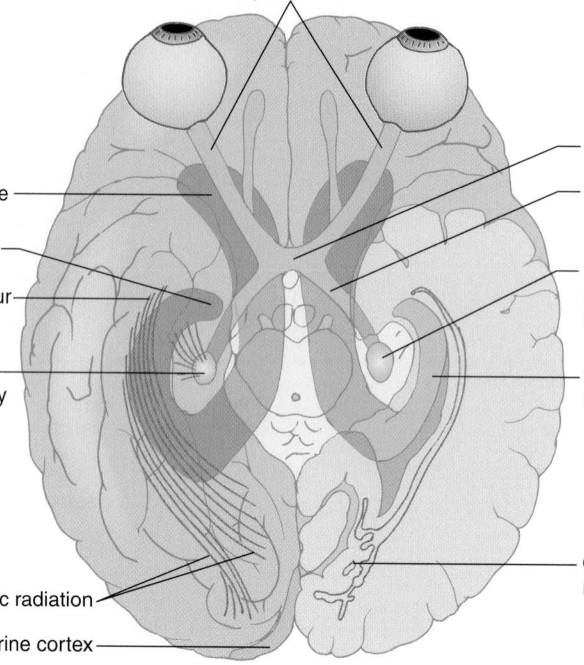

FIGURE 3-6. The visual pathway from the retina to the calcarine area, as seen from below.

III. THE VISUAL FIELD

The visual field is… "an island of vision surrounded by a sea of blindness."

—**Harry Traquair**

A. Definition of the visual field

Cover one eye and stare fixedly straight ahead. The entire area of vision is the *visual field* of that eye.

B. Duality of the visual field

1. The entire visual field consists of a *central* field and a *peripheral* field, based on the duality of the cone and rod receptors of the retina.
2. If a patient (Pt) reported decreasing visual acuity and had no opacities such as a cataract, the lesion would most likely affect the ❒ cones/❒ rods in the retina or their pathway to the cerebrum.

☑ **cones**

3. If a Pt reported decreasing ability to see in dim light but acuity was preserved, the lesion would most likely affect the ❒ central/❒ peripheral part of the retina that contains the ❒ rods/❒ cones.

☑ **peripheral;** ☑ **rods**

C. Self-demonstration of the central field of vision

1. **Do this experiment to demonstrate the surprisingly limited field of central vision:** The central field extends only about 30 degrees, whereas the total field of peripheral vision when you look straight ahead is nearly 180 degrees wide.
   a. Position yourself 1 m from a long row of books or get closer to a short row, so that the books extend beyond the limit of your peripheral vision.
   b. Stare fixedly at the title of a book in the middle of the row. Without moving your eyes at all, can you read more than one book title on either side? ❒ Yes/❒ No.

☑ **No.** If you could read more than one, you shifted fixation. Repeat the experiment.

2. **Do this experiment to demonstrate color vision in the central field:**
   a. Fixate on the same book in the middle of the row. Be sure to position yourself so that the row of books extends to the peripheral limit of your field.
      i. While staring at the book directly in front of you, try to determine the color of the most distant book that you can see in the periphery. Do not shift your vision.
      ii. After trying to determine the color, shift your gaze to look straight at the book. How does the color of the book differ when seen by your central field of vision as contrasted to its color when seen in the peripheral field? __________

Peripherally, the book is drab, nearly colorless. With central vision it immediately becomes bright and vivid.

3. **Now do this experiment concerning color vision:**
   a. Hold out, at the periphery of your temporal field, a colored pen, preferably red, or any other small, colored item.
   b. Stare fixedly straight ahead and move the colored item until it is in line with your central vision. How does the color differ as the item moves from peripheral to central vision? __________

The more central the item, the brighter the color.

4. **Self-demonstration of the perimeter of the peripheral fields.**
   a. Close or cover one eye and fixate straight ahead with the other. Extend the arm that is *ipsilateral* to the fixating eye straight out to the side and point your index finger up. Now, keeping the elbow extended, rotate the arm forward from the shoulder. The point at which you first see the finger defines the temporal perimeter of your visual field.
   b. Repeat the experiment, fixating with the same eye and closing the other. This time extend the arm that is *contralateral* to the fixating eye and rotate the arm forward until your finger just becomes visible. Did you have to move it farther forward than the ipsilateral arm? __________.

Do the experiment.

   c. Ostensibly the nose would seem to limit the nasal part of the visual field. Phylogenetically this may be true, but the extent of the retina itself limits the extent of the nasal field.
   d. To locate the vertical perimeter of the visual field, fixate straight ahead with one eye and bring your index finger down from above and then up from below. What structure limits the height of the visual field? __________.

The eyebrow or the eyelid, if it is ptotic. If the Pt has ptosis, lift up the lid while testing the visual fields.

5. **The importance of testing central and peripheral vision:** Diseases, such as retinitis pigmentosa and glaucoma, and some drugs, such as vigabatrin, affect the rods first and cause constriction of the peripheral fields. Other disorders, such as the macular degeneration of aging, impair the cones and cause loss of central vision, and yet other diseases affect both rods and cones and cause loss of central and peripheral vision. Hence, the examiner (Ex) must test for these two types of visual loss.

D. Nomenclature for the visual fields and visual field defects

1. Learn the nomenclature of the visual fields in Fig. 3-7.

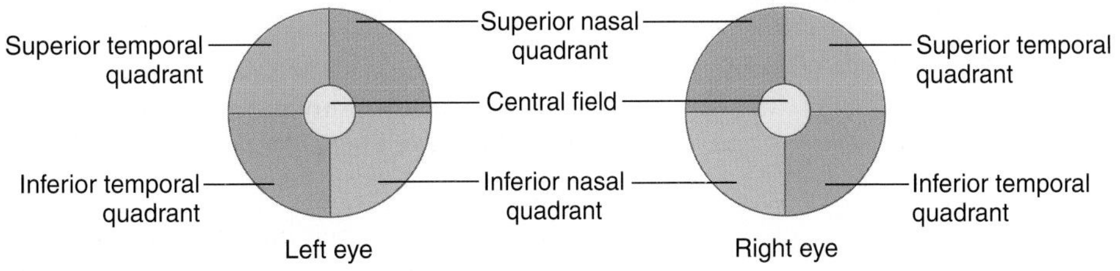

FIGURE 3-7. Nomenclature of the normal visual fields.

2. Visual field defects tend to fall into patterns of one-quarter or one-half of the visual fields (Figs. 3-4 and 3-8). Blindness in one-quarter of a field is called *quadrantanopia* (literally: *quadrans* = one-quarter; *an* = without; *opia* vision). Because of complete blindness in the superior temporal quadrant, as shown in Fig. 3-8A, the full name is *complete left superior temporal* ________________.

quadrantanopia

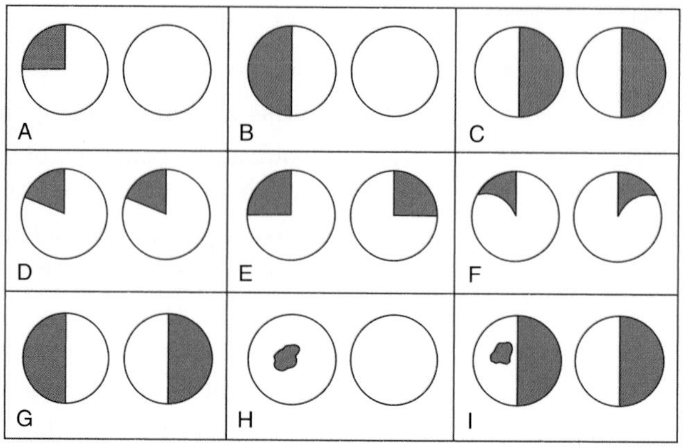

FIGURE 3-8. Patterns of visual field defects (A–I). The darkened area is the area of blindness. The patient's left eye is to the reader's left. Imagine that you are looking through the patient's eyes.

3. Blindness in one-half of a field, or a hemidefect, as in Fig. 3-8B, would be called *hemianopia*. The complete name for the field defect is *complete temporal hemianopia* of the left eye.

4. With involvement of corresponding quadrants or halves of the fields, e.g., the right halves, the defect is termed *homonymous,* and described as *right* or *left*. Give the complete name for the field defect shown in Fig. 3-8C.________________.

Complete right homonymous hemianopia

5. The terms *homonymous* or *corresponding* as applied to visual field defects mean that the defect corresponds to the way the visual pathways represent the retinal and visual images of the right and left visual fields during binocular vision. Refer to Fig. 3-4. When the Pt with a complete right homonymous hemianopia looks straight ahead, he would be blind in the ❒ right/❒ left half of space and see in the ❒ right/❒ left half.

☑ right; ☑ left

6. Name the defect shown in Fig. 3-8D.

________________________________.

Incomplete left superior homonymous quadrantanopia

7. Non-corresponding field defects are sometimes called *heteronymous* to contrast them with homonymous (Fig. 3-8E). It is simpler to describe them directly. Thus, the defect shown in Fig. 3-8E would be called complete superior bitemporal ________________.

quadrantanopia

8. The defect shown in Fig. 3-8F is called

________________________________.

incomplete superior bitemporal quadrantanopia

9. The defect shown in Fig. 3-8G is called________________

________________.

complete bitemporal hemianopia

10. Why would the field defects shown in Figs. 3-8E to 3-8G not be homonymous?________________.

The defect is not in corresponding parts of the fields according to the way the visual pathways represent the right and left halves of space (Fig. 3-4).

11. An irregular field defect not approximating a quadrantic defect is called a *scotoma*. A scotoma may be *central, centrocecal, paracentral,* or *peripheral*. The defect shown in Fig. 3-8H would be called a ________________ scotoma of the left eye.

central

12. A central scotoma that blends with the blind spot is called a *centrocecal scotoma* (*caecum* = blind). A *paracentral* defect would be near the point of central vision but detached from it.

E. Review of the anatomic basis of visual field defects

Return to Fig. 3-4 and use these instructions to learn it thoroughly.

1. Review and learn the names down the right side of Fig. 3-4.
2. Notice that light rays from the right half of space fall on the nasal side of the right retina and on the temporal side of the left retina.
3. At the chiasm, axons from the nasal half of the right retina decussate to travel through the optic tract with the axons from the temporal half of the left retina.
4. The retinal axons synapse on neurons of the lateral geniculate body, a thalamic nucleus that relays sensory impulses to the cerebral cortex. The tract of axons formed by geniculate body neurons is called the *optic radiation* or *geniculocalcarine tract*.
5. Using a colored pencil, draw in Fig. 3-4 the retinal pathway from the nasal half of the left retina and temporal half of the right. Include the geniculate body synapse. Make sure you draw a mirror image of the corresponding axons already in the drawing.
6. The bars drawn across the optic pathways at A to G of Fig. 3-4 simulate lesions at various sites. At the left, label the field defects resulting from the lesions.
7. Note that lesions of the inferior fibers, E, of the geniculocalcarine tract in Fig. 3-4 cause contralateral superior homonymous quadrantanopia (Ebeling and Reulen, 1988; Hughes et al., 1999; Lepore, 2001). Study Fig. 2-27 in relation to Fig. 3-5B to understand this finding.
8. Practice drawing the entire optic pathway from the retina to the occipital cortex.
9. Figures 3-5A and 3-6 show the actual course of the optic pathways through the cerebrum. Note that visual field testing assays the integrity of large parts of the temporal and occipital lobes and the inferior margin of the parietal lobe.
10. To test whether you have mastered the anatomy of the visual fields and the hemisected eyeball mnemonic, move the eyeball well forward over the temporal lobe and reason out the field defect that interruption of the anterior part of loop of the geniculocalcarine tract would cause. Remember that the upper half of the visual field falls on the lower half of the retina.________________ ____.

Contralateral homonymous superior quadrantanopia

IV. CLINICAL TESTING OF CENTRAL VISION

A. Tests of visual acuity

1. For crude screening of visual acuity, have the Pt read newsprint held at an arm's length. Test each eye separately. The Pt keeps eye glasses on. Although glasses improve acuity by correcting for a refractive error, they do not improve acuity impaired by opacities of the refracting media of the eye or retinal or optic nerve lesions.
   a. If the history or screening test suggests a visual complaint, use a Snellen or Jaeger chart or a Rosenbaum Pocket Vision Screener for a numerical evaluation of acuity and consider referring the Pt to an ophthalmologist for visual field testing, as explained below.
   b. For a small child or mentally impaired Pt, use a large **E** printed on a card and have the Pt point in the direction that the cross bars point after you direct **E** *up* and *down* and *right* and *left*.
2. Test the acuity of partially blind Pts by having them count the number of fingers held up at various distances. If the Pt cannot see to count fingers, find out whether the Pt can see hand movements. If this fails, see if light perception remains. That is to say, push the analysis to the limit. If the Pt cannot see even a bright light, the vision in the involved eye is *NLP* (no light perception).
3. The standard neurologic examination does not include color testing. If necessary, use Ishihara or similar color vision cards.

B. Screening central vision with an Amsler grid

1. With each eye separately, the Pt fixates on a dot in the center of a grid work held about 30 cm away (Fig. 3-9).

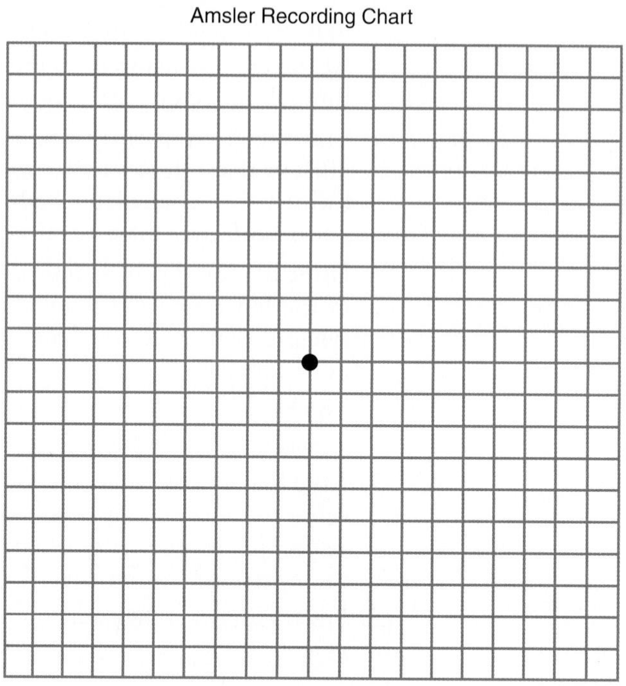

FIGURE 3-9. Amsler grid for screening for scotomas in the central visual fields.

2. The Ex asks whether the Pt can see each of the four corners and whether any of the squares in the grid are missing or distorted.

C. Tangent screen testing of central vision

1. The Amsler grid serves as a quick screening test, but the tangent screen maps out field defects precisely.
2. The Pt sits 1 or 2 m away from a black screen 1 or 2 m^2 while fixating on its center (with the other eye covered).
3. The Ex moves a 1- to 5-mm white body through the field of vision. After mapping the physiologic blind spot, the Ex systematically searches the central field for pathologic blind spots, called *scotomas*. The chart becomes part of the medical record (Fig. 3-10).

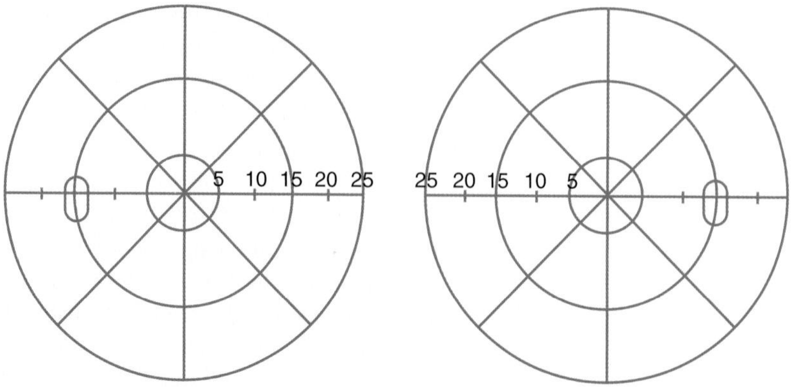

FIGURE 3-10. Chart for recording the central portion of the visual fields, as determined by tangent screen examination.

4. When no tangent screen is present, at the bedside or clinic, the Ex may select a fixation point on the wall and use a laser pointer as a substitute for the white spot.

D. Mapping the physiologic blind spot

1. Do this experiment with Fig. 3-11.

FIGURE 3-11. Demonstration of the blind spot. L = left; R = right.

a. Hold the page about 30 cm away.
b. Cover your left eye.
c. Fixate on the left cross. Make sure you keep fixating on the left cross all of the time, but you should also attend to the right cross.
d. As you maintain fixation on the left cross and continue to attend to the right cross, move your face slowly toward the page.
e. At a point with your eye a few inches from the page, the right cross disappears. As you continue to move closer, it reappears. If this does not happen, you broke your fixation on the left cross—try again.
f. Again cover your left eye, fixate on the left cross, and position your head so that the right cross disappears. Put your pencil point in the blind spot and move it very slowly toward the left cross. Make a mark on the paper when the point just becomes visible. By working around the blind spot, you can map out its perimeter. Be careful: If your fixation wavers, your blind spot will have irregular borders. The blind spot or other scotomas are mapped more accurately on a distant tangent screen than with the short target distance of this experiment.

2. Get a partner. Draw a small **X** on a piece of paper to fixate on and fasten the paper to a wall, making your own tangent screen. Seat the partner 100 cm away and map out the blind spot, moving the test object from the far right through the blind spot, toward the fixation point. Then work from the center of the blind spot to its periphery to outline it.
3. We do not ordinarily recognize our own blind spots. We attend to the fixation point of the visual axes and ignore it.
4. The absence of receptor neurons at the optic papilla or optic nerve head causes the blind spot. Normally the diameter of the blind spot depends on the diameter of the optic disc (Fig. 3-12).
5. **Effect of papilledema on the size of the blind spot:** Swelling of the optic papilla increases the size of the blind spot because the swelling impairs the function of the retina that surrounds the papilla (see Section VII, Ophthalmoscopy).

E. Location of lesions that cause scotomas or quadrantic/hemianopic field defects

1. Retinal lesions such as hemorrhages or exudates block penetration of light rays to the receptor neurons or destroy them. The scotoma produced depends on the size and location of the lesion.
2. Although in theory retinal or optic nerve lesions might cause quadrantic or hemianopic field defects; in practice, this virtually never occurs. Retinal or optic nerve

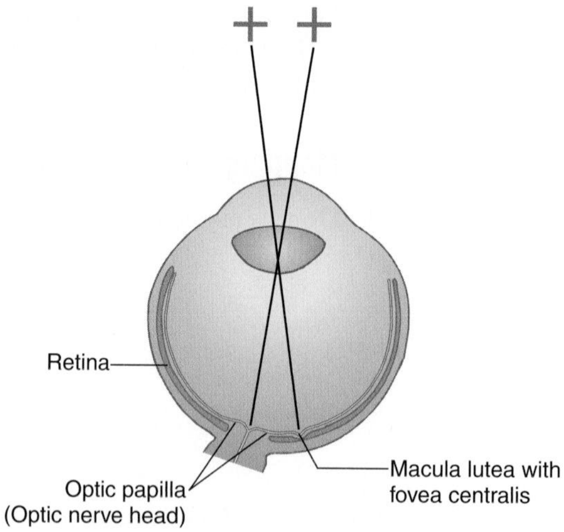

FIGURE 3-12. Horizontal section of the right eye to explain the blind spot.

lesions generally cause *central scotomas, centrocecal* (a central scotoma connected to the blind spot), or *paracentral scotomas.* The Pt with these scotomas loses acuity and color vision.

3. Lesions of the chiasm, optic tract, geniculocalcarine tract, or occipital lobe usually are the cause of hemianopic or quadrantanopic field defects (Fig. 3-4).
4. From the chiasm on back to and including the calcarine cortex, the more posterior the lesion in the optic pathway, the more congruent the field defect in the two eyes.
5. A Pt who suddenly lost visual acuity without blindness would most likely have a macular lesion, if the lesion affects the retina. If the scotoma is large, the Ex can detect it by carefully moving a pencil tip or small white object, the size of a small pearl, very slowly through the central field. Ophthalmoscopic examination, of course, will disclose many retinal lesions. With an acute lesion in the optic nerve, the retina may look normal for some weeks before optic atrophy becomes visible. Demonstration of a scotoma by tangent screen examination would establish an organic cause for the loss of acuity.
6. Figure 3-8I shows the visual fields of a 53-year-old hypertensive Pt who complained of headaches, sudden loss of vision on the right side, and blurring of vision in the left eye. Write out the name of the defects.________________________
____
____________________.

Complete right homonymous hemianopia with left superior quadrant paracentral scotoma. The Pt had an infarct of the left occipital lobe, causing the right hemianopia, and a recent hypertensive hemorrhage in the left retina, causing the scotoma.

F. Generalized constrictions of the visual field

In addition to the patterned field defects already discussed, some Pts have a generalized constriction of the visual field. The most common causes are

1. Hysteria (see Fig. 14-6)
2. Malingering
3. Optic disc drusen
4. Post-papilledema optic atrophy
5. Retinitis pigmentosa (degeneration of the periphery of the retina, as contrasted to macular degeneration

BIBLIOGRAPHY · Visual Fields

Bender MB, Bodis-Wollner I. Visual dysfunctions in optic tract lesions. *Ann Neurol* 1978;3:187–193.

Brazis PW, Masdeu JC, and Biller J. *Localization in Clinical Neurology, 5th ed* Philadelphia: Lippincott Williams and Wilkins, 2007, pp. 131–168.

Ebeling U, Reulen HJ. Neurosurgical topography of the optic radiation in the temporal lobe. *Acta Neurochir* 1988;92:29–36.

Hughes TS, Abou-Khalil B, Lavin PJM, et al. Visual field defects after temporal lobe resection. A prospective quantitative analysis. *Neurology* 1999;53:167–172.

Lepore FE. The preserved temporal crescent: clinical implications of an "endangered" finding. *Neurology* 2001;57:1918–1921.

Trobe JD, Acosta PC, Krischer JP, et al. Confrontation visual field techniques in the detection of anterior visual pathway lesions. *Ann Neurol* 1981;10:228–234.

V. TECHNIQUE FOR CONFRONTATION TESTING OF THE PERIPHERAL VISUAL FIELDS

A. Positioning of examiner and patient

1. Confront the Pt by stationing yourself directly in front. Start with your *left* eye directly in line with the Pt's *right* eye, at a distance of about 50 cm—eye to eye but not breath to breath. The Pt covers the left eye with the left hand (Fig. 3-13).

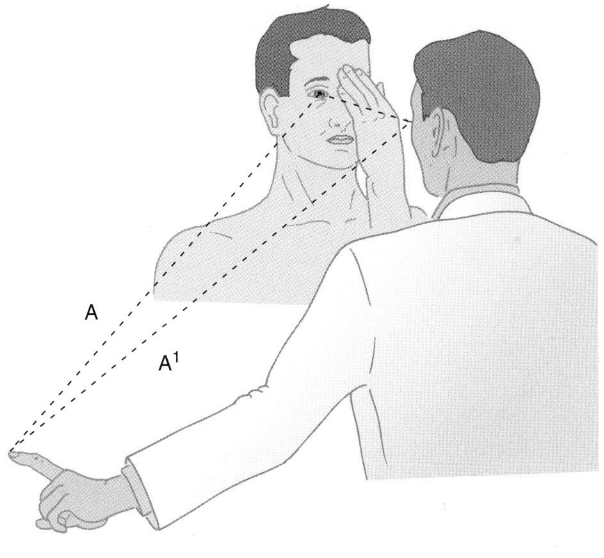

FIGURE 3-13. Position of doctor and patient for testing the visual fields by confrontation. Distance A = A′.

2. Hold up your left index finger just outside your own peripheral field, in the inferior temporal quadrant. Hold the finger about equidistant between your eye and the Pt's, as shown in Fig. 3-13, A = A′. Ideally the finger should extend beyond the perimeter of the field. Wiggle the finger slowly and move it very slowly toward the central field. Request the Pt to say "now" as soon as the wiggling finger is seen. Try to match the perimeter of the Pt's visual field against your own. Test all quadrants of each eye separately, each time starting at the limit of the field.
3. After surveying the visual field by the wiggling finger, you can refine the test by asking the Pt to count the number of fingers presented in each of the four quadrants of the visual field of each eye. Have the Pt close or cover the eye not being tested. Then randomly hold up one, two, or five digits (three or four is too complicated) in each quadrant for the Pt to count.
4. As a further refinement, the Ex may present the fingers for counting simultaneously in two separate quadrants of one eye or present wiggling fingers to each field.

5. In addition to testing the periphery of each quadrant, the Ex may use the finger-counting technique for the inner part of each quadrant, within the central 10 degrees (Bender and Bodis-Wollner 1978; Trobe et al., 1981).

B. Technical pointers for confrontation testing

Point 1: Position yourself and the Pt comfortably.

Point 2: State clearly what you want the Pt to do. The best instructions are: "I want you to look directly into my eye. Don't look away. Now I want to find out how far you can see out of the corner of your eye. Say, 'Now' as soon as you see my finger wiggle." Instruct the Pt not to look at your nose. The Pt's eyes will converge, and your fields will not match the Pt's. Try to fit or titrate your island of vision against the Pt's.

Point 3: Test the midpoint of the quadrants, about 45, 135, 225, and 315 degrees (Fig. 3-14) rather than 0, 90, 180, and 270 degrees. If you test along the vertical or horizontal axis, you may miss a full quadrant defect, because of the intact fields on the border of the defect. See the left eye in Fig. 3-8A.

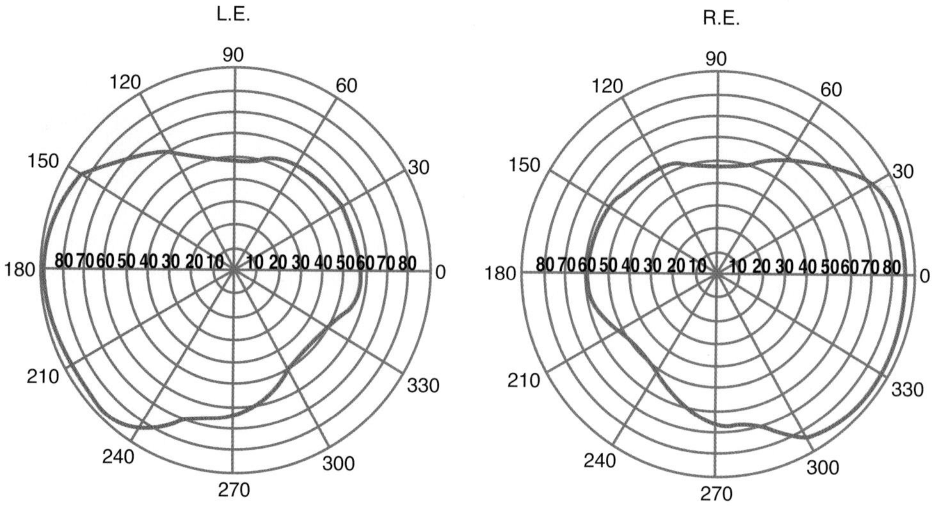

FIGURE 3-14. Actual outline of visual fields charted by perimetry. The numbers are readings in degrees from the center. L.E. = left eye; R.E. = right eye.

Point 4: Confrontation is suitable for detecting large erosions of the island of vision by the sea of blindness. Practice testing the visual fields on a normal person. The combination of acuity testing, Amsler grid, and confrontation testing, all of which you can complete in a few minutes, will usually disclose visual defects or at least disclose the need for further testing by tangent screen and perimetry.

C. Quantitative mapping of the visual fields and blind spot

1. Detailed mapping of the peripheral fields requires perimetry by an ophthalmologist or neurologist. Accurate plotting of the fields discloses the somewhat irregular outline in Fig. 3-14, rather than being exactly round as the text depicts them. The tangent screen and perimeter, although valuable in themselves, only extend, but do not supplant, confrontation and the other visual tests by the attending physician.
2. Perimetry by the Goldmann manual kinetic perimeter or automated static perimetry of the central visual field can extend the tangent screen and confrontation test. Of the two, the Goldmann test includes more of the temporal field, whereas the automated tests include only the central 30 degrees of the visual field (Lepore, 2001).

VI. SUPPRESSION OF VISION

A. Do this experiment to demonstrate physiologic suppression of vision

☑ one eye open

1. Fixate on a distant point straight ahead. Place your palm on your forehead with your wrist directly between your eyes, while maintaining fixation on a distant point. Close one eye and then open it. Under which condition do you see more of your wrist? ❒ one eye open/❒ both eyes open
2. By closing one eye, you prove that the light rays from the wrist are striking photosensitive areas of the retina, yet the wrist, although visible with one eye open, nearly vanishes with both eyes open. The experiment shows that the medial, overlapping portions of the visual fields undergo suppression during binocular vision (Fig. 3-15). This physiologic suppression of the overlapping fields of the two eyes rids the visual image of confusing elements.

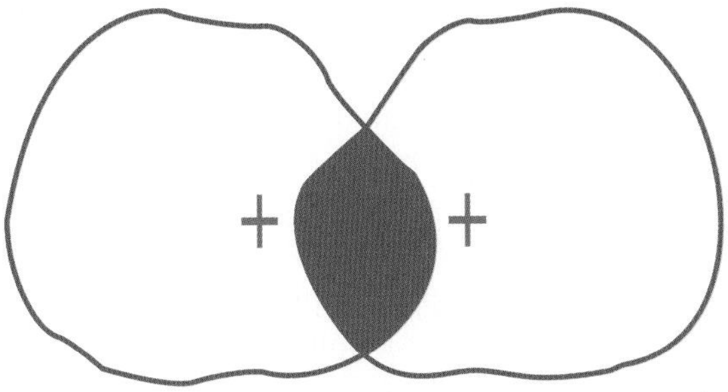

FIGURE 3-15. The overlapping, shaded area of the visual fields undergoes physiologic suppression.

B. Pathologic suppression of vision

1. **Suppression amblyopia (amblyopia ex anopsia):** If one eye in an infant turns in or out, the infant learns to suppress the image from the errant eye. If suppression continues for the first few years of life, the Pt ultimately becomes completely blind in the deviating eye, even though the retina and visual pathways remain structurally intact.
2. **Visual inattention or visual extinction to double simultaneous stimulation:**
   a. Fixate straight ahead.
   b. Hold your arms out to the sides, in the upper or lower quadrant, with your index finger pointing up.
   c. Rotate your arms forward until your index fingers just come into view in each eye. Notice that you can make out both fingertips at the periphery of your fields, even though you are looking straight ahead. The presentation of two stimuli, such as the two fingers, on opposite sides, is called *double* or *simultaneous stimulation*.
   d. **Technique for simultaneous stimulation of visual fields:** Assume the same position as for regular confrontation, but with the Pt keeping both eyes open. Extend your fingers into your inferior temporal quadrants, near, but not beyond, the periphery of your own visual fields. Wiggle one finger and request the Pt to point to the finger that moves. Then wiggle both fingers simultaneously and ask the Pt to point to any finger that moves. The normal person, perceiving both stimuli, points to both fingers. Repeat the test in the upper temporal quadrants and then simultaneously stimulate upper and lower nasal and temporal quadrants of one eye at a time.
   e. **Results and interpretation of inattention to simultaneous stimulation**
      i. Patients with parietal or parieto-occipital lobe lesions, usually on the right side of the cerebrum, will not attend to the stimulus from the contralateral side when presented with simultaneous stimuli on both sides. In the usual case, when the Pt does not attend to stimuli from the left half of space, the lesion is in the ❒ right/❒ left parietal lobe.

☑ right

ii. However, when tested by confrontation with one finger in the left visual field, no defect is demonstrated. The Pt is then said to have visual inattention for the left side of space.

simultaneous (or double)

f. Hemianopia is detected by using one stimulus, whereas visual inattention is detected by using ____________________ stimuli.

hemianopia; visual inattention

g. Blindness in one-half of the visual field is called ____________. If the Pt fails to recognize a stimulus in one-half of a visual field when both halves are stimulated, it is called ____.

Hemianopia means that the Pt is blind for single and double stimuli in one visual field. *Visual inattention* means that the Pt does not perceive one of simultaneous right- and left-sided stimuli but has no hemianopia when tested with a single stimulus.

h. Explain the difference between hemianopia and visual inattention.________ ____ ______________________________.

i. Patients with right parietal lobe lesions also may fail to attend to auditory or tactile stimuli from the left side (Chapter 10).

C. Neuro-ophthalmologic findings in cortical blindness (double hemianopsia)

1. Bilateral destruction of the visual cortex, as from infarction including hypoperfusion-related watershed infarcts, hypoxia, preeclampsia-eclampsia, posterior reversible encephalopathy syndrome (PRES), mitochondrial encephalomyopathy, lactic acidosis with stroke-like episodes (MELAS), or trauma, results in *cortical blindness*, characterized by:
   a. Complete blindness, with no light perception and no response to a menacing gesture.
   b. Loss of smooth pursuit of the Ex's moving finger in testing the range of eye movements but preservation of volitional movements.
   c. No optokinetic nystagmus.
   d. Normal pupillary reactions, funduscopic examination, and no nystagmus.
   e. Sometimes the Pt will deny the blindness and will claim that vision is present (Anton's syndrome).
2. Magnetic resonance imaging will confirm the bi-occipital lesions.

BIBLIOGRAPHY

Acheson JF, Sanders MD. Vision. *J Neurol Neurosurg Psychiatry* 1995;29:4–15.

Bender MB, Bodis-Wollner I. Visual dysfunctions in optic tract lesions. *Ann Neurol* 1978;3:187–193.

Brazis PW, Masdeu JC, and Biller J. *Localization in Clinical Neurology, 5th ed.* Philadelphia: Lippincott Williams and Wilkins, 2007, pp. 131–168.

Gross CG. Leonardo da Vinci on the eye and brain. *Neuroscientist* 1997;3:347–354.

Harrington D. *The Visual Fields: A Textbook and Atlas of Clinical Perimetry*, 2nd ed. St. Louis, C.V. Mosby, 1971.

Lepore FE. The preserved temporal crescent: clinical implications of an "endangered" finding. *Neurology* 2001;57:1918–1921.

Liu GT, Volpe NJ, Galetta SL. *Neuro-ophthalmology.* Philadelphia, W.B. Saunders, 2001.

Shingleton BJ, O'Donoghue MW. Blurred vision. *N Engl J Med* 2000;343:556–562.

Trobe JD, Acosta PC, Krischer JP, et al. Confrontation visual field techniques in the detection of anterior visual pathway lesions. *Ann Neurol* 1981;10:228–234.

VII. OPHTHALMOSCOPY

A. Introduction

1. By now, you know what we would ask you do to learn ophthalmoscopy. Sit down with a normal person and, using colored pencils, draw the optic fundus and its vessels. Draw them faithfully, precisely, and in exquisite detail. You will never do

competent ophthalmoscopy unless you can draw the fundus. Moreover, you often should use drawings in your clinical notes rather than laborious written descriptions.

2. Making a drawing forces you to search the fundus systematically.

B. Technique of ophthalmoscopy

1. Remove your and the Pt's glasses, unless one or both of you have a severe refractive error. The closer you can get your eye to the ophthalmoscope and the closer the scope to the Pt's eye, the larger the area of fundus visible.
2. Darken the room, leaving only a little background illumination.
3. Ask the Pt to fixate on a specific point straight ahead.
4. Instruct the Pt to blink as needed and breathe normally, but the Ex should avoid exhaling in the Pt's face. Both Pt and Ex should be in a comfortable position. Establish a "proprioceptive circuit" to steady the Pt's head and your hand (Fig. 3-16).

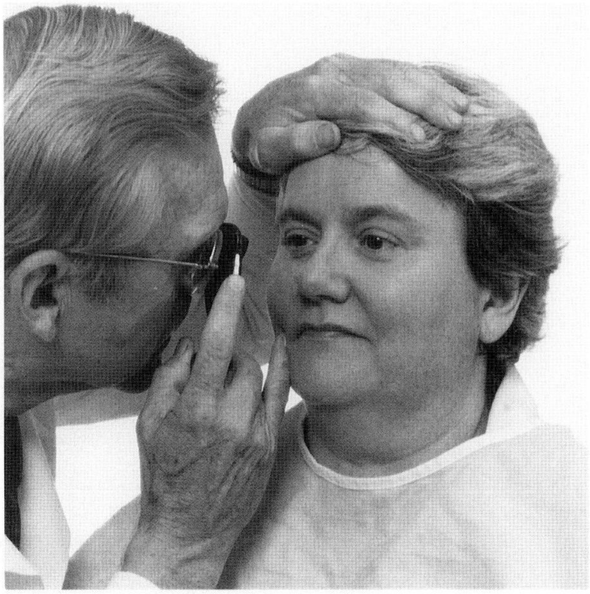

FIGURE 3-16. "Proprioceptive link" to steady the patient and examiner for ophthalmoscopy. The link is between the examiner's two hands and the patient's head.

5. Turn the rheostat on the ophthalmoscope down a little to avoid too strong a beam of light. With too bright a light, the pupil constricts strongly, thus reducing the view of the retina, and photophobic Pts will flinch to avoid discomfort.
6. Hold the ophthalmoscope in your right hand and move your right eye to the Pt's right eye; hold the scope in your left hand and move your left eye to the Pt's left eye. Otherwise you are nose to nose. When looking through the scope, keep both eyes open. Attend only to the image from the eye that looks through the scope. Learn this art. It well repays the time required because it will enable you to relax during the procedure. Start with the ophthalmoscope 10 to 15 cm from your partner's eye and, with a strong positive lens, focus on the media in succession from cornea to lens to vitreous, using successively weaker lenses. Inspect the cornea with and without the scope for opacities and for a circular ring near the limbus, which, if grayish-white, is an *arcus senilis,* or, if greenish-brown, a *Kayser-Fleischer ring* pathognomonic of Wilson hepatolenticular degeneration.
7. Next focus on a retinal vessel by using whatever lens setting, from 0 to a strong plus or minus that is required to overcome refractive errors. After locating a retinal vessel, follow it along until you find the optic disc (optic papilla). Now study Figs. 3-3, 3-17, and 3-18A before continuing.

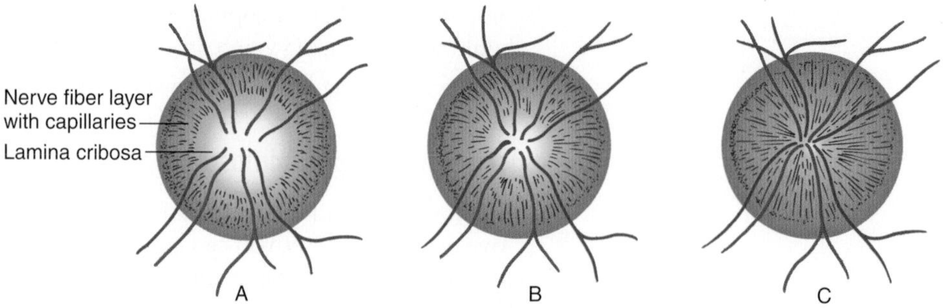

FIGURE 3-17. Normal variation in the size of the physiologic cup of the optic papilla. The cup size depends on whether the nerve fibers perforate the lamina cribrosa at its periphery (A) or all over its surface (C). (A) Large cup. Notice the large white ring of lamina cribrosa between the nerve fibers and the central vessels. Notice the spread of the vessels where they perforate the lamina cribrosa. (B) Medium-size cup. Notice the small white ring and the more compact relation of the vessels. (C) Absence of a physiologic cup in an otherwise normal disc. The vessels originate as from a point. The disc appears like this in pseudopapilledema.

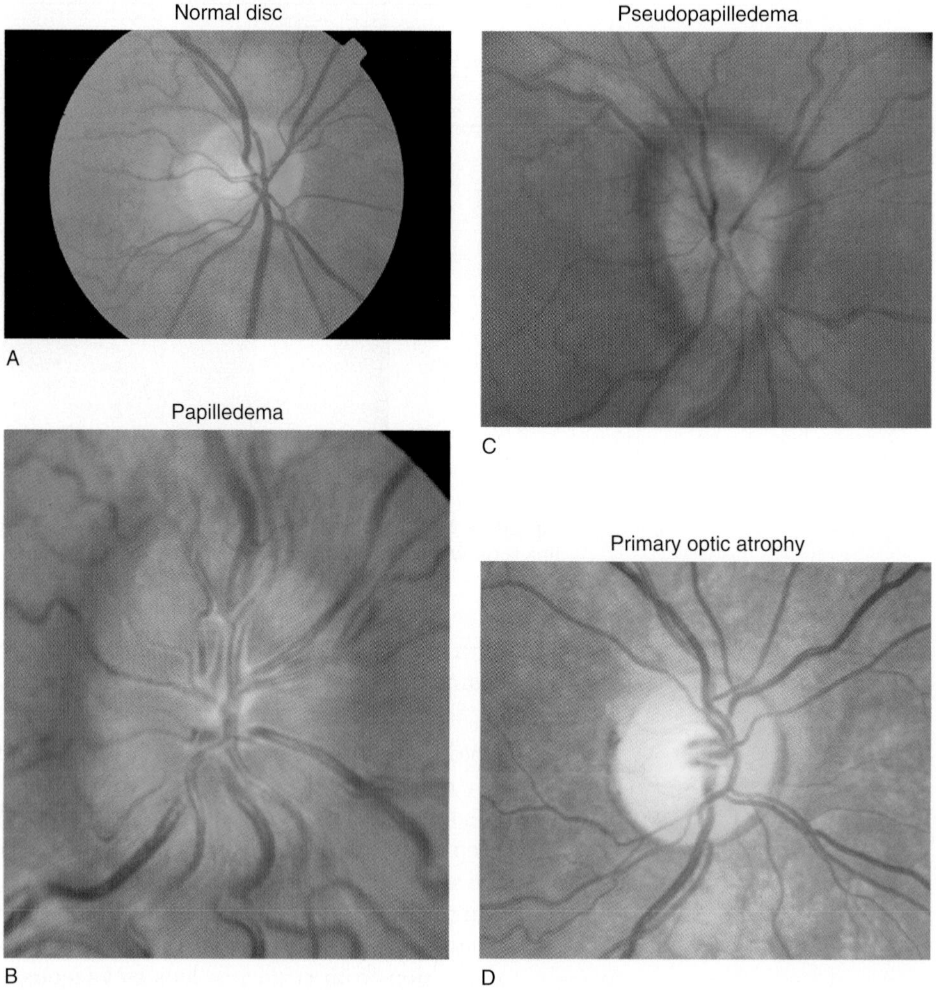

FIGURE 3-18. Photographs of optic papilla in various conditions. (courtesy of Drs. Kathleen B. Digre and James J. Corbett. Reproduced from KB Digre, JJ Corbett. Practical Viewing of the Optic Disc. Boston: Butterworth Heinemann, 2003). (A) Normal. (B) Papilledema. Notice how the edematous swelling engulfs and obscures the proximal segments of many vessels. (C) Pseudopapilledema. (D) Primary optic atrophy. (E) Secondary optic atrophy. (F) Large physiologic cup, a normal variation.

Secondary optic atrophy

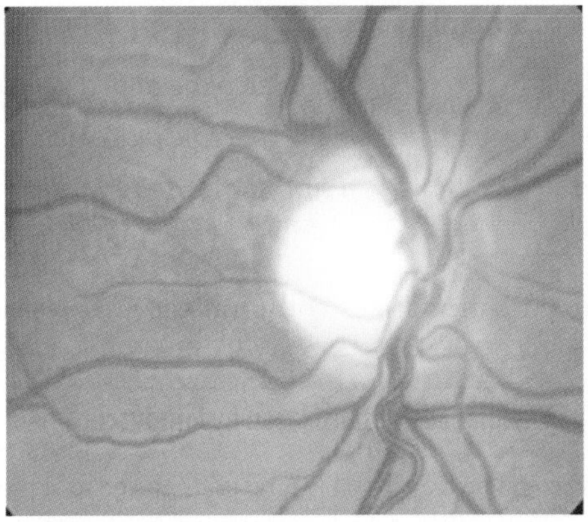

E

Large physiologic cup

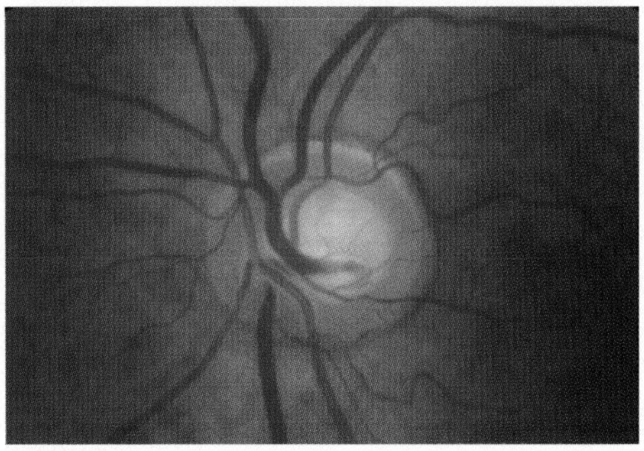

F

FIGURE 3-18. (Continued)

8. Next, identify the pigment ring around the disc, note the disc color, and the presence or absence of a physiologic cup. If present, the physiologic cup is white as compared with the rest of the disc. Identify the arteries, the thin, brighter appearing vessels, and the thicker, duller appearing veins.
9. Look for venous pulsations where the veins bend over the edge of the physiologic cup. Venous pressure slightly exceeds the intraocular pressure. Visible pulsation occurs in nearly 90% of normal Pts when both eyes are examined (Levin, 1978). Venous pulsations disappear at intracranial pressures above 190 mm H_2O. Because of the absence of visible pulsations in some normal persons, the presence of pulsation is more important than its absence.
10. Follow each artery out as far as possible. Locate the macula, a darker, avascular area two disc diameters lateral to the disc. Note the pearl of light reflecting from the *fovea centralis,* the center of the macula. This light reflection fades in older persons.
11. Now make a drawing of your partner's fundus. To check how observant you have been, answer questions 11a to 11l. Write your answers in the left-hand margin, and you will have created your own program.
    a. What is the normal ratio of arterial to venous diameter?
    b. What is the width of the stripe of light reflection from the arteries?
    c. Do the arteries normally nick or indent the veins where they cross?
    d. Between the superior and inferior temporal branches of the retinal artery, how many blood vessels can you count coursing over the disc? Be sure to have the disc sharply in focus.
    e. Which margin of the disc shows the most pigment?
    f. Which borders of the disc—the superior, inferior, nasal, or temporal—normally look more blurred than the other borders?
    g. What is the normal color of the disc?
    h. Which half of the disc, nasal or temporal, is the palest?
    i. What is the range of normal variability in the diameter of the physiologic cup? (Answer only after you have looked at several eyes.)
    j. How many disc diameters lateral to the disc is the macula?
    k. Describe the macula.
    l. Does the fundus appear perfectly smooth or does it have a leathery texture?
12. Now, after trying to answer the questions, decide whether you should repeat the drawing. The questions cannot be bluffed. Either you know the answers or

you don't. Should you try again? While wrestling with your conscience, listen to Walt Whitman:

Failing to fetch me at first keep encouraged,
Missing me one place, search another,
I stop somewhere waiting for you.

13. Table 3-1 summarizes common vascular lesions visible by funduscopy.

TABLE 3-1 · Vascular Lesions Disclosed by Funduscopy

Emboli: talc/corn starch emboli in IV drug users; Hollenhorst plaques: yellow cholesterol emboli in retinal arterioles; fibrin–platelet emboli: white emboli in arterioles; septic emboli: small retinal hemorrhages with a central white spot (Roth's spots)
Trauma/subarachnoid hemorrhage: subhyaloid hemorrhages between the retina and the vitreous, characteristic of battered infants
Central retinal artery occlusion: pale retina, attenuated arterioles, and red macula (cherry-red spot)
Central retinal vein occlusion: widespread intraretinal hemorrhages and dilated retinal veins
Hypertensive retinopathy: "copper or silver wire" arteries, A-V nicking, flame hemorrhages, "cotton-wool" exudates, and papilledema
Diabetic retinopathy: microaneurysms, "hard" exudates, retinal hemorrhages; vitreous hemorrhage

ABBREVIATIONS: A-V = arterial to venous diameter ratio; IV = intravenous.

C. Papilledema

1. **Definition:** *Papilledema* means a blurred or elevated optic papilla (optic nerve head or optic disc) resulting from edema fluid in the nerve fibers as they cross the disc to perforate the lamina cribrosa and enter the optic nerve. Papilledema is classed as early, fully developed, chronic, and chronic atrophic.
2. **Pathophysiology:** Most often, papilledema results from transmission of increased intracranial pressure into the eye via the subarachnoid space, which extends out along the optic nerve (Fig. 3-19). Other causes include direct pressure on the optic nerve from retrobulbar lesions.

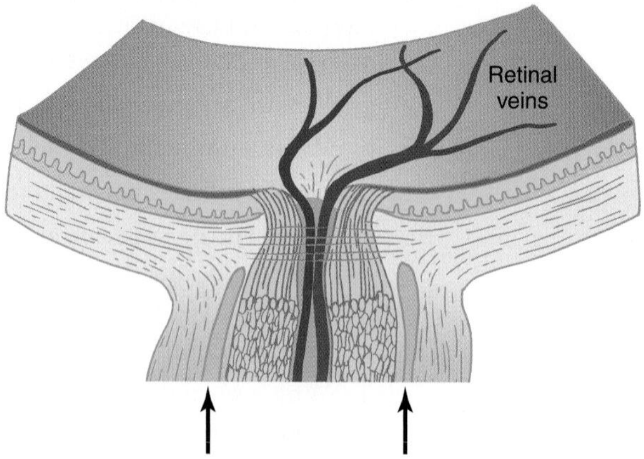

FIGURE 3-19. Section of optic papilla and optic nerve. The arrows show how the subarachnoid space extends around the optic nerve.

a. The retinal veins converge on the optic papilla to form the ophthalmic vein, which enters the retinal end of the optic nerve. If the pressure around it increases, the ophthalmic vein, being thin walled, collapses, obstructing the retinal veins (Fig. 3-19).
b. The retinal veins and papillary capillaries distend and leak fluid into the nerve fibers on the optic papilla and into the surrounding retina. The veins may rupture, causing visible hemorrhages on or around the papilla.

3. **Ophthalmoscopic features of progressive papilledema are as follows:**
   a. Engorged veins cause hyperemia (increased redness) of the disc and loss of venous pulsations.
   b. The nerve fibers blur as they converge on the disc. Then the blurred margins become elevated. To see the elevation, start with a positive lens (+8) in the ophthalmoscope, find the disc, and focus on it by reducing the power of the lens. The upper and lower poles of the disc blur first, then the nasal side of the disc, and then the lateral. Some blurring of the upper and lower poles is normal, particularly in emmetropic or hyperopic eyes. After focusing on the elevated disc, focus on the retina.
   c. As the disc elevates, the physiologic cup obliterates. Linear, peripapillary hemorrhages and splinter and flame-shaped retinal hemorrhages and cotton-wool exudates then appear.
   d. As the edema spreads from the papilla outward, peripapillary folds may also appear in the retina adjacent to the elevated disc.
   e. From Fig. 3-18, pick out the retina that shows papilledema (and one hemorrhage): ❒A/❒B/❒C/❒D/❒E/❒F.

☑ **B.** The linear peripapillary hemorrhage is at the vein bifurcation, just superior to the optic disc.

D. Differential diagnosis of papilledema, other disc lesions, and pseudopapilledema

1. Table 3-2 lists some conditions that resemble papilledema.
2. **Differential diagnosis of true and pseudopapilledema.**
   a. Perhaps 5% of normal individuals have some blurring and even slight elevation of the optic papilla, a condition called *pseudopapilledema*, that has to be distinguished from early papilledema. The experienced Ex readily recognizes advanced papilledema when it shows extreme papillary swelling, venous congestion, and hemorrhages. Pseudopapilledema often may lead to unnecessary tests when, in most instances, careful clinical observations, based on drawings and periodic assessment of the disc, would lead to the correct, benign diagnosis of pseudopapilledema.

TABLE 3-2 · Optic Disc Anomalies Confused with Papilledema

Medullated nerve fibers: a whitish-yellow patch of fibers that radiates into the retina from the disc
Congenital vascular anomalies of the vessels with glial overgrowth
Small scleral aperture: the disc appears protruded; usually seen in a hyperopic eye with a short sagittal axis
Drusen (waxy-appearing bodies that push up from beneath and may protrude through the disc)
Pseudopapilledema and papillitis: see later sections

   b. In pseudopapilledema, the disc margins look blurred, but the central rather than the peripheral portion of the disc protrudes, as in true papilledema, and the vessels show preretinal branching (Fig. 3-20).

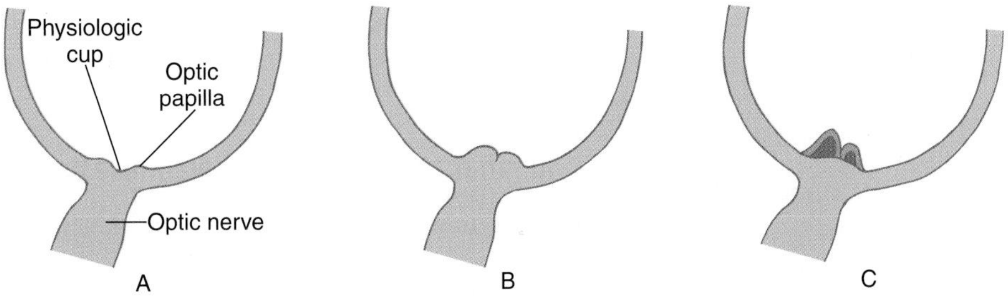

FIGURE 3-20. Optic papilla in horizontal sections of the eye. (A) Normal optic papilla, showing slight elevation of the papillary margins and normal depth of the physiologic cup. (B) Early true papilledema, showing elevation of the papillary margins and beginning obliteration of the physiologic cup. (C) Pseudopapilledema, showing preretinal branching of the vessels, central elevation of the optic papilla, and absence of a physiologic cup.

c. The elevated disc of pseudopapilledema in some Pts may come from *drusen* (hyaloid bodies) pressing up from beneath the nerve fiber layer.

d. Drusen and pseudopapilledema most frequently affect blond Caucasians and hyperopic rather than myopic Pts. If you suspect pseudopapilledema in a blond Caucasian or hyperopic Pt, inspect the fundi of family members. The answer becomes clear if other family members also have blurred discs. From Fig. 3-18, select the disc which shows pseudopapilledema: ❐A/❐B/❐C/❐D/❐E/❐F.

☑ C

3. **Two further tests help identify papilledema in doubtful cases:** Measurement of the blind spot size and the fluorescein dye test:

   a. **Measurement of the blind spot**

      i. Edema from the swollen disc enlarges the blind spot. In pseudopapilledema caused by drusen, the blind spot also increases.

      ii. What type of visual field examination would best measure the blind spot? ❐ confrontation/❐ perimetry/❐ tangent screen

      ☑ tangent screen

      iii. Although papilledema increases the size of the blind spot, papilledema per se does not generally impair visual acuity until later, after weeks to months.

   b. **The fluorescein dye test:** After injection of fluorescein into an arm vein, the fundus is photographed. In papilledema, fluorescein passes through the leaky walls of the distended retinal vessels into the optic papilla.

   c. Name the two tests in addition to ophthalmoscopic examination to diagnose papilledema? ________________________________.

   Measurement of the blind spot and the fluorescein dye test.

4. **To summarize the differential diagnosis of papilledema and pseudopapilledema, complete** Table 3-3. Place a + or 0 in the right-hand columns.

TABLE 3-3 · Differentiation of True Papilledema and Pseudopapilledema

	Papilledema	Pseudopapilledema
DISC CHARACTERISTICS		
Hyperemic, pink color (vascular distention)	___	___
Physiologic cup present (early)	___	___
Sparing of temporal margin (early)	___	___
High point of elevation central (see Fig. 3–20B)	___	___
Drusen (hyaline bodies) submerged in children, exposed in adults, gray-yellow translucent color of disc; applies only to blond Caucasians	___	___
VESSEL CHARACTERISTICS		
Dilated veins	___	___
Venous pulsation present	___	___
Disc obscures origin of vessels	___	___
Arteries appear tortuous, show preretinal branching; disc does not obscure the origin of the vessels	___	___
Prominent choroidal vessels (from lack of retinal pigment)	___	___
HEMORRHAGES	___	___
HYPEROPIA	___	___
ENLARGED BLIND SPOT	___	___
FLUORESCEIN DYE TEST: shows leaky vessels	___	___

Answers (margin):

+	0
+	0
+	0
0	+
+	0
0	+
+	0
0	+
0	+
+	0
0	+
+	0*
+	0

*if drusen cause pseudopapilledema

E. Summary of procedures to diagnose papilledema

1. Make drawings or photographs and keep careful clinical notes that describe the retina:

   a. The color of the disc.

   b. Degree of blurring of disc margins and location of blurring. Record any measurable elevation of the disc as the diopter difference between the elevation of the disc margin and the adjacent retina.

c. Presence or absence of the physiologic cup.

d. Venous congestion and pulsation.

e. Peripapillary wrinkles and folds.

f. Hemorrhages or exudates

2. Measure the Pt's visual acuity. It is generally preserved in early papilledema, but the Pt may complain of *obscurations of vision*, episodic blurring of vision or blindness lasting seconds. Disc swelling from optic neuritis or papillitis causes severe central visual loss and is generally unilateral, whereas papilledema is usually bilateral.
3. Chart the blind spot in the visual field.
4. Consider the anomalies confused with papilledema (Table 3-2).
5. Make careful serial examinations.

F. Optic atrophy, primary and secondary

1. **Definition:** *Optic atrophy* means degeneration and disappearance of the optic axons that originate in the ganglion cell layer of the retina and penetrate the optic disc.
2. **Pathogenesis of optic atrophy (anterograde or retrograde axonal degeneration)**

   a. If a retinal lesion destroys neurons of the ganglionic layer of the retina or interrupts the axons *before* they penetrate the lamina cribrosa, the axons undergo *Wallerian (anterograde) degeneration* and disappear.

   b. If a lesion interrupts optic axons *behind* the optic papilla, in the optic nerve, chiasm, or tract, the axons undergo *retrograde degeneration* that also causes them to disappear from the optic papilla and retina. Thus, after retinal or optic nerve lesions, the optic disc becomes denuded of axons and appears white, which brings us to a profound secret: The optic axons and retinal neurons are transparent and colorless. Why then doesn't the optic disc normally appear white, being backed by the white lamina cribrosa of the sclera? The physiologic cup appears white because no optic axons perforate the white lamina cribrosa at the site of the physiologic cup.

   i. One theory proposed that the capillaries that accompany and nourish the nerve fibers cause the pinkish color of the disc. When the axons, the parenchyma, atrophy, so do the capillaries that give the axonal layer its color. The loss of capillarity in optic atrophy reflects a general rule: whenever the parenchymatous elements of an organ degenerate, so does its blood supply. Compare the capillarity of the pre- and postmenopausal ovary. With optic atrophy or retinal destruction, the arteries and veins also become smaller.

   ii. Another theory holds that the loss of axons changes the refraction of light at the disc, causing the pallid appearance.

3. **Primary optic atrophy:** Depletion of the optic axons and capillaries exposes the full extent of the chalk-white lamina cribrosa, which then appears as a flat white disc with a cookie-cutter sharp border against the retina, a condition called *primary optic atrophy.* In Fig. 3-18, select the disc showing primary optic atrophy: ❐A/❐B/❐C/❐D/❐E/❐F.

☑ D

4. **Secondary optic atrophy:** This follows longstanding disc lesions, such as chronic papilledema or papillitis. The optic nerve fibers disappear, but connective tissue proliferation incited by the lesion causes the disc to become gray with shaggy, ragged borders due to glial scarring. In primary and secondary optic atrophy, the nerve fibers crossing the disc disappear, but connective tissue proliferates on the disc only in ❐ primary/❐ secondary optic atrophy.

☑ secondary

5. Table 3-4 summarizes the differential features of primary and secondary optic atrophy.
6. From Fig. 3-18, select the disc that shows secondary optic atrophy: ❐A/❐B/❐C/❐D/❐E/❐F.

☑ E

TABLE 3-4 · Differentiation of Primary and Secondary Optic Atrophy

Primary optic atrophy	Secondary optic atrophy
Follows acute or chronic lesions of optic nerve or retina	Follows chronic lesion of optic papilla, usually papilledema or papillitis
Disc is chalk-white with cookie-cutter sharp borders	Disc is gray with shaggy borders from connective tissue proliferation
Lamina cribrosa exposed	Lamina cribrosa obscured
Arteries and veins reduced in size if optic atrophy is severe and prolonged	Arteries thin; veins may be dilated
May affect only one sector of the disc	Not limited to a sector-affects entire disc

7. **Two conditions to distinguish from optic atrophy are**
   a. A very *large physiologic cup* that occupies much of the disc.
   b. *Optic nerve hypoplasia*, a congenitally small optic disc and nerve, often associated with underdevelopment of septal region, hypothalamus, and pituitary gland, a condition called *septooptic dysplasia*.

G. Differential diagnosis of papilledema, papillitis, and acute retrobulbar neuritis

1. Inflammatory or toxic processes may attack the optic papilla, causing *papillitis*. Inflammatory, toxic, or demyelinating processes may affect the optic nerve behind the eyeball (where the optic axons become myelinated), causing *acute retrobulbar neuritis* (Fig. 3-21C). The Pt loses visual acuity and color vision with acute retrobulbar neuritis.

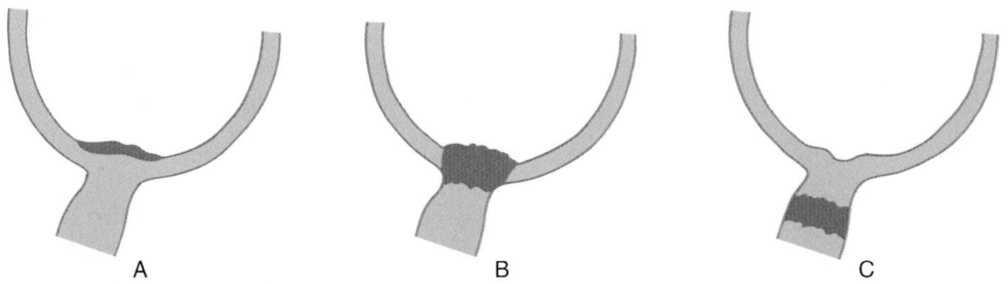

FIGURE 3-21. Sites of lesions affecting the optic papilla and nerve. (A) Papilledema. (B) Papillitis. (C) Retrobulbar neuritis.

2. With the ophthalmoscope alone, the Ex may not be able to distinguish papillitis from papilledema. With papillitis, the Pt loses vision early; with papilledema, the Pt retains vision until late in the disease.
3. With acute retrobulbar neuritis, the disc and vessels look normal early in the course, but if the process destroys optic axons in the optic nerve, what happens to the nerve fibers and capillaries on the disc?____.

   The nerve fibers and capillaries degenerate and disappear.

   a. The optic disc then has the ophthalmoscopic appearance called __________________________ optic atrophy.

   primary

4. **Note this critical fact:** The degeneration of optic nerve fibers and capillaries takes several weeks. Thus, the Ex will not see optic atrophy early in acute retrobulbar neuritis. Even though the Pt lacks vision, the optic disc may look normal: The Pt sees nothing and neither does the Ex.
5. **Mnemonic for differential effects of papilledema, papillitis, and acute retrobulbar neuritis on appearance of the disc and visual acuity.**
   a. If the Ex sees a swollen disc and the Pt sees as usual, it's papilledema.
   b. If the Ex sees a swollen disc and the Pt doesn't see well, it's papillitis.

c. If the Ex sees nothing abnormal and the Pt doesn't see well or is blind, it's acute retrobulbar neuritis.

Mnemonic for differentiating papilledema, papillitis, and acute retrobulbar neuritis

1. If both the Ex and Pt see something, the diagnosis is____________________.
2. If the Ex sees something and the Pt doesn't, the diagnosis is____________________.
3. If neither Ex nor Pt sees anything, the diagnosis is____________________.

papilledema

papillitis

acute retrobulbar neuritis

6. Many conditions damage the optic nerve and give a clinical picture of optic neuritis. Those conditions include methanol intoxication, collagen-vascular disease, and autoimmune diseases such as multiple sclerosis.
7. A notable exception to preserved vision with papilledema is ischemic optic neuropathy. It leads to a sequence of sudden onset of blindness, optic disc swelling, and secondary optic atrophy. It is relatively common in Pts older than 50 years, but it also affects children (Chutorian et al., 2002).

H. Summary of causes for blurred discs

See Fig. 3-22.

BIBLIOGRAPHY · Ophthalmoscopy

Chutorian AM, Winterkorn JMS, Geffner M. Anterior ischemic optic neuropathy in children: case reports and review of the literature. *Pediatr Neurol* 2002;26:358–364.

Kaufman PL, Alm A. *Adler's Physiology of the Eye,* 10th ed. St. Louis, C.V. Mosby, 2002.

Levin BE. The clinical significance of spontaneous pulsations of the retinal vein. *Arch Neurol* 1978;35:37–40.

VIII. SUMMARY OF CLINICAL AND ANCILLARY TESTS OF VISION, THE VISUAL FIELDS, AND THE OPTIC DISCS

A. Routine tests: visual acuity, direct ophthalmoscopy, Amsler grid, and confrontation testing of visual fields

B. Special ancillary tests: fluorescein angiography, blind spot measurements

See Section III D of Chapter 5 and Table 5-7 for a complete summary of ancillary tests for the optic system.

BIBLIOGRAPHY · General References

Acheson JF, Sanders MD. Vision. *J Neurol Neurosurg Psychiatry* 1995;29:4–15.

Bender MB. Rudolph SH, Stacy CB. The Neurology of the visual and oculomotor systems. In Joynt RJ, ed. *Clin Neuro*. Philadelphia, J.B. Lippincott, 1990, Chap. 12, pp. 1–132.

Brazis PW, Masdeu JC, and Biller J. *Localization in Clinical Neurology, 5th ed.* Philadelphia: Lippincott Williams and Wilkins, 2007, pp. 131–168.

Digre KB, Corbett JJ. Practical Viewing of the Optic Disc. Boston: Butterworth Heinemann, 2003. Amsterdam, Boston, London, Oxford, New York, Paris, San Diego, San Francisco, Singapore, Sydney, Tokyo.

Gross CG. Leonardo da Vinci on the eye and brain. *Neuroscientist* 1997;3:347–354.

Liu GT, Volpe NJ, Galetta SL. *Neuro-ophthalmology.* Philadelphia, W.B. Saunders, 2001.

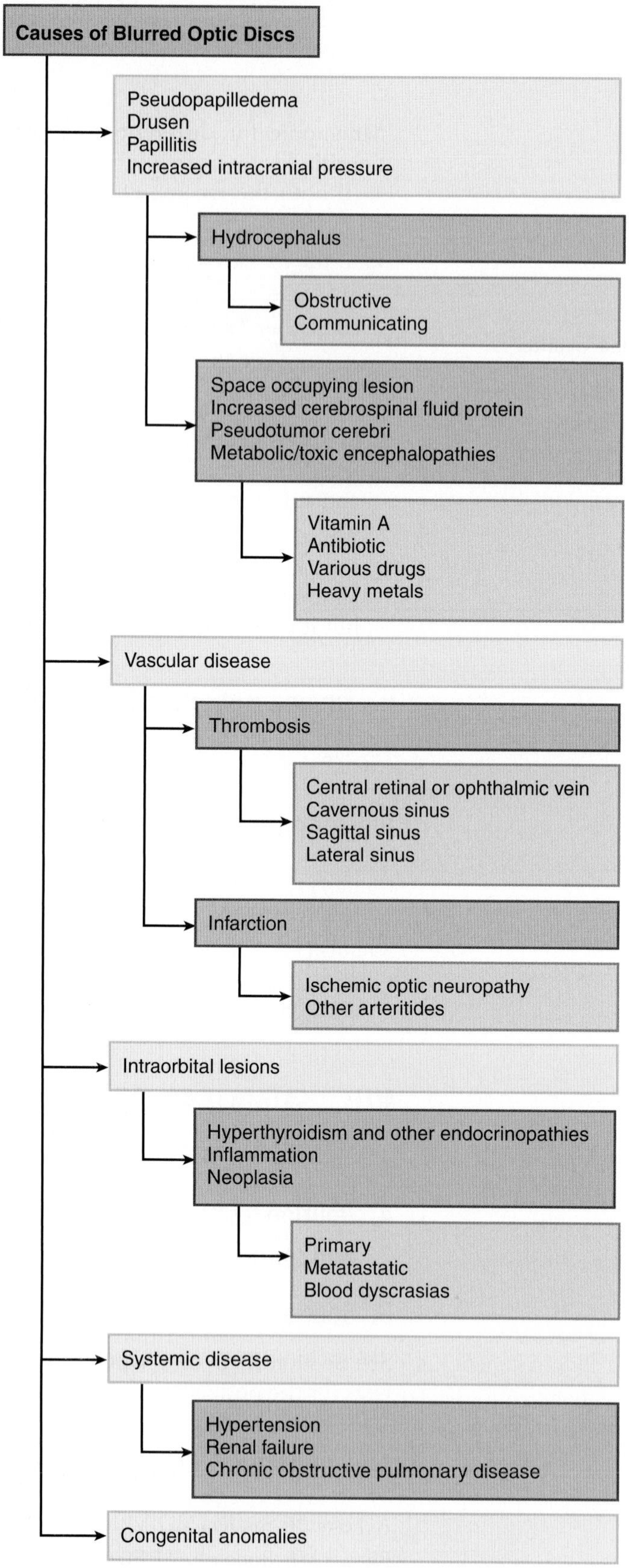

FIGURE 3-22. Dendrogram listing common causes for blurred optic discs.

Learning Objectives for Chapter 3

I. ANATOMY OF THE EYEBALL

1. Make a drawing of a cross section of the eyeball at the level of the optic disc and fovea centralis (Fig. 3-1).

II. DUAL ORGANIZATION OF THE OPTIC SYSTEM

1. State which nerves provide afferent fibers for vision and somatic sensation from the eye.
2. Describe some ocular-related functions of CrN V.
3. Describe the visual pathway from the receptor to the receptive cortex.
4. Distinguish between the retinal image and the visual image (Fig. 3-2).
5. Describe the meaning of the law that the mind projects the visual image to the usual site of origin of the light rays that strike the retina. Give some examples of this law.
6. Describe the receptors for the macula and the periphery of the retina and state the functions of these two parts of the retina.
7. Recite the mnemonic of the C's to remember macular function.
8. Describe the retinal origin of the axons in one optic tract (Fig. 3-4).
9. Describe the terminations of the optic tract.
10. Trace a nerve impulse from its origin to its termination in sensory cortex (Fig. 3-4).
11. Describe how to use the "set the eyeball on the occipital pole" mnemonic to remember the topographic termination of the retina on the occipital cortex and the representation of the visual fields (Fig. 3-5B).

III. THE VISUAL FIELDS

1. Describe a simple method for self-demonstration of the limited field of central vision for acuity and color vision.
2. Describe how to locate the perimeter of your own peripheral visual field and state which part of the peripheral visual field has the greatest extent.
3. State which anatomic structure limits the height of the visual field.
4. Diagram the visual pathway from the retinas of the two fields to the cortex.
5. Recite the nomenclature for the quadrants of the normal visual fields (Fig. 3-7).
6. Assume lesions at various sites along the visual pathway and describe the resulting visual field defect. Use Fig. 3-4.
7. State how a tumor expanding upward against the center of the chiasm from the pituitary fossa would affect the visual fields.
8. Describe the effect of an anterior temporal lobe lesion on the visual fields.

IV. CLINICAL TESTING OF CENTRAL VISION

1. Describe how to test central vision at the bedside in a cooperative, normal older child or adult and in young children or mentally retarded Pts.
2. Describe the use of the Amsler grid (Fig. 3-9).
3. State the indication for a tangent screen examination and demonstrate how to do it (Fig. 3-10).
4. Describe the difference between a scotoma and a patterned visual field defect.
5. Describe how to demonstrate your own blind spot in the visual field (Fig. 3-11).
6. Explain what causes the blind spot (Fig. 3-12).
7. Distinguish between a central scotoma, centrocecal scotoma, and a paracentral scotoma.
8. Name for common causes for generalized constriction of the visual fields.

Learning Objectives for Chapter 3

V. TECHNIQUE FOR CONFRONTATION TESTING OF THE PERIPHERAL VISUAL FIELDS

1. Demonstrate how to test the peripheral visual fields by confrontation (Fig. 3-13).
2. Explain why the Ex tests the extent of the peripheral fields by placing the finger at the midpoint of the quadrants, rather than exactly on the vertical or horizontal axes.

VI. SUPPRESSION OF VISION

1. Describe how to demonstrate physiologic suppression of vision in the overlapping nasal fields of the two eyes (Fig. 3-15).
2. Explain the cause and prevention of suppression amblyopia (amblyopia ex anopsia).
3. Distinguish between visual inattention (suppression) on simultaneous bilateral stimulation and a hemianopic visual field defect.
4. State the site of the lesion usually responsible for visual inattention.
5. Describe the neuro-ophthalmologic findings in cortical blindness, the site of the lesion, and the radiographic procedure of choice to identify the lesion.

VII. OPHTHALMOSCOPY

1. Make and label a drawing of the normal optic fundus as seen through an ophthalmoscope (Figs. 3-3 and 3-18A).
2. Explain why the Ex, when facing the Pt, looks through the ophthalmoscope with the right eye into the Pt's right eye but uses the left eye in testing the extent of the visual field of the Pt's right eye.
3. Describe how to use a "proprioceptive link" to steady the Pt and the Ex for ophthalmoscopy.
4. State what type of lens is used to see the surface of the cornea and the superficial media of the eye.
5. Name two types of rings seen around the periphery of the cornea.
6. Make drawings to show the extreme variations in the size of the physiologic cup in normal individuals (Fig. 3-17).
7. Explain why the central part of the normal optic disc (the physiologic cup) appears white, whereas the periphery appears orange-pink.
8. Describe how to distinguish retinal arteries from veins.
9. State the normal ratio of arterial to venous diameter in the retina.
10. State the ratio of the width of the stripe of light reflection from the artery to the width of the artery.
11. State which border of the optic disc usually shows the most pigment.
12. State which border of the optic disc normally appears sharper than other borders.
13. State which part, the medial or lateral, of the optic papilla normally appears paler than the other.
14. Describe how to locate the macula and fovea centralis and describe their normal appearance.
15. Describe the texture of the normal retina as seen through the ophthalmoscope.
16. Describe the anatomic feature that enables increased intracranial pressure to cause papilledema (Fig. 3-19).
17. Describe the changes that occur in the fundus as papilledema begins and evolves.

Learning Objectives for Chapter 3

18. Contrast papilledema and pseudopapilledema and pick them out from a series of fundus photographs (Table 3-3 and Fig. 3-18).
19. Name anatomic lesions of the optic papilla that need to be differentiated from papilledema (Table 3-2).
20. Describe procedures other than ophthalmoscopy to detect true papilledema.
21. Contrast primary and secondary optic atrophy and pick them out from a series of fundus photographs (Table 3-4 and Fig. 3-18).
22. Describe the ophthalmoscopic findings in papilledema, optic neuritis, and acute retrobulbar neuritis and state the effect each lesion has on vision (Fig. 3-21).
23. State the time required for optic atrophy to become evident by ophthalmoscopy after a retrobulbar lesion or compression of the optic nerve or chiasm.
24. Discuss the effect of partial or incomplete optic nerve lesions on visual acuity, color vision, visual fields, and the appearance of the optic disc.
25. Recite the categories of disorders that cause blurred optic discs (Fig. 3-22).

4 Examination of the Peripheral Ocular Motor System

In examining and treating motor anomalies (of the eye), one never loses an uneasy feeling of incompetence until he has become thoroughly familiar with the physiologic fundamentals from which the signs and symptoms of those anomalies are to be derived. Therefore, a discussion of motor anomalies of the eyes should begin with a synopsis of the physiology of the sensorial and motor apparatus of the eyes.

—Alfred Bielschowsky (1871–1940)

I. OCULAR ALIGNMENT AND DIPLOPIA

A. The goals of the ocular motor system

1. The ocular motor system *finds, fixates, focuses*/aligns on, and *follows* visual targets. In a word, the system *f*oveates. To foveate means to align each eye so as to cause the central light ray to fall on the fovea and the entire retinal image to fall on corresponding retinal points of both eyes (Figs. 4-1 and 4-3).
2. The eyes must continually foveate whether the target remains fixed or moves or whether the eyes remain fixed or move in any direction: horizontal, vertical, rotatory, and vergences (convergence and divergence). Foveation promotes visual acuity and a single (fused) mental image and secures the advantages of binocular stereoscopic vision for survival.

B. Ocular alignment, the visual axes, and diplopia

1. To examine ocular alignment, start with the patient (Pt) looking straight ahead, the so-called *primary position* of the eyes. Theoretically, the point of fixation in the primary position is at infinity (Fig. 4-1).
2. A line drawn from the fovea centralis of one eye to the center of its visual field defines the *visual axis*. This line runs through the center of the media of the eye, striking the fovea centralis without undergoing any refraction. It is the "line of sight" of that eye. In Fig. 4-1, line F-∞ defines the ______________ of the eye.

visual axis (or line of sight)

3. With the eyes in the primary position, fixating on infinity, the visual axes are ❒ convergent/❒ essentially parallel/❒ divergent.

☑ **essentially parallel** (Fig. 4-1)

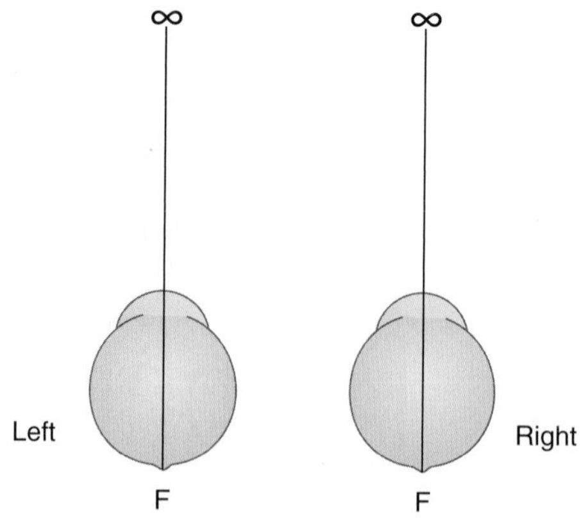

FIGURE 4-1. Visual axes with the eyes in the primary position, fixating on infinity distance. F = fovea.

4. In Fig. 4-2, draw the visual axes where the eyes fixate on a point closer than infinity.

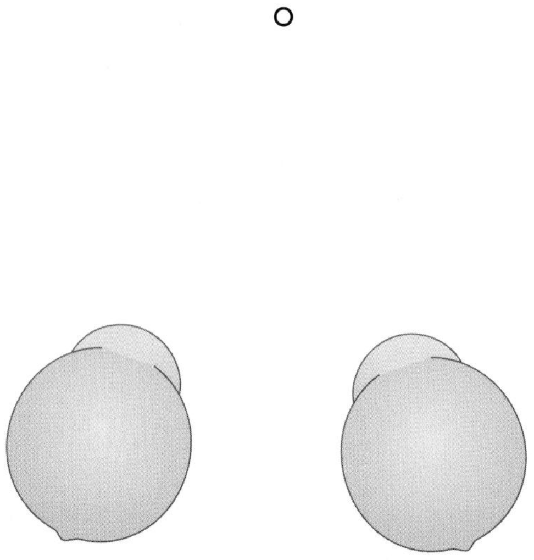

FIGURE 4-2. Blank for drawing the visual axes when the eyes fixate on a near point.

5. When looking at a near point, the eyes converge (*ad*duct). Because each eye adducts, the central light ray from the fixation point remains on the fovea, the region of maximum visual acuity.
6. In Fig. 4-3 draw in the visual axes (from the fovea centralis to the center of the arrow). Study Fig. 4-3 to understand how binocular fixation brings the retinal images onto corresponding parts of the two retinas. To prove you understand the drawing, reproduce it sight unseen.

C. Self-demonstration of the visual axis of the dominant eye

1. With both eyes open, fixate strongly on a doorknob across the room. Then place your index fingertip 20 cm away from your eye, so that the knob appears to rest on the fingertip. Be sure to maintain fixation on the doorknob but see the fingertip secondarily.
2. Alternately, wink the right and then the left eye as you fixate on the doorknob. (If you can't wink each eye independently, cover one and then the other with your free hand.) What happens to the image of the finger?________________

It shifts to one side after closing one eye but does not shift when closing the other eye (if you strictly maintain your original fixation on the doorknob).

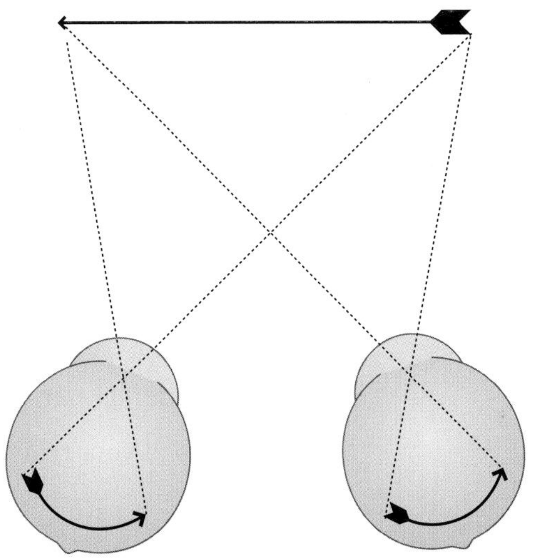

FIGURE 4-3. Binocular retinal image formed when the visual axes of the two eyes align properly on the center of the target. Rays along the visual axes strike the foveae. The remainder of the image falls on corresponding (but not precisely identical) temporal or nasal parts of the retina.

3. **Explanation of the shifting image:** The shift occurs because you fixate primarily along the visual axis of the dominant eye; the other eye angles secondarily onto the target.

D. Self-production of physiologic diplopia

1. With both eyes open, first strongly fixate on the doorknob, and then hold up your fingertip to make the doorknob seem to balance on it. Then fixate strongly on your fingertip but secondarily attend to the doorknob. Alternate focusing strongly on one target while you attend to the other target.
2. What happens to the appearance of the doorknob when you strongly focus on the fingertip or to the fingertip when you strongly focus on the doorknob? ______________________________

The object appears double when you shift from one to the other.

3. **Figure 4-4 explains why the previous experiment disclosed physiologic diplopia.**

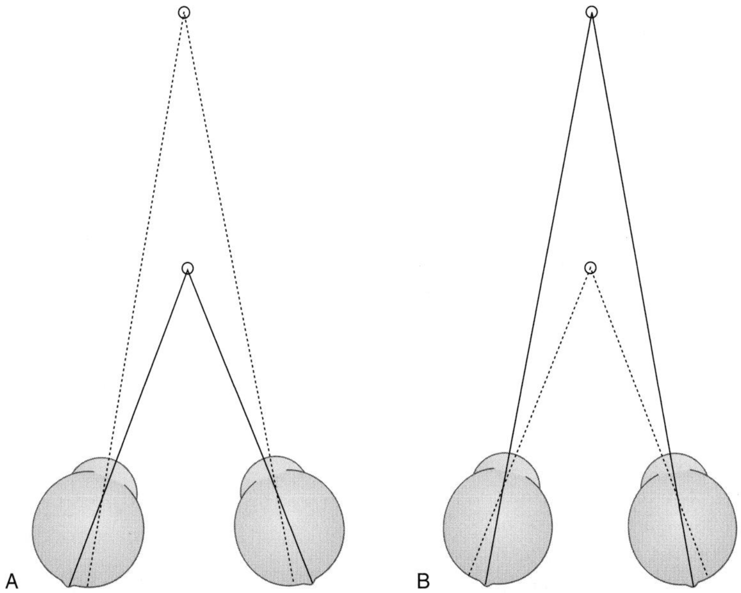

FIGURE 4-4. Changes in the angulation of the visual axes (solid lines) when the eyes diverge from a near fixation point (A) to a distant one (B). The rays from any other point in the visual field (dotted lines) fall off the fovea and macula and cause diplopia when attended to.

a. In Fig. 4-4, rays from only one distance, the fixation point, strike the fovea. All other rays deviate from the fovea in proportion to their distance from the fixation point. Only the rays coming in along the visual axes strike correspondingly on the fovea centralis of each eye.

b. Why don't we have diplopia all the time? Recall that you had to consciously attend to the point of non-fixation to get diplopia. Ordinarily, we have learned to suppress physiologic diplopia. It only appears when we make a determined effort to break through its physiologic suppression. We attend only to the non-diplopic images.

E. Self-production of pathologic diplopia by canthal compression

1. Place the tip of your right index finger on your right lateral canthus, as shown in Fig. 4-5.

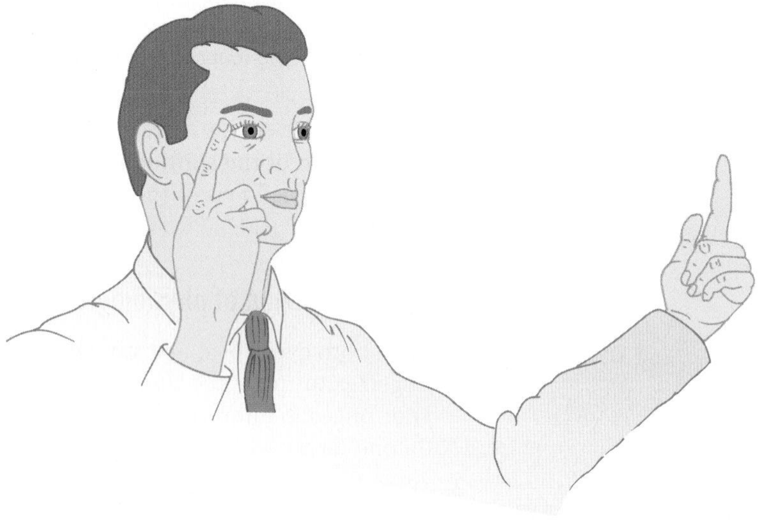

FIGURE 4-5. Position of finger for lateral canthus compression to produce diplopia when gazing at the opposite finger.

2. Hold up your left index finger at arm's length and fixate on it.
3. While fixating, press very gently on your right eyelid just above the canthus with your right index finger. By changing the pressure, you should experience diplopia. If you fail to produce diplopia when looking at your finger, look across the room at a distant object.
4. Repeat the experiment but this time hold the outstretched finger horizontally. With the finger properly angled, you should get diplopia. It may be greater with the finger in one position than another, and it may change each time you try the experiment, depending on the deviation of the eyeball.
5. **Identifying the faulty image in diplopia:** While your right finger compresses your right lateral canthus, choose the best angle of the left finger to get diplopia.

   a. While experiencing diplopia, try to identify the faulty image. You can identify it by:

      i. Alternating the pressure on the eye, causing the faulty image to move while the other image remains on target.

      ii. Winking the displaced eye.

      iii. Noticing which image is the sharpest. Can you explain why the image from the displaced eye is not as sharp as that from the non-displaced eye?

      ____

The non-displaced eye receives the central rays from the visual target directly on the cones, the site of sharpest vision. The retinal image in the displaced eye falls off the macula, onto the rods (Fig. 4-6). You have mechanically interfered with its foveation.

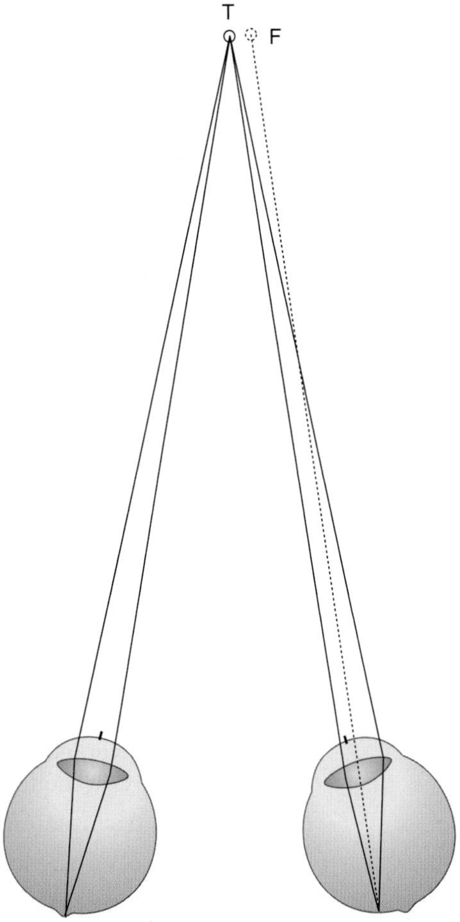

FIGURE 4-6. Diagram explaining projection of the false image to the right when the right eye fails to abduct. With a colored pencil, draw the visual axis of each eye, from the fovea through the corneal center to the target region. Notice how much the visual axis from the right eye misses the target, T. F = false image; T = true image.

b. While producing diplopia, move your left finger to the right. What happens to the distance between the diplopic images as you move your target finger away from its starting position?

____

The distance between the diplopic images increases.

6. **Explanation for diplopia produced by canthal compression.**

   a. For description, the visual image of the aligned eye is called the *true* image, and that of the misaligned eye is called the *false* image. Of course, one image is no more "true" or "false" than the other, because both are visual images that the mind imposes on the afferent data.

   b. Consider now the diplopia produced with the target finger vertical. (Even if you failed to get diplopia this way, you can follow the explanation.) With the finger vertical in the midline, you obtained one or, with practice, two results: one image was projected to the *right* or to the *left* of the true position of the finger. The direction of displacement of the eyeball determines the direction of projection of the false image. Study Fig. 4-6.

7. Explain why the false image appears to the right of the true image in Fig. 4-6.

____

____

____

Because the right eye fails to *ab*duct to align with the left as it *ad*ducts, the retinal image of the right eye falls on the *nasal* half of the retina; by learning, the mind projects the visual image to the right (temporal) side.

8. The eyeball displacement experiment shows that both eyes have to align properly to bring the retinal images onto the corresponding retinal areas, thus avoiding the penalty of diplopia and decreased visual acuity.

II. THE ACTIONS OF THE INDIVIDUAL EXTRAOCULAR MUSCLES

Note: Every general physician must learn to detect ocular malalignment. First learn that the lateral rectus muscle has only one action, *ab*duction of the eye, and the medial rectus has only one action, *ad*duction. All other extraocular muscles (EOMs) have multiple actions, depending on the position of the eye. If the time allotted to study the neurologic examination (NE) is short, photocopy Fig. 4-18, which summarizes these actions, paste it in your handbook for reference, and skip to Section II, J and K. *If you wish to* **understand** *the actions of the EOM, work through the text, which calls for you to make two simple models enabling you to reason out the actions and recall them as needed.*

I find that many students automatically reject model-making as a waste of time. Let me say this: You will never really understand the ocular rotations unless you experience these actions by seeing them happen and feeling them with your own fingers. It might interest your skeptics to know that Leonardo da Vinci (1452–1519), who dissected many human bodies to learn about the actions of muscles, devised the method of tugging on tapes attached to the insertion of muscles to teach himself how the muscles worked. To experience the actions of the muscles, get these materials to make the two models:

1. To make an **axial rotation model** get:
   a. A small ball of clay, a piece of a kitchen sponge, or even a wad of gum
   b. Three toothpicks or, better, thin round applicator sticks
2. To make an **eyeball rotation model** get:
   a. A soft, sponge rubber ball, 2 to 3 in. in diameter, that you can stick pins into
   b. Several straight pins, preferably with large heads
   c. A piece of leather (from the tongue of an old shoe) or plastic
   d. Scissors

A. Model 1: Axial rotation of the eyeball around three axes

1. Each eye has to aim its visual axis at any point within the perimeter of movement. To achieve infinitely variable movement within that perimeter, the eyeball rotates *axially* around three axes: a vertical axis, a lateral axis, and an anteroposterior axis (A-P; Fig. 4-7).
2. To visualize the axial rotation of the eyes, reproduce Model 1 as shown in Fig. 4-7B and label the axes. Rotate each of the three sticks around the *vertical, lateral,* and *A-P axes*. Actually hold the stick between your thumb and forefinger and spin the model. Then and only then, as you see it and your fingers feel it, will you understand that ocular rotation is *axial* rotation, not eccentric rotation. In Fig. 4-8 check the eye which shows the correct, axial rotation.

B. Model 2: Eyeball rotation model to demonstrate the pull of the extraocular muscles

1. On your rubber ball, draw a pupil and an iris. Then place dots for the points of emergence of the three axes and label them (Fig. 4-9).
2. Cut two strips of leather. Mark them MR and LR for the medial and lateral rectus muscles, respectively. Consider this model as the **right** eyeball.
3. Draw an arrow along the strips to represent the vector or line of pull of the contracting muscle (see the arrow in Figs. 4-9 and 4-11).

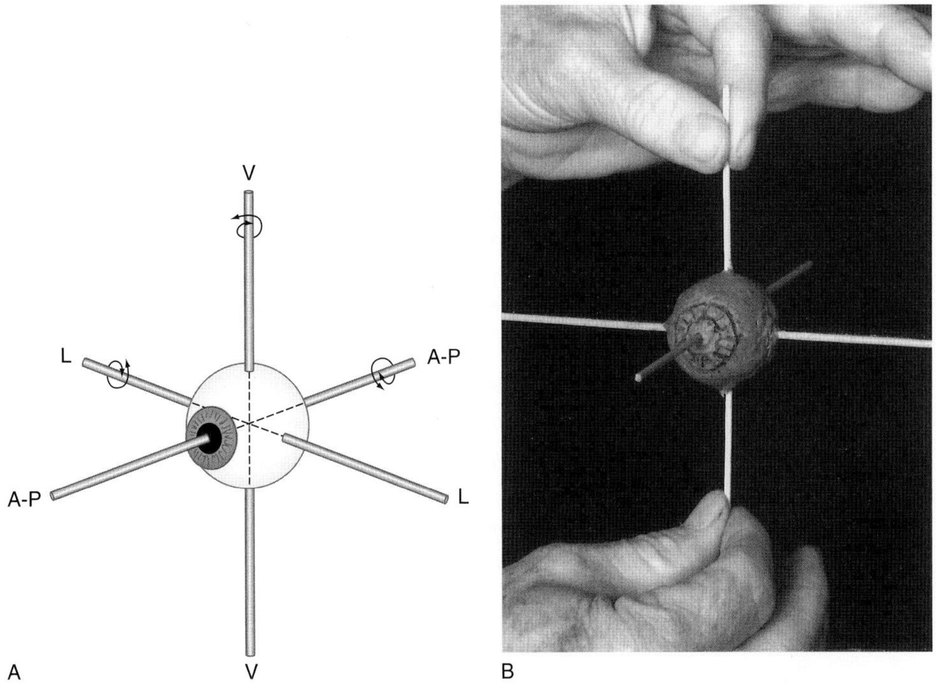

FIGURE 4-7. (A) The three rotational axes of the eye. A-P = anteroposterior; L = lateral; V = vertical. (B) Holding the model as shown, spin it on each of its three axes. You must make the model and spin it between your fingers to fully appreciate the meaning of axial rotation around three axes.

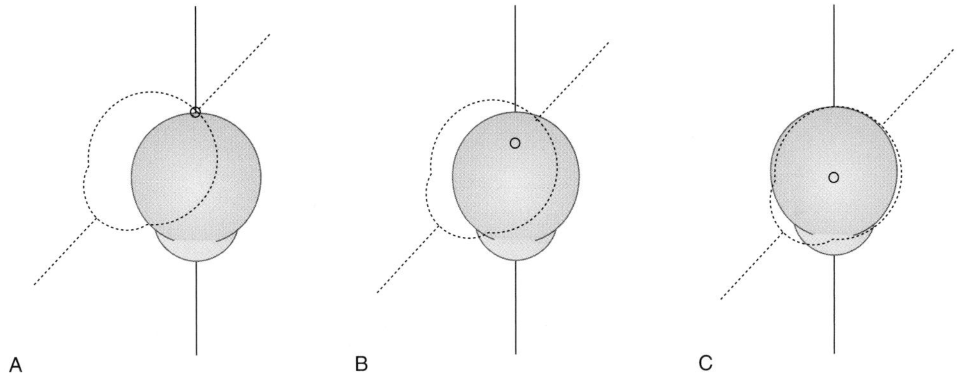

FIGURE 4-8. Diagram showing the alternative ocular rotations. Select the correct *axial* rotation: ❐A/❐B/❐C.

☑ C

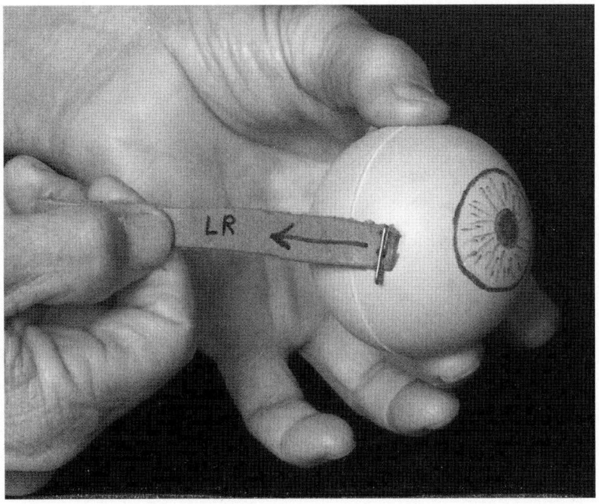

FIGURE 4-9. Ball with leather strip pinned in place to simulate the right eye. The left hand holds the ball with the thumb and second digit pinching the vertical axis. When the right hand pulls back on the LR, the eyeball will rotate to the right around the vertical axis (abduct). LR = lateral rectus muscle.

4. Stick a pin through the anterior end of each strip and into the ball. **Stick the pin anterior to, but exactly in line with, the lateral axis.** If you insert the pin posterior to the lateral axis, the muscles would retract, not rotate, the eyeball (Fig. 4-9).
5. Although in vivo the muscular actions differ somewhat from a mechanical model, the model provides valuable insights with regard to these actions.

C. Types of eye movements and nomenclature

1. The eyeball can rotate laterally or medially around its vertical axis, upward or downward around its horizontal axis, and torsionally (rotate in or out) around its A-P axis.
2. *Ductions* are monocular rotations when the opposite eye is covered, e.g., adduction.
3. *Versions* are binocular parallel rotations to the sides, up, or down.
4. *Vergences* are binocular non-parallel rotations, e.g., convergence or divergence.

D. Action of the medial and lateral rectus muscles

1. The simplest way to move the eyes around two axes is by four muscles (Fig. 4-10). Label the axes in Fig. 4-10 and learn the names of the four rectus muscles. Especially note their insertion anteriorly on the eyeball.

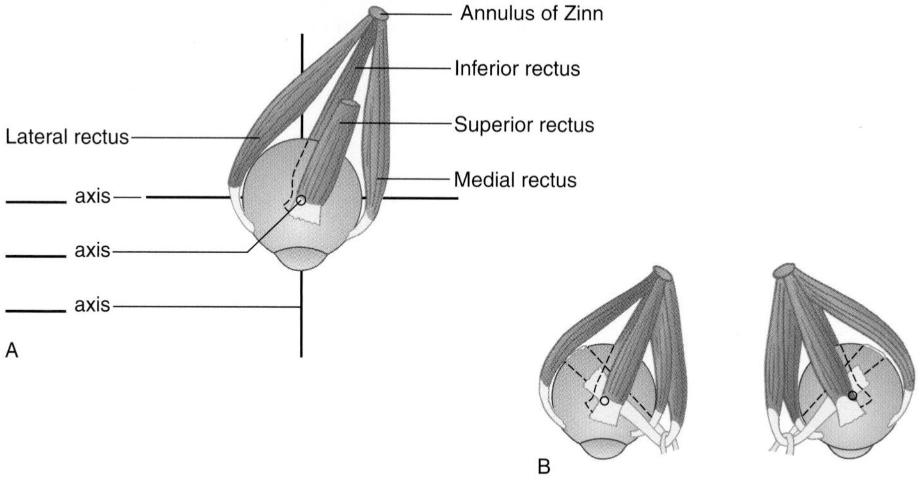

FIGURE 4-10. Origin and insertion of the ocular muscles. (A) Right eye, superior view, showing the origin and direction of insertion of the four recti with the eye in the primary position. (B) Both eyes, showing all six ocular rotatory muscles.

2. While holding the rubber ball with your index finger on the top of the vertical axis and your thumb on the bottom (pincer's grasp), pull straight back on the lateral rectus strip with your other hand. Alternately pull the medial or lateral recti strips and observe the exact axial rotation of the ball around the vertical axis. Study Fig. 4-11 and label the axes.
3. Only from your model will you fully appreciate this fact: You have to pull exactly straight back on the strips that represent the medial and lateral recti, along the vector arrow shown in Fig. 4-11, or the eye will wobble around rather than demonstrating precise axial rotation around the vertical axis.
4. Because the medial and lateral recti pull exactly straight "on center," they have one and only one action: to *ad*duct or *ab*duct the eye. The actions of the medial and lateral recti rotate the eye around the ____________ axis. Because the other ocular rotatory muscles pull off center in relation to the ocular axes, they display more than one effective action.

vertical

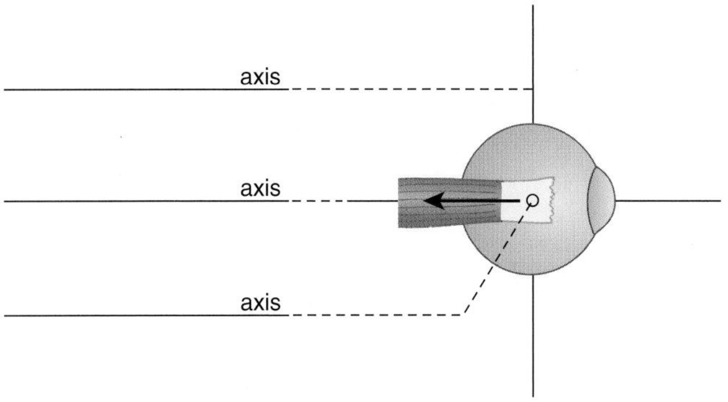

FIGURE 4-11. Lateral view of the right eye showing the direct pull of the lateral rectus muscle over the lateral axis (rotation around the vertical axis).

E. Action of the superior rectus muscle

lateral

1. Attach another leather strip, label it SR for superior rectus, and draw an arrow to represent its vector or line of pull. Figure 4-12B shows that contraction of the superior rectus would rotate the eye *upward* around the ___________ axis. Reproduce this action by holding the rubber ball with its lateral axis between your thumb and second finger. This is the primary action of the muscle.

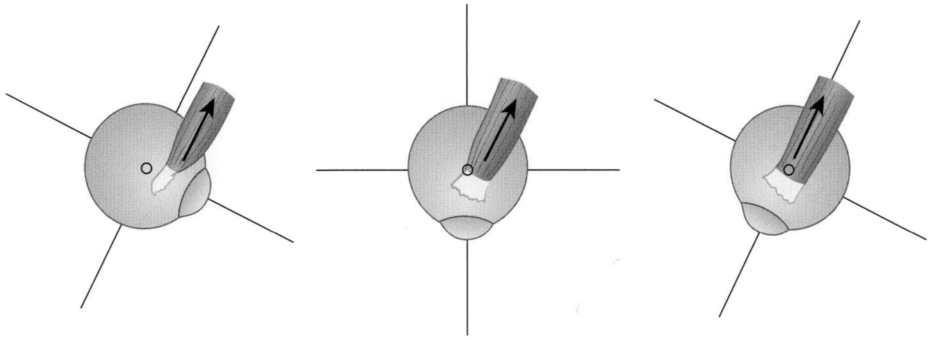

FIGURE 4-12. Right eye and superior rectus muscle, superior view (A–C). Notice how the position of the eye changes the relation of the muscle insertion to the vertical axis and, hence, changes the effective action of the muscle.

2. The angulation, or "off center" pull, of the superior and inferior recti causes a difference in the strength of the primary action and permits secondary and tertiary actions, depending on the position of the eye. To understand how the actions of some ocular muscles change as the eyes rotate, you must know the origin and insertion of the muscles in relation to the axes of the eyeball.

☑ laterally

3. The recti all originate from the *annulus of Zinn,* a cuff that encircles the optic foramen. In Fig. 4-10 (top view of the right eye), note that from their origin the recti angle ❒ laterally/❒ medially.

☑ medial to

4. Figure 4-12B shows that, with the eyes in the primary position, the superior rectus runs somewhat ❒ medial to/❒ lateral to the vertical axis.

upward

   a. We have already seen that the superior rectus has the primary action to rotate the eye _________________ around the lateral axis.
   b. To analyze the other actions of the superior rectus, angle the strip along the normal line of pull of the muscle, as in Fig. 4-12B. Now hold the eyeball by its *vertical* axis and notice that the ball rotates *medially* when you pull back on the strip.

medial; adduction

c. Because its line of pull runs slightly medial to the vertical axis, the superior rectus has a secondary action to rotate the eye *medially* around the vertical axis. The muscle whose sole action is medial rotation of the eye is the ________________ rectus. This action is termed _____ duction.

5. To better visualize the secondary and tertiary actions of the superior rectus, imagine the eye in a position of extreme *ad*duction, as in Figs. 4-12A and 4-13. Hold the ball by the A-P axis and pull on the superior rectus strip after the ball has been turned medially, as in Fig. 4-13. You will find that it rotates *inward*.

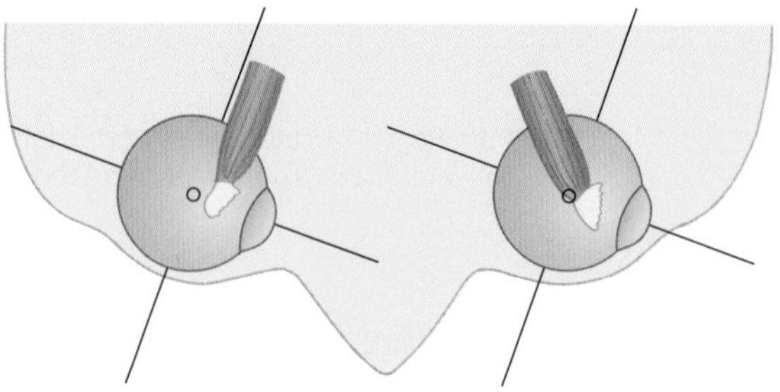

FIGURE 4-13. Superior view of the eyes illustrating the relation of the pull of the superior rectus muscle to the ocular axes when the eyes rotate to the left (rotation exaggerated).

6. Now you have observed that the superior rectus can *elevate* the eye, *ad*duct it, and *tilt the vertical axis inward*. Inward tilting of the vertical axis is called **intorsion,** as shown in Fig. 4-14.

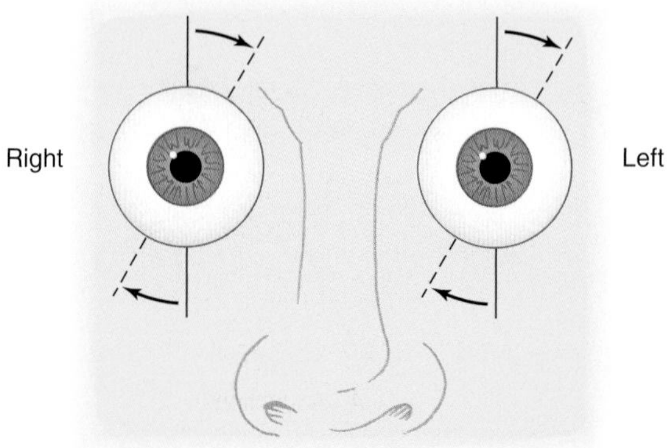

FIGURE 4-14. Torsion of the eyes. The right eye shows *in*torsion, and the left shows *ex*torsion. Naming the torsions depends on whether the top of the vertical axis tilts *in*(intorsion = medially) or *out* (extorsion = laterally).

☑ intorsion

extorsion

A-P

7. In Fig. 4-14, the right eye has rotated around the A-P axis, tilting the top of the vertical axis *in*. This action is called ☐ intorsion/☐ extorsion.

8. In the left eye of Fig. 4-14, the top of the vertical axis tilts *out*. Therefore, it is called _____torsion.

9. The torsions involve rotation of the eye around the _____ axis.

10. When the eye is *ab*ducted, the point of insertion of the tendon of the superior rectus shifts *laterally* in relation to the vertical axis, as shown in Fig. 4-12C. The vector (arrow) now pulls directly over the vertical axis.

See next frame.

11. Would the superior rectus act to *ad*duct or intort when the eye is *ab*ducted? ☐ Yes/☐ No.

☑ abducted

Adduction

12. With the eye *ab*ducted, the superior rectus pulls directly over the vertical axis. It dissipates none of its strength in *ad*duction or intorsion. Therefore, the superior rectus elevates the eye most strongly when the eye is ☐ adducted/☐ straight ahead/☐ abducted.

13. In what position of the eye would the superior rectus have the weakest action of elevation? ___________

elevation; abducted

14. In summary, the primary action of the superior rectus is ____________ of the eye. This action is strongest when the lateral rectus has ____________ the eye.

adduction; intorsion

a. The secondary and tertiary actions of the superior rectus are ____________ and ____________ of the eye.

b. What direction would you ask the Pt to look to test the *strongest* elevating action of the right superior rectus?

Up and to the right

____

F. Action of the inferior rectus muscle

☑ depress

1. The *inferior rectus* muscle has the same direction of origin and insertion as the superior rectus (Fig. 4-10). The primary action of the inferior rectus is to ❐ depress/❐ elevate the eye.

adduct

2. Its secondary action would be to ____________ the eye.

☑ externally

3. To analyze the tertiary inferior rectus action, pin another strip to the rubber ball to represent the inferior rectus. Hold the ball by the A-P axis and consider the inferior rectus action with the eye *ad*ducted. Then, when the inferior rectus contracts, the top of the vertical axis should tilt ❐ internally/❐ externally.

extorsion; intorsion

4. External tilting of the vertical axis is called ________________. Internal tilting is called ________________.

Adduction

5. What is the only eye position in which the superior and inferior recti could rotate the eye in the same direction? ____________________________

6. The superior and inferior recti are ineffective *ad*ductors until the medial rectus muscle, the most critical muscle for *ad*duction, has already begun to act.

7. To test the strongest action of the right inferior rectus as a depressor, in what direction would you ask the Pt to look?

Down and to the right (down and out)

____.

8. In summary, list the primary and two supplementary actions of the inferior rectus muscle.

Depress; adduct; extort

____

G. Action of the superior oblique muscle

1. The superior oblique originates from the lesser wing of the sphenoid bone, just above the annulus of Zinn. Its tendon runs through a trochlea (pulley) attached to the rim of the bony orbit (Fig. 4-15A). When the tendon runs to the eye, it inserts *posteriorly* to allow the superior oblique to have an effective pull when contracting. In so attaching, the tendon runs somewhat *medial* to the vertical axis, like the superior and inferior recti. Cut another strip, label it SO (superior oblique), and draw an arrow to represent its vector along the line of the tendon.

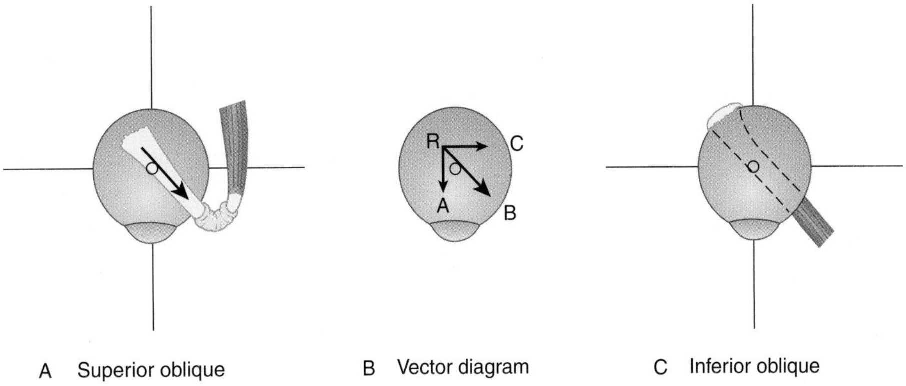

FIGURE 4-15. Right eye, superior view, showing the actions of the superior and inferior oblique muscles (A–C). (A) The arrow represents the line of pull of both muscles. This vector runs somewhat medial to the vertical axis. Notice that vector R-B originates at R, posterolateral to the vertical axis.

2. The vector diagram of Fig. 4-15B resolves arrow R-B into effective components.
   a. Vector R-A ❒ depresses/❒ elevates the eye around the ____________ axis.
   b. Vector R-C ❒ abducts/❒ adducts the eye around the ____________ axis and ❒ intorts/❒ extorts the eye around the ____________ axis.
   c. Therefore, vector R-B acts to ____________ the eye, ____________ the eye, and ____________ the eye.

☑ depresses; lateral

☑ abducts; vertical; ☑ intorts; A-P

depress; abduct; intort

3. **To recapitulate:** Contraction of the superior oblique, when the eye starts in the primary position, causes:
   a. A primary action to ❒ depress/❒ elevate the eye.
   b. A secondary action to ❒ adduct/❒ abduct/❒ elevate the eye.
   c. A tertiary action to ❒ intort/❒ extort the eye.

☑ depress

☑ abduct

☑ intort

4. With the eye in the primary position, the line of pull of the superior oblique tendon runs *medial* to the vertical axis (arrow in Fig. 4-15A). Complete Fig. 4-16 to show the relation of the vertical axis of the eye to the line of pull of the superior oblique tendon when the eye is *ad*ducted.

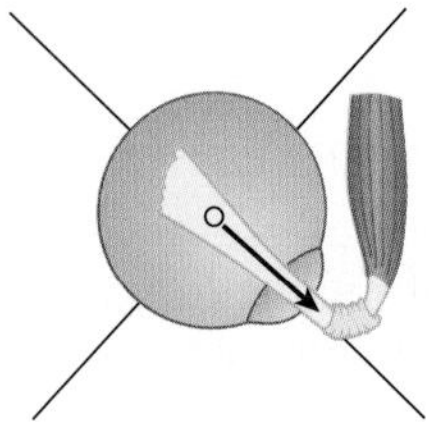

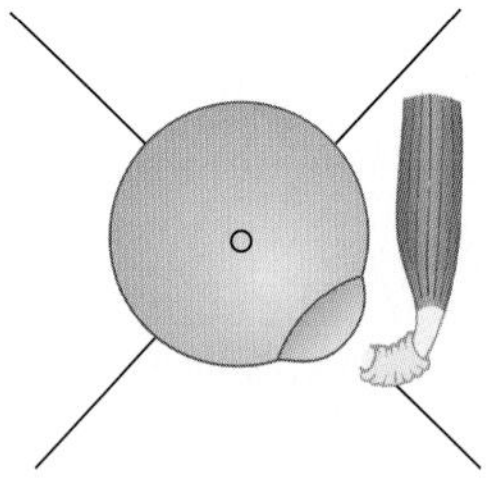

FIGURE 4-16. Blank to be completed to show the relation of the line of pull of the superior oblique tendon to the vertical axis when the eye is adducted.

5. When the eye is *ad*ducted, the tendon of the superior oblique pulls directly over the vertical axis. Therefore, none of the depressor action of the muscle is dissipated in the other actions, which are to ____________ and to ____________ the eye.

abduct; intort

6. In what position of the eye does the superior oblique show the strongest *primary* action of downward rotation of the eye? ____________

Adduction

7. Hence, the clinical test for the strongest action of the superior oblique is to ask the Pt to look ____.

in and down

H. Action of the inferior oblique muscle

1. The inferior oblique muscle, in contrast to the other ocular muscles, originates from the medial inferior rim of the bony orbit. **No other ocular muscle originates anteriorly.** In inserts on the posterior part of the eyeball. To attain sufficient resting length, it wraps further around the eye than the other muscles.
2. The inferior oblique passes posteriorly, somewhat *medial* to the vertical axis. Its obliquity and alignment with the vertical axis matches the superior oblique (Figs. 4-15A and 4-15C).
   a. The *primary* action is exactly antagonistic to the superior oblique. The inferior oblique acts to ____________________ the eye.
   b. The *secondary* action is to ____________________ the eye, acting in harmony with the superior oblique.
   c. The *tertiary* action is to _____ the eye, antagonistic to the superior oblique.
   d. The one direction in which the superior and inferior obliques rotate the eyeball the same way is ____________________.

elevate

abduct

extort

abduction

3. The obliques can abduct strongly only after the lateral rectus has already started to rotate the eye laterally. After lateral rectus paralysis, the obliques cannot initiate abduction and the eye cannot be abducted. We run squarely into a problem. Intorsion, the so-called tertiary action of the superior oblique, is clinically one of its most important actions. Therefore, in classifying intorsion as a tertiary action, we do not dismiss it as a negligible action.

I. A vector diagram of ocular muscle action

1. In the blanks of Fig. 4-17, place the initials of the muscles represented by the vector arrow numbers.

1. LR
2. IR
3. SR
4. MR
5. IO
6. SO

1. ________
2. ________
3. ________
4. ________
5. ________
6. ________

A

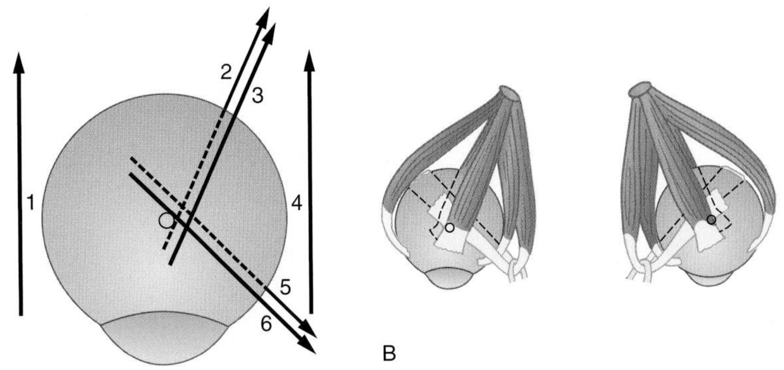

FIGURE 4-17. Eyes viewed from above. (A) Composite vector diagram showing the effective direction of pull of the muscles with the right eye in the primary position. Fill in blanks 1 to 6 with initials corresponding to the muscle represented by the vector. (B) Composite drawing of all six ocular rotatory muscles. Match them with the vectors shown in A.

lateral rectus

2. The vector diagram combined with a knowledge of the origin and insertion enable you to remember forever the actions of the ocular muscles. We can state that, when the eye is in the primary position, the pull or vector of all the ocular muscles is *medial* to the vertical axis except for the ____________________ muscle.

superior and inferior obliques and the superior and inferior recti

3. Because four of the ocular muscles pull "off center," i.e., medial to the vertical axis, they display their particular secondary and tertiary actions. The four muscles that pull off center when the eye is in the primary position are the ____ ____.

medial and lateral recti

4. The two muscles that always pull "on center" and therefore have only primary actions are the ____________________.

5. Cover the answers in Table 4-1 and recite them. Use drawings or the ball model, when necessary, to deduce the answers.

TABLE 4-1 · **Summary of Actions of the Individual Extraocular Muscles**

Muscle	Primary action	Secondary	Tertiary
Medial rectus	Adducts		
Lateral rectus	Abducts		
Superior rectus	Elevates	Adducts	Intorts
Inferior rectus	Depresses	Adducts	Extorts
Superior oblique	Depresses	Abducts	Intorts
Inferior oblique	Elevates	Abducts	Extorts

J. Mnemonic summary of the actions of the ocular rotatory muscles

The only action of the **medial** and **lateral recti** is to rotate the eyeballs **medially** and **laterally,** respectively.

The **superior** and **inferior recti** rotate the eyeball **superiorly** and **inferiorly,** respectively, as their primary actions when the eyes are turned **outward.** Hence, all recti primarily rotate the eyeball in the direction of the adjective component of their names.

With the eyes turned in the, **superior** and **inferior obliques** rotate the eyeballs **inferiorly** and **superiorly,** respectively, as their primary actions, an action opposite to the adjective component of their names.

The **superior oblique intorts** the eye, except when the eye looks in.

The **inferior oblique extorts** the eye, except when the eye looks in.

K. Yoking of ocular muscles

Note: If you did not do Sections II, A to J, use Table 4-1 and Fig. 4-18 for the following frames:

1. SR 4. IO 7. SR

2. LR 5. MR 8. LR

3. IR 6. SO 9. IR

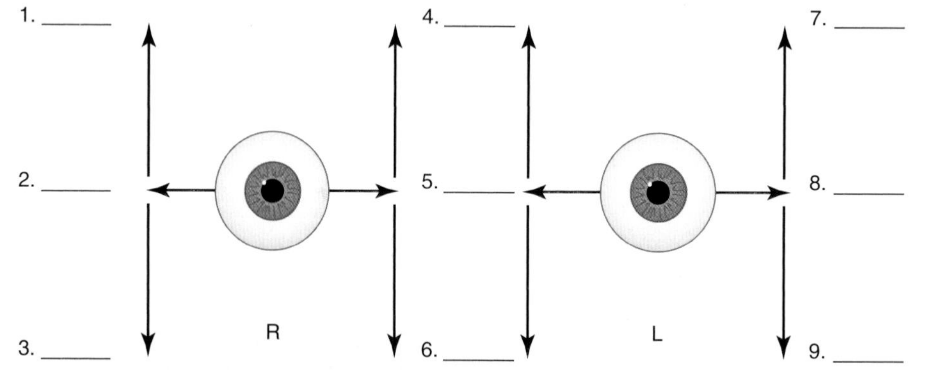

FIGURE 4-18. Yoking of the strongest actions of ocular muscles in moving the eyes in the cardinal directions of gaze. In blanks 1 to 9, place the initials of the muscle whose strongest action is indicated by the arrow. Then read across the diagram, e.g., 1 to 4 to 7, to see which muscles pair up. Thus, in looking to the right and up, the superior rectus muscle (1) of the right eye is yoked with the inferior oblique muscle (4) of the left eye. L = left; R = right.

1. The ocular muscles of the two eyes collaborate with each other to keep the eyes aligned. If a Pt has diplopia when looking to the left, you would suspect weakness of the *ab*ductor of the left eye or the *ad*ductor of the right eye.
   a. The strongest *ab*ductor of the left eye is the muscle whose only function is abduction, the ____________________ muscle.

   lateral rectus

   b. The strongest *ad*ductor of the right eye is the muscle whose only function is *ad*duction, the ____________________ muscle.

   medial rectus

   c. When muscles of the two eyes act in unison for conjugate gaze, we say that they are **yoked.**
2. Suppose a Pt complains of diplopia only when looking *up* and to the *left*.
   a. When the left eye is *ab*ducted, the strongest elevator is the ____________________ muscle.

   superior rectus

   b. When the right eye is *ad*ducted, the elevating power of its superior rectus is diverted to the secondary action of the muscle, ____________________, and to the tertiary action of the muscle, ____________________.

   adduction; intorsion

inferior oblique

c. As the superior rectus loses its elevator strength during *ad*duction, the muscle that converts its action solely to elevation is the ________________.

☑ decreases; ☑ increases

d. During *ad*duction of an eye, the elevator action of the superior rectus ❐ decreases/❐ increases, and the elevator action of the inferior oblique simultaneously ❐ decreases/❐ increases.

superior rectus; inferior oblique

e. Thus for upward gaze to the left, the muscle that elevates the left eye, the ________________ muscle, is yoked to a muscle of the right eye. The yoked muscle of the right eye that replaces the vanishing elevator action of the right superior rectus as the eye *ad*ducts is the ________________ muscle.

Superior oblique

f. Which muscle has the strongest *depressant* action when the eye is *ad*ducted? ________________

inferior rectus

g. The muscle with the strongest depressor action with the eye *ab*ducted is the ________________.

inferior rectus; superior oblique

h. A Pt looking to the right has diplopia when he looks down. Which of the yoked muscles should you suspect of weakness: the ________________ muscle of the right eye or the ________________ muscle of the left eye.

During conjugate eye movements, the yoke muscles (the muscles of the two eyes that rotate the eyes in the same direction) receive equal stimulation.

3. **Hering's law (Ewald Hering, 1834–1918) of equal stimulation of the yoke muscles.** The law states that the muscles yoked for conjugate eye movements receive *equal* stimulation by the nervous system. Thus, if the *right* lateral rectus is stimulated to rotate the right eye to the right, the *left* medial rectus receives equal stimulation. This principle is called *Hering's law*. State Hering's law in your own words.

____

4. **A summary of the yoke muscles.** If you studied pages 130–139, complete Fig. 4-18 by writing in the initials of the muscles **most important** for the movement indicated by the arrows. If you did not read those pages, simply copy in the correct initials for reference.

L. Oppositional action of pairs of ocular muscles of one eye and the tonic innervation of the extraocular muscles

1. The medial and lateral recti of one eye exemplify a general law of the EOMs: The muscles of one eye act in agonist and antagonist pairs. For each direction of eye movement, one or more muscles act in exactly the opposite direction.
2. An electromyographic needle inserted into the EOMs records a continuous play of nerve impulses called **tonic innervation** that maintains light tension in the muscles with the eyes still and in the primary position. Other skeletal muscles are electrically silent when the part they move is at rest. During conjugate movement of the eyes, Sherrington's law of reciprocal inhibition holds: The muscle or muscles in one eye that cause the rotation are actively innervated, whereas the antagonists are inhibited. After the eye movements stop, tonic innervation resumes.
3. Because each agonist–antagonist pair of EOMs receives a tonic, equal play of nerve impulses, the pull of one muscle balances the pull of the other, like opposing rubber bands under slight tension. Thus, **the position of the eyes is always positively determined.**
4. After paralysis of one EOM, the eye deviates in the direction of pull of the intact, oppositional muscle, which continues to receive its tonic innervation. After paralysis of the lateral rectus muscle (VI nerve palsy), tonic innervation of the medial rectus causes the eye to rotate ❐ inward/❐ outward.

☑ inward

M. Review of actions of the extraocular muscles

1. List the six ocular rotatory muscles and their origins and insertions in relation to the axes of ocular rotation.
2. The muscles (or tendons in the case of the superior obliques) all insert *distal* to the way they approach the globe (Fig. 4-17).

3. With the eyes in the primary position, the vector of only one muscle, the lateral rectus, pulls *lateral* to the vertical axis (Fig. 4-17).
4. Only one muscle, the inferior oblique, originates anteriorly, and only one muscle, the superior oblique, runs through a trochlea (pulley).
5. Reason out the position of the eye when only one muscle is paralyzed. The eye turns away from the pull of the paralytic muscle because the intact muscles act unopposed.
6. Reason out the position of the eye when only one nerve is intact.
7. Distinguish between the *possible* movements of the muscle according to the mechanics of origin and insertion and the *strongest* movements of the muscle when the eye is rotated into the optimum position.

III. CLINICAL TESTS FOR OCULAR MALALIGNMENT AND THE RANGE OF EYE MOVEMENTS

A. Initial inspection of the relation of the limbus to the eyelid

Initially inspect the relation of the limbus to the lid margins as the Pt gazes straight ahead. Then look for gross malalignment of the eyes but beware of first impressions, particularly if the Pt has asymmetrical eyelids or canthus dystopia, as many young children do. Depend on the corneal reflection test as the best test for ocular malalignment.

B. Technique for the corneal light reflection (Hirschberg's) test

Use a partner, if available, but the instructions assume that you have no partner and will use a hand mirror.

1. Darken the room and locate one distant light source such as a light bulb or an otoscope light.
2. Face the light source and gaze straight ahead into the mirror while holding it as far away as possible to avoid convergence. Observe that one bright diamond of light reflects off each cornea. By slight mirror movements, try to center these diamonds simultaneously on the two corneas. What is the exact location of the corneal light reflection with respect to the true geometric center of each cornea?

____

____

After being centered as carefully as possible, the points of corneal light reflection fall slightly medial to the true corneal centers. The visual axis does not quite coincide with the geometric anteroposterior axis, which diverges slightly (Fig. 4-19).

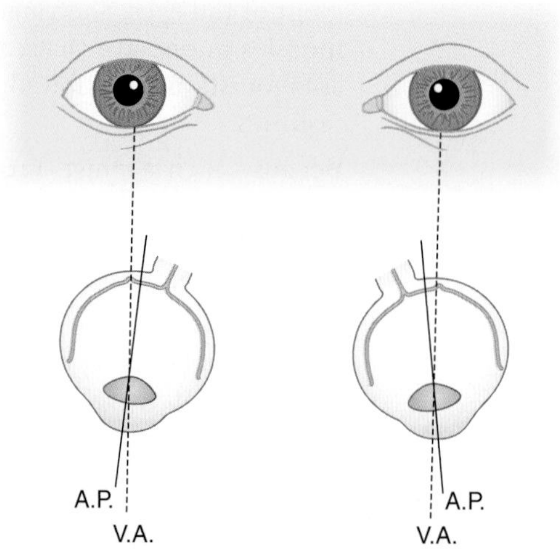

FIGURE 4-19. Diagram to show why the corneal light reflections are slightly medial to the true geometric centers of the corneas. The patient is looking straight ahead. The fixation reflexes have automatically aligned the visual axes parallel to each other, to bring the parallel light rays from infinity onto the foveae. The true, geometric A.P. axes of the eyes now diverge slightly. A.P. = anteroposterior axis; V.A. = visual axis.

3. While watching your corneal light reflections, move the mirror slightly to one side (or have your partner move his eyes). The points of light reflection from each cornea then displace the same distance from the corneal centers, to end on corresponding corneal points, if ocular alignment is normal in all fields of gaze. Move your mirror around full range, chasing the points of reflection over the surfaces of the corneas and noting the correspondence of the points of each eye.
4. Thus, the examiner (Ex) checks for ocular malalignment in two ways:
   a. Abnormal relation of the corneal limbus to the margins of the eyelids.
   b. Non-correspondence of the points of corneal light reflection
5. Why do you look for *non*-correspondence of the corneal light reflections and *ab*normality of the limbus relation rather than for correspondence and normality?
____
____

As a first principle of physical diagnosis, expect every finding to be abnormal until proven otherwise. If you missed this answer, review page 38.

C. Technique for evaluating the range of movement of the eyes

1. During the history, the Ex judges the range of volitional eye movements.
2. Start the formal examination with the Pt sitting. Gently press on top of the Pt's head with one hand and fix the head in position by a "proprioceptive link" between yourself and the Pt, permitting only the eyes to move. Mentally retarded or demented Pts have difficulty separating eye and head movements.
3. Ask the Pt to fixate on your finger, which you hold up in the midline, about 50 cm away, at station 1 in Fig. 4-20.

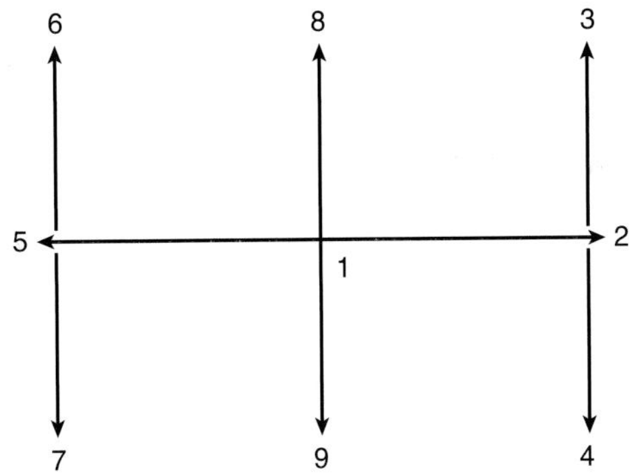

FIGURE 4-20. The H-shape through which the examiner moves his finger to test ocular motility.

4. Request the Pt to follow your finger horizontally with the eyes to station 2, the extreme end of lateral gaze. For testing *horizontal* eye movements and vergences, hold the finger *vertically;* for testing *vertical* movements, hold the finger *horizontally*. Then the Pt can more easily follow the finger and better appreciate any minimal separation of diplopic images that might occur.
5. Hold the finger at station 2 and inspect the corneal light reflections and the relation of the limbus to the lid margins, canthi, and caruncles. Look for nystagmus (discussed in Chapter 5).
6. Next, move to stations 3 and 4 at the extremes of lateral upward and downward gaze. Repeat the observations of step 4.
7. Move your finger back to the horizontal plane and across to station 5 and repeat all observations and maneuvers at stations 6 and 7.
8. Move your finger back to station 1 and say, "Look right at my finger," as you move it in to touch the bridge of the Pt's nose. Look for convergence and the accompanying pupilloconstriction. Usually, one eye breaks off convergence when the finger is several centimeters away from the nose.
9. Finally hold your finger horizontally and ask the Pt to follow it to stations 8 and 9.

10. Figure 4-21 shows the normal range of eye movements in millimeters. Notice that upward gaze has the least range. Diffuse brain disease impairs the relatively restricted upward movements more than other movements, but midbrain lesions can selectively impair upward or downward movements or both.

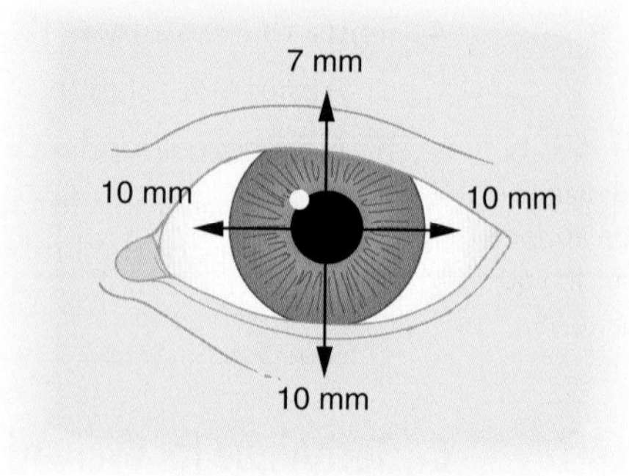

FIGURE 4-21. Range of ocular rotations, in millimeters.

11. Because the Pt may have experienced diplopia while observing your finger, ask the Pt about it. Select the best-phrased question:
    a. ❒ You are seeing two fingers instead of one, aren't you?
    b. ❒ Do you have diplopia?
    c. ❒ Do you see one or two fingers?

☑ c

12. Students frequently make type a and b errors. The first question may force an erroneous answer, because the Pt expects the doctor to know what will happen. The second question uses a technical term, *diplopia*, unfamiliar to the Pt. Make a general rule about phrasing such questions.

____

Avoid questions that imply the answer or that use technical terms. Ask questions that allow Pts to report freely and as exactly as possible whatever they experience.

13. If the Pt reports double vision, darken the room and watch the corneal light reflections as the Pt pursues a tiny light, such as an otoscope lamp, through the configuration shown in Fig. 4-20.

D. The cover-uncover test for ocular malalignment

After inspecting the eyes in the primary position and through the whole range of movement, do the **cover-uncover test** (Fig. 4-22).

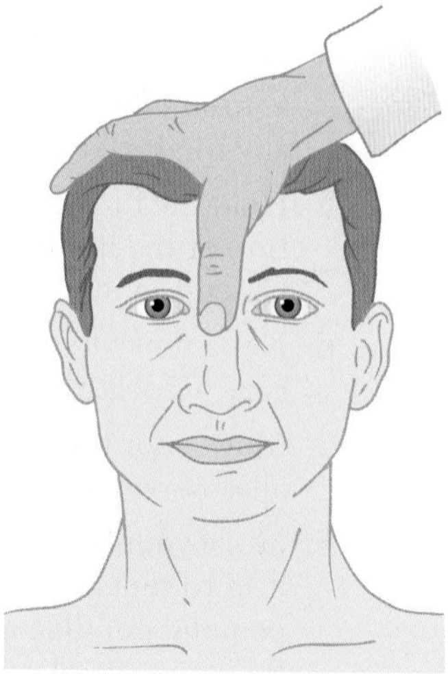

FIGURE 4-22. Resting position of the examiner's thumb for the cover-uncover test.

1. **Place your thumb between the Pt's eyes, as shown in Fig. 4-22.**
2. **Instruct the Pt to stare at a distant point.** Admonish the Pt to maintain fixation on the distant point, which is essential.
3. **Move your thumb first in front of one eye, then back to the bridge of the nose, and then over the other eye.** The thumb does not have to occlude all vision, only *central,* that is, *foveal* vision. Look for deviation of one or both eyes and for the corneal light reflections as you move the thumb from station to station.
4. **Interpretation of the cover-uncover test:** Covering one eye requires the other eye to foveate. When both eyes are locked together in fixation, neither eye moves: **the Pt has no ocular malalignment.** Movement of an eye after occlusion of central vision means a defective alignment lock of the eyes.

E. The heterotropias: naming overt ocular deviations

1. Medical terms for overt ocular malalignments are *heterotropia* and *strabismus*. The ophthalmologist speaks of "heterotropia," and the neurologist speaks of "strabismus." The layman speaks of "squints" or "cross-eyed" for convergent strabismus or "wall-eyed" for divergent strabismus.
2. **Definition of heterotropia:** Heterotropia (overt strabismus) is any ocular deviation detected by observing non-correspondence of the corneal light reflections with the eyes in any position. This is an ❒ operational/❒ interpretational definition. Explain.

____

☑ **operational**. Heterotropia is defined in terms of the maneuver or operation by which you can identify it. An operational definition states what operations you do, the actual steps and actions required, to personally verify something through your own senses.

   a. Suppose we stated that "Heterotropia is any overt deviation of the visual axis of an eye from the fixation point." This would be an ❒ operational/❒ interpretational definition.

      This definition, based on an imaginary "visual axis" is an interpretational definition. It does not state the operations by which the observer may personally discover heterotropia.

☑ **interpretational**

   b. The physician must clearly distinguish operational from interpretational definitions. Most dictionary definitions uncritically mix operation and interpretation. Suppose you wish to find the length of a meter. Some dictionaries will advise you that a meter is one ten-millionth of the distance between the equator and the poles, measured on a meridian of the Earth. Well, don't try to step that off. That obviously *interprets* the length of a meter in terms of something else. Try this definition: "A meter is the distance between two transverse lines on a platinum-iridium bar kept at the National Bureau of Standards, when the bar is at 0°C." The definition implies the operation required to discover the length of a meter: you lay your own bar down beside the meter bar and mark the distance on it. Now that simple operation enables you to derive, verify, and actually experience the length of a meter. In other words, if you do *this,* you will find out *that.*
   c. As operationally defined by the best test for it, heterotropia means any overt ocular deviation detected by ____ ____________.

inspecting the eyes for non-correspondence of the corneal light reflections when the eyes are in any position

3. The heterotropias are named according to the direction of deviation of the errant eye:

   Exotropia: eye deviates outward (laterally)

   Esotropia: eye deviates inward (medially)

   Hypertropia: eye deviates upward

   Hypotropia: eye deviates downward
4. To give the full name, designate the right or left eye. Thus, left exotropia means that the left eye deviates ❒ in/❒ out/❒ up/❒ down.
5. If both eyes deviate outward, the Pt would have bilateral __________.

☑ **out**
exotropia

6. The Pts shown in Figs. 4-23A to 4-23D fixate straight ahead in each case. In deciding whether the right or left eye is affected, remember that you face the Pt. In most ocular illustrations, the eyes will face you or face downward on the page to simulate the actual circumstance of looking at a Pt.

A. R esotropia

B. L esotropia

C. L exotropia

D. R hypertropia

A. ______

B. ______

C. ______

D. ______

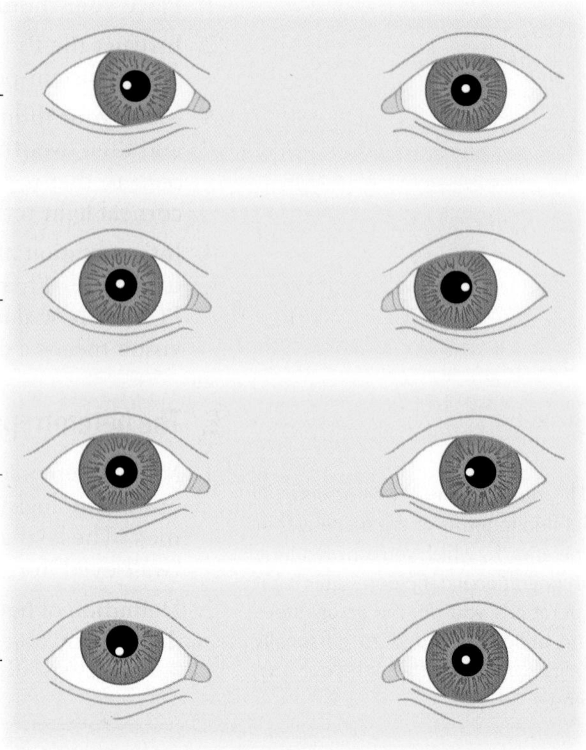

FIGURE 4-23. Location of the corneal light reflections in heterotropia. Write your diagnoses in blanks A to D and designate whether the abnormal eye is right or left.

F. Analysis of the cover-uncover test in monocular heterotropia

☑ right esotropia

1. Start with Fig. 4-24A, step 1 at the bottom of the figure. The Pt was instructed to look straight ahead. Being allowed free vision, the Pt fixates with the left eye, the dominant eye. This Pt appears to have the ocular malalignment called ❒ right/❒ left/❒ ____.

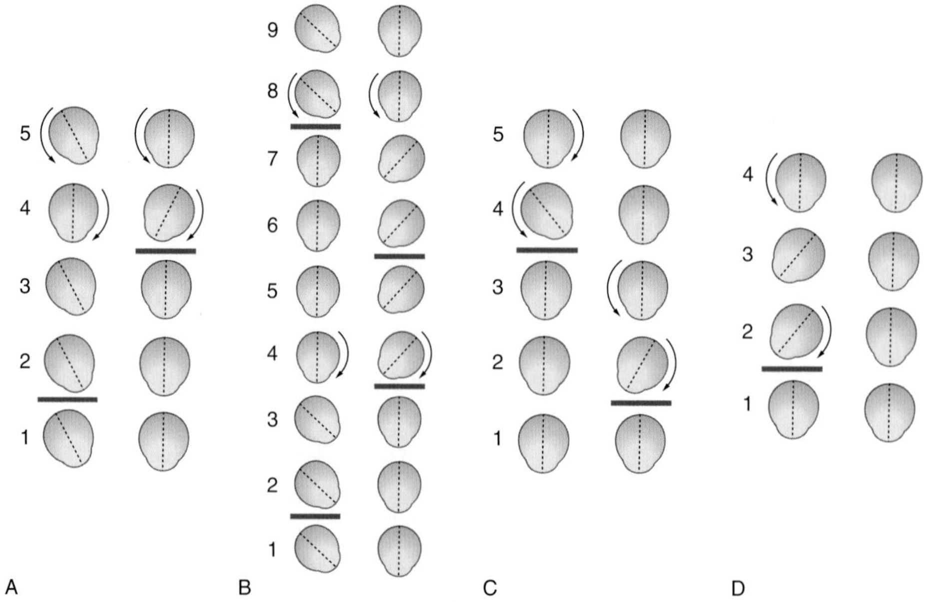

FIGURE 4-24. Results of the cover-uncover test for ocular malalignment. See text for explanation. (Adapted with permission from Jampolsky A. Strabismus. In Holt L, ed. *Pediatric Ophthalmology.* Philadelphia, Lea & Febiger, 1964, Chap. 20, pp. 210–259.)

2. In step 2, the Ex's thumb occludes central vision of the right eye. The ocular alignment of neither eye changes.
3. In step 3, the Ex replaces the thumb on the bridge of the Pt's nose. The eyes maintain the same angulation of the visual axes.
4. In step 4, the Ex re-instructs the Pt to maintain fixation on the original distant point and covers the Pt's left eye. The Pt's right eye then shifts to bring the central light ray onto the fovea, and the left eye rotates inward (as explained later).
5. In step 5, the Ex replaces the thumb on the bridge of the Pt's nose. The eyes shift to return fixation to the dominant left eye.
6. A Pt with right exotropia instead of esotropia would show a similar sequence of events. If you would like, draw the events of right exotropia alongside Fig. 4-24A, steps 1 to 5. In any event, work through Fig. 4-24A without using the instructions in the text.

G. Analysis of the cover-uncover test in alternating heterotropia

1. Work through Fig. 4-24B. In steps 1 and 2 the Pt ostensibly has the ocular malalignment called ❐ right/❐ left ____tropia.

☑ right esotropia

2. Subsequent steps in Fig. 4-24B show that the Pt alternates fixation when allowed free vision. In step 1 the Pt fixates with the left eye, and in step 5 the Pt fixates with the right eye. In contrast, Fig. 2-24A shows that the Pt always returns to fixation with the left eye when allowed free vision. Because the right and left eyes of the Pt in Fig. 2-24B alternately deviate inward, the heterotropia is called *alternating* ____________________.

esotropia

3. Work through Fig. 4-24B, imagining that the Pt's eyes deviated *out* rather than *in*. This heterotropia would be called ____________________.

alternating esotropia

H. The cover-uncover test for heterophorias, the latent rather than the overt ocular deviations

1. When a normal person looks at infinity, the visual axes are parallel. The two retinal images "fuse" into one mental image. Binocular vision requires fusion of central vision and develops as the infant matures. Fusion and fixation reflexes operate to keep both eyes "on target" whenever the normal person's eyes are open.
2. In some Pts, the eyes appear straight during preliminary testing and show normal motility, but upon blocking central vision in one eye, the eye deviates. After removal of the cover, thus reestablishing central vision, the fusion-fixation reflexes immediately realign the eye. Ocular deviations appearing *only* when central vision is blocked and disappearing when central vision is reestablished are **heterophorias.**
3. An ocular deviation apparent when the Pt is permitted free central vision is called hetero____________________, whereas a deviation apparent *only* after occlusion of central vision is called hetero____________________.

tropia; phoria

4. The critical operation of the cover-uncover test is to __________ central vision.

block (cover or occlude)

5. Which maneuver must always restore ocular alignment to distinguish heterophoria from heterotropia? ____________________

Uncovering the occluded eye to allow free vision.

6. *Inward* deviation, or *ad*duction, of the eye only during occlusion of central vision is called ❐ exophoria/❐ hyperphoria/❐ esophoria.

☑ esophoria

7. Overt in-turning of an eye when the Pt has free central vision is called ____________________.

esotropia

8. *Ab*duction of an eye *only* during occlusion of central vision is called ____________________.

exophoria

9. Upward deviation of an eye only during occlusion of central vision is called ____________________.

hyperphoria

> **Mnemonic:** If you have trouble keeping your tropias and phorias straight, try to remember **t** for **t**ropia for overtly **t**urned eye.

esophoria (Because esophoria virtually always involves both eyes, the adjective *alternating* is actually unnecessary.)

10. Fig. 4-24C depicts the cover-uncover test in heterophoria. Work through it. The latent deviation in Fig. 4-24C is called alternating _______________.

☑ right

   a. Suppose in step 5 of Fig. 4-24C that the right eye had not returned to proper alignment on removal of the cover. Such an overt inward deviation, not corrected all of the time by central vision, would be called ❐ right/❐ left esotropia.

☑ intermittent

   b. If one of the Pt's eyes aligns sometimes after removal of the cover, but does not align at other times, the condition is called ❐ intermittent/❐ alternating heterotropia.

11. Complete the definitions in 11a and 11b by stating the clinical maneuvers that disclose heterophoria and heterotropia:

☑ overt

   a. Heterotropia is an ❐ overt/❐ latent ocular deviation as detected by inspection for _______________________________________.

      Non-corresponding corneal light reflections and abnormal relation of the corneal limbus to the eyelid margins.

☑ latent

   b. Heterophoria is an ❐ overt/❐ latent ocular deviation detected by _______________________________________.

      Seeing the eye shift when its central vision is blocked during the cover-uncover test and returning to alignment with restoration of central vision.

intermittent right exotropia

12. Now try to name the abnormality shown in Fig. 4-24D. Pay particular attention to step 3. Because the Pt starts and finishes with apparently straight eyes, the deviation of one eye is only intermittent. Therefore, the abnormality in Fig. 4-24D is called _______________________________.

the right eye remains overtly deviated even after restoration of central vision

13. The abnormality in Fig. 4-24D is a *tropia* rather than a *phoria* because _______________________________________ _______________________________________.

I. Clinical classification of heterotropia

1. To determine the cause of heterotropia, try to classify it into one of two types:
   a. The **paralytic** type, caused by a neuromuscular lesion.
   b. The **non-paralytic** type, usually caused by lesions that impair central vision in one eye and therefore impair fixation: refractive errors, opacification of the cornea or lens (refracting media), or macular lesions.
2. Effect of paralytic heterotropia caused by nerve or muscle lesions on yoke muscles.

☑ away from

   a. After paresis or paralysis of an ocular muscle, the intact muscles act unopposed. Hence, the eye deviates ❐ away from/❐ toward the direction of pull of the afflicted muscle.

☑ increases

   b. When the Pt looks in the direction of pull of the afflicted muscle, the normal eye moves more than the afflicted eye. Hence, the degree of heterotropia and diplopia ❐ increases/❐ decreases when the Pt looks in the direction of action of the afflicted muscle.

☑ left; see next frame

   c. When turning in the direction of pull of a weak muscle, the eye rotates too little, whereas the *normal* eye may rotate too far as the brain strives to move the laggard eye. With a lateral rectus paralysis on the *right*, the Pt's ❐ right/❐ left eye would *ad*duct too far when the Pt looks to the right. Explain this result by Hering's law. _______________________________________ _______________________________________.

   d. Hering's law states that **the nervous system stimulates the yoke muscles equally.** If a muscle is weak, the Pt automatically overstimulates in an attempt to rotate the afflicted eye. The normal yoke muscle receives the same excessive stimulus and contracts too strongly.

3. **Use of the cover-uncover test to analyze neuromuscular heterotropia.** Study Richard Scobee's lucid description to understand primary and secondary deviations of the eyes when the paretic eye and the sound eye are alternately covered or uncovered.

Primary deviation is the deviation of the eye with the paretic muscle when the sound eye is fixing. Secondary deviation is the deviation of the sound eye when the eye with the paretic muscle is fixing. In paresis, secondary deviation is greater than primary deviation.

As an example of primary deviation, suppose the left lateral rectus is paretic, right eye dominant, and the Pt fixes upon some object straight ahead with the right eye. The right medial rectus and the right lateral rectus are normal muscles and require but a normal innervation to maintain fixation with the right eye. According to Hering's law, similar normal innervations go to the yoke muscles of the right lateral rectus and the right medial rectus—to the left medial rectus and the left lateral rectus. The left lateral rectus is paretic and responds in subnormal fashion to normal stimuli; the left medial rectus is normal and thus not properly opposed by the subnormal tonus of its paretic antagonist. The left medial rectus will, therefore, seem to overact since it will pull the left eye inward toward the nose in adduction. The deviation produced is small but definite and is a left esotropia. This is deviation of the paretic eye with the sound eye fixing—primary deviation.

As an example of secondary deviation, suppose the left lateral rectus is paretic, left eye dominant, and the Pt fixes upon some object straight ahead with the dominant left eye. The left lateral rectus, in order to perform its usual functions, must be excessively innervated because it is paretic; its yoke muscle, the right medial rectus, receives the same excessive innervation according to Hering's law. The right medial rectus is a normal muscle receiving an excessive innervation and it makes an excessive response, pulling the right eye well inward in adduction. This is a deviation of the sound eye with the paretic eye's fixing—secondary deviation. In paresis, secondary deviation is greater than primary deviation and the reason should now be obvious.

—Richard Scobee

---

4. The primary and secondary deviations exemplify this law: **The fixating eye, the one that foveates, determines the amount of innervation to both eyes.** This is a straightforward application of a previous law stated in this chapter, namely ________________ law.

Hering's

To encourage the weak muscle to act when fixating, the central nervous system (CNS) sends out a strong stimulus that only the intact eye responds fully to.

5. **Effect of neuromuscular (paralytic) heterotropia on head position**
   a. To avoid diplopia, the Pt tends to compensate for a paretic eye muscle by turning or tilting the head. A **face turn** implies a horizontally acting muscle palsy, **chin elevation** or **depression** implies a vertically acting muscle palsy, and a **head tilt** implies a torsional acting muscle palsy.
   b. The Pt moves the head *toward* the action of the weak muscle. To avoid diplopia, a Pt with a right lateral rectus palsy would tend to keep the head turned to the right. Then the left eye *ab*ducts, lining up better with the in-turned right eye.
   c. With a right superior oblique palsy, the Pt has weakness of ❒ intorsion/❒ extorsion of the right eye, an action for which the superior oblique is mainly responsible.

   ☑ intorsion

   d. The unopposed action of the extortors would cause extorsion of the eye. In compensation, therefore, the Pt with a right superior oblique palsy tilts his or her head to the ❒ right/❒ left to prevent diplopia.

   ☑ left (If the answer is unclear, review Figs. 4-12 and 4-14.)

e. A persistent head tilt or turn is called **torticollis.** Oblique muscle palsy is only one of its many causes. With a unilateral acute or acquired superior oblique muscle palsy, the Pt will tilt the head to the side opposite the paralytic muscle, turn the face to the same side, and keep the chin depressed—actions all designed to minimize the use of the superior oblique muscle (Brazis et al., 2007).

6. **Effect of neuromuscular heterotropia on vision in infants:** suppression amblyopia.
   a. Infants with heterotropia learn to suppress the image from the errant eye, a condition called **suppression amblyopia** or **amblyopia ex anopsia.** If suppression continues for the first years of life, the deviant eye may become completely blind, even though the retina and visual pathways remain structurally intact. The strength of the suppressive forces that rid the visual image of confusing elements may prevent the child from ever recovering vision.
   b. **Suppression amblyopia** is a preventable cause of monocular blindness, treated by the simple expedient of placing a patch intermittently over the sound eye to require the Pt to use the errant eye.
   c. Suppression amblyopia occurs not only with heterotropia but also with many monocular disorders of retinal image formation—refractive errors, opacification of the refracting media, or retinal lesions.
   d. Never neglect ocular deviations or other impediments to vision because of a naive expectation that the infant will simply "grow out" of it. The infant may grow more and more "into" it. A complete eye examination of every infant will disclose this preventable cause of blindness.

J. Non-paralytic or concomitant heterotropia versus paralytic heterotropia

1. Of the two varieties of eye deviation, a concomitant heterotropia, has the same amount of deviation in both eyes in all directions of gaze, but in non-concomitant heterotropia, the angle of deviation changes with the position of the eyes.
2. With muscular paresis or paralysis, the eyes do not move concomitantly; one eye moves *more* or *less* than the other. Hence, we can classify paralytic heterotropia as non-concomitant. In concomitant heterotropia or nonparalytic heterotropia, the eyes display the same degree of malalignment in all positions when both eyes are open, but each eye has vision and a normal range of movement (ductions) at monocular testing.
3. The Ex should complete the cover-uncover test in the nine cardinal directions of gaze (Fig. 4-20). If the eyes maintain the same degree of deviation in all directions of gaze, the heterotropia is ❒ concomitant/❒ non-concomitant.

   ☑ **concomitant**

4. Concomitant heterotropia may be intermittent, but when present, the deviation is the same in all directions of gaze. What happens to the angulation of the eyes in heterotropia due to neuromuscular lesions when the eyes move? ______________________

   The angle of deviation of the two eyes increases when the eyes move in the direction of action of the afflicted muscle.

5. Concomitant heterotropia usually results from a disturbance in image formation in one macula—cloudiness of the cornea, a severe refractive error, a cataract, or a macular lesion. It seems as if the retina establishes a new macula, off center from the true macula, and then the visual axis aligns on the new macula.
6. The Pt alternates in fixating with the normal eye and the abnormal one. The Pt learns to suppress vision from whichever eye that is not in use at the moment for fixation, much as you can learn to use a monocular microscope or an ophthalmoscope with both eyes open. Thus, the Pt alternately fixes with one eye and suppresses vision from the other eye. When fixation alternates between the two eyes, suppression amblyopia does not occur.
7. **The clinical characteristics of concomitant heterotropia:**
   a. The deviation of the eyes is ❒ the same/❒ different for the primary position and in all directions of gaze.

   ☑ **the same**

   b. In contrast to non-concomitant heterotropia, the primary and secondary deviations disclosed by the cover-uncover test are ❒ equal/❒ unequal in concomitant heterotropia.

   ☑ **equal**

If they weren't equal at all times, the Pt would have non-concomitant heterotropia.

c. When either eye fixates alone, it shows a full range of motility. None of the individual muscles is paralyzed.

☑ non-concomitant

8. The term *paralytic heterotropia* is essentially synonymous with ☐ concomitant/☐ non-concomitant heterotropia.

concomitant

9. The term *non-paralytic heterotropia* is essentially synonymous with ____________________ heterotropia.

10. Complete Table 4-2 by making a check mark in the proper column.

P	N-P
✓	
	✓
✓	
	✓
	✓
✓	
✓	

TABLE 4-2 · Differential Diagnosis of Paralytic and Non-Paralytic Heterotropia*

Clinical characteristic	Paralytic (non-concomitant)	Non-paralytic (concomitant)
Ocular deviation changes with eye movement		
Full movement when each eye is tested after covering the other		
Secondary deviation is greater than primary deviation		
Secondary and primary deviations are equal		
Frequently has opacity or severe refractive error in one eye		
Has diplopia if heterotropia occurs after young age		
Often has compensatory head turning or tilting		

*These rules apply to most patients. With longstanding heterotropia, fibrosis, contractures, and eccentric fixation or fusional problems at the cortical level may confound the diagnosis.

K. The laws of diplopia and the clinical analysis of diplopia

1. Repeat the canthal compression experiment and obtain diplopia with the finger vertical. Move the finger to the right and to the left while studying the distance between the true and false images. Identify the false image by its haziness. This is one law of diplopia: **The aberrant or "false" image is always hazier than the "true" image.**

a. If the false image projects to the right of the target finger (from weakness of the right lateral rectus muscle), the distance between the images increases as you move the target finger to the ☐ left/☐ right side (see Fig. 4-25).

☑ right

b. If the false image projects to the *left*, the distance between the images increases as you move the target finger to the ☐ left/☐ right side.

☑ left

c. If your eyes follow the images too far laterally, one disappears. Can you discover an explanation (look for the simplest one).

The nose blocks the light rays from entering one eye. The brain no longer receives two confusing images.

☑ **increases.** Go to the next frame for the explanation, unless you would like to try to work it out yourself.

2. As you move your finger away from the midpoint, the distance between the true and false images ☐ increases/☐ decreases/☐ stays the same.

3. **Explanation for the increasing distance between the diplopic images:**

a. In Fig. 4-25A, the left eye, aligned on target, receives the real image on its fovea. The mind projects the visual image back to the true target position (T_1). The deviated right eye receives the real image on the nasal side of the fovea. The mind projects the visual image to the right of the true target position (F_1).

b. In Fig. 4-25B, the mobile left eye follows the target to the right (T_2). The paralytic right eye remains stuck in its original position, and, as the target moves

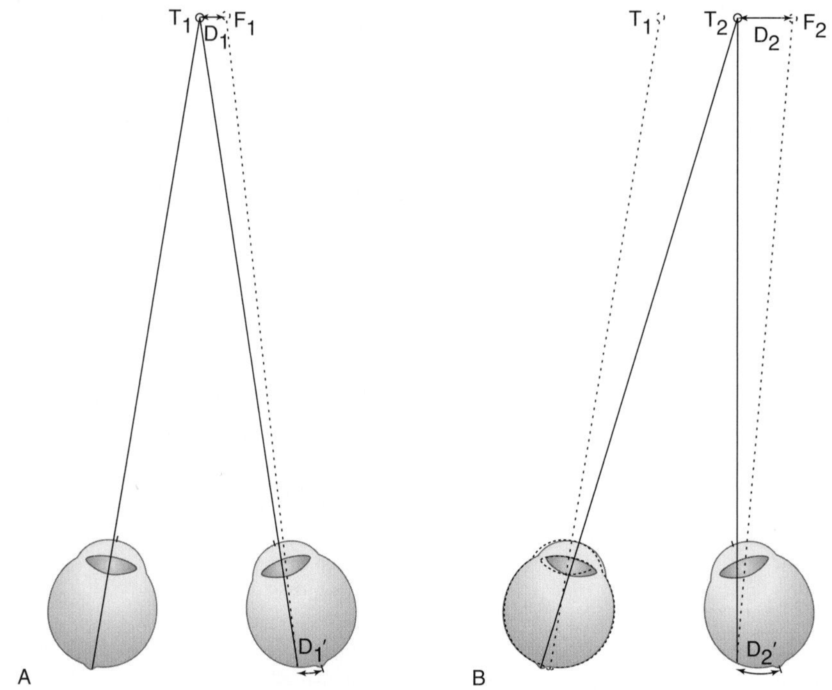

FIGURE 4-25. Illustration of a law of diplopia: the distance between the true and false images increases when the Pt looks in the direction of projection of the false image. The target has moved from site T_1 to site T_2, but the paralytic right eye has not moved. D_1 = distance 1; D_2 = distance 2; F_1 = false image; T_1 = true image.

rightward, the real image moves leftward (nasally) on the retina. The mind projects the visual image more and more rightward. Thus, $D_2 > D_1$.

4. No matter which way the false image deviates, it moves away from the true image. The true image remains centered on target. This is another law of diplopia: **The false image appears peripheral to the true image.**

5. If the false image is to the right of the true image, as in Fig. 4-25A, the eye is deviated to the left (or has not rotated sufficiently to the right). The false image projects in the ❒ same/❒ opposite direction of the eye deviation.

   ☑ **opposite**

   a. If the false image projects above the true image, the afflicted eye deviates ❒ upward/❒ downward.

   ☑ **downward**

   b. If the false image is to the left, the afflicted eye is deviated to the ❒ right/❒ left.

   ☑ **right**

6. This is another law of diplopia: **the false image projects in the ❒ same/❒ opposite direction as the direction of eye deviation.**

   ☑ **opposite**

7. In Fig. 4-25, with projection of the false image to the right, the right eye has failed to *ab*duct to center its visual axis on target. Thus, the diagram depicts paralysis of the ______________________________ muscle.

   lateral rectus

8. This is another diplopia law: **The false image projects ❒ toward/❒ away from the normal direction of pull of the paretic muscle.**

   ☑ **toward**

9. Thus, when the Pt looks in the direction of pull of the paretic muscle or the visual target moves in that direction, the distance between the diplopic images ❒ increases/❒ decreases.

   ☑ **increases**

10. Summarize the four laws of diplopia with respect to image projection:

    a. The law stating whether the true or false image is the sharpest: ______________________________.

    see frame K1

    b. The law of peripheral projection: ______________________________.

    see frame K4

    c. The law of direction of projection with respect to eye deviation: ______________________________.

    see frame K6

See frame K8

d. The law relating the projection of the false image in relation to the pull of the paretic muscle:

____

11. In summary, the use of the corneal light reflection test and the laws of diplopia permit you to diagnose the faulty muscle. Don't memorize these laws. Recover them whenever needed by pressing on your lateral canthus, your Aladdin's lamp, and thinking through the foregoing exercises, particularly Fig. 4-25.

L. A summary of the clinical tests for diplopia

1. **Observe the corneal light reflections:** Locate them when the eyes look straight ahead and when held in the various directions of gaze (Fig. 4-20).
2. **Identify the position of maximum diplopia:** As you move your finger for examining light through all fields of gaze, have the Pt report when the two images are maximally separated. A red glass placed over one eye (by convention placed over the right eye) helps to keep track of the two images during motility testing. The point of maximum separation identifies the action of the weak muscle.
3. **Identify the eye which produces the false image:** The eye that produces the false image has the faulty muscle. The false image is the peripheral image. Identify it by occluding vision alternately in the two eyes. After occlusion of the normal eye, the sharp, central image disappears. After occlusion of the abnormal eye, the hazy, peripheral image disappears.
4. **Reason out the muscle responsible for the deficient ocular action** (Fig. 4-18 and Tables 4-1 and 4-4).

M. Analyze these patients

1. This Pt complains of double vision when looking to the left. Gazing to the left causes the greatest separation of the images.

   medial rectus; lateral rectus

   a. The muscle pairs responsible for left lateral gaze are the ______________ muscle of the right eye and the ______________ muscle of the left eye.

   ☑ left; ☑ left; lateral rectus

   b. On occlusion of the right eye, the central image (true image) disappears. On occlusion of the left eye, the peripheral image (false image) disappears. Therefore, the afflicted eye is the ❒ left/❒ right eye and the afflicted muscle is the ❒ right/❒ left ______________ muscle.

2. The next Pt complains of double vision when looking up. The images separate greatest when the Pt looks up and to the left.

   superior rectus; inferior oblique

   a. The most important muscle for this action of the left eye is the ______________ muscle and that of the right eye is the ______________ muscle.

   ☑ left; ☑ left; superior rectus

   b. On occlusion of the right eye, the central image disappears. On occlusion of the left eye, the peripheral image disappears. Therefore, the afflicted eye is the ❒ right/❒ left and the afflicted muscle is the ❒ right/❒ left ______________.

N. Localizing the lesion by thinking along the course of the ocular motor nerve

1. The lesion that interrupts an ocular motor nerve or any nerve causes different signs if it affects the central or peripheral course. Always start at the nucleus of origin of the nerve and think through to its termination.
2. A central lesion will usually also affect long tracts:

   a. A lesion of cranial nerve (CrN) III in the midbrain will cause ataxia if the dentatothalamic tract is interrupted, contralateral tremor if the lesion also affects the region around the red nucleus, disturbances in vertical gaze if the lesion is dorsomedial to the red nucleus (Chapter 5), or hemiplegia if the lesion affects the midbrain basis (Fig. 2-18).

b. A lesion of CrN VI in the basis pontis will cause contralateral hemiplegia because that is where CrN VI comes into conjunction with the pyramidal tract (Fig. 2-16).

3. Peripherally each nerve generally comes into conjunction with another nerve or structure, and the lesion will affect more than one structure.
   a. In the region of the cavernous sinus, CrNs III, IV, V, and VI and the carotid sympathetic nerve are related in different ways (Section VIII).
   b. Within the orbit, a lesion will cause a different set of signs involving several of the same nerves. Brazis et al. (2007) succinctly review the syndromes encountered by lesions along the course of the ocular motor nerves.
4. Remember the many diseases that can cause diplopia and ocular palsies but do not directly interrupt ocular motor nerves: myasthenia gravis, hyperthyroidism, botulism, diabetes, arteritides, aneurysms, inflammation, and primary or metastatic neoplasms. Therefore, the "thinking through" process must also include the neuromyal junction, the muscles themselves, the adjacent anatomical structures, and the whole person: systemic disease.

BIBLIOGRAPHY · General References

Brazis PW, Masdeu JC, Biller J. *Localization in Clinical Neurology*. 5th ed. Philadelphia: Lippincott Williams & Wilkins, 2007.

Shaunak S, O'Sullivan E, Kennard C. Eye movements. *J Neurol Neurosurg Psychiatry* 1995;59:115–125.

Clinical Tests for Ocular Malalignment and the Range of Eye Movements

Helveston E. A two-step test for diagnosing paresis of a single vertically acting extraocular muscle. *Am J Ophthalmol* 1967;64:914–915.

Keane JR. Fourth nerve palsy: historical review and study of 215 inpatients. *Neurology* 1993;43:2439–2443.

Von Noorden GK. *Binocular Vision and Ocular Motility*. 5th ed. St. Louis: Mosby, 1996.

IV. REFRACTION AND ACCOMMODATION

A. Refraction by negative and positive lenses

1. To understand lenses, start with the law of the prism: **A prism bends light rays toward its base** (Fig. 4-26A).

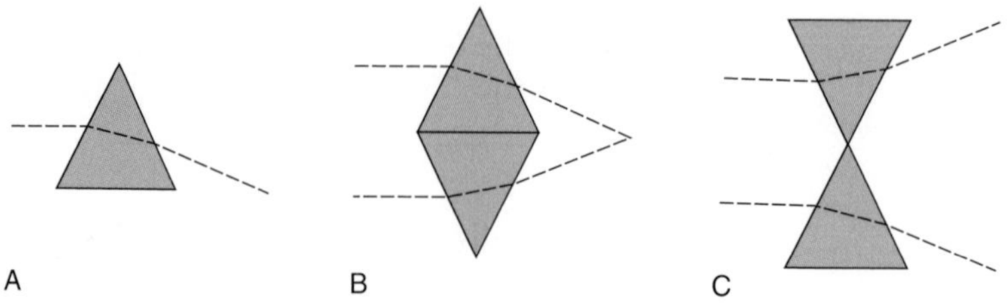

FIGURE 4-26. The law of the prism states that a prism refracts light toward its base. Two prisms base to base make a converging, positive lens or, if apex to apex a diverging, a negative lens.

   a. Two prisms, placed base *in*, form a *positive* or *converging* lens (Fig. 4-26B).
   b. Two prisms placed base *out* form a *negative* or *diverging* lens (Fig. 4-26C).
   c. Rounding of the sides of the prism into the familiar lens shape reduces chromatic and spherical aberrations.

2. In bending light rays, a prism or lens bends violet more than red, thus causing **chromatic** aberration because the rays do not fall on one focal point but are spread out. Any defect in the curvature of the lens causes **spherical** aberration (astigmatism).
3. A pinhole aperture screens out the more peripheral light rays, which must undergo more refraction than the central rays, thus reducing chromatic and spherical aberrations (Fig. 4-27D).

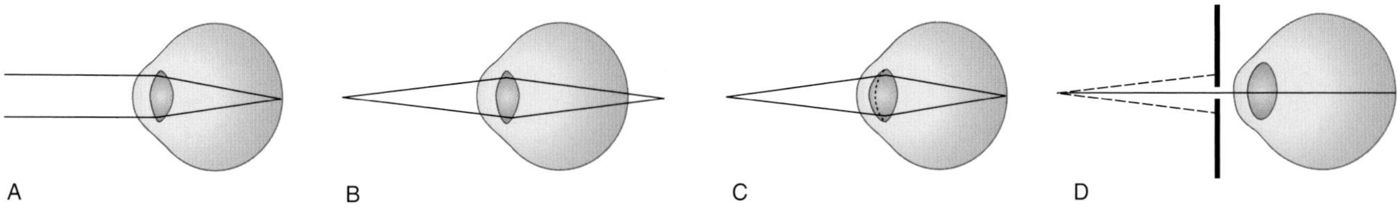

FIGURE 4-27. Schematic cross sections of the eye to show the focal point of light rays in various conditions of refraction. (A) Emmetropic eye. Parallel rays from a distant object focus on the retina. (B) Emmetropic eye has not adjusted to accommodate for near vision. The light rays from the near point diverge as they travel to the eye; hence, they focus behind the retina. (C) Emmetropic eye accommodated for near vision. The lens has thickened, increasing its power of refraction. The divergent rays now focus on, rather than behind, the retina. (D) Pinhole effect. The pinhole allows the central non-refracted rays to pass to the retina but blocks the more peripheral rays.

B. Light refraction by the normal eye

The refracting media of the eye includes the cornea and lens. Learn Figs. 4-27A to 4-27D.

C. The accommodation reflex

1. Accommodation for near vision requires three muscles to complete three actions:
   a. **Convergence:** medial recti (skeletal)
   b. **Pupilloconstriction:** pupilloconstrictor muscle of the iris (smooth muscle, parasympathetic)
   c. **Lens thickening:** ciliary muscle (smooth muscle, parasympathetic)
2. **Functions of the three actions:**
   a. Convergence by the **medial rectus muscles** aims the visual axes onto the near fixation point (Fig. 4-3).
   b. Pupilloconstriction by the **pupilloconstrictor muscle** of the iris causes cormiosis (pinhole effect; Fig. 4-27D), reducing spherical and chromatic aberrations.
   c. Lens thickening increases its ability to refract the more divergent rays coming from the near fixation point. Contraction of the **ciliary muscle,** a sphincter, relaxes the suspensory ligament of the lens, allowing it to thicken by its natural elasticity.
3. Thus, during the accommodation reflex for near vision, three distinct events occur: The visual axes ________________ onto the fixation point; the pupils ________________, and the lens ________________.

converge; constrict; thicken

4. Although volition initiates the act of looking at a near target, neural mechanisms lock the three events of accommodation into a single **accommodation reflex.** Thus, whenever a person voluntarily converges the eyes, neural circuits automatically cause pupilloconstriction and lens thickening. Complete Table 4-3.

TABLE 4-3 · The Accommodation Reflex and the Muscles Responsible

List the three events of the accommodation reflex	List the responsible muscles
	(skeletal)
	(smooth)
	(smooth)

convergence; medial recti
cormiosis; pupilloconstrictor muscle
lens thickening; ciliary muscle

D. Myopia and hyperopia

1. Learn Fig. 4-28.

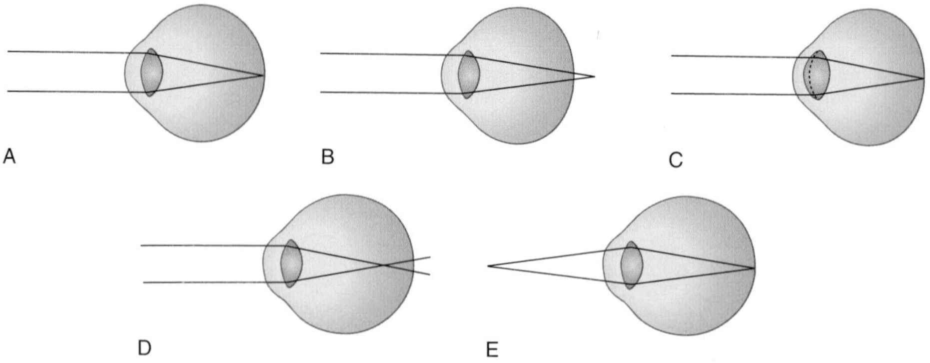

FIGURE 4-28. Focal point of light rays relative to the anteroposterior diameter and refractive power of the eye. (A) Emmetropia. The refracting power and the diameter of the normal eye match. Parallel rays from a distant source focus on the retina without accommodation. Divergent rays from a near source will require lens thickening to focus on the retina. (B) Hyperopia. The diameter of the eye is too short relative to its refracting power. Parallel rays focus behind the retina. (C) Hyperopia with accommodation. The lens of the hyperopic eye must thicken, thus increasing its focusing power, to bring parallel rays to focus on the retina. When looking at a near object, the hyperopic person has no accommodation reserve. (D) Myopia. The diameter of the eye is too long relative to its refracting power. Parallel rays focus in front of the retina. (E) Myopic eye focusing on near object. Divergent rays from the near object focus properly on the retina with little or no accommodation.

2. A person with sharp vision for objects that are far away *and* close is ☐ emmetropic/☐ myopic/☐ hyperopic.

☑ **emmetropic**

3. For far vision, the emmetropic person's muscles of accommodation are ☐ active/☐ relaxed.

☑ **relaxed**

4. A person with sharp vision for far objects, but blurred vision for close objects, is called *farsighted*. The technical term for farsightedness is ☐ emmetropia/☐ myopia/☐ hyperopia.

☑ **hyperopia**

5. The hyperopic eye focuses parallel rays ☐ behind/☐ in front of/☐ on the retina.

☑ **behind** (Fig. 4-28B)

   a. The hyperopic Pt requires some activity of the accommodation reflex to thicken the lens ☐ only when viewing far objects/☐ only when viewing close objects/☐ when looking at close and far objects.

   ☑ **when looking at close and far objects**

   b. Normally, however, the accommodation reflex should act only during near vision. The hyperopic Pt requires some degree of accommodation at all times to bring the focal point forward onto the retina.

6. A person with blurred vision for distant objects but sharp vision for near objects is *nearsighted*. The technical term for nearsightedness is ☐ emmetropia/☐ myopia/☐ hyperopia.

☑ **myopia**

   a. The myopic eye focuses parallel rays from far objects ☐ in front of/☐ on/☐ behind the retina.

   ☑ **in front of**

   b. Which of the three events of the accommodation reflex actually work against the myopic Pt who is attempting to look at a near object? Explain.

   ____

   ____

   Lens thickening works against the myope. The near object's rays diverge more before striking the lens and, hence, move the focal point backward, nearer to the desired focal point on the retina. Lens thickening, however, moves the focal point *forward*.

7. On scrap paper, draw three eyeballs and show the focal points of parallel rays in emmetropia, hyperopia, and myopia. Compare with Figs. 4-28A, 4-28B, and 4-28D.

E. Relation of refractive errors to heterotropia and heterophoria

1. During the first months of life, infants must develop binocular fixation and fuse the images from the two eyes. The infant's eyeball is too short relative to its refracting power. With maturation, the eyeball expands.

2. With the eyeballs too short in relation to the focal point of the lens, the infant is basically ❒ myopic/❒ emmetropic/❒ hyperopic.

☑ Hyperopic. However, the smallness of the eyeball means that the infant lacks sharp vision for far objects.

3. As the eyeball increases in diameter with maturation, the hyperopia tends to change to emmetropia. If the child is more nearly emmetropic at birth, instead of hyperopic, he would become ________________ as the diameter of the eye increases with growth.

myopic

4. Because of the small diameter of the eyeball relative to the focusing power of the lens, infants tend to keep their lenses thickened. In other words, they tend to accommodate all of the time. Detailed inspection of near objects places extra demands on the accommodation mechanism of the infant's eyes. The need for accommodation may overcome the hyperopic child's capacity for it.

   a. Because one of the accommodation mechanisms is convergence of the eyes, the hyperopic child at first will show only a latent tendency to crossing of his eyes, that is, ❒ esotropia/❒ esophoria/❒ exotropia/❒ exophoria.

☑ esophoria

   b. With severe hyperopia, the esophoria may convert to an overt internal deviation of an eye, which is called ________________.

esotropia

   c. Thus, refractive errors or neuromuscular lesions may cause crossed eyes. Two eyelid anomalies in children may give a false impression of crossed eyes because the medial margin of the limbus appears to be too close to the medial eyelid margins. Name these two anomalies.

Dystopic canthi and epicanthal folds (Fig. 1-6)

5. Consider the infant who will become myopic at maturity. As his eyeball enlarges with age, he becomes ❒ more/❒ less myopic. Therefore, the nervous system adjusts by reducing accommodation.

☑ more

   a. With an underactive accommodation mechanism, the child's eyes would tend to ❒ drift apart/❒ converge too much.

☑ drift apart

   b. At first the eyes might show only a latent tendency to drift apart, which would be called ________________, or later, if overt, ________________.

exophoria; exotropia

6. Tropias and phorias commonly accompany refractive errors.

   a. Esophoria or esotropia in a child would raise the suspicion of a refractive error called ❒ myopia/❒ emmetropia/❒ hyperopia.

☑ hyperopia

   b. Exophoria or exotropia in a child would raise the suspicion of ❒ myopia/❒ emmetropia/❒ hyperopia.

☑ myopia

7. Which child would experience increasing inability to read the chalkboard at school, requiring differentiation of neurologic and ophthalmologic causes for blurred vision, the ❒ myope or ❒ hyperope?

☑ myope

F. Presbyopia, blurred vision, myopia, and hyperopia

1. At the age of approximately 42 years, normal adults experience blurred vision when they try to read newsprint or look at near objects. The differential diagnosis then involves a neurologic versus an ophthalmologic disorder.

2. Because of aging, the lens loses its elasticity. It will no longer thicken to increase its refractive power during accommodation, a condition called **presbyopia.**

   a. Who would suffer blurred near vision first and foremost from presbyopia, the ❒ hyperope or the ❒ myope? Explain.

   ____

   ____

☑ **hyperope.** The presbyopic hyperope suffers first and foremost from blurred near vision, because the hyperope is already straining the accommodation mechanism. Any loss of elasticity will reduce refraction and thus blur close objects. The myope doesn't need much accommodation and therefore doesn't suffer much when it fails.

3. Would placing a pinhole in front of the eye of the presbyopic hyperope improve near vision and help differentiate the visual blurring from presbyopia from blurring due to a lesion of the macula or optic nerve? ❒ Yes/❒ No. Explain.

   ____

   ____

☑ **Yes.** A pinhole will block off the more peripheral rays from the near object, thus allowing only the central rays to reach the retina. The pinhole acts as a tiny pupil. The pinhole eliminates the need to increase refraction by lens thickening. Hence, restoration of visual acuity by the pinhole establishes a disorder of refraction, not a retinal or optic nerve lesion.

4. **The parallax test for positive or negative corrective lenses**

   a. The **parallax test** provides a quick way to test whether the Pt's glasses correct for hyperopia or myopia. For the parallax test, hold the glasses over any vertical line, about a foot away, and slowly move the glasses to the right and left alternately.

☑ **backward** (remember the law of the prism, Fig. 4-26).

b. With a *divergent (negative) lens,* the line will appear to move *in the direction* that you move the glasses. Myopia requires a *divergent* or *negative* lens to move the focal point ❐ backward/❐ forward onto the retina.

c. With a *convergent (positive) lens,* the line will appear to move in the *opposite* direction to the movement of the glasses. Hyperopia requires a *convergent* or *positive* lens to bring the focal point forward onto the retina.

d. In summary:

i. If the lens corrects for myopia, the image will appear to move in the direction that you moved the eyeglasses.

ii. If the lens corrects for hyperopia, the image will appear to move in the opposite direction.

5. If you understand all of this, explain why a presbyopic myope removes his glasses to read newsprint, whereas a presbyopic hyperope (who previously had fairly adequate accommodation) puts his glasses on to read but removes them for far vision. The question is: Which, the presbyopic myope or the presbyopic hyperope, benefits from half-frame or bifocal positive lens?

At some point, the teacher and the text must fade away. If you understand the text, you can figure out the answer.

G. Some commoner causes of blurred vision/blindness

1. Various ages: malformations, infections, vascular proliferative or occlusive disease, retinitis pigmentosa and other CNS degenerative diseases (some with cherry red macula), diabetes mellitus, neoplasia, retinal detachment, trauma, migraine, and toxic (methanol) (Miller et al., 2005; Shingleton and O'Donoghue, 2000).
2. Selected age-related causes of blurred vision/blindness.

a. Birth through childhood: opacities of the media, astigmatism, and refractive errors:

20/300–400	Birth, eyeball too short
20/40–60	1 y
20/30	3 y
20/20	5 y

b. In later childhood, ages 5 to 7 years, the myopic child has to sit closer and closer to blackboard as the eyeballs continue to grow, and the child becomes increasingly nearsighted.

c. Young adults: optic neuritis Leber hereditary optic neuropathy and other neuropathies/neuritides.

d. At ages 40 to 45 years:

i. **Presbyopia:** The lens loses its elasticity to focus on near objects (the "arms are too short" for the Pt to hold the newspaper far enough away to read the print).

ii. **Glaucoma:** Signs include high intraocular pressure, optic disc cupping, pupillodilation, and constricted peripheral fields.

e. Older than 50 years:

i. Cataracts and macular degeneration (Fine et al., 2000), both diagnosable by ophthalmoscopy.

ii. Central serous retinopathy.

iii. Temporal arteritis and ischemic optic neuropathy (Chutorian et al., 2002).

BIBLIOGRAPHY · Blurred Vision and Blindness

Chutorian AM, Winterkorn JMS, Geffner M. Anterior ischemic optic neuropathy in children: case reports and review of the literature. *Pediatr Neurol* 2002;26:358–364.

Fine SL, Berger JW, Maguire MG, et al. Age-related macular degeneration. *N Engl J Med* 2000;342:483–491.

Miller NR, Newman NJ, Biousse V, Kerrison JB, eds. *Walsh and Hoyt's Clinical Neuro-ophthalmology*, 6th ed. Philadelphia: Lippincott Williams & Wilkins, 2005.

Shingleton BJ, O'Donoghue MW. Blurred vision. *N Engl J Med* 2000;343:566–562.

V. INNERVATION OF THE OCULAR MUSCLES

A. Classification of ocular muscles into intraocular and extraocular

1. Each eye has 11 ocular muscles: four smooth muscles and seven striated muscles. Because they derive from somites, the striated muscles receive somite CrNs III, IV, and VI. Learn Fig. 4-29.

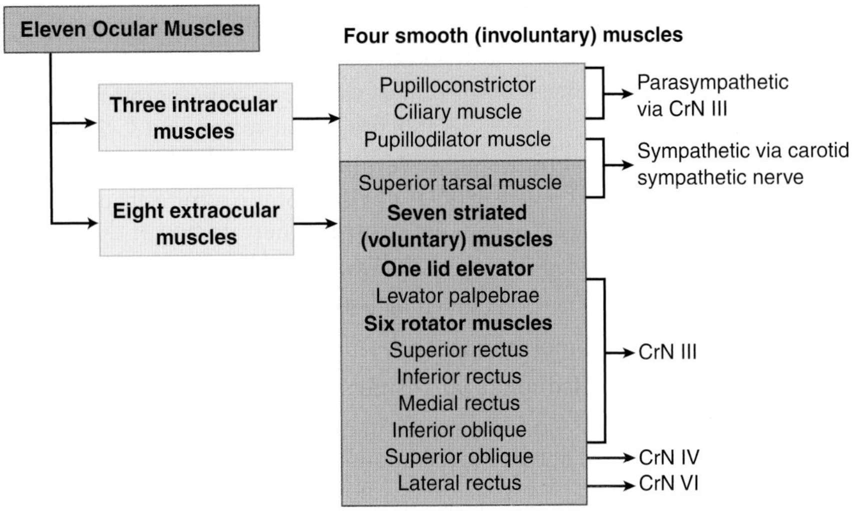

FIGURE 4-29. Classification of the 11 ocular muscles according to type and innervation. Note that the superior tarsal muscle is both a smooth and an extraocular muscle, the only one so classified.

2. One ocular-related muscle, the orbicularis oculi, a sphincter that closes the eyelids, derives from a brachial arch and belongs to the facial muscles, innervated by CrN VII.

B. Peripheral innervation of the extraocular muscles

Six nerves innervate the eye, four motor and two sensory (Table 4-4).

TABLE 4-4 · Afferent and Efferent Innervation of the Eye by Its Six Nerves

Number (name) of nerve	Innervation	Clinical effects of interruption of nerve
Efferent		
CrN III (oculomotor nerve)	Striated muscle: superior, medial, and inferior recti; inferior oblique	Diplopia, eye abducted and turned down
	Levator palpebrae	Ptosis (paralysis of volitional lid elevation)
	Smooth muscle: pupilloconstrictor; ciliary muscle	Pupil dilated and fixed to light; loss of lens thickening
CrN IV (trochlear nerve)	Striated muscle: superior oblique	Diplopia, most severe on looking down and in; eye extorted; head tilted to side opposite paralyzed eye
CrN VI (abducens nerve)	Striated muscle: lateral rectus	Diplopia, most severe on looking to side of paralysis; eye turned in (adducted)

(*Continued*)

TABLE 4-4 · **Afferent and Efferent Innervation of the Eye by Its Six Nerves (Continued)**

Number (name) of nerve	Innervation	Clinical effects of interruption of nerve
Carotid sympathetic nerve	Smooth muscle: superior tarsal and pupillodilator	Horner syndrome (ptosis, miosis, hemifacial anhidrosis, vasodilation)
Afferent		
CrN II (optic nerve)	Visual afferents	Blindness
CrN V (trigeminal nerve)	Corneal/conjunctival afferents Proprioceptive afferents	Corneal anesthesia of cornea; loss of corneal reflex No known clinical effect

ABBREVIATION: CrN = cranial nerve.

1. Of the four essentially motor nerves, three convey somatic efferent fibers: CrNs III, IV, and VI.
   a. Two of the three somatomotor nerves serve only one EOM: CrN VI innervates the lateral rectus, and CrN IV innervates the superior oblique. CrN III serves the remaining EOMs and two of the three intraocular muscles.
   b. Only CrN III of the somite group also conveys parasympathetic (GVE) fibers. These fibers innervate two of the three intraocular smooth muscles, the pupilloconstrictor and ciliary muscles.
2. The fourth motor nerve of the eye, the **carotid sympathetic nerve,** innervates the third intraocular muscle, the **pupillodilator** muscle and one clinically important EOM, the **superior tarsal.** The carotid sympathetic nerve travels from the carotid artery at the level of the cavernous sinus into the superior orbital fissure and to the eyeball by hitchhiking along other orbital nerves (Fig. 4-31).
3. **Test your knowledge of Table 4-4 by completing frames 4-12.**
4. CrN III
   a. CrN III is called the ______________ nerve.
   b. The EOMs innervated by III are ______________ ______________.
   c. CrN III innervates two intraocular muscles and all EOMs, except for ______________.
   d. In addition, CrN III innervates a muscle that elevates the eyelid, the ______________ muscle.
5. CrN IV
   a. CrN IV is named the ______________ nerve.
   b. CrN IV innervates the only EOM to have a trochlea, the ______________ muscle.
   c. The superior oblique has three actions: ______________, ______________, and ______________.
6. CrN VI
   a. CrN VI is named the ______________ nerve. It innervates the ______________ muscle.
   b. The only action of the lateral rectus is to ______________ the eye.

Answers (margin):

oculomotor

medial, superior, and inferior recti, inferior oblique, and levator palpebrae

lateral rectus and superior oblique

levator palpebrae

trochlear

superior oblique

depression; abduction; intorsion

abducens; lateral rectus

abduct

VI. EXAMINATION OF THE PUPILS

A. Technique of pupillary examination

1. Start with normal illumination of the room, with no direct sunlight. Ask the Pt to gaze at a distant point to avoid pupilloconstriction from the accommodation reflex.

a. The pupils should appear black, equal in size, perfectly round and react to light and to accommodation. Normal pupils appear almost exactly centered in the iris, or very slightly inferomedially placed. A non-black pupil, usually a whitish one, indicates an opacification of the cornea or lens.

b. Compare the size of the two pupils and record the pupillary size in millimeters. To measure pupillary diameter, compare the pupil with a series of circles graded in millimeters (Litvan et al., 2000) (Fig. 12-30).

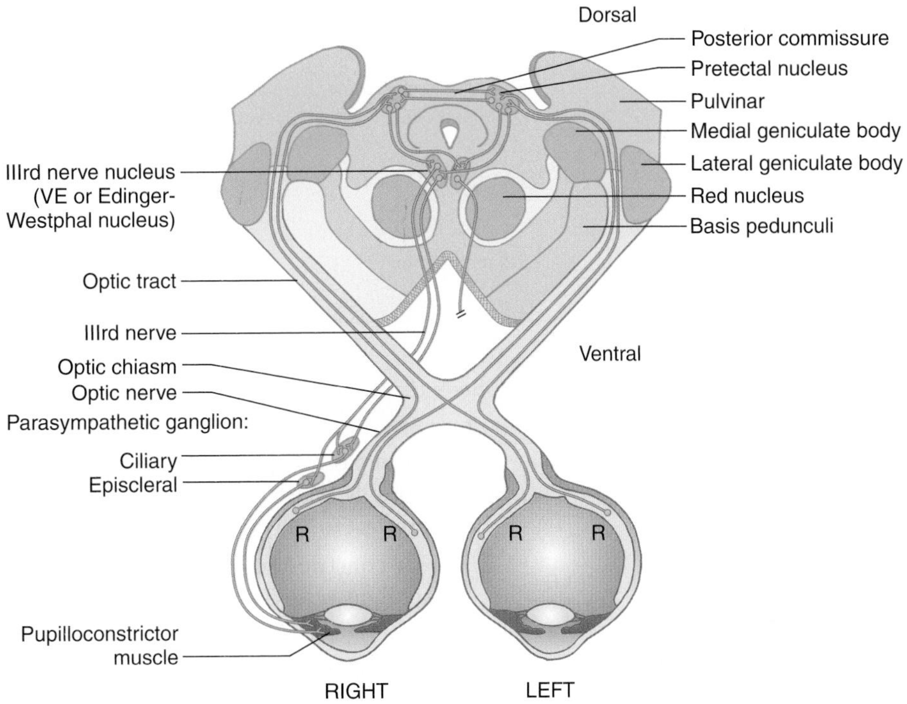

FIGURE 4-30. Diagram of afferent (optic nerve) and efferent (III nerve) pathways for pupilloconstriction. The mesencephalon has been transected through its rostral part, encroaching on the geniculate bodies and pulvinar nuclei of the diencephalon. Learn this diagram. R = receptor in the retina. (Adapted with permission from Crosby E, Humphrey T, Lauer E. *Correlative Anatomy of the Nervous System.* New York, Macmillan Company, 1962.)

i. Look for anisocoria. Benign congenital anisocoria in which both pupils react normally is relatively common.

ii. Look for faint rapid oscillations of the pupillary margins, called **hippus.** Although often benign, hippus may accompany a metabolic encephalopathy.

c. Inspect the limbus for a Kayser-Fleischer ring or an arcus senilis. The latter may indicate hyperlipidemia.

2. **Check for pupillodilation and a dilation lag.**

a. Dim the room lights and inspect the pupils immediately and after 5 to 15 seconds.

b. Normal pupils dilate promptly, within 5 seconds of dimming the light, because of activation of the pupillodilator fibers by the sympathetic nervous system.

c. A dilation lag of seconds to minutes indicates a lack of sympathetic innervation (Horner syndrome) or a myotonic pupil (Adie pupil; Table 4-5).

TABLE 4-5 · Differential Diagnosis of Argyll Robertson and Adie Pupils

Characteristic	Argyll Robertson pupil	Adie tonic pupil/syndrome
Laterality	Usually bilateral	Usually unilateral (anisocorial)
Size	Cormiosis	Mild corectasia
Pupillary outline	Irregular	Regular (normal circle)
Iris atrophy	Present	Absent
Response to light	None (neither direct nor consensual)	Very slow direct and consensual response; remains myotonically contracted if light is removed
Response to dark	No pupillodilation	Slow pupillodilation; delayed constriction on re-exposure to light
Response to accommodation	Constricts	Constricts very slowly and remains myotonically constricted after relaxation of accommodation
Response to mydriatics	Poor or none	Responds normally
Other neurologic features	Virtually pathognomonic of syphilis; if tabes dorsalis is present, the patient will have dorsal column signs and no muscle stretch reflexes	Benign disorder, often associated with absent muscle stretch reflexes; no dorsal column signs: Adie's syndrome
Sex predeliction	More men than women have neurosyphilis	70% women/30% men

3. Check the *direct* and *consensual* pupillary light reflexes.
   a. Instruct the Pt to look at a distant point across the room. Beam a flashlight slowly in from the sides to illuminate each eye separately. Observe whether both pupils constrict promptly and equally to unilateral illumination. After the prompt initial constriction, the pupils normally dilate slightly.
   i. Direct constriction of the pupil in the eye stimulated by light is called the **direct light reflex.**
   ii. The consensual constriction of the opposite pupil when light stimulates only one eye is the **consensual light reflex.** Normally, the direct and consensual pupillary responses are equal.
   b. Do not shine the flashlight abruptly into the Pt's eyes from directly in front, for two reasons:
      i. The Pt will automatically look at the light and accommodate for near vision.
      ii. The bright light will cause discomfort, particularly if the Pt has photophobia, mental retardation, or dementia.
4. For the **swinging flashlight test,** alternately swing the light from one eye to the other and hold it on the new eye for 3- to 5-second intervals. Watch for equal reactions of both pupils. If the Pt has an afferent defect in one optic nerve (e.g., due to optic neuritis), the pupils will dilate as the light swings from the normal to the affected eye (Marcus-Gunn pupil or relative afferent pupillary defect) rather than maintaining the same degree of constriction.
5. While the room is dimly lit, do the ophthalmoscopic examination.
6. Whenever a question exists about the duration of an ocular finding, such as anisocoria or ptosis, ask the Pt to bring in an old facial photograph.
7. Rehearse the foregoing steps of the pupillary examination (steps V-A-3 and 4 of the Standard NE).
8. In recording the pupillary reactions, many Ex's write **PERLA** as shorthand for "pupils equal and react to light and in accommodation." We often find that **PERLA** actually means "**p**upillary **e**xamination **r**eally **la**x." But if the note says, "pupils 3 mm, equal, centered, react to light and in accommodation and dilate promptly in dim light," the reader can trust in a meticulous examination. Such a baseline note in the chart is indispensable for the acutely ill hospitalized Pt whose neurologic signs may change abruptly and for the chronic Pt whose signs may change subtly over time.

B. Pathway for the pupillary light reflexes

1. Learn the pathway for the pupillary light reflex as if your life depended on it: someone else's may. Evaluation of the pupillary reflexes is critical in coma, cerebrovascular disease, brain tumors, and head injuries. Study Fig. 4-30 this way:
   a. Learn the names on the left-hand side. Those on the right are for general orientation.
   b. As typifies reflex arcs, the pupillary reflex arc has a *receptor, an afferent limb, central nuclear synapse(s), an efferent limb,* and *an effector*. Start at R, the receptors for light, the rods and cones. Always start at the receptor to analyze any reflex. Trace the path of impulses through the brain stem and back to the effector muscles.
   c. Notice the alternate ipsilateral–contralateral course of axons through the optic chiasm.
   d. Notice that, after the nerve impulses reach the mesencephalon, they are distributed bilaterally to the parasympathetic (GVE) nucleus of CrN III, called the **Edinger-Westphal nucleus.** Hence, light stimulation in one eye will constrict both pupils equally. The consensual pupillary constriction equals the direct constriction.
   e. Efferent axons travel to the eye via both III nerves. Notice that, according to the general plan of the parasympathetic system, the ganglion of synapse of the GVE axon, the **ciliary or episcleral ganglion,** is near the end organs, the ciliary and pupilloconstrictor muscles. The same efferent pathway serves pupilloconstriction to light and in accommodation.
2. On scrap paper draw the axonal pathways for the pupillary light reflex and check your drawing against Fig. 4-30.
3. **Patient analysis:** A Pt has equal pupils and no direct light reflex in the left eye but has a consensual light reflex on the left when the right eye is illuminated. The lesion is in the ❒ right optic tract/❒ left III nerve/❒ left optic nerve.

☑ left optic nerve

4. **Describe the result of the swinging flashlight test in the foregoing Pt.**

___

See frame A4

C. Physiology and pharmacology of the pupils

1. **The eyeball contains three intraocular muscles, all smooth muscles: the pupillodilator, the pupilloconstrictor, and the ciliary muscles.**
   a. The pupilloconstrictor and pupillodilator muscles of the iris adjust the diameter of the pupil.
      i. The pupillodilator muscle fibers run radially from the pupillary margin, like spokes in a wheel.
      ii. The pupilloconstrictor muscle fibers form a sphincter around the pupillary opening.
   b. The ciliary muscle is likewise a sphincter, adjusting the diameter of the lens by relaxing its suspensory ligament, to allow the lens to thicken by its own elasticity. The ciliary muscle does not control the pupils.
2. **Role of smooth muscle in the tubular viscera:** Smooth muscle adjusts the diameters of the apertures and lumens of the tubular viscera, the bowel, bronchi, blood vessels, ureters, bladder, etc. Curiously, however, the heart, the one viscus that functions solely to change its diameter, is made of striated, not smooth, muscle. Striated muscle is specialized for quick, powerful phasic contractions, smooth muscle for slow, tonic contractions.
3. Tonic opposition of the pupilloconstrictor and pupillodilator muscles
   a. Like the EOMs that act in tonically innervated, oppositional pairs, the pupilloconstrictor and pupillodilator muscles actively oppose each other to adjust the pupillary size.

b. The pupilloconstrictor muscle is *parasympathetic* and *cholinergic;* the pupillodilator is *sympathetic* and *adrenergic* (Low, 2008). Normally the outflow of tonic innervation by sympathetic and parasympathetic impulses balances out. After the pupil adopts any new size, the vector acting to increase pupillary diameter equals the vector acting to decrease it. Thus, a tug-of-war between the constrictor and dilator muscles always positively determines pupillary size.

c. If a lesion or drug blocks one system, sympathetic or parasympathetic, the other acts unopposed. The pupil assumes the size dictated by the tonic innervation that reaches the intact muscle.

☑ **pupillodilation (corectasia, mydriasis)**

☑ **pupilloconstriction (cormiosis)**

i. Parasympathetic denervation of the eye results in ❒ pupillodilation/ ❒ pupilloconstriction.

ii. Sympathetic denervation results in ❒ pupilloconstriction/❒ pupillodilation.

4. **Pupillodilation (mydriasis)**

☑ **sympathetic;**

☑ **parasympathetic**

a. The ophthalmologist never presumes to do a complete funduscopic examination without dilating the pupil. Pharmacologically, pupillodilation can result from mimicking the ❒ sympathetic/❒ parasympathetic nervous system or by blocking the ❒ sympathetic/❒ parasympathetic nervous system.

☑ **parasympathetic**

b. After sympathomimetic or parasympathetic blocking drugs have dilated the pupil, exposure to light will make the Pt uncomfortable, a symptom called **photophobia.** Which drug would also interfere with lens thickening by paralyzing the ciliary muscle (cycloplegia): ❒ sympathomimetic or ❒ parasympathetic blocking agent?

c. Although pupillodilator drugs (mydriatics) cause temporary blurring of vision, they are necessary to see the periphery of the fundus. The pupils of infants and deeply pigmented irises respond slowly to mydriatics.

i. For infants use cyclopentolate (Cyclogyl) in a 1% ophthalmic solution, two drops in each eye every 15 minutes for three doses or 1% tropicamide (Mydriacyl), ophthalmic solution or 2.5% phenylephrine (Neo-Synephrine), ophthalmic solution. To reduce burning and tearing, you can pretreat with a topical anesthetic, proparacaine, ophthalmic solution.

ii. For older Pts use one or two drops in each eye. Repeat in 15 to 20 minute.

d. Because pupillodilation increases intraocular pressure, check the intraocular pressure of adults older than 40 years by tonometry before instilling mydriatics. Two percent of all adults older than 40 years have glaucoma. The danger of precipitating acute glaucoma with mydriatics is greater for the hyperopic Pts.

5. **Determinants of pupillary size in addition to light**

a. Local disease of the eye and iris.

b. Local ocular or systemic drugs affecting the autonomic nervous system.

c. Emotionality: sympathetic nervous system predominance causing pupillodilation and tachycardia.

d. Sleep and drowsiness: parasympathetic nervous system predominance during sleep causes pupilloconstriction and bradycardia.

e. Age: The pupils of the fetus are large and fail to react to light until the 30 to 32 weeks of gestational age (Isenberg and Vasquez, 1994). Then at term birth the pupils are small ("Gee, its bright out here"). The pupils enlarge through adolescence (the so-called "wide-eyed" innocent look). The size and reactivity then gradually diminish until senility when the pupils again become small and poorly reactive. Small pupils give the person a "flinty-eyed" miserly look, whereas large pupils are considered sexy and receptive; hence, the use of atropine by women who wanted to be *la belladonna* (the beautiful lady).

D. Patient analysis

A 51-year-old woman was admitted to the hospital because of high blood pressure. She had no visual complaints, and the intern recorded a normal ocular examination. Her examination a few hours after the initial examination by the intern disclosed a dilated right pupil, but no eyelid ptosis, heterotropia, fundus lesions, visual field defects, or other ocular signs. She had no direct or consensual pupillary light reflex on the right and no pupilloconstriction in accommodation. The direct and consensual response of the left pupil to light was normal, and it constricted during accommodation. The best inference is

1. ❒ The Pt is blind in the right eye and has a right CrN III lesion.
2. ❒ The Pt has an intact right optic nerve but has interruption of the right CrN III.
3. ❒ The Pt has had eye drops placed into the right eye to dilate the pupil.

☑ 3. See the next frame

1. Alternative 1 is excluded because the presence of sight in both eyes, and the presence of the consensual reflex in the left pupil prove that the right optic nerve, the afferent pathway, from the right retina is intact. Alternative 2 is excluded by lack of ptosis or ocular malalignment. Alternative 3 is all that remains.
2. The previous frame emphasizes that a common cause of dilated, non-reactive pupils in medical student practice in teaching hospitals is that the intern or resident has previously (and properly) instilled eye drops to dilate the pupil for an adequate funduscopic examination. However, the intern erred in not recording the use of a mydriatic drug. The more general implication of the frame is that in "thinking through" a reflex arc, you must include the neuromyal junction **and** the effector as way stations in the reflex arc. The final lesson is: Always record on the chart that you have dilated the pupils.

E. Patient analysis

1. This 24-year-old man is drowsy because of a head injury, but he can be aroused. His left eye is turned down and out and does not turn in reflexly or on command, although the other eye moves on command. When the Pt attempts to look to the right and down, the left eye intorts strongly but remains turned down and out. The left pupil is dilated and fixed (non-reactive) to light or in accommodation. No eye drops were used. The right pupil shows a direct and a consensual response to light and reacts normally in accommodation. This Pt most likely has a lesion of his ❒ left optic nerve/❒ right optic nerve/❒ left CrN IV only/❒ left CrN III/❒ a lesion of one nerve cannot explain the ocular findings.

☑ left CrN III

2. Should you instill mydriatics in a Pt with a head injury? ❒ Yes/❒ No. Explain.

____

____

☑ No
Because of the importance of pupillary signs in monitoring acute changes, avoid mydriatic eye drops in Pts with impaired consciousness.

3. List two contraindications to pupillodilator drugs.

____

Glaucoma and impaired consciousness

F. The syndrome of parasympathetic paralysis of the eye (internal ophthalmoplegia)

1. The muscles innervated by the GVE, parasympathetic axons of CrN III, are ❒ intraocular/❒ extraocular and ❒ smooth/❒ skeletal.

☑ intraocular; ☑ smooth

2. The GVE axons of CrN III constitute the only efferent pathway for active pupilloconstriction. Because the GVE and GSE axons of CrN III originate from the same nuclear region and travel in the same peripheral nerve, lesions affecting CrN III generally involve both sets of axons, but important exceptions occur. State the symptoms and signs that would be caused by a pure parasympathetic paralysis of the eye.

____

Blurring of near vision (ciliary muscle paralysis) and dilated pupil, not reactive to light or in accommodation (pupilloconstrictor muscle paralysis).

3. Apart from head injuries, causes of III nerve palsies include ischemia, as in diabetic III nerve palsy, an aneurysm of the circle of Willis, neoplasm, or inflammation. Often ischemic III nerve palsy spares the pupil, whereas aneurysmal III nerve palsy virtually always affects the pupil (Brazis et al., 1991).

G. The syndrome of sympathetic paralysis of the eye and face: Bernard-Horner or Horner syndrome

1. **The sympathetic pathway to the eye:** This pathway displays the typical features of all sympathetic innervation.
   a. The upper motoneuron pathway begins in hypothalamic neurons and descends through the brainstem tegmentum to the spinal cord. Learn Fig. 4-31.

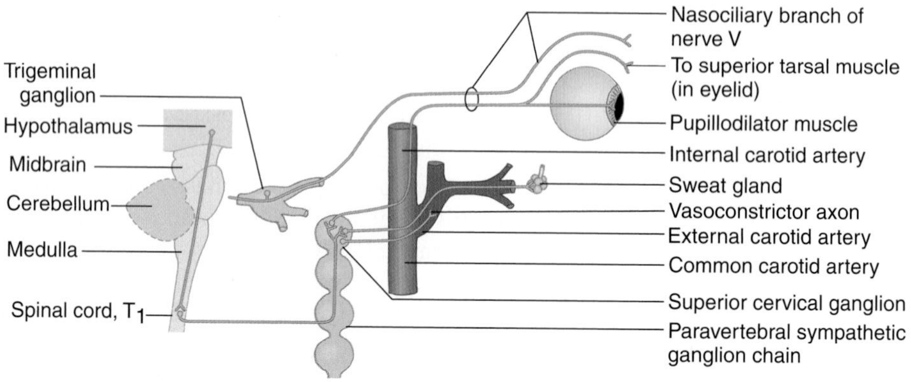

FIGURE 4-31. Diagram of the sympathetic pathway from the hypothalamus (part of the diencephalon) to the pupillodilator and superior tarsal muscles, sweat glands of the face, and the smooth muscle of the carotid arteries.

   b. The upper motoneuron pathway synapses on the GVE lower motoneurons of the intermediolateral cell column of the spinal cord gray matter.
      i. The sympathetic visceral efferent column extends in the spinal cord from T1 to L2 and L3.

Mnemonic: T1-L2-3.

      ii. Axons to the eye derive from T1 and T2 (also called the *ciliospinal center of Budge*).
   c. As is also typical, the sympathetic GVE axons, the second-order neurons in the sympathetic pathway, exit with a spinal nerve to synapse in a paravertebral ganglion.
   d. From the paravertebral ganglion, the superior cervical for the carotid sympathetics, the third-order axons, then hitchhike as a plexus along blood vessels or nerves to their effectors.
   e. The carotid sympathetic nerve innervates the smooth muscles of the vessels of the entire internal and external carotid systems.
      i. The external carotid artery carries sympathetic axons to the sweat glands of the face.
      ii. The internal carotid artery carries the sympathetic axons to the ocular smooth muscles and the sweat glands of the forehead.

superior tarsal; pupillodilator

   f. The sympathetic axons innervate two ocular muscles, ________________ (extraocular) and ________________ (intraocular).
   g. **Note:** The sympathetic and parasympathetic systems differ in the location of the ganglion containing the secondary axon.
      i. The ganglia of the sympathetic nervous system are located in the paravertebral chain.
      ii. By contrast, the ganglia of the parasympathetic nervous system are located in or near the effector innervated.

2. **Patient analysis:** A 21-year-old man has suffered a stab wound in the neck interrupting the sympathetic innervation to one side of his face. Run down the right-hand labels of Fig. 4-31 to compile a list of signs that would occur.

____

Ipsilateral ptosis, pupilloconstriction (cormiosis), anhidrosis, and flushing (vasodilation)

3. These four features of sympathetic facial denervation constitute the **Bernard-Horner** or **Horner syndrome.** Although enophthalmos is also described as part of this syndrome in humans, it is more apparent, because of ptosis, than real.
   a. Explain why miosis occurs after sympathetic denervation of the eye.

   ____

   The pupillodilator and pupilloconstrictor muscles tonically oppose each other. After pupillodilator muscle paralysis, the pupilloconstrictor muscle acts unopposed.

   b. After sympathetic paralysis, the miotic pupil will constrict further in response to light or accommodation, because the muscle receives an additive constrictor stimulus rather than simply a "tonic" stimulus.
   c. A diagnostic feature of unilateral Horner syndrome is an increase in the degree of the anisocoria just after dimming the room light. Pupillodilation in the first 5 seconds depends on sympathetic activation. The normal pupil will dilate within 5 seconds, whereas the abnormal pupil has a **dilation lag** and briefly remains the same size. The anisocoria lessens in 15 to 20 seconds because of a decrease in parasympathetic innervation to the abnormal eye.
   d. In bright light the miosis of the normal pupil will cause it to approximate the Horner pupil. Thus, the miosis may be missed without examining the Pt in a darkened room.
4. **Separation of the components of Horner syndrome:** The number of signs of sympathetic facial denervation varies depending on the location of the lesion along the sympathetic pathway:
   a. If the lesion interrupts the sympathetic pathway *distal* to the origin of the external carotid artery, the only sympathetic denervation signs the Pt will show are ________________ and ________________.

   ptosis; cormiosis

   b. If the lesion interrupts the sympathetic pathway *proximal* to the external carotid artery (between hypothalamus and external carotid artery), the Pt will show, in addition to ptosis and cormiosis, the other two features of Horner syndrome: ________________ and ________________.

   hemifacial (ipsilateral) anhidrosis; vasodilation

   c. The vasodilation is best seen in the conjunctival vessels.
   d. With a congenital unilateral Horner syndrome, such as with an Erb brachial plexus injury, the ipsilateral iris often becomes heterochromic.
5. **Clinical testing of the ocular sympathetic pathway to the eye:** the faciociliary or spinociliary (ciliospinal) reflex.
   a. To test the sympathetic pathway to the eye, pinch the skin over the face (CrN V afferent) or neck (C2 or C3 afferent) firmly for 5 seconds. Both pupils should dilate briskly—the *faciociliary reflex* or the *spinociliary (ciliospinal) reflex.*
   b. Should you do the test in a darkened or a brightly lit room and with the Pt looking at a near or distant target? Explain.

   ____

   Do the test in dim light and with the Pt looking in the distance, to avoid the strong pupilloconstriction due to light and accommodation that could mask the pupillodilation of the sympathetic reflex.

6. **Causes of Horner syndrome:** Apart from direct trauma, important causes include brainstem infarction that interrupts the descending axons from the hypothalamus (Fig. 4-31 and see Table 10-4); neoplastic or inflammatory masses in the lung apex, neck, base of the skull or orbit; and vascular diseases of the carotid artery, such as cervicocephalic arterial dissections, or aneurysms. A newly acquired Horner syndrome requires a search for such lesions.

H. Abnormal pupillary reflexes with absent muscle stretch reflexes

1. **Tabes dorsalis** with an **Argyll Robertson pupil** (Sir Douglas Argyll Robertson, 1837–1909) caused by neurosyphilis and **Adie tonic pupil** syndrome (William Adie, 1886–1935) feature absent muscle stretch reflexes and abnormal pupillary responses (Table 4-5).

2. The neuropathy of diabetes mellitus may also cause abnormal pupillary reflexes and absence of muscle stretch reflexes. The Argyll Robertson pupil may also occur in neurosyphilis without tabes dorsalis. Table 4-5 shows why you test pupillary constriction to light and in accommodation.

BIBLIOGRAPHY · Examination of the Pupils

Brazis PW. Localization of lesions of the oculomotor nerve: recent concepts. *Mayo Clin Proc* 1991;66:1029–1035.

Isenberg SJ, Vazquez M. Are the pupils of premature infants affected by intraventricular hemorrhage? *J Child Neurol* 1994;9:440–442.

Litvan I, Saposnik G, Maurino J, et al. Pupillary diameter assessment: need for a graded scale. *Neurology* 2000;54:530–531.

Low PA, Benarroch EE, eds. *Clinical Autonomic Disorders*. 3rd ed. Philadelphia, Lippincott Williams & Wilkins, 2008.

VII. CLINICAL EVALUATION OF PTOSIS

A. Elevation of the eyelid

1. Two muscles elevate the eyelid and, hence, adjust the vertical diameter of the palpebral fissure: the **superior tarsal (Muller's) muscle** and the **levator palpebrae muscle.**
   a. The superior tarsal muscle, a smooth muscle, acts *tonically* to elevate the eyelid. It is innervated by the ______________________.
   b. The levator palpebrae muscle, a skeletal muscle, acts *tonically* and *phasically* to elevate the eyelid. It is innervated by ______________.

carotid sympathetic nerve

CrN III

2. **Try this experiment to understand eyelid elevation.**
   a. Look straight ahead into your mirror. The combined tonic action of the superior tarsal muscle and the levator palpebrae muscle sets the height of your palpebral fissure. Elevate and lower the mirror while observing the rise and fall of your upper lids, but do not allow your head to move.
   b. Now try to elevate and lower your eyelids without moving your eyes and try to elevate and lower your eyes without allowing your upper lid to move. Can you separate the eyeball and eyelid movements? ❒ Yes/❒ No
   c. Activation of the levator palpebrae muscle causes the quick or phasic rise and fall of the eyelid during vertical eye movements. Although eyelid elevation is linked automatically as an associated movement to the ocular muscles that elevate the eyeball, the levator palpebrae is a skeletal muscle. Inhibition of its action in the CNS allows the lid to follow the eyeball when it rotates down.

By now you know not to look here for answers that you should work out for yourself.

3. Levator palpebrae paralysis causes:
   a. Severe ptosis, greater than with superior tarsal ptosis.
   b. Paralysis of lid elevation during upward gaze.
4. Will the lid elevate when the Pt with sympathetic ptosis looks up? ❒ Yes/❒ No. Explain. ______________________________
5. **Differentiation of sympathetic and III nerve ptosis:** Complete Table 4-6 by placing a plus sign in column 2 or 3.

☑ **Yes.** The levator palpebrae is intact and will automatically elevate the lid when the eye rotates up.

B. The causes of ptosis (blepharoptosis)

1. Sometimes ptosis comes neither from a III nerve lesion nor from sympathetic denervation. In myasthenia gravis, levator palpebrae weakness results from defective cholinergic transmission at the neuromyal junction. Ptosis from nerve or neurohumoral transmission lesions is **neuropathic** ptosis. Ptosis from muscular dystrophies is **myopathic** ptosis. Sometimes ptosis is congenital and may or may not accompany other anomalies. After injury or inflammation, lid edema may

III	Sympathetic
	+
+	
	+
+	
	+
+	

TABLE 4-6 · Differential Diagnosis of III Nerve and Sympathetic Ptosis

Feature	Present with IIIrd nerve lesion	Present with sympathetic pathway lesion
Cormiosis		
Corectasia		
Reaction to light and accommodation		
Usually have heterotropia		
Elevation of eyelid on upward gaze		
Normal sweating		

cause ptosis. The point is this: In analyzing ptosis or any other neurologic sign, you must "think through" the possible lesion sites, down to and including the effector, and integrate each sign with other physical signs and the history. The lesion causing the ptosis may be:

a. **Central:** at the hypothalamus, brainstem, or spinal cord.

b. **Peripheral:** along the course of the III or sympathetic nerves.

c. **Neuromyal:** at the nerve-muscle junction.

d. **Local in the muscle itself:** myopathic, congenital, inflammatory, or traumatic.

e. Other causes include edema of the eyelid and dehiscence of the levator muscle aponeurosis.

2. In Bell's facial palsy from interruption of CrN VII, the eyelid may droop to the degree that it covers the eye. Normally frontalis contraction elevates the eyebrow. In Bell's palsy, the drooping of the eyelid occurs because of paralysis of the frontalis muscle, which inserts into the eyebrow. Proof of the nature of this form of ptosis comes from the eyebrow-lifting test. Lifting of the eyebrow by the Ex corrects the ptosis in a VII nerve palsy, but it remains in a III nerve palsy (Ohkawa et al., 1997).
3. **Cerebral ptosis:** Pts with acute strokes may have unilateral or bilateral ptosis in association with hemiparesis. The lesion will be in the right cerebral hemisphere more often than in the left. The ptosis may appear ipsilateral to the lesion. The mechanism of this ptosis is uncertain. The development of complete bilateral ptosis may predict brain herniation (Averbuch-Heller et al., 2002).
4. The ptosis with myasthenia gravis will often fluctuate or fatigue throughout the examination and may become more evident on one side when the fellow lid is manually elevated (**enhanced ptosis**). Also an **ice-bag test** may improve the ptosis in patients with myasthenia gravis. In this test, an ice pack is held over one eye (both lids closed) for two minutes and afterwards the position of the lid is observed. Lessening of the degree of ptosis often may occur in myasthenic patients probably due to improved neuromuscular transmission.
5. Thus ptosis, like all signs and symptoms, poses a puzzle to be solved. Every sign generates many diagnostic possibilities that the Ex must systematically sort through. Two important points of distinction for neuropathic ptosis are

   a. Other signs of interruption of CrN III usually accompany ptosis from levator palpebrae paralysis.

   b. Other signs of interruption of the carotid sympathetic nerve usually accompany ptosis from superior tarsal muscle paralysis.

BIBLIOGRAPHY · Ptosis

Averbuch-Heller L, Leigh RJ, Mermelstein V, et al. Ptosis in patients with hemispheric stroke. *Neurology* 2002;59:620–624.

Ohkawa S, Yamasaki H, Osumi Y, et al. Eyebrow lifting test: a novel bedside test for narrowing of the palpebral fissure associated with peripheral facial nerve palsy. *J Neurol Neurosurg Psychiatry* 1997;63:256–257.

VIII. CONJUNCTION SYNDROMES OF THE CRANIAL NERVES

A. Conjunctions of cranial nerves with pathways of the central nervous system

1. The lesion that interrupts an ocular motor nerve (or any other nerve) causes different signs if it affects the central or peripheral course of the nerve. When considering a lesion of a specific nerve, always start at the nucleus of origin of the nerve and think through to its termination.
2. A central lesion will almost always also affect a neighboring long tract in addition to the CrN.
   a. A midbrain lesion that causes a III nerve palsy lesion may interrupt the dentatothalamic tract and cause contralateral ataxia and tremor; or, if it affects the region dorsomedial to the red nucleus, it will paralyze down gaze; or, it will cause hemiplegia, if the lesion affects the midbrain basis (Fig. 2-18).
   b. A contralateral hemiplegia usually will accompany a VI nerve lesion in the basis pontis because of the conjunction of CrN VI with the pyramidal tract at that site (Fig. 2-16).

B. Eponymic conjunction syndromes of the peripheral parts of ocular motor cranial nerves

1. CrN II, the ocular motor CrNs III, IV, and VI, CrN V, and the carotid sympathetic nerve runs through the region of the cavernous sinus, the tip of the petrous bone, and the superior orbital fissure. Notice in Fig. 4-32 that CrNs III and IV and two sensory branches of CrNs V, V1 and V2 run in the lateral wall of the cavernous sinus and that CrN VI runs through the lumen. The lumen also contains the siphon of the internal carotid artery. The optic chiasm (not shown) sits just above the stalk of the pituitary gland.

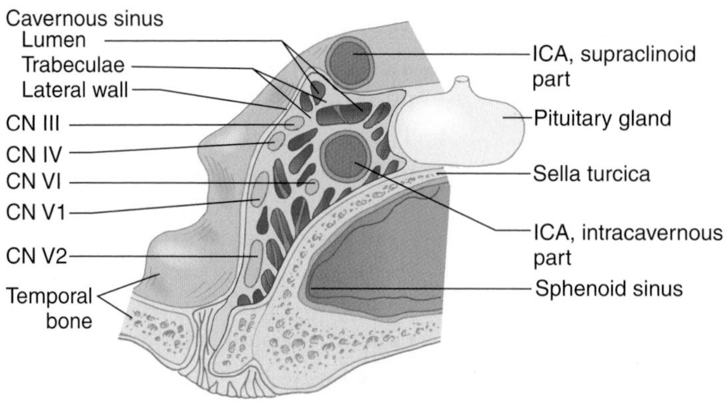

FIGURE 4-32. Coronal section through the cavernous sinus and pituitary gland. CN = cranial nerve. ICA = internal carotid artery; V = sensory divisions of CN V1 and V2.

2. The symptoms and signs consist of pain or numbness in the ophthalmic division of CrN V, palsies of the ocular motor nerves, with ptosis, either sympathetic or III nerve in origin, and visual defects from involvement of CrN II or the chiasm. A carotid-cavernous fistula adds proptosis. A painful ophthalmoplegia plus or minus sympathetic paralysis is the core feature. Depending on the particular combinations of nerves affected, the syndrome is called Gradenigo's, Tolosa-Hunt (Brazis et al., 2007), or Raeder's paratrigeminal (Goadsby, 2002). Typically the cause is inflammation, neoplasm, trauma, or an internal carotid artery fistula or aneurysm.

3. Remember that many diseases can cause diplopia and ocular palsies that do not directly interrupt optomotor nerves: myasthenia gravis, hyperthyroidism, botulism, and myopathies. Therefore, the "thinking through" process of differential diagnosis must also include the neuromyal junction, the muscles themselves, the adjacent anatomical structures, and systemic disease such as endocrinopathies.

C. Other cranial nerve conjuction syndromes

1. A single lesion in the cerebellopontine angle frequently affects CrNs VII and VIII at the internal auditory meatus and sometimes adjacent CrNs VI, and IX and others. Review Fig. 2-20.
2. CrNs IX, X, and XI come into conjunction at their exit site at the jugular foramen. Review Table 2-4.

BIBLIOGRAPHY · Eponymic Conjunction Syndromes

Brazis PW, Masdeu JC, Biller J. *Localization in Clinical Neurology,* 5th ed. Philadelphia: Lippincott Williams & Wilkins, 2007.

DeMyer W. *Neuroanatomy*. Baltimore: Lippincott Williams & Wilkins, 1998.

Goadsby PJ. "Paratrigeminal" paralysis of the oculopupillary sympathetic system. *J Neurol Neurosurg Psychiatry* 2002;72:297–299.

D. Patient analysis

1. The 34-year old woman in Fig. 4-33A suddenly noticed double vision.

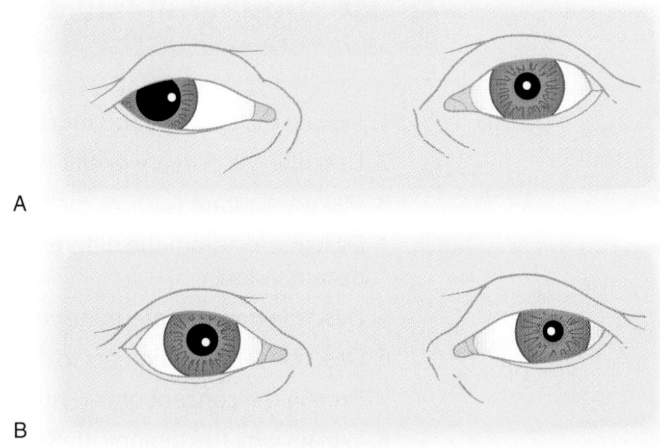

FIGURE 4-33. (A, B) Two Pts with ocular abnormalities.

right III nerve (Cerebral angiograms showed an aneurysm of the right posterior communicating artery, which had compressed the III nerve just after its exit from the midbrain.)

2. She was unable to adduct, elevate, or depress her right eye, but it did intort when she attempted to look down and to the left. The right eyelid did not elevate on volitional upward gaze. The right pupil neither reacted directly nor consensually to light. The left pupil did react directly and consensually. All other neurologic functions were intact. These findings indicated a lesion affecting the ________________________.

E. Patient analysis

1. The 21-year-old woman in Fig. 4-33B complained of deep pain behind her left eye for several weeks. She also noticed diplopia when looking far to the left. For some weeks her left eyelid had drooped. Examination showed ptosis that was corrected on upward gaze, miosis, and mild weakness of abduction of the left eye; however,

The Pt had sympathetic ptosis, minimal lateral rectus palsy, suggesting involvement of CrN VI, and pain suggesting involvement of CrN V. See next frames.

the corneal light reflections remained aligned when she had her eyes in the primary position. She had no other neurologic abnormalities. At her doctor's request, the Pt brought in old facial photographs that proved that the ptosis was new. Does the lesion localize to one nerve? If not, what nerves are implicated? ______________________________.

2. Because this Pt had only ptosis and miosis without hemifacial anhidrosis, the lesion must have affected her sympathetic pathway distal to the origin of her external carotid artery.
3. The conjunction site of the sympathetic pathway and the VI nerve is at the cavernous sinus region. This region receives its sensory innervation from CrN V. Hence, some lesion was progressively attacking successive sensory and motor nerves at the base of the skull.
4. Inspection of the nasopharynx disclosed a soft tissue mass. Radiographs of the skull base showed bony erosion. A biopsy disclosed a nasopharyngeal carcinoma. It had infiltrated the base of the skull and cavernous sinus and encircled the internal carotid artery, where it had interrupted the carotid sympathetic and VI nerves. Painful ophthalmoplegia of this type is called the **Tolosa-Hunt syndrome.**

IX. SUMMARY OF THE EXAMINATION FOR VISION AND THE PERIPHERAL OCULAR MOTOR SYSTEM

Now return to the Standard NE and rehearse Part VA15.

Learning Objectives for Chapter 4

I. OCULAR ALIGNMENT AND DIPLOPIA

1. Explain the concept and function of foveation.
2. Describe the primary position of the eyes.
3. Make a diagram to show the visual axis of a normal eye (Fig. 4-1).
4. Describe/diagram the difference in the visual axes of the eyes during near and distant vision.
5. Describe how to determine your dominant eye.
6. Describe self-experiments to demonstrate physiologic and pathologic diplopia.
7. Explain the concept of true and false images in diplopia.
8. Explain why the diplopic (false) image produced by displacing your eyeball by compression of your lateral canthus was less sharp than the (true) image from the non-displaced eye.

II. ACTIONS OF THE INDIVIDUAL EXTRAOCULAR MUSCLES

1. Describe the three axes of rotation of the eyeball and distinguish axial from eccentric rotation.
2. Define ductions, versions, and vergences.
3. List the EOMs (extraocular muscles), their origins and insertions and, by means of a ball model, demonstrate their actions (Fig. 4-9).
4. Make a diagram that shows the difference in the actions of the superior rectus and the superior oblique muscle when the eye is adducted, straight ahead, and abducted (Figs. 4-12 and 4-15).
5. Make a composite vector diagram to summarize the line of pull of the EOMs of one eye according to the law that the line of pull runs medial to the vertical axis for all EOMs, except the lateral rectus (Fig. 4-17).

Learning Objectives for Chapter 4

6. Make a tabular summary of the ocular rotatory muscles and list their primary, secondary, and tertiary actions (Table 4-1).
7. Recite the mnemonic that states how the adjective of the name of a rectus muscle aids in remembering the action of the muscle.
8. Explain the concept of yoking of ocular muscles, state Hering's law, and draw a figure summarizing the yoke muscles (Fig. 4-18).
9. Name the muscle that turns the adducted eye up and the muscle that turns the abducted eye up.
10. Explain why an eye deviates in a predictable direction after paralysis of one of its EOMs.

III. CLINICAL TESTS FOR OCULAR MALALIGNMENT AND THE RANGE OF EYE MOVEMENTS

1. Describe and demonstrate how to check the corneal light reflections.
2. Explain why the corneal light reflections fall a little to the medial side of the true geometric center of the corneas with the eyes in the primary position (Fig. 4-19).
3. Explain why inspecting the corneal light reflections is a more reliable test for ocular malalignment than inspecting the relation of the limbus to the lids.
4. Describe and demonstrate how to test the range of eye movements (Fig. 4-20).
5. State which direction of movement has the weakest range normally and declines most in aging or diffuse brain disease (Fig. 4-21).
6. Describe and demonstrate how to do the cover-uncover test for ocular malalignment (Fig. 4-22).
7. Explain and give examples of the difference between an operational and an interpretational definition.
8. Give an operational definition of heterotropia and outline the terms used to describe the various directions of eye deviation.
9. Name the type of heterotropia by inspecting the corneal light reflections of a series of illustrations (Fig. 4-23).
10. Describe and interpret the results of the cover-uncover test from a series of diagrams of the results (Figs. 4-24A to 4-24D).
11. Distinguish between heterotropia and heterophoria.
12. Explain why the Pt shows a greater ocular deviation when fixating with the paretic eye than when fixating with the sound eye (explain why the secondary deviation is greater than the primary deviation).
13. Describe the effects of heterotropia on vision in infants and head position.
14. Define suppression amblyopia (amblyopia ex anopsia). Describe how it may arise and how to prevent it.
15. Describe the direction of the head tilt to compensate for weakness of intorsion and minimize the diplopia from a right superior oblique muscle palsy.
16. Describe the clinical differentiation between paralytic (non-concomitant) and non-paralytic (concomitant) heterotropia (Table 4-2).
17. Explain these laws of diplopia:
    a. The false image is fuzzier than the true image.
    b. The false image projects peripheral to (or away from) the true image.
    c. The false image projects *opposite* to the direction of deviation of the paralytic eye.
    d. The false image projects *toward* the direction of action of the paralytic muscle.
    e. The distance between the true and false images increases as the eyes move in the direction of action of the paralytic muscle (Fig. 4-25).

Learning Objectives for Chapter 4

IV. REFRACTION AND ACCOMMODATION

1. Make a diagram to show the action of negative and positive lenses, thus illustrating the law of the prism (Fig. 4-26).
2. Describe the three actions of the accommodation (near) reflex.
3. Name the muscles that produce each of these actions (Table 4-3).
4. Make a diagram showing the point of focus of parallel light rays in the myopic, emmetropic, and hyperopic eye (Fig. 4-27).
5. Describe the relation between myopia and hyperopia and eso- and exophorias and eso- and exotropias.
6. Describe the age of onset of presbyopia and its differential affect on vision in myopes and hyperopes.
7. Describe the effect of a pinhole aperture on myopia, hyperopia, and presbyopia.
8. Explain why a pinhole aperture would correct blurred vision from presbyopia or a refractive error but not from a macular or optic nerve lesion.
9. Describe how to use the parallax test to determine whether the Pt's glasses correct for hyperopia or myopia.
10. Explain why a presbyopic myope removes eyeglasses to read newsprint, whereas a presbyopic emmetrope and in particular a presbyopic hyperope must put eyeglasses on for near vision.
11. Recite several causes of blurred vision related to the age of the Pt.

V. INNERVATION OF THE OCULAR MUSCLES

1. Name and classify the 11 intra- and extraocular muscles (Fig. 4-29).
2. Give the name and number of the CrNs that innervate the ocular muscles. Reason out and describe the clinical deficits due to interruption of each of these nerves (Table 4-4).
3. Name the nucleus of origin for each of the CrNs that innervates eye muscles and state which division of the brainstem it is located in.

VI. EXAMINATION OF THE PUPILS

1. Explain why a Pt should look at a distant point when you tests the pupillary light reflexes.
2. Describe the size and shape of the normal pupils.
3. Demonstrate how to examine the pupils.
4. Contrast the Argyll Robertson and Adie tonic pupils. Use the left column of Table 4-5 as a "prompt."
5. Define the direct and consensual pupillary light reflexes.
6. State whether in a normal person the direct and consensual pupilloconstrictions are equal or unequal.
7. Explain why the Ex should not abruptly shine the flashlight into the Pt's eyes from directly in front.
8. Describe the effect of interruption of one optic nerve or one III nerve on the direct and consensual pupillary light reflexes in the swinging flashlight test.
9. Recite what to write in the chart to document a thorough pupillary examination.
10. Diagram the pathways of the pupillary light reflex (Fig. 4-30).
11. Name the intraocular muscles and their nerve supply.
12. Name the pharmacologic class of the neurotransmitter for each intraocular muscle.

Learning Objectives for Chapter 4

13. Describe what happens to pupillary size after interruption or blocking of the parasympathetic or sympathetic nervous system and explain why this change in size occurs.
14. State whether a sympathomimetic or parasympathetic blocking drug will affect accommodation and explain why.
15. Explain why a mydriatic is used in the examination of the eye and describe the effect on the Pt's vision.
16. State the effect of a pupillodilator drug on intraocular tension. State the age range of Pts most likely to suffer from this effect.
17. Describe several determinants of pupillary size, including age.
18. Diagram the parasympathetic pathway from the brain to the intraocular muscles. State the clinical deficits resulting from the internal ophthalmoplegia due to interruption of this pathway (Fig. 4-30).
19. Diagram the sympathetic pathway to the eye and contrast the location of the parasympathetic and sympathetic ganglia (Fig. 4-31).
20. Describe Horner syndrome and the differences in signs dependent on interruption of the sympathetic pathway at various sites between the CNS and the orbit.
21. Describe the spinociliary (ciliospinal) reflex.
22. What are some important causes of acquired Horner syndrome?
23. Name three disorders characterized by abnormal pupils and absent muscle stretch reflexes.
24. Explain why you should test for pupilloconstriction to light and in accommodation in the routine examination.

VII. CLINICAL EVALUATION OF PTOSIS

1. Name the two muscles that elevate the eyelid and their nerve supply.
2. Describe the clinical features that differentiate III nerve from sympathetic ptosis (Table 4-6).
3. Describe how to "think through" the efferent pathway in analyzing ptosis.

VIII. CONJUNCTION SYNDROMES OF THE CRANIAL NERVES

1. Explain the concept of "conjunction syndromes" as a localizing technique in clinical neurology.
2. Name the CrNs that come into conjunction at the base of the forebrain and pituitary fossa, in the region of the cavernous sinus (Fig. 4-32).
3. Describe the core clinical features of the conjunction syndromes caused by lesions of the cavernous sinus.
4. Recite the common causes for the cavernous sinus conjunction syndromes.
5. Recite the CrNs involved in the conjunction syndromes at the cerebellopontine angle and the jugular foramen.

5 Examination of the Central Ocular Motor Systems

I. CENTRAL SYSTEMS FOR THE CONTROL OF EYE MOVEMENTS

A. The eyes move at two speeds, fast and slow (Dell'Osso and Daroff, 1999)

1. Physiologic fast eye movements, *saccades*, include:
   a. All voluntary horizontal and vertical eye movements
   b The kickback phase of jerk nystagmus, whether pathologic or physiologically induced by caloric or optokinetic stimuli
   c. Rapid eye movements in sleep
2. Pathologic fast eye movements, *opsoclonus* and *ocular flutter*, are faster than any saccades that the person can produce by volitional eye movements and are described later.
3. Slow eye movements include:
   a. Smooth pursuit
   b. Vergences (convergence/divergence)
   c. The deviation phase of vestibular and optokinetic nystagmus

B. The five eye movement systems tested by the neurologic examination

Five central systems control *voluntary* and *reflex* eye movements. Voluntary selection of a visual target requires saccadic action to move the eyes to the target. After that, *fixation*, *fusion*, *following*, and *focusing* (vergences and the control of refraction) proceed more or less automatically (Table 5-1).

1. **Saccadic system:** saccade = to *jerk* or *reign* in. Saccadic movement describes eye movements by increments or jerks, like a ratchet (Kennard et al., 1994).
   a. **Self-demonstration of saccades:**
      i. Look straight ahead. Then, while keeping your head completely still, move your eyes all the way to the right and hold them there.
      ii. With your head still, very slowly try to move your eyes as continuously and smoothly as possible *all* the way from the right to the left. Attend to how your eyes move. Do they move continuously and smoothly or by incremental jerks? ______________________

You will experience your eye movements as jerks, that is, saccades. Try this experiment on other people and observe their saccades.

   b. You cannot move your eyes smoothly voluntarily. **All volitional eye movements require saccades.**
   c. Frontotegmental corticobulbar pathways are thought to mediate all such saccades (Fig. 5-1).
   d. The supplementary motor area, substantia nigra, superior colliculus, vermis, fastigial nucleus, reticular formation, and vestibular system play roles in saccadic production and accuracy.

TABLE 5-1 · The Five Major Eye-Movement Systems

System	Function or characteristic
Saccadic system	Produces all volitional movements and the fast phase of reflex eye movements (frontal lobe)
Fixation (position maintenance system)	Fixates and maintains eyes on target and locks them in unison to fuse the two retinal images into one visual image (occipital lobe)
Smooth pursuit system	Keeps eyes on moving target (occipital lobe)
Vergence system	Converges or diverges eyes for near or distant targets (occipital lobe)
Counter-rolling system	Vestibular and neck proprioceptive system: counter-rolls the eyes to keep them fixed on the visual target in compensation for head movement

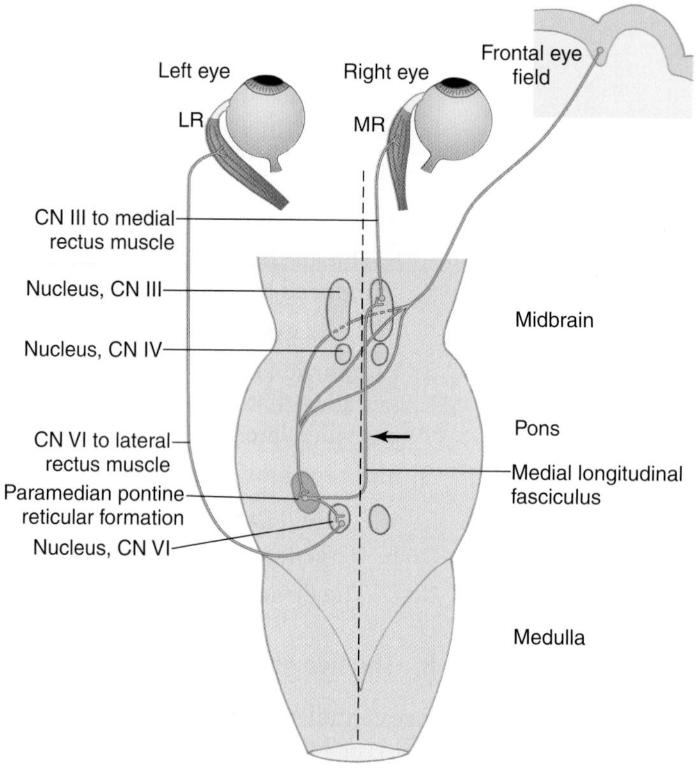

FIGURE 5-1. Dorsal view of the brainstem to show corticobulbar pathways for voluntary conjugate lateral eye movements.

e. **To test for saccadic accuracy:** Hold up your index fingers about 18 in. apart and ask the patient (Pt) to look at one and then the other. Move the targets around to require the Pt to look at different sites. Saccadic accuracy depends on connections in the dorsal part of the cerebellar vermis and the fastigial nuclei.

2. **Fixation (position holding) system**

a. After you choose a visual target and voluntarily saccade onto it, fixation reflexes hold the eyes on the target and promote fusion of both retinal images into one sharp visual image. Breaking away from the chosen target requires generation of another saccade to jerk the eyes away and onto a new visual target. Fixation reflexes tend to keep the eyes on target when the head moves.

b. Retino-geniculo-occipito-tegmental and retino-occipito-fronto-tegmental pathways mediate fixation and fusion.

3. **Smooth pursuit system**
   a. **Self-demonstration of smooth pursuit:**
      i. Keep your head still and facing straight ahead throughout this exercise.
      ii. Move your eyes all the way to the right, but this time hold up your finger about 30 cm away, fixate on it, and move it slowly all the way across from right to left. Allow only your eyes to pursue it. If you actually keep your head still and keep your eyes fixed on the moving finger, you will experience *smooth* rather than *saccadic* movement.
      iii. Practice eliciting smooth pursuit on another person.
   b. The smooth pursuit system keeps the eyes on target when the target moves. Drug intoxication, including alcohol, causes irregular or jerky rather than smooth pursuit of a moving object.
   c. Retino-geniculo-occipito-parieto-frontal-tegmental pathways mediate smooth pursuit.
4. **Vergence system**
   a. This system *converges* or *diverges* the eyes to ensure fusion of the two retinal images and appropriate refraction when the person looks at a near or distant visual target. It also keeps the eyes on target as the target moves toward or away from the person. This system mediates the accommodation reflex.
   b. The vergence system depends on retino-geniculo-occipito-tegmental pathways.
5. **The counter-rolling system of the eyes**
   a. **Self-demonstration of counter-rolling of the eyes:**
      i. Hold up your finger at arm's length, directly in front of you. Then, while holding your finger still, fixate on it and move your head horizontally and vertically.
      ii. Your eyes will reflexly *counter-roll* against the direction of head movement to maintain fixation on the chosen visual target.
   b. In the alert Pt, two systems collaborate to hold the eyes on target:
      i. The **ocular fixation system.**
      ii. The **proprioceptive system.** It arises in the vestibule and neck. It counter-rolls the eyes, an action called the *vestibulo-ocular reflex* (VOR).
   c. In the comatose Pt who cannot fixate, the examiner (Ex) can move the Pt's head (doll's eye maneuver) to test the counter-rolling reflex (VOR). See VOR in Chapters 9 and 12. Absence of fixation during coma makes counter-rolling depend on the VOR.
6. **In summary**
   a. If the visual target moves, the smooth pursuit system holds the eyes on target.
   b. If the Pt is conscious and if the head moves, the fixation reflexes and VOR keep the eyes on a target that is still.
   c. If the Pt is unconscious, only the proprioceptive reflexes can act, because the Pt cannot fixate.
7. Now, I haven't just loaded on you five more things to memorize. If you did the exercises, the following mnemonic will work:

A mnemonic to recall the five eye-movement systems.

1. Hold up your finger and choose to look at it. Your **saccadic system** will move your eyes onto the target. You have tested the frontotegmental pathways.
2. Your **fixation system** will lock the eyes on target until something, a saccade or a reflex, moves them off. You have tested the retino-geniculo-occipitotegmental pathways.

3. Move your finger *right or left* or *up or down*, and the **smooth pursuit system** will maintain fixation on the target. You have tested the horizontal conjugate movement and the vertical conjugate movement pathways.
4. Hold your finger still and move your head *right or left* or *up or down*, and the **counter-rolling system** will maintain fixation on the target. You have tested the vestibular and neck proprioceptive and fixation pathways.
5. Move your finger toward or away from your eyes. The **vergence system** then angles the eyes to keep them foveated on target and at the same time initiates the accommodation reflex. You have tested the retino-geniculo-occipito-tegmental pathways.

8. The foregoing exercises involved a still head or a still target. If the head and eyes both move toward a target, the counter-rolling by the VOR opposes the head and eye movement and undergoes suppression.

C. The corticopontine pathway for voluntary conjugate horizontal eye movements

1. Different pathways mediate conjugate *vertical* and *horizontal* eye movements. The pathway for voluntary conjugate horizontal eye movements begins in the cortex of the posterior-inferior part of the frontal lobe and runs to the pontine tegmentum (Fig. 5-1).
2. This cortical pathway terminates in the **paramedian pontine reticular formation** (PPRF) near the midline of the pons and responsible for generating horizontal eye movements. This region sends fibers to the ipsilateral abducens nucleus. The abducens nucleus sends fibers via cranial nerve VI to the ipsilateral lateral rectus muscle and, via the medial longitudinal fasciculus (MLF), also sends fibers that cross to the opposite medial rectus subnucleus. The medial rectus subnucleus innervates the medial rectus muscle. Thus, stimulation of the right PPRF or right abducens nucleus will make the eyes deviate conjugately to the right. (Frohman et al., 2001; Fig. 5-1).
3. **Effects of interruption of the horizontal gaze pathway**
   a. Interruption of the cortical efferent pathway for horizontal movements *rostral* to its decussation results in deviation of the eyes *ipsilateral* to the lesion (the eyes "look toward the lesion"), because the opposite pathways are intact and continue to convey tonic innervation.
   b. Interruption *caudal* to the decussation results in deviation to the side *contralateral* to the lesion.
4. **Effects of interruption of one MLF**
   a. After interruption of one MLF, say the right (tip of the arrow in Fig. 5-1), the right eye will not *ad*duct when the Pt attempts to look to the left (Ross and DeMyer, 1966).
   b. In addition to adductor paralysis on left lateral gaze, the Pt's left eye undergoes oscillations, a feature that you cannot deduce from the diagram. Such ocular oscillations are called **nystagmus.** Hence, a second sign of the MLF syndrome is monocular nystagmus of the *ab*ducting eye. At rest the eye has no nystagmus. It occurs only during *ab*duction. The symptoms accompanying the eye movements are **diplopia** and **oscillopsia** (oscillating vision).
   c. These two signs, paralysis of the *ad*ducting eye and nystagmus of the *ab*ducting eye, appear only on gaze to the opposite side of the MLF lesion.
      i. The eyes *ad*duct normally on convergence.
      ii. The corticobulbar pathways for convergence and vertical eye movements run directly into the mesencephalon to the LMNs of the III and IV nuclei, rather than looping down into the pons and returning in the MLF.

d. After a *left*-sided MLF lesion, what would be the only direction of gaze that would cause diplopia and heterotropia? (To reason out the answer from Fig. 5-1, draw in the pathway from the left cerebral hemisphere with colored pencil) ❒ looking right/❒ looking left/❒ looking straight ahead

☑ **looking to the right**

e. **Summary of the signs and symptoms of the MLF syndrome**

i. The *signs* of a unilateral MLF lesion consist of *heterotropia* and *monocular nystagmus*. They appear only when the Pt attempts to look away from the side of the interruption of the MLF. Other eye movements, including conjugate vertical gaze and pupillary responses remain normal.

ii. The *symptoms* of a unilateral MLF lesion may include *diplopia* and *oscillopsia*.

iii. During horizontal gaze the Pt cannot ❒ abduct/❒ adduct the eye ipsilateral to the lesion and shows monocular nystagmus of the contralateral, ❒ abducting/❒ adducting eye.

☑ **adduct;** ☑ **abducting**

f. Describe the signs of a bilateral MLF lesion at the level of the arrow in Fig. 5-1.

____

____

Monocular nystagmus of the leading (abducting) eye on attempted gaze to either side. Paralysis of adduction of the following (adducting) eye on attempted gaze to either side. The other eye movements and pupillary responses remain.

g. Would the eyes of a Pt with a bilateral MLF lesion converge during accommodation? ❒ Yes/❒ No. Explain.

____

☑ Yes. The convergence pathways run directly into the midbrain without involving the MLF.

D. Bilateral destruction of the frontal corticotegmental pathway for horizontal gaze (supranuclear paralysis of gaze)

1. If bilateral lesions destroy the pathway to the brainstem from the frontal eye fields, the Pt cannot produce saccades to voluntarily move the eyes to either side, but the vestibular counter-rolling reflexes can still move the eyes to the sides. Some weakness of vertical gaze is present or will develop because the Pt often has a progressive dementia or severe bilateral cerebrovascular disease.
2. After paralysis of voluntary movements, the vestibulo-ocular and fixation reflexes tend to become overly active ("released"). Indeed the full movement of the eyes by reflexes establishes that the LMNs of the ocular motor system are intact and that the cause for the paralysis of eye movements is supranuclear, in the UMNs. The Pt cannot voluntarily break fixation by moving the eyes and must blink or jerk the head to interrupt the afferent arc that maintains the fixation reflex. This condition when seen congenitally in children is called **Cogan's syndrome of oculomotor apraxia.**
3. The slow deviation phase of calorically induced or optokinetic nystagmus remains but the saccadic kickback fails, because the saccades depend on the integrity of the frontal eye fields.
4. Another form of progressive supranuclear palsy, called the **Steele-Richardson-Olszewski syndrome,** affects vertical movements first, usually the downward before the upward (Liu et al., 2001; Steele, 1994), and then horizontal movements. The lesion responsible affects the midbrain and basal forebrain structures.

E. Cortical pathway for vertical eye movements

1. Pathways for *vertical* eye movements arise diffusely from frontal and parietal cortices. Like the convergence pathways, they project directly to the midbrain, without looping down into the pons and reflecting back in the MLF.
2. The cortical pathway for conjugate *upward* eye movements runs in the tegmentum *dorsal* to the pathway for *downward* movements (Bhihdayasiri et al., 2000).
   a. **Parinaud's syndrome:** Dorsal compression of the midbrain, as from a pineal tumor, mesencephalic hemorrhage or obstructive hydrocephalus, will selectively impair *upward* vertical movements (Parinaud's syndrome) before affecting downward gaze. Convergence palsy and light-near dissociation of the pupils are commonly present also.

b. **Bell's phenomenon** (Sir Charles Bell, 1774–1842)

i. When most persons attempt to close their eyes, the eyeballs automatically rotate upward and somewhat outward. This associated eyeball movement, called **Bell's phenomenon,** occurs during voluntary eyelid closure or sleep, but closure of the eyelid by the orbicularis oculi muscle obscures it.

ii. In a Pt with UMN paralysis of voluntary elevation of the eyes, the presence of Bell's phenomenon proves that the midbrain and LMNs for the eye elevation are intact.

iii. The Ex will most easily see Bell's phenomenon if interruption of the facial nerve paralyzes the face, preventing eyelid closure. Idiopathic interruption of the facial nerve is called **Bell's palsy** (Chapter 7).

3. The cortical pathway for conjugate *downward* eye movements runs into the midbrain tegmentum dorsomedial to the red nucleus, where a lesion may selectively affect it, sparing vertical and horizontal eye movements (Bhihdayasiri et al., 2000). The lesion interrupts connections with the rostral interstitial nucleus of the MLF (riMLF), the saccadic brainstem center for vertical eye movements (Fig. 5-2), just as the PPRF is a brainstem center for horizontal saccades (see Fig. 5-1).

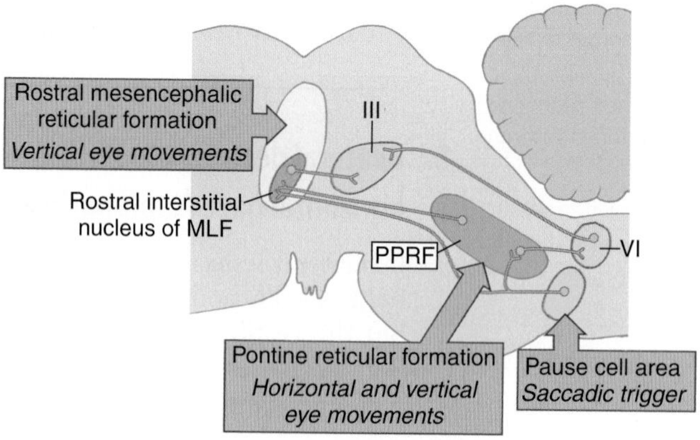

FIGURE 5-2. Sagittal section of the brainstem. The riMLF and the PPRF act as brainstem centers for the generation of saccades. The riMLF mediates vertical saccades and the PPRF mediates the horizontal. Lesions of these regions or their cortical input pathways impair the saccadic actions necessary for volitional vertical and horizontal gaze. PPRF = paramedian pontine reticular formation; riMLF = rostral interstitial nucleus of the medial longitudinal fasciculus. (Reproduced with permission from Kennard C, Crawford TJ, Henderson L. A pathophysiological approach to saccadic eye movements in neurologic and psychiatric disease. *J Neurol Neurosurg Psychiatry* 1994;57:881–885.)

F. Comparison of the LMN (nuclear), internuclear, and UMN (supranuclear) lesions of the ocular pathways

1. Interruption of LMNs of cranial nerve (CrN) III, IV, or VI paralyzes individual extraocular muscles (EOMs) or sets of muscles. No reflex or voluntary act can activate a muscle affected by LMN paralysis. The Pt suffers diplopia and strabismus.

2. Interruption of *internuclear* pathways, such as the MLF, paralyzes only movements mediated through that pathway. Other reflexes or voluntary pathways can still activate the ocular muscles. The Pt has diplopia only when that pathway should participate, as in the MLF syndrome.

3. Interruption of *supranuclear* pathways, the UMNs of the ocular motor system, impairs voluntary conjugate eye movements, not the actions of the individual EOMs. Reflexes can still activate the muscles. The Pt does not have diplopia. We can conclude that ocular movements illustrate the previously announced epigram that UMN lesions paralyze ☐ movements/☐ muscles, whereas LMN lesions paralyze ☐ movements/☐ muscles.

☑ movements
☑ muscles

4. In fact, the MLF syndrome helps to emphasize the principle that, when a muscle is paralyzed for only one movement and participates in others, the responsible lesion cannot be at the LMN level.

G. The concept of a head- and eye-centering center

1. **Self-demonstration of the head- and eye-centering tendency:** You can stare straight ahead, more or less vacantly or vapidly for some period, with no discomfort. Such staring spells, trances, or "tuning out" spells are common, even in infants, and especially in many retarded and learning-disabled children. But if you stare fully to one side, or up or down, discomfort soon demands that you return to the neutral, primary position. To *experience* the centering demand do this:
   a. Seat yourself comfortably. Pick out a target far to your left, almost behind you. Then turn your head and *especially your eyes* to the left and keep them there as long as possible, gazing at the target. Blink as necessary but do not break fixation. As you keep the eyes deviated, attend to your own sensations. Time how long you can maintain the deviated position. Now do the experiment.
   b. After some period of increasing discomfort as you keep your head and eyes deviated, a physiologic imperative will demand that you return them to the primary position, sometimes after as little as 30 seconds. You may feel the discomfort as anxiety, vertigo, blurred vision, or even headache. In any event, notice that you felt a considerable relief when you returned to the primary position. **Something about the organism wants its eyes and head straight ahead.** In fact, many brain-impaired Pts cannot sustain deviation for even 30 seconds, a sign called **motor impersistence.**
   c. Deviation of the eyes for any reason, voluntary or reflex, triggers a saccade that kicks the eyes back to the primary position, unless overridden by volition, as in the previous experiment. Inhibiting the saccadic kick-back reflex requires some of voluntary effort in the eye deviation experiment as does overcoming visco-elastic forces in the eye socket consequent to deviating the eyes.
2. **Many vectors compete to determine the position of the head and eyes at any given instant.**
   a. The will or intent of the bearer of the eyes, the emotional state, the survival requirements and advantage-seeking possibilities of the circumstances, and the attractiveness of the visual display.
   b. The position of the head in relation to space, movement, gravity, and the activity of the vestibular system.
   c. The illumination and conditions of vision.
   d. The refractive capability of the eyes and the distance of the visual target.
   e. The demands of binocular fixation and image fusion.
3. **Origin of vectors that determine head and eye position:** Vectors competing for the control of the head and eyes originate at every level of the neuraxis: posterior frontal cortex (Gaymard et al., 2000), basal motor nuclei, diencephalon, reticular formation, cerebellum, and even the rostral part of the spinal cord. Hence, lesions at any of these levels can more or less influence the movement and position of the head and eyes.
   a. For each head and eye position, vectors act to keep them there and others to move them away. In the aggregate, these opposing vectors result in **tonic innervation.** The continuous active contraction of the intraocular muscles and EOMs maintains them in a state of oppositional tension that positively determines eye position. The head and eyes seek the null, primary position, not because of the absence of stimulation but because all vectors balance out.
   b. To avoid chaos, some circuitry must integrate and balance these vectors. Although no head- and eye-centering center exists as such in one specific site, the concept of a head- and eye-centering center that balances the *right* and *left* vectors and the *up* and *down* vectors explains a number of clinical phenomena.
4. **A tale of opposing vectors**
   a. Normally the *right* cerebral hemisphere tends to drive the head and eyes to the *left*, balanced by the left hemisphere trying to drive them to the right. The vectors from the two hemispheres actively oppose and counterbalance each other. Study Figs. 5-3A to 5-3C.

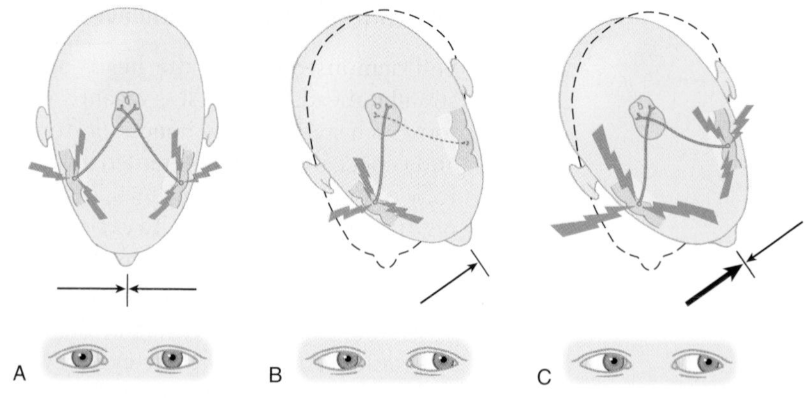

FIGURE 5-3. A head- and eye-turning center (conjugate gaze center) occupies the posterior part of the frontal lobe (zigzag lines). The arrows beneath A through C represent the strength of a vector originating on one side, acting to turn the head and eyes contralaterally. Notice the corticobulbar pathway to the pons and that it decussates. Relate this pathway to Fig. 5-1. (A) Normal resting condition. The vectors are equal and the head and eyes remain straight ahead. (B) A lesion has destroyed the left conjugate gaze center. The vector from the right center acts unopposed, deviating the head and eyes to the left. (C) An epileptogenic lesion has caused an excessive discharge of impulses from the right conjugate gaze center. The vector from the right hemisphere overpowers the one from the left. The head and eyes deviate to the left but for an entirely different reason than in B.

b. The corollary is that **any persistent conjugate deviation of the eyes or head and eyes in any direction means some disorder of the CNS pathways.** If only one eye deviates, the lesion affects the LMNs or neuromuscular level.

H. Effect of destructive cerebral lesions on the position of the eyes and head

1. A sudden massive lesion of one cerebral hemisphere, say the *right*, will interrupt the corticobulbar and corticospinal tracts, causing a complete *left* hemiplegia. This lesion also nullifies the vector arising in the *right* hemisphere that should continually strive to turn the eyes and head to the *left* (Fig. 5-3B).
2. What would you expect the position of the head and eyes to be in the foregoing Pt? ☐ midline/☐ turned to the left/☐ turned to the right. Explain.

____

____

☑ **turned to the right.** The lesion has eliminated the vector from the right hemisphere that always tries to turn the head and eyes to the left. The vector from the left hemisphere acts unopposed. Therefore, the head and eyes turn to the right, toward the side of the lesion and opposite to the hemiplegic side.

3. The head and eye deviations are most prominent in the acute phase of the lesion (Tijssen et al., 1991). The head- and eye-centering mechanisms reset themselves quickly, but the hemiplegia endures.

I. Effect of irritative lesions on the position of the head and eyes

1. Some cerebral lesions irritate cortical neurons, causing them to fire excessively. Such an irritative lesion initiates epileptic seizures. Electrical stimulation of the cortex has the same effect. Suppose a Pt has a focal epileptic seizure that begins by turning the head and eyes to the *right*. You would anticipate that the Pt had an epileptogenic focus in the ☐ right/☐ left frontal lobe (Fig. 5-3C).

☑ **left**

2. *During* the epileptic discharge, the excess of impulses on the left side overcomes the normal vector from the right. *After* the epileptic cataclysm has subsided, the excessive discharge has metabolically exhausted the neurons in the seizure focus, rendering them temporarily nonfunctional. Immediately *after* an epileptic seizure caused by a left-sided cerebral lesion, to which side would the head and eyes be turned? ☐ right/☐ left. Explain.

____

____

☑ **left.** Because the *left* eye- and head-turning center is exhausted, the *right* acts unopposed. The head and eyes turn to the *left, opposite* to the direction that they turned during the seizure.

J. The rostral midbrain syndrome (Sylvian aqueduct syndrome; pretectal syndrome)

1. Many nuclei and pathways that control the actions of the eyes and pupils surround the rostral part of the Sylvian aqueduct, in the midbrain tectum, pretectum, tegmentum, and periaqueductal gray matter. The actions controlled include upward and downward gaze, vertical ocular alignment, pupillary size, palpebral fissure height, vergences, and the movements mediated by CrN III (Table 5-2).

TABLE 5-2 · Rostral Midbrain Syndrome (Sylvian Aqueduct Syndrome; Pretectal Syndrome)

Pupillary changes: anisocoria, corectasia, corectopia, absence of constriction to light or dissociated reactions to light and accommodation
Eyelid abnormalities: eyelid retraction (Collier's sign), lid lag, reptilian stare or conversely ptosis.
Supranuclear upward or downward gaze palsy, or combined palsy of upward and downward gaze
Convergence/accommodation paralysis
Nystagmus: convergence nystagmus or convergence-retraction nystagmus, vertical nystagmus on attempted upward gaze, see-saw nystagmus
CrN III palsy
Strabismus: III nerve or pseudoabducens palsy, thalamic esotropia, skew deviation
Head tilt
Oculogyric crises: forceful deviation of the eyes, common in parkinsonism

ABBREVIATION: CrN = cranial nerve.

2. Pure paralysis of upward gaze is known as **Parinaud's syndrome**
3. Midbrain signs in addition to the Sylvian aqueduct syndrome per se include:
   a. Oculogyric crises
   b. Minimal to severe impairment of consciousness
   c. Hemiparesis or quadriparesis
   d. Decerebrate rigidity
   e. Central neurogenic hyperventilation
   f. Tremor or ataxia
4. The **top of the basilar syndrome** is caused by infarction in the terminal branches of the basilar artery, the posterior cerebral arteries. These arteries irrigate the midbrain-diencephalic junction and the inferomedial aspect of the temporo-occipital region. Infarction may cause any combination of midbrain, posterior thalamic, or temporo-occipital region signs, including loss of consciousness, depending on the location of the occlusion, the extent of the thrombus, and the collateral flow.

BIBLIOGRAPHY · Central Systems for the Control of Eye Movements

Bender MB. Brain control of conjugate horizontal and vertical eye movements. A survey of the structural and functional correlates. *Brain* 1980;103:23–69.

Bender MB, Rudolph SH, Stacy CB. The neurology of the visual and oculomotor systems. In Joynt RJ, Griggs RC, eds. *Clinical Neurology.* Philadelphia, Lippincott Williams & Wilkins, 1998, Vol. 1, Chap. 12, 1–132.

Bhihdayasiri R, Plat GJ, Leigh J. A hypothetical scheme for the brainstem control of vertical gaze. *Neurology* 2000;54:1985–1993.

Brazis PW, Masdeu JC, Biller J. *Localization in Clinical Neurology.* 5th ed. Philadelphia: Lippincott Williams and Wilkins, 2007.

Frohman EM, Zhang H, Kramer PD, et al. MRI characteristics of the MLF in MS patients with chronic internuclear ophthalmoparesis. *Neurology* 2001;57:762–768.

Gaymard B, Siegler I, Rivaud-Pechoux S, et al. A common mechanism for the control of eye and head movements in humans. *Ann Neurol* 2000;46:829–822.

Kennard C, Crawford TJ, Henderson L. A pathophysiological approach to saccadic eye movements in neurologic and psychiatric disease. *J Neurol Neurosurg Psychiatry* 1994;57:881–885.

Leigh, RJ, Zee, DS. *The Neurology of Eye* Movements, 4th ed. New York, Oxford University Press, 2006.

Liu GT, Volpe NJ, Galetta SL. *Neuro-ophthalmology. Diagnosis and Management*. Philadelphia, W.B. Saunders, 2001.

Pullicino P, Lincoff N, Truax BT. Abnormal vergence with upper brainstem infarcts: pseudoabducens palsy. *Neurology* 2000;55:352–358.

Ross A, DeMyer W. Isolated syndrome of the medial longitudinal fasciculus in man. *Arch Neurol* 1966;15:203–205.

Steele JC. Historical notes [on progressive supranuclear palsy]. *J Neurol Transm* 1994;suppl 42:3–14.

Tijssen CC, van Gisbergen JAM, Schulte BPM. Conjugate eye deviation: side, site, and size of the hemispheric lesion. *Neurology* 1991;41:846–850.

K. The asymmetric tonic neck reflex (ATNR; Magnus-deKleijn reflex): integration of the contralateral visual field, proprioception, touch, the grasp reflex, and voluntary eye movements, or how the infant discovers its own hand

1. **Technique to elicit the ATNR**

   a. With the infant supine and quiet, gently and slowly turn the infant's head to one side and hold it there for at least 30 seconds. Then turn the infant's head back fully to the opposite side (Fig. 5-4).

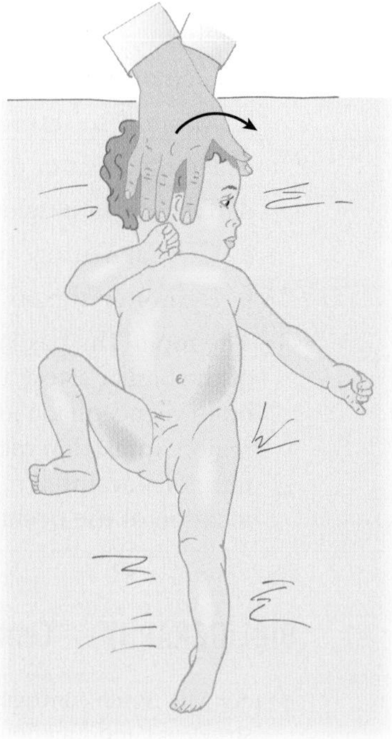

FIGURE 5-4. Demonstration of the tonic neck reflex. Turning of the infant's head to one side (in this case by the examiner) causes the ipsilateral extremities to straighten and the opposite to flex.

   b. Normally the infant *extends* the arm and leg on the side to which the head is turned and *flexes* the contralateral extremities. **As the head looks to one side, the hand extends into that visual field (Magnus, 1926).**

   c. Normal infants 2 to 4 months of age spend much time in the ATNR posture, but they can readily escape from it. During this period, the infant learns to fixate on and to reach for objects and to convert the primitive grasp reflex to volitional grasping of objects.

2. **Physiology of the asymmetric tonic neck reflex:** The slow head turning stimulates position sense receptors in the neck (fast head turning elicits a counter-rolling vestibular reflex). The afferent pathway runs rostrally into the brainstem reticular formation. Reticulospinal pathways complete the reflex.
3. **Interpretation of the ATNR**
   a. Because the head and eyes look to the extended hand, the TNR may serve as the forerunner of eye and hand coordination. By sight and proprioception, the infant discovers its own extending hand. If the hand touches an object, the grasp reflex closes the fingers on it. The eyes then learn to direct, via the pyramidal tract, the hand as it explores space and learns to grasp visual targets. The ATNR demonstrates the unity of a visual field, proprioception, touch, and contralateral movement control. The sequence marvelously expresses the **law of contralateral cerebral sensorimotor innervation** (Chapter 2).
   b. Primitive behaviors such as the ATNR and the grasp reflex disappear as cerebral pathways establish dominance according to the normal developmental timetable. Undue persistence of the ATNR posture, when spontaneously assumed by the infant or induced by an Ex, predicts poor motor development. The more obligatory the ATNR and the longer it persists in infancy, the more abnormal the infant. When strong and persistent, it interferes with sitting and voluntary movement.
4. The ATNR may sometimes reappear in older children or adults who suffer high brainstem or cerebral lesions interrupting corticobulbar and other descending motor pathways: cerebral dominance over the brainstem is lost. Other primitive reflexes also may reappear in aging and dementia (Chapter 11).
5. **Summary of the ATNR**
   a. When the head of a young infant turns to one side, the *ipsilateral* extremities tend to ❒ flex/❒ extend, whereas the *contralateral* extremities tend to ❒ flex/❒ extend.
   b. The foregoing definition is ❒ operational/❒ interpretational. An operational definition states a fact or an agreed upon procedure by which a phenomenon is disclosed.
   c. Give an interpretational definition of the TNR.

   ____
6. What is the prognostic significance of undue persistence of the TNR or any primitive reflex after the first months of life?

   ____

   ____

☑ extend; ☑ flex

☑ operational

The TNR is a primitive brainstem reflex that promotes the development of normal eye and hand (visuomotor) coordination in infants.

Persistence of the TNR indicates that UMN dominance over the brainstem reflexes is lagging behind the developmental timetable. The infant usually shows permanent deficits in UMN control of movement.

BIBLIOGRAPHY · Asymmetric Tonic Neck Reflex

Magnus R. Cameron Prize Lectures on some results of studies in the physiology of posture. *Lancet* 1926;2:531–536, 585–588.

II. NYSTAGMUS

A. Definition

Nystagmus consists of involuntary, rhythmic oscillations of the eyeballs. Nystagmus can be physiologic or pathologic.

1. *Physiologic* nystagmus is triggered by:
   a. Spinning (merry-go-round)
   b. Focusing on stripes on a rotating drum (optokinetic nystagmus)
   c. Endpoint gaze

2. *Pathologic* nystagmus arises most commonly from lesions located in:
   a. The media, retina or optic nerve or optic chiasm that interfere with vision.
   b. Vestibular end organ or nerve.
   c. The brainstem tegmentum and cerebellum (Leigh and Zee, 2006).
3. Diencephalic or cerebral lesions infrequently cause nystagmus. Thalamic lesions or in infants retinal or hypothalamic lesions, such as optic nerve hypoplasia or gliomas, can cause mixed forms of nystagmus. Cerebral lesions may cause a type of gaze paretic nystagmus. Although the clinical findings usually suffice to diagnose the cause of nystagmus, magnetic resonance imaging examination of the brain often is necessary.

B. Symptoms of nystagmus

1. Symptoms may accompany nystagmus:
   a. **Oscillopsia:** apparent oscillation of objects viewed.
   b. **Vertigo:** a sensation of movement, generally a feeling of rotation or spinning of self or the environment (Chapter 8).
   c. **Nausea:** with or without vomiting
   d. **Blurred vision**
2. The presence of symptoms depends on the rapidity of onset and the duration and site of the lesion. Just as heterotropia of congenital or early origin usually does not cause diplopia, nystagmus of congenital or early origin may not cause symptoms.

C. The signs of nystagmus

If you can describe the Pt's nystagmus well, you need not memorize its endless kinds and causes. Dendrograms (Figs. 5-6 and 5-7) based on the clinical features listed in Table 5-3 will lead to the probable diagnosis. Begin by describing the *plane*, the *type* (jerk or pendular), and the *direction*, if a jerk nystagmus.

1. **Note the plane of eye movements** (Table 5-3)
   a. **Horizontal:** eyeball oscillates around the vertical axis.
   b. **Vertical:** eyeball oscillates around the lateral axis.
   c. **Rotatory (torsional):** eye oscillates around the anteroposterior (A-P) axis.
   d. **Mixed.**

TABLE 5-3 · Steps in the Clinical Analysis of Nystagmus

1. Note the *plane* of eye movements (horizontal, vertical, torsional or mixed), *type* (jerk or pendular), and *direction* (unidirectional or bidirectional), if it is a jerk nystagmus.
2. Note the type of nystagmus, pendular or jerk.
3. Note the direction of the fast movement of the nystagmus, if the Pt has jerk nystagmus.
4. Note the amplitude and rate.
5. Note whether the nystagmus is binocular and symmetrical, monocular, or dissociated (different amplitude in the two eyes or different directions).
6. Note whether the nystagmus occurs in the primary position or the eccentric positions and the effect of eye movements in the cardinal directions of gaze (Figs. 5-6 and 5-7).
7. Look for a null point where bidirectional nystagmus is minimal or absent.
8. Test for the effects of changes in head position or posture on nystagmus.
9. Test for latent nystagmus by covering each eye separately and inspecting the other eye with magnification provided by the ophthalmoscope.
10. Look for associated rhythmic movements of the lids, face, jaw, tongue, palate, pharynx, neck, or limbs (palatal and ocular myoclonus).
11. In selected Pts, test for optokinetic nystagmus, the Romberg fall, and past-pointing and do caloric irrigation.
12. Consider electronystagmography and radiographic imaging.

ABBREVIATION: Pt = patient.

Mnemonic to remember the planes of nystagmus: Name the *possible* planes of eye movement as related to the three axes of rotation of the eye, the A-P, lateral, and vertical axes.

vertical

lateral

A-P

horizontal

vertical

rotatory (torsional)

mixed

i. In *horizontal* (lateral) nystagmus, the eyeball rotates around the _______ axis.

ii. In *vertical* nystagmus, the eyeball rotates around the _________ axis.

iii. In *rotary nystagmus* (torsions), the eyeball rotates around _____ the axis.

e. Hence, the planes of nystagmus are (order unimportant)

i. __________

ii. __________

iii. __________

iv. __________

2. **Note the** ***type*** **of nystagmus,** ***pendular*** **or** ***jerk:***
   a. *Jerk nystagmus* has *fast* and *slow* components.
   b. *Pendular nystagmus* resembles a pendulum or metronome. The eyeballs show an equal to-and-fro, metronomic oscillation.
   c. If *to* equals *fro,* the Pt has __________ nystagmus.
   d. If *to* does not equal *fro,* the Pt has __________ nystagmus.

pendular

jerk

3. **Note the** ***direction*** **of the fast movement of the nystagmus, if the Pt has jerk nystagmus:**
   a. The *direction* of jerk nystagmus means the direction of movement of the fast component.
   b. If the nystagmus jerks to the right side, we say the direction is to the __________________.
   c. If the fast component always jerks in one direction, the nystagmus is **unidirectional.** If the direction of the jerk changes with the direction of eye movements, the nystagmus is **bidirectional.** Look for a neutral zone in which the nystagmus changes direction.
   d. **Nomenclature note on designating the direction of jerk nystagmus:** Custom dictates naming jerk nystagmus by the direction of the fast movement, but the important event is the deviation or slow phase (Leigh and Zee, 2006). The slow movement initiates nystagmus by triggering a saccadic jerk, a kickback reflex. Slow velocity systems include smooth pursuit and optokinetic nystagmus, vergences, and the slow phase of nystagmus induced by vestibular stimulation. Pathologic nystagmus reflects an imbalance in these slow velocity systems that normally should hold the eyes steadily on the visual target (gaze-holding mechanisms).

right

4. **Note the amplitude and rate.**
5. **Note whether the nystagmus is binocular and symmetrical, monocular, or dissociated. Dissociated nystagmus shows different amplitudes in the two eyes or different directions** (Shawkat et al., 2001).
6. **Note whether the nystagmus occurs in the primary position or the eccentric positions and the effect of eye movements in the cardinal directions of gaze** (Fig. 4-20). Determine whether the nystagmus changes in rate, amplitude, or direction as the eyes fixate in the primary position and move through the various fields of gaze, including convergence. Jerk nystagmus increases when the Pt looks in the direction of the fast phase (Alexander's law), because the volitional and reflex saccades add up.
7. **Look for a null point where bidirectional nystagmus is minimal or absent.**

8. **Test for the effect of changes in head position or posture on nystagmus:**
   a. Make quick, rotations of the Pt's head over a short distance and try the Dix-Hallpike maneuver (Chapter 9).
   b. Test for cancellation of the vestibulo-ocular reflex by the eye-to-thumb rotation test. The Pt sits on a revolving stool, extends an arm, holds the thumb vertically, and maintains fixation on the thumb. The Ex rotates the Pt's head, body, and thumb as a unit to the right and left. If eyes break away from the thumb and show nystagmus, the Pt may have a lesion of the cerebellum or central vestibular pathways. Try this simple test yourself.
9. **Test for latent nystagmus by covering each eye separately and inspecting the other eye with magnification provided by the ophthalmoscope.** By removing fixation, this maneuver releases nystagmus.
10. **Look for associated rhythmic movements of the lids, face, jaw, tongue, palate, pharynx, neck, or limbs (palatal and ocular myoclonus).**
11. **In selected Pts, test for optokinetic nystagmus, the Romberg fall (Chapter 10), past pointing, and caloric irrigation.**
12. **Consider electronystagmography and radiographic imaging.**

D. The laws of nystagmus

These general laws are subject to exceptions but have practical value.

1. **Jerk nystagmus**
   a. Central and peripheral vestibular lesions may cause jerk nystagmus.
   b. Unidirectional jerk nystagmus is always vestibular in origin.
   c. Acquired bidirectional horizontal nystagmus is almost always central in origin and usually indicates a brainstem lesion or toxic/metabolic state.
   d. Alexander's law: Looking in the direction of the fast phase of a jerk nystagmus increases its amplitude.
   e. Jerk and pendular nystagmus may have a rotatory component.
2. **Peripheral versus central origin of nystagmus**
   a. The two cardinal features that distinguish peripheral from central vestibular nystagmus are unidirectionality and inhibition of peripheral nystagmus by visual fixation. Fixation has little effect on central nystagmus (Hotson and Baloh, 1998).
   b. Peripheral nystagmus, particularly when vertical has a torsional component, but a pure vertical or pure torsional nystagmus, is always central in origin.
   c. Acquired pendular nystagmus usually is caused by brainstem or cerebellar strokes, neoplasms, or multiple sclerosis.
   d. Positional nystagmus may occur with peripheral vestibular or central lesions.
   e. Acquired peripheral nystagmus is short lasting, and central is long lasting.
3. **Nystagmus with posterior fossa/cerebellar disease**
   a. Cerebellar lesions or drugs characteristically cause bidirectional gaze-evoked nystagmus, deficient smooth pursuit, impaired saccadic accuracy, and slow initiation of saccades.
   b. Visual suppression of nystagmus is minimal or absent with cerebellar as with any central nystagmus.
   c. Flocculus and paraflocculus lesions cause downbeat nystagmus-deficient smooth pursuit, gaze-evoked nystagmus, and rebound nystagmus.
   d. Upbeat and downbeat nystagmus, especially in the primary position, indicate a posterior fossa lesion (Hirose et al., 1998; Janssen et al., 1998).
   e. Downbeat nystagmus, characterized by slow upward drifts and fast downward phases, may indicate a foramen magnum lesion such as the Chiari malformation (Wagner et al., 2008).
   f. Torsional nystagmus may arise from medullary lesions.

4. **Miscellaneous laws**
   a. The characteristics of the nystagmus do not differentiate congenital nystagmus without afferent defect from nystagmus with afferent defect.
   b. Gaze-evoked nystagmus may occur with CNS or neuromuscular lesions that cause weakness of eye movements.
   c. Some types of nystagmus stay horizontal on upward gaze: congenital, peripheral vestibular, and periodic alternating.
   d. Cold water irrigation of the horizontal canal of one ear reproduces the effect of an acute vestibular lesion on that side, e.g., fast phase and vertigo to the opposite side, the Romberg fall, and past-pointing to the same side (Chapter 9).

E. Diagnostic dendrograms for specific types of nystagmus

1. Summarize the nystagmus with regard to *plane* (form), *type,* and *direction* (if a jerk type) according to Fig. 5-5.

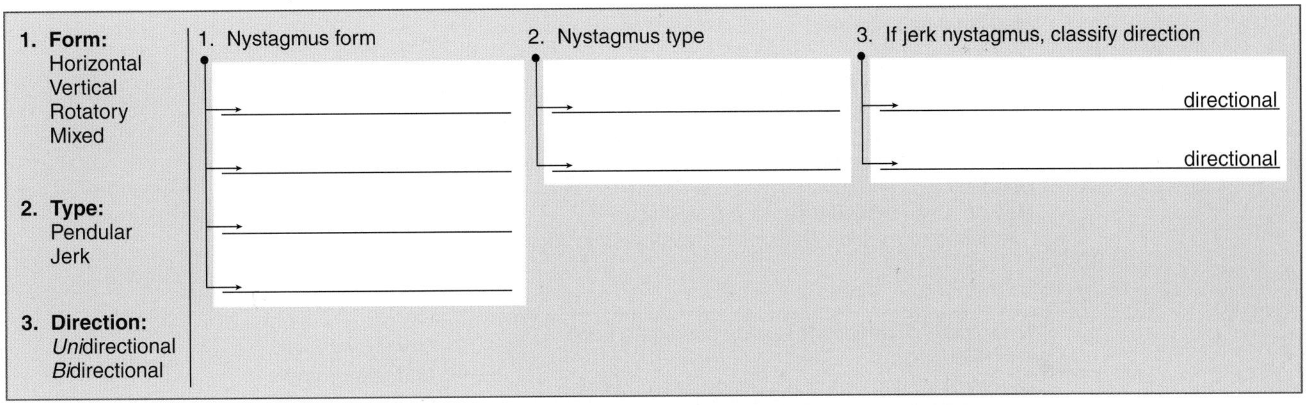

FIGURE 5-5. Classification of nystagmus as to form, type, and direction.

2. The data from Table 5-3 and Fig. 5-5, when integrated with the history, permits you to enter the dendrograms of Figs. 5-6 and 5-7. Read through the dendrograms for familiarity but do not memorize them. Notice that *pendular* nystagmus implies an ocular cause or central lesion. Unidirectional jerk nystagmus implies a lesion of the peripheral vestibular system or the immediate central connections.
3. **Differentiation of spontaneous peripheral and central vestibular nystagmus** (Table 5-4).
4. **Differentiation of positional vestibular nystagmus** (Table 5-5)

See Chapter 9 for positional maneuvers and the Romberg test.

F. Some uncommon non-nystagmoid repetitive eye movements

1. **Ocular bobbing:** A type of eye movement resembling downbeat nystagmus likewise shows a fast downward movement and slow drift back to the primary position, but it differs from nystagmus in being arrhythmic and having a low frequency of 2 to 12 per minute. The lesion, usually vascular (often a hemorrhage), inflammatory, neoplastic, traumatic, or demyelinating, affects the pons, but it also may occur with cerebellar lesions compressing the pons. The Pt is usually comatose and quadriplegic and lacks other spontaneous or induced eye movements.

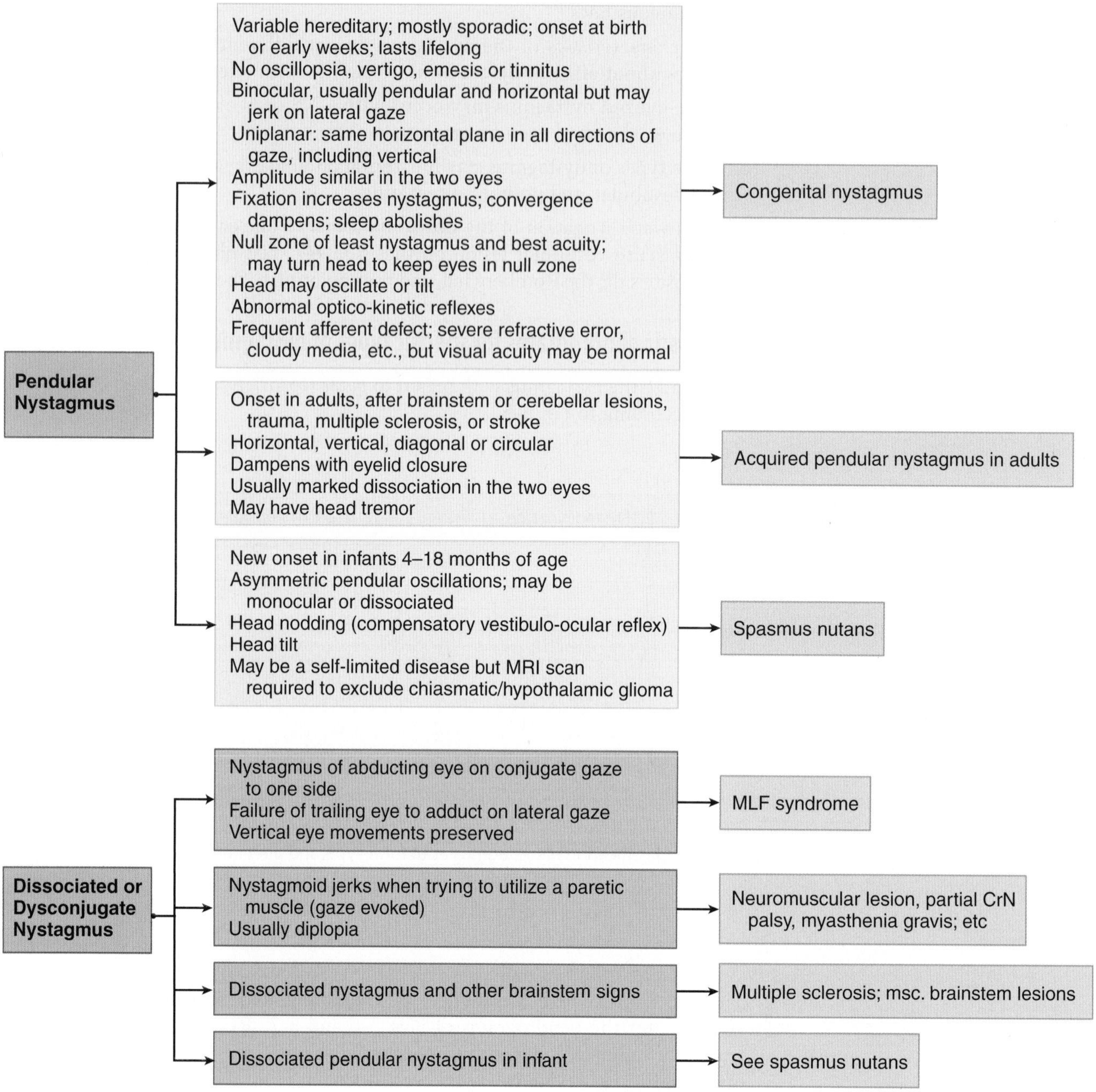

FIGURE 5-6. Differential diagnostic dendrogram for pendular nystagmus.

2. **Ocular flutter** describes intermittent bursts of lightning-fast eye movements. It may precede or accompany **opsoclonus,** defined as rapid, chaotic, and more or less continuous non-rhythmic lightning jerks of the eyeballs in various directions ("saccadomania").
   a. Flutter and opsoclonus may be sporadic or associated with neuroblastoma in children or visceral carcinoma in adults.
   b. They belong to types of rapid eye movements without a slow component, whereas nystagmus in general reflects disorders of slow eye-movement systems.
3. **Voluntary "nystagmus":** Some Pts with Munchausen's syndrome or pseudoseizures can make rapid shuddering or shimmering ocular movements that resemble nystagmus but consist of back-to-back saccades (Davis, 2000; remember, all voluntary movements are saccadic). Diagnostic features are

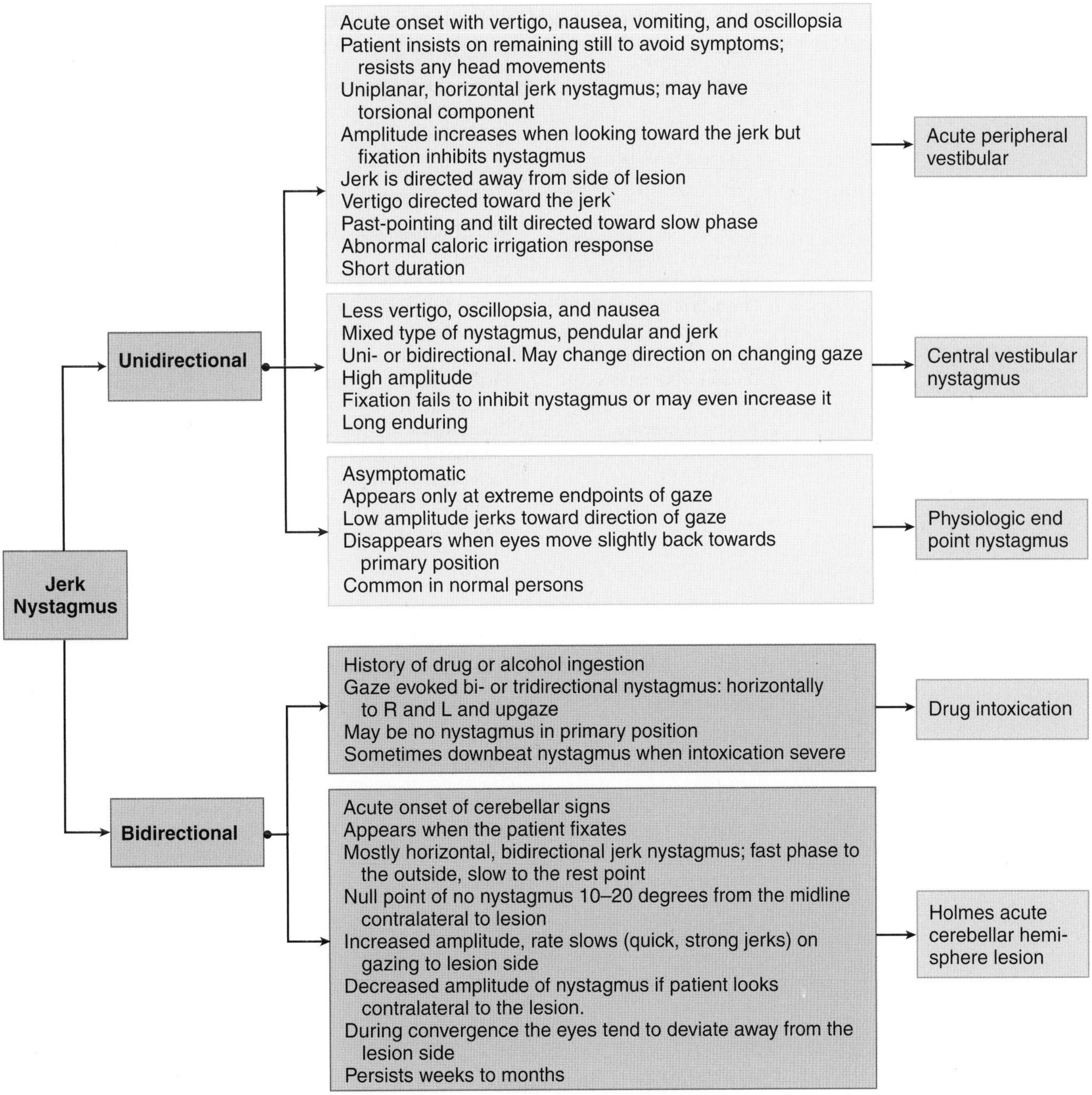

FIGURE 5-7. Differential diagnostic dendrogram for jerk nystagmus.

a. The movements are horizontal and equal in excursion.

b. Sustainable only for short periods, usually less than 15 to 30 seconds, because they require extreme concentration.

c. Best accomplished with slight convergence.

d. The Pt frequently blinks and closes the eyes.

e. Nystagmus stops by having the Pt change the direction of gaze.

G. Electronystagmography

Electronystagmography, as done by neuro-ophthalmologists or ear, nose, and throat specialists, provides a visual quantitative record for the analysis of nystagmus waveforms (Dell'Oss and Daroff, 1999).

TABLE 5-4 · Differentiation of Peripheral and Central Vestibular Nystagmus

Symptoms or signs	Peripheral (end organ)	Central (nuclear)
Direction of nystagmus	Unidirectional; fast-phase opposite lesion	Bidirectional or unidirectional
Purely horizontal nystagmus without torsional component	Uncommon	Common
Vertical or purely torsional nystagmus	Never present	May be present
Visual fixation	Inhibits nystagmus and vertigo	No inhibition
Severity of vertigo	Marked	Mild
Direction of spin	Toward fast phase	Variable
Direction of past-pointing	Toward fast phase	Variable
Direction of the Romberg fall	Toward fast phase	Variable
Effect of head turning	Changes the Romberg fall	No effect
Duration of symptoms	Finite (minutes, days, weeks) but recurrent	May be present
Tinnitus or deafness	Often present	Usually absent
Common causes	Infection (labyrinthitis), Ménière's disease, neuronitis, vascular disorders, trauma,toxicity	Vascular, demyelinating, and neoplastic disorders

TABLE 5-5 · Differentiation of Peripheral and Central Positional Nystagmus

Symptoms or signs	Peripheral (extra-axial)	Central (intra-axial)
Latency	2–20 s	None
Persistence	Disappears within 50 s	Lasts longer than 1 min
Fatigability	Disappears on repetition	Repeatable
Positions	Present in one position	Present in multiple positions
Vertigo	Always present	Occasionally absent, with only nystagmus present
Direction of nystagmus	Unidirectional	Changes directions in different positions
Incidence	Common (85% of all cases)	Uncommon (10–15% of all cases)

BIBLIOGRAPHY · Nystagmus

Brazis PW, Masdeu JC, Biller J. *Localization in Clinical Neurology,* 5th ed. Philadelphia, Lippincott Williams & Wilkins, 2007.

Davis BJ. Voluntary nystagmus as a component of a non-epileptic seizure. *Neurology* 2000;55:1937.

Dell'Osso LF, Daroff RB. Nystagmus and saccadic intrusions and oscillations. In Glaser JS, ed. *Neuro-ophthalmology,* 3rd ed. Philadelphia, Lippincott Williams & Wilkins, 1999, Chap. 11, pp. 369–400.

Hirose G, Ogasawara T, Shirakawa T, et al. Primary position upbeat nystagmus due to unilateral medial medullary infarction. *Ann Neurol* 1998;43:403–406.

Hotson JR, Baloh RW. Acute vestibular syndrome. *N Engl J Med* 1998;339:680–685.

Janssen JC, Larner AJ, Morris H, et al. Upbeat nystagmus: clinicoanatomical correlation. *J Neurol Neurosurg Psychiatry* 1998;65:380–381.

Leigh RJ, Zee, DS. *The Neurology of Eye Movements,* 4th ed. New York, Oxford University Press, 2006.

Shawkat FS, Kriss A, Russell-Eggitt I, et al. Diagnosing children presenting with asymmetric pendular nystagmus. *Dev Med Child Neurol* 2001;43:622–627.

Wagner JN, Glaser M, Brandt T, et al. Downbeat nystagmus: aetiology and comorbidity in 117 patients. *J Neurol Neurosurg Psychiatry* 2008;79:672–677.

III. SUMMARY OF THE LAWS OF OCULAR MOTILITY FOR THE CLINICAL EXAMINATION

A. Laws governing the actions of the ocular muscles

1. **The law of axial rotation of an eyeball:** The six EOMs rotate the eyeball around one of its three axes: A-P, vertical, or horizontal (Fig. 4-1).
2. **The law of on-center/off-center pull of the extraocular muscles:** The ocular muscles that pull only "on center" have one primary rotary action, whereas those that pull "off center" cause primary, secondary, and tertiary rotations. The line of pull or vector of all EOMs runs *medial* to the vertical axis, except for the lateral rectus muscle (Fig. 4-17). **Corollary:** The muscles that pull off center change their actions depending on the position of the eye when the muscle acts (Figs. 4-12 to 4-16).
3. **The law of positive tonic oppositional innervation of the intra- and extra-ocular muscles**
   a. The intraocular and extraocular muscles of one eye act in oppositional sets that receive equal tonic innervation. (The ciliary muscle ostensibly seems to be an exception, but the elasticity of the lens acts as its opponent.)
   b. Tonic innervation positively holds the eye in position. When the eyes are still, the pull of one muscle balances out the pull of the other.
      i. After paralysis of a muscle, the eye assumes the position, or the pupil assumes the size, dictated by the pull of the intact, tonically innervated, oppositional muscle.
      ii. A nuclear, nerve, or neuromuscular lesion paralyzes individual ocular muscles, causing strabismus and diplopia.
      iii. Persistent monocular deviation arises peripherally, whereas persistent conjugate (binocular) deviation arises centrally.

B. Laws governing the central control of eye movements

1. **The law of conjugate ocular fixation and conjugate movement:** The eyes fixate and move conjugately, except during vergences. **Corollary:** Failure of conjugate fixation and conjugate movement is always abnormal.
2. **Hering's law of equal innervation of the corresponding EOMs:** The muscles that collaborate to move the two eyes in a given direction receive equal innervation. This law ensures that the two eyes move equally and remain aligned in all directions of gaze, with the retinal images on corresponding sites to avoid blurred vision and diplopia.
3. **The law of different pathways for horizontal and vertical conjugate eye movements:** The supranuclear pathway for volitional conjugate *horizontal* eye movements arises in the posterior-inferior frontal cortex and loops down into the pontine tegmentum and back up to the midbrain through the MLF (Fig. 5-1). In direct contrast, the pathways for *vertical* movements arise more diffusely from the cortex and run directly into the pretectum and midbrain without looping down into the midbrain.
   a. The pathway for conjugate *upward* eye movements courses into the midbrain dorsal to the pathway for conjugate *downward* movements.
   b. **Corollary:** Focal lesions may selectively paralyze horizontal or vertical gaze and may selectively paralyze upward or downward gaze.
4. **The law of control of saccades by the frontoparietal tegmental pathway:** The frontoparietal ocular motor pathways mediate all saccadic eye movements. Saccadic movements include those that move the eyes voluntarily or restore them to the primary position after deviation by vestibular or optokinetic reflexes and during rapid eye movement of sleep. **Corollary:** Because fast and slow movements (slow pursuit and vestibular deviation) arise in different pathways, focal lesions may affect the pathways selectively.

5. **The law of a positive head- and eye-centering mechanism**
   a. Each side of the brain tonically produces vectors that tend to drive the head and eyes to the opposite side. *Upward* and *downward* vectors arise bilaterally from the cortex.
   b. Normally, the vectors that try to drive the head and eyes in opposite directions cancel out. The eyes tend to remain in the primary position or, if moved from it, tend to return to the primary position because of active centering vectors (Fig. 5-3).
   c. If the eyes deviate from the primary position for any reason, saccadic kickback tends to restore the eyes to the primary position. **Corollary:** Any *persistent* deviation of the eyes horizontally or vertically indicates an unbalanced drive caused by interruption of, or excessive drive from, one of the centering systems.
      i. *Destruction* of one supranuclear pathway for eye movements results in persistent conjugate deviation of the eyes in the direction dictated by the intact pathway (Fig. 5-3B).
      ii. *Irritation* of one supranuclear pathway for eye movements results in persistent conjugate deviation of the eyes in the same direction dictated by that pathway (Fig. 5-3C).
6. **The law of occipito-parietal control of visually mediated reflexes**
   a. Visually mediated, clinically testable ocular motor reflexes are **fixation, fusion, pursuit, vergences,** and **optokinetic nystagmus.**
   b. All require an intact afferent arc starting with the retina and mediated through the geniculo-occipito-parieto-tegmental and occipito-parietofronto-tegmental pathways.
7. **The law of competition between reflex and volitional control of eye movements:** Fixation, fusion, following, vergences, and optokinetic nystagmus operate reflexly, but the normal person can override the reflexes by volition. After bilateral interruption of the voluntary pathways, the fixation reflexes may become tenacious or "hyperactive," and then the Pt cannot move the eyes from the target without blinking or moving the head.
8. **The counter-rolling law:** When the head moves, proprioceptive reflexes, arising in the vestibular system and neck, and fixation reflexes hold the eyes on target by counter-rolling the eyes against the direction of head movement, thus keeping the eyes locked on the visual target. **Corollary:** Failure of the eyes to counter-roll indicates failure of one or more of these systems. When unconsciousness negates voluntary movements and fixation, failure of the eyes to counter-roll in response to vestibular stimulation by head turning (doll's eye test) or caloric irrigation means interruption of the vestibular system peripherally or in the brainstem tegmentum.

C. Review the five eye systems mnemonic (pages 179–180 and Table 5-1)

D. Table 5-6 outlines the clinical tests for central eye-movement disorders

E. Summaries of the eye examination

1. Five parts of the routine clinical eye examination:
   a. Visual acuity and fields: Snellen, Rosenbaum, and Amsler grids.
   b. Peripheral visual field: confrontation.
   c. Eye movements: test cardinal directions of gaze and the five eye-movement systems (Table 5-1).
   d. Pupils: reaction to light and accommodation.
   e. Ophthalmoscopy.
      i. Anterior segment: external eye to lens.
      ii. Posterior segment: vitreous, retina, and optic nerve head.

TABLE 5-6 · Outline of Clinical Tests for Central Eye-Movement Disorders

Type of eye movement	Method of examination
Spontaneous movements during ordinary behavior and ordinary environmental stimuli	Inspection while taking the history. Look for misalignment, range, and persistence of eye movements, and for hyperkinesias such as nystagmus.
Volitional fixation and volitional movements	Examiner observes steadiness and range of eye movements after commanding the patient to fixate on a distant object straight ahead and then to move the eyes to the *right, left, up,* and *down.*
Visual reflex ocular movements Smooth pursuit	The patient's eyes pursue the examiner's finger as it moves through the full range of ocular movements.
Vergences	The examiner directs the patient to look at near and distant objects and to follow the examiner's finger as it moves toward the patient's nose.
Reflex fixation	The patient fixates straight ahead and the examiner turns the patient's head slowly to the right, left, up, and down.
Alignment lock	As the patient fixates straight ahead, the examiner alternately covers and uncovers one and then the other eye and looks for deviation in alignment after monocular occlusion of vision (cover-uncover test).
Optokinetic nystagmus	Patient fixates on a rotating drum or a moving striped strip.
Non-visual reflex ocular movements	
Caloric nystagmus*	Irrigation of ears with hot or cold water.
Positional nystagmus*	Placing the patient's head in various positions.
Contraversive eye-turning test (doll's eye test)*	Quick turning of the patient's head by the examiner's hands (used in comatose patients).
Associated eye movement (Bell's phenomenon)	The examiner holds the patient's eyelids open and observes the involuntary upward movement of the eyes that occurs when the patient attempts to close the lids.

*Discussed in Chapter 9.

2. Table 5-7 summarizes the ancillary procedures used to supplement the routine eye examination.

IV. REHEARSAL OF THE EYE EXAMINATION

Now we have to unite the individual fragments of the eye examination into a coherent routine. We could easily convince you to practice if you were a tennis player wanting to improve your strokes or an actor. A great actor, preparing to play the role of a physician, would practice hour after hour to capture the exact nuances of professional behavior. Ours, too, is a performing art. If you want to offer a professional performance to your Pts, practice Part V, steps 1 to 5, of the Standard Neurologic Examination (NE). Practice until the steps unite into one beautiful, flowing sequence for testing CrNs II, III, IV, and VI and their central pathways. Then you can say with Blaise Cendrars:

I have deciphered all the confused texts of the wheels and I have assembled the scattered elements of a most violent beauty.

The five steps that you have just rehearsed from the Standard NE constitute a minimum routine examination. Patients with ocular complaints may need more thorough study. Use Table 5-7 as a reference to supplement Part V A of the basic examination.

TABLE 5-7 · Ancillary Tests for Examination of the Optic System

Test	Purpose
Indirect ophthalmoscopy	Broader view of retina
Slit-lamp microscopy	Visualize corneal surface and ocular media
Tangent screen	Tests central vision
Perimetry	Tests central and peripheral vision
Optokinetic nystagmus	Tests pathway between the retina, occipitoparietal cortex, and brainstem tegmentum
Maddox rod	Detection of ocular deviation
Red-glass test	Detection of diplopic image
Prisms	Quantify ocular misalignment
Forced ductions	Test for mechanical restrictions of EOMs
Edrophonium (tensilon) test or ice-bag test	Detection of myasthenia gravis
Fluorescein angiography	Differentiation of papilledema from pseudopapilledema; occult macular lesions
Positional changes	Test of vestibular system function
Caloric irrigation	Test of vestibular system function
Rotation	Test of vestibular system function
Ultrasonography	Measures diameter of eyeball
Electronystagmography	Records waves forms of nystagmus
Electro-oculography	Records eye movements
Electroretinography	Measure function of retinal layers
Visual evoked responses	Tests retino-geniculo-calcarine pathway
Electroencephalogram	Record visual-related occipital electrical activity
CT/MRI	Anatomic visualization of orbit
MRI of brain	Anatomic visualization of optic pathways

ABBREVIATIONS: CT = computed tomography; EOMs = extraocular muscles; MRI = magnetic resonance imaging.

Learning Objectives for Chapter 5

I. CENTRAL SYSTEMS FOR THE CONTROL OF EYE MOVEMENTS

1. Define a saccade and list the eye movements that are saccadic.
2. State the five major eye-movement systems and the pathways involved. (Mnemonic: hold up your finger and choose to look at it.)
3. Diagram the pathway for voluntary conjugate horizontal eye movements, from cortex to ocular muscles (Fig. 5-1).
4. Describe the clinical findings after interruption of the right MLF.
5. Explain why an eye that fails to adduct because of an MLF lesion will adduct during convergence.
6. Describe the effect on eye movements of bilateral interruption of the corticobulbar pathway for voluntary horizontal conjugate gaze.
7. Contrast the pathways for voluntary vertical eye movements and convergence with the horizontal movement pathway.
8. Describe the difference in the location of pathways for upward gaze and downward gaze at the pretectal-midbrain level.
9. Describe Parinaud's syndrome and associated findings.
10. Describe how to interpret the presence of Bell's phenomenon in a Pt with paralysis of voluntary upward gaze.
11. Explain how the aphorism that UMN (supranuclear) lesions paralyze movements, whereas LMN lesions paralyze muscles, applies to the optomotor system.
12. By means of a vectors, explain the concept of a head- and eye-centering center.

Learning Objectives for Chapter 5

13. Explain the effect of an acute destructive lesion of a cerebral hemisphere on the position of the head and eyes as contrasted to an irritative, epileptogenic lesion of the same hemisphere (Fig. 5-3).
14. Describe several neuro-ophthalmologic findings that would suggest a lesion in the pretectal-tectal-tegmental region surrounding the Sylvian aqueduct (Sylvian aqueduct syndrome).
15. Describe how to elicit the ATNR, the response expected, and the clinical interpretation of the results (Fig. 5-4).
16. Explain how the ATNR reflects the law of contralateral cerebral sensorimotor innervation.

II. NYSTAGMUS

1. Define nystagmus.
2. State the symptoms that often accompany acquired nystagmus.
3. Classify nystagmus as to plane (form), type, and direction.
4. State which type of nystagmus implies an ocular lesion and which type implies a vestibular or neurologic lesion.
5. Describe several maneuvers to induce eye movements after UMN paralysis to prove that the LMNs are intact. (**Hint:** Table 5-6 contains several of them, although not formally listed as such.)
6. Decide, depending on your field of medicine, how much of the information presented on nystagmus you need to carry with you and rehearse that material. If you want to do neurology, it's a lot; for pediatrics or general practice, it's a fair amount; but if you incline toward orthopedics or dermatology, it's a little.

III. SUMMARY OF THE LAWS OF OCULAR MOTILITY FOR THE CLINICAL EXAMINATION

1. Explain the clinical applications of each of the laws of ocular motility listed in Section III, A and B.
2. Demonstrate the Standard NE of vision and ocular motility (Section F of the Standard NE and Table 5-5).
3. Describe several maneuvers to induce eye movements after paralysis of volitional movements to prove that the LMNs are intact.

6 Examination of the Motor Cranial Nerves V, VII, IX, X, XI, and XII

To those I address, it is unnecessary to go farther, than to indicate that the nerves treated of in these papers are the instruments of expression, from the smile upon the infant's cheek to the last agony of life.

—**Sir Charles Bell (1774–1842)**

I. V CRANIAL NERVE MOTOR FUNCTION: CHEWING

A. Functional anatomy of chewing

1. **Motor-wise, cranial nerve (CrN) V only** chews. Its motor axons innervate *all* and, for clinical purposes, *only* the chewing muscles: **masseter, temporal,** and **lateral and medial pterygoids.** CrN V conveys no efferents to glands or smooth muscle and no special sensory afferents (Table 2-7).
2. **Jaw closure**
   a. Place your fingertips about 2 cm above and in front of the angle of your mandible. Bite hard and relax several times. The muscle felt, the **masseter,** is the easiest of the chewing muscle to palpate.
   b. The other jaw-closing muscles are the **temporalis muscles** that originate in the temporal fossa and insert on the mandible and the **medial pterygoid muscle.**
3. **Lateral jaw movement:** Move your jaw from side to side. Chewing requires not only jaw closure but also a lateral, grinding action and jaw opening, caused by the **lateral pterygoid muscles.**
   a. In Fig. 6-1 notice that the lateral pterygoid muscle originates from the skull base and *inserts* near the mandibular condyle.
   b. Because the skull base is fixed, only the mandible moves when the pterygoids contract. Equal contractions of right and left pterygoids pull the mandible straightforward (Fig. 6-1).
   c. If only the *right* lateral pterygoid muscle contracts, the mandibular tip moves to the ❒ right/❒ left.
   d. If the patient (Pt) can move the jaw to the right but not to the left, the lateral pterygoid muscle on the ❒ right/❒ left is paralyzed.
   e. As a second action, the lateral pterygoid muscles act to open the jaw because they insert on the neck of the mandible (Fig. 6-2).

☑ left

☑ right

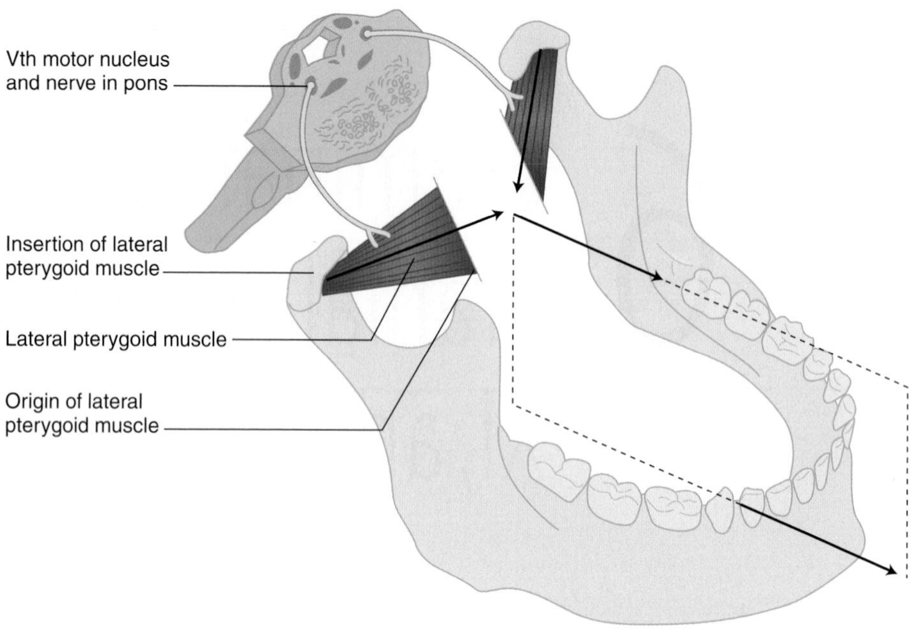

FIGURE 6-1. Innervation and action of the lateral pterygoid muscles. If both muscles contract equally, the tip of the mandible moves straight forward. If one muscle contracts, the tip moves forward and to the opposite side. Study the vector diagram (arrows between the muscles).

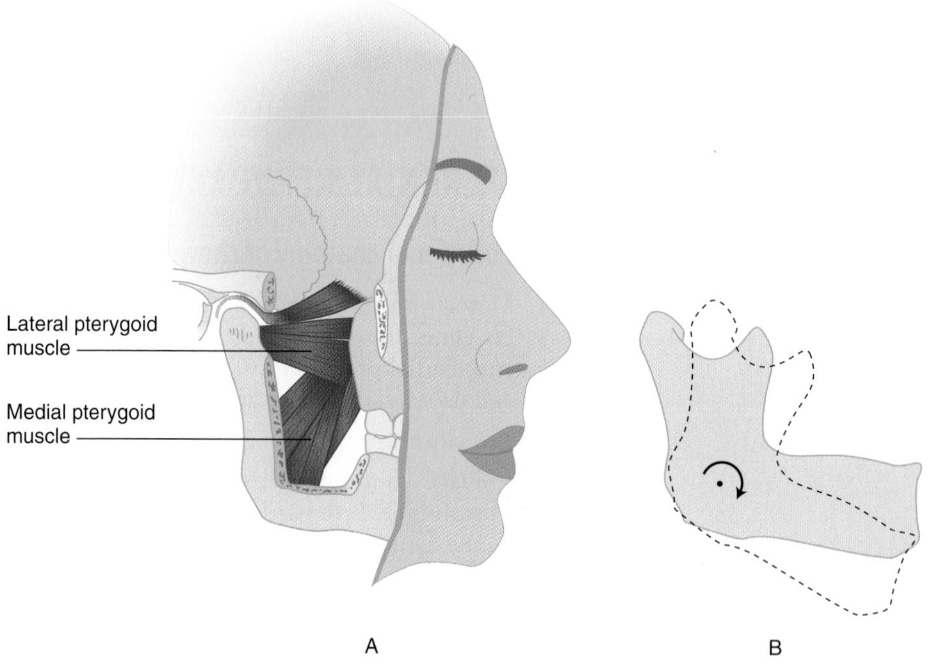

FIGURE 6-2. (A) Action of lateral pterygoid muscles to depress the tip of the mandible when the patient forcefully opens the jaw. The forward pull of the lateral pterygoid muscles also opens the jaw because the jaw is suspended to rotate around a lateral axis. (B) Arrow indicates the rotation.

lateral pterygoid

f. If the Pt's mandible moves forward and down in the midline on jaw opening, both _______________ muscles have contracted equally.

☑ right; ☑ down

g. If the *left* lateral pterygoid muscle contracts, the tip of the mandible moves not only to the ❒ right/❒ left but also ❒ up/❒ down.

Lateral movement and opening of the jaw

4. Name the two major actions of the lateral pterygoid muscles.

____

Masseter, temporal, and medial pterygoid

5. The remaining mandibular muscles innervated by CrN V all close the jaw. Name these muscles.

____

B. Lower motoneuron lesions of cranial nerve V

1. Unilateral destruction of the perikarya or axons of CrN V causes complete paralysis of all ipsilateral chewing muscles.
2. The denervated muscle undergoes atrophy. **Atrophy** and **paralysis** are the two outstanding signs of lower motoneuron (LMN) lesions. Which chewing muscle can you most readily palpate to check for atrophy? _____________

Masseter

C. Upper motor neuron innervation of cranial nerve V

1. Pursuant to general principles, one cerebral hemisphere sends upper motoneuron (UMN) axons to the contralateral V nerve nucleus. However, the contralateral innervation law requires some qualification. Compare your inability to contract half of your anal sphincter or half of your throat with the ease with which you flex a finger. **These proximal (axial) muscles, such as those for trunk extension, chewing, and swallowing, that customarily act symmetrically much of or all the time usually receive about the same number of crossed and uncrossed UMN axons.** The law of contralateral innervation holds best for independent unilateral movements, such as those of the hand. Hence, we find that:
   a. Many *proximal* (axial) muscles that ordinarily contract symmetrically have ❐ mostly ipsilateral/❐ bilateral/❐ mostly contralateral UMN innervation.
   b. The *distal* (appendicular) muscles that ordinarily contract unilaterally have mainly ❐ ipsilateral/❐ bilateral/❐ contralateral UMN innervation.
2. Because of bilateral UMN innervation, unilateral UMN lesions do not cause a severe or enduring unilateral paralysis of the chewing muscles (Willoughby and Anderson, 1984). UMN lesions, as a rule, do not selectively paralyze individual muscles or sets of muscles innervated by one peripheral nerve.

☑ bilateral

☑ contralateral

D. Clinical tests of cranial nerve V motor function

Note: Do these tests on yourself as they are described.

1. **Inspection:** Inspect the temples and cheeks for atrophy of the temporalis and masseter muscles. The temporal muscle fills out the temple. Even when the Pt bites, the muscle is difficult to palpate, but after temporalis muscle atrophy, the temple sinks in. In myotonic dystrophy, the chewing muscles and sternocleidomastoid muscles atrophy. Review Fig. 1-13I. The masseters of some individuals undergo hypertrophy and stand out strongly.
2. **Palpation:** To test for masseter atrophy, ask the Pt to clench the teeth together strongly and unclench several times, while you simultaneously palpate the muscles of the two sides as they mound up and relax under your fingertips.
3. **Testing for weakness of jaw closure**
   a. Ask the to Pt clench the teeth strongly.
   b. Place the heel of one palm on the tip of the Pt's mandible and the other hand on the Pt's forehead. Press hard on the tip of the mandible. You must brace the Pt's head with your opposite hand because jaw closure is a very strong movement and you do not want to test the strength of the neck muscles and jaw closure at the same time. **The principle is to test the strength of one muscle or one limited set of muscles at one time.**
   c. If the Pt complains of fatigability when chewing, as in myasthenia gravis, have the Pt chew for a period before testing.
4. **Testing for weakness of the lateral pterygoid muscles**
   a. Ask the Pt to forcefully open the jaw. Note whether its tip aligns with the crevice between the upper, medial incisor teeth. Weakness of one lateral pterygoid muscle would cause the jaw to deviate to the ❐ ipsilateral/❐ contralateral side.

☑ ipsilateral (Fig. 6-2)

b. Then ask the Pt to move the jaw from side to side.

c. Ask the Pt to hold the jaw forcefully to the side as you try to push it back to the center with the heel of your palm. Brace the Pt's head by pressing your other hand against the opposite cheekbone.

5. **A word of caution:** Do not jerk or apply sudden force in testing jaw muscles, particularly in elderly or edentulous Pts. The temporomandibular joint may dislocate.

6. To ensure that you can do it, test V nerve motor function on yourself and on a partner. Don't just sit there: get up and do it! The text cannot substitute for the proprioceptive experience provided by using your own hands.

E. Analyze this 46-year-old man's difficulty in chewing

Examination disclosed atrophy and paralysis of the left temporal and masseter muscles. When he opened his jaw, it deviated to the left. He could not move it forcefully to the right. No other muscles were weak. The evidence points to ❒ an LMN/❒ a UMN lesion on the ❒ right/❒ left/❒ both sides. Explain.

☑ a LMN; ☑ left.

____

____

____

The paralysis affects the muscles of one nerve, CrN V. The paralysis is complete, and the muscles are atrophic. Because the atrophic and paralyzed muscles are on the left, the lesion interrupts the left V nerve.

II. VII CRANIAL NERVE MOTOR FUNCTIONS

A. Functional anatomy of facial movements

1. Except for the mandible and eyelid elevation, CrN VII innervates every other movement that the face can make. (For now study only the LMNs of VII in Fig. 6-3.)

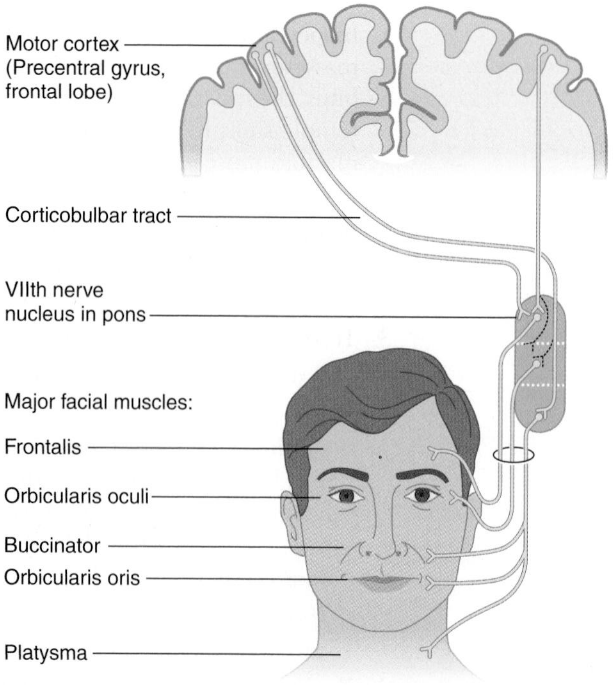

FIGURE 6-3. Upper and lower motoneuron innervations of the facial muscles. The dotted lines indicate that the number of crossed and uncrossed axons to the orbicularis oculi muscles vary from person to person. Therefore, the degree of weakness of the muscle differs after upper motoneuron lesions.

2. Look into a mirror and make every possible facial movement, including wiggling your nose and ears. (Which CrN do you suppose your dog uses to perk up his ears?)
3. **Work through Table 6-1.** Look into the mirror as you follow the commands the examiner (Ex) uses to test the facial muscles.

TABLE 6-1 · Summary of Tests of the Facial Muscles Innervated by Cranial Nerve VII

Examiner's command	Observation	Muscle tested
"Wrinkle up your forehead" or "Look up at the ceiling"	Inspect for asymmetry	Frontalis
"Close your eyes tight and don't let me open them"	Inspect for asymmetry of wrinkles; try to pull eyelids apart	Orbicularis oculi
"Pull back the corners of your mouth, as in smiling"	Inspect for asymmetry of nasolabial fold	Buccinator
"Wrinkle up the skin on your neck" or "Pull down hard on the corners of your mouth"	Inspect for asymmetry	Platysma

4. **Functions of the facial muscles**
   a. Expression of emotions, such as when frowning and smiling.
   b. Compression of lips for whistling, blowing, and spitting; labial sounds of speech; swallowing and other feeding actions.
   c. Controlling and protecting the facial apertures: the palpebral fissures, oral fissure, nares, lips, and external auditory canals.
   d. Dampening excessive movement of the ossicles by stapedius muscle contraction during loud sounds. After stapedius paralysis, ordinary sounds may seem uncomfortably loud, a symptom called **hyperacusis.**

B. Intra- and extra-axial anatomy of cranial nerve VII

1. Learn Fig. 6-4 and compare it with the generalized brainstem section in Fig. 2-14.

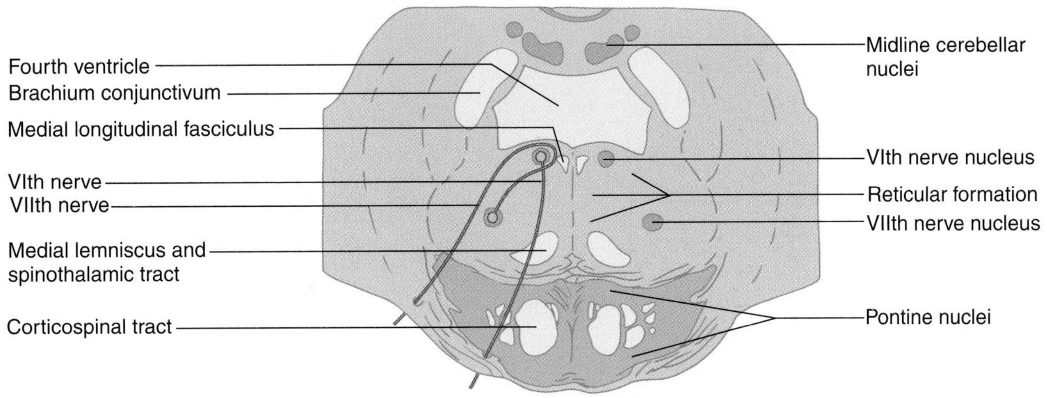

FIGURE 6-4. Transverse section at the caudal level of the pons that includes cranial nerve VI and VII nuclei.

2. Notice the peculiar internal loop of CrN VII around the VI nerve nucleus. Use a colored pencil to draw in the course of CrNs VI and VII on the opposite side of Fig. 6-4.

V; VI; VII (Fig. 2-21)

3. The pontine tegmentum contains motor nuclei for three CrNs: ____, ____, and ____.

corticospinal (pyramidal tract)

4. Through the basis of the pons run the ________________ tracts to the LMNs of the spinal cord.

VI

5. Before exiting from the pons, the VII nerve fibers loop around the nucleus of the ____th CrN.

VI; VII; VIII (review Fig. 2-20 if you erred)

6. Three CrNs exit at the pontomedullary sulcus. In ventrodorsal order, these nerves are ____, ____, and ____.
7. As typifies peripheral nerves, the VII nerves do not cross the midline.

ipsilaterally

8. If a lesion destroys the VII nerve nucleus, the intra-axial course of the axons, or the peripheral nerve trunk, the result is paralysis of *all* facial muscles ❒ ipsilaterally/❒ contralaterally.
9. The only sensory function of CrN VII tested clinically is taste (Chapter 8).
10. **Mnemonics for remembering CrN VII functions:** At first glance, mastery of CrN VII seems hopeless. See Fig. 6-5.

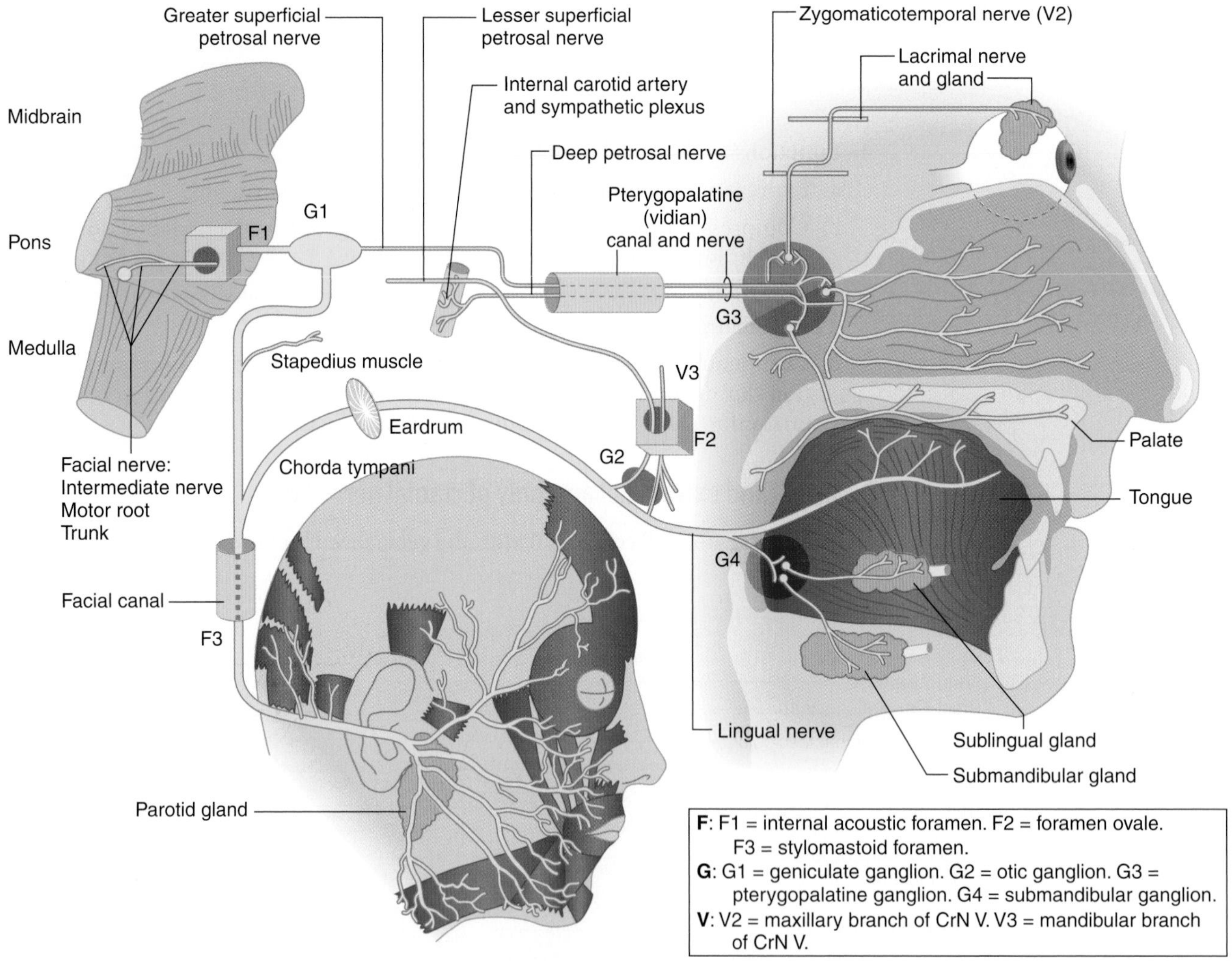

FIGURE 6-5. Diagram of the complete distribution of cranial nerve VII. (Reprinted with permission from DeMyer W. *Neuroanatomy,* 2nd ed. Baltimore: Williams & Wilkins, 1998.)

a. Salvation comes from considering CrN VII as three nerves, a bran-chiomotor nerve (Fig. 6-6A), a secretomotor nerve (Fig. 6-6B), and a taste nerve (Fig. 6-6C).

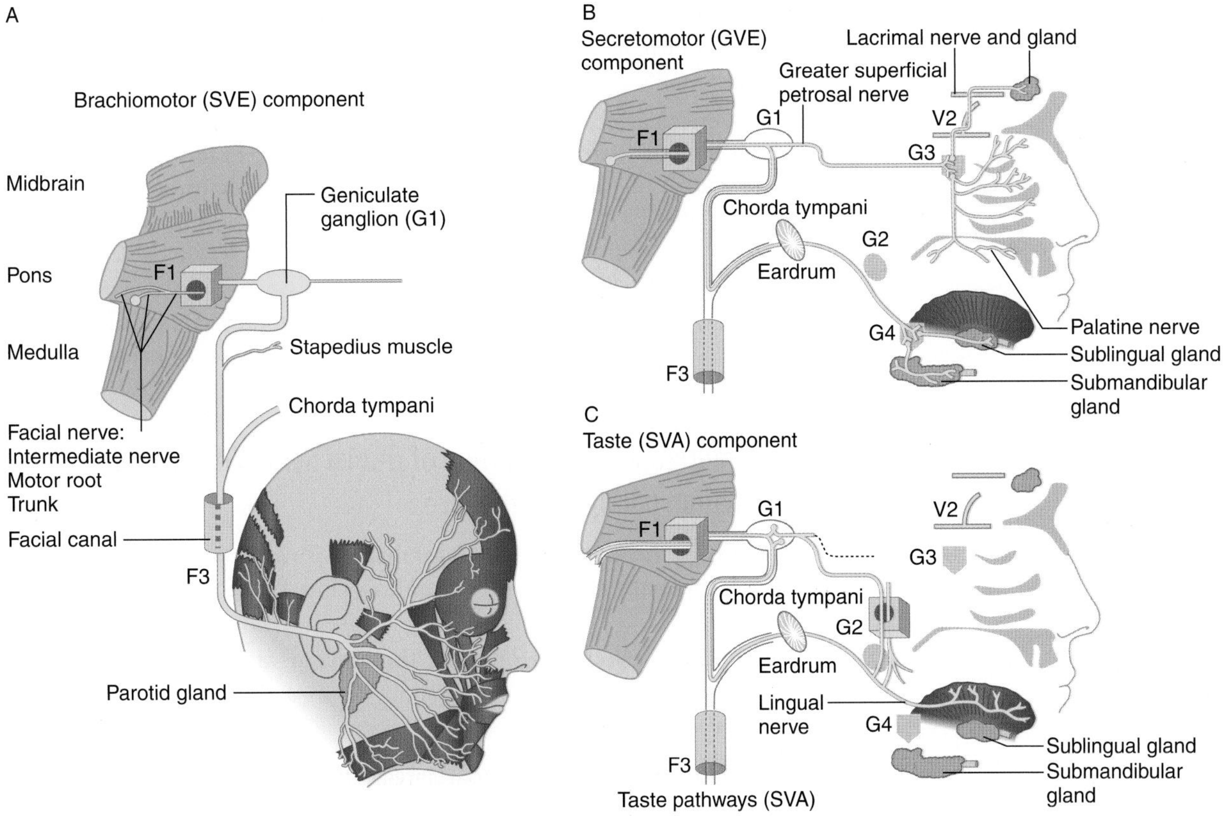

FIGURE 6-6. Diagram of cranial nerve VII as composed of three nerves: (A) a branchiomotor nerve, (B) a secretomotor nerve, and (C) a taste nerve. (Reprinted with permission from DeMyer W. *Neuroanatomy,* 2nd ed. Baltimore: Williams & Wilkins, 1998.)

b. Remember that, in addition to moving the face, CrN VII innervates:
   i. Tasting: taste from the anterior two-thirds of the tongue via the geniculate ganglion
   ii. Snotting: parasympathetic axons to the nasal mucosa via the pterygopalatine ganglion
   iii. Tearing: parasympathetic axons to the lacrimal gland via the pterygopalatine ganglion
   iv. Salivating: parasympathetic axons via the submandibular ganglion.

Mnemonic summary of the clinically important functions of CrN VII: It *tears,* snots, tastes, salivates, *moves the face,* and *dampens sounds.*

Cranial Nerve Seven

This is the nerve that lets you cry
And wets your mouth when it is dry
Dampens noise when you are young
Tastes on two-thirds of your tongue
And lastly—now, just let me think
Lets you give a smile—and wink!

—Meredith Rose Golomb, MD

c. Complete interruption of CrN VII proximally causes ipsilateral facial paralysis, xerophthalmia, loss of nasal secretions, loss of taste, xerostomia, and hyperacusis.

d. Lesions can affect various sites distally along the course of CrN VII, causing the clinical signs to differ. The Ex can reason out the lesion site by "thinking along" the course of the VIIth nerve. For example, interruption of CrN VII at the facial canal (see facial canal in Fig. 6-5) would cause ipsilateral facial paralysis, but not the other clinical signs of a proximal lesion. LMN paralysis of the facial muscles is called **Bell's palsy.**

e. In the Guillain-Barré syndrome (GBS), a bilateral LMN facial palsy may occur (facial diplegia). Sarcoidosis and Lyme disease also may cause bifacial palsy of the LMN type.

C. Upper motoneuron innervation of cranial nerve VII and upper motoneuron paralysis of the face

1. By knowing the degree of unilaterality of various facial movements, you can unravel the pattern of UMN paralysis and fix it in your memory forever (Fig. 6-3).
2. As you watch in your mirror, make the movements listed in Table 6-2.

TABLE 6-2 · Tests for Unilaterality of Facial Movements

Movement	Result
Retract one corner of your mouth at a time.	Every normal person can do it; the movement is unilateral.
Wink one eye at a time; watch in your mirror for simultaneous contraction of the opposite orbicularis oculi muscle.	Most can do it, but some cannot wink one eye without the other; when one eye winks, the opposite orbicularis oculi contracts to some degree.
Elevate one eyebrow at a time.	Few can do it unilaterally, but everyone can elevate them together; the movement is essentially *bilateral.*

☑ lip retraction

a. The freest unilateral facial movement normally is ❒ forehead elevation/❒ eyelid closure/❒ lip retraction.

☑ forhead elevation

b. The least free unilateral facial movement normally is ❒ forehead elevation/❒ eyelid closure/❒ lip retraction.

c. The utility of the various facial movements explains the gradient of unilaterality. Notice when eating that you make unilateral movements to manipulate food and clear it from your cheeks (buccinator muscle). Indeed a major discomfort of a facial palsy is that food lodges in the cheek. Unilateral forehead movements offer no such utility, and we usually activate both sides of the forehead equally. Although the eyes usually blink together, sometimes you do need to close only one. Thus, the utility of unilateral eyelid action falls between that of mouth retraction and forehead wrinkling.

☑ mainly from the contralateral hemisphere

3. Body parts such as the hand and lip that have the freest, most independent unilateral movements receive their UMN innervation ❒ equally from each hemisphere/❒ mainly from the contralateral hemisphere/❒ mainly from the ipsilateral hemisphere.
4. Proximal, customarily symmetrical movements, such as chewing and swallowing, receive about the same number of UMN axons from each hemisphere, let us say 50/50.
5. The freest, independent unilateral movements are innervated by crossed and uncrossed UMN axons in a ratio of, let us say, 90/10. For movements with an intermediate degree of unilateral independence, the ratio might be 60:40, and so on.

☑ lip retraction ☑ forehead wrinkling

6. Now predict the pattern of facial muscle weakness after unilateral destruction of one corticobulbar pathway. The Pt would show *most* paralysis of ❐ forehead wrinkling/❐ eyelid closure/❐ lip retraction and *least* paralysis of ❐ forehead wrinkling/❐ eyelid closure/❐ lip retraction.

7. **Facial weakness after acute, severe interruption of UMNs**
   a. After a large, acute UMN lesion, such as a massive cerebral infarct, eyelid closure is usually paretic (incomplete paralysis), along with paralysis of lip retraction. Rarely, even the frontalis muscle is somewhat paretic. Because such a Pt has weakness of eyelid closure, the Ex who does not understand the gradient of unilaterality of facial movement may erroneously diagnose a lesion of the *ipsilateral* facial nerve rather than the *contralateral* corticobulbar tract.
   b. In the *acute* phase, shortly after a severe UMN lesion, lip retraction contralateral to the lesion will be paralyzed during volitional movement **and** during emotional expression, such as smiling.
   c. In the *chronic* phase of the UMN lesion, especially if the Pt has bilateral UMN lesions, lip retraction may remain weak during volitional action but may be prominent or even exaggerated during emotional expression (Monrad-Krohn phenomenon). See *pseudobulbar palsy* in Section VIII of this chapter.

D. Clinical testing of cranial nerve VII motor function

1. Facial inspection begins upon meeting the Pt and continues while taking the history.
   a. Notice the overall play of facial muscles during speech and emotional expression. The face may move too much or too little. Many disorders, such as muscular dystrophy (Fig. 1-13I), parkinsonism, and depression, reduce all facial movements, a condition called **masked facies,** as if the Pt wore an immobile mask.
   b. Excessive or involuntary movements seen on inspection of the face include **blepharospasm,** which may close the eyelids so tightly that the Pt cannot see; **hemifacial spasm,** in which all the muscles innervated by one of the VII nerves twitch; and **tics, chorea,** and **athetosis,** as described in Chapter 7.
   c. Next, search for asymmetry of facial movements, asymmetry of blinking, and asymmetry of the movement and depth of the nasolabial skin creases. The nasolabial creases begin just lateral to the lips and bow upward to the nares. To detect mild unilateral weakness of lip retraction after partial UMN lesions, watch for asymmetry of the depth and movement of these creases. Using your mirror, observe these two creases when your lips are at rest, when you smile, and when you speak (say *EEE* loudly). Slight congenital asymmetries are common.
2. Work through Table 6-1 with a partner. Often it's quicker to demonstrate the desired movements and give the commands. In working through Table 6-1, pay particular attention to the strength of eyelid closure. Can you open your partner's eyelids against a maximum effort at closure?

____

Don't go to Aristotle for the answer: Get it from your own experience on your partner or yourself.

E. Analysis of patients with facial weakness

1. The Pts shown in Figs. 6-7 and 6-8 were asked to pull back the corners of their mouths, as in smiling, and simultaneously to close their eyes tightly. Make sure that you understand that the side that shows the action, that "draws to one side," is the normal one. The side that fails to move is the abnormal one. The Pt with a facial palsy may state in the history that the face "draws to one side," as if that were the abnormality. Especially compare both sides of each face for asymmetry of facial movement and for differences in the bulk of the chewing muscles.
2. Describe the abnormalities of the Pt in Fig. 6-7. Be sure that you start at the hair and systematically examine every facial contour and feature.

____

____

See next frame

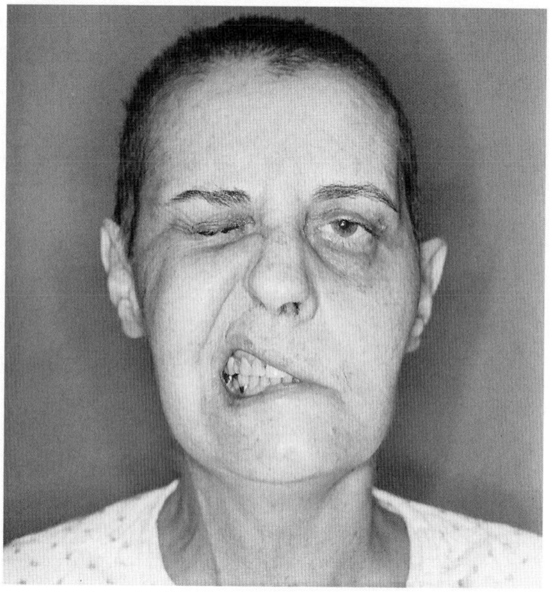

FIGURE 6-7. Patient 1 with facial palsy. She was asked to close her eyes tightly and to pull back the corners of her mouth, as in smiling.

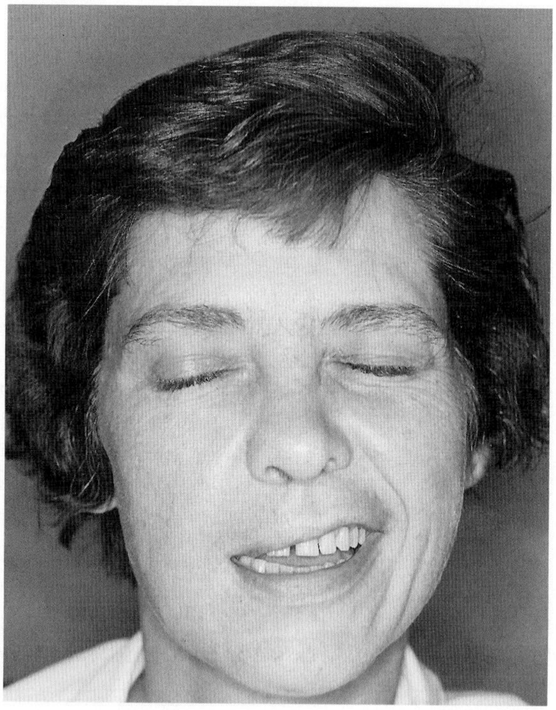

FIGURE 6-8. Patient 2 with facial palsy. She was asked to close her eyes tightly and to pull back the corners of her mouth, as in smiling.

☑ left VII nerve

a. In Fig. 6-7 the Pt has weakness of eyelid closure on the left, as shown by lack of contraction of the orbicularis oculi muscle and absence of any "crow's feet" wrinkles around the eye. The mouth retractors on the left are paralyzed. When this Pt looked up, the left half of her forehead failed to wrinkle. This pattern of total paralysis of all facial muscles on the left side implicates a lesion of the ❒ right/❒ left VII nerve or the ❒ right/❒ left corticobulbar tract.

V

b. The *cognoscente* of physical diagnosis will also have detected the hollowing of the Pt's left temporal fossa and the concavity over the left masseter muscle, indicating atrophy of the chewing muscles and thus a lesion of CrN _____.

c. If you missed this finding, remember that you must compare both halves of the body, specifically looking for just such asymmetries. The patient in Fig. 6-7 had undergone surgery to remove an acoustic nerve tumor, a neurinoma. The tumor, expanding in the cerebellopontine angle, had already destroyed CrNs V and VII, but full abduction of her left eye indicated sparing of CrN ________.

VI

d. Did you also wonder about her very short hair? It was just growing back after having been shaved off for the operation.

e. This Pt was one of a minority who fail to show Bell's phenomenon when attempting to close the eyelids. If Bell's phenomenon had occurred, the eye would have turned ________________________________ ________________.

upward and somewhat outward (Chapter 4)

3. Describe the abnormalities of the Pt shown in Fig. 6-8.

____

____.

See next frame

a. In Fig. 6-8, the right side of the Pt's mouth failed to retract, and eyelid closure on the right was weak, as shown by the wider exposure of the upper eyelid and lack of wrinkling around the right eye. This "crow's feet" wrinkling on the normal side resulted from the purse-string, sphincter action of the orbicularis oculi muscle. When the Pt in Fig. 6-8 looked up, her forehead acted equally on both sides. Thus, on the right side of her face, the Pt had *active* forehead movements, *weak* eyelid closure, and *paralysis* of mouth retraction. This gradient of facial weakness on the right side of the Pt's face indicates a lesion of the ❒ right/❒ left facial nerve or the ❒ right/ ❒ left corticobulbar tract.

☑ left corticobulbar tract

b. The Pt shown in Fig. 6-8 had a UMN facial palsy after an occlusion of her left middle cerebral artery had caused infarction of her left cerebral hemisphere.

BIBLIOGRAPHY · Cranial Nerve VII

May M, Schaitkin BM. *The Facial Nerve, 2nd ed.* New York, Thieme Medical Publishers, 1999.

III. CRANIAL NERVE IX AND X MOTOR FUNCTIONS

A. Peripheral distribution of cranial nerves IX and X

Learn Figs. 6-9 and 6-10.

B. LMN innervation of the pharynx and larynx by cranial nerves IX and X

1. The skeletal muscles supplied by CrNs IX and X originally came from branchial arches. The branchial efferent nucleus for IX and X, the **nucleus ambiguus,** is in the ❒ mesencephalon/❒ pons/❒ medulla.

☑ medulla(Fig. 2-14)

2. CrN IX supplies only one muscle exclusively (stylopharyngeus). Because this muscle aids in swallowing, its isolated function cannot be tested clinically. The remaining branchial efferent fibers of CrNs IX and X supply the pharyngeal constrictors. Because they act as a unit in swallowing, the isolated function of the individual constrictors cannot be tested at the bedside.

3. **Mnemonic for the skeletal muscle innervated by CrN X:** It innervates the **palatal** muscles, aided by CrN V, the **pharyngeal constrictors,** aided by CrN IX, and the **laryngeal muscles** unaided: the **palate, pharynx,** and **larynx**, in rostrocaudal order.

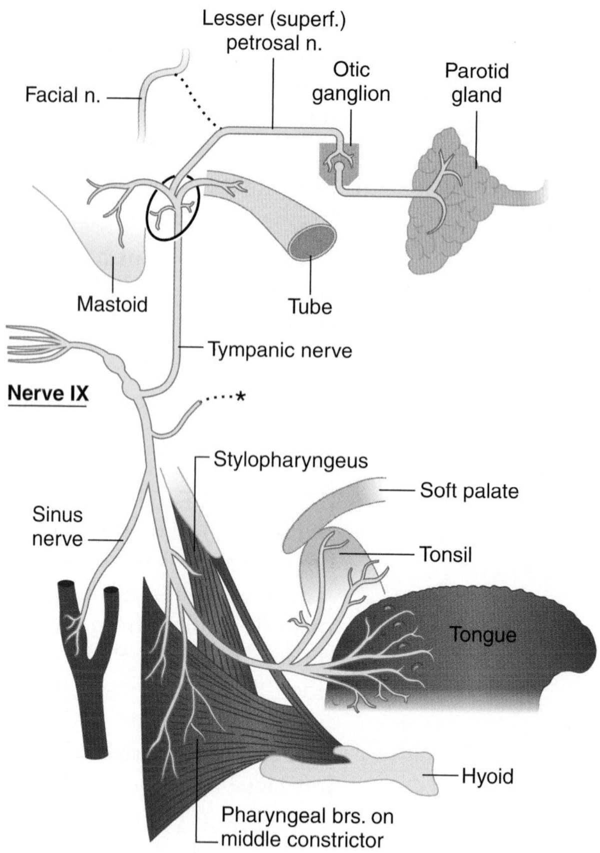

FIGURE 6-9. Innervation of the palate, tongue, and pharynx by cranial nerve IX. Motor axons innervate the stylopharyngeus and middle pharyngeal constrictor muscles. Sensory axons mediate taste from the tongue, the gag reflex, and the vasomotor, cardioinhibitory, and respiratory reflexes of the carotid body and sinus. (Reproduced with permission from Grant JCB. *An Atlas of Anatomy,* 6th ed. Baltimore, Williams & Wilkins, 1972.)

IX; X

4. Because even complete interruption of CrN V has little clinical effect on palatal function, we can say that the motor functions of the palate, pharynx, and larynx are innervated by CrNs _______ and _______.

X

5. CrNs IX and X mediate sensation from the palate and pharynx and CrN X alone from the larynx. Hence, CrNs IX and X are the *motor* and *sensory* sentinels of the palatal orifice and pharynx, but CrN ___ alone is the sensorimotor nerve of the larynx.
6. CrN IX also carries afferents from the carotid sinus that mediate baroceptive reflexes and from the carotid body that mediates baroceptive and chemoceptive reflexes.

C. Normal swallowing

1. Swallowing requires precise coordination of bulbar and respiratory muscles by a distributed network of neural connections involving the posterior inferior frontal gyrus, anterior insular region, basal motor nuclei, diencephalon, reticular formation, and cerebellum (Newton et al., 1994; Zald and Pardo, 1999). Lesions at various sites in this network may cause dysphagia. Unilateral lesions in the lowest part of the precentral gyrus and posterior part of the inferior frontal gyrus may impair swallowing without causing dysarthria (Wiles, 1991), although the two frequently coexist.

XII

2. The tongue initiates the act of swallowing by voluntarily throwing a bolus of food back into the palatal archway. Tongue movements are innervated exclusively by CrN _____. (If you don't know, sort through CrNs I to XII to find right one.)

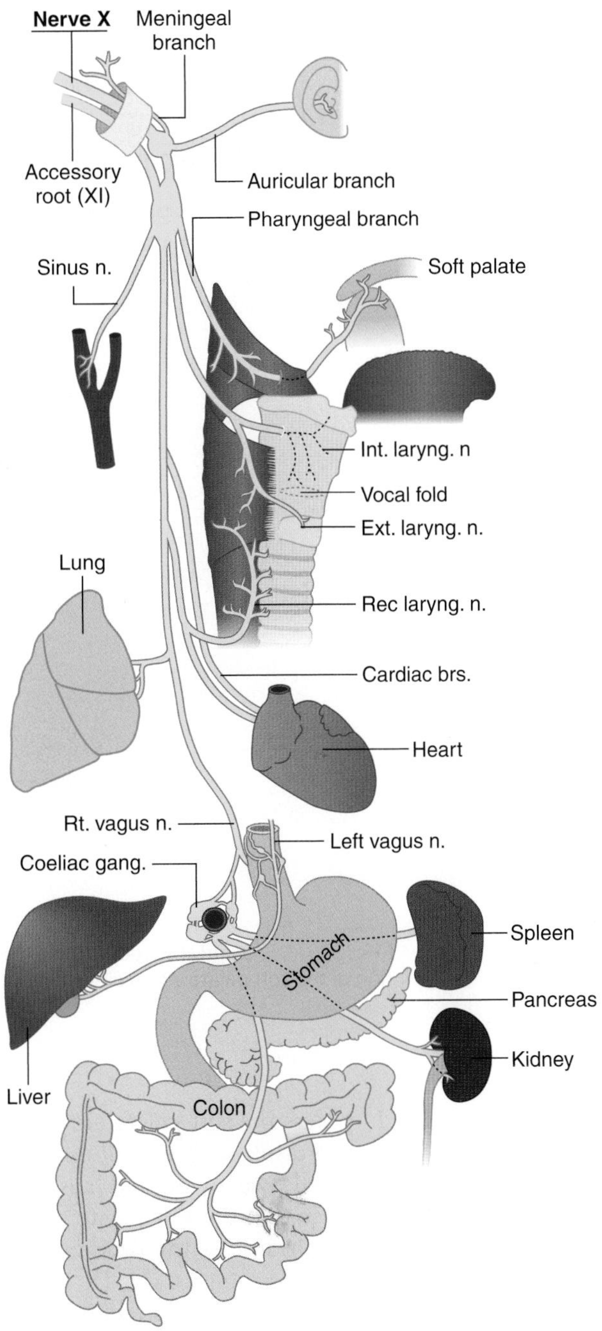

FIGURE 6-10. Innervation of the palate, pharynx, larynx, and thoracicoabdominal viscera by cranial nerve X. The palatal branch innervates the levator veli palatini muscle. The pharyngeal and laryngeal branches mediate sensory and motor functions of these structures. (Reproduced with permission from Grant JCB. *An Atlas of Anatomy,* 6th ed. Baltimore, Williams & Wilkins, 1972.)

3. Afferents from the palate via CrN IX then complete the act reflexly (Perlman and Schultze-Delrieu, 1997). The bolus stimulates the palate to elevate and deflect the bolus from the nasopharynx into the oropharynx. The pharyngeal constrictors contract, the larynx elevates, and the vocal cords close.
4. Swallowing requires afferent information via CrNs V, IX, and X, and motor actions are mediated by CrNs V, VII, IX, X, and XII. Connections in the region of the nucleus of the tractus solitarius in the medulla, in proximity to the respiratory center, act as a swallowing center. It coordinates the actions of swallowing and breathing to avoid aspiration (Newton et al., 1994; Section IV G describes clinical testing for disordered swallowing, i.e., dysphagia).

V; VII

5. Hold your jaw open and try to swallow with your lips open. You may succeed after a struggle, but normal swallowing requires sealing of the lips and closure of the jaw. CrN ___ innervates jaw closure and CrN ___ innervates lip closure.

D. Clinical physiology of the soft palate

1. The levator veli palatini muscle, innervated via the pharyngeal plexus by CrN X, swings the soft palate upward and backward to contact the posterior wall of the pharynx. This action seals off the *naso* pharynx from the *oro* pharynx. See Figs. 6-11A and 6-11B.

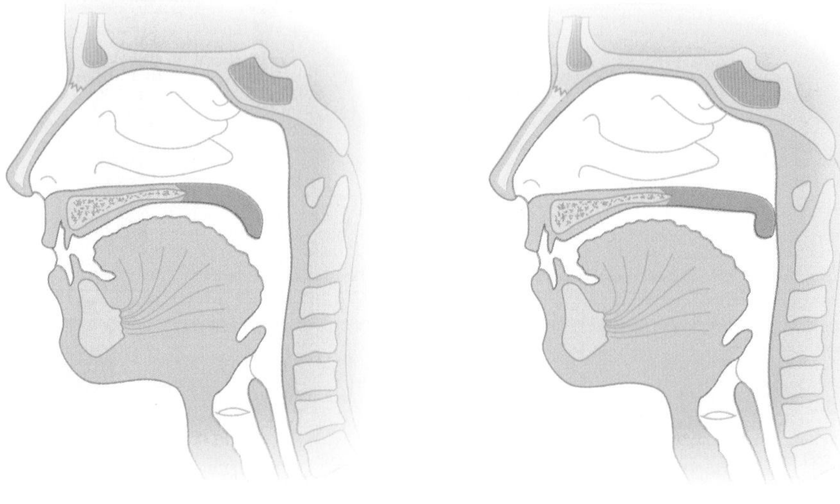

FIGURE 6-11. Sagittal section of the head. (A) Position of the soft palate when relaxed. (B) Position of the soft palate when elevated, occluding the nasopharynx from the oropharynx.

V; VII

2. Unless the soft palate elevates properly, *liquid* will escape into your nose when you drink, and *air* will escape into your nose when you speak. The results are "nasal" swallowing and "nasal" speech. Because liquids and gases are fluids, we can agree that the soft palate and other branchial muscles of the throat control the fluid traffic at the oropharyngeal, nasopharyngeal, esophageal, and laryngotracheal openings. CrNs IX and X innervate, guard, and control the internal apertures of the head much as CrNs ___ (sensory) and ___ (motor) innervate the external apertures (eyes, mouth, ears, and nares).
3. The nasopharyngeal airway remains open until the palate elevates. The palate elevates as required to block anything in your oropharynx from entering your nasopharynx. Thus, the palate elevates when you:
   a. Swallow
   b. Whistle or trumpet
   c. Make certain speech sounds

E. Upper motor neuron innervation of cranial nerves IX and X

equal (50/50)

1. The palate, pharynx, and vocal cords act with bilateral synchrony. By knowing this fact, you can predict that the number of crossed and uncrossed UMN fibers from each cerebral hemisphere would be about ___________.
2. Because of the usual bilateral UMN innervation, unilateral UMN lesions that cause hemiplegia only rarely cause unilateral weakness of the palate (Willoughby and Anderson, 1984), but Pts with acute hemiplegia frequently show mild dysarthria (about 60%).

BIBLIOGRAPHY · Cranial Nerves IX and X, Swallowing, and Dysphagia

Groher ME. *Dysphagia. Diagnosis and Management*, 3rd ed. Boston, ButterworthHeinemann, 1997.

Newton HB, Newton C, Pearl D, et al. Swallowing assessment in primary brain tumor patients with dysarthria. *Neurology* 1994;44:1927–1932.

Perlman AL, Schultze-Delrieu KS. *Deglutition and Its Disorders: Anatomy, Physiology, Clinical Diagnosis, and Management*. San Diego, Singular Publishing Group, 1997.

Smith Hammond GA, Goldstein LB, et al. Cough and aspiration of food and liquids due to oral-pharyngeal dysphagia ACCP evidence based guidelines. Chest 2006; 129 (Suppl): 154S-N168S.

Wiles CM. Neurogenic dysphagia. *J Neurol Neurosurg Psychiatry* 1991;57:1037–1039.

Willoughby EW, Anderson NE. Lower cranial nerve motor function in unilateral vascular lesions of the cerebral hemisphere. *Br Med J* 1984;289:791–794.

Zald DH, Pardo JV. The functional neuroanatomy of swallowing. *Ann Neurol* 1999;46: 281–286.

IV. ROLE OF CRANIAL NERVES IN SPEECH

A. The basic physiology of speech

1. Speech requires a *bellows*, ergo lungs and respiratory muscles, that express a stream of air through the larynx and upper airway.
2. Speech requires a *vibrator for phonation*, ergo the vocal cords.
3. Speech requires *articulation*, ergo palate, tongue, lips, and mandible.
4. Speech requires *resonance*, ergo pharyngeal, oral, and nasal passages and cavities. The nasal passages resonate only three sounds of the English language: *m*, *n*, and *ng*.
5. Speech requires *neural control*, ergo UMNs to LMNs. Chapter 11 discusses cerebral circuits and cerebral disorders of speech.

B. Phonation: role of cranial nerve X

Galen (A.D. 130–200) of Pergamum was troubled by the squealing of piglets during surgical experiments. But his curiosity drove him to continue his investigations. Because he had no anesthetic, he eliminated the squealing and satisfied his curiosity with one stroke. After verifying the origin of the voice in the larynx, he found that he could silence it by cutting the recurrent laryngeal nerves, and that is how we learned what these nerves do.

C. Articulation of speech

1. **Phonation versus articulation:** After the larynx phonates, articulation shapes the sounds into speech. **By whispering this sentence, you can clearly separate phonation from articulation.** When whispering, you do not phonate at all, but you still articulate every word with perfect clarity. Articulate speech consists of a mixture of voiced and non-voiced sounds.
2. **Labial sounds:** While watching your lips in a mirror, recite loudly each letter of the alphabet, but then try to repeat each letter without any lip movement. In Table 6-3, check the sounds that require strong labial action.
3. **Lingual sounds:** Complete Table 6-4 by reciting the alphabet loudly and checking the sounds that require strong lingual actions.
4. **Vowel sounds**
   a. Compare the tongue actions when making *D*, *G*, and *J* sounds, strong linguals, with those needed to make the vowel sounds *A*, *E*, *I*, *O*, and *U*. To understand tongue action during vowel sounds, press down on your tongue with a tongue blade as you recite the vowels.

TABLE 6-3 · Letter Sounds Requiring Strong Lip Action (Labials)

	Strong labial		Strong labial
A		N	
B		O	
C		P	
D		Q	
E		R	
F		S	
G		T	
H		U	
I		V	
J		W	
K		X	
L		Y	
M		Z	

TABLE 6-4 · Letter Sounds Requiring Strong Tongue-Tip Elevation (Linguals)

	Strong lingual		Strong lingual
A		N	
B		O	
C		P	
D		Q	
E		R	
F		S	
G		T	
H		U	
I		V	
J		W	
K		X	
L		Y	
M		Z	

b. Vowels require palatal elevation. The palate does not completely seal off the nasopharynx during most speech sounds. Instead, it reduces the nasopharyngeal aperture, thereby detouring most of the air through the mouth, the path of least resistance. Only a few sounds require complete palatal closure:

i. **Plosives:** *K* or hard *G*, as in *good*.

ii. **Vowels:** sustained *EEEEE*... or *Ah*...

c. Clinicians traditionally test for palatal elevation by asking the Pt to say, *Ahh* ... The vowel *E* requires tighter palatal closure, but the Pt can say *Ah* more easily with the mouth open to permit palatal inspection. As a test for palatal function, ask the Pt to repeat: "We see three gray geese."

5. **Plosive sounds**

a. Plosives require momentary impounding of air and sudden release. Try this experiment: cup your palm and hold it about just in front of your lips. Loudly say, *Puh, puh, puh; M, M, M;* and *kuh, kuh, kuh.*

b. With two of these sounds, you felt a strong puff of air in your palm. The sound not requiring forceful air expulsion and therefore not a plosive was ________________.

M ("em")

c. To divert all air through your mouth, for plosives, the palate must effectively seal the nasopharynx off from the oropharynx. Therefore, if the Pt articulates vowels and plosives well, the velopharyngeal (palatal) valve closes well.

6. **Sibilants and fricatives**

Try it yourself.

   a. **Sibilants** are hissing or whistling sounds. Cup your palm over your mouth and sustain a forceful *SSS*… or a prolonged *Hisssss*… Do you feel a stream of air against your palm? ❒ Yes/❒ No.
   b. **Fricatives** are high-frequency frictional or rustling sounds. Cup your hand to your mouth and forcefully pronounce *V, V, V*…; *Z, Z, Z*…; and *F, F, F*…
   c. Try the sibilants and fricatives again, without using tongue or lips at all. Can you say them?
   d. To produce sibilants and fricatives, you must force a strong stream of air through a small aperture formed by lips, tongue, and teeth. To divert air from the nose into the mouth, the velopharyngeal valve must close more or less completely.

7. **Voiceless consonants:** Many speech sounds, such as sibilants and plosives, require no phonation. As examples of such voiceless consonants, say *Shhhh, P, T,* and *K*. Hence, all speech sounds require ❒ articulation/❒ phonation, but not all speech sounds require ❒ articulation/❒ phonation.

☑ articulation; ☑ phonation

D. Nomenclature for disorders of speech

1. **Mutism** means the inability or refusal to speak. Neuromuscular disorders may cause mutism, but commonly it implicates a block at the level of the cerebrum or mind, as in dementia or **hysterical** mutism, or an afferent block, as in **deaf** mutism. In **elective** mutism a child, for example, may refuse to speak at all in public or at school but talks readily at home. Acute injury to the mid portion of the cerebellum, with or without nuclear involvement, can cause a spectrum of speech disturbances, including transient mutism as observed in certain cases following posterior fossa surgery (mostly tumors) in children (Jones et al. 1996).
2. **Dysphonia** means a disorder of phonation (in the sounds of speech produced by the larynx), such as hoarseness or spasmodic dysphonia.
3. **Dysarthria** means only faulty articulation of speech sounds. It does not refer to the content of speech, the words, syntax, rhythm, and the vocabulary. It may result from central lesions of the brain or cerebellum, intoxications (such as alcohol), or neuromuscular disorders. It commonly occurs with lesions along the course of the pyramidal tract, in which case the Pt usually has other pyramidal tract signs. The extent of associated pyramidal signs in stroke Pts varies from dysarthria and UMN facial palsy, to dysarthria and clumsy hand syndrome, dysarthria and ataxic hemiparesis, or dysarthria and hemiparesis, and most lesions are on the left side of the cerebrum or brainstem (Okuda and Tachibana, 2000; Urban et al., 2001). Chapter 11 discusses **dysprosody** and **aphasia.**

E. Hyponasal and hypernasal speech

1. In **hyponasal** speech, too little air escapes through the nose.
   a. Pinch your nostrils together and say "Good morning."
   b. Lack of nasal escape of air transforms "Good morning" into "Good bordig," as when a cold causes swelling of the nasal mucous membranes. This would be ❒ hypernasal/❒ hyponasal speech.

☑ hyponasal

2. In **hypernasal** speech, too much air escapes through the nose. Because of muscular weakness or mechanical defects, such as a cleft palate, the palate fails to seal off the oropharynx, a condition called **velopharyngeal incompetence** (*velum* curtain soft palate). A Pt with *hyper*nasal speech would have ❒ velopharyngeal incompetence/❒ nasal obstruction, whereas a Pt with *hypo*nasal speech would have ❒ velopharyngeal incompetence/❒ nasal obstruction.

☑ velopharyngeal incompleteness;
☑ nasal obstruction

3. An unfortunate, common, but preventable error

   a. Failure to distinguish between hyper- and hyponasal speech leads to serious errors in treatment. When the palate elevates, it contacts the dorsal pharyngeal wall (Fig. 6-11). In children, the adenoid tissue, which occupies the posterior pharyngeal wall, may hypertrophy and then bulge forward into the pharyngeal lumen. Hypertrophy of the adenoid would cause ❐ hyponasal/❐ hypernasal speech.

☑ hyponasal

   b. Some Pts with neurogenic palatal weakness or submucous palatal clefts will have hypernasality, but the Ex may conclude that enlarged adenoids are at fault. Actually, the adenoids *reduce* the need for velopharyngeal closure. Removal of the adenoids of a Pt with hypernasal speech will make it ❐ better/❐ worse. Explain. ____.

☑ worse

   Removal of the adenoid tissue increases the distance the palate has to close to shut off the nasopharynx. A weak palate is now even less capable of preventing nasal escape of air.

F. Stuttering: involuntary pauses and repetitions interrupt the smooth flow of words and sentences

1. All of us have brief pauses and repetitions when we speak, the toddler more than the adult, but the stutterer's pauses and repetitions impede communication. The Pt usually falters and repeats the first syllable of words, sometimes the middle or last syllables.
2. Although emotional stress worsens stuttering, the cause of stuttering is still unknown. The standard bedside neurologic examination (NE) of stutterers discloses no evidence of neurologic dysfunction per se.

G. Testing the motor function of cranial nerves IX and X

1. **Speech**

   a. During the history, the Ex appraises the Pt's speech almost automatically. Perfectly normal articulation requires no formal testing. Otherwise, test the articulation mechanisms individually.

   b. Test articulation by the soft tissues, the soft palate, tongue, and lips, with the **KLM** test. *Kuh, Kuh, Kuh* tests the function of the ____________; *La, La, La* tests the ________________; and *Mi, Mi, Mi* tests the ________________.

soft palate (velopharyngeal valve); tongue (linguals); lips (labials)

   c. Most infants or young children with delayed speech or dysarthria require a thorough audiologic examination.

2. **Difficulty swallowing (dysphagia)**

   a. To test for mild to moderate dysphagia, give the Pt a glass containing 150 mL of tap water. The Pt should swallow it at a rate exceeding 10 mL/s (Nathadwarawala, 1992).

   b. Any Pt with dysphagia may aspirate food or fluids into the lung, causing aspiration pneumonitis. Avoid the timed swallowing test if the Pt gives a history of aspiration or obvious difficulty swallowing saliva. Deficits in coughing maybe as important as the impaired swallowing in determining aspiration risk. (Smith Hammond et al., 2006).

3. **Neurologic examination of the palate and larynx**

   a. As the Pt says *Ahh*, inspect the tonsillar pillars for asymmetry as they arch upward and medially to form the palate. Look at the arch, the arch above, not the uvula. Study your own palatal action in the mirror.

   b. Students commonly mistake an asymmetrically hung uvula for palatal palsy. Let the uvula hang as it will. Look for asymmetry of the palatal arch. See Figs. 6-12A and 6-12B.

   c. Fig. 6-12A shows a normal person saying *Ahh* ..., and Fig. 6-12B shows a palatal palsy. Which side is paralyzed in B? ❐ right/❐ left.

☑ right(the right side has failed to elevate)

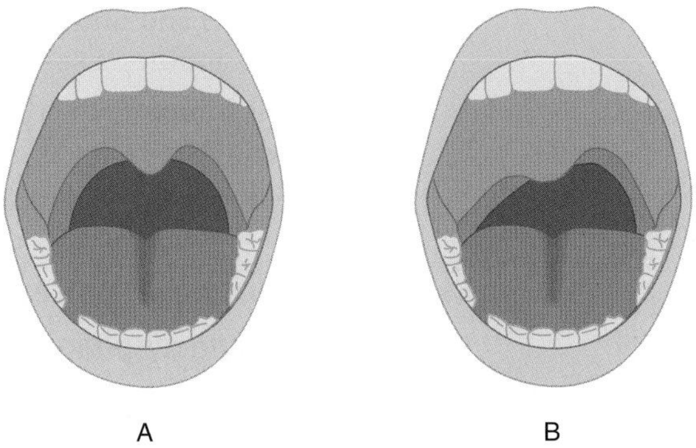

FIGURE 6-12. Palatal arch. (A) Symmetrical elevation of the palatal arch when a normal subject says *Ah*. . . . (B) Asymmetrical elevation of the palatal arch when a Pt with unilateral palatal weakness says *Ah*. . . ., indicating a weak levator veli palatini muscle.

IX; X

☑ UMNs

d. The **gag reflex** is an additional test for palatal elevation. Touch one tonsillar pillar and then the other with a tongue blade. The afferent arc of the gag reflex is primarily CrN ___. The efferent arc is CrN ___.

e. If the palate fails to elevate when the Pt says *Ah* but does elevate during the gag reflex, the Pt would have a lesion of the ❒ UMNs/❒ LMNs/❒ muscles.

f. If the history and examination disclose no evidence of dysarthria or dysphagia, omit the gag reflex. It is uncomfortable and unnecessary. Furthermore, the gag reflex may be absent in a large number of healthy elderly people.

g. Causes of incompetent palatal elevation include UMN or LMN lesions, congenital malformations such as cleft palate, myopathies, or local lesions in the soft tissue, and palatopharyngeal discrepancy in size. Palatal incompetence is not one thing or another. Like every sign, it poses a puzzle to be solved.

4. **Hoarseness and unilateral vagal lesions**

   a. Many mechanical or neurogenic disorders of the larynx can cause hoarseness. Vocal cord paralysis may cause hoarseness but not in all Pts. Therefore, in addition to listening to the voice and looking at the palate, vocal cords may need to be inspected by laryngoscopy.

   b. Unilateral vocal cord paralysis usually causes a breathy, raspy voice or a voice flutter, because of vibration of the flaccid cord, and may cause stridor and anoxia.

      i. In addition, paralysis of the cricothyroid muscles, the pitch adjustor muscles (innervated by the superior laryngeal nerve), results in a monotone sound without changes in pitch.

      ii. Interruption of the entire vagus nerve results in dysphagia and dysphonia, because of paralysis of the pharyngeal constrictors.

5. After listening to many Pts, you will come to recognize disorders in rhythm and force (dysprosody) and timber of the voice. The speech affliction is often characteristic and even pathognomonic of the underlying disease.

   a. In **cerebral palsy,** the cry or the speech has a characteristic slow, ratchet-like onset and a harsh, tight, and irritating dysphonic quality that is diagnosable without even seeing the Pt.

   b. In the **cat's cry syndrome** (*cri du chat*), the infant's cry is high-pitched and sounds like the chromosome 5p deletion syndrome, (also called 5p minus syndrome). The Pt's karyotype confirms the diagnosis: the fifth chromosome lacks a short arm.

   c. In **hypothyroidism,** the voice is deep and raspy.

   d. In **paralysis agitans** (parkinsonism), the muscular rigidity dampens the normal inflections and modulations of the Pt's voice: The sound is all on one plane, i.e., "plateau speech." **Cerebellar disease** causes the opposite: The Pt overaccentuates some sounds and underaccentuates others; the voice scans from one peak of volume to another, a so-called scanning speech.

e. The most common dysarthria of all is slurring due to intoxication with alcohol and other drugs.

f. Table 6-5 presents a classification of speech disorders.

H. Ancillary diagnostic procedures for mutism, dysphonia, dysarthria, and dysphagia

Whenever the Pt, in particular infants or children, presents with disorders in speaking or swallowing, consider these tests:

1. Audiologic investigation: The Pt who does not hear correctly does not speak correctly.
2. Direct laryngoscopy.
3. Plain radiographs of the oropharyngeal airway.
4. Radiographic cinematography, often with a "barium swallow," to visualize the palate and pharynx in action.

TABLE 6-5 · Classification of Speech Disorders

Dysphonia: disorder in the pitch, quality, or volume of the voice
Spasmodic dysphonia
Hoarseness
Pubertal "squeaks"
Vocal tics (Tourette's syndrome)
Dysarthria: disorder in the articulation of sounds
Palatals
Linguals
Labials
Fricatives and sibilants
Plosives
Dysprosody: disorder in the melody, stress, rhythms and inflections that give shades of meaning to speech
Aphasia: inability to express or receive words as symbols for communication
Broca
Wernicke
Conduction
Global
Transcortical motor
Transcortical sensory
Mixed transcortical
Anomic
Striatocapsular
Thalamic
Mutism
Elective
Hysterical
Deaf
Echolalia: stereotyped, non-communicative repetition of words or sentences heard
Developmental disorders
Pervasive developmental disorders (lack of communicative speech): mental retardation and autism
Stammering: blocking or involuntary pauses in speech
Stuttering: repetitions, prolongations, and interjections of syllables or whole words
Cluttering: rapid speech characterized by dropping of syllables
Speech disorders caused by lesions of specific motor system
Ataxic speech (drunk-man speech): cerebellar lesions
Spastic dysarthria (pseudobulbar speech): bilateral corticobulbar tract lesions
Plateau speech: parkinsonism/substantia nigra lesion
Bradylalia, choreiform, dystonic and athetoid speech: extrapyramidal lesions

BIBLIOGRAPHY · Speech, Dysphonia, and Dysarthria

Aronson AE. *Clinical Voice Disorders,* 3rd ed. New York, Thieme Medical Publishers, 1990.

Jones S, Kirollos RW, Van Hille PT. Cerebellar mutism following posterior fossa tumor surgery. *Br J Neurosurg* 1996;10(2):221–224.

Nathadwarawala KM, Nicklin J, Wiles CM. A timed test of swallowing capacity for neurological patients. *J Neurol Neurosurg Psychiatry* 1992;55:822–825.

Okuda B, Tachibana H. Isolated dysarthria. *J Neurol Neurosurg Psychiatry* 2000;68:119–120.

Pollack MA, Shprintzen RF, Zimmerman-Manchester KL. Velopharyngeal insufficiency. The neurological perspective. A report of 32 cases. *Dev Med Child Neurol* 1979; 21:194–201.

Urban PP, Wicht S, Vukurevic G, et al. Dysarthria in acute ischemic stroke. Lesion topography, clinicoradiologic correlation, and etiology. *Neurology* 2001;56:1021–1027.

V. CRANIAL NERVE XI MOTOR FUNCTIONS

A. Functional anatomy of cranial nerve XI

spinal accessory

1. CrN XI has two parts, **spinal** and **accessory.** Hence, its full name is the ______________________________ nerve.
2. The **spinal** part supplies the **sternocleidomastoid** (SCM) and rostral portions of the **trapezius** muscles.
3. The **accessory** part is accessory to the vagus. The accessory fibers arise in the nucleus ambiguus of the medulla and merely hitchhike along the proximal part of CrN XI before joining CrN X for distribution to the pharynx and larynx. The NE tests the spinal part.

B. The sternocleidomastoid muscle

1. Study Fig. 6-13.

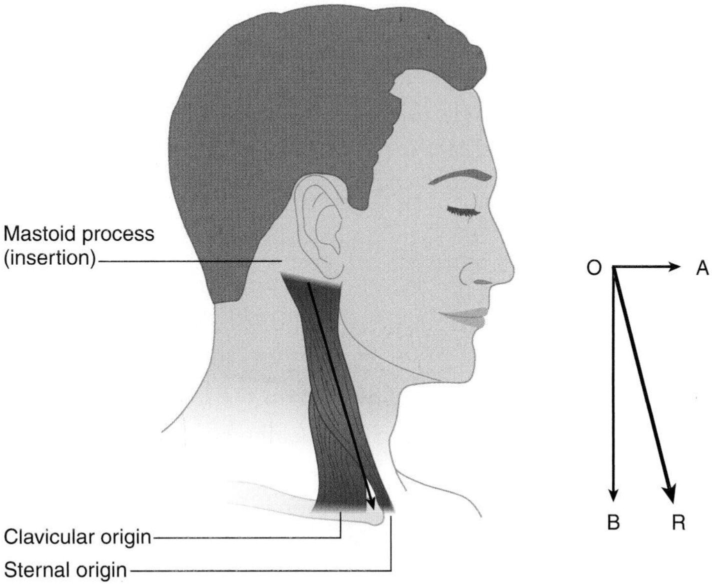

FIGURE 6-13. Origin and insertion of the sternocleidomastoid muscle. The oblique arrow in the vector diagram (O-R) is the actual line of pull. It resolves into a *horizontal* vector (O-A) that thrusts the head forward and turns it to the opposite side and into a *vertical* vector (O-B) that tilts the head to the same side as the muscle.

sternum; clavicle; mastoid

2. The SCM *originates* from the ________________ and the ____________ *inserts* into the ______________ process.

3. **Mnemonic:** To remember once and for all the actions of the SCM muscle, make a C with your thumb and forefinger and place it on your SCM muscles (Fig. 6-14A).

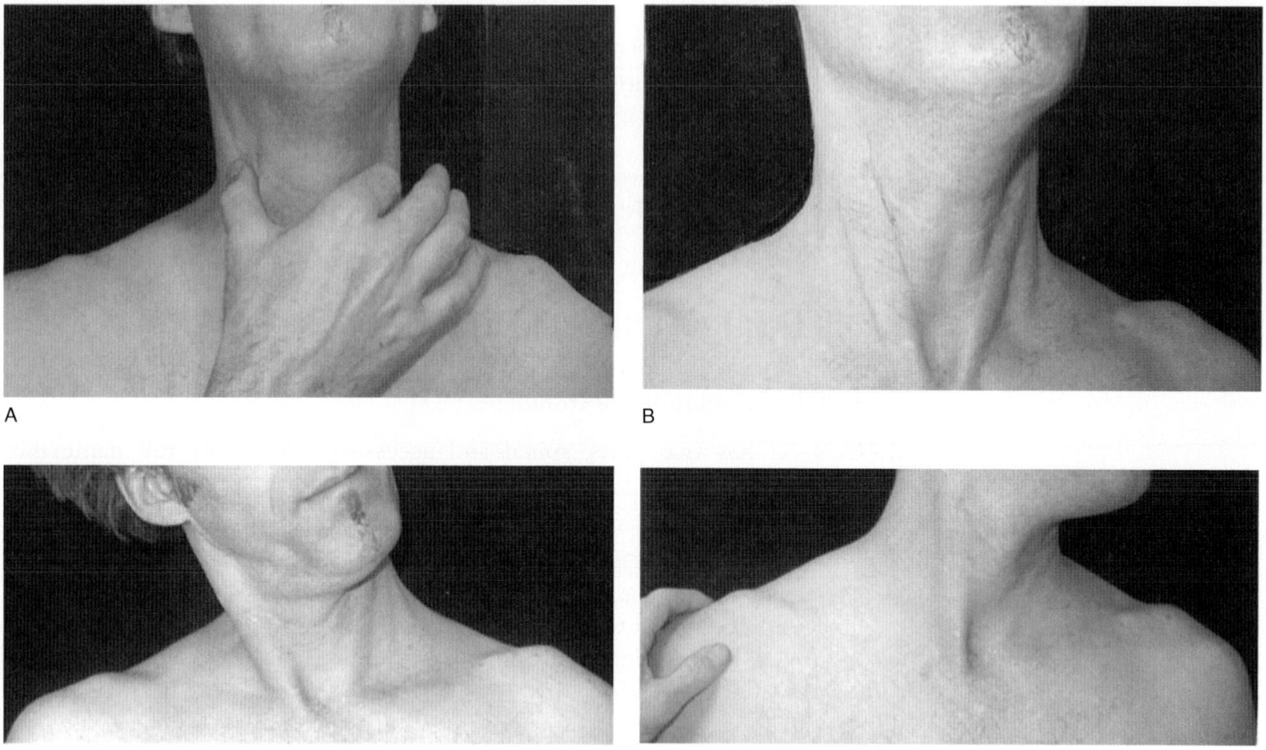

A B C D

FIGURE 6-14. Mnemonic for remembering the actions of the SCM muscles. (A) Make a *C* of the thumb and forefinger and place it on the SCMs. (B) Press the head forward against the opposite hand, and the *C* fingers will feel the SCMs contract bilaterally. The hand is removed in Figs. 6-14B to 6-14D to expose the muscular contractions, but keep your hand in place as in step (A) to feel your own muscles act. (C) Tilt the head to the right (tilt, not turn) and feel the right SCM contract. (D) Turn the head to the left (turn, not tilt) and feel the right SCM contract. Thus the SCM acts to thrust the head forward, tilt it ipsilaterally, and turn it contralaterally. SCM = sternocleidomastoid.

a. Now start with your head in the neutral position and, while palpating your own SCM, place your other hand on your forehead and press *back* on it while you press your head *forward*. You will feel both SCM muscles contracting strongly (Fig. 6-14B).

b. Return your head to the neutral position and then *tilt* (tilt, not turn) your head fully to the right. You will feel your *right* SCM spring into action (Fig. 6-14C).

c. Next try turning (turning, not tilting) your head strongly to the left. You will feel your *right* SCM contract strongly (Fig. 6-14D).

☑ forward

d. SCM *thrusts* the head ❒ forward/❒ backward.

☑ opposite

e. SCM *turns* the head to the ❒ same/❒ opposite side.

☑ same

f. SCM *tilts* the head to the ❒ same/❒ opposite side.

☑ away from

g. The action of one SCM in turning the head, like the action of one lateral pterygoid muscle in turning the mandible, results in turning ❒ toward/ ❒ away from the side of the muscle that is contracting.

4. **Mnemonic for the actions of the SCM muscle:** Make a C with your thumb and forefinger and place it on your SCM muscles. Then *thrust* your head forward against your other hand, *turn* your head, and *tilt* it.

C. The trapezius muscle

1. The trapezius muscle *originates* in the midline from the occiput and the spinous processes of all cervical and thoracic vertebrae. It *inserts* into the clavicle and scapula.
2. CrN XI innervates only the rostral part of the trapezius muscle, the part that lifts the shoulders. The cervical plexus innervates the rest of the muscle.

D. Clinical testing of muscles supplied by cranial nerve XI

1. Inspect the SCM and trapezius muscles for size and asymmetry.
2. Next palpate the muscles at rest and as they exert their actions.
3. To test the strength of SCM and trapezius muscles, try the maneuvers listed in Table 6-6 on another person.

TABLE 6-6 · Clinical Tests of the Motor Function of Cranial Nerve XI

Command to patient	Examiner's maneuver
1. "Turn your head to the left. Do not let me push it back."	Place your right hand on the left cheek of the patient, your left hand on his right shoulder to brace him, and try to force his head to the midline. Repeat with the patient's head turned to the right. With the patient's head turned to the left, you test the ❒ right SCM/ ❒ left SCM/ ❒ trapezius muscle when you try to return the head to the midline.
2. "Push your head forward as hard as possible."	Place one hand on the patient's forehead and push backward. What do you do with your other hand to brace the patient? In this maneuver you test the action of the ❒ SCM/ ❒ trapezius muscles, which thrust the head forward.
3. "Try to touch your ears with the tips of your shoulders. Hold them there and don't let me push them down."	Place your hands on both of the patient's shoulders and press down. Observe from the front and back and watch for scapular winging that may occur with trapezius or serratus anterior weakness.

ABBREVIATION: SCM = sternocleidomastoid.

☑ right SCM

Press forward on vertebrae prominens (C7)

☑ SCM

4. In step 1, why should you press on the Pt's cheek, rather than on the mandible?

____

____

You do not want to test the lateral pterygoid and the SCM at the same time. Test one muscle at a time whenever possible. Moreover, strong lateral pressure on the jaw may dislocate the temporomandibular joint, particularly in an edentulous or elderly Pt.

E. Upper motoneuron innervation of cranial nerve XI

1. An acute severe hemispheric lesion that interrupts the UMNs (the pyramidal tract) will cause contralateral hemiplegia. The Pt's head turns to the side of the lesion because of assumed weakness of the SCM *ipsilateral* to the lesion. However, muscles which are ipsilateral may play a greater note in head turning than the contralateral SCM (Fitzgerald, 2001). Caudal to the brainstem, on the hemiplegic side, the SCM (and perhaps other cervical muscles that turn the head) are the *only* muscles that retain their strength (Willoughby and Anderson, 1984). In contrast, the trapezius muscle is paralyzed like the remaining muscles on the hemiplegic side. Thus these paralyzed muscles receive the classic *contralateral* UMN innervation.
2. The course of the UMN axons to the SCM is still unclear. The clinical evidence suggests that the UMN fibers to one SCM derive mainly from the *ipsilateral* hemisphere and that they run directly without decussating to the LMNs for the SCM or that the fibers undergo a double decussation to end up ipsilateral to the hemisphere that activates them (Gandevia and Applegate, 1988; Marcus, 1989). However, transcranial magnetic stimulation studies suggest that innervation is predominantly contralateral, and there is minimal ipsilateral innervation.

BIBLIOGRAPHY · Cranial Nerve XI

Fitzgerald T. Sternocleidomastoid Paradox. *Clin Anat* 2001;14:330–331.

Gandevia SC, Applegate C. Activation of neck muscles from the human motor cortex. *Brain* 1988;111:801–813.

Marcus JC. The spinal accessory nerve in childhood hemiplegia. *Arch Neurol* 1989;46:60–61.

Thompson ML, Thickbroom GW, Mastaglia FL. Corticomotor representation of the sternocleidomastoid muscle. *Brain* 1997;120:245–255.

VI. XII CRANIAL NERVE MOTOR FUNCTIONS

A. Functional anatomy of the tongue

hypoglossal

1. CrN XII controls tongue movements. Because XII runs under the tongue, it is named the _________________ nerve.
2. **Action of the genioglossus muscle**
   a. To understand how XII nerve lesions affect tongue movements, learn the action of the genioglossus muscles. Notice in Fig. 6-15 the triangular shape of each genioglossus muscle.

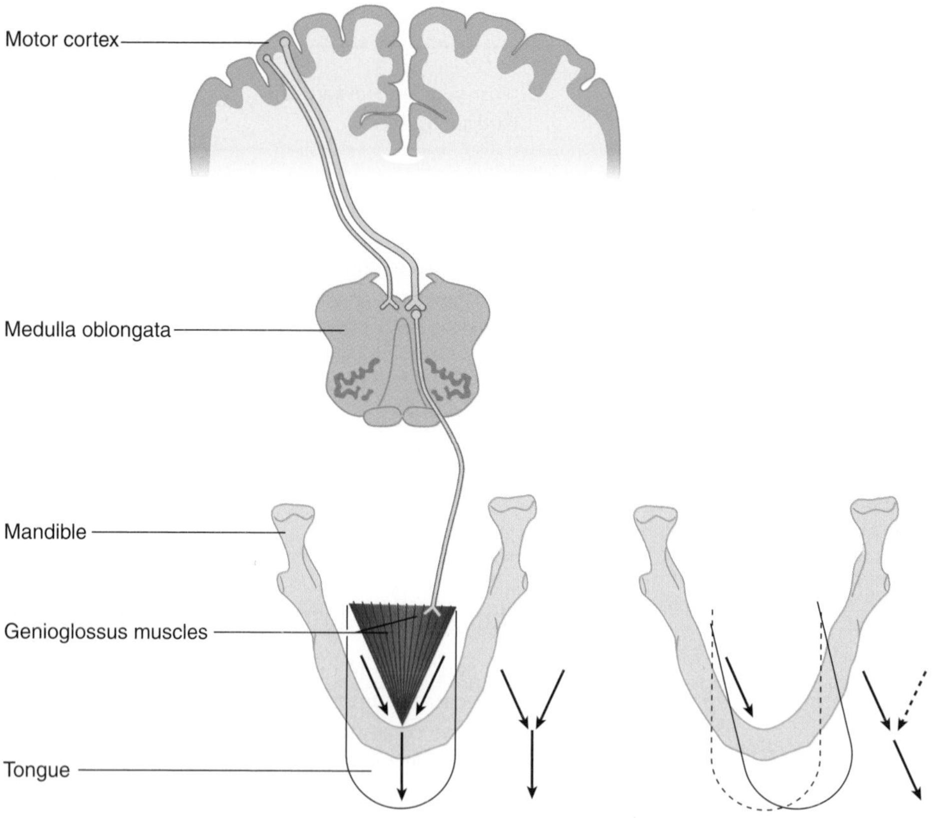

FIGURE 6-15. Innervation and action of the genioglossus muscle. The diagram to the right shows that, when only the right genioglossus muscle contracts, it pulls the right-sided *base* of the tongue forward, thereby protruding and deviating the *tip* of the tongue to the left.

i. Its **apex** originates from the apex of the mandible, which is hard, un-yielding, and immobile.

ii. Its **base** fans out to insert into the base of the tongue, which is soft, fleshy, and mobile. Symmetrical genioglossus contraction, therefore, must pull the base of the tongue ❒ forward/❒ backward.

☑ forward (Fig. 6-15)

genioglossus

b. If the tongue protrudes in the midline, right and left ________________ muscles contract equally.

☑ right

c. If the Pt attempts to protrude the tongue in the midline, and it deviates to the right, the weakness affects the ❐ right/❐ left genioglossus muscle.

☑ opposite

3. Compare the action of genioglossus in Fig. 6-15 with that of the lateral pterygoid muscle in Fig. 6-1. Clearly the mechanics of tongue and jaw protrusion are identical. Midline protrusion results from symmetrical muscular action. Compare the action of these two muscles with the SCM. All three muscles, when contracting unilaterally, turn the part they operate to the ❐ same/❐ opposite side.

☑ left; genioglossus

4. The muscle that turns the tongue to the *right* is the ❐ right/❐ left ____________________________ muscle.

☑ right; lateral pterygoid

5. The muscle that turns the mandible to the *left* is the ❐ right/❐ left ____________________________ muscle.

☑ left; SCM

6. One visible muscle that turns the head to the *right* is the ❐ right/❐ left ____________________________ muscle.

7. With the tongue inside the mouth, the Pt can deviate the tip of the tongue to the non-paralyzed side but not to the paralyzed side, in contrast to its deviation to the paralyzed side when outside the mouth. The genioglossus, an extrinsic muscle, acts on the protruded tongue, whereas intrinsic muscles cause lateral movement of the tip of the non-protruded tongue (Riggs, 1984).

B. Lower motoneuron lesions of cranial nerve XII

Notice in Fig. 6-15 that each XII nerve innervates one-half of the tongue. Although we have mentioned only the genioglossus, the bulk of the tongue is muscle. After interruption of the XII nerve, the muscle fibers on the *ipsilateral* half of the tongue undergo atrophy. Therefore, the signs of XII nerve interruption are **ipsilateral atrophy** and **ipsilateral deviation** of the tongue on attempted midline protrusion.

C. Upper motoneuron innervation of cranial nerve XII

☑ eyelid closure

1. Figure 6-15 shows that one hemisphere sends crossed and uncrossed axons to the hypoglossal nucleus. Using a colored pencil, draw in the UMN and LMN innervations from the *left* motor cortex. Notice the somewhat thicker line representing crossed fibers, indicating a slightly greater percentage of decussated corticobulbar fibers. In this respect, the UMN innervation of the tongue most closely resembles the innervation of ❐ forehead elevation/❐ eyelid closure/❐ lip retraction.

☑ left

2. In 10% to 15% of Pts, the tongue deviates after a unilateral corticobulbar lesion. Thus, if the tongue deviates after a *right* hemisphere lesion, the tongue would deviate to the ❐ right/❐ left when protruded; use Fig. 6-15 to reason out the answer.
3. In hysterical hemiplegia, if the tongue deviates, it typically deviates to the side *opposite* to the putatively paralyzed extremities (Keane, 1986).
4. Because the corticobulbar fibers for branchial nuclei and the corticospinal fibers run more or less together through the brainstem, isolated interruption of just the corticobulbar fibers to the tongue is unlikely. Thus, if a UMN lesion affects tongue movements, the Pt usually shows a UMN type of facial palsy and frank hemiplegia.

D. Clinical testing of cranial nerve XII

1. **Inspection of the tongue at rest**
   a. Inspect the tongue for the most reliable sign of a XII nerve lesion, hemiatrophy. However, diseases that affect LMNs bilaterally, such as amyotrophic lateral sclerosis, result in bilateral tongue atrophy.
   b. Palpation may help resolve questionable hemiatrophy. While wearing a rubber glove, palpate each half of the tongue between your thumb and index finger.

2. **Testing tongue motility and deviation**
   a. Say to the Pt, "Stick your tongue straight out as far as possible and hold it there." Check for alignment of the median raphe of the tongue with the crevice between the medial incisor teeth. Check the alignment of your own tongue in a mirror.
   b. Then, if the history or findings suggest a bulbar problem, ask the Pt to move the tongue alternately to the right and to the left and to try to touch the tip of the tongue to the tip of the nose and then to the tip of the chin. On protrusion the tongue tip should extend well beyond the teeth. Many disorders may impair tongue motility:
      i. Weakness due to UMN or LMN interruption
      ii. Myopathy
      iii. Rigidity, as in parkinsonism
      iv. Apraxia (Chapter 11), mental retardation, dementia, or a major mental illness such as depression or schizophrenia
3. **Tongue strength:** Tongue strength per se is hard to evaluate. Have the Pt press the tongue against the cheek while you press your finger against the cheek. Keep your tongue in your cheek while you evaluate this rather unreliable test.
4. **Involuntary movements of the tongue**
   a. Rippling of a normal tongue frequently indicates incomplete relaxation. Ask the Pt to make some tongue movements and then inspect it again after the Pt relaxes it. Rippling of one half of the tongue, if that half is weak and atrophic, suggests fasciculations (see Chapter 7), which supports the diagnosis of an LMN lesion, but pathologic fasciculations and normal rippling are difficult to distinguish by clinical inspection.
   b. Patients with involuntary movements such as chorea or athetosis (Chapter 7) cannot keep a protruded tongue still. Ask the Pt to hold the tongue protruded and still for 30 seconds.
   c. Infants with mental retardation or cerebral palsy often display an action called **tongue thrusting.** Whenever the mother puts food into the infant's mouth, the tongue thrusts it back out, impairing nutritional input.
5. **Dysarthria:** Interruption of the UMN pathway to the tongue, the corticolingual pathway, causes dysarthria. Usually weakness of the lower part of the face on one side or frank hemiparesis accompanies the dysarthria. Occasionally an isolated lacune (a small infarct) will interrupt the corticolingual fibers from the motor cortex, causing dysarthria, but with no other signs of hemiparesis (Urban et al., 2001).

E. Distinguishing unilateral upper from lower motoneuron weakness of the tongue

1. If the tip of the protruded tongue deviates, the Pt has a *UMN* or an *LMN* lesion. Suppose the tongue deviates to the *left*. If the lesion is UMN, it involves the ❒ right/❒ left hemisphere. The weakness is usually ❒ severe/❒ moderate.

☑ right; ☑ moderate

2. The clinical distinction between unilateral UMN and LMN weakness of the tongue rests on supporting evidence of UMN signs in other movements or on positive evidence of LMN involvement. What would be the best evidence of a unilateral, LMN XII nerve lesion?

____

Ipsilateral atrophy and considerable ipsilateral deviation on protrusion.

F. Patient analysis

1. The Pt shown in Fig. 6-16 was asked to stick out his tongue straight out. Describe any abnormalities.

____

____

The tongue shows right-sided atrophy and deviation of the tip to the right.

2. These clinical findings indicate interruption of the ❒ right/❒ left ❒ XII nerve/❒ corticobulbar tract.

☑ right; ☑ XII nerve

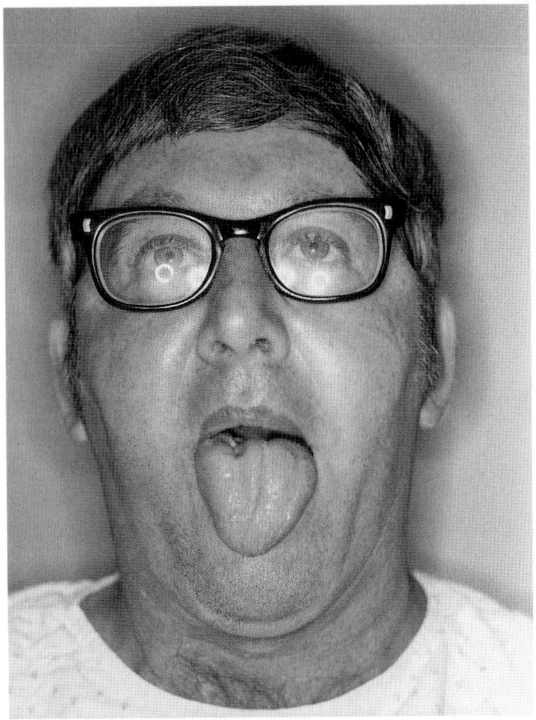

FIGURE 6-16. This patient was asked to stick his tongue straight out.

3. The Pt shown in Fig. 6-16 had a glioma of the medulla oblongata that destroyed the fibers of CrN XII in their intra-axial course.

BIBLIOGRAPHY · Cranial Nerve XII

Keane JR. Wrong-way deviation of the tongue with hysterical hemiparesis. *Neurology* 1986;36:1406–1407.

Riggs JE. Distinguishing between extrinsic and intrinsic tongue muscle weakness in unilateral hypoglossal palsy. *Neurology* 1984;34:1367–1368.

Urban PP, Wicht S, Vukurevic G, et al. Dysarthria in acute ischemic stroke. Lesion topography, clinicoradiologic correlation, and etiology. *Neurology* 2001;56:1021–1027.

VII. MULTIPLE CRANIAL NERVE PALSIES, PATHOLOGIC FATIGABILITY, AND MYASTHENIA GRAVIS

A. Signs and symptoms of multiple cranial nerve palsies

If a Pt has diplopia, dysphagia, dysphonia, or dysarthria, particularly if these complaints are intermittent, or if the Ex finds an unexplained ocular, facial, or bulbar palsy, such as ptosis, strabismus, or mild hypernasal speech, suspect myasthenia gravis. Myasthenics may have little or no deficit when rested, as when first arising in the morning, but as the day wears on, or as they use their CrN muscles to look, talk, swallow, or chew, the weakness gets worse. Symptoms are often worsened by a rise in body temperature and often improved by cold. This **pathologic fatigability** of muscles, particularly of CrN muscles, is virtually pathognomonic of myasthenia gravis. Myasthenic Pts have a deficit in cholinergic transmission at the motor end plates of skeletal muscles. The diagnosis depends on clinical demonstration of the pathologic fatigability, repetitive nerve stimulation that shows a decrementing response, restoration of strength by giving a cholinergic drug, and demonstration of antibodies that block acetylcholine receptors at motor end plates of the skeletal muscles or IgG antibodies against the muscle-specific kinase (MuSK) in cases of seronegative myasthenia gravis.

B. Bedside tests for pathologic fatigability of cranial nerve muscles

1. The Ex chooses for testing the particular muscles implicated by the Pt's history or that have displayed weakness during the NE. If the Pt complains of double vision or ptosis, select the eye muscles; if the complaint involves dysphagia, dysarthria, or dyspnea, select the oropharyngeal and breathing muscles. To bring out latent weakness of such muscles or of a muscle not overtly weak, require the Pt to make repetitive or prolonged contractions. Make sure that you enlist the Pt's full cooperation and effort.
2. To test for ptosis or diplopia, carefully measure the height of the palpebral fissure and record the range of eye movements. Pay particular attention to the range of upward eye movement, the ocular movement that has the least range. Ask the Pt to follow your finger up and down through a full range of movement. Then measure the height of the palpebral fissure and again record the range of eye movements. The ice pack test may also be useful in cases of eyelid ptosis due to myasthenia gravis (Chatzistefanou et al., 2009). Test lateral eye movements by noting the distance between the limbus and lateral or medial canthi before and after repetitive exercise, or have the Pt hold the eyes in a deviated position for a timed period. Test oropharyngeal function by actually timing how long the Pt can read or count aloud without weakness of the voice, and then have the Pt try to swallow a glass of water (Section IV G 3). Test fatigability of the tongue by having the Pt waggle it from side to side. For masseter weakness, request the Pt to chew gum or paraffin a given number of times. Test palatal function by timing how long the Pt can sustain an EEEE°. Test breathing by measuring vital capacity before and after a timed period of hyperventilation. As a quick, quantitative, apparatus-less test for breathing insufficiency, useful in myasthenia or other neurologic disorders in lieu of spirometry, ask the Pt to take a full, deep breath and to count aloud softly from 1 up. Control the rate of counting by tapping your finger at the rate of one per second. The average adult Pt should reach at least 25. Try this test yourself. The point of the foregoing tests is to select some quantifiable or measurable end point to prove that repetitive use of the muscle causes pathologic fatigability or that cholinergic medication restores strength.

C. Electrical tests for pathologic fatigability in myasthenia gravis

Electrical testing for myasthenia includes repetitive stimulation of a peripheral nerve while recording the amplitude of the action potentials generated in the muscle fibers. Myasthenics show a decrement in the amplitude of muscular contraction after repetitive electrical stimulation of the nerve. The repetitive nerve stimulation test (Jolly's test) provides entirely objective data. It eliminates the need for the Pt's active participation, as required by the repetitive exercise tests. Single muscle fiber analysis also aids in establishing the diagnosis.

BIBLIOGRAPHY · Myasthenia Gravis

Chatzistefanou KI, Kounis T, Iliakis E, et al. The ice pack test in the differential diagnosis of myasthenic diplopia. *Opthalmology* 2009;116:2236–2243.

D. Summary of common causes for multiple cranial nerve palsies or weakness of multiple ocular and faciobulbar muscles

1. Myasthenia gravis
2. Landry-Guillain-Barré-Strohl polyradiculopathy syndrome (including the C. Miller Fisher variant)
3. Chronic basilar meningitis
4. Diabetes mellitus
5. Neoplasms along the base of the skull and nasopharynx
6. Botulism

7. Myotonic dystrophy (diffuse weakness of all CrN muscles with predilection for temporal, masseter, and SCM muscles and relative sparing of extraocular muscles; Fig. 1-13I)

VIII. PSEUDOBULBAR AND BULBAR PALSY: UPPER VERSUS LOWER MOTONEURON PALSIES OF THE CRANIAL NERVES

A. Bulbar paralysis

Clinicians use many different terms for UMN and LMN paralysis, terms that bear the imprint of medical history. The older anatomists visualized the medulla as a bulb-like expansion of the spinal cord. Thus, they called the medulla "the bulb." They called LMN paralysis from a lesion of the bulb or its nerves, IX, X, and XII, "bulbar paralysis." They called paralysis of speech and swallowing after UMN lesions "pseudobulbar," or "false bulbar" paralysis, because the lesion was not truly in the bulb or its nerves. The UMNs to the bulb were called "corticobulbar fibers." By usage, the term **corticobulbar fibers** has expanded to include *all* cortical efferent fibers to the brainstem, in particular to the LMNs of CrNs III through XII. But we limit the term **bulbar paralysis** to LMN paralysis of bulbar CrNs IX, X, and XII. Well, "A foolish consistency is the hobgoblin of little minds" (Ralph Waldo Emerson, 1803–1882). Thus, *bulbar paralysis* refers to an ❒ LMN/❒ UMN lesion of CrNs ❒ IX to XII/❒ III to XII.

☑ LMN; ☑ IX to XII

B. The syndrome of pseudobulbar palsy

1. After acute, bilateral interruption of the corticobulbar fibers, as after bilateral cerebral infarction, the Pt becomes obtunded or comatose, mute, or severely demented, and loses all ability to speak or swallow. In the recovery phase or with gradual lesions of the corticobulbar tracts, the Pt shows a characteristic, virtually pathognomonic syndrome termed **pseudobulbar palsy.**
   a. The Pt initiates speaking or swallowing very slowly, if at all, and has severe dysarthria or near mutism.
   b. The voice has a peculiar strained pitch and quality.
   c. The Pt may swallow or chew reflexly but cannot initiate these acts volitionally and may yawn automatically but cannot open the mouth volitionally.
   d. The Pt exhibits extreme emotional lability by crying one moment and laughing the next, like turning on and off a faucet. The face appears immobile most of the time, as though it were a wooden mask, but when the Pt cries or laughs, the facial movements expressing the emotion become exaggerated; strangely, when queried, the Pt may not feel the emotion that the behavior of crying or laughing expresses (Lieberman and Benson, 1977). Sometimes the syndrome expresses itself by uncontrollable burst of inappropriate laughter, called *fou rire prodromique* (Parvizi et al., 2009). The most common causes in adults are bilateral strokes, amyotrophic lateral sclerosis, or other degenerative diseases (Wortzel et al., 2008). Gelastic seizures are another cause, and most commonly result from hypothalamic hamartomas.
   e. The pseudobulbar syndrome occurs in children who have bilateral perisylvian opercular and insular lesions from congenital malformations, hypoxiaischemia, or encephalitis (Christen et al., 2000; Grattan-Smith et al., 1989).
2. Thus, the UMN pathways that activate the muscles for emotional expression differ from those for volitional movement, but we do not know their exact course. The motor pathways for behavioral expression of emotion can thus operate separately from the limbic pathways that produce the experience of emotion.
   a. LMN lesions of CrNs would cause loss of ❒ emotional movements only/❒ volitional movements only/❒ volitional and emotional movements.
   b. Acute bilateral UMN lesions would cause loss of volitional and emotional facial movements initially, but in the chronic stage emotional expression may be ________________.

☑ volitional and emotional movements

exaggerated

Check against frame B1. Did you include everything?

c. Summarize the clinical features of pseudobulbar palsy and state the pathways affected.

____.

3. Table 6-7 lists the many different terms for UMN and LMN paralysis. Clearly, the terms *UMN* and *LMN* convey the concept concisely and informatively.

TABLE 6-7 · Synonyms or Near Synonyms for Muscular Paralysis from UMN and LMN Lesions

UMN paresis or paralysis	LMN paresis or paralysis
Central	Peripheral
Pseudobulbar	Bulbar
Suprasegmental	Segmental/nuclear
Supranuclear	Infranuclear

ABBREVIATIONS: LMN = lower motoneuron; UMN = upper motoneuron.

BIBLIOGRAPHY · Pseudobulbar Palsy

Christen H-J, Hanefeld F, Kruse E, et al. Foix-Chavany-Marie (anterior operculum) syndrome in childhood: a reappraisal of Worster-Drought syndrome. *Dev Med Child Neurol* 2002;42:122–123.

Grattan-Smith PJ, Hopkins IJ, Shield LK, et al. Acute pseudobulbar palsy due to bilateral focal cortical damage: the opercular syndrome of Foix-Chavany-Marie. *J Child Neurol* 1989;4:131–136.

Lieberman A, Benson DF. Control of emotional expression in pseudobulbar palsy. *Arch Neurol* 1977;34:717–719.

Parvizi J, Coburn KL, Shillcutt SD, et al. Neuroanatomy of pathological laughing and crying: a report of the American Neuropsychiatric Association Committee on Research. *J Neuropsychiatry Clinc Neurosci* 2009;21:75–87.

Wortzel HS, Oster TJ, Anderson CA, et al. Pathological laughing and crying. Epidemiology, pathophysiology and treatment. *CNS Drugs* 2008;22 (7);531–545.

IX. THE NEUROLOGY OF BREATHING

A. Four functions of the breathing apparatus

1. **Gas exchange for respiration**
   a. Homeostatic control of blood gases and pH
   b. Clearing the airway by coughing, sniffing, and sneezing
2. **Sucking and blowing**
3. **Emotional expression:** sighs, laughter, crying, exclamations, hissing, breath-holding, hyperventilation
4. **Speech**

B. The neuroanatomy of breathing

1. **Origin of the drive to breathe:** The drive to breathe arises from two sources: the **forebrain** and the **brainstem** reticular formation. The isolated spinal cord by itself cannot produce any drive to breathe. That drive must descend from the brain. Thus separation of the spinal cord from the brain by transection at the medullocervical junction causes complete and irreversible apnea.
2. **The forebrain and the control of volitional and emotional breathing**
   a. The forebrain mediates the **volitional** control of breathing via the pyramidal tracts, particularly for speech.
   b. The forebrain also mediates the **emotional** control of breathing, in particular for laughing and crying, through descending pyramidal and nonpyramidal pathways. Other common examples of emotional expression through control of breathing are hyperventilation attacks in anxiety, breath-holding spells in infants, and sighing.

3. **The reticular formation and the control of automatic breathing**

   a. Reticulospinal tracts, arising in the medullary reticular formation, control **automatic,** essentially homeostatic, breathing for the control of blood gases and pH.

   b. The **caudal** half of the reticular formation, from the mid-pons to the medullocervical junction, generates the rhythmic drive to breath and controls the related reflexes served by the caudal CrNs (swallowing, chewing, rooting, sucking, coughing, and hiccoughing) and mediates the control of blood pressure and pulse. Bilateral permanent lesions of the caudal reticular formation permanently impair or abolish breathing and the related reflexes.

   c. The medullary reticular formation provides the single most important pathway for survival, the **reticulospinal pathway.** It activates the LMNs of the muscles of respiration, essentially the diaphragm and intercostal muscles. The reticulospinal tracts decussate at the medullocervical junction, just ventral to the obex, and descend in the ventrolateral quadrants of the spinal cord to activate the phrenic and intercostal motoneurons (Fig. 6-17).

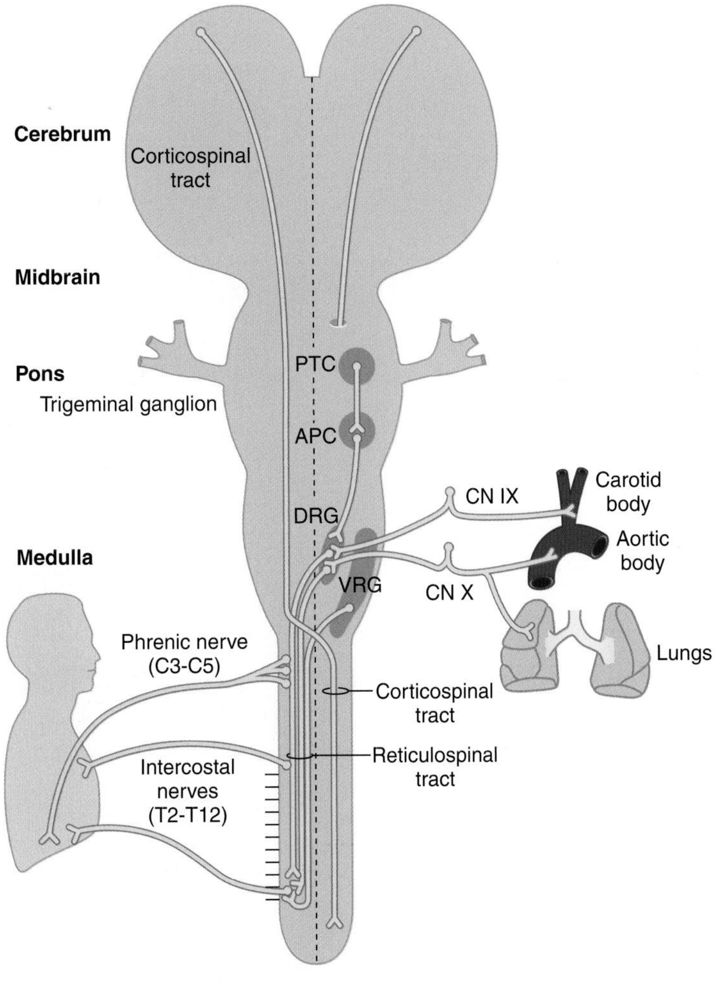

FIGURE 6-17. Neuroanatomy of breathing. By stimulating motoneurons in the spinal cord from C3 to T12, the corticospinal tracts control volitional breathing, and the reticulospinal tracts control automatic breathing. APC = apneustic center; CN = cranial nerve; DRG = dorsal respiratory group of neurons, mainly inspiratory, associated with the dorsal motor nucleus of the vagus nerve; PTC = pneumotaxic center; VRG = ventral respiratory group of mixed inspiratory and expiratory neurons associated with the nuclei ambiguus and retroambigualis. (Reproduced with permission from DeMyer W. *Neuroanatomy,* 2nd ed. Baltimore, Williams & Wilkins, 1998.)

   d. The **phrenic nerves** are the most important nerves in the body. With intact phrenic nerves and the drive to breathe descending through the reticulospinal tracts, the Pt can maintain life by diaphragmatic action alone, even after spinal cord transection caudal to the phrenic level (C3 to C5) paralyzes all the intercostal muscles. Transcutaneous stimulation of the phrenic nerves and electromyographic recording of the diaphragm can directly access the LMNs for breathing (Markand et al., 1983).

e. Figure 6-18 shows an infant who suffered spinal cord transection during a breech delivery. The infant shows dorsiflexed wrists secondary to intact extensor muscles and paralyzed flexors. The spared extensor muscle motoneurons are slightly rostral to the level of the flexors. The lesion has spared the phrenic nerve, which arises from C3 to C5, but has interrupted all ascending and descending spinal pathways at the C7 level, thus depriving the intercostal muscles of pyramidal and reticulospinal activation. Because of the descent of the diaphragm without intercostal action, the chest sucks in and the abdomen protrudes when the infant inspires, the so-called abdominal breathing (Fig. 6-18). The legs show the characteristic flexed posture that follows chronic spinal cord transection (paraplegia in flexion; Figs. 6-18A and 6-18B).

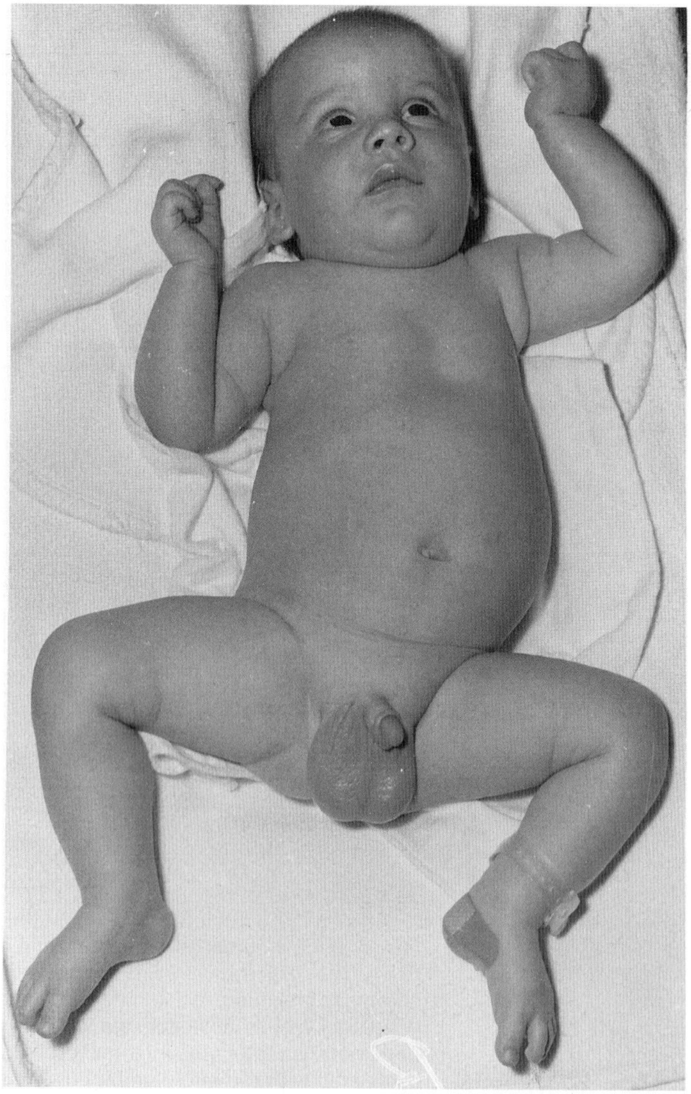

A

FIGURE 6-18. Eight-week-old infant showing the characteristic posture and breathing action after spinal cord transection at level C7 due to a breech delivery. (Reproduced with permission from DeMyer W. Anatomy and clinical neurology of the spinal cord. In Joynt RJ, ed. *Clinical Neurology,* rev. ed. Philadelphia, Lippincott, 1990, Vol. 3, Chap. 43, pp. 1–32.)

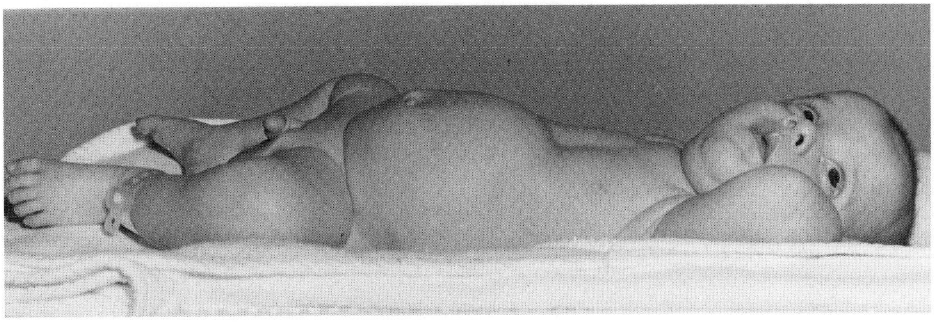

B

FIGURE 6-18. (Continued)

4. **Coughing**

   Another breathing-related function of the caudal reticular formation is coughing, which depends on the abdominal muscles for the explosive expulsion of air. Coughing is an important protective reaction to clear the airway in response to irritant gases, vomitus, or foreign bodies. Many diseases of the central and peripheral nervous systems impair coughing by interrupting the afferent or efferent arc or causing paralysis, thus leading to pneumonia. The Ex should record whether any Pt with respiratory difficulty can cough. Quantitative measurement of air flow is the most reliable way to assess the neuromuscular sufficiency for coughing (Smith Hammond, 2001).

C. Ondine's curse and the dichotomy between volitional and automatic breathing

1. Consider a Pt with intact pyramidal tracts but interruption of the reticulospinal pathways. Such a condition may arise from any of the following conditions:
   a. Bilateral destruction of the medullary reticular formation
   b. Interruption of the reticulospinal tracts at the obex (Fig. 6-17)
   c. Interruption of the reticulospinal tracts as they descend in the ventro-lateral quadrants of the spinal cord white matter (Fig. 2-12C)
2. The Pt without a reticulospinal pathway lacks automatic breathing but continues to breathe while awake because of the respiratory drive generated in the waking forebrain, transmitted through the pyramidal tracts. Sleep removes the respiratory drive arising in the forebrain. Thus with no automatic breathing to take over, the Pt becomes apneic when going to sleep and may die. This condition, **Ondine's curse,** condemns the Pt to death if he goes to sleep. To breathe and, hence, to live, the Pt must remain perpetually awake, never to enjoy Keats' "sleep full of sweet dreams and quiet breathing."
3. By contrast, interruption of the pyramidal tracts, with the reticulospinal tracts intact, abolishes volitional control of breathing, but automatic breathing, via the reticulospinal tracts, keeps the Pt alive, whether awake or asleep. Such Pts with bilateral pyramidal tract destruction also show the pseudo-bulbar palsy syndrome described in Section VIII.

D. Hypoventilation in hemiplegia

Hemiplegia causes paresis of respiratory actions. Because some Pts have a larger number of decussating axons in the pyramidal tract than others, the effects of UMN lesions may vary somewhat from Pt to Pt. Interruption of the pyramidal tract reduces diaphragmatic and intercostal actions contralaterally during voluntary breathing but not during automatic breathing (Polkey et al., 1999).

BIBLIOGRAPHY · Breathing

Markand O, Kincaid JC, Pourmand R, et al. Electrophysiologic evaluation of diaphragm by transcutaneous phrenic nerve stimulation. *Neurology* 1984;34:604–614.

Polkey MI, Lyall RA, Moxhan J, et al. Respiratory aspects of neurological disease. *J Neurol Neurosurg Psychiatry* 1999;66:5–15.

Smith Hammond CA, Goldstein LB, Zajac DJ, et al. Assessment of aspiration risk in stroke with quantification of voluntary cough. *Neurology* 2001;56:502–506.

X. LOCALIZING DIAGNOSTICON FOR BRAINSTEM SYMPTOMS AND SIGNS

Figure 6-19 summarizes the clinical effects of brainstem lesions. One important, classic localizing combination is paralysis of a CrN in the midbrain, pons, and medulla *ipsilateral* to the lesion and motor or sensory signs *contralateral* to it due to interruption of a decussating tract, i.e., right VI nerve palsy and left-sided pyramidal signs caused by a lesion of the basis pontis.

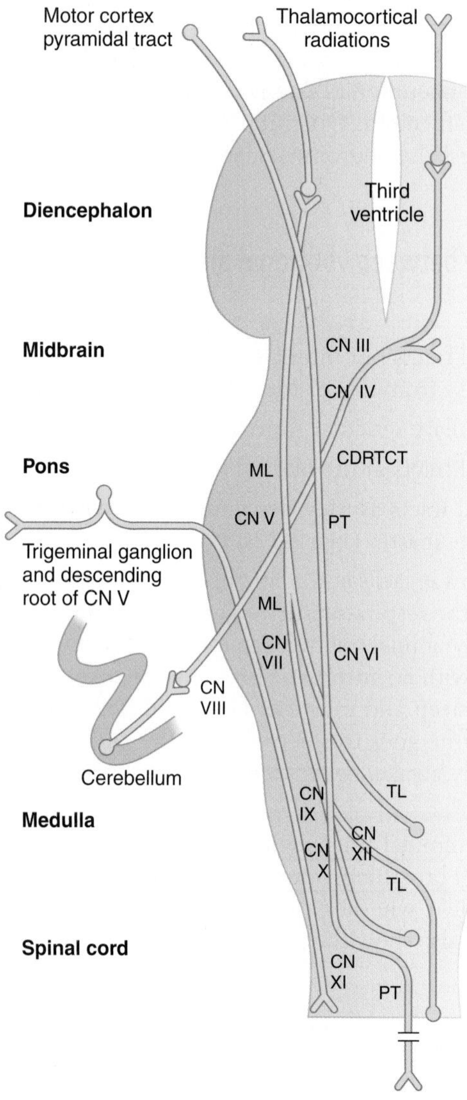

Clinical findings after destructive lesions

Diencephalon

Unilateral lesions: Contralateral hemisensory loss, including face (ML and its terminal nucleus {posterior ventral nucleus}); contralateral involuntary movements, especially hemiballism (subthalamic nucleus and rubrosubthalamic connections)

Bilateral lesions: Akinesia, unconsciousness; Cheyne-Stokes respiration, especially if lesion extends bilaterally into cerebrum

Midbrain

Unilateral lesions: Ispilateral cranial nerve (III) palsy, corectasia; intention or postural tremor (CDRTCT) or contralateral hemiballism, hemiplegial (PT), and hemisensory loss, including face (ML)

Bilateral lesions:
In basis: Quadriplegia, pseudobulbar palsy
In tegmentum: Unconsciousness, hyperventilation, decerebrate rigidity; parkinsonism (SN)

Pons

Unilateral lesions: Ipsilateral cranial nerve (V, VI, or VII) palsy, no corneal reflex; Loss of pain and temperature sensation (descending root of CN V); contralateral hemiplegia (PT) and hemisensory loss (ML) in face and body, depending on involvement of descending root of CN V or trigeminal lemniscus; nystagmus, vertigo and nausea (VP and RF)

Bilateral lesions:
In basis: Quadriplegia (locked-in syndrome)
In tegmentum: Unconsciousness if in rostral half of pons; apneustic or cluster breathing if in caudal half; nystagmus, vertigo, nausea and vomiting (VP and RF)

Medulla

Unilateral lesions: Ipsilateral cranial nerve palsy: of pharynx (IX, X), palate (X), or tongue (XII); Horner's syndrome; dysphagia; hiccups; loss of corneal reflex (sometimes); loss of pain and temperature sensation on face (descending root of CN V); contralateral hemiplegia (PT), hemisensory loss on body (ML); nystagmus, vertigo, nausea and vomiting (VP and RF)

Bilateral lesions: Quadriplegia; ataxic breathing or apnea; hypotension

FIGURE 6-19. Localizing diagnosticon for brainstem lesions (exclusive of central ocular pathways). CDRTCT = cerebello-dentato-rubro-thalamo-cortical tract; CN = cranial nerve; ML = medial lemniscus; PT = pyramidal tract; TL = trigeminal lemniscus; RF = reticular formation; SN = substantia nigra; VP = vestibular pathways. (Reproduced with permission from DeMyer W. *Neuroanatomy,* 2nd ed. Baltimore, Williams & Wilkins, 1998.)

XI. SEQUENTIAL SCREENING EXAMINATION OF THE MOTOR FUNCTIONS OF ALL CRANIAL NERVES

A. Preliminary observations

And now the crucial test: Can you actually and systematically examine CrN motor function? If you did your job when taking the history, you have already observed the Pt's eye movements and blinking; noted the degree and symmetry of other facial movements; inspected the relation of the eyelids to palpebral fissures; looked for enor exophthalmos; listened to phonation and for the articulation of labials, linguals, and palatals; and noted the spontaneous swallowing of saliva. If these are all normal, the Pt cannot have too much wrong with CrN motor function, but you must do a minimum formal examination anyhow.

B. Motor examination of all of the cranial nerves in 45 seconds

The formal examination of CrN motor function begins with the eyes. The NE outline at the beginning of the text lists motility last in the ocular sequence for a reason. The Ex can then flow smoothly through the entire CrN motor examination, yes, III to XII, in just 45 seconds, in a normal cooperative Pt. No, the 45 seconds is not a misprint. Get a partner and rehearse the commands and observations listed in Table 6-8 until you meet the 45-seconds criterion.

TABLE 6-8 · Rapid Sequential Screening of the Motor Function of the Cranial

Nerves	Commands to patient Nerves by examiner	Observations and tests by examiner
III, IV, VI	"Follow my finger"	Move finger through the pattern described in Chapter 4 and pictured in Fig. 4-20 and watch for asymmetrical corneal light reflections, lid-limbus relations, nystagmus, and pupilloconstriction during convergence. Inquire about diplopia.
	"Look up at the ceiling"	Watch for asymmetry or absence of forehead wrinkling and eyebrow elevation.
	"Close your eyes tight and don't let me open them"	Look for asymmetry of wrinkles radiating from lateral canthi and try to force lids open with your fingers.
VII	"Draw back the corners of your mouth" or "Smile"	Look for asymmetry of the nasolabial folds. Have patient make labial sounds if speech sounded abnormal.
	"Draw down the corners of your mouth hard"	Look for asymmetry of movement and for wrinkling of skin on neck from platysma action.
V	"Bite your jaws together hard"	Palpate the masseter muscles.
	"Open your jaw as wide as possible"	Look for deviation of the tip by sighting on the notch between the medial two incisors.
	"Hold your jaw to one side"	Try to push it back. Repeat test to the opposite side.
XII	"Stick out your tongue as far as possible"	Look for deviation, atrophy, and fasciculations. Test for lingual articulations if speech sounded abnormal.
	"Move your tongue from side to side"	Look for weakness or slowness of movement.
X	"Say *Ah*"	Look for asymmetrical palatal elevation. Test for palatal articulations and do gag reflex if speech or swallowing were abnormal.
XI	"Turn your head to one side and don't let me push it back"	Try to push head back to midline. Inspect and palpate stenocleidomastoid muscles. Repeat maneuver to opposite side.
	"Touch your ears with your shoulders"	Try to press the patient's shoulders back down.

BIBLIOGRAPHY · The Cranial Nerves

DeMyer W. *Neuroanatomy.* Baltimore, Williams & Wilkins, 1998.

Samii M, Jannetta PJ, eds. *The Cranial Nerves*. New York, Springer-Verlag, 1981.

Wilson-Pauwels L, Akesson EJ, Stewart PA, et al. *Cranial Nerves in Health and Disease.* Philadelphia, BC Decker, 2002.

Learning Objectives for Chapter 6

I. CRANIAL MOTOR V FUNCTION: CHEWING

1. State in one word the motor function of CrN V.
2. Name the chewing muscles innervated by CrN V.
3. Describe the actions of the lateral pterygoid muscles and describe the effect of paralysis of one lateral pterygoid muscle on jaw movement (Figs. 6-1 and 6-2).
4. Describe the UMN (corticobulbar) innervation of the V nerve nucleus.
5. Demonstrate the steps in the clinical examination of the chewing muscles.
6. Demonstrate how to place your hands to test the strength of the lateral pterygoid muscle.
7. Describe a complication of improper technique in testing the jaw strength of an elderly, edentulous Pt.
8. Describe the clinical findings on inspection, palpation, and strength testing of a Pt after complete unilateral interruption of the motor division of CrN V.

II. CRANIAL NERVE VII MOTOR FUNCTIONS

1. List the major movements of your own face (exclusive of the mandible) and name the muscles responsible (Table 6-1 and Fig. 6-3).
2. Recite the commands for testing the actions of the facial muscles (Table 6-1).
3. On a cross-section drawing of the pons, show the origin and intra-axial course of CrNs VI and VII (Fig. 6-4).
4. Describe the effect of proximal interruption of CrN VII on hearing.
5. Describe how to break CrN VII into three nerves as a mnemonic (Fig. 6-6).
6. Recite the mnemonic for all of the clinically important functions of CrN VII. (**Hint:** It begins with *tears*.)
7. State which facial movements a normal person can most easily make unilaterally and which least easily (Table 6-2). Relate this observation to the degree of unilaterality or bilaterality of the UMN innervation of the movements.
8. Describe the pattern of facial muscle paralysis after a CrN VII (LMN) lesion as contrasted to a corticobulbar tract (UMN) lesion. Relate the side of the paralysis to the side of the LMN or UMN lesion.
9. Explain why an acute UMN lesion will sometimes cause paresis of the orbicularis oculi muscle along with paralysis of the lower part of the face.
10. Describe the clinical observations you make to detect mild UMN palsy of the face.
11. Describe whether it is easy or difficult to open a normal person's forcefully closed eyelids.
12. Describe the discrepancy between volitional and emotional facial movements, such as smiling, often seen in the chronic stage after UMN lesions affecting the face.
13. Describe *masked facies* and mention some disorders that cause it.
14. List several types of involuntary movements seen by inspecting the Pt's face.
15. Make a diagram of CrN VII and recite the different clinical effects of lesions at various sites along its course (Figs. 6-5 and 6-6).

Learning Objectives for Chapter 6

III. CRANIAL NERVE IX AND X MOTOR FUNCTIONS

1. State which CrNs provide clinically significant motor and sensory nerve fibers for the palate, pharynx, and larynx. Use the mnemonic in III B 3, if you wish.
2. Describe the sequence of the act of normal swallowing. State which CrNs participate and the actions of the muscles they innervate.
3. Describe the action and functions of the soft palate (Fig. 6-11) and state which CrN is mainly responsible for its action.
4. Produce two sounds that require complete palatal closure.
5. State whether severe and enduring unilateral palatal palsy would implicate a UMN or an LMN lesion and explain why.

IV. ROLE OF CRANIAL NERVES IN SPEECH

1. Distinguish between *phonation* and *articulation*.
2. Demonstrate on yourself how to recall the sounds that require strong labial or lingual action.
3. Produce a fricative, sibilant, voiceless consonant and a plosive.
4. Recite a vowel sound that requires complete palatal closure.
5. Define *aphonia/dysphonia, anarthria/dysarthria,* and *aphagia/dysphagia*.
6. Distinguish between *hypernasal* and *hyponasal* speech and relate them to the size of the nasopharyngeal opening.
7. Explain why removal of adenoid tissue may worsen the speech of a Pt who has hypernasal speech.
8. Recite three sounds that you ask the Pt to make that respectively test palatal, lingual, and labial articulations.
9. State which CrNs innervate the muscles responsible for labial, lingual, and palatal sounds.
10. Describe a quantitative bedside test for dysphagia.
11. Make a drawing to show the appearance of the palate of a Pt with a unilateral palatal palsy. State which sound the Pt should make when you inspect the palatal arch for weakness (Fig. 6-12).
12. Describe how to elicit the gag reflex. State which CrNs mediate the afferent and efferent arcs of the reflex.
13. Describe the effects of unilateral vocal cord paralysis on the Pt's voice and the nerve that innervates laryngeal muscles except for the cricothyroid.
14. State the nerve that innervates the cricothyroid muscle and the effects of its interruption.
15. State several neurologic, neuromuscular, or anatomic causes for deficient velopharyngeal closure.
16. State the only way to conclusively identify paralysis of a vocal cord.
17. State which sensory CrN you must always test in an infant or young child with delayed speech or significant dysarthria.

V. CRANIAL NERVE XI MOTOR FUNCTIONS

1. Explain why CrN XI is called the *spinal accessory* nerve.
2. Name the two clinically testable muscles innervated by CrN XI.
3. Describe the actions of the sternocleidomastoid muscle and demonstrate how to use the *C* mnemonic on yourself to remember these actions.
4. Demonstrate the clinical examination of the SCM and trapezius muscles (Table 6-6).

Learning Objectives for Chapter 6

5. Explain whether to press on the Pt's cheek or mandible to test the strength of head rotation by the SCM muscle.
6. Describe the effect of hemiplegia on the action of the SCM muscles on the two sides.

VI. CRANIAL NERVE XII MOTOR FUNCTIONS

1. By means of a vector diagram, explain the action of the genioglossus muscle (Fig. 6-15).
2. Explain this statement: "The lateral pterygoid, sternocleidomastoid, and the genioglossus muscles all turn the part they operate to the opposite side."
3. State the typical signs of LMN XII nerve palsy and the findings that distinguish LMN from UMN weakness of the tongue.
4. Demonstrate the steps in the clinical examination of the motor functions of the tongue.

VII. MULTIPLE CRANIAL NERVE PALSIES, PATHOLOGIC FATIGABILITY, AND MYASTHENIA GRAVIS

1. Describe the most frequent presenting symptoms of Pts with pathologic fatigability of multiple CrN muscles.
2. Name the neuromuscular disease you should suspect when the Pt has these complaints.
3. Describe the neurochemical defect in myasthenia gravis.
4. Describe how to decide which muscles to test for pathologic fatigability in a Pt suspected of myasthenia gravis.
5. Describe in principle the clinical, electrical, and pharmacologic tests for pathologic fatigability of muscles.
6. Describe several quantitative bedside tests for pathologic fatigability.
7. Describe a simple, quantitative, apparatus-less bedside test for respiratory insufficiency.
8. State the pharmacologic action of edrophonium.
9. Describe the procedure for the edrophonium test and state what precautions you should take to ensure the Pt's safety and comfort during the edrophonium test.
10. Describe the symptoms and signs that may occur during an edrophonium test. Describe the mnemonic or organizing principles for remembering these effects.
11. Describe the end points you use to decide how much edrophonium to give and when to terminate the test. Explain why you titrate the dose of edrophonium to one of these end points rather than giving a preset dose.
12. Recite a number of diseases that can cause multiple cranial nerve palsies.

VIII. PSEUDOBULBAR AND BULBAR PALSY: UPPER VERSUS LOWER MOTONEURON PALSIES OF THE CRANIAL NERVES

1. Explain the term *bulbar palsy*.
2. Describe the effect of pseudobulbar palsy on the Pt's emotional expression.
3. Describe the effect of pseudobulbar palsy on speaking, swallowing, and volitional facial movements.

IX. THE NEUROLOGY OF BREATHING

1. State the functions of the breathing apparatus.
2. Describe the origins of the drive to breathe.
3. Give examples of the expression of emotions that employ the breathing apparatus.

Learning Objectives for Chapter 6

4. Contrast the major functions of the rostral half of the reticular formation with the caudal half.
5. Describe the role of the pontomedullary reticular formation in breathing and list the breathing-related reflexes mediated through it and the medullary CrNs.
6. Describe the origin, course, and LMNs of termination of the reticulospinal pathways for breathing (Fig. 6-17).
7. Name the single most important peripheral nerve for the maintenance of breathing and the spinal cord segments from which it arises.
8. Describe a laboratory test to assess directly the integrity of the phrenic nerve and diaphragm.
9. Describe the pathways that mediate automatic and volitional breathing.
10. Describe which pathway is responsible for automatic breathing during sleep and describe the nature of Ondine's curse.
11. Describe the posture of a Pt with a C7 level cord transection and the characteristic action of the chest and abdomen when such a Pt breathes (Fig. 6-18).

X. A LOCALIZING DIAGNOSTICON FOR BRAINSTEM SYMPTOMS AND SIGNS

1. List in rostrocaudal order the three parts of the brainstem and the CrN motor nuclei contained in each (Fig. 6-19).
2. Commencing with the midbrain and working caudally, describe the typical unilateral and contralateral signs seen after unilateral lesions of the midbrain, pons, and medulla (Fig. 6-19).

XI. SEQUENTIAL SCREENING EXAMINATION OF THE MOTOR FUNCTIONS OF ALL CRANIAL NERVES

1. Starting with the ocular movements, recite the commands and demonstrate the maneuvers used to screen the motor functions of all CrNs (III to XII) in serial order in less than 1 minute in a normal, cooperative Pt (Table 6-8).

7 Examination of the Somatic Motor System (Excluding Cranial Nerves)

But the expression of a well-made man appears not only in his face,
It is in his limbs and joints also, it is curiously in the joints of his hips and wrists.
It is in his walk, the carriage of his neck, the flex of his waist, and knees...
To see him pass conveys as much as the best poem, perhaps more.

—Walt Whitman (1819–1892)

I. INSPECTION OF THE BODY CONTOURS, POSTURES, AND GAIT

A. Initial inspection

1. The motor examination begins the instant you meet the patient (Pt). Study every activity: How the Pt sits, stands, walks and gestures; the postures; and the general activity level. Unobtrusive observation of the Pt's spontaneous activity often discloses more than formal tests, particularly in infants or mentally ill Pts.
2. For the formal examination, the Pt undresses and stands under an overhead light. Underclothes remain in place, in deference to modesty, but at some time you must look under them. If you leave one-third of the body covered, you can do only two-thirds of an examination. Before the cock crows, one of you will violate this commandment: thou shalt undress every Pt. Your own anxieties about viewing nudity may exceed those of the Pt about being viewed nude. After all, the Pt came to you expecting an examination.
3. Next, ponder, yes **ponder,** the Pt's somatotype or body build. Compare the Pt's contours and proportions with those of a standard normal person of like age and sex and with those of family members. From abnormalities in the Pt's *Gestalt*, sometimes from just a glance at the silhouette, the examiner (Ex) can diagnose an immense number of syndromes, such as arachnodactyly, achondroplastic dwarfism, and Down's syndrome.
4. Next, scrutinize the size and contours of the Pt's muscles, looking for atrophy or hypertrophy, body asymmetry, joint malalignments, fasciculations, tremors, and involuntary movements. Proceed in an orderly, rostrocaudal, face-neck-shoulder-arm-forearm-hand-chest-abdomen-thigh-leg-foot-toe sequence and continually compare right and left sides.

B. Station and gait testing

1. Next, observe the Pt's **station,** the steadiness and verticality of the standing posture. Then test the **gait** by asking the Pt to walk freely across the room. Look for unsteadiness, a broad-based gait, and lack of arm swinging. Ask the Pt to walk on the toes, heels, and in tandem (from heel to toe along a straight line). Request a deep knee bend. Ask a child to hop on each foot and to run. **Watching the Pt walk is the single most important part of the entire neurologic examination.** An essay at the end of Chapter 8 details gait analysis, after you have a better concept of what to look for.
2. Now, rehearse the five steps of Section VI A of the Standard Neurologic Examination (NE). Yes, I'll ask you to demonstrate them by and by.

II. PRINCIPLES OF STRENGTH TESTING

Note: Do the strength tests on another person. How else can you learn to match your strength against another's?

A. The matching principle

Select those movements that just about match your arm and hand strength. Even if an iron bar loses much of its strength, it may remain too strong for your hands to bend. Conversely, wet tissue paper offers too little resistance. To gauge strength accurately, select movements that are neither too strong for you to possibly overcome nor too weak for you to judge their resistance.

B. The length–strength principle

Under the conditions of clinical testing, the muscles are strongest when acting from their *shortest* position and have little or no strength when acting from their *longest* position.

1. To understand the length-strength law, work through Figs. 7-1A to 7-1B to test biceps and triceps strength. **You must do the exercises the text calls for. You will find yourself hesitant and clumsy at first—that's why you have to practice, to get a "feel" or sympathy for the task.** In all strength tests, the participants should exert maximum power, but they should pull to a peak in a slow crescendo, without jerking.
2. The biceps pull test, biceps against biceps, perfectly exemplifies the matching principle, when the Pt and Ex match muscle to muscle.
3. Relate the strength of the biceps and triceps muscles to their length: these muscles are strongest when acting from their ❒ shortest/❒ intermediate/❒ longest position.

   ☑ shortest
4. Now test the flexor and extensor strength of your partner's neck. In testing these movements, place one hand on the Pt's forehead or occiput and the other on the front or back of the Pt's chest to provide bracing and counterpressure.
5. To test the strength of the neck flexors, start with your partner's head strongly extended. Then you resist the neck flexion with your hands. Next test the neck flexor strength when your partner starts with the head tightly flexed, chin on chest. Then you try to extend it. The neck flexors are strongest with the neck ❒ flexed/❒ extended, in which position the flexor muscles are ❒ shortest/❒ longest.

   ☑ flexed; ☑ shortest
6. Next compare the maximum strength of the neck extensors with that of the neck flexors. One action, extension or flexion, by far exceeds the strength of the other. Determine which.
7. To see whether we have discovered a general length-strength law, test the quadriceps femoris and hamstring muscles with the knee fully flexed and then fully extended. With the knee fully extended, the quadriceps femoris muscle is ❒ strongest/❒ weakest and ❒ shortest/❒ longest.

   ☑ strongest; ☑ shortest (thus confirming the length-strength law)

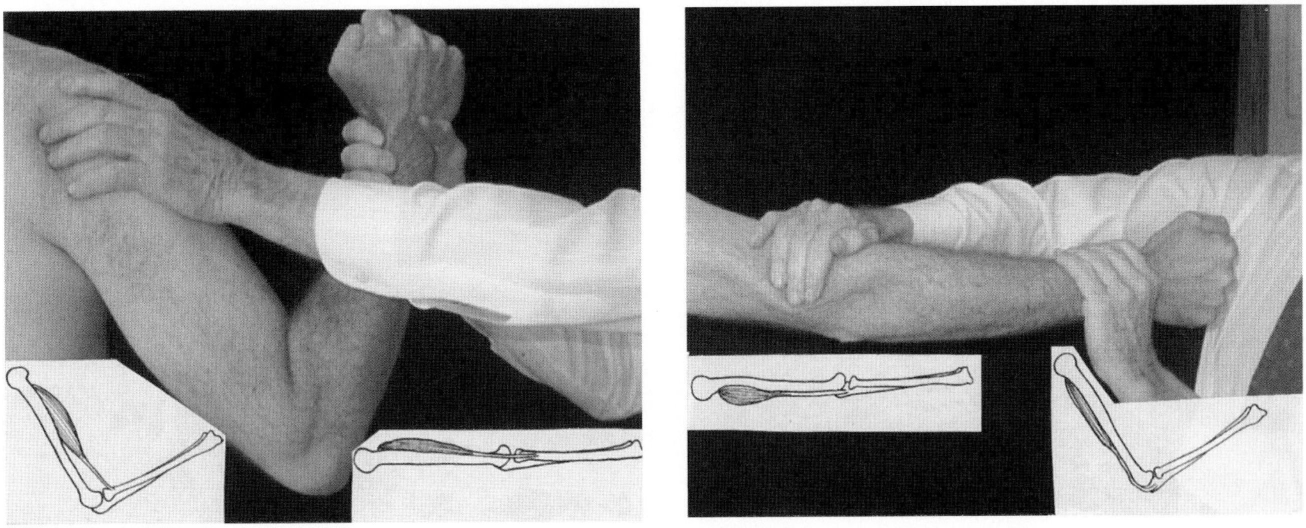

A B

FIGURE 7-1. Relation of length to strength of muscles. The examiner pulls or pushes on the patient's wrist with one hand while stabilizing the patient's elbow or shoulder with the other hand. (A) Position of examiner's hands to test biceps strength. The examiner pulls with the right hand, exactly matching strength with the patient's biceps. The left hand braces the patient. The left insert shows the biceps flexed, at its shortest and therefore strongest position. The right insert shows the biceps in its longest therefore weakest position. (B) Position to test triceps strength. The examiner presses just above the patient's elbow with the right hand and presses in the opposite direction with the left. The inserts show the length of the triceps with the arm extended or flexed. You must actually do these tests on another person with the arms extended and flexed to appreciate the great difference in strength in the two positions.

Note: The kinesiologist's length-strength law that the skeletal muscles are strongest when shortest differs from Starling's law of the heart that the output of cardiac contraction increases as the resting length of the cardiac muscle fibers increases.

☑ fully bent

With the elbow bent, the triceps is longest and therefore weakest.

8. In general, to test muscles of weak or modest strength more accurately, start with the Pt in a position of strength, e.g., neck flexed. But to test very strong muscles, place them at a disadvantage to bring them within your range of strength. Thus, to reduce the strength of the normally powerful triceps muscle to bring it within the testing range, test the Pt with the elbow ❒ fully bent/❒ fully extended. Explain.

____

____

9. With the elbow extended, the triceps is far too strong for the Ex to overcome. It can lose considerable strength and still offer strong resistance.

C. The antigravity muscle principle: how to remember the strongest sets of muscles

1. Muscles work in opposing, *agonist-antagonist* pairs (Basmajian, 1985). One of the opposing pairs is immensely stronger than the other, e.g., neck extension is far stronger than flexion. Without a general law to recall the strongest of opposing sets of muscles, you face the oppressive task of memorizing each set individually. If we look at a quadruped, or better, at a man in quadrupedal position, the solution leaps out at us (Fig. 7-2). The immensely powerful muscles all belong to the postural antigravity system of a quadruped.
2. Stand up and assume the postures shown in Figs. 7-2A and 7-2B. Of particular importance, assume the posture shown in Fig. 7-2B. Notice then how the triceps muscle locks the upper extremities against collapse from the pull of gravity and how

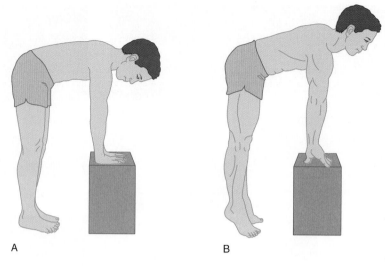

FIGURE 7-2. Man in quadruped posture. (A) Relaxed. (B) Rising on fingers and toes.

the quadriceps femoris similarly locks the lower extremities. The neck extensors erect the head. Buttocks and back extensors erect the trunk, holding it from collapse by gravity when the person stands or, equally important, when leaping or locomoting. When a person leaps or locomotes, the hands and feet lever *downward*. The muscles that support or lock the standing posture against collapse by the pull of gravity and that leap against gravity and propel or locomote constitute the **antigravity muscle system.** Invariably, the strength of these antigravity muscles greatly exceeds that of their antagonists.

3. Using the principle of the superior strength of the antigravity locking, locomoting, and leaping muscles, predict the strongest of these opposing movements: wrist ❑ extension/❑ flexion; trunk ❑ extension/❑ flexion; foot ❑ dorsiflexion/❑ plantar flexion; toe ❑ extension/❑ flexion.

☑ flexion; ☑ extension; ☑ plantar flexion; ☑ flexion

4. Confusion may arise when applying the antigravity theory to some actions such as arm abduction. When abducting, the arm acts against the pull of gravity, but the abductor muscles do not support the standing skeleton against collapse by gravity when the animal stands, leaps, or locomotes; hence, the arm elevators and abductors are not postural antigravity muscles and, quite to the contrary, their opponents are. Consider as examples of postural antigravity muscles the pectoral and latissimus dorsi muscles. The pectoral muscles prevent the forelimbs from straddling out when the animal stands. (Imagine the leverage acting to spread a giraffe's legs.) The latissimus dorsi muscles pull the forelimbs backward, thrusting the shoulders forward and upward, i.e., against gravity, when the quadruped leaps or locomotes. Consequently, the strength of these adductor and flexor muscles acting at the shoulder far exceeds their opponents, the abductor-extensor muscles. Applying this consideration to the hip, which would be stronger? ❑ hip abductors/❑ hip adductors. Explain.

____

____

☑ hip adductors

Read the last paragraph again if you can't explain the answer. As another example, consider the action of dorsiflexing and plantar flexing the foot when walking. The dorsiflexors lift the foot against the pull of gravity, but merely act to clear the toes and set the foot in place again so that the powerful plantar flexors can again act to support the posture, leap, or locomote.

5. The antigravity theory predicts not only the strongest muscles but also how much stronger they are. Your arm and hand strength cannot even begin to overcome the antigravity muscles when set in their strongest positions, with fingers, feet, and toes flexed (Fig. 12-13). But your arm and hand strength just about equals or barely overcomes the non-antigravity muscles when set in their strongest position, with the head flexed, jaw open, arms abducted, hips flexed, and wrists and feet dorsiflexed.
6. As a final bonus, the antigravity theory explains the very important posture called **decerebrate rigidity,** seen in the comatose Pt, when the Pt assumes the position dictated by contraction of the entire system of antigravity muscles (Fig. 12-13).

D. The engagement principle

This is the most commonly neglected technique. For all strength testing and the entire NE, the Ex must engage the Pt's competitive spirit to get maximum effort (Chapter 1, Section IX C 4; DeMyer, 1998). Challenge the Pt to a game: "I am trying to test how strong you are. Do your best on each test. *Don't let me win.*"

III. TECHNIQUE OF TESTING FOR MUSCULAR WEAKNESS

A. The rostrocaudal sequence

1. Test the muscles in the natural rostrocaudal order because it requires no memorization. After testing cranial nerve muscles, simply continue in the neck-shoulder-arm-forearm-hand-chest-abdomen-thigh-leg-foot-toe sequence and continually compare right and left sides.
2. Before testing strength, the Ex has an opportunity to test for range of motion of the joints, if the history suggests a need to do so. To test range of motion, ask the Pt to move the joint actively through its full range of motion, and then you attempt to passively manipulate the joint.

B. Testing for weakness of neck flexors and extensors

1. Neck extensors are far too strong for the Ex's arm and hand strength.
2. In what position does the Ex ask the Pt to place the head to bring the strength of the relatively weak neck flexors up into the best range to test? ____.

Flexion

C. Testing for weakness of shoulder girdle muscles

1. The *trapezius* was tested with the cranial nerves (CrNs).
2. Test shoulder and arm movements by having the Pt extend the arms forward, to the sides, and then over the head. Inspect from front and back. Have the Pt stand directly under an overhead light that will cast a shadow of the scapular border. Look for scapular movement, in particular winging of the dorsal border away from the rib cage. Have the Pt lean forward against a wall with the arms extended to exaggerate scapular winging.
3. After testing **free movement** of arm abduction and elevation, test the **strength** of these movements. Have your Pt (or partner) hold the arms straight out to the sides (abducted). Push down on the arms as the Pt resists. Where do you push? That depends. If you are a strong man and the Pt a woman, push down *proximally* at the elbows to *reduce* your leverage. If you are a woman and the Pt a man, push down *distally* on the forearms or wrists to *increase* your leverage. Select a point where your strength in pushing down about equals that of the standard person of the height, weight, age, and sex of your Pt. Here you must build your own catalog of experience. Work through Table 7-1.
4. Arm abduction is complex, requiring *supraspinatus* action to initiate the act, *deltoid* action to carry the arm to shoulder height, and *scapular* rotation to continue the elevation to the vertical position. The serratus anterior and trapezius muscles hold the scapula in place against the chest wall. Serratus anterior paralysis (long thoracic nerve) results in winging of the scapula away from the chest wall.
5. Test for latissimus dorsi strength by starting with the Pt's arms extended to the sides. The Ex applies upward pressure on the elbows. This is a very strong muscle, but it is easily felt and seen. Also, to test for the action of the muscle, the Ex may palpate it while the Pt makes a strong voluntary cough. This test is helpful in Pts with hysterical paralysis of the arm because the action is automatic.

TABLE 7-1 · Method of Testing Shoulder Girdle Strength

Action	Commands and maneuvers
Arm elevation	Request the patient to hold the arms straight out to the sides. Press down on both arms at a point where you expect your strength to approximate the patient's.
Arm adduction downward	With the arms extended to the sides, the patient resists your efforts to elevate them.
Arm adduction across the chest (pectoralis muscles)	With the arms extended straight in front, the patient crosses the wrists. You try to pull them apart.
Scapular adduction	With the hands on the hips, the patient forces the elbows backward as hard as possible. Standing behind the patient, the examiner tries to push them forward.
Scapular winging	Have the patient try a push-up or lean forward against a wall, supporting the body with outstretched arms.

D. Testing for weakness of upper arm muscles: flexion and extension of the elbow

1. **Elbow flexors:** The Pt tightly flexes the forearm. Brace one hand against the Pt's shoulder. With the other hand, grasp the Pt's wrist and attempt to straighten the Pt's forearm. This matches your biceps against the Pt's. When an average person competes with another average person of the same age and sex, the battle is a deadlock and, hence, ideal for testing (Fig. 7-1A).
2. **Elbow extensors:** If you give the matter no thought, you might try to test the triceps with the elbow locked in extension. But the triceps, an antigravity muscle, is tremendously strong, and with an average person against another average person, the locked-out elbow wins easily. Conversely, if the Pt's locked-arm yields, the Pt's triceps is significantly weak. For a subtler test, start with the Pt's elbow flexed, as in testing the elbow flexors, but this time grasp the wrist and oppose extension of the forearm by the Pt. This maneuver puts the triceps at a disadvantage, and average person against average person; the Ex will win, but barely. Because this test pits nearly equal strengths, it discloses slight loss of triceps power better than the arm-extended position.

E. Testing for weakness of forearm muscles: wrist flexion and extension

1. **Wrist flexors:** The Pt makes a fist and holds the wrist flexed against your efforts to extend it. By hooking your fingers around the Pt's fist and flexing your own wrist, you can pit your own wrist flexion against the Pt's. Brace the Pt's wrist with your other hand. Other forms of manual opposition will not overcome the wrist flexors, because they are very strong antigravity muscles. (Visualize a quadruped leaping [Fig. 7-2B].)
2. **Wrist extensors:** For support, rest the Pt's forearm flat on his thigh or a tabletop. The Pt then holds the wrist forcefully cocked-up (dorsiflexed) as you try to press it down with the butt of your palm on the Pt's knuckles. With the Pt's wrist in extension, the relatively weak wrist extensors just about match your arm and hand strength.

F. Testing for weakness of finger muscles

1. Carefully inspect and palpate the thenar and hypothenar eminences for size and asymmetry. Look for atrophy of interosseous muscles. Elderly people show obvious interosseous atrophy.
2. **Abduction-adduction of the fingers:** Test by carefully figuring out how to match your strength against the Pt's.

a. Start with the first dorsal interosseous muscle. Palpate it in your own hand as the mass of soft tissue alongside the second metacarpal bone, in the web between your thumb and index finger. The first dorsal interosseous muscle moves the index finger *away* from the middle finger and *toward* the thumb. Palpate your own muscle during that action.

b. To test a Pt's dorsal interosseous muscle, press the terminal phalanx of your *right* index finger alongside the resisting terminal phalanx of the Pt's *right* index finger, matching muscle to muscle, which is an ideal test (Fig. 7-3).

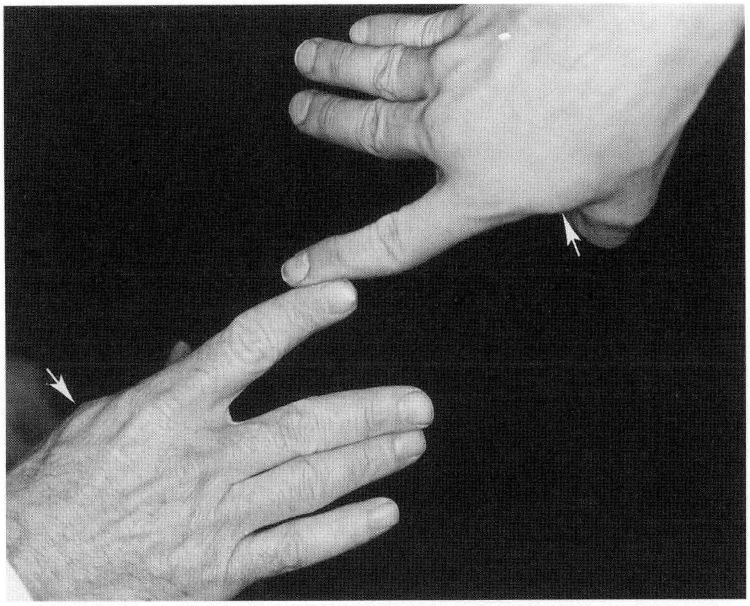

FIGURE 7-3. Method of matching the examiner's finger strength against the patient's. Notice the bulging first dorsal interosseous muscle in the examiner and the patient (arrows).

c. Work through the fingers, learning how to match your finger abductors and adductors against the Pt's.

3. **Finger extension:** The Pt holds out the hands with palms down and fingers hyperextended. Simply turn your hand over so that the dorsum of your fingernail presses against the dorsum of the Pt's. Then you can carefully match the extensor strength of each of your own fingers against the Pt's.

4. **Finger flexion:** Strength of the grip as a whole.

a. **Ask the Pt to squeeze your fingers:** Grasp the Pt's wrist with one hand to steady the arm and offer two fingers of your other hand for the Pt to grasp. To add an element of fun and competition to the test, particularly with a child, and to keep the Pt working at top strength, say, "Don't let my fingers get away," as you try to extract your fingers from the Pt's grasp.

b. **Try this experiment:** Grip a pencil as tightly as possible in your fist. Notice that your wrist automatically *dorsiflexes* slightly. Have your partner try to pull the pencil out of your grip when your hand is in the normal position it automatically assumes when you tighten your grip. Then hold your wrist *flexed* as strongly as possible and *dorsiflexed* as strongly as possible, and ask your partner to pull the pencil out of your grip in each instance. Finger flexion is strongest when the wrist is ❐ strongly flexed/❐ partly dorsiflexed/❐ completely dorsiflexed.

☑ partly dorsiflexed

c. **This experiment shows that partial dorsiflexion of the wrist allows the strongest grip:** Partial dorsiflexion is the **functional position of the hand,** the position to select when putting a cast on the forearm or wrist to treat a fracture or when splinting the wrist to maintain optimum hand position while the Pt recovers from paralysis. This so-called *functional position of the hand* is the position of complete shortening of the finger flexor muscles and therefore the position that allows them to exert the strongest grip. Further flexion of the wrist merely slackens the flexor tendons of the fingers without further shortening of the finger flexor muscles. Hence, this action of the hand does not contradict the law that the muscles are strongest from their shortest position. Now if you understand all of this, state into which position you would try to force an assailant's wrist to cause him to drop a knife? Explain.

____

____

Force the assailant's wrist into flexion. First, your hands have a chance to overpower the assailant's wrist extensors; second, the assailant's flexed wrist can no longer grip the knife strongly, and it may fall out of his hand.

G. Testing for abdominal muscle weakness

1. **Position:** With the Pt supine (face up), ask for a sit-up or for the Pt to elevate the legs or the head. At the same time, watch the umbilicus as the abdominal muscles contract.
2. **Try this experiment:** While lying supine, stick your index finger in your own umbilicus to palpate it during the foregoing actions. If the muscles of all four quadrants have equal strength, the umbilicus will remain centered. When the Pt attempts to raise the head or legs, what would happen to the position of the umbilicus if the lower abdominal muscles were weak and the upper muscles were intact? The umbilicus would migrate ❐ upward/❐ downward.

   ☑ upward (the intact muscles pull the umbilicus in their direction)

   a. In general, if some abdominal muscles are weak, the umbilicus will migrate ❐ toward/❐ away from the pull of the intact muscles during strong abdominal contraction.

   ☑ toward

   b. The umbilical migration test aids greatly in localizing the level of spinal cord lesions. The umbilicus corresponds to the X thoracic segment of the spinal cord (Fig. 2-10). Spinal cord transection at the T10 level paralyzes all muscles *caudal* to that level. Because of paralysis of the lower abdominal muscles, when a Pt with a T10-level cord lesion contracts the abdominal muscles, the umbilicus migrates ❐ upward/❐ downward (Beevor's sign).

   ☑ upward

H. Testing for weakness of the large back muscles

The average Pt's back is far too strong for the Ex to test by manual opposition. Two tests can be done:

1. With the Pt prone, ask the Pt to arch the back and rock on the stomach. Inspect and palpate the paraspinal muscles.
2. Have the Pt bend forward at the waist and straighten up. If you try to oppose the Pt's straightening up from a bent waist, you may cause a back sprain or herniation of an intervertebral disc.

I. Testing for weakness of the hip girdle

1. **Hip flexion:** With the patient sitting, ask the Pt to lift a knee off of the table surface and to hold the thigh in a flexed position. With the butt of your palm, try to push the knee back down. The flexors are relatively weak, non-antigravity muscles. Give them the advantage of a flexed position.
2. **Thigh abduction and adduction:** With the Pt sitting, have the Pt hold the legs *abducted* as you try to press them together with your hands on the lateral sides of the knees. Then have the Pt try to hold the legs *adducted* (squeezed together) as you place your hands on the medial sides of the knees to try to pull the knees apart. It is inconvenient for the Ex to try to test adductor strength when starting with the Pt's legs apart.

3. **Hip extension:** With the Pt prone, have the Pt lift the knee from the table surface and hold it up. Place your hand on the popliteal space and try to press the knee back down.

J. Testing for weakness of the thigh muscles

1. **Knee extensors**
   a. The deep knee bend has already tested the quadriceps, an immensely powerful antigravity muscle that ordinarily is too strong to test by manual opposition if it acts from the strongest position. To test the quadriceps, place it at a mechanical disadvantage, starting with the knee ❒ flexed/❒ intermediate/❒ straight.
   b. With the Pt prone, have the Pt try to touch the heel to the buttock to induce extreme flexion of the knee. Grasp the Pt's ankle and oppose extension. Compare the extensor strength of the two legs.
2. **Knee flexors (hamstrings):** The Pt holds the knee at an angle of 90 degrees, while you try to straighten it by grasping the Pt's ankle.

☑ flexed

K. Testing for weakness of ankle and toe movements

1. Have the Pt *dorsiflex*, *invert*, and *evert* the feet. Inspect, palpate the leg, and check for the strength of these movements by manual opposition.
2. **Plantar flexion** of the foot is ordinarily too strong to test by manual opposition. Because the Pt walked on the balls of the feet during the gait examination, you already know that the plantar flexors can lift the entire body weight of the Pt.
3. The Pt holds the toes *flexed* or *extended* as the Ex attempts to press them back to the neutral position. Which action of the big toe is strongest, ❒ extension/❒ flexion? Explain.

____

____

☑ flexion

Of course, flexion! Which action leaps or locomotes and which action merely lifts the foot into place for another leaping or locomoting action (Fig. 7-2)?

L. Screening tests for muscle weakness during the routine physical examination versus a complete examination

1. Testing for weakness of every muscle in every Pt would be a waste of time. For the screening NE, sample a few selected movements, as outlined in Section VI, step C of the Standard NE. Rehearse it.
2. Patients with neurologic symptoms and signs require a much more extensive examination. From the history and initial appraisal, the Ex selects the critical muscles for testing and the conditions under which to do the tests. For example, if the Pt complains of weakness after exertion, have the Pt climb stairs before testing. If the Pt's muscles "freeze up" when cold, put the arm in ice water and ask the Pt to make repetitive contractions. If the muscles cramp when the Pt writes, have the Pt write. Always reproduce any conditions that trigger symptoms.
3. The diagnosis of specific nerve injuries and entrapment neuropathies requires detailed testing of individual muscles and comparison with charts of segmental versus peripheral nerve innervation patterns (Table 2-1 and Figs. 2-10 and 2-11). Of the guides to muscle testing, the little pamphlet entitled *Aids to the Examination of the Peripheral Nervous System* fits easily in your bag (see also Jenkins, 2002; Sunderland, 1978). For entrapment neuropathies, see Dawson et al. (1998) and Kopell and Thompson (1987).

M. Recording the strength examination

1. Table 2-1 lists muscles or movements usually tested. The Ex may use a word scale, such as *paralysis, severe weakness, moderate weakness, minimal weakness,* and *normal* or a numerical scale from 0 to 5 (Table 7-2). Disease-specific gradings are also available (Armon and Ponraj, 1996; Mathieu et al., 2001).

TABLE 7-2 · **Numerical Scale to Record Muscle Strength (British Medical Research Council)**

Score	Description
5	Normal strength
4	Moves joint through full range against resistance greater than gravity but examiner can overcome the action (make a percentage estimate of strength to compensate for broad range of this number)
3	Moves part full range against gravity but not against any resistance
2	Moves part only when positioned to eliminate gravity
1	Only a flicker of contraction of muscle but cannot move joint
0	Complete paralysis

2. A hand-held myometer or dynamometer objectively quantifies strength (Lanska, 2000; Goonetilleke et al., 1994; Thijs et al., 1998; van der Ploeg et al., 1991; Wiles et al., 1990), but remember the principle of full engagement, which states that the Pt's effort is the limiting factor in accuracy.
3. Record in the Pt's chart the movements or muscles actually tested. If the Pt displays weakness on a later visit, the record will provide reliable documentation for comparison.

N. Review

Rehearse Section VI A, B, and C of the Standard NE. **Do you remember the steps? No? That's the reason to rehearse them now.**

BIBLIOGRAPHY · The Strength Examination

Armon C, Ponraj E. Comparing composite scores based on maximal voluntary isometric contraction and on semiquantitative motor testing in measuring limb strength with ALS. *Neurology* 1996;47:1586–1587.

Basmajian JV, De Luca CL. *Muscles Alive,* 5th ed. Baltimore, Williams & Wilkins, 1985.

Dawson DM, Hallett M, Millender LH. *Entrapment Neuropathies,* 3rd ed. Boston, Little, Brown and Company, 1998.

DeMyer W. Pointers and pitfalls in the neurologic examination. *Semin Neurol* 1998; 18:161–168.

Goonetilleke A, Madarres-Sadeghi H, Guiloff RJ. Accuracy, reproducibility, and variability of hand-held dynamometry in motor neuron disease. *J Neurol Neurosurg Psychiatry* 1994;57:326–332.

Guarantors of Brain. *Aids to the Examination of the Peripheral Nervous System,* 4th ed. Philadelphia, W.B. Saunders, 2000.

Jenkins DB. *Hollinshead's Functional Anatomy of the Limbs and Back,* 8th ed. Philadelphia, W.B. Saunders, 2002.

Lanska DJ. William Hammond, the dynamometer, and the dynamograph. *Arch Neurol* 2000;57:1649–1653.

Mathieu J, Boivin H, Meunier M, et al. Assessment of disease-specific muscular impairment rating scale in myotonic dystrophy. *Neurology* 2001;56:336–340.

Thijs RD, Notermans NC, Wokke JHJ, et al. Distribution of muscle weakness of central and peripheral origin. *J Neurol Neurosurg Psychiatry* 1998;65:794–796.

van der Ploeg RJO, Fidler V, Oosterhuis HJGH. Hand-held myometry: reference values. *J Neurol Neurosurg Psychiatry* 1991;54:244–247.

Wiles CM, Karni Y, Nicklin J. Laboratory testing of muscle function in the management of neuromuscular disease. *J Neurol Neurosurg Psychiatry* 1990;53:384–387.

IV. RESULTS OF DIRECT PERCUSSION OF MUSCLE

It will not surprise the *cognoscente* in physical diagnosis that percussion belongs in the sequence of inspection, palpation, and strength testing of muscle.

A. Self-demonstration of percussion irritability of muscle

1. Bare your biceps muscle and strike its belly a sharp blow with the point of your reflex hammer (tomahawk type). You will see a faint dimple or ripple at the percussion site. Strike a crisp blow and jerk the hammer out of the way because the ripple is very transient.
2. The contraction of muscle fibers in response to a direct blow demonstrates the intrinsic irritability of the muscle fibers themselves. It is not a reflex and not dependent on innervation (Brody and Rozear, 1970). In fact, percussion irritability remains, and may even increase, after denervation of the muscle, because the denervated muscle fibers become hyperirritable (Cannon's law of hypersensitivity of denervated structures, Walter Cannon, 1871–1945).

B. Percussion myoedema

Sometimes a tiny hump, called **myoedema,** appears at the percussion site. The sarcoplasmic reticulum is slow in the reuptake of calcium. Myoedema occurs in some normal people and often in debilitation or dysmetabolic states such as uremia and myxedema.

C. Percussion myotonia

Place your hand, palm up, on the table. Crisply percuss your thenar eminence with the point of your percussion hammer. Normally the thumb bounces up a little due to percussion irritability, but if your thumb slowly rises up from your palm and holds up, you have got problems. You have **percussion myotonia.**

D. Muscle contraction myotonia

1. Ask the Pt to make a tight fist, hold it for 10 seconds, and flip the fingers open as quickly as possible on command. The myotonic Pt cannot flip the fingers open rapidly, and the wrist involuntarily flexes because of sustained "after contraction" or delayed relaxation of the flexors.
2. Ask the Pt to close the eyelids as tightly as possible for 5 seconds. When the Pt attempts to open the eyelids, the myotonia keeps them closed (Dyken, 1966).
3. Myotonia occurs in myopathies such as myotonia dystrophica (Harper, 2001), myotonia congenita, paramyotonia congenita, certain channelopathies, and in some types of periodic muscular paralysis associated with a disturbance in potassium metabolism (Dubowitz, 1995).

E. Summary of muscle responses to percussion

1. List the three muscular responses to direct percussion: percussion ________________, percussion ________________, and percussion ________________.

irritability; myoedema; myotonia

2. Normal persons show percussion ________________ of their muscles.

irritability

3. Some normal persons show percussion ________________.

myoedema

4. No normal persons show percussion ________________. It indicates a primary disease of the muscle, hence, a myopathy.

myotonia

5. Apart from the myotonic myopathies, percussion of most myopathic muscles, as in Duchenne's muscular dystrophy, after disease has impaired the contractile properties of muscle, demonstrates little or no contraction. Percussion irritability of muscle is reduced or absent in those myopathies that do not have myotonia, but increases in muscle after denervation.

BIBLIOGRAPHY · Muscle Diseases (Myopathies)

Brody JA, Rozear MP. Contraction response to muscle percussion: physiology and clinical significance. *Arch Neurol* 1970;23:259–265.

Dubowitz V. *Muscle Disorders in Childhood*, 2nd ed. London, W.B. Saunders, 1995.

Dyken P. Extraocular myotonia in families with dystrophia myotonica. *Neurology* 1966;16:738–740.

Harper PS. *Myotonic Dystrophy,* 3rd ed. Philadelphia, W.B. Saunders, 2001.

Jones HR, DeVivo DC, Darras BT. *Neuromuscular Disorders of Infancy, Childhood, and Adolescence. A Clinicians Approach.* Philadelphia: Butterworth-Heinemann, 2002.

Karpati G, Hilton-Jones D, Griggs RC. *Disorders of Voluntary Muscle.* New York, Cambridge University Press, 2001.

Katirji B, Kaminski HJ, Preston DC, et al, eds. *Neuromuscular Disorders in Clinical Practice.* Boston, Butterworth-Heinemann, 2002.

Koppel HP, Thompson WAL, *Peripheral Entrapment Neuropathies.* Baltimore, Williams & Wilkins, 1987.

Sunderland S, *Nerves and Nerve Injuries.* 2nd ed. London, Churchill Livingston, 1978.

V. EXAMINATION OF MUSCLE STRETCH REFLEXES

A. Physiology of the muscle stretch reflexes

1. Evolution has perfected muscle fibers as contractile engines. Whatever the stimulus—a nerve impulse, chemical agent, electricity, or mechanical deformation, such as by percussion—the fiber responds by contracting.
2. Stretch of the entire muscle causes reflex contraction of the entire muscle, as contrasted to percussion irritability of individual muscle fibers. The stretch-sensitive receptors for the muscle stretch reflexes (MSRs) are the **muscle spindles,** which consist of small bags of small muscle fibers (Lance and McLeod, 1981).

Mnemonic: Remember muscle spindles as "muscles within a muscle" (Fig. 7-4).

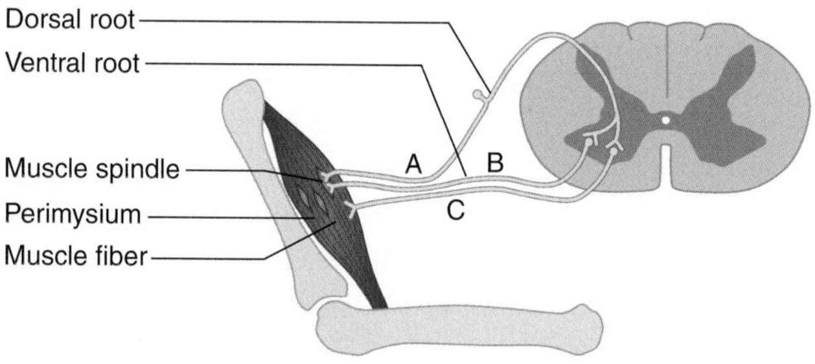

FIGURE 7-4. Muscle spindle innervation. The muscle spindles are tiny bags of specialized muscle fibers, located in the equatorial plane of the muscle. They have afferent (A) and efferent (B) axons. The regular muscle fibers receive only efferent axons (C).

3. **Effects of stretch on the muscle spindles**
   a. The muscle fibers of the spindle originate and insert into the perimysial connective tissue, which ultimately is continuous with the tendons. If the joint shown in Fig. 7-4 *extends,* the tendon pulls on the perimysium and stretches the muscle spindles. Flexion of the joint causes relaxation of the muscle spindles.
   b. To reset themselves to remain sensitive to stretch throughout the entire range of muscle length, the muscle spindles must readjust their length whenever the muscle length changes.
   c. Flexion of a part momentarily relaxes the spindle tension. The muscle fibers of the spindles respond by contracting slightly to maintain their original tension.
   d. During extension of the part, the spindles adjust to maintain their original tension by lengthening slightly.
4. **Innervation of the muscle spindles**
   a. Each muscle spindle has its own afferent and efferent axons that maintain its constant tension; see afferent axon A and efferent axon B in Fig. 7-4. The

regular muscle fibers, outside the spindle, have only efferent axons, depicted by axon C.

b. In response to stretch, the spindles send an afferent volley into the neuraxis by axon A. In response to slow stretch, the spindles signal intermittently and asynchronously. The spindles quickly adapt to the new length and resume a baseline level of activity.

c. If the stretch is rapid, essentially instantaneous, all spindles of the muscle, numbering hundreds, synchronously send a strong afferent volley into the central nervous system (CNS). The strong afferent volley stimulates the lower motor neurons (LMNs) of the regular muscle fibers. The resultant discharge of the LMNs causes a clinically evident muscular contraction, the **muscle stretch reflex.** Axon C in Fig. 7-4 is the efferent axon.

d. The event that initiates the MSR is stretch of the ❒ muscle spindles/❒ regular muscle fibers, but the resultant twitch of the entire muscle is the result of contraction of the ❒ muscles spindles/❒ regular muscle fibers.

☑ muscle spindles; ☑ regular muscle fibers

5. When the MSR acts, the muscular contraction pulls the two ends of the muscles closer together. The tension on the muscle spindles is momentarily ❒ reduced/❒ increased. Hence, the spindles cease firing abruptly, and the MSR ends abruptly.

☑ reduced

6. When the muscle comes to rest at a new length, what adjustment takes place in the tension of the muscle spindles?

____

They reset their tension to their baseline level.

7. Explain why only a quick stretch elicits an MSR.

____

____

All spindles must fire rapidly and synchronously to discharge the LMNs. If the stretch is too slow, the spindles fire slowly and asynchronously, and they adapt to the new resting length without sending a sufficiently strong volley to discharge the LMNs.

8. Muscle fibers contract in response to stimulation of the muscle membrane by direct percussion. This phenomenon is called _______________ irritability of the muscle.

percussion

9. In contrast to percussion irritability, reflex irritability of muscle depends on a strong volley of afferent impulses initiated by the stretch of the specialized stretch receptors called _______________________.

muscle spindles

10. After interruption of all efferent axons to a muscle, what would be lost, percussion irritability or the MSRs? Explain.

____

____.

Denervation of a muscle abolishes the MSRs, which depend on the integrity of the reflex arc (Fig. 7-4). Percussion irritability depends on the intrinsic property of muscle fibers. It remains or increases after denervation (Cannon's law of hypersensitivity of denervated end organs).

11. To elicit an MSR and avoid percussion irritability, the Ex stretches the muscles by percussing tendons, not the muscles directly. Direct percussion of the muscle not only causes direct contraction of the muscle fibers but also stretches spindles. The muscle twitches in either case, but clinically the Ex cannot distinguish the cause. The tap on the tendon can elicit contraction only by stretching the muscle spindles.

BIBLIOGRAPHY · Physiology of Muscle Stretch Reflexes

Lance JW, McLeod JG. *A Physiological Approach to Clinical Neurology,* 3rd ed. London, Butterworth, 1981.

Swash M, Kennard C. *Scientific Basis of Clinical Neurology.* Edinburgh, Churchill-Livingstone, 1985.

B. Technique for eliciting muscle stretch reflexes

1. **Holding the percussion hammer and delivering the blow**

a. A percussion hammer permits you to strike a rapid blow, producing the instantaneous stretch of the muscle spindles necessary to elicit an MSR. To deliver a crisp stimulus, you must learn how to swing a hammer, not peck with it. The same technique applies whether you use the Taylor tomahawk hammer pictured in this text or the long Tromner or Babinski hammer (Lanska, 1999). I prefer the tomahawk-type hammer because hammers with longer handles cannot be used readily on tiny babies in bassinets or threaded easily between the wiring and tubing of a Pt in intensive care. The hammer handle should have convex sides to accommodate the tip of the thumb and forefinger, thus allowing the Ex to hold it loosely to deliver a brisk blow. Hammers with round or octagonal handles, like those given away free by drug companies, will fly out of your hand unless you grip them too tightly, which means you will have to peck rather than percuss.

b. Hammer pecking is the wrong way to elicit MSRs. Consider first the wrong technique, hammer pecking. The novice grips the hammer tightly with all of the fingers and pecks at the target without using wrist action. Recall how a baby holds a rattle tightly in its fist and bangs or pecks, using all arm action and no wrist action. Grip the handle of your reflex hammer tightly and peck the table-top in this incorrect manner. (Go ahead, do it. If you know what's wrong, you will appreciate what's right. Pecking is the most common error students make.)

c. Hammer swinging is the right way to elicit MSRs. Dangle the hammer handle loosely between the thumb and forefinger, allowing it to swing like a pendulum. Think of the hammer handle as a bird: hold it too tightly and you crush it to death; hold it too loosely and it flies away. Figure 7-5 shows how a loose

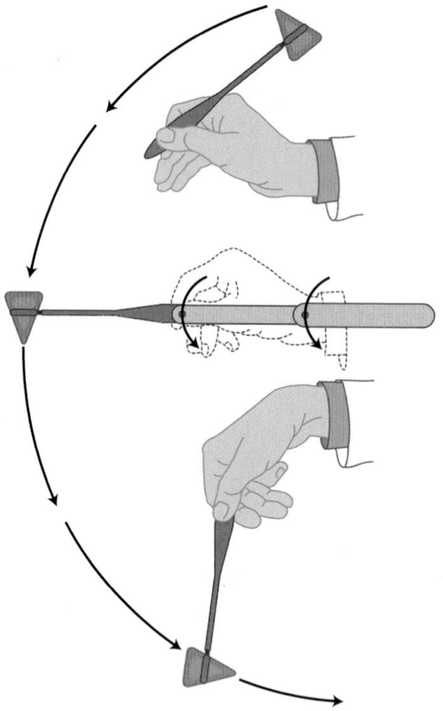

FIGURE 7-5. Technique for striking a crisp blow with a reflex hammer. Notice the loose, double pivot action at the wrist and fingers.

wrist and loose finger grip impart the maximal terminal velocity to the hammer head by literally throwing it without actually releasing it.

i. Simultaneous extension of the elbow added to the wrist swing adds further velocity to the tip of the hammer, thus delivering the crisp blow that instantaneously and simultaneously stretches all spindles to successfully elicit the MSR.

ii. Practice by holding your wrist a foot above a hard tabletop. Starting with the handle of the hammer lying back across the web between your thumb and forefinger (Fig. 7-5), whiplash the hammer head against the tabletop. **If the velocity of the hammer head is great enough and the wrist and grip loose enough, the hammer head bounces all the way back up and falls backward across the crevice between your thumb and forefinger, thus returning to the starting position shown in Fig. 7-5**. Practice until you can get this limp-wrist, whiplash feeling of literally throwing or swinging the hammer tip, but without actually releasing the handle. As a loose-wrist hammer swinger, you will proudly elicit MSRs when your tight-fisted colleagues, with their incorrect hammer-pecking style, fail.

2. **Eliciting the MSRs in the NE**
   a. Have the Pt sit or recline. The Pt places the part to be tested at rest, with the muscles relaxed. Usually the best position is intermediate between full extension and full flexion. The response of the muscle and the mechanics of the tap with the hammer will depend on the joint angle (Lin et al., 1997). About 90 degrees for the elbow, knee, and ankle joints is a standard angle.
   b. Work through Figs. 7-6 to 7-18, testing the reflexes on yourself where possible and on a partner. Do the reflexes in pairs, directly comparing right and left sides.

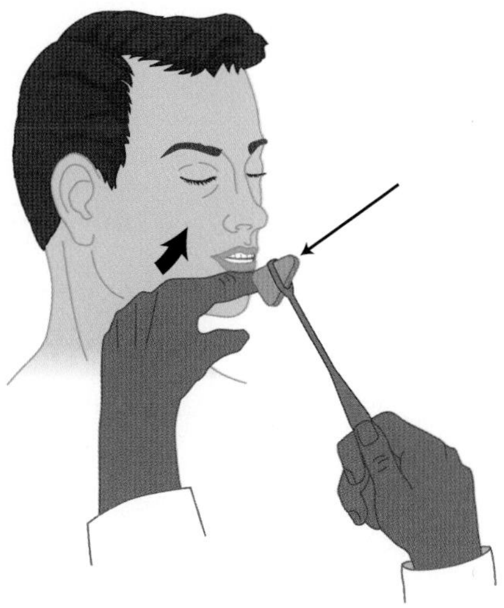

FIGURE 7-6. Jaw reflex. With the patient's jaw sagging loosely open, the examiner rests a finger across the tip and strikes it a crisp blow. In Figs. 7-6 to 7-18, the thin arrow shows the direction of the percussion hammer blow, and the thick arrow shows the response.

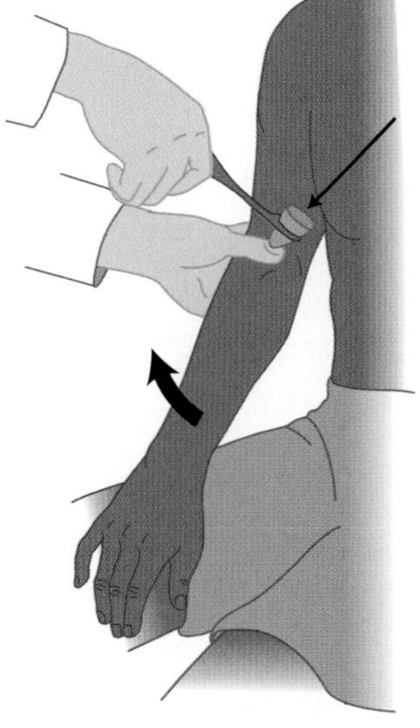

FIGURE 7-7. Biceps reflex. The examiner's thumb places slight tension on the patient's biceps tendon and the bicipital aponeurosis. The examiner strikes his thumbnail a crisp blow.

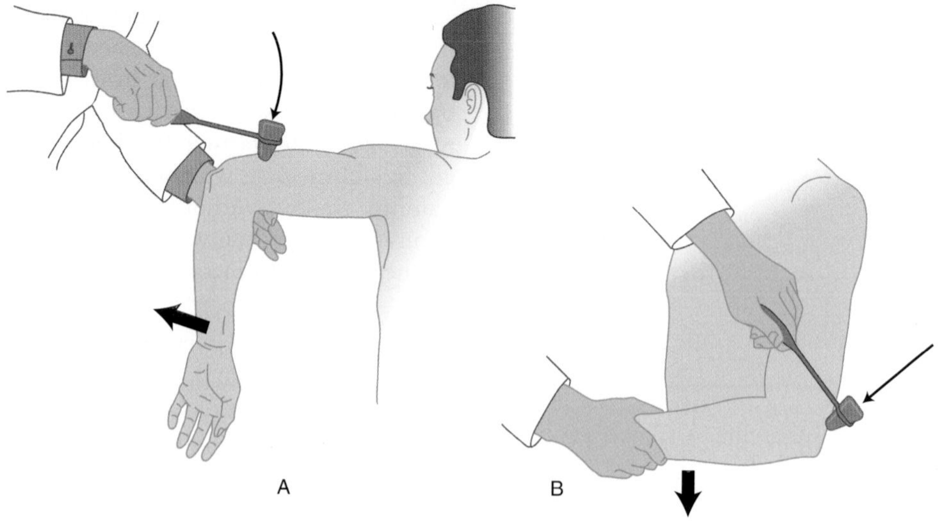

FIGURE 7-8. Triceps reflex. (A) Dangle the patient's forearm over your hand and strike the triceps tendon. (B) Cradle the patient's forearm in your hand and strike the triceps tendon.

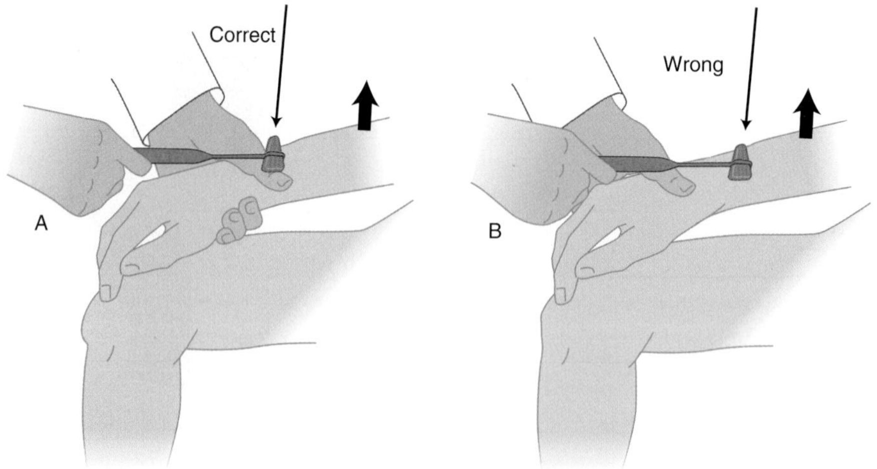

FIGURE 7-9. Brachioradialis reflex. Cradle the patient's forearm in one hand, placing the thumb on top of the radius. (A) The hammer strikes the examiner's thumbnail rather than the patient's radius. (B) Don't whack away on the patient's unprotected bone. The examiner may cradle both forearms side by side for accurate comparison of the responses of the two arms.

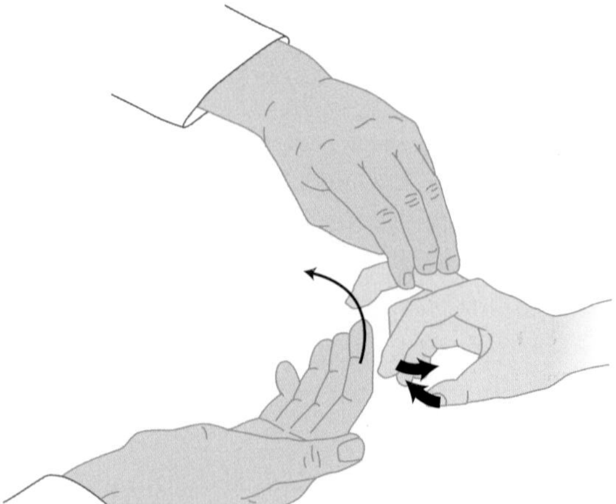

FIGURE 7-10. Finger flexion reflex (Tromner's method). The examiner supports the patient's completely relaxed hand and briskly flips the patient's distal phalanx upward, as though to flip a handful of water high into the air. The patient's fingers and thumb flex in response to the stretch of the finger flexor muscles.

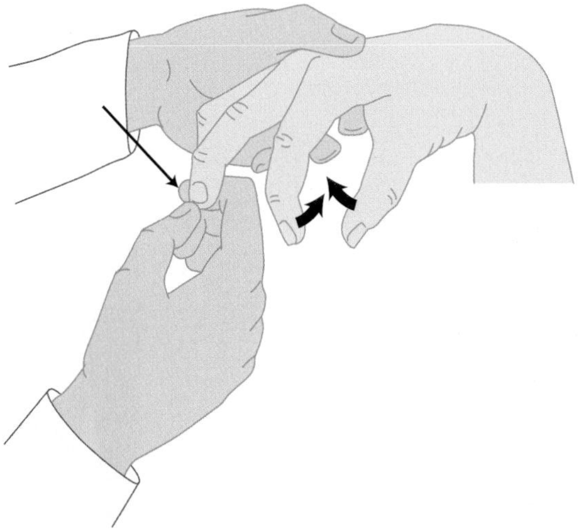

FIGURE 7-11. Finger flexion reflex (Hoffman's method). The examiner depresses the distal phalanx and allows it to flip up. The extension of the phalanx stretches the flexor muscles, causing the fingers and thumb to flex. This method is effective only with very brisk muscle stretch reflexes.

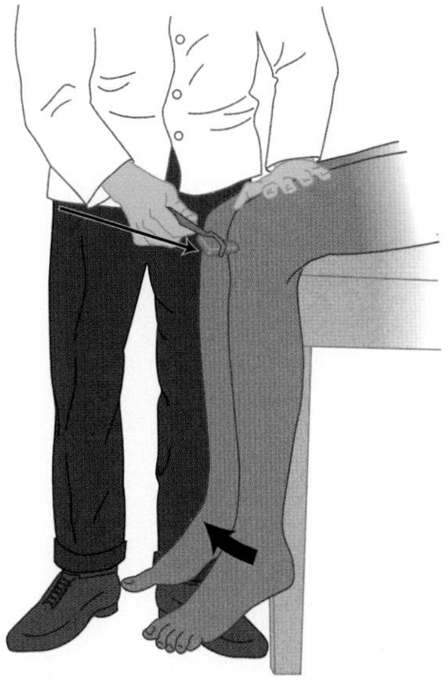

FIGURE 7-12. Quadriceps femoris reflex, with the patient sitting. The examiner strikes the patellar tendon a crisp blow. By placing a hand on the patient's knee, the examiner feels and sees the magnitude of the response.

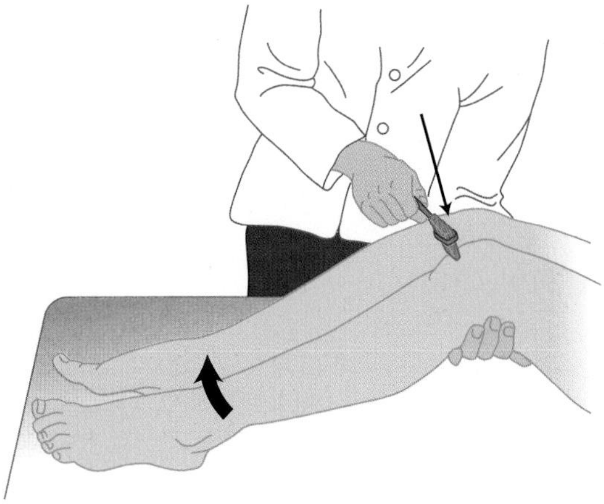

FIGURE 7-13. Quadriceps femoris reflex, with the patient supine. The examiner bends the patient's legs to place slight tension on the patellar tendon. The blow then will deform the tendon and transmit a stretch to the muscle.

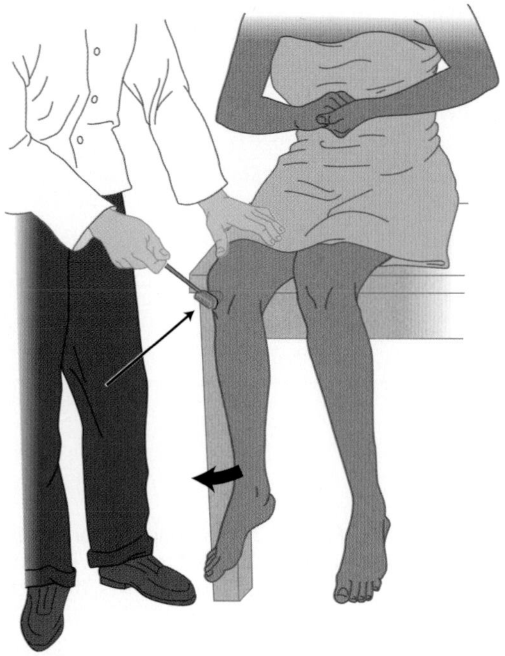

FIGURE 7-14. Pull method (of Jendrassik) for reinforcing the quadriceps reflex. The patient locks the hands and pulls apart hard while the examiner strikes the tendon.

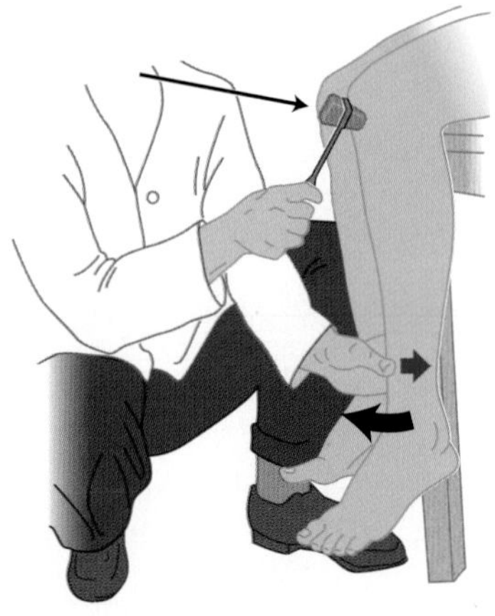

FIGURE 7-15. Counterpressure method for the quadriceps reflex. The examiner applies slight thumb pressure (small arrow) against the patient's tibia. The patient counteracts the thumb pressure by slight tension in the quadriceps femoris muscle. Then the examiner strikes the quadriceps tendon.

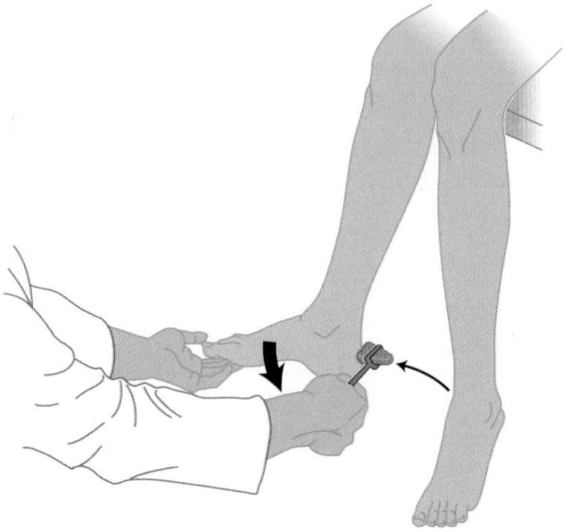

FIGURE 7-16. Triceps surae reflex, with the patient sitting. The patient completely relaxes the leg. The examiner dorsiflexes the foot to place slight tension on the triceps surae muscle. Try reinforcement if no reflex occurs.

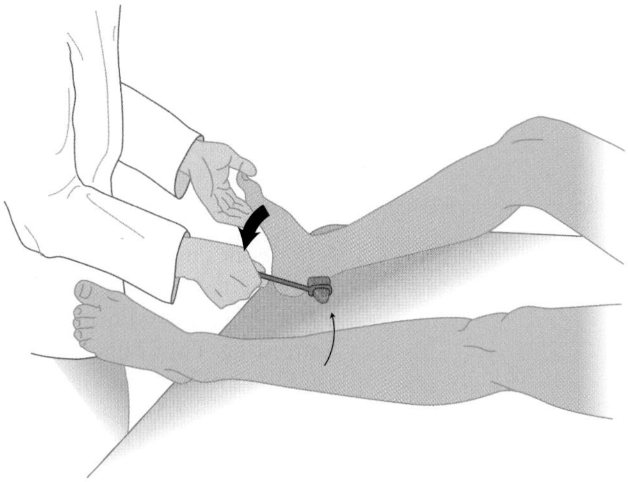

FIGURE 7-17. Triceps surae reflex, with the patient supine. With the patient's knee bent and relaxed, the examiner dorsiflexes the patient's foot to place slight tension on the triceps surae muscle. Try reinforcement if no reflex occurs.

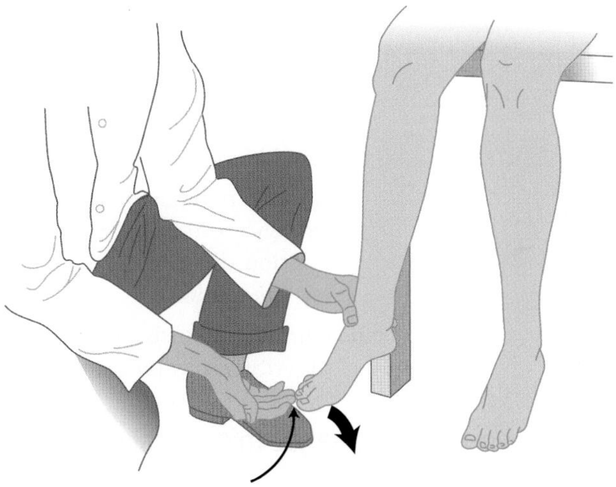

FIGURE 7-18. Toe flexion reflex (Rossolimo's sign), a muscle stretch reflex. The maneuver is identical with the finger flexion method shown in Fig. 7-9. Tapping the ball of the foot also elicits toe flexion.

c. In testing the knee jerks (quadriceps reflex), have the Pt sit with the legs dangling over the edge of a table. The Ex can then observe the degree of pendulousness, which usually amounts to three after-swings before the leg stops swinging. Normally the foot swings back and forth in an exact straight line. Spasticity diminishes the amplitude and number of after-swings (Fowler et al., 2000) and causes the foot to swing in irregular, rotatory, or sidewise arcs (Wartenberg, 1953).

3. In hypothyroidism, the quadriceps reflex has a "hung-up" appearance when tested with the Pt's legs dangling over table edge. At the end of its extension, the leg appears to pause briefly before dropping into the flexed position. Hung-up reflexes can also be seen in hypothermia, diabetes mellitus, treatment with beta-blockers and complete heart block. Chorea may results in apparently "hung-up" reflexes.
4. The latencies of the MSRs can be recorded by electromyography (EMG) and used in the differential diagnosis of demyelinating and axonal polyneuropathies (van Dijk et al., 1999).

C. What to do if your first attempts to elicit a muscle stretch reflex fail

1. **Strike a crisper blow:** Make sure you have *swung* the hammer, not pecked with it.
2. **Change the mechanical tension on the muscle:** Flex or extend the joint somewhat to alter the tension on the tendon. Compress the tendon slightly more, or slightly less, with your thumb (Fig. 7-7).
3. **Try reinforcement**
   a. **Jendrassik's maneuver for reinforcing an MSR:** Slight innervation of the muscle being tested increases the excitability of the LMNs for the MSR. For this purpose, have the Pt make a strong voluntary contraction of a muscle you are not testing. Thus failing to get a quadriceps femoris reflex after several trials, ask the Pt to lock the fingers together and pull hard as you tap the quadriceps tendon (Fig. 7-14). In this, the **Jendrassik maneuver,** the voluntary upper motor neuron (UMN) innervation of the arm muscles "overflows" to increase the excitability of the LMN pool of the lower extremities (Gasser and Diamantopolous, 1964; Hagbarth et al., 1975; Lance and McLeod, 1981; Stam et al., 1989; Wartenberg, 1945).
   b. **The counterpressure method of reinforcement:** If Jendrassik's maneuver fails, ask the Pt to tense very slightly the muscle being tested. Ask the Pt to just counterbalance the slight pressure you apply against the action of the muscle, as shown in Fig. 7-15. Too much tension in the muscle keeps the hammer from stretching the muscle spindles.
4. **Absence of MSRs:** If all maneuvers fail, conclude that the MSRs are absent, which usually indicates a pathologic condition, with some exceptions:
   a. In infants or girls, the lack of prominent tendons may make it difficult to elicit some MSRs, such as the biceps.
   b. Lack of patellar development in infants makes it mechanically difficult to stretch the tendon of the quadriceps femoris muscle by tapping its tendon. Position the infant's leg nearly straight, with the infant recumbent, and then tap the tendon.
   c. During diaschisis or neural shock, such as after acute spinal cord transection, the MSRs may be inactive.

D. Analyze this clinical problem in eliciting muscle stretch reflexes

1. You wish to elicit the biceps reflex of a 38-year-old conscious woman who is seated. Her arm should be positioned ______________________________.

partly bent across her thigh (Fig. 7-7)

2. If you have struck a crisp blow but noted no MSR, list the maneuvers you must try before concluding that the Pt has no biceps MSR.
____
____

Change the thumb pressure on the tendon. Reposition the elbow at a slightly different angle. Ask her to "tense" her leg muscles (extend her legs) for reinforcement. (The counterpressure method of reinforcement is inconvenient for arm reflexes.)

3. In the same Pt, you could not elicit the quadriceps and triceps surae MSRs when the Pt was sitting. What maneuvers do you try before concluding she has no quadriceps MSR?
____
____

Above all, strike the tendon a crisp blow. Next, request the Pt to lock her hands and pull as you strike the quadriceps tendon; then ask the Pt to counterbalance the slight pressure you apply against the tibia. These are examples of the **pull** method (Jendrassik's maneuver) and **counterpressure** methods of reinforcement.

4. For the triceps surae MSR, use Jendrassik's maneuver and then the counterpressure maneuver by having the Pt slightly plantar flex the foot as you press up on the sole with your finger and tap the Achilles tendon with the other hand. If these maneuvers fail to elicit quadriceps or triceps surae MSRs, place the Pt supine and try different positions of flexion of the legs or have the Pt kneel on a chair.

E. Nomenclature for the muscle stretch reflexes

1. Name the MSRs according to the muscles that respond or to the part that moves, e.g., the quadriceps MSR or the knee jerk (Fig. 7-12), or the triceps surae MSR, or ankle jerk (Fig. 7-16).

2. The fact that tendon percussion elicited the MSR led to the archaic, misleading term of "deep tendon reflexes" for the MSRs. This name implied that the tendons contain the receptor. In fact, the tendon receptors inhibit the MSR. Robert Whytt in 1763 had recognized that stretch was the adequate stimulus for muscle contraction (Pearce, 1997). In 1885, Sir William Gowers (1845–1915) stated:

> It seems, therefore, most desirable to discard the term "tendon reflex" altogether. The phenomena are, according to the explanation above given, dependent on a "muscle reflex" irritability, which has nothing to do with the "tendon-muscular phenomena," but the intervention of tendons is not necessary for their production; the one condition which all have in common is that passive tension is essential for their occurrence, and they may more conveniently be termed **myotatic contractions** [*myo* = muscle; *teinein* to stretch]. The irritability, on which they depend, is due to and demonstrative of a muscle reflex action which depends on the spinal cord.

3. Gowers synthesized a complex body of knowledge into a single word, *myotatic,* but his plea for rational, informative terminology has fallen unheeded. Each class of medical students learns about the "deep tendon reflexes" and almost universally fails to understand the spindle mechanism and the adequate stimulus required to elicit the MSRs.

F. Scaling and recording muscle stretch reflexes by using a stick figure

1. Grade the MSRs on a scale of 1 to 4. (Table 7-3) Some Exs require clonus for a score of 4 (Bradley, 1994) but not others (Hallett, 1993; Litvan et al., 1996). Some Exs prefer a verbal description rather than numbers (Manschot et al., 1998).

TABLE 7-3 · Grading of Muscle Stretch Reflexes

0	Areflexia
1	Hyporeflexia
2	Normal
3	Hyperreflexia
4	Clonus present

2. Because of the wide range in normal persons, the absolute value assigned to the MSR is less important than asymmetry, or a discrepancy between one part of the body and another. A stick figure displays the MSRs and, as shown later, other reflexes for interpretation at a glançe. Notice in Fig. 7-19A, which shows a normal subject, that the finger and toe flexion MSRs (Figs. 7-10, 7-11, and 7-18) may not be obtainable.

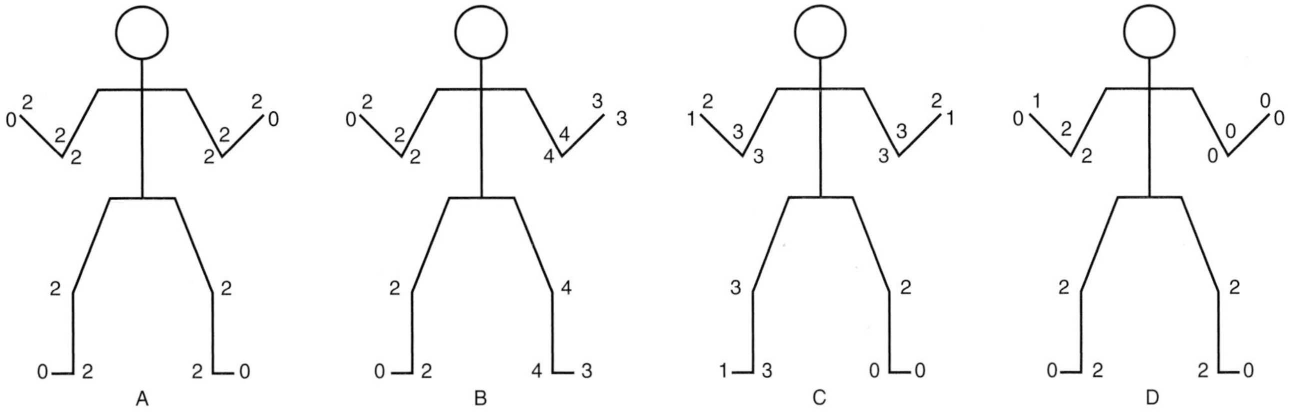

FIGURE 7-19. Stick figure method of recording muscle stretch reflexes.

Hyperreflexia on the left.

Quadriceps hyporeflexia, triceps surae, and toe areflexia on the left.

Areflexia of the left arm.

a. Describe the reflex pattern shown in Fig. 7-19B. ____________________
b. Describe the reflex pattern shown in Fig. 7-19C.
____
_________________________________.
c. Describe the reflex pattern shown in Fig. 7-19D.
____

3. Quantification of the MSRs by use of a mechanical hammer linked to EMG recording may refine the grading and interpretation of subtle reflex differences (Cozens et al., 2000; van Dijk et al., 1999).

BIBLIOGRAPHY · Muscle Stretch Reflexes

Bradley WG. Myotatic reflex scale. *Neurology* 1994;44:1984.

Cozens JA, Miller S, Chambers IR, et al. Monitoring of head injury by myotatic reflex evaluation. *J Neurol Neurosurg Psychiatry* 2000;68:581–588.

Fowler EG, Nwigwe AI, Ho TW. Sensitivity of the pendulum test for assessing spasticity in persons with cerebral palsy. *Dev Med Child Neurol* 2000;42:182–189.

Gasser M, Diamantopoulos E. The Jendrassik maneuver. I. The pattern of reinforcement of monosynaptic reflexes in normal subjects and patients with spasticity or rigidity. *Neurology* 1964;14:555–560.

Gowers W. *Diagnosis of Diseases of the Brain and of the Spinal Cord.* New York, William Wood, 1885.

Hagbarth KE, Wallin G, Burke D, Lofstedt L. Effects of the Jendrassik maneuver on muscle spindle activity in man. *J Neurol Neurosurg Psychiatry* 1975;38:1143–1153.

Hallett M. Myotatic reflex scale. *Neurology* 1993;43:2723.

Lance JW, McLeod JG. *A Physiological Approach to Clinical Neurology,* 3rd ed. London, Butterworth, 1981.

Larner AJ. Normalisation of slow-relaxing tendon reflexes (Woltman's sign) after cardiac pacing for complete heart block. Br J of Clinical Practice 1995; 49: 331–332.

Lanska DJ. The Babinski reflex hammer. *Neurology* 1999;53:655.

Lanska DJ, Lanska MJ. John Madison Taylor (1855–1931) and the first reflex hammer. *J Child Neurol* 1990;5:38–39.

Lin JP, Brown JK, Walsh EG. Soleus muscle length, stretch reflex excitability, and the contractile properties of muscles in children and adults: a study of the functional joint angle. *Dev Med Child Neurol* 1997;39:469–480.

Litvan I, Mangone CA, Werden W, et al. Reliability of the NINDS myotatic reflex scale. *Neurology* 1996;47:969–972.

Manschot S, van Passel L, Buskens E, et al. Mayo and NINDS scales for assessment of tendon reflexes: between observer agreement and implications for communication. *J Neurol Neurosurg Psychiatry* 1998;64:253–255.

Pearce JMS. Robert Whytt and the stretch reflex. *J Neurol Neurosurg Psychiatry* 1997; 62:484.

Sadjapour K. Loss of ankle reflex. *Arch Neurol* 1983:40:64.

Stam J, Speelman HD, van Crevel H. Tendon reflex asymmetry by voluntary mental effort in healthy subjects. *Arch Neurol* 1989;46:70–73.

van Dijk GW, Wokke JHJ, Notermans NC, et al. Diagnostic value of myotatic reflexes in axonal and demyelinating polyneuropathy. *Neurology* 1999;53:1573–1576.

Wartenberg R. *Diagnostic Tests in Neurology.* Chicago, Year Book Medical Publishers, 1953.

Wartenberg R. *The Examination of Reflexes*. Chicago, Year Book Medical Publishers, 1945.

VI. CLINICAL AND ELECTROMYOGRAPHIC SIGNS ACCOMPANYING AREFLEXIA AND HYPOREFLEXIA AFTER INTERRUPTION OF THE REFLEX ARC

A. Areflexia and the reflex arc

1. **Areflexia** is pathologic, except in toe and finger MSRs and in some particular muscles in infants and females who lack prominent tendons. Some persons with

generalized hyporeflexia (or hyperreflexia) merely fall at one end of the normal range. These persons will have muscles of normal size and strength, and sensation will be normal. Ballet dancers and women who wear very high-heeled shoes may lose their quadriceps and triceps surae stretch reflexes (Sadjapour, 1983). In deciphering the cause of areflexia or hyporeflexia, you must think through the afferent and efferent limbs of the reflex arc (Fig. 7-4).

2. To think through a reflex arc, start with the stimulus and the receptor. The adequate stimulus is sudden stretch of the muscle. If you get no response, then ask this question: Was the stimulus adequate? Outline the clinical maneuvers to elicit a reflex when your first attempt fails.

   ____

   ____

Deliver a crisper blow, alter tendon tension by finger pressure or repositioning the part, and try reinforcement.

3. The two methods of reinforcement are:
   a. To have the Pt contract ❒ strongly/❒ weakly a set of muscles *not* being tested (method of Jendrassik).
   b. To have the patient contract ❒ strongly/❒ weakly the muscle being tested (counterpressure method).

☑ strongly

☑ weakly

4. Having applied the proper stimulus for the MSR, the next step in thinking through the reflex arc is to consider the integrity of the muscle spindles and afferent limb. We cannot directly check the integrity of the muscle spindle clinically, but we can test the afferent limb as a whole.
   a. Interruption of the nerve or dorsal root conveying spindle afferents would also interrupt other sensory afferents. Hence, areflexia from interruption of the afferent arc causes loss of sensation.
   b. Would interruption of sensory afferents from the muscle cause paralysis? ❒ Yes/ ❒ No. Explain.

   ____

   ____

☑ No

As long as UMN and LMN pathways to the regular muscle fibers are intact, movement is possible. In tabes dorsalis, for example, the axons of the dorsal roots selectively degenerate. Because the afferent axons from the muscle spindles are lost, the Pt has areflexia and has sensory ataxia but can move.

5. Knowing that the stimulus is proper and that the afferent arc is intact, consider next the LMN and the efferent side of the arc. (We do not consider the synapses of the afferent axon on the LMNs because we cannot evaluate them clinically.) The term *LMN* includes the cell *body* of the neuron and its *axon*. Many diseases attack the bodies of LMNs. Poliomyelitis, one of the most specific, destroys LMNs, with less effect on the dorsal horns or afferent fibers. A Pt with poliomyelitis loses MSRs because of destruction of the efferent arc but retains sensation.

6. After the LMN cell body, consider the *efferent axon* through the ventral root and peripheral nerve. The efferent axon may be interrupted by mechanical lesions such as cuts or compression. Many toxic and metabolic disorders, such as lead poisoning, may predominantly affect efferent axons, causing a **motor neuropathy.** Other toxins, such as arsenic, regularly affect afferent and efferent axons, causing a **sensorimotor neuropathy.** Irrespective of cause and irrespective of involvement of the afferent system, a lesion of the LMN cell body or axons has essentially the same effect on the muscle: weakness, atrophy, and loss of MSRs.

7. Consider next in the efferent arc the *neuromyal junction*. Two diseases of the neuromyal junction that cause defective impulse transmission are **myasthenia gravis** and **botulism.** Myasthenia is a disease of fluctuating intensity. Complete areflexia is unusual. Other major disorders of the neuromuscular junction include Lambert—Eaton myasthenic syndrome (LEMS) and several other congenital (end plate acetylcholinesterase deficiency, acetylcholine receptor deficiency, slow channel syndrome, fast channel syndrome), and several other autoimmune, genetic, toxic and drug related conditions (Conville and Vincent, 2002).

8. The final level of the reflex arc is the *effector*, the *muscle*. Many *myopathies*, including the muscular dystrophies and myositides, may cause areflexia (Karpati et al., 2001; Katirji et al., 2002). The afferent and efferent limbs of the reflex arc are preserved, but the diseased muscle cannot respond.

Receptor, afferent axons, LMN (including efferent axon), neuromyal junction, and effector (muscle) (Fig. 2-5).

9. List the clinically significant stations in a reflex arc, beginning with the stimulus.
____
____

BIBLIOGRAPHY

Karpati G, Hilton-Jones D, Griggs RC. *Disorders of Voluntary Muscle*. New York, Cambridge University Press, 2001.

Katirji B, Kaminski HJ, Preston DC, et al, eds. *Neuromuscular Disorders in Clinical Practice.* Boston, Butterworth-Heinemann, 2002.

Jacob S, Viegas S, Lashley D, Hilton-Jones D. Myasthenia gravis and other neuromuscular junction disorders. *Pract Neurol* 2009;9:364–371.

Conville JMc, Vincent A. Diseases of the neuromuscular junction. *Current Opinion in Pharmacology* 2002;2(3):296–301.

B. Effects of neuromuscular disease on muscle size

1. **Use hypertrophy and disuse atrophy of normal muscle**
   a. The size of normal muscle depends on use. If used, a muscle undergoes **use hypertrophy**—witness weightlifters. If not used, muscle undergoes **disuse atrophy.** For example, the muscles of a limb immobilized in a cast begin to undergo disuse atrophy within 24 hours. After removal of the cast, the muscles resume their work, undergo use hypertrophy, and regain their normal size.
   b. UMN lesions that result in paresis or paralysis reduce muscle use. Therefore, the muscles undergo some degree of disuse atrophy, but the atrophy is slight in relation to the effect of LMN lesions or myopathies.
   c. If deprived of axons by LMN lesions, muscle fibers undergo **denervation atrophy,** a severe atrophy ending in death of the muscle fibers, unless reinnervation occurs.
   d. A normal muscle put at rest for prolonged periods undergoes ________________ atrophy, whereas a muscle deprived of its nerve supply undergoes ________________ atrophy.

disuse; denervation

2. Myopathies, primary diseases of muscle, also may result in death of muscle fibers. This atrophy is called **myopathic atrophy.** List the three types of muscular atrophy:
   a. From prolonged inactivity, ________________ atrophy.
   b. From LMN lesions, ________________ atrophy.
   c. From primary diseases of muscle, ________________ atrophy.
   d. In some myopathies, notably Duchenne's muscular dystrophy, some muscles go through a stage of pseudohypertrophy, appearing enlarged for the first years before undergoing atrophy.

disuse; denervation; myopathic

3. **Differentiation of aplasia, hypoplasia, and atrophy**
   a. **Aplasia** (amyoplasia) means that the muscle has failed to develop. **Hypoplasia** means that the muscle has failed to develop to its normal size.
   b. **Atrophy** of whatever type (disuse, denervation, or myopathic) means that the muscle once had a normal size and then lost its bulk.
   c. These various terms enable the Ex to designate the mechanism of the reduction in muscle bulk.
4. **Circumferential measurement of the extremities:** If the history or examination suggests a disorder that could affect muscle size, measure the greatest circumference of the part for documentation in the chart and to compare the right and left sides.

C. Neuromuscular disease, motor units, and electromyography

1. **Definition of a motor unit:** A **motor unit** is one LMN, its axon, and all of the muscle fibers it innervates.

a. Each efferent axon from a motoneuron may innervate one or more muscle fibers. In some small muscles, such as the extraocular, each motor axon is thought to innervate only one muscle fiber. In large muscles, such as the gluteus maximum or quadriceps femoris, each motor axon may innervate hundreds of muscle fibers. Learn Fig. 7-20.

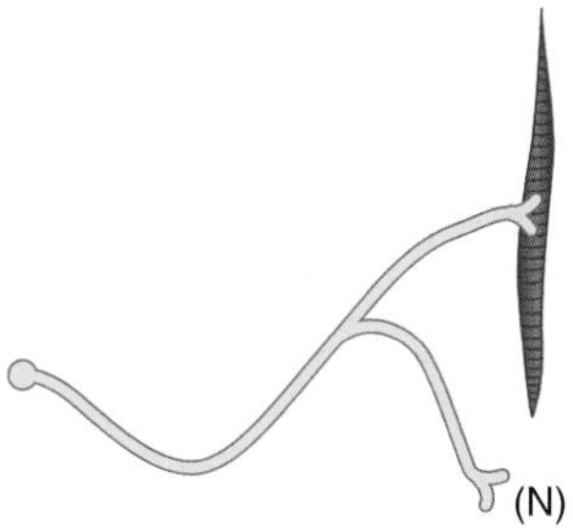

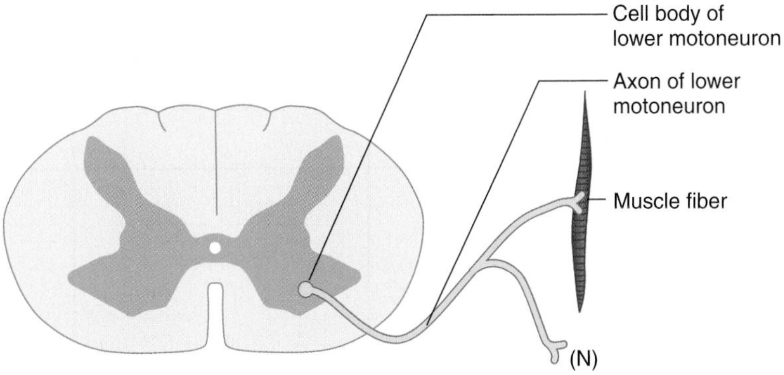

FIGURE 7-20. Cross section of spinal cord and motor unit. The motor unit consists of a motoneuron body, its axon, and all of the muscle fibers innervated by the axon. N varies from zero to hundreds of additional muscle fibers. The larger muscles have larger values of N. Encircle the portion of Fig. 7-20 that defines the motor unit and compare it with the drawing in the answer column.

☑ all

b. If a normal LMN discharges a nerve impulse, ❐ some/❐ all/❐ none of the muscle fibers of the motor unit would be expected to contract.

2. **Motor units and fasciculations**

a. The muscle fibers of the motor units are grouped together in a fascicle (fasciculus) of the muscle. If a single motor unit fires, the Ex can see the contraction of the fascicle of muscle fibers as a small ripple or twitch under the Pt's skin. Such a twitch is a **fasciculation.** You have all probably experienced twitching of an eyelid: that is a fasciculation. The Ex can see fasciculations, and the Pt can see and feel them.

An LMN, its axon, and all the muscle fibers it innervates.

b. Define a motor unit.

____

A small muscular twitch called a *fasciculation*.

c. If one motor unit discharges, what would the Ex see and what is the technical name for it? ______________________________

3. **Myokymia:** When motor units discharge abnormally in groups for prolonged periods, they cause a visible, rippling, worm-like action of the muscle called **myokymia.** The muscles go into more or less continuous spasm that may appear focally or segmentally and may affect at times only the facial muscles or even the ocular muscles. In the "stiff-man" or, better said "stiff-person," syndrome of Isaacs, the myokymia affects widespread muscle groups.

4. **Cramps:** Cramps are sustained contractions that last seconds to minutes, often brought on by exercise and relieved by stretching the muscle. The EMG shows high-frequency motor unit discharges of 200 to 300 impulses/s.

5. **Electromyography**

a. Normally motor units discharge only when stimulated by UMNs or other afferents. A needle inserted into a normal resting muscle and wired to an amplifier and oscilloscope records no electrical activity in most skeletal muscles at rest. When the motor units discharge, the oscilloscope screen displays numerous electrical potentials caused by depolarization of muscle fibers. The recording of this electrical activity from muscle is called **electromyography** (Aminoff, 1999). See Fig. 7-21.

b. The surface membrane of a diseased LMN becomes unstable. The neuron may then discharge spontaneous, random impulses, rather than discharging only in response to appropriate stimuli. All the muscle fibers connected to the

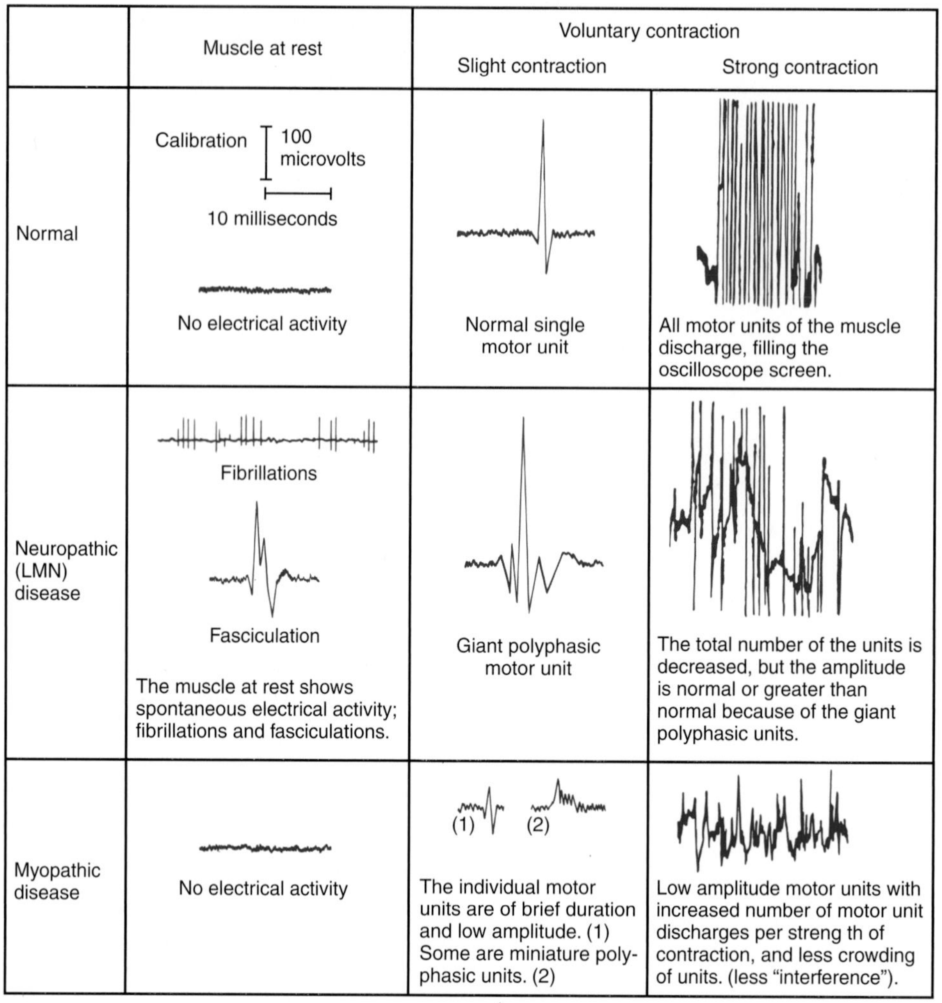
Muscle at rest
Voluntary contraction
Slight contraction
Strong contraction
Normal
Calibration
100 microvolts
10 milliseconds
No electrical activity
Normal single motor unit
All motor units of the muscle discharge, filling the oscilloscope screen.
Neuropathic (LMN) disease
Fibrillations
Fasciculation
The muscle at rest shows spontaneous electrical activity; fibrillations and fasciculations.
Giant polyphasic motor unit
The total number of the units is decreased, but the amplitude is normal or greater than normal because of the giant polyphasic units.
Myopathic disease
No electrical activity
(1)
(2)
The individual motor units are of brief duration and low amplitude. (1) Some are miniature poly-phasic units. (2)
Low amplitude motor units with increased number of motor unit discharges per streng th of contraction, and less crowding of units. (less "interference").

FIGURE 7-21. Electromyographic (oscilloscopic) tracings of the electrical activity recorded from muscle. (Courtesy Dr. Mark Dyken.)

axon of the motoneuron contract, resulting in spontaneous fasciculations (Fig. 7-21B). Some normal individuals who do not have neuronal disease show **benign fasciculations,** particularly after exercise.

6. **Wallerian degeneration and the EMG of denervation**
   a. If the neuronal perikaryon dies, its axon dies. The axon also dies after complete separation from its perikaryon. The process of dissolution of the dead axon and its myelin sheath is called **Wallerian degeneration** (August Waller, 1816–1870). See Fig. 7-22.

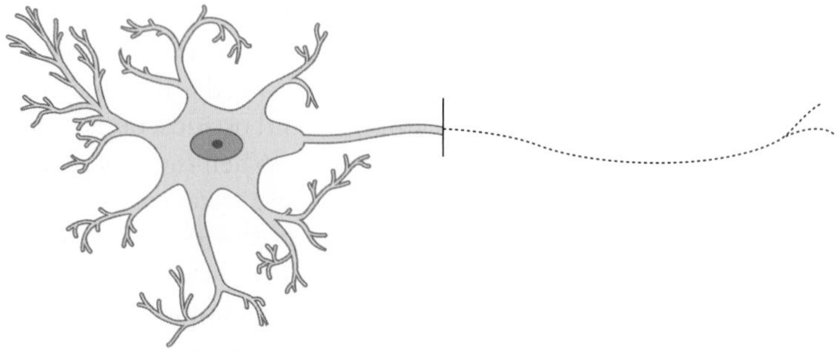

FIGURE 7-22. Neuron and axon to show Wallerian (anterograde) degeneration of the distal, severed part of the axon that has lost contact with the metabolic machinery in the perikaryon.

b. After axonal severance and Wallerian degeneration, the denervated muscle fibers will not contract in response to volition, afferent stimuli, or direct electrical stimulation of the peripheral nerve trunk. The Ex can still elicit a twitch of the denervated muscle fibers by direct percussion until they ultimately die.

7. **Fibrillations**

a. **Definition:** A **fibrillation** is a random, spontaneous contraction of an individual denervated muscle fiber. After denervation by Wallerian degeneration of the motor axon, the muscle fiber undergoes a period of hyperexcitability (*Cannon's law of hypersensitivity of denervated structures*). It seems as if the muscle fibers attempt to compensate for the lack of nerve impulses by discharging more easily. Thus, the membrane of the individual muscle fiber depolarizes spontaneously and the fiber contracts. Because of the small size of single muscle fibers, the Ex cannot see fibrillations, but an oscilloscope can record them (Fig. 7-21).

b. Spontaneous depolarization of the membranes of diseased LMNs causes visible muscular twitches called ______________, whereas spontaneous depolarization of individual denervated muscle fibers causes ______________________________.

fasciculations; fibrillation

c. The Ex can see the motor unit twitches called ______________, but the oscilloscope is required to "see" the individual muscle fiber contractions called ______________.

fasciculations; fibrillations

8. After the death of LMNs, fasciculations cease. They occur only during the period when the neurons, although abnormal, remain intact. Fibrillations begin about 3 weeks after denervation and continue for as long as the denervated muscle fibers remain alive, until the final stage of denervation atrophy, when the muscle fibers die.

9. **Define fasciculations and fibrillations.** Include the operations by which they are detected and their pathophysiology.

____

____

____

____

Fasciculations are contractions of muscle fascicles, detected by clinical inspection or by characteristic EMG waves. They indicate a hyperexcitable state of the cell membrane of the LMNs, which depolarize spontaneously, causing contraction of all muscle fibers of the motor unit. **Fibrillations** are spontaneous contractions of individual denervated muscle fibers, detected by characteristic EMG waves. They indicate a state of hyperexcitability of the muscle fibers after denervation.

10. **Giant polyphasic motor units:** As recorded by EMG, giant polyphasic waves have a greater amplitude and more complex form than do normal motor units (Fig. 7-21). Denervated muscle fibers induce sprouting of new axonal terminals from a neighboring intact axon. When that axon fires, it activates not only its original number of muscle fibers but also the previously denervated adjacent muscle fibers. The larger number of muscle fibers firing causes the polyphasic giant EMG potentials.

11. Magnetic resonance imaging with gadolinium enhancement also provides diagnostic information about denervated and dystrophic muscles (Bendszus and Koltzenburg, 2000).

D. Summary of the clinical and electromyographic syndrome of lower motoneuron lesions

1. The *clinical syndrome* of LMN lesions consists of **paresis** or **paralysis, atrophy, fasciculations,** and **areflexia** of the affected muscles, summarized in Table 7-7.

2. The *EMG syndrome* of LMN lesions consists of spontaneous individual motor unit discharges called ______________________, spontaneous contractions of individual muscle fibers called ______________________, and the appearance of ______________________ motor units on EMG.

fasciculations; fibrillations; giant polyphasic *motor units*

BIBLIOGRAPHY · Electromyography and Nerve Conduction Velocity Studies

Aminoff MJ, ed. *Electrodiagnosis in Clinical Neurology*, 4th ed. New York, Churchill Livingstone, 1999.

Bendszus M, Koltzenburg M. Visualization of denervated muscle by gadolinium-enhanced MRI. *Neurology* 2000;57:1709–1711.

Dumitru D, Amato AA, Zwarts MJ. *Electrodiagnostic Medicine*. New York, Williams & Wilkins, 2001.

E. Differentiation of lesions at various sites in the reflex arc

Note: More than one answer may be correct in the next frames.

☑ LMN lesions and ☑ myopathies

1. Paresis or paralysis would accompany which one or more of the following? ❐ dorsal root lesions/❐ LMN lesions/❐ myopathies

☑ LMN lesions

2. Denervation atrophy occurs with which one or more of the following? ❐ dorsal root lesions/❐ LMN lesions/❐ myopathies

☑ dorsal root lesions

3. Loss of sensation occurs with which one or more of the following? ❐ dorsal root lesions/❐ LMN lesions/❐ myopathies

all three

4. Absence of MSRs occurs with which one or more of the following? ❐ dorsal root lesions/❐ LMN lesions/❐ myopathies
5. Complete Table 7-4 to differentiate the various neuromuscular syndromes associated with lesions of the reflex arc. Notice that hypotonia (loose floppy limbs) occurs with lesions at any level of the reflex arc.

TABLE 7-4 · Clinical Signs and Probable Diagnoses of Lesions at the Level of the Reflex Arc*

Answer	Clinical signs	Probable diagnosis: Dorsal root lesion	LMN lesion	Myopathy
1 ☑	Areflexia, hypotonia, loss of sensation. No atrophy, weakness, or EMG abnormalities.	1 ❐	2 ❐	3 ❐
2 ☑	Weakness, areflexia, atrophy, hypotonia, fasciculations, and fibrillations. No sensory loss.	1 ❐	2 ❐	3 ❐
1 ☑; 2 ☑	Weakness, areflexia, atrophy, fasciculations, fibrillations, hypotonia, and loss of sensation.	1 ❐	2 ❐	3 ❐
3 ☑	Weakness, areflexia, atrophy, and hypotonia. No sensory loss, fasciculations, or fibrillations.	1 ❐	2 ❐	3 ❐
3 ☑	Weakness, hyporeflexia, atrophy, hypotonia, percussion myotonia. No sensory loss, fasciculations, or fibrillations.	1 ❐	2 ❐	3 ❐

*The correct answer may require checking more than one of the three choices in the columns.
ABBREVIATIONS: EMG = electromyographic; LMN = lower motoneuron.

F. Consider this patient

Three weeks before hospitalization, a 52-year-old man became violently ill with nausea, vomiting, and bloody diarrhea. The gastrointestinal symptoms receded, but 4 days before admission, he began to have severe pain in his extremities and some leg weakness. Examination showed intact cranial nerves. He had slight paresis of his hand muscles and severe leg weakness, most pronounced distally. He was hyporeflexic in the arms and areflexic in the lower extremities. He had difficulty recognizing pinprick and light touch over his hands, and his feet were almost anesthetic. He had no muscular atrophy on admission, but it became evident in 10 days. An EMG on admission disclosed no spontaneous activity indicative of fasciculations or fibrillations. A second

EMG, done 3 weeks after hospitalization, disclosed fasciculations and numerous fibrillations in the muscles that were clinically weak and areflexic.

☑ a combined sensorimotor

1. This Pt had ❐ only a motor/❐ only a sensory/❐ a combined sensorimotor neuropathy.

symptoms of severe pain, distal sensory loss, and areflexia

2. From the history and examination, the evidence for sensory neuropathy was (review the case protocol to sift out the answers): ______________________.

initially, weakness and areflexia; later, atrophy, fasciculations and fibrillations

3. The evidence for motor neuropathy was ______________________.
4. A neuropathy after a severe gastrointestinal upset suggests poisoning. The neuropathy may lag behind the toxic exposure by days or weeks. The Pt's urine had high arsenic levels, the result of rat poison given by his wife.
5. The onset of the Pt's fasciculations and fibrillations 3 weeks after the first clinical signs of neuropathy is the usual time required for these denervation signs to appear. Even if a knife severs a nerve, fibrillations do not appear until 3 or more weeks. Complete Table 7-5.

☑ No. Atrophy, fasciculations, and fibrillations indicate an efferent lesion.

6. Would a lesion confined to the afferent axons, cause muscular atrophy, fasciculations, and fibrillations? ❐ Yes ❐ No. Explain. ______________________

BIBLIOGRAPHY · Arsenic Poisoning

Goebel HH, Schmidt PF, Bohl J, et al. Polyneuropathy due to acute arsenic intoxication: biopsy studies. *J Neuropathol Exp Neurol* 1990;49:137–149.

VII. CLINICAL ANALYSIS OF HYPERACTIVE MUSCLE STRETCH REFLEXES AND CLONUS

A. Causes of hyperreflexia

1. Hyperreflexia has many causes. Figure 7-23 illustrates that each sign generates many diagnostic possibilities.

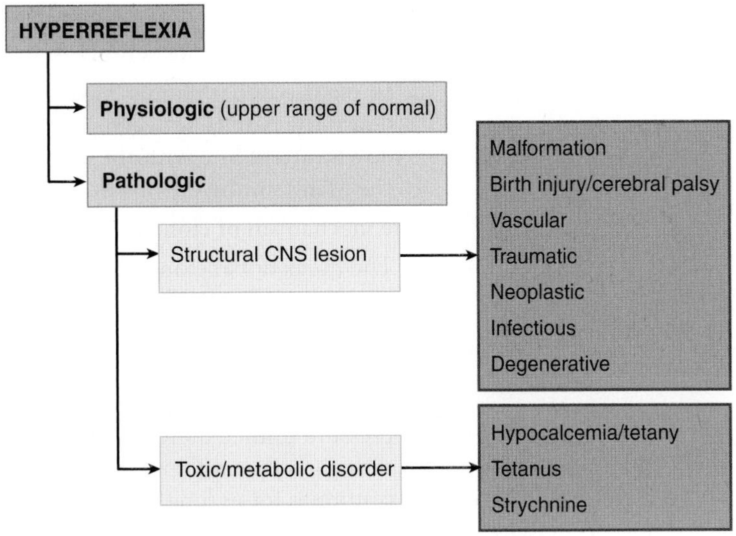

FIGURE 7-23. Dendrogram of common causes for hyperreflexia.

2. To analyze any finding, first ask, "Is it merely a normal variation?" Very brisk MSRs may fall within the wide range of normal variation. The most common cause of pathologic hyperreflexia is interruption of UMN pathways between the cerebrum and the LMNs. When UMN lesions increase MSRs on one side, the Ex should also find weakness on that side, i.e., a hemiparesis. The syndrome or pattern of signs integrated with the history produces the diagnosis.

B. Clonus

1. **Definition:** Clonus is a to-and-fro, 5- to 8-cycles per second (cps), rhythmic oscillation of a body part, elicited by a quick stretch. Clonus is another way to demonstrate hyperactive MSRs after interruption of the UMNs. With extremely brisk MSRs, noxious stimuli and cold elicit clonus (Dimitrijevic et al., 1980).
2. **Technique for eliciting clonus**
   a. Induce the Pt to relax completely. To elicit ankle clonus, flex the Pt's knee slightly to relax the triceps surae muscle.
   b. Hold the Pt's foot as shown in Fig. 7-24. Gently but briskly jerk the foot upward and a little outward. After the upward jerk, maintain finger pressure against the

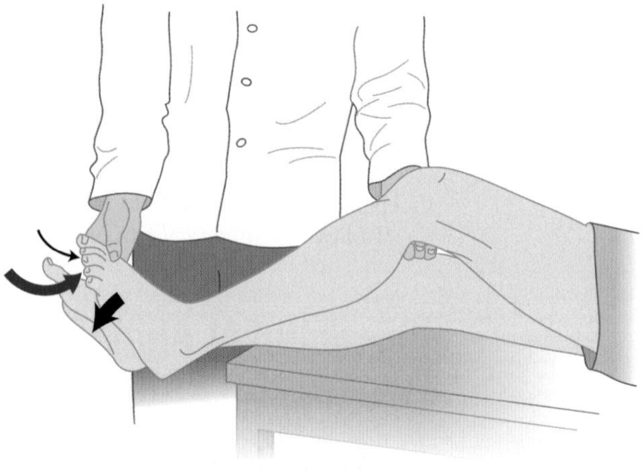

FIGURE 7-24. Method for eliciting ankle clonus. The examiner jerks upward and a little outward on the patient's foot (thin arrow). The thick arrow represents the downward response.

sole of the Pt's foot. If the foot oscillates between flexion and extension for as long as you maintain pressure, the Pt has the sustained type of clonus.
   c. To elicit wrist clonus, simply jerk quickly up on the Pt's hand.
   d. To elicit patellar clonus, have the Pt's lower extremity straight and relaxed. Grasp the patella between your thumb and index finger and displace it briskly downward in line with the Pt's thigh, stretching the quadriceps femoris muscle. Maintain the downward pressure to sustain the clonus.
3. **The mechanism of clonus**
   a. The quick dorsiflexion of the Pt's foot stretches the muscle spindles of the triceps surae (Fig. 7-25A). The triceps surae responds with a single MSR, causing the foot to plantar flex (Fig. 7-25B, thick arrow).
   b. The Ex continues to apply light finger pressure against the ball of the Pt's foot throughout. When the plantar flexion stops from the first MSR, the finger pressure immediately dorsiflexes the foot again (Fig. 7-25C, thin arrow). This action elicits another MSR from the triceps surae muscle, and the sequence continues for as long as the Ex maintains finger pressure.
   c. With pathologic hyperreflexia, the Ex can easily sustain the clonus by continued finger pressure.

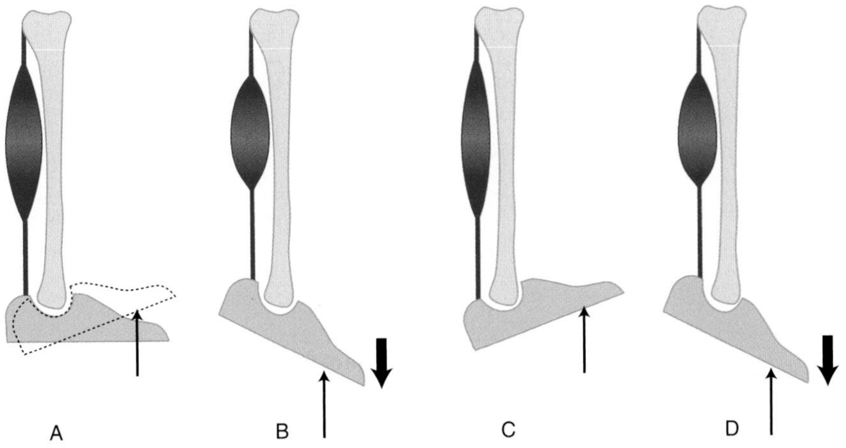

FIGURE 7-25. Mechanism of ankle clonus. The thin arrow represents the light pressure applied by the examiner to the ball of the patient's foot, and the thick arrow indicates the response.

The muscle spindles have to be stretched briskly to initiate an afferent volley.

4. The same technique of applying a quick jerk elicits wrist, finger, or jaw clonus.
5. Explain why the Ex must jerk the part briskly to elicit clonus?

____

6. **Clinical interpretation of clonus**
   a. Some normal individuals with physiologic hyperreflexia will have a few clonic jerks, and this condition is called **abortive clonus.** In mature individuals, only sustained clonus qualifies as abnormal.
   b. Some normal neonates with extreme physiologic hyperreflexia exhibit sustained clonus set off by movement and gravity (Shuper et al., 1991). It will affect the jaw and the limbs. Simply eliciting an MSR by tendon percussion, jarring the bed, or spontaneous movements of the infant may initiate a train of clonic after-jerks. The proof that the action is clonus comes from immediately arresting it by holding the part to prevent the succession of stretches. Maneuvers of that type do not cause tremors and seizures to stop.

Clonus is a series of to-and-fro rhythmic oscillations of a part generally initiated by a quick jerk that stretches a muscle.

7. Give an operational definition of clonus, i.e., describe the maneuvers and responses.

____

____

Clonus is a series of repetitive MSRs initiated by stretching the muscle spindles and is indicative of interruption of UMNs (the pyramidal tract).

8. Give a pathophysiologic definition of the mechanism and clinical interpretation of sustained clonus.

____

____

Newborn and young infants

9. At what age do many normal individuals show clonus? ____________.

Note: The definition of clonus given here does not apply to the use of the term in describing generalized motor seizures, as in the phrase *tonic-clonic seizures*. The cause of the to-and-fro movements in seizures is an abnormal hypersynchronous discharge of central neurons, not a perpetuated MSR.

BIBLIOGRAPHY · Clonus

Dimitrijevic MR, Nathan PW, Sherwood AM. Clonus: the role of central mechanisms. *J Neurol Neurosurg Psychiatry* 1980;43:321–332.

Shuper A, Zalaberg J, Wertz R. Jitteriness beyond the neonatal period: a benign movement pattern in infancy. *J Child Neurol* 1991;6:243–245.

VIII. DISORDERS OF MUSCLE TONE: HYPERTONIA AND HYPOTONIA

Note: As developed to this point, the syndrome of UMN lesions consists of paresis or paralysis, hyperreflexia, and clonus. Understanding spasticity, yet another component of the full UMN syndrome (Table 7-5), requires a general discussion of muscle tone.

☑ Early
☑ Intermediate
☑ Late

TABLE 7-5 · **Time of Onset of Neurologic Signs in Acute Motor Neuropathies**

	Early	Intermediate (days)	Late
Paresis, paralysis, and areflexia	❐	❐	❐
Atrophy	❐	❐	❐
Fibrillations and fasciculations	❐	❐	❐

A. Definition

Muscle tone is the muscular resistance that the Ex feels when manipulating a Pt's resting joint (apart from gravity or joint disease).

B. Self-demonstration of muscle tone

1. Place your right forearm across your thigh with your wrist dangling freely. Supinate your forearm to place your radius up. After relaxing this arm completely, grasp its hand with your left hand and flex and extend the wrist as fully as possible.
2. As your active hand moves your relaxed hand, the active hand will feel slight resistance. This slight resistance to passive movement is normal muscle tone. The ligaments set the ultimate range of joint movement.
3. Try now to relax your elbow and, with your other hand, flex and extend your forearm, but now you have to contend with gravity. Try these exercises with a partner.
4. These exercises serve two purposes: to provide proprioceptive experience in judging muscle tone and to provide insight into the difficulty in relaxing a part completely. Do not lose patience when your Pts fail to relax. Keep working patiently to get the part completely relaxed before judging tone.

C. Origin of muscle tone

Normally, the resistance of the muscle to passive movement has two components:

1. The elasticity of the muscle, which ordinarily is slight unless the muscle is fibrotic.
2. The number and rate of motor unit discharges, which is the critical variable. The number and rate of motor unit discharges depend on:
   a. The stimulation of LMNs by muscle spindles and other receptors in skin, tendons, joints, and bone.
   b. Stimulation or inhibition of LMNs by pyramidal and extrapyramidal pathways. Thus muscle tone depends on the activity of motor units as determined by the algebraic sum of diverse excitatory and inhibitory impulses from the peripheral nervous system and CNS on the LMNs.
   c. Because numerous pathways affect tone and the theories about it are complex and conflicting, we will content ourselves with the operational findings and their clinical analysis. We thus avoid the error of giving priority to explanations and interpretations at the expense of operational techniques.
3. You can easily surmise that the two possible alterations of tone are too much tone, **hypertonia,** and too little tone, **hypotonia.**

D. Hypertonia

1. The two most common hypertonic states are **spasticity** and **rigidity.** Less common is **paratonia** (*Gegenhalten*).
2. **Spasticity:** As operationally defined, spasticity is an initial catch or resistance and then a yielding when the Ex briskly manipulates the Pt's resting extremity. The catch-and-yield sequence resembles pulling the blade of an ordinary pocketknife open. When first opened, the blade resists but quickly yields as it straightens out. The similar phenomenon in muscle tone is called **clasp-knife spasticity** (Fig. 7-26).

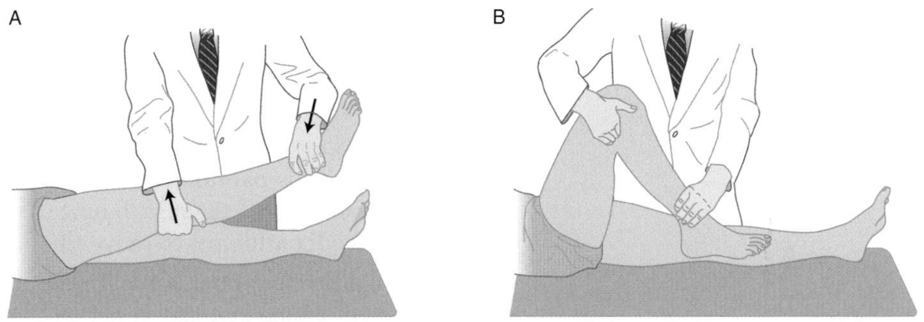

FIGURE 7-26. Method for eliciting clasp-knife spasticity. (A) The examiner lifts the patient's leg with one hand, placing the other under the patient's knee. As briskly as possible, in fact with a jerk, the examiner simultaneously pushes *down* with the ankle hand and *up* with the other. (B) The spastic leg catches and then molds to the flexed position, like a clasp-knife closing.

   a. The brisk movement required to elicit clasp-knife spasticity suggests that the stimulus has to engage the muscle spindles. According to this interpretation, the resistance felt is simply an MSR, which then fades out as the muscle spindles readjust. Increased sensitivity of the MSR arc is the fundamental change, of which hyperreflexia, clonus, and spasticity are derivative. Although hyperreflexia, clonus, and clasp-knife spasticity usually parallel each other in intensity, occasionally one feature predominates out of proportion to the others. The pathophysiology of these variations is unknown. Clasp-knife spasticity is generally greater in the *flexors* of the upper extremities and *extensors* of the lower.

   b. The three phenomena presented to this point, which indicate a pyramidal tract or UMN lesion and act through an oversensitive MSR arc, are ____.

   hyperreflexia, clonus, and clasp-knife spasticity

   c. On the assumption that the UMN denervation of the spinal reflex arcs causes spasticity, various therapies have attempted to relieve spasticity by interrupting the arc peripherally and in the spinal cord itself (Goldstein, 2001).

3. **Rigidity:** As operationally defined, rigidity is an increased muscular resistance felt throughout the entire range of movement when the Ex slowly manipulates a Pt's resting joint. The steady resistance feels like bending solder or a lead pipe. Hence, its name, **lead-pipe rigidity.** It involves the agonists and antagonists at the joints.

   a. The presence of lead-pipe rigidity indicates an extrapyramidal lesion in the basal motor circuitry, more specifically in the dopaminergic projection from the substantia nigra to the striatum in parkinsonism. The pathophysiology of lead-pipe rigidity is uncertain.

   b. A **cogwheel phenomenon** often occurs with the rigidity of parkinsonism. The Ex feels the rigidity as a series of ratchet-like catches while slowly moving the elbow or wrist through its range of motion. It apparently reflects the superimposed beats of the parkinsonian tremor, even though the tremor may not be otherwise obvious.

c. In testing for increased tone, the voluntary movement of a part not under manipulation will increase the tone (Froment's maneuver; Pryse-Phillips, 1995). For example, the Ex asks the Pt to turn the head back and forth while testing tone in the elbow or observing for rest tremor.

4. **Paratonia** (*Gegenhalten: gegen* = against or toward; *halten* = to hold; therefore to hold against or resist).

   a. **Definition:** Paratonia is the resistance, equal in degree and range, that the Pt presents to each attempt of the Ex to move a part in any direction. It is a *pari passu* response.

   b. **Self-demonstration of paratonia:** Press your palms together and, while maintaining the palms in contact with constant slight pressure, move both hands to the right and left and then up and down. Imagine one hand as the Pt's and the other as the Ex's. If one hand increases pressure, speeds up, or detours, so does the other in equal degree. It is like leading and following in ballroom dancing. The balanced, proprioceptive resistance or opposition of one hand in pursuit of another hand is **paratonia.** The Pt is not necessarily rigid at rest. The Ex feels the paratonia as a slight stiffening of the Pt's limb in response to the contact when the Ex attempts to move the Pt's extremity.

   c. **Clinical significance of paratonia:** Paratonia occurs in dementia, often in combination with abulia and gait apraxia (Chapter 11). Some otherwise normal persons who cannot relax completely for testing muscle tone show a paratonia-like resistance to passive movement of their parts by the Ex.

E. Review of spasticity and rigidity

1. Give an operational definition of clasp-knife spasticity.

____

____

See frame D 2

2. Give an operational definition of lead-pipe rigidity.

____

____

See frame D 3

3. Clasp-knife spasticity indicates a lesion of the ❐ pyramidal tract/❐ extrapyramidal tracts, whereas lead-pipe rigidity indicates a lesion of the ❐ pyramidal tract/ ❐ extrapyramidal tracts.

☑ pyramidal tract; ☑ extrapyramidal tracts

4. Check the signs that require a brisk stimulus to elicit.

   a. ❐ Clasp-knife spasticity

   b. ❐ Lead-pipe rigidity

   c. ❐ Hyperactive MSR

   d. ❐ Clonus

   e. ❐ Paratonia

☑ a; ☑ c; and ☑ d

5. Why do the signs checked in frame 4 require a brisk stimulus to elicit them?

____

____

To activate a strong afferent volley from muscle spindles and to fire the LMNs before the spindles adjust to their new length.

F. Differentiation of spasticity and rigidity

Lesions can affect pyramidal and extrapyramidal pathways, causing mixtures of spasticity and rigidity, especially in cerebral palsy. Usually the Ex can differentiate the two (Table 7-6).

BIBLIOGRAPHY · Spasticity and Rigidity

Goldstein EM. Spasticity management: an overview. *J Child Neurol* 2001;16:16–23.

Pryse-Phillips W. *Companion to Clinical Neurology.* Boston, Little, Brown and Company, 1995.

TABLE 7-6 · Clinical Differentiation of Spasticity and Rigidity

Spasticity*	Rigidity†
Clasp-knife phenomenon in hemiplegic, quadriplegic, monoplegic, or paraplegic distribution	Lead-pipe phenomenon, often with cogwheeling and tremor at rest; usually in all four extremities but may have a "hemi" distribution
The examiner elicits the clasp-knife phenomenon, a catch-and-yield sensation, by a quick jerk of the resting extremity	The examiner elicits the lead-pipe resistance of rigidity by making a relatively slow movement of the patient's resting extremity
Clonus and hyperactive MSRs	No clonus; MSRs not necessarily altered
Extensor toe sign	Normal plantar reflexes
Tends to predominate in one set of muscles, such as flexors of the upper extremity, the extensors of the knee, and plantar flexors of the ankle	Tends to affect antagonistic pairs of muscles about equally
EMG inactive with the muscle at complete rest	EMG tends to show electrical activity with the muscle as relaxed as the patient can make it

*A component of pyramidal syndromes.
†A component of extrapyramidal syndromes.
ABBREVIATIONS: EMG = electromyography; MSR = muscle stretch reflex.

G. Hypotonia (flaccidity)

1. **Definition:** Hypotonia is a decreased resistance the Ex feels when manipulating a Pt's resting joint. Hypotonic Pts generally show an increased range of joint movement, as with hyperextensible knees (*genu recurvatum*) or flaccid heel cords.
2. **Causes of hypotonia** (Fig. 7-27)
3. Hypotonia from lesions at the level of the reflex arc or peripheral neuro-muscular system. Review Fig. 7-4.
   a. Interruption of afferent fibers in peripheral nerves or dorsal roots reduces muscle tone by removing the inflow of excitatory afferent impulses. In fact, dorsal rhizotomy is done therapeutically in some spastic Pts to reduce muscle tone.
   b. Manifestly, section of *ventral* roots would cause hypotonia because no nerve impulses could reach the muscles. *Primary myopathies* cause hypotonia by reducing the ability of the muscles to respond to tonic nerve impulses.
4. **Differentiation of peripheral causes for hypotonia:** As usual, clinical differentiation depends on fitting the constellation of findings into a syndrome, as outlined in Table 7-4.
5. **Central causes of hypotonia** (Fig. 7-27): Although cerebral, cerebellar, and brainstem lesions sometimes cause hypotonia, the pathophysiology is elusive. Many congenital brain disorders, such as Down's syndrome and Prader-Willi syndrome, cause profound hypotonia. Patients with spastic cerebral palsy may present as hypotonic infants before spasticity evolves, or they may remain hypotonic.
6. **Hypotonia from cerebral or spinal (neural) shock**
   a. **Definition:** Neural shock is a stage of hypotonic total paralysis and total areflexia that immediately follows an acute, severe UMN lesion. Typically Pts with slowly evolving UMN lesions display the standard syndrome of hypertonia, hyperreflexia, and paralysis, in more or less parallel degree. The term *shock* in this context designates the disastrous disorganization of the acutely injured nervous system. Depending on the lesion site, the Ex may specify **cerebral** or **spinal shock.**
   b. **Diaschisis:** The concept of neural shock of the motor system merges with the general concept of diaschisis. After any acute lesion, the signs and symptoms often exceed what we can understand by the actual tracts interrupted or neurons destroyed. For example, acute, strictly unilateral occipital lobe infarction, may result in complete (bilateral) cortical blindness for a period of hours or

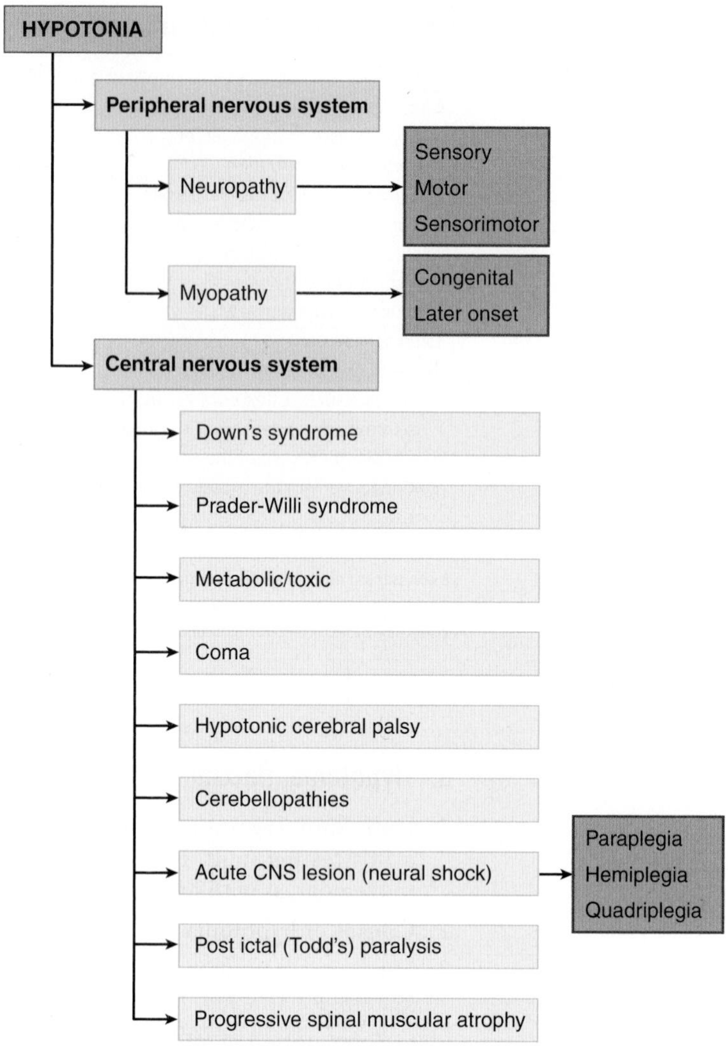

FIGURE 7-27. Dendrogram of common causes for hypotonia.

days, particularly if the Pt is somewhat obtunded. After that period, the Pt will show only the expected hemianopia dictated by the unilateral destruction of the visual cortex. Constantin von Monakow (1853–1930) named this distant impairment of function, beyond the confines of the acute lesion, **diaschisis** (Nguyen and Botez, 1998).

c. **Causes of neural shock or diaschisis:** Inciting lesions are large, acute, and catastrophic, including trauma, spinal cord transection, and large brain infarcts or hemorrhages.

d. If a Pt originally in a stage of neural shock begins to recover movement, the recovery usually parallels the emergence of the MSRs, spasticity, and clonus. After most UMN lesions of slow onset, most Pts show increased MSRs, clonus, and spasticity early in the course, without going through a hypotonic phase. Thus, the clinical signs of UMN lesions depend on:

  i. The rapidity of onset.

  ii. The size of the lesion.

  iii. The stage in the recovery of the CNS after an acute lesion.

H. Testing range of motion

1. The Ex observes the range of motion during the Pt's active free movements of the extremities when testing muscle strength. To test muscle tone, the Pt remains

completely relaxed while the Ex moves the Pt's joints slowly through their entire allowable range.

a. With hyperreflexia and spasticity, the range is reduced. With hypotonia and hyporeflexia or areflexia, it is increased.

b. Normally you can extend and flex the Pt's wrist to about 90 degrees to the forearm or dorsiflex the foot to nearly a 45-degree angle with the shin.

c. The range of motion varies with the Pt's age and sex. The newborn infant's foot can be dorsiflexed to contact the shin. Women have slightly more joint excursions than men, and the elderly tend to lose some range of motion.

2. If a joint shows a restricted range of movement, you should continue to apply pressure, taking care not to cause pain. The joint may then yield further.

a. If it does not yield, it is a **fixed** contracture.

b. If it does yield, it is a **dynamic** contracture.

3. Record range of motion by degrees, using a goniometer or protractor for precision.

BIBLIOGRAPHY · Diaschisis

Nguyen DK, Botez MI. Diaschisis and neurobehavior. *Canad J Neurol Sciences* 1998;25:5–12.

IX. EXAMINATION OF THE SUPERFICIAL REFLEXES (SKIN-MUSCLE REFLEXES)

Note: Do the next part of the text at home to test your own bare foot. Get a reflex hammer and a broken wooden tongue blade to use as stimulating objects.

A. Superficial versus deep reflexes

1. Because stimulation of receptors deep to the skin elicits the MSRs, the MSRs are classed with the **deep reflexes**. Stimulation of receptors in skin and mucous membranes elicits *superficial* or **skin-muscle reflexes.** By stimulating deep or superficial receptors with stimuli of appropriate quality and site (Vlach, 1989), the Ex can elicit a response from each muscle. In addition to causing hyperactive MSRs, spasticity, and clonus, UMN lesions alter the superficial reflexes in characteristic ways.

2. The superficial skin-muscle reflexes commonly elicited in the NE consist of:

a. Corneal reflex

b. Gag reflex

c. Abdominal skin-muscle reflexes

d. Anal wink and bulbocavernosus reflexes

e. Plantar reflex (the most important of all reflexes)

B. Standard technique for eliciting the plantar reflex

1. Place the Pt supine with the limbs completely relaxed and symmetrically arranged, and with the knees straight or slightly flexed, with knees slightly turned out. The feet should be warm.

a. Using the serrated, broken end of a tongue blade, a key, or the butt of a reflex hammer, the Ex strokes the *lateral* side of the sole (Fig. 7-28).

b. If the plantar stroke has the correct *length*, *velocity*, and *pressure*, the large toe normally flexes. After UMN interruption, the toe extends at the metatarsophalangeal joint, a phenomenon called the **Babinski sign** (Joseph Babinski, 1857–1932; Babinski, 1896, 1898; van Gijn, 1996a, 1996b; Fig. 7-33).

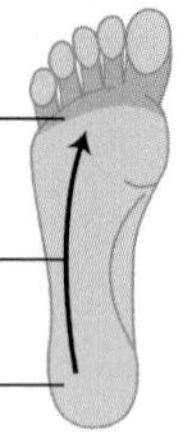

FIGURE 7-28. Sole of the right foot. The arrow marks the plantar stroke. Notice that it stops short of the shaded zone, the base of the toes.

☑ d

Statement **a** ensures that a child or adolescent will giggle and pull the foot away. Statement **b** will not be welcomed by a Pt who has a burning painful neuropathy or an elderly demented Pt. Statement **c** uses technical jargon and does not inform the Pt of what you propose to do. Statement **d** is correct.

2. Because the sole is ticklish or sensitive, the Pt, especially if senile, demented, or paranoid, may view the act of plantar stimulation as unnecessary, ludicrous, or even hostile. Critique each of the following statements and check the statement that best ensures the Pt's relaxation and cooperation.
   - ❐ a. "Hold still while I tickle the bottom of your foot."
   - ❐ b. "I am going to scratch the bottom of your foot. Hold it still."
   - ❐ c. "Hold still while I stimulate your sole."
   - ❐ d. "I am going to press gently on your foot. If it's unpleasant, tell me."
3. Next, hold the Pt's ankle with one hand to keep the foot in place and control the pressure of the plantar stroke.

☑ lateral margin

4. Place the stimulus object at the Pt's heel and stroke it slowly along the sole (Fig. 7-28). Make the path along the ❐ medial margin/❐ lateral margin/❐ center of the foot.
5. **Characteristics of the plantar stimulus**
   a. *Length* is only one of the significant variables of the plantar stimulus. Figure 7-28 shows that the plantar stroke stops short of the base of the toes. Extending the stroke to the base of the toes produces unpredictable toe movements.
   b. Another variable is the amount of *pressure* applied.
   c. A third variable of the plantar stroke is its *velocity*.
   d. Hence, the three important variables of the plantar stroke are the ______________, ______________, and ________________.

length; pressure; velocity

6. **Self-demonstration of the plantar reflex**
   a. Test your own foot and, if available, another person's. Try different velocities, pressures, and lengths, always stopping the stroke short of the base of the toes.
   b. In applying the plantar stimulus to yourself, what errors in the instructions given in B 1 for positioning did you have to make?
   ____
   ____

All of them! You were sitting, your leg was flexed, many of your muscles were contracting, and you had a bent trunk and asymmetrical posture. Reread frame B 1 if you missed this answer.

   c. By stroking your own foot, you will learn to apply the plantar stroke with slight pressure. Patients with sensory neuropathy who have extremely tender soles (hyperesthesia) find the slightest plantar stimulus intolerable. Thus, always begin with very slight pressure or even apply the stroke first to the *lateral* aspect of the foot (Chaddock's maneuver; Fig. 7-34B), a region less sensitive than the sole.

C. The criterion for success in eliciting a reflex

1. A reflex, by definition, consists of a relatively invariant response to a specified stimulus. Reproducibility is the goal in eliciting any reflex, either toe flexion or extension in the case of the plantar reflex. If no response or inconstant responses occur, your stimulus is probably wrong. Try again.
   a. Consider length first. Having already started at the heel, you can't get much more length and remain on the sole. You must avoid the base of the toes. What remains to increase length is to swing the stroke across the ball of the foot.

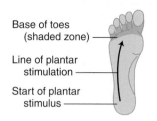

b. If you fail to get reproducible responses after changing the length, change the velocity of the stroke.

c. If changing the length and velocity of the stroke and using gentle pressure fails, increase the pressure but remain short of pain and within the Pt's limit of tolerance.

2. State the criterion that proves that you have applied the plantar stimulus correctly.

Reproducibility of toe movement, either flexion or extension.

D. Summary of the standard method for plantar stimulation

1. Write a statement to forewarn the Pt before a plantar stimulus.

Well, would your statement put *you* at ease?

2. Describe the correct position of the Pt for the plantar stimulus.

Supine, relaxed, all body parts symmetrical, legs extended or knees slightly flexed and turned out, foot relaxed.

3. Why stop the plantar stroke short of the base of toes?

It produces unpredictable toe movements.

4. If you obtain no response or variable responses, what is the most likely explanation?

The stimulus was improper with respect to length, velocity, or pressure.

E. Anatomy of the plantar reflex arc

1. The *reflexogenous zone,* the zone from which a reflex can be elicited, is the first sacral dermatome (S1) for the normal plantar reflex. Study the area of the S1 dermatome and its relation to lumbar dermatomes 4 to 5 (L4 to L5) in Fig. 7-29.

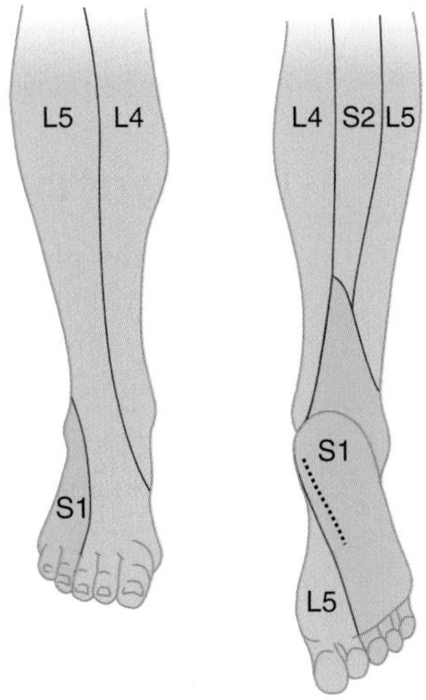

FIGURE 7-29. Dermatomes for the foot.

2. Cover Fig. 7-29 and shade in the S1 dermatome in Fig. 7-30.

3. Clinical analysis of any reflex requires "thinking through" the reflex arc. According to first principles of thinking through a reflex arc, we begin at the ________________.

receptor

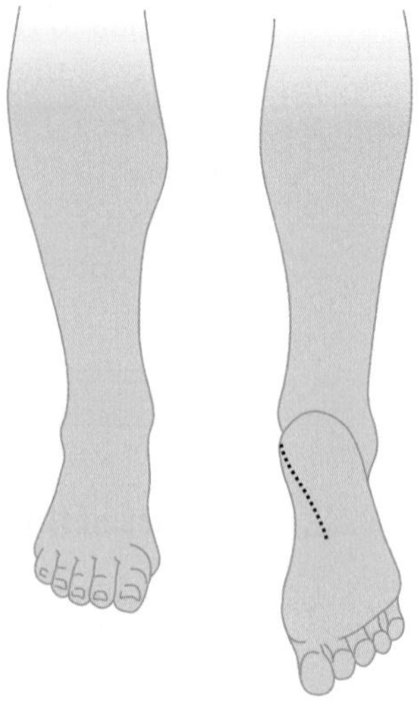

FIGURE 7-30. Blank for shading the S1 dermatome.

☑ superficial

4. Because the skin contains the receptor nerve endings, the plantar reflex is classed as a ❒ superficial/❒ deep reflex.

5. Learn Fig. 7-31 and then answer frames a to f.

S1

a. The reflexogenous zone for the plantar reflex is the ______________ dermatome.

sciatic

b. The *afferent* nerve, or *tibial* nerve, is a branch of the ______________ nerve.

lumbar (L4 to L5); sacral (S1 to S2)

c. Mediating the plantar reflex are the IV and V segments of the __________ level of the spinal cord and the I and II segments of the ______________ level.

tibial; peroneal

d. The sciatic nerve divides into two large branches just proximal to the knee. The branch to the toe *flexors* is the ______________ nerve, and the branch to the *extensors* is the ______________ nerve.

sciatic

e. The major nerve that divides into tibial and peroneal branches is the _________ nerve.

Tibial

f. What nerve, if cut, would interrupt the *afferent* and *efferent* arcs of the normal plantar response, leaving the toe extensor muscles innervated? ______________

F. Physiology of the plantar stimulus

1. **Pain and the plantar reflex:** The plantar stimulus results in a somewhat noxious feeling of tickling, pressure, and pain. The effective plantar stimulus presumably acts mainly through the *pain* receptors in the skin. However, one cannot safely infer from the subjective component of the reflex precisely which receptors elicited the response, because the stimulus activates several types of afferent endings.

2. **Summation and the plantar reflex**

a. Figure 7-32 shows the oscilloscopic patterns of electrical shocks applied to a Pt's nerve. The brief shock illustrated in Fig. 7-32A did not elicit a response. Increasing only the *duration* of the shock elicited a response (Fig. 7-32B).

b. A stimulus that requires increasing application to elicit a response is said to **summate** or to undergo **summation.** A certain minimum number of afferent impulses has to add up, or summate, to fire the LMNs to the muscles. When, as in Fig. 7-32, a stimulus must act over a finite time to cause the reflex, we say that **temporal summation** has occurred.

☑ spatial

c. Suppose a person fails to feel movement when an object moves a distance of 500 μm across the skin. Then, while keeping the time the same, the Ex moves the object 1000 μm, and the person does feel movement. The response occurs because the object acts on an increased area of skin. This exemplifies ❒ spatial/❒ temporal summation.

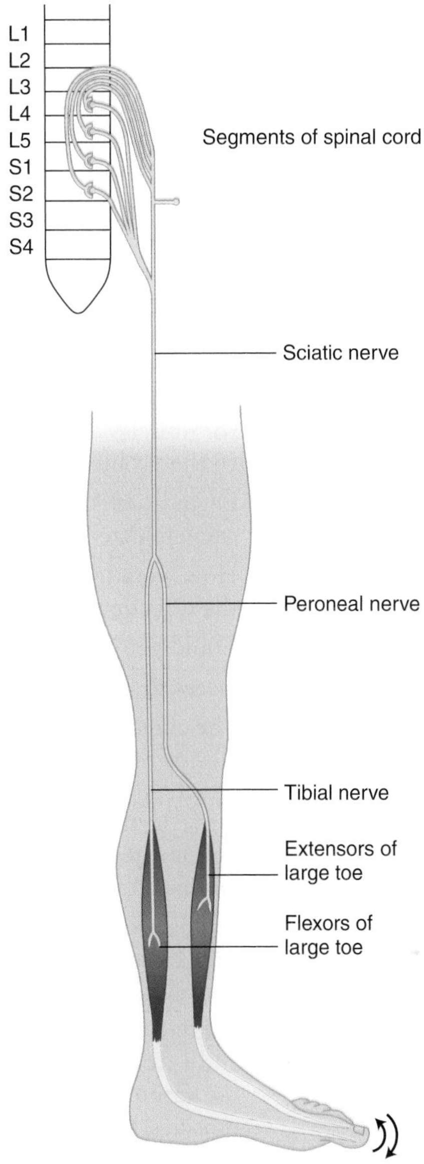

FIGURE 7-31. Reflex arc for plantar reflexes. For simplicity, the diagram shows the flexor hallucis brevis in the calf rather than in the foot.

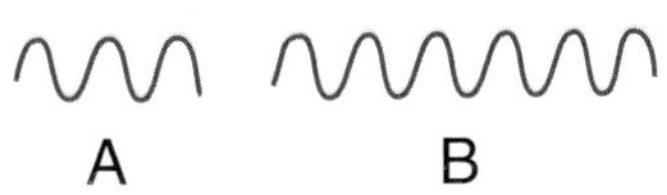

FIGURE 7-32. Oscilloscopic pattern of electrical stimuli.

3. When the Ex elicits a plantar reflex, the toe may not move until the object reaches the instep or ball of the foot. This delay in the response indicates that some type of summation has occurred.
   a. The fact that moving the object from the heel to the instep requires a finite amount of time suggests that ____________ summation is necessary.
   b. The fact that the moving object stimulated successively more receptors also suggests that ____________ summation may have occurred.
4. Thus, to get the muscles of the toes to contract, the central excitatory state of the motoneurons was increased by ____________ and ____________ summation.

temporal

spatial

temporal; spatial

G. The role of agonist-antagonist contraction in the plantar reflex

1. Reflexes differ greatly regarding the adequate stimulus, the number of muscles acting, and overall complexity. The relatively simple MSR involves a limited muscular contraction. In some reflexes, the simultaneous contraction of the *antagonist* opposes the prime mover, the *agonist.* In other reflexes, the contraction of the agonist inhibits the antagonist (Sherrington's law of reciprocal inhibition).
2. In the normal plantar reflex, we know that the toe flexors contract because we can see the toe flex. Occasionally the first response to the plantar stimulus is slight toe flexion that then reverts to extension. The question is whether the toe extensor muscles co-contract in opposition to the flexors and are simply overpowered by the flexors, or whether the toe extensors contract at all. What pathologic conditions or laboratory experiments would prove that the toe extensor and flexor muscles contract simultaneously in the plantar reflex? If you need help to solve the problem, try one of the hints below:
   a. Begin by "thinking through" the reflex arc (Fig. 7-31). Would a lesion, or procaine injected at a particular site, help answer the question?
   b. How would you detect extensor muscle contractions even if the toe moved in the direction of the flexors?
   c. Could you use EMG?
3. **Answers to frame 2**
   a. The clinically minded investigator would look for Pts in whom the flexor muscles of the toe were paralyzed, leaving the afferent impulses from the sole intact. Such a situation might occur by interruption of the motor branch of the nerve to the flexor muscles, a muscle injury, or by a disease such as anterior poliomyelitis that might happen to destroy the LMNs supplying the flexors, leaving all *afferent* axons from the sole and *efferent* axons to the extensors intact.
   b. The laboratory-minded investigator would make simultaneous EMG recordings from the flexors and extensors during the application of the plantar stimulus.
   c. Landau and Clare (1959) concluded from their EMG study that flex-ors and extensors of the toe both contract simultaneously in response to a plantar stimulus, with the outcome a mechanical competition between these muscles, but van Gijn (1976 a & b) disagreed. At the spinal cord level, however, some integrative mechanism must determine whether flexion or extension will occur.

H. Normal variations and flexion synergy in response to a plantar stimulus

1. **Flexion synergy**
   a. *Some* normal persons will show little or no toe or leg movement after a plantar stimulus, a so-called **mute sole.** Arthritic changes, trauma, or previous toes surgery may prevent movement of the toe. Palpate for the action of the extensor hallucis longus tendon, if mechanical factors prevent toe movement.
   b. *Most* normal persons tend to withdraw their feet from a plantar stimulus and flex the great toe. The withdrawal movement, like the response to stepping on a tack, consists of dorsiflexion of the ankle and flexion of the knee and hip, a **triple flexion synergy** (Walshe, 1956; van Gijn, 1996a, 1996b). The tensor fasciae latae, hamstrings, and tibialis anterior muscles visibly and palpably contract during this triple flexion synergy. Watch for these actions as you apply the plantar stimulus. Since Babinski's original description, the synergistic extension of the great toe and triple flexion of the ankle, knee, and hip have been considered integral parts of the planter reflex (Babinski, 1896, 1898).
2. The small toes may fan, but this does not constitute a consistent or clinically important part of the plantar reflex.

I. Pathologic variations in the plantar reflexes

1. After interruption of the UMNs to the lumbosacral cord, the great toe extends instead of flexing, a result called an **extensor plantar response, extensor toe sign,** or **Babinski sign** (Fig. 7-33A).

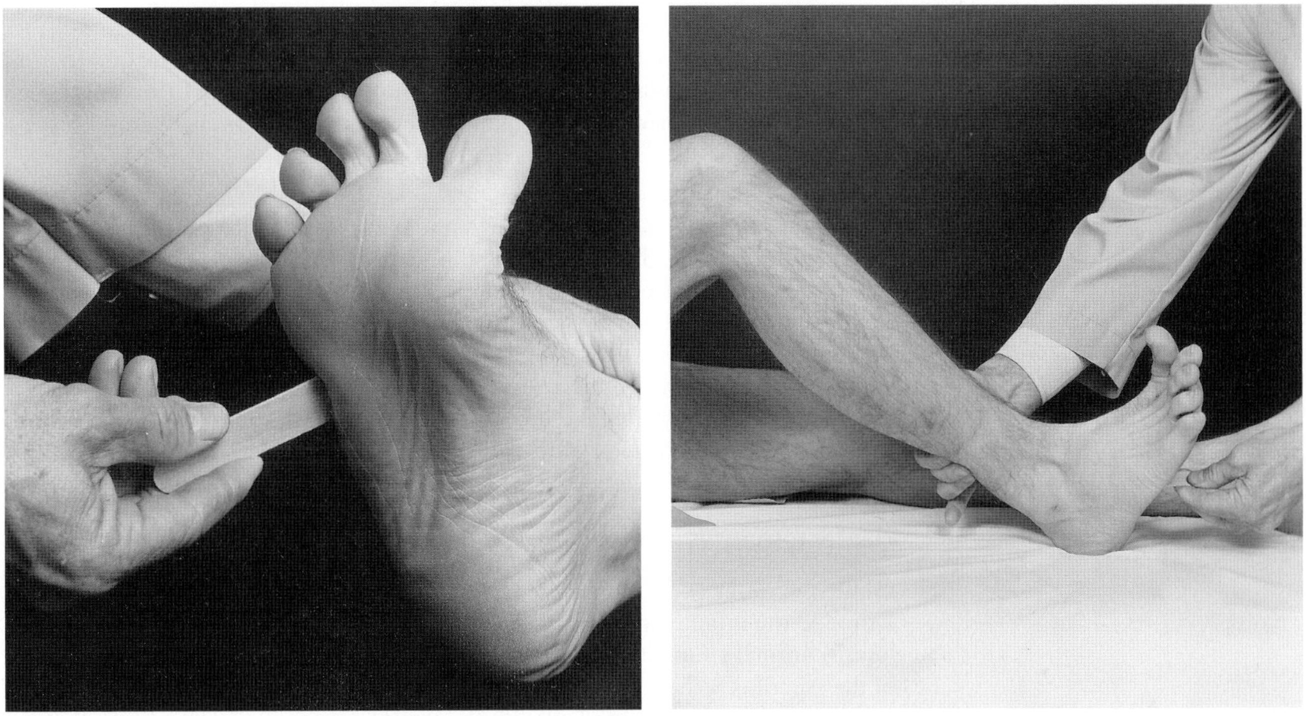

A B

FIGURE 7-33. Abnormal responses to a plantar stimulus. (A) Extension (dorsiflexion) of the great toe in response to a plantar stimulus in a patient with an upper motoneuron lesion. (B) Flexor withdrawal reflex (triple flexion reflex) consisting of dorsiflexion of the ankle and flexion of the knee and hip in response to plantar stimulus.

2. For best communication, simply state that the Pt has a *flexor plantar response* or an *extensor plantar response,* whichever occurred. If you report a Babinski sign, don't redundantly say that the Pt has a positive Babinski sign. There is no negative Babinski sign. The sign, dorsiflexion of the toe, is either present or not.
3. The flexor synergy that tends to withdraw the leg of a normal person after a plantar stimulus usually becomes more prominent and stereotyped in the presence of an extensor toe sign. Although anatomically the upward toe movement is called *extension* and is mediated by the extensor hallucis longus, physiologically the movement shortens the joint angle and, hence, is regarded as flexion, and the movement belongs to the overall flexion synergy of the leg (Fig. 7-33B).
4. Some Pts voluntarily extend or wiggle the big toe, making the response un-readable. After admonishing the Pt to relax, try again. A struggling child or some Pts with involuntary movement disorders or cerebral palsy may inadvertently or spontaneously dorsiflex the great toe and may hold it tonically extended. To identify a true extensor toe sign, carefully notice the relation of the toe extension and the flexion synergy to the plantar stimulus. A true extensor toe sign meets four criteria:
   a. The toe usually begins to extend only *after* the plantar stroke has moved a few centimeters along the sole to produce spatial and temporal summations. In

some Pts, in particular paraplegics, a very slight or brief stimulus, even a puff or air, may provoke extension.

b. The toe remains tonically extended as the plantar stroke continues.

c. Just after release of the stroke, the toe then promptly but slowly returns to the neutral position ("floats" back into neutral position). The mode of return of the toe is as important as the mode of extension in determining the nature of the response.

d. Some degree of a triple flexion synergy always occurs, best monitored by inspection or palpation of the tensor fascia lata muscle.

5. Thus, **the Ex must confirm that the behavior of the toe is indeed related to, provoked by, and dependent on the plantar stimulus, and that any flexion of the leg displays a similar correlation.** To qualify as a reflex, the response should show a "machine-like fatality," to use Sherrington's words.

6. Clinicians interpret the extensor toe response as a sign of *anatomic* or *pathophysiologic* interruption of the pyramidal tract (van Gijn, 1996a, 1996b; Walshe, 1956). No other hypothesis fits the facts as well. Reversible pathophysiologic conditions that result in transient extensor toe signs, with or without the other features of the UMN syndrome, include toxic-metabolic coma, postictal hemiparesis after epileptic seizures (Todd's paralysis), trauma with concussion or contusion, transient ischemic attacks, and hemiplegic migraine. The Pt's prompt and full recovery provides the proof of a transient pathophysiologic state rather than anatomic interruption of the pyramidal pathway (Walshe, 1956).

J. Plantar responses in infants

1. Observers differ as to the frequency of the extensor response in young infants. Examine the infant supine, awake but not crying, and with the head in the midline. **In normal young infants, the toe response varies, depending on the qualities of the stimulus.** When you next examine a young infant, apply a very light stroke with the tip of your fingernail, merely a caress. The toe extends. Then, with the pad of your thumb (not the nail), apply pressure on the ball of the foot. The toe flexes. Neither stimulus will cause any discomfort. The thumb pressure will cause a plantar grasp reflex that competes with toe extension. Then apply a standard plantar stimulus. The response elicited, extension or flexion, depends in large degree on the nature of the stimulus imposed, whether nociceptive, a simple touch or pressure, and the object used to apply the stimulus (Bodensteiner, 1992).

2. Hence, the extension of the great toe, although pathologic in older Pts, does not indicate that the young infant has a UMN lesion. In general, the closer the Pt's age to 1 year, the more constant the flexor response (Zafeiriou et al., 1999).

3. By including the test for the plantar grasp reflex, the Ex adds significant information. It should be active and demonstrable in normal infants. Its absence in the first 6 months correlates with poor neurologic development (Futagi et al., 1999).

Normal infants variably show extensor or flexor toe responses, depending on the nature of the stimulus. In older persons, consistent extensor responses indicate a UMN lesion.

4. Contrast the clinical significance of an extensor toe response in infants and older subjects.

____

____

K. Changes in the stimulus and reflexogenous zone for the plantar reflex after upper motoneuron lesions

1. To elicit a plantar response requires a combination of *site, length, velocity,* and *pressure* of the stimulus. The usual reflexogenous zone for a plantar reflex, either normal or pathologic, is the __________ dermatome. Draw a foot, shade this dermatome, and check it against Fig. 7-29.

S1

2. After severe structural lesions, such as complete spinal cord transection, the extensor toe sign and leg withdrawal lose all local signature or local specificity.

Almost any stimulus of any part of the skin caudal to the level of the lesion results in toe extension, with a strong flexor synergy or flexor spasms.

3. **Additional maneuvers for eliciting superficial toe reflexes**

   a. Many other eponymic maneuvers besides Babinski's elicit toe movement from superficial stimuli (Ghosh and Pradhan, 1998; van Gijn, 1996b). These maneuvers, in particular those outside the S1 dermatome, generally are less effective than stimuli within the S1 dermatome. In normal persons, these stimuli usually fail to elicit toe flexion, but after UMN lesions, they may elicit toe extension, just as with Babinski's maneuver (Fig. 7-33). Ghosh and Pradhan (1998) found that the maneuver of Gonda (Fig. 7-34G) elicits toe extensions more readily than planter stimulation in children with spastic cerebral palsy.

   b. The multitude of eponyms implies that the maneuvers represent different phenomena, but physiologically, as stimuli, the maneuvers betray a unifying simplicity. Do the maneuvers shown in Fig. 7-34 on yourself and a partner, paying attention to the stimulus properties of each maneuver.

Descriptive Name	Eponym	Maneuver
A. Plantar toe reflex	Babinski	Move an object along the lateral aspect of the sole.
B. None	Chaddock	Move an object along the lateral side of the foot.
C. Achilles-toe reflex	Schaeffer	Squeeze hard on the Achilles tendon.
D. Shin-toe reflex	Oppenheim	Press your knuckles on the patient's shin and move them down.
E. Calf-toe reflex	Gordon	Squeeze the calf muscles momentarily.
F. Pinprick-toe reflex	Bing	Make multiple light pinpricks on the dorsolateral surface of the foot.
G. Toe-pull reflex	Gonda, Stransky	Pull the fourth toe outward and downward for a brief time and release suddenly.

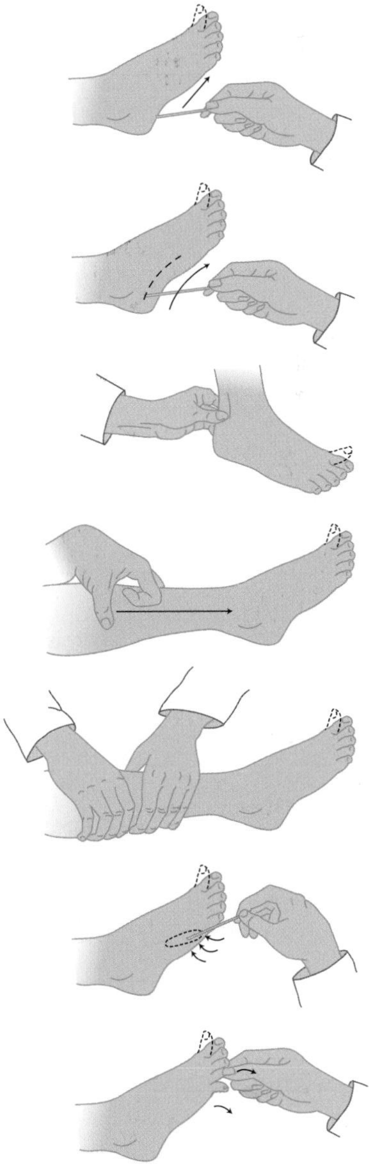

FIGURE 7-34. Methods for eliciting the extensor toe sign.

In each maneuver, the stimulus acts over a certain interval of time, stimulates more than one point of skin, and causes a noxious or uncomfortable sensation. We can infer that these maneuvers act through a spatially and temporally summated, somewhat noxious superficial stimulus to elicit the plantar response (Roby-Brami et al., 1989).

c. Can you recognize the common physiologic features of the stimuli used in Fig. 7-34?

____

____

____

d. You can now discover new signs yourself. Run your thumbnail down your shin: You have now discovered a new sign. Squeeze on a corn (a very effective way to elicit an extensor toe response) and you have another sign, and so on. The response from the S1 dermatome is the most constant and useful. If stimulation of the S1 dermatome produces a convincing, reproducible response, the other maneuvers are superfluous. Sometimes, after an equivocal response to plantar stimulation, doing another maneuver, such as Oppenheim's or Gordon's, simultaneously with the plantar stimulus may enhance toe dorsiflexion.

e. If you want to know all the eponyms to feel educated, try the following mnemonic.

Mnemonic: Eponymic ways to produce an extensor toe sign (Fig. 7-34):
B is for Babinski, stimulate the ***bottom*** of the foot.
C is for Chaddock, stimulate the lateral ***side*** of the foot.
G is for Gonda, ***grasp*** the IV digit.
Go is for Gordon, ***grip*** the calf.
O is for Oppenheim ***on*** the shin maneuver.
S is for Schaeffer, ***squeeze*** the Achilles tendon.

BIBLIOGRAPHY · Extensor Toe Sign and Plantar Responses

Babinski J. Sur le réflexe cutané plantaire dans certains affections organiques du systéme nerveux central. *Compt Rendu Soc Biol* 1896;48:207–208.

Babinski J. Du phénoméne des orteils et de sa valeur sémiologique. *Semin Med* 1898;18:321–322.

Futagi Y, Suzuki, Y, Goto M. Clinical significance of plantar grasp response in infants. *Pediatr Neurol* 1999;20:111–115.

Ghosh D, Pradhan S. Extensor toe sign: by various methods in spastic children with cerebral palsy. *J Child Neurol* 1998;13:216–220.

Lance JW. The Babinski sign. *J Neurol Neurosurg Psychiatry* 2002;73:360–362.

Landau W, Clare M. The plantar reflex in man, with special reference to some conditions where the extensor response is unexpectedly absent. *Brain* 1959;82:321–355.

Roby-Brami A, Ghenassia JR, Bussel B. Electrophysiological study of the Babinski sign in paraplegic patients. *J Neurol Neurosurg Psychiatry* 1989;52:1390–1397.

van Gijn J. *The Babinski sign: a centenary*. Utrecht, Universiteit Utrecht, 1996a.

van Gijn J. The Babinski sign: the first hundred years. *J Neurol* 1996b;243:675–683.

Vlach V. Evolution of skin reflexes in the first years of life. *Dev Med Child Neurol* 1989;31:196–205.

Walshe FMR. The Babinski plantar response, its forms and its physiological and pathological significance. *Brain* 1956;79:529–556.

Zafeiriou D, Tsikoulas IG, Kemenopoulous GM, et al. Plantar response profile of high-risk infants at one year of life. *J Child Neurol* 1999;14:514–517.

L. Reasons for the otherwise puzzling absence of extensor toe signs in patients with upper motoneuron lesions, or how to avoid being fooled

1. **Analysis of a Pt**

A 24-year-old man struck his head on the bottom of a swimming pool when he dove in. The impact forced his head sharply backward. Examination shortly after his neck injury disclosed complete paralysis, absence of all superficial and deep reflexes, and complete anesthesia caudal to C5. Breathing was solely diaphragmatic.

spinal (or neural)

a. Such a phase of complete paralysis, hypotonia, and areflexia after an acute, severe spinal cord injury is called ____________ shock.

b. Within 8 days, his MSRs returned and became very hyperactive. Extensor toe signs appeared and sensation started to return. Within 15 days after injury, the full UMN syndrome was present, but some weak voluntary movements had returned. Eight weeks after the injury, he was able to move all extremities. Six months after the injury, he had slight hyperreflexia of the left leg and a suggestive extensor toe sign on the left, but otherwise walked fairly normally.

c. A contusion of the Pt's spinal cord had temporarily interrupted all impulse transmission through the lesion site. After recovery, he still had residual signs indicating permanent destruction of some UMN axons on the left side of the cord.

d. Thus one reason for absence of an extensor toe sign after UMN lesions is the stage of spinal or cerebral (neural) shock.

2. **Compression damage to the common peroneal nerve**

a. Compression neuropathy of the common peroneal nerve may account for absence of a Babinski sign by interrupting the innervation of the toe extensor muscles. Patients paralyzed from any cause, UMN or LMN, may suffer from compression damage to the common peroneal nerve because the paralyzed leg may rest in outward rotation, in the same position, for long periods. The nerve then gets compressed between the fibular head and the bed surface or bed rail (Fig. 7-35).

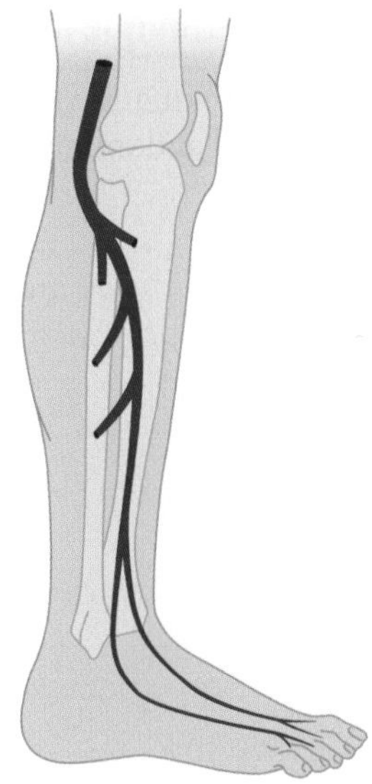

FIGURE 7-35. Course of the common peroneal nerve. Notice how it runs superficial to the fibula, where it is exposed to injury.

b. Feel the head of your fibula. Move your fingertip a half a centimeter or so distally. To feel your common peroneal nerve, press fairly hard and move your fingertip back and forth across the fibula. Because the nerve angles obliquely downward and forward across the fibula (Fig. 7-35), you should feel it slip back and forth under your fingertip.

3. **Common peroneal palsy and foot drop**

a. The common peroneal nerve warps around the fibular head and passes into the "fibular tunnel" (between the peroneus longus muscle and the fibula). Damage to the common peroneal nerve causes a foot drop because it supplies all foot and toe extensors. The Pt cannot dorsiflex the foot and toes, and the toes will drag when the Pt walks. If the Pt recovers from UMN paralysis, such a remaining peroneal palsy precludes a satisfactory gait. The physician has to ensure proper measures to protect the peroneal nerve, ulnar nerve, and other nerves of paralyzed Pts and when applying casts for fractures.

b. **Crossed knee peroneal palsy:** The superficial position of the nerve accounts for a common cause of foot drop, the so-called **crossed knee palsy.** The Pt compresses the nerve when sitting with one knee crossed over the other. Cross your legs and notice how the peroneal nerve may be entrapped between the fibula and the patella and lateral condyle of the opposite knee.

Spinal or cerebral shock; a lesion of the reflex arc, such as peroneal nerve injury; loss of afferent impulses from sensory neuropathy; etc.

4. **Give two basically different reasons for the absence of an extensor toe sign after an undoubted UMN lesion.**

____

____

5. Even after exclusion of all of the foregoing explanations, some Pts with UMN lesions will fail to show an extensor toe sign or other features of the UMN syndrome. Then we have to invoke "biologic variability" but do so only after careful analysis of all the possible pathogenic factors.

BIBLIOGRAPHY · Peroneal Neuropathy

Sourkes M, Stewart JD. Common peroneal neuropathy. A study of selective motor and sensory involvement. *Neurology* 1991;41:1029–1033.

M. Technique for eliciting the superficial abdominal and cremasteric reflexes

1. Stroking the skin of the abdominal quadrants or inner thighs elicits the superficial abdominal and cremasteric reflexes (Fig. 7-36).

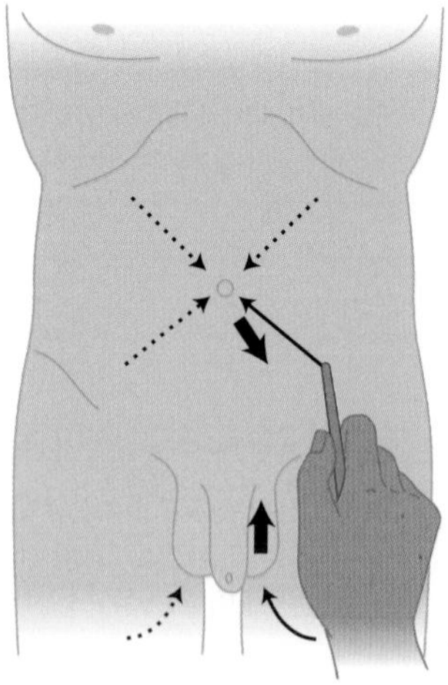

FIGURE 7-36. Method for eliciting the superficial abdominal and cremasteric reflexes. The thin arrows represent the direction of the examiner's stroke. The thick arrows indicate the direction of the response. The umbilicus twitches in the direction of the quadrant stimulated.

2. Using a broken tongue blade, a key, or the blunt end of a reflex hammer, practice obtaining the superficial abdominal reflexes on yourself and a partner. In contrast to the plantar reflex, the stimulus may have to move a little faster, almost a whisk action of the wrist, to elicit the twitch of the umbilicus toward the quadrant

stimulated. The partner may sit or recline. You may be unable to obtain the reflex on yourself, but by trying, you will learn two important things:

a. The stimulus is somewhat unpleasant.

b. Excessive tension in the abdominal muscles obscures the abdominal skin-muscle reflexes. Because you will have to flex or raise your head, you may tense your muscles too much. However, slight abdominal tension may reinforce the response.

3. Normally in response to abdominal skin stimulation, the umbilicus twitches ❒ toward/❒ away from the quadrant stimulated.

☑ toward

4. Normally in response to thigh stimulation of a male, ❒ elevation/❒ depression of the ❒ ipsilateral/❒ contralateral/❒ both testicle(s) occurs. Females, of course, do not exhibit this reflex.

☑ elevation; ☑ ipsilateral

5. The abdominal stimulus has the same properties as the plantar stimulus. If perceived by the Pt, the stimulus is felt as ______________, and it requires ______________ and ______________________ summation.

unpleasant (noxious); spatial; temporal

6. Therefore, in deference to the Pt's comfort, apply the first abdominal stimulus gently.

7. **Effect of UMN lesions on the abdominal and cremasteric reflexes:** These superficial reflexes disappear, at least temporarily, after UMN lesions.

8. **Natural history of the abdominal and cremasteric reflexes**

a. You may find it difficult to elicit abdominal reflexes in normal young infants. The individual, whether infant or adult, has to relax to tolerate the somewhat uncomfortable or tickling sensation produced. Abdominal tension obscures the response. As the infant matures, the abdominal reflexes appear.

b. In normal elderly or obese Pts or in multiparous women with lax abdomens, the abdominal reflex is often absent.

c. In the acute phase of an UMN lesion, the abdominal and cremasteric reflexes are usually absent. Later they may recover. If the brain lesion occurs early in life, as in cerebral palsy, these reflexes regularly return.

9. What two normal features of the superficial reflexes in young infants would indicate UMN interruption in a more mature patient?

____

Extensor toe responses and absence of abdominal reflexes.

N. Anal wink (S2, S3, S4) and bulbocavernosus reflexes (S3, S4)

1. Pricking the skin around the anus causes a quick, twitch-like constriction of the anal sphincter, the so-called **anal wink.** The anal reflex is the first spinal reflex to return after spinal shock (Pedersen et al., 1978).
2. Pricking the glans penis causes reflex contraction of the bulbocavernosus muscle, detected by pressing a (gloved) finger against the Pt's perineum. The pinprick may also elicit an anal wink.
3. Perform these tests to investigate symptoms such as incontinence or impotence that suggest a lesion of the lumbosacral cord, cauda equina, or lumbosacral plexus, not as part of the routine NE. EMG studies of the anal sphincter and anal wink reflex are also helpful (Pedersen et al., 1978).

BIBLIOGRAPHY · Anal Reflexes

Pedersen E, Harving H, Klemar B, et al. Human anal reflexes. *J Neurol Neurosurg Psychiatry* 1978;48:813–818.

O. Recording the reflexes

1. A stick figure conveniently displays several routinely elicited reflexes (Fig. 7-37). Record the MSRs as 0 to 4+; the toe response with an up or down arrow; the

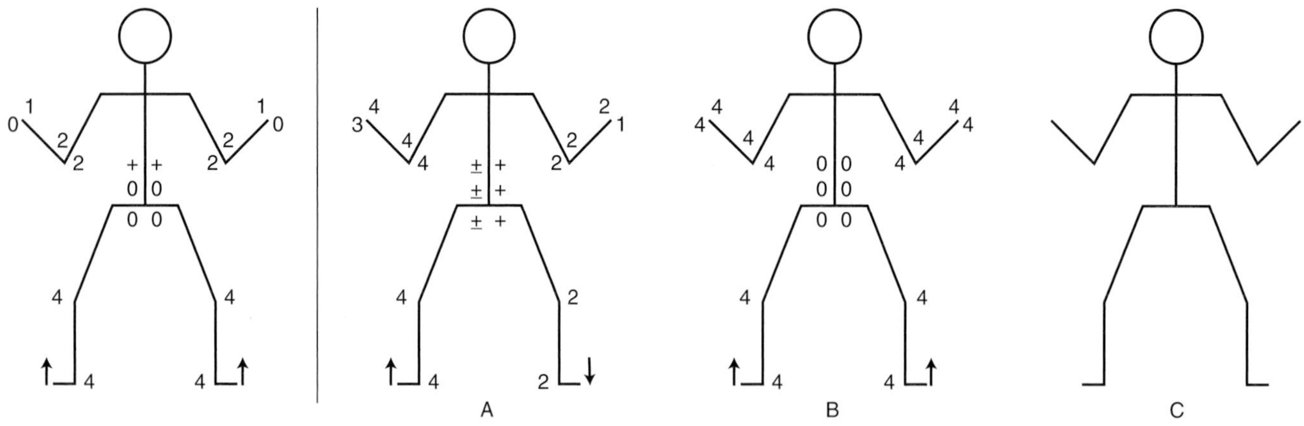

FIGURE 7-37. Recording of reflex changes after upper motoneuron lesions.

abdominal and cremasteric reflexes with a 0 if absent, ± if equivocal or barely present, and + if normally active.

☑ hemiplegia

2. Figure 7-37A depicts ❐ hemiplegia/❐ quadriplegia/❐ paraplegia.

☑ quadriplegia

3. Figure 7-37B depicts ❐ hemiplegia/❐ quadriplegia/❐ paraplegia.
4. **Patient analysis:** Consider a paraplegic Pt with spinal cord transection at the X thoracic level. The IX and X thoracic segments innervate the upper half of the abdomen, the XI and XII the lower. Thus the UMN signs appear only distal to T10. Fill in Fig. 7-37C to show the reflex pattern expected.

The umbilicus would migrate upward (Beevor's sign) because the rectus muscles of the upper part of the abdomen would contract, but the muscles of the lower abdomen would be paralyzed.

5. What direction would the Pt's umbilicus in Fig. 7-37C move if he were supine and attempted to elevate his head and shoulders? Explain.

____

____

6. The Ex can also use the MSR of the abdominal muscles to localize a lesion at T10. Place a finger in each of the four quadrants and tap it briskly, as in eliciting the brachioradialis reflex (Fig. 7-9). The hyperactive response from the two lower quadrants will contrast with the normal or negligible response from the upper two quadrants.

X. SUMMARY OF THE STANDARD "TEXTBOOK" SYNDROMES OF UPPER AND LOWER MOTONEURON LESIONS AND THEIR VARIATIONS

A. Complete Table 7-7 to contrast the typical findings with a chronic upper motoneuron lesion and a chronic lower motoneuron lesion.

B. Clinical variations in the pyramidal (upper motoneuron) syndrome

The level of the lesion along the course of the pyramidal tract (Fig. 2-29) determines the distribution of the weakness and other UMN signs. For the effect on the gait, see the gait essay at the end of Chapter 8.

1. **Standard hemiplegic distribution:** Unilateral interruption of the pyramidal tract at any level from the cortex to the pontomedullary junction causes weakness of the contralateral side of the body, from the lower facial muscles on down (Fig. 6-8B).
   a. The *degree* of paralysis depends on how many of the million or so axons of the pyramidal tract (DeMyer, 1959) the lesion interrupts, and the individual variation in the number of crossed and uncrossed axons.

UMN	LMN
✓	
	✓
✓	
	✓
	✓
✓	
	✓
✓	
	✓
	✓
✓	
✓	

TABLE 7-7 · Clinical Syndrome of UMN versus LMN Lesions

UMN	LMN	Characteristic
		Paralyzes movements in hemiplegic, quadriplegic, or paraplegic distribution, not in individual muscles
		Paralyzes individual muscles or sets of muscles in root or peripheral nerve distributions
		Atrophy of disuse only (late and slight)
		Atrophy of denervation (early and severe)
		Fasciculations and fibrillations
		Hyperactive MSRs
		Hypoactive or absent MSRs
		Clonus
		Clasp-knife spasticity
		Hypotonia
	*	Absent abdominal-cremasteric reflexes
		Extensor toe sign

*Direct disease of the LMNs to the abdominal muscles abolishes these reflexes but disease confined to other LMNs does not.

ABBREVIATIONS: LMN lower motoneuron; MSR muscle stretch reflex; UMN upper motoneuron.

b. The *gradient* and *distribution* of weakness are highly characteristic, essentially pathognomonic, of pyramidal tract interruption at cerebral, midbrain, and pontine levels. The weakness or paralysis involves the contralateral lower facial muscles and the contralateral extremities. Medullary level lesions usually spare the face. In the extremities, the distal muscles are more affected than the proximal, and the finger movements suffer most of all. Unilateral paralysis of the tongue, palate, pharynx, and larynx is unusual, but the ipsilateral sternocleidomastoid is affected (Chapter 6). The opposite hemidiaphragm is weak during volitional breathing but acts bilaterally during automatic breathing (Chapter 6). UMN interruption equally paralyzes flexor and extensor muscles, contrary to traditional opinion (Thijs et al., 1998).

2. **Monoplegia:** A small lesion of the motor cortex or internal capsule, where the pyramidal fibers have a discrete somatotopic arrangement, may cause contralateral weakness of one arm or one leg or, rarely, just one or a few finger movements (Kim, 2002; Takahashi et al., 2002). A lesion of the leg area of its projection fibers will cause a contralateral lower extremity monoplegia. Interruption of the pyramidal tract on one side of the thoracic spinal cord causes a monoplegia of the ipsilateral leg.
3. **Double hemiplegia:** The lesion interrupts both pyramidal tracts somewhere rostral to the pontomedullary junction. The lower part of the face and all four extremities are paralyzed bilaterally. The Pt also shows pseudobulbar palsy.
4. **Spastic diplegia:** Bilateral pre- or perinatal cerebral lesions may result in a bilateral pyramidal syndrome, but with the legs more affected than the arms, and the bulbar muscles relatively spared. This reverses the arm-leg gradient of the weakness of double hemiplegia. Spastic diplegics often display involuntary movements such as athetosis.
5. **Pseudobulbar palsy:** Bilateral interruption of the corticobulbar component of the pyramidal tract (or all of the tract, at cerebral or brainstem levels) causes bilateral weakness of the oropharyngeal muscles with dysphagia, dysarthria, and spastic dysphonia, but the Pt shows exaggerated smiling and crying (Chapter 6).
6. **Locked-in syndrome:** Bilateral interruption of the pyramidal tracts in the basis pontis or cerebral peduncles causes UMN paralysis of all volitional movements except vertical eye movements. The Pts remain conscious and not demented but are "locked-in" to themselves by the paralysis. See Chapter 12.
7. **Quadriplegia (tetraplegia):** Bilateral interruption of the pyramidal tracts in the caudal medulla or cervical region spares the face but paralyzes the volitional movements of the trunk and all four extremities. The Pt loses volitional bladder and bowel control and volitional control of breathing. The lesion spares those corticobulbar fibers to the face and bulbar muscles that depart rostral to the medullary level (Chokroverty et al., 1975; Ropper et al., 1979).

8. **Paraplegia:** Bilateral interruption of the pyramidal tracts caudal to the cervical region spares the arms but causes paralysis of the legs, with loss of bladder and bowel control.

C. A warning about the presence or absence of muscle stretch reflexes in relation to upper and lower motoneuron lesions

1. Although the general rule that LMN lesions cause hyporeflexia or areflexia and UMN lesions cause hyperreflexia holds, you now know that, in the acute phase of UMN lesions, the MSRs may be temporarily absent.
2. In the Guillain-Barré (Landry-Guillain-Barré-Strohl) syndrome of polyneuropathy, the Pt typically suffers an ascending flaccid paralysis, beginning in the lower extremities. Typically also the Pt has the expected areflexia. In some Pts with the axonal form of this neuropathy, the MSRs are preserved or even hyperactive (Yuki and Hirata, 1998). Thus the distinction between a central or peripheral paralysis, that is, between a *neuropathy* and a *myelopathy*, becomes difficult on clinical grounds alone. The EMG aids materially in the differential diagnosis by placing the lesion in the peripheral nervous system and in differentiating the demyelinating from axonal forms of the syndrome (Van Dijk et al., 1999).

D. Review of paralysis and sensory deficits immediately after acute spinal cord transection

1. Spinal cord transection at the medullocervical junction or at segments C1 to C3 (Fig. 2-5) results in complete apnea, complete quadriplegia, and complete anesthesia caudal to the lesion. The Pt dies of hypoxia within minutes unless given artificial respiration. The blood pressure also drops because interruption of the reticulospinal tracts stops the down flow of vasoconstrictor tone to the preganglionic sympathetic neurons in the intermediolateral column of the spinal cord. The sensorimotor deficits affect only the trunk and legs if the lesion is caudal to T1 (paraplegia).
2. During the stage of spinal shock, the Pt loses all somatomotor and most visceromotor responses caudal to the level of the lesion. The Pt shows flaccid paralysis of somatic muscles and sphincters and flaccid (atonic) bladder and bowel paralysis, with incontinence. All superficial and deep reflexes and most autonomic reflexes are abolished. If any visceral-related function remains, it is usually anal sphincter tone.
3. Gradually the classic UMN signs of increased MSRs, spasticity, and extensor toe signs will appear, as will reflex emptying of the bladder and bowel. In contrast, slowly evolving spinal cord compression results in spastic paralysis from the start. The Pt does not go through a phase of spinal shock.
4. After the phase of spinal shock, the transected spinal cord, isolated from the brain, can mediate simple actions such as MSRs and flexor withdrawal reflexes. It can also mediate reflex sweating, piloerection, micturition, defecation, and ejaculation (although the Pt feels no sensation), but it cannot produce any voluntary movements, respiratory drive, or respiratory-related reflexes such as coughing, sneezing, and hiccoughing. These reflexes require coordination of bulbar and spinal muscles. In summary, the isolated spinal cord can reflexly twitch some muscles, sweat, ejaculate and reflexly eliminate urine and feces, but the isolated spinal cord cannot breathe or make voluntary movements. These actions require intact reticulospinal and corticospinal tracts from the brain.

E. Patient analysis

1. **Medical history:** This 61-year-old man awakened one morning with double vision and inability to move his right side. He noticed mild numbness and tingling of his right side. When he called to his wife, he noticed slurring of his speech. He had been diabetic and hypertensive for many years.

2. **Physical findings:** The Pt was conscious, cooperative, and intact mentally. His left eye turned down and out, and the pupil was dilated. He could not adduct it. He had mild dysarthria. He had severe weakness of the right extremities, including the lower part of his face on the right. His right extremities were flaccid and somewhat hyporeflexic. He had a flexor plantar response on the left but little response at all on the right. He responded somewhat less to pain and touch on the right side.

3. **Lesion localization**

   a. Before continuing with the text, you may want to propose where and what the lesion is. It may help you to review the brainstem cross sections shown in Figs. 2-15 to 2-18.

   b. In localizing a single lesion to explain the Pt's findings, first assemble the data that require explanation. The flaccidity and weakness, in a hemiplegic distribution, indicates interruption of the pyramidal tract in the acute stage of shock. The slight sensory findings suggest some involvement of a sensory pathway. The pupillodilation, down and out position of the left eye, and inability to adduct it indicates a III nerve palsy. Therefore the Ex should "think circuitry" by visualizing the course of the pyramidal tract to try to locate a site where it comes into anatomic relation with a somatosensory pathway and CrN III.

   c. The association of an LMN III nerve palsy on the *left* and *hemiplegia* of the *right* extremities suggests a lesion in the basis of the ❐ mesencephalon/ ❐ pons/❐ medulla on the ❐ right/❐ left side.

☑ mesencephalon; ❐ left (Fig. 2-16)

   d. Slight involvement of the medial lemniscus on the left could explain the sensory deficit on the right and indicate extension of the lesion from the basis into the tegmentum.

   e. Magnetic resonance imaging showed patchy lucencies in the midbrain tegmentum and an overt infarct in the midbrain basis, where CrN III runs through it medially. At the midbrain level, the pathway for somatic sensation via the medial lemniscus had crossed the midline. Review Fig. 2-18 to see how a midbrain lesion could explain the III nerve palsy, right-sided pyramidal tract signs, and right-sided sensory findings. The Pt had the classic localizing findings of a brainstem lesion: a cranial nerve palsy on one side, and long tract signs on the other (Fig. 6-19).

   f. What normal findings in this Pt would indicate that the lesion for the most part spares the dorsal part of the midbrain? (**Hint:** Review Figs. 2-18 and Fig. 6-19 to see what structures would have caused clinical signs if they had been destroyed. Does he show signs of the rostral midbrain syndrome (Table 5-2), or cerebellar signs in the left extremities?)

   ____

   ____

Extensive, particularly bilateral midbrain tegmental lesions would cause ataxia or tremor of the left extremities, palsy of CrN III on the left, disturbances of vertical gaze, convergence nystagmus, worse sensory loss, or coma.

4. **Clinical course:** After several days the MSRs on the right became hyperactive, and spasticity, clonus, and a classic extensor toe sign appeared. The Pt did not regain any useful movements of his arm or fingers and could only walk when he wore a brace to support his knee. The III nerve palsy improved, but he remained with diplopia. The sensory loss disappeared, indicating only a transient ischemia of the medial lemniscus.

5. **Course of corticobulbar fibers to the facial nucleus**

   a. Because the Pt's hemiparesis included his face, the corticobulbar axons must have been in the basis of the midbrain. Infarcts of the basis pontis typically affect the face. The much rarer infarcts of the basis of the medulla (the medullary pyramids) often spare the face. What do these facts tell you about how far down the brainstem the fibers to the face travel?

   ____

   ____

The corticobulbar fibers generally accompany the other pyramidal tract fibers to the caudal end of the pons before departing for the CrN VII nucleus in the pontine tegmentum. Medullary pyramid lesions usually spare the UMN facial fibers, because they have already left the tract (Ropper et al, 1979).

BIBLIOGRAPHY · The Pyramidal Tract

Bodensteiner JB. Plantar responses in infants. *J Child Neurol* 1992;7:311–313.

Chokroverty S, Rubino F, Haller C. Pure motor hemiplegia due to pyramidal infarction. *Arch Neurol* 1975;32:647–648.

DeMyer W. Number of axons and myelin sheaths in adult human medullary pyramids. *Neurology* 1959;9:42–47.

Jagiella WM, Sung JH. Bilateral infarction of the medullary pyramids in humans. *Neurology* 1989;39:21–24.

Kim JS, Chung JP, Ha SW. Isolated weakness of the index finger due to small cortical infarction. *Neurology* 2002;58:985–986.

Lenn NJ, Freinkel AJ. Facial sparing as a feature of prenatal-onset hemiparesis. *Pediatr Neurol* 1989;5:291–295.

Nyberg-Hansen R, Rinvik E. Some comments on the pyramidal tract with special reference to its individual variations in man. *Acta Neurol Scand* 1963;39:1–30.

Paulsen GW, Yates AJ, Paltan-Ortiz JD. Does infarction of the medullary pyramid lead to spasticity? *Arch Neurol* 1986;43:93–95.

Ropper AJ, Fisher CM, Kleinman GM. Pyramidal infarction in the medulla: a cause of pure motor hemiplegia sparing the face. *Neurology* 1979;29:91–95.

Takahashi N, Kawamura M, Araki S. Isolated hand palsy due to cortical infarction; motor hand area. *Neurology* 2002;58:1412–1414.

Thijs RD, Notermans NC, Wokke JHJ, et al. Distribution of muscle weakness of central and peripheral origin. *J Neurol Neurosurg Psychiatry* 1998;65:794–796.

Walshe F. On the role of the pyramidal system in willed movements. *Brain* 1947;70:329–354.

Yuki N, Hirata K. Preserved tendon reflexes in Campylobacter neuropathy. *Ann Neurol* 1998;43:546–547.

XI. THE CONCEPT OF DEFICIT AND RELEASE PHENOMENA AFTER LESIONS OF THE MOTOR PATHWAYS

Upon this gifted age, in its dark hour,
Rains from the sky a meteoric shower
Of facts... they lie unquestioned, uncombined,
Wisdom enough to leech us of our ill
Is daily spun, but there exists no loom
To weave it into fabric, ...

—Edna St. Vincent Millay (1892–1950)

A. The theory of deficit and release phenomena

By this time, the array of positive and negative effects of neurologic lesions may seem puzzling, but we can subsume them under a theory of deficit and release phenomena.

1. **Deficit phenomena** are sensorimotor functions that the Pt loses after a neurologic lesion, e.g., loss of movement or loss of vision.
2. **Release phenomena** are sensorimotor functions that increase or first emerge after a neurologic lesion. The release phenomenon may consist of an exaggeration of a normal action, e.g., hyperactive MSRs, or a new response, e.g., the change in the behavior of the large toe from flexion to extension (Babinski sign).

B. Deficit and release phenomena after upper motoneuron (pyramidal) lesions

1. Review the components of the UMN syndrome (Table 7-7) and list the deficit and release phenomena seen in the classic or chronic stage.
   a. Deficit phenomena:

   ____

   ____

Paresis or paralysis, mild disuse atrophy, and absence of abdominal and cremasteric reflexes that may return.

Hyperactive MSRs, clonus, spasticity, and an extensor toe sign.

b. Release phenomena:

____

____

☑ release
It is a new behavior or response not present before the UMN lesion and is unmasked or released by the UMN lesion.

2. The extensor toe sign would be classed as a ❐ deficit/❐ release phenomenon because

____

____

☑ deficit; ☑ release

3. In the acute phase after pyramidal tract interruption, particularly after spinal cord transection, the Pt may show only ❐ deficit/❐ release and no ❐ deficit/❐ release phenomena.

C. Pathophysiology of release phenomena

1. Release phenomena appear because the lesion has interrupted connections that presumably inhibited or suppressed the overactive function and because some intact pathway positively drives the overactivity.
2. Whether interruption of the pyramidal tract alone accounts for all of the release phenomena of the UMN syndrome remains unclear, but the clinician will make few errors in localization by assuming that pyramidal tract interruption is a necessary and sufficient condition for the full UMN syndrome to appear. However, involvement of other sensory and motor pathways may condition the expression and degree of the various components of the UMN syndrome.

D. Deficit and release phenomena after lower motoneuron lesions

By a stretch of the imagination, we can extend the deficit-release concept to the peripheral nervous system and even the sensory pathways.

1. **Deficit phenomena** after LMN lesions consist of:
   a. Paresis or paralysis of individual muscles in a segmental or peripheral nerve distribution.
   b. Decreased or absent MSRs.
   c. Denervation atrophy (early and severe atrophy).
2. **Release phenomena** after LMN lesions consist of:
   a. Fasciculations.
   b. Fibrillations.
3. Regarding fasciculations, the disease of the LMN "releases" the depolarization mechanism of its own neuronal membrane, allowing the motor unit to fire randomly. In the case of fibrillations, the denervation "releases" the depolarization mechanism of the individual muscle fibers, allowing them to fire randomly.

E. Deficit phenomena after interruption of autonomic motor axons

1. Paralysis and atony of smooth muscle, thus abolishing peristalsis, propulsion, and emptying.
2. Vasomotor paralysis, with vasodilation, orthostatic hypotension, and impotence.
3. Anhidrosis.
4. Trophic changes consisting of hair loss, atrophy of skin, and dystrophy of nails.

F. Autonomic release or irritative phenomena after peripheral nerve lesions

In certain instances, lesions of peripheral nerves (or spinal cord lesions) release autonomic signs consisting of hyperhidrosis or vasoconstriction, rather than anhidrosis and vasodilation (see causalgia in Chapter 10).

G. Deficit and release phenomena after lesions of the basal motor nuclei

See Section M, page 303.

XII. INVOLUNTARY MOVEMENT DISORDERS

A. Introduction to the concept of voluntary and involuntary movements and the notion of free will

1. We experience ourselves as having free will. This experience leads us to classify behaviors intuitively as *voluntary* and *involuntary*. But then we must puzzle over behaviors such as breathing, bladder and bowel emptying, and postural reflexes that straddle the voluntary-involuntary dichotomy. For example, you can freely will yourself to hold your breath for a period of time, but ultimately you simply have to breathe. You have no choice. The physiologic imperative to act (i.e., to emit a certain behavior) overpowers the will. Mentally ill Pts often experience their behaviors and even their very thoughts as involuntary or directed by external forces. Thus, Pts come to the physician because they experience behaviors and thoughts that they cannot willfully control.
2. By virtue of operational definitions, we can identify certain movements and behaviors that we can agree to class as voluntary or involuntary.

B. Working definition of voluntary and involuntary movements (behaviors)

1. A **voluntary** movement is one that the standard normal person can start or stop at the person's own command or an observer's command.
2. An **involuntary** movement is one that the standard normal person does not start and cannot stop at the person's own or an observer's command.
   a. As strictly construed by neurologists, *involuntary movements* mean those patterns of muscle contractions (tremors and other movement sequences) caused by identifiable structural or biochemical lesions in the circuitry of the basal motor nuclei, reticular formation, and cerebellum.
   b. Broadly construed, the concept of *involuntary movements* can also include the gamut of muscle fiber contractions of peripheral and central origins, extending from fibrillations to epileptic seizures.
3. Write out the definition of behavior given in Chapter 1, page 1:

   ____

   ______________________________.
4. Reread the statements in B1 to 2 a and 2b above and substitute the word *behavior* for *movement*. It will give you a different feeling for the definition of behavior.

C. Clinical operations for identifying voluntary and involuntary movements

Neurologic lesions result in patterns of involuntary movements, recognizable from the history, inspection, and sometimes requiring laboratory tests, as for fasciculations. The operations for clinical analysis of involuntary movements follow.

1. Find out when the movements started, what conditions trigger or alleviate the movements, their relation to sleep and emotion, and their evolution over time. In other words, what is the history?
2. Describe the pattern of the movements, their distribution, rate, amplitude, and force. In other words, what are the physical findings?
3. Inspection is pivotal, allowing recognition without recourse to the Pt's testimony, in most cases. To see is to diagnose, because most involuntary movements fall into stereotyped, identifiable patterns (Fig. 15-4).

D. Some normal involuntary movements

1. **Physiologic synkinesia (*syn* = with; *kinesis* motion)**: A **synkinesis** is an involuntary or automatic movement that accompanies a voluntary movement. If you voluntarily close your eyes, your eyeballs automatically roll up (Bell's phenomenon).

Walk and your arms swing. Lean forward and your leg muscles automatically brace. Use these examples to identify other synkinesias (**Hint:** What about convergence of the eyes?). The degree of volition in the synkinesias varies. You can't stop Bell's phenomenon, but you can stop your arms from swinging when you walk.

2. **Myoclonic jerks**
   a. Myoclonic jerks are sudden, brief, shock-like, involuntary twitches of individual muscles or sets of muscles. A myoclonic twitch may appear in a single muscle, such as the biceps, perhaps after unaccustomed work. Or a more widespread startle response may cause an upright jerk of the head as when the person is falling asleep. A sudden discharge in the reticular activating system of the brainstem causes the lightening, myoclonic jerk of the head and the sudden restoration of consciousness. Myoclonus may occur at rest or provoked by voluntary action (action myoclonus), or triggered by diverse stimuli (stimulus-sensitive or reflex myoclonus).
   b. Epileptic myoclonic jerks, often refractory to treatment, occur in many CNS diseases. What is *physiologic* under one circumstance is *pathologic* under another.
   c. Myoclonic jerks are separate from fasciculations. Define a fasciculation.
   ____
   ____

   A fasciculation is a muscular twitch caused by random discharge of an LMN and its fascicle of muscle fibers (a motor unit discharge).

   d. A twitch of the entire muscle or groups of muscles is called a ______________ jerk, whereas a twitch of a single fascicle of muscle is called a ______________.

   myoclonus; fasciculation

3. **Benign fasciculations**
   a. Fasciculations appear in some normal persons, particularly after exercise. If the person has no weakness or other signs of LMN disease, the diagnosis is *benign fasciculations*. Twitching of an eyelid is an example.
   b. What clinical and EMG findings would differentiate pathologic from benign fasciculations?
   ____
   ____

   If LMN disease causes the fasciculations, the Ex should find the full syndrome of LMN disease: weakness, hypoor areflexia, hypotonia, and denervation atrophy, as supported by fibrillations and giant polyphasic motor units in the EMG.

4. **Physiologic tremor:** See next section.

E. Tremors

1. **Definition:** Tremors are rhythmic, involuntary, oscillations of one or more regions of the body (Fig. 7-38).
2. **Clinical characteristics of tremors:** Types of tremors differ in *distribution*, *rate*, and *amplitude* and whether they occur at *rest* or during *voluntary muscular contractions*. They also differ in response to drugs, in response to sleep and emotion, and in pathogenesis.
   a. **Distribution:** Tremors most commonly affect the head, jaw, tongue, palate, and hands but may affect the trunk or legs.
   b. **Rate:** Tremors vary in rate between 3 and 12 cps.
   c. **Amplitude:** Tremors vary from barely perceptible to gross.
   d. **Relation to rest and volitional muscular contractions:** Tremors dichotomize into two main groups: *rest* tremor and *action* tremors. Action tremors appear during voluntary muscular contractions, either to move a part or to maintain a voluntary posture. Action tremors include postural, kinetic, isometric, and task-specific types (Fig. 7-38).
   e. **Response of tremors to drugs:** Drugs may increase or decrease tremor. Tremors commonly accompany lithium treatment. Anticholinergic drugs or dopamine decrease the tremor of parkinsonism. Alcohol and propranolol decrease physiologic or essential tremor, whereas adrenalin increases them. Tremors, "the shakes," commonly follow withdrawal from alcohol and other drugs.

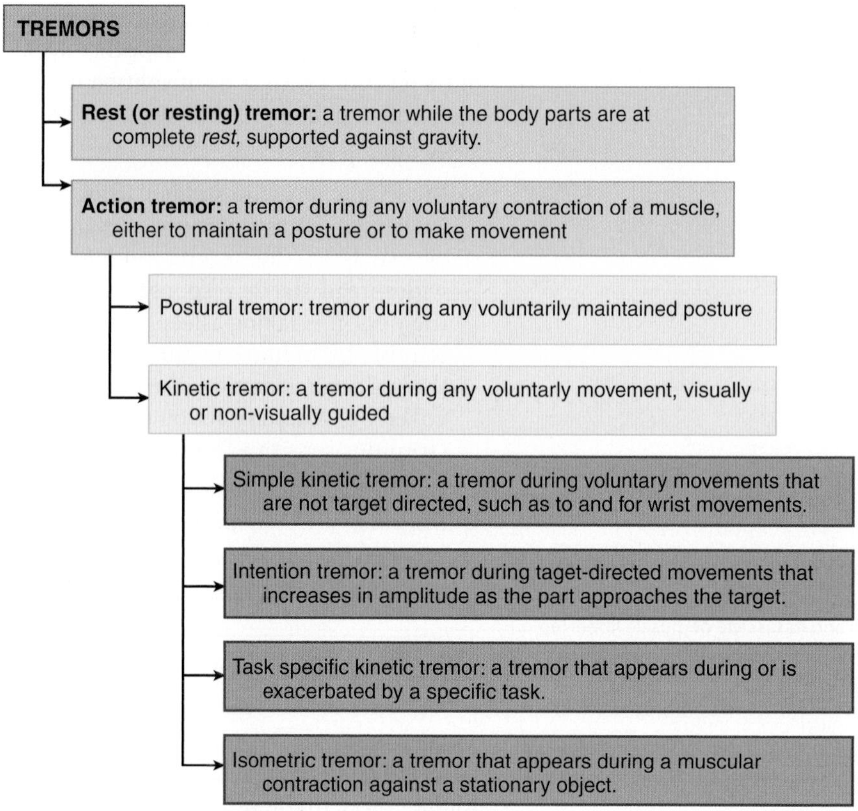

FIGURE 7-38. Classifications of tremors.

f. **Response of tremors to sleep and emotion:** Like virtually all involuntary movements, tremors generally increase during emotional stress but dampen or disappear during tranquility and cease during sleep (Chokroverty et al., 2002).

g. **Lesion site for tremors:** No single "tremorogenic" center exists. Tremors generally arise from disruption of the feedback circuits of the basal motor nuclei (Fig. 2-31), inferior olivary nucleus, and the cerebellum. Occasionally tremors occur with peripheral neuropathies.

3. **Clinical characteristics of tremor types:** Inspect the Pt for tremors under three conditions: *rest, maintaining a posture,* and *during movement* (Bain, 2002).

a. **Rest (or resting) tremor** is a tremor when the body parts are at complete *rest,* supported against gravity. Have the Pt sit with the arms relaxed and the forearms supported by the thighs or recline. Look for a tremor of the fingers and hands.

i. Rest tremor generally *disappears* during voluntary movement but *increases* during mental stress such as counting backward or when walking or moving another body part.

ii. The Ex can bring out a minimal or inapparent tremor or increase the amplitude of a rest tremor of the hands by having the Pt move the head from side to side (Froment's maneuver).

iii. Rest tremor is highly characteristic of parkinsonism.

b. **Postural or position maintenance tremor** occurs during the maintenance of any intentional posture, such as holding the head up, the trunk erect, or the arms out stretched. Postural tremor qualifies as an *action tremor* (Fig. 7-38) because the "action" refers to the sustained volitional contraction to hold the part in position. The hands, when extended in front, show a regular, rhythmic tremor of several cycles per second. If the Pt brings the finger in to touch his nose, intention tremor may appear. As the finger approaches the nose and the Pt attempts to stop the finger to maintain a position, the tremor reappears or heightens as an *end point* or *terminal tremor*. When the finger actually touches the nose, the tremor may or may not dampen. When the Pt returns his hands to his lap, at rest, any such action tremor disappears.

c. **Kinetic tremor** or **intention tremor** (also called *ataxic tremor*) may appear during any voluntary movement. At rest, the hand remains still, but upon movement, as when the Pt does the finger-to-nose test, mild to moderate deviations detour the part from a straight line path. *Intention* and end-point *tremor* appear in various degrees and combinations. They implicate a lesion of the cerebellum or its efferent pathways.

d. **Task-specific tremors** appear during defined tasks, such as writing. An **orthostatic tremor,** a very fine, rapid, 16-cps tremor of the legs appears mainly when the Pt stands, usually combined with a general feeling of unsteadiness. Some patients experience sudden falls. Listening to the muscles with the bell of the stethoscope may demonstrate the tremor (Gershlager et al., 2004). **Isometric tremor** appears during a sustained muscular contraction against a stationary object.

e. **Mixed tremors:** A particular type of mixed tremor that appears at rest, while maintaining a posture, and that becomes severe during voluntary movement often follows trauma to the midbrain or other midbrain lesions (Samie et al., 1990). Because the lesion affects the region of the red nucleus, this mixed type of tremor is called **rubral** or **Holmes' tremor,** implying a lesion of the dentatorubral or dentatothalamic tract, in the superior cerebellar peduncle pathway (Samie et al., 1990). Holmes' tremor mainly involves the hand and proximal arm, and is mostly unilateral. Dystonic tremor is a postural and kinetic tremor, usually not present at rest, and typically involving the body part affected by dystonia (Deuschl, 2003).

F. Kymographic records of tremors

1. From these kymographic recordings, identify the type of tremor and the pathophysiologic basis:

   a. The Pt is sitting quietly in a chair. An accelerometer attached to a hand records this tremor (Fig. 7-39).

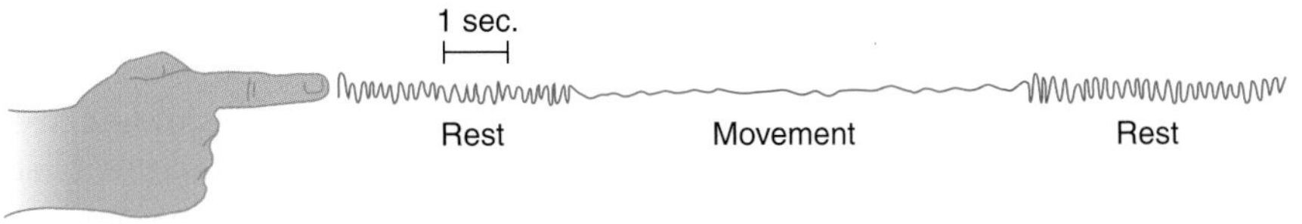

FIGURE 7-39. Kymographic record of tremor.

5 or 6

   b. The rate of the tremor is about ____ cps.

☑ rest

   c. Because the tremor occurs at rest but disappears during intentional movement, it qualifies as a ❒ rest/❒ intention/❒ postural tremor.

parkinsonism

   d. This type of tremor signifies a lesion of the extrapyramidal pathways and is characteristic of the disorder called ________________ (eponym).

2. The next Pt was sitting quietly, holding her arms extended in front, at shoulder level. Only a faint instability appeared. Figure 7-40 shows the tremor when the Pt attempted to touch her index finger to her nose. After she reached her nose, the tremor increased somewhat.

kinetic, intention, or ataxic

   a. The tremor illustrated in Fig. 7-40 is called ________________ tremor.

☑ cerebellar

   b. It signifies a lesion of the ❒ pyramidal/❒ basal ganglia/❒ cerebellar pathways.

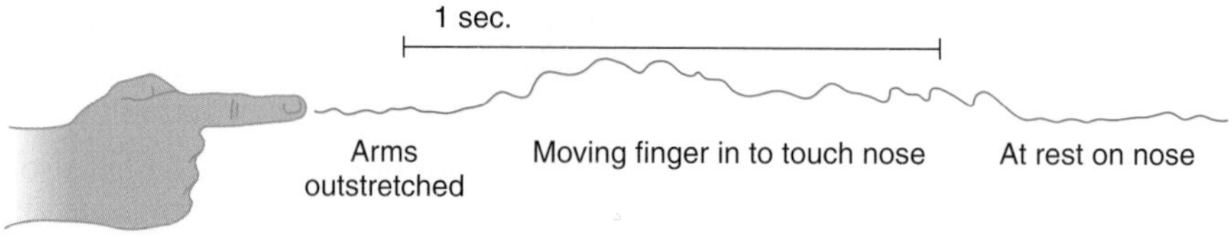

FIGURE 7-40. Kymographic record of tremor.

☑ postural

3. The next Pt had no tremor when sitting still, but when she held her arms straight out, a tremor appeared (Fig. 7-41).
   a. After she reached her nose, the tremor was accentuated. The tremor shown in the initial phase (Fig. 7-41), when the Pt was holding her arms extended and still, is called ❐ resting/❐ physiological/❐ postural tremor.

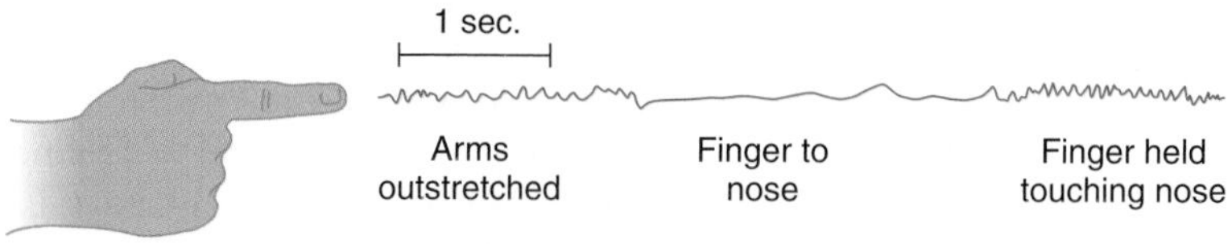

FIGURE 7-41. Kymographic record of tremor.

cerebellum

☑ parkinsonian

Parkinsonian tremor appears at rest, has a low amplitude and a regular frequency of around 5 cps, disappears during intentional movement and sleep, and increases during emotional stress.

   b. It signifies a lesion of the ________________ or its efferent pathways.
   c. Because it may dampen during movement, postural tremor is like ❐ parkinsonian/❐ intention/❐ essential tremor.
   d. Give the full clinical characteristics of parkinsonian tremor.

   ____

   ____

G. Clinical features of several common tremor syndromes

1. **Physiologic tremor**
   a. **Self-demonstration of physiologic tremor:** Insert a large sheet of paper between your index finger and the adjacent finger and hold your arm straight out in front of you. The rustling of the paper demonstrates *physiologic tremor*. The tremor has a frequency of about 10 cps.
   b. Physiologic tremor is generally low in amplitude, relatively rapid (6 to 13 cps), and is most evident during movement or when a part sustains a posture. It varies from 6 cps in childhood, to 8 to 13 cps in adulthood, and back to around 6 cps in senility.
   c. Physiologic tremor arises from a combination of neurally mediated oscillations and the ballistic effects of respiratory and cardiac actions (ballistocardiogram). Thus, it has neurologic and mechanical origins.
2. **Emotional tremor,** a normal phenomenon, to be distinguished from psychogenic tremor, is an enhanced physiologic tremor. It occurs at rest, but it worsens during volitional movement: Witness the quivering knees and quivering voice of the novice orator. From personal experience you know that emotional tremor is ❐ rapid/❐ very slow and of ❐ very great/❐ relatively low amplitude.

☑ rapid; ☑ relatively low

3. **Essential (familial) tremor**
   a. This autosomal dominant or sporadic disorder resembles physiologic tremor in frequency, with a range of 4 to 12 cps, but has a greater amplitude.

b. It affects the hands predominantly but may affect the head, bulbar muscles, and voice (Lou and Jankovic, 1989; Louis, 2001). It typically appears during a sustained posture but may appear during voluntary movements. It generally dampens or disappears with the Pt at rest. Tremors involving the tongue, trunk and lower limbs are rarely encountered.

c. The lesion site is unknown (Rajput et al., 1991).

4. **Essential palatal tremor versus symptomatic palatal tremor (palatal myoclonus)**

a. Palatal tremor has the characteristics of essential tremor. The Pt may experience an audible click. The tremor disappears during sleep.

b. A disorder formerly called *palatal myoclonus* has a frequency of 110 to 160 beats/min. It may affect other bulbar muscles derived from the branchial arches. It violates the law of disappearance of involuntary movements during sleep because it persists. It follows, with variable delays, lesions in the triangle between the cerebellum red nucleus, central tegmental tract, and inferior olivary nucleus (Mollaret's triangle).

5. **Senile tremor** has a frequency of about 6 to 10 cps. Senile and familial tremors merge in their clinical manifestations, but senile tremor, although frequently familial, may result from nonfamilial lesions of aging.

6. **Parkinsonian tremor** (Jankovic and Tolosa, 1998)

a. Parkinsonian tremor has a frequency of 3 to 6 cps and low to moderate amplitude. Drum your fingertips on the table, timing 25 beats per 5 seconds, to observe two features of this tremor: moderate frequency and relatively low amplitude. It appears when the part is at rest, increases during mental and emotional tension, but disappears or dampens during intentional movement, and is absent during sleep. Often it appears asymmetrically. Typically affecting the hands and digits, the rustling of the thumb against the pads of the fingers resembles pill-rolling; hence its name, *pill-rolling tremor*. Voluntary head movements enhance the tremor (**Froment's maneuver**).

b. A 4- to 8-cps postural tremor occurs also about as often as the classic rest tremor (Brooks, 2002).

c. Degeneration of the dopaminergic pathway that runs from the substantia nigra of the midbrain to the striatum causes parkinsonism, but other neurons also degenerate. The parkinsonian triad of *rest tremor, lead-pipe rigidity,* and *hypokinesia* may appear as an entity or with associated widespread neuronal degeneration, known as the **Parkinson plus syndromes** (Victor and Ropper, 2001).

d. Parkinsonian tremor differs from most tremors by ❐ increasing/❐ decreasing during volitional movement, and resembles other involuntary movements by ❐ increasing/❐ decreasing during emotional stress and ❐ increasing/❐ disappearing during sleep.

☑ decreasing; ☑ increasing; ☑ disappearing

e. The rest tremor of parkinsonism, a hyperkinesia, contrasts with a reduction in the overall mobility of the Pt, called **bradykinesia** or **hypokinesia.** Paradoxically, an irresistible need to move, a physiologic imperative called **akathisia** (see Section XII P) also plagues the Pt, requiring abrupt, restless shifts of position against the background of bradykinesia and muscular rigidity. In a given Pt, one or more of the signs may predominate. Thus, one Pt displays mainly tremor and the next mainly rigidity. The basic motor signs of parkinsonism include a quatrain of:

i. Rest tremor

ii. Lead-pipe rigidity, often with a "cogwheeling," ratchet-like yielding due to the superimposition of the beats of the tremor

iii. Overall bradykinesia

iv. Postural instability

f. Derivative signs of the rigidity of the laryngeal muscles are loss of inflections of the voice, resulting in a characteristic monotonous tone, i.e., *plateau speech*, and words running together (Caekebeke et al., 1991). Rigidity of the facial muscles results in an absence of emotional expression, i.e., a *masked face*.

g. **Oculogyric crises** are spasms of upward deviation of the eyes or of the eyes and head. Common in post-encephalitic parkinsonism, oculogyric crises may occur in other disorders of the basal motor nuclei. Summarize for yourself the motor manifestations of parkinsonism.

h. Neurologic evaluation scales for following the course of parkinsonism document changes in their status (Gollomp, 2002; www.wemove.org).

7. **Neuropathic tremor:** This tremor, usually an action type, occurs with a variety of acquired or hereditary peripheral neuropathies, more commonly with demyelinating than with axonal types (Bain, 2002). The tremors are mainly postural and action tremors.

8. **Drug-induced and toxic tremors:** A number of tremors, as with hyperthyroidism, lithium treatment, delirium, and drug over dosage or withdrawal (including alcohol), share features of one or more of the foregoing types of tremors or come from an enhancement of physiologic tremor.

9. **Psychogenic tremors** have inconsistent, complicated patterns that change with circumstances (Koller et al., 1989). Most of these tremors are action tremors. They often develop suddenly and sometimes have spontaneous remissions. The tremor decreases during distraction or volitional movement of the contralateral hand. When the Ex tests for muscle tone, the Pt shows resistance to passive movement of the joint, indicating increased tone of the part, and the tremor stops briefly, which is known as the **coactivation sign** (Deuschl et al., 1998). See Chapter 14 for other clinical features of psychogenic disorders.

H. Disorders to differentiate from tremors

1. **Clonus** is a repetitive MSR.

2. **Asterixis** consists of sudden lapses of a sustained posture, which may have a periodic or pseudo-rhythmic frequency. To elicit asterixis, ask the Pt to extend the arms straight out, with the wrists dorsiflexed. The wrist will then periodically drop and immediately re-extend. First described in hepatic encephalopathy, it also appears in other metabolic-toxic encephalopathies and after structural lesions of the cerebello-thalamo-cortical circuits (Victor and Ropper, 2001; Kim, 2002).

3. **Myoclonus**

   a. **Myoclonus** means shock-like, lightning fast contractions of parts of muscles or groups of muscles. Individual movements are very brief but may be repetitive. They are irregular in rate and amplitude and symmetric or asymmetric (Victor and Ropper, 2001).

   b. When restricted to one group of muscles, it is called segmental **myoclonus clonus** or **myoclonus simplex**.

   c. When widespread, the movements are **myoclonus multiplex** or **polymyoclonus**.

   d. Myoclonus appears in a large number of metabolic, toxic, and degenerative diseases and types of epilepsy and may arise from lesions at the spinal level. Many different disorders that do not belong together are semantically linked by the term **myoclonus**.

   e. The distinction between polymyoclonus, chorea, severe ataxia, hyperexplexia, and multiple tics is sometimes difficult.

   f. A distinctive syndrome of opsoclonus and polymyoclonus affects children as an autoimmune disorder and as a distant effect of neuroblastoma. Personality changes are usual, particularly irritability.

4. **Rhythmic myoclonus versus so-called cortical tremor:** The Pt shows intermittent brief jerks, irregular or rhythmic, of slow frequency and often limited to segmental levels (Deuschl et al., 1998). Cortical tremor consists of high-frequency jerks (7 to 18 cps) similar to high-frequency postural tremor. Epileptiform discharges appear in the electroencephalogram (EEG).

5. **Partial continual epilepsy (of Kozhevnikoff/Kojewnikow):** The Pt shows continuous low-frequency jerks of one muscle group days and nights for weeks, months to years. The EEG shows focal epileptiform discharges.

I. Review of tremors

Before proceeding with the text, review the tremor hyperkinesias by actually acting them out (Figs. 7-38 to 7-41). If you feel the need to, organize your own table or make a personal differential diagnostic dendrogram.

BIBLIOGRAPHY · Tremor and Parkinsonism

Bain PG. The management of tremor. *J Neurol Neurosurg Psychiatry* 2002;72 (suppl 1): i3–i9.

Brooks DJ. Diagnosis and management of atypical parkinsonism syndromes. *J Neurol Neurosurg Psychiatry* 2002;72 (suppl 1):i10–i16.

Caekebeke JFV, Jennekens-Schinkel A, van der Linden ME, et al. The interpretation of dysprosody in patients with Parkinson's disease. *J Neurol Neurosurg Psychiatry* 1991;54:145–148.

Chokroverty S, Hening WA, Walters AS, et al, eds. *Sleep and Movement Disorders.* Philadelphia, Butterworth-Heinemann, 2002.

Deuschl G, Bain P, Brin M, Ad Hoc Scientific Committee. Consensus statement of the Movement Disorder Society. *Mov Disord* 1998;13(suppl 3):2–23.

Deuschl G, Dystonic tremor. Revue Neurologique 2003;159:900–905.

Gershlager W, Munchau A, Katzenschlager R, et al. Natural history and syndromic association of orthostatic tremor: a review of 41 patients. Movement Disorders 2004;19(7):788–795.

Jankovic J, Tolosa E. *Parkinson's Disease and Movement Disorders,* 3rd ed. Hagerstown, Lippincott Williams & Wilkins, 1998.

Koller W, Lang A, Vetere-Overfield B, et al. Psychogenic tremors. *Neurology* 1989;41:234–238.

Lou JS, Jankovic J. Essential tremor: clinical correlates in 350 patients. *Neurology* 1989;39:1094–1099.

Louis ED. Essential tremor. *N Engl J Med* 2001;345:887–891.

Rajput AH, Rozdilsky B, Ang L, et al. Clinicopathologic observations in essential tremor: report of six cases. *Neurology* 1991;51:1422–1424.

Samie MR, Selhorst JB, Koller WC. Post-traumatic midbrain tremors. *Neurology* 1990;40:62–66.

Victor M, Ropper AH. *Adams and Victor's Principles of Neurology.* 7th ed. New York, McGraw-Hill, 2001.

J. Non-tremor types of hyperkinesias

1. Several hyperkinesia display characteristic clinical features that predict the lesion site (Table 7-8). (Chokroverty, 1990; Klawans et al., 1988; Lang and Weiner, 1992).

TABLE 7-8 · Clinicopathologic Correlations Between Movement Disorders and Lesions of the Basal Motor Nuclei

Movement disorder	Classic lesion site
Chorea: multiple, quick, random movements ("the fidgets") usually most severe in the appendicular muscles	Striatum, atrophy, autoimmune disease; may also occur after lesions in a subthalamic red nucleus lesion
Athetosis: slow, writhing movements most severe in the appendicular muscles	Diffuse hypermyelination of the corpus striatum and thalamus, as in cerebral palsy
Dystonia: long, sustained twisting movements most severe in axial muscles	Genetic, acquired, or pharmacologic lesion of basal motor nuclei
Hemiballismus: wild, flinging movements of half of the body	Hemorrhagic lesion of contralateral subthalamic nucleus, usually in a hypertensive patient
Parkinsonism (paralysis agitans): pill-rolling rest tremor of 5–6 cycles/s of the fingers, lead-pipe rigidity, and akinesia	Degeneration of the substantia nigra
Rest, postural, and terminal tremor ("rubral" or Holmes tremor)	Midbrain lesion, in the region of the red nucleus and superior cerebellar peduncle, often post-traumatic

2. **Chorea** refers to incessant, random, moderately quick movements—a grimace, elevation of a finger or arm, a misstep when walking, an interruption when speaking. Overall, chorea resembles the "fidgets." One part or another of the body is flickering into motion all of the time. The movements resemble a choreographer working out the movements for a dance or, perhaps better described, they simulate fragments of normal movements. For instance, at one time or another, after you start to make an inappropriate movement (perhaps reaching up to pick your nose), you may suddenly decide to arrest it midway. Or after starting such a movement, you may have diverted it to brushing back your hair. Patients with chorea may employ this ruse. Nevertheless, an observer can perceive the stoppage or the diversion in the continuity of the initial movement.
3. **Athetosis** refers to slow, writhing movements of the fingers and extremities. If severe, athetosis affects speech and some proximal movements. These movements wax and wane and generally do not hold the part in a fixed posture. Athetosis often accompanies or follows partial interruption of the pyramidal tracts, particularly in Pts with cerebral palsy and spastic quadriplegia or diplegia. The quick random fidgety movements, called ________________, contrast with the slow writhing distal movements, called __________________.

chorea; athetosis

4. **Dystonia** refers to prolonged, slow, alternating contraction and relaxation of agonists and antagonists. The prolonged muscular contractions hold the part in one position for periods and may lead to pretzel-like body positions with fixed scoliosis and fixed contractures of joints.
   a. **Focal dystonia,** such as spasmodic torticollis and writer's cramp, may affect more or less restricted groups of muscles.
   b. The sustained postural deviations of dystonia differ from the quick movements of chorea and the slower writhing, mainly distal movements called __________________.

athetosis

   c. Although dystonia is traditionally classed as an extrapyramidal movement disorder, the lesion site and pathophysiology of the hereditary form are unknown (Zeman and Dyken, 1968), but dystonia can result from known, acquired lesions of the basal motor nuclei (Zeman and Whitlock, 1968).
5. **Hemiballismus** refers to violent flinging movements of one-half of the body. *Ballista* means to throw, as in *ballistics*. The Pt's arm thrashes about as if it were trying to fling away a handful of snakes. Hemiballismus usually appears abruptly in elderly hypertensive Pts. The lesion is predictable. A peculiar, sharply delimited hemorrhage destroys the contralateral subthalamic nucleus of Luys or its immediate surrounding pathways. This almond-sized and almond-shaped diencephalic nucleus belongs to the basal motor nuclei. Hemiballismus may also result from lesions in the caudate, putamen, globus pallidus, precentral gyrus, or thalamic nuclei.
6. **Tics** are quick, lightning fast, stereotyped, involuntary movements of face, tongue, upper extremities, or phonations. (Jankovic and Tolosa, 1998). In contrast to the preceding hyperkinesias, the sequence of movements is identical each time if the Pt has one type of tic. However, the Pt may have multiple kinds of tics. All of us display minor tics: wrinkling of the forehead, followed by blinking the eyes, or hitching up the trousers, or a shrug of the shoulder. Athletes display a number of tic-like maneuvers, as when a basketball player prepares to shoot a free throw, or a tennis player prepares to serve. Tics increase during emotional stress, are less prominent during periods of concentration, and often abate during sleep. Although mostly of low amplitude, tics, when violent, may throw the Pt to the floor, thus resembling an exaggerated startle response called **hyperexplexia.** Of the movement disorders discussed, tics, being quick and usually of low to moderate amplitude, most closely resemble ❒ chorea/❒ athetosis/❒ hemiballismus.

☑ chorea

7. **Multiple tic syndrome of Gilles de la Tourette:** Some tics are regarded as psychogenic, but they figure prominently in an organic disorder called **Tourette's syndrome,** which has three major features:
   a. Multiple tics that change from time to time.

b. Involuntary respiratory actions and vocalizations with squawks, barks, howls or sniffs, humming, and sometimes the involuntary utterance of expletives.

c. Personality traits: sometimes rigid, obsessive-compulsive, or abrasive (Kurlan, et al., 2002; Leckman and Cohen, 1999) and attention deficit hyperactivity disorder (Tourette's Syndrome Study Group, 2002).

K. Continuum between the named types of hyperkinesias

Dystonia, athetosis, chorea, and tics represent way stations along a continuum of involuntary movements, not necessarily discrete entities. They differ perhaps more in their speed than in any other way. Tics and chorea are the fastest, with each movement measured in a second or even less. Next comes athetosis, lasting just a little longer, in seconds. Then comes dystonia, which lasts many seconds to minutes or even longer, as in spasmodic torticollis, a form of dystonia in which the head remains deviated for long periods.

As an oversimplified, 1, 2, 3 mnemonic, think of each tic as shorter than 1 second (but the same tic may be repetitive), individual choreiform movements as lasting 1 second, athetosis as lasting 1 to 3 seconds (but the movements may flow into one another), and dystonia as lasting from 3 seconds to minutes or longer.

Hemiballismus differs from chorea in its more violent amplitude and unilaterality. Hemichorea may occur, but it is most frequently bilateral, as in Huntington's or Sydenham's chorea.

L. Drug-induced extrapyramidal movement syndromes and the tardive dyskinesias

Various tranquilizers, antipsychotics, and antidepressant drugs alter the balance of neurotransmitters in the basal motor circuits (Yassa et al., 1990). These chemical lesions mimic the effect of anatomic lesions in producing hypo- and hyperkinesias, ranging from parkinsonism to dystonia. The involuntary movements often predominately affect facial, oral, buccal, and pharyngeal movements, with dysphonia and dysphagia (Meige's syndrome; Lang and Weiner, 1992). Unfortunately, tardive dyskinesia may be permanent and very resistant to therapy. Levodopa, used to treat parkinsonism, also produces dyskinesias (Olanow, 2000).

M. The concept of deficit and release phenomena after lesions of the basal motor connections

For general discussion, see Section XI of this chapter.

1. **Deficit phenomena** after lesions of the basal motor circuitry include overall bradykinesia, gait impairment, masked facies, and loss of voice inflection.
2. **Release phenomena** include the hypertonia called lead-pipe rigidity, tremor (generally tremor of the part at rest), akathisia, and the patterned hyperkinesias such as tics, chorea, athetosis, dystonia, and hemiballismus. Whether the concept of release phenomena applies to these phenomena requires some stretch of the imagination. Even less does the concept apply to the other syndromes of excessive behavior, such as hyperactivity.

N. Rating scales for involuntary movement disorders

Various rating scales such as the Abnormal Involuntary Movement Scale enable the Ex to quantify various involuntary movements to determine the degree of disability, to follow the course of the disease, and to document the effects of treatment (Gollomp, 2002; Herndon, 1997; Marsden and Fahn, 1984, 1987, 1994).

O. Some simple, general tests for motor dysfunction: writing, finger-tapping speed, the Archimedes spiral, and activities of daily living

These tests are useful in analyzing most motor disorders, especially in Pts with hemiparesis, tremor, rigidity, or ataxia, not only for differential diagnosis but also to appreciate functional disability.

1. **Writing:** Watch the Pt write spontaneously and, if a motor disorder or cerebral disorder is suspected, write a sentence to dictation. Like the gait, most motor disorders affect writing. The ataxic dysgraphia of cerebellar disease, the micrographia of rigidity, and the tremulous dysgraphia of essential tremor stand out vividly from each other.
2. **Finger-tapping speed**
   a. **Technique:** For a convenient bedside test in lieu of an actual counter, place an ordinary audiocassette on the table and have the Pt grasp it between the thumb and third digit, leaving the index finger free to tap (Fig. 7-42). Ask the Pt to

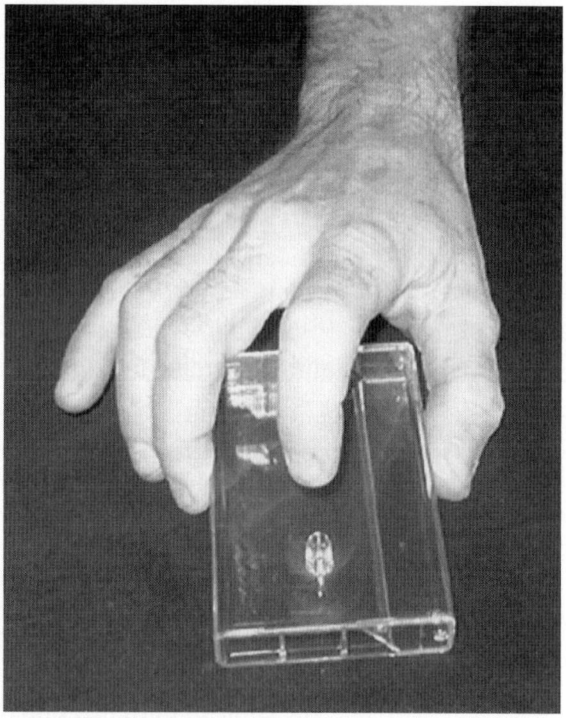

FIGURE 7-42. Position of the patient's hand for tapping on a plastic audiotape box. The examiner listens for the rate and rhythm of the taps.

tap as rapidly as possible for several seconds. The Ex should demonstrate the test first. Normal subjects tap at rate of around 50 taps per 10 seconds. Children and the aged tap at slower rates.

   b. The cassette serves three purposes:
      i. The Ex will quickly learn about the Pt's fine motor skills.
      ii. The dyspraxic Pt has difficulty assuming the position or even in picking up and arranging the box.
      iii. Most important, the cassette amplifies the sound so that the Ex can estimate the speed and the rhythm. The ear can detect subtle differences between the right and left hands far better than the eye.
   c. Because the test engages the entire central and peripheral motor systems, spasticity, rigidity, ataxia, and neuromuscular disorders will slow finger-tapping speed discernibly, and the Ex will easily hear the disturbance in rhythm of the cerebellar Pt.

BIBLIOGRAPHY · Finger Tapping

Blessing W. Alternating two finger tapping as part of the neurological motor examination. *Aust N Z J Med* 2000;30:506–507.

Cousins MS, Corrow C, Finn M, et al. Temporal measures of human finger tapping: effects of age. *Pharmacol Biochem Behav* 1998;59:445–449.

Moritz CH, Haughton VM, Cordes D, et al. Whole-brain functional MR imaging activation from a finger-tapping task examined with independent component analysis. *Am J Neuroradiol* 2000;21:1629–1635.

3. **Archimedes spiral**
   a. **Technique:** The Pt places a pen in the middle of a sheet of paper and makes a spiral line encircling the center point, making several winds of the pen, out to the periphery.
   b. The difference in rigidity that narrows the spiral but leaves its lines fairly regular, ataxia in which the spiral's lines irregularly weave in and out, and the continuous wavering of lines of essential tremor are striking.
4. **Tasks of daily living:** Frequently the Ex should elect to watch the Pt button, use scissors, tie shoelaces, drink a glass of water, and arrange clothes as if to put them on.

P. Akathisia, restless legs, and hyperactivity: the urge to move

1. **Akathisia** refers to motor unrest manifested by continual shifting of positions and sometimes by restlessly moving about. When questioned, Pts often report an actual feeling in their muscles of an urge to move (Sachdev, 1995). Akathisia appears typically in Parkinson's disease, in other diseases of the basal motor nuclei, and with psychotropic medications.
2. **Restless-legs syndrome** (Ekbom's syndrome; Chokroverty and Jankovic, 1999; Ekbom, 1960): When attempting to rest or sleep, these Pts feel an irresistible urge, a necessity, to move their legs around. No force of will can hold the legs still against the pathophysiologic imperative, and the aimless, incessant wandering of the legs prevents the onset of sleep. Symptoms are partially or totally relieved by movements such as walking or stretching (Allen et al., 2003). Exhaustive exercise or some drugs, such as antihistamines, may induce restless legs.
3. **The hyperactive child:** Hyperactive children display incessant, rapidly changing motor activity, often starting in infancy. Their driven, inappropriate, and usually annoying activity consists of fidgeting, pushing, pulling, banging, rummaging, clamoring, whining, and running. The hyperactivity continues with little regard for other people, danger, and reward and punishment. Rather than a standard, stereotyped pattern like athetosis or dystonia, the disorder consists of the sheer quantity of activity. Usually these children are so clamorous that my secretary can already diagnose them by the noise they make as they clatter down the long hall to my office. By stretching the imagination, we might think of restless legs as a localized type of akathisia and of childhood hyperactivity as its generalized childhood counterpart. No specific known brain lesion underlies hyperactivity, but many hyperkinetic children have other subtle or overt evidence of brain damage or frank mental retardation. The foregoing syndromes of driven behavior border on a variety of cursive states such as compulsive walking or running and cursive epilepsy. All have in common an irresistible drive, a pathophysiologic imperative, to move.
4. **Self-mutilation:** The Pt compulsively inflicts self-injury by biting, scratching, or pounding despite punishments or rewards. The head-banging infant or child particularly distresses parents. Although generally seen in mentally retarded Pts, some individuals with normal intelligence scratch, bite fingernails, pick their nose or lips, or otherwise injure themselves compulsively (neurodermatitis) in response to some pathophysiologic imperative that overcomes willpower. Smoking with its intermittent irritation of the lungs may fall into the same category. The Pt scratches, as it were, the respiratory mucosa, but of course chemical addiction belongs to the scenario.

5. **Stereotyped behavioral mannerisms:** Many retarded, autistic, and some otherwise normal children and psychotic adults display repetitive behaviors, including spinning, rocking, patting, touching, grimacing, licking, and mouthing. Repetitive back arching and thigh squeezing may act as masturbatory equivalents. Children with Rett's syndrome display a characteristic hand wringing. Where these behaviors, in addition to so many of the behaviors discussed above, fall in the scale between voluntary and involuntary further stretches the notion of free will.

Q. Epilepsy

1. **Definition:** Epilepsy is any change in the mental, motor, or sensory state of the Pt caused by an abnormal hypersynchronous discharge of neurons.
2. Involuntary epileptic motor activity may consist of tonic or clonic spasms and myoclonic jerks that affect all or part of the body or of complex automatisms with laughter and cursive states during complex partial (psychomotor) seizures.
3. If epilepsy causes the abnormal motor activity, the Pt usually will lose consciousness and have amnesia for the episode, and EEG monitoring usually will record epileptiform activity. However, during some epileptiform movements, the Pt retains consciousness (see Chapter 13).

R. Avoiding pitfalls (pratfalls) in distinguishing psychogenic from organic motility disturbances

1. Hysterical movement disorders or malingering may imitate organic movement disorders. See Chapter 14.
2. Anxiety or emotional tension makes virtually all hyperkinesias worse, but most dampen or disappear when the Pt is relaxed or asleep. Only a few abnormal involuntary movements occur during sleep: sleep myoclonus, palatal myoclonus (actually palatal tremor), somnambulism, and some epileptic seizures.
3. During the evolution of one illness, the form of the hyperkinesias or the degree of hypo- or hypertonia may change. Hence, what starts as a flaccid hemiparesis may end as spastic hemiparesis. Simple athetosis may end as dystonia or so-called **tension athetosis,** in which the Pt's efforts to make a voluntary movement is paralleled by the degree of an athetoid or dystonic spasm. Torsion dystonia and tension athetosis are classic examples of pathophysiologic imperatives that determine the contraction of the muscles, rather than the Pt's "will."
4. Psychotropic medications, alcohol, and street drugs frequently cause hypokinetic or hyperkinetic movement disorders. Consider drugs in the differential diagnosis of tremors or any other movement disorder of new onset.
5. Mothers of hyperactive children invariably appear distraught, depressed, and defeated by their inability to cope with their children. Usually the child's hyperactivity discloses itself by the slapdash, frenetic way the child executes the Ex's requests. If, however, the child appears calm during the period of examination, as a few will, the Ex may mistakenly conclude that the mother is "overanxious." The usual problem is an underanxious physician, not an overanxious mother. Thus the immediate inspection of the Pt, which serves so well to recognize the standard hyperkinesias of extrapyramidal origin, may, on some occasions, fail in recognizing the hyperactive child if the observation period is too brief. On the next visit, detain the child in the waiting room for a considerable period before the appointment. Then, after the child has defaced your office décor, scattered the toys all over the reception room (without actually playing with any), exasperated your other Pts, and driven your receptionist mad, you will understand the mother's plight.

S. Patient analysis

The Pt is a mentally normal 47-year-old woman who was born with mild spastic cerebral palsy. Her motor disorder has not changed in the decades since childhood.

athetosis

For the serial photographs, she was requested to extend her arms out in front of her and to hold them as still as possible. Similar movements appear when she is at rest or walking. The individual movements last 2 to 3 seconds and have low to moderate force and amplitude, but may merge with each other in a continuous pattern. The movements shown in Fig. 7-43 would best be classified as ________________.

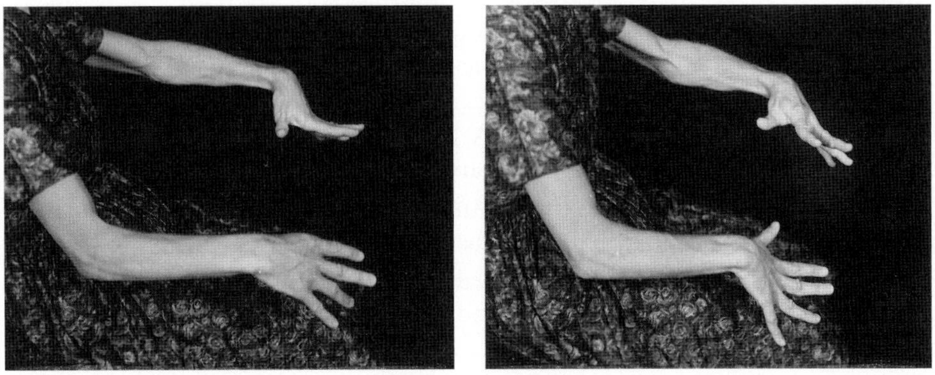

FIGURE 7-43. Action sequence of involuntary movements.

T. A summary of involuntary movements (hyperkinesias) by operational definition

1. For clinical diagnosis, I have defined hyperkinesias broadly to include *any* extra muscular activity of peripheral or central origin caused by a lesion of the nervous system.
2. For the clinical characteristics in frames *a* to *v*, write down the proper descriptive diagnosis in the blank. Where possible, act out the motility disorder described.

fibrillations

a. Spontaneous random contractions of denervated muscle fibers detected by EMG: ________________.

fasciculations

b. Spontaneous random twitches of small parts of muscles detected by clinical inspection and EMG: ________________.

myoclonic jerks

c. Sudden spontaneous contraction of a muscle or group of muscles, which may simulate a startle reaction: ________________.

tics

d. Spontaneous stereotyped sequence of muscular contractions, most prominent in facial muscles, in patients with obsessive-compulsive personality traits: ________________.

epilepsy

e. Spontaneous tonic or clonic jerking of the body, often accompanied by loss of consciousness: ________________.

chorea

f. Spontaneous, quick movements simulating fragments of normal movements, usually most prominent in extremities: ________________.

athetosis

g. Spontaneous, writhing movements of fingers and extremities that may affect facial and axial muscles: ________________.

dystonia

h. Spontaneous, long-sustained deviations of appendicular and axial parts, with alternating agonist-antagonist contractions, that may ultimately lead to fixed deformities: ________________.

hemiballismus

i. More or less incessant (during waking hours), wild, flinging movements of one-half of the body, seen usually in elderly hypertensive patients: ________________.

oculogyric crisis

j. Spontaneous upward deviation of the eyes and head, seen usually with rest tremor and lead-pipe rigidity: ________________.

restless-legs syndrome of Ekbom	k. Irresistible wandering of the legs, especially when the patient tries to rest or to sleep: ______________________.
hyperkinesia	l. Incessant, driven, usually annoying or aggressive behavior in a child: ______________________.
parkinsonian (rest) tremor	m. A tremor at rest of 6 cps, which dampens or disappears on intentional movement: ______________________.
intention (ataxic) tremor	n. Irregular tremor of a movement in progress, but no tremor at rest: ______________________.
postural tremor	o. Rapid tremor of an outstretched hand that dampens when a movement is in progress and reappears when a new posture is held: ______________________.
familial (essential) tremor	p. A 10-cps tremor of the hands that often has an autosomal dominant hereditary pattern: ______________________.
senile tremor	q. An 8-cps tremor of the head or of the head and hands occurring in an elderly patient: ______________________.
tardive dyskinesia	r. A therapy-resistant hyperkinesia usually with predominant face, lip, and tongue movements that appear after prolonged ingestion of psychotropic medications: ______________________.
akathisia	s. A state of motor unrest in a parkinsonian Pt characterized by irresistible restless shifting of postures: ______________________.
asterixis	t. Sudden yielding of a sustained posture, as of the dorsiflexed wrist with the arms extended: ______________________.
myokymia	u. Prolonged rippling or undulating, worm-like contractions of muscles, distributed focally or in widespread groups, associated with repetitive discharges of groups of motor units: ______________________.
polymyoclonus	v. Irregular, quick, low amplitude, widespread movements of trunk and extremities, often associated with opsoclonus: ______________________.

BIBLIOGRAPHY · Involuntary Movements

Allen RP, Picchietti D, Hening WA, et al. Restless legs syndrome: diagnostic criteria, special considerations, and epidemiology. A report from the restless leg syndrome diagnosis and epidemiology workshop and the National Institutes of Health. Sleep Medicine 2003; 4:101–119.

Chokroverty S. *Movement Disorders.* Great Neck, PMA Publishing Corp., 1990.

Chokroverty S, Jankovic J. Restless legs syndrome. A disease in search of identity. *Neurology* 1999;52:907–910.

DeMyer W. Spasmodic torticollis, status marmoratus and status dysmyelinatus. Consensus statement of the Movement Disorder Society. *Mov Disord* 1998;13(suppl 3):2–23.

Ekbom K. Restless legs syndrome. *Neurology* 1960;10:868–873.

Gollomp S. Track Parkinson's progression with this handy tool. *Practical Neurol* 2002;1:42–51.

Herndon RM, ed. *Handbook of Neurologic Rating Scales*. New York, Demos Vermande, 1997.

Klawans HL, Goetz CG, Tanner CM. *Common Movement Disorders.* New York, Raven, 1988.

Kurlan R, Como PG, Miller B, et al. The behavioral spectrum of tic disorders. A community-based study. *Neurology* 2002;59:414–420.

Lang AE, Weiner W. *Drug-induced Movement Disorders*. Mount Kisco, Futura Publishing, 1992.

Leckman JF, Cohen DJ, eds. *Tourette's Syndrome—Tics, Obsessions, Compulsions: Developmental Psychopathology and Clinical Care.* New York, John Wiley & Sons, 1999.

Marsden CD, Fahn S, eds. *Movement Disorders.* 3 vols. Oxford, Butterworth-Heinemann, 1984, 1987, 1994.

Meyers R. Ballismus. In: Vinken PJ, Bruyn GW, eds. *Handbook of Clinical Neurology.* Vol 6. Amsterdam: North-Holland, 1968; 476–490.

Olanow CW, ed. Levodopa-induced dyskinesias. *Ann Neurol* 2000;47(suppl 1):S1–S203.

Sachdev P. *Akathisia and Restless Legs.* New York, Cambridge University Press, 1995.

Sawle G, ed. *Movement Disorders in Clinical Practice* [with CD-ROM]. Oxford, Isis Medical Media Ltd, 1999.

Tourette's Syndrome Study Group. Treatment of ADHD in children with tics. *Neurology* 2002;58:527–536.

Vitek JL, Giroux M. Physiology of hypokinetic and hyperkinetic movement disorders: model for dyskinesia. *Ann Neurol* 2000;47(suppl 1):S131–S140. Also see: http://www.wemove.org.

Yassa R, Nair NPV, Iskandar H, et al. Factors in the development of severe forms of tardive dyskinesia. *Am J Psychiatry* 1990;147:1156–1163.

Zeman W, Dyken P. Dystonia musculorum deformans. In Vinken PJ, Bruyn GW, eds. *Diseases of the Basal Ganglia. Handbook of Clinical Neurology,* vol. 6. Amsterdam, Elsevier, 1968.

Zeman W, Whitlock C. Symptomatic dystonias. In Vinken PJ, Bruyn GW, eds. *Diseases of the Basal Ganglia. Handbook of Clinical Neurology,* vol 6. Amsterdam, Elsevier, 1968.

XIII. SUMMARY OF THE SOMATIC MOTOR SYSTEM EXAMINATION

Demonstrate the motor examination, commencing with the initial inspection for gait, posture, tremors, and abnormal movements; followed by palpation, strength testing, and muscle tone; and proceeding through the deep reflexes, percussion, and superficial reflexes.

Learning Objectives for Chapter 7

I. INSPECTION OF BODY CONTOURS, POSTURES, AND GAIT

1. Describe the initial steps in appraising the Pt's motor system before formal testing of individual parts and muscles (Section VI A of the Standardized NE).
2. Describe the lighting and initial observations to start the motor examination.
3. Describe what comparisons to make to decide whether a body part or an observation is abnormal.
4. State a principle that ensures an *orderly* inspection of the skeleto-muscular system.
5. Demonstrate and describe the sequence and observations for gait testing.

II. (a) TECHNIQUE OF TESTING FOR MUSCULAR WEAKNESS

1. Explain which option offers the best test of muscle strength: a movement that the Ex can very easily overcome, a movement that the Ex can just about match, or a movement that is much stronger than the Ex's.
2. Relate the strength of a muscle to its length (length-strength law) as applied to clinical testing (Fig. 7-1).
3. Demonstrate how to use the length-strength law to minimize the strength of a very strong muscle or to maximize the strength of a weak one so that their strengths more closely match the Ex's arm and hand strength.
4. Describe which movements at the jaw, neck, trunk, shoulder, elbow, wrist, fingers, hip, knee, and ankle are the strongest, and explain how the quadrupedal posture (Fig. 7-2) and the concept of postural anti-gravity muscles provide an easy way to remember the relative strength of these movements.
5. Explain why the dorsiflexors of the foot do not qualify as antigravity muscles, even though they lift the foot against gravity in walking.
6. State the principle for remembering which movements or positions of a normal person the Ex can just about match with hand and arm opposition and which the Ex cannot even begin to overcome by manual opposition.

Learning Objectives for Chapter 7

III. (b) TECHNIQUE OF TESTING FOR MUSCULAR WEAKNESS

1. State the principle that guides the order of testing muscles.
2. Demonstrate how to test the strength of the muscles acting at the shoulders, elbows, wrist, and hand joints.
3. Demonstrate how to match finger strength with the Pt (Fig. 7-3).
4. Demonstrate how to test the strength of the Pt's grip and explain the concept of the functional position of the hand.
5. Demonstrate how to test the strength of the abdominal muscles.
6. Describe the results of the umbilical migration test (Beevor's sign) in a Pt who has a transverse spinal cord lesion at the X thoracic level.
7. Demonstrate how to test the strength of the muscles of the back and those acting at the hip, knee, ankle, and foot joints. Describe the relative strength of the agonist-antagonist actions at these joints.
8. Demonstrate the entire screening examination for muscle strength (exclusive of cranial nerves; Section VI C of the Standardized NE).
9. Describe quantitative scales for recording the strength examination in the clinical record.

IV. RESULTS OF DIRECT PERCUSSION OF MUSCLES

1. Define and describe percussion irritability of muscle, percussion myoedema, and percussion myotonia. State whether these are normal or pathologic and, if pathologic, what they may indicate.
2. Demonstrate some different ways to elicit myotonia.
3. Describe the differences in the responses of normal, denervated, and myopathic muscles to direct percussion.

V. EXAMINATION OF MUSCLE STRETCH REFLEXES

1. Name the receptor for the MSR.
2. Draw a diagram showing the innervation of the muscle spindle and of the regular muscle fibers (Fig. 7-4).
3. Describe the response of the muscle spindles to lengthening or shortening of the muscle.
4. Explain why only a quick stretch of a muscle elicits an MSR.
5. Contrast the effect of section of the efferent nerve to a muscle on percussion irritability and the MSR.
6. Explain why the Ex percusses tendons, not the muscle itself, to elicit the MSRs.
7. Describe and demonstrate the proper technique for eliciting an MSR with a percussion hammer, differentiating between *swinging* the hammer and *pecking* with the hammer (Fig. 7-5).
8. Describe the effect of spasticity on the swing of the leg after the Ex has elicited the quadriceps reflex.
9. Demonstrate the sequence used to elicit the MSRs in the routine NE (Figs. 7-6 to 7-18).
10. Demonstrate how to prevent hurting the Pt in eliciting the brachioradialis reflex.
11. Describe the procedure to go through when you fail to obtain an MSR on your first attempt.
12. Describe two methods of reinforcing an MSR.
13. Describe some conditions or circumstances when the Ex may fail to elicit an MSR, even though the reflex arc is anatomically intact.

Learning Objectives for Chapter 7

14. Describe the position of an infant's leg to elicit a quadriceps reflex.
15. Explain why the traditional term *deep tendon reflex* is a misnomer for an MSR.
16. By means of a stick figure, record typical MSR responses as elicited from a normal person and give the normal range of the grading system (Fig. 7-19 and Table 7-2).
17. Explain why a right-to-left comparison of the magnitude of MSRs is more informative than the absolute value assigned to the response.

VI. CLINICAL AND ELECTROMYOGRAPHIC SIGNS ACCOMPANYING AREFLEXIA AND HYPOREFLEXIA AFTER INTERRUPTION OF THE REFLEX ARC

1. Describe how to "think through" the reflex arc (Fig. 7-4) to analyze hyporeflexia or areflexia.
2. Describe the major differences in the sensory and motor findings when the lesion interrupts only the afferent or only the efferent limb of the reflex arc.
3. Explain the difference between *disuse* atrophy of muscle, *denervation* atrophy, and *myopathic* atrophy.
4. Define so as to distinguish *atrophy, aplasia,* and *hypoplasia* of muscle.
5. Draw and define a motor unit (Fig. 7-20).
6. Define a fasciculation and its clinical expression.
7. Define myokymia.
8. Define cramps.
9. Describe electromyography.
10. Define Wallerian degeneration (Fig. 7-22).
11. Define a fibrillation and describe how it is detected.
12. Differentiate fasciculations from fibrillations.
13. Recite the general law used to explain fibrillations.
14. Describe the pathogenesis and detection of giant polyphasic motor units.
15. Name a radiographic procedure that visualizes denervated or dystrophic muscles.
16. Describe how various combinations of sensory loss, areflexia, hypotonia, fasciculations, fibrillations, and percussion myotonia localize the lesion to the dorsal root, LMN, peripheral nerve, or muscle (Table 7-4).
17. Describe the relative time of appearance of weakness, areflexia, atrophy, and fibrillations after the acute onset of an LMN lesion (Table 7-5).

VII. CLINICAL ANALYSIS OF HYPERACTIVE MUSCLE STRETCH REFLEXES AND CLONUS

1. Outline the common causes for hyperreflexia (Fig. 7-23).
2. Describe the difference in the effect of UMN and LMN lesions on the magnitude of MSRs.
3. Demonstrate how to elicit clonus and discuss its clinical implication (Fig. 7-24).
4. Explain why the Ex must make a very brisk initial movement to elicit clonus.
5. Distinguish between non-pathologic (unsustained or abortive) and pathologic (sustained) clonus.
6. Describe how to abort physiologic clonus of the newborn to distinguish the oscillatory action from a tremor or seizure.

Learning Objectives for Chapter 7

VIII. DISORDERS OF MUSCLE TONE: HYPERTONIA AND HYPOTONIA

1. Give an operational definition of muscle tone.
2. State the two major factors that cause muscle tone.
3. Give operational definitions of spasticity and rigidity and demonstrate how to elicit them (Fig. 7-26 and Table 7-6).
4. Describe the cogwheel phenomenon and contrast it with the clasp-knife phenomenon.
5. Describe the difference in the pathways implicated in causing spasticity and rigidity.
6. Describe the difference in the speed of the movements required to elicit spasticity and rigidity.
7. Describe some disorders of the peripheral nervous system and CNS that may cause hypotonia (Fig. 7-27).
8. Define neural shock (diaschisis, cerebral, or spinal shock) and describe what that state implies about the severity and rapidity of onset of the lesion.
9. Contrast the usual motor signs of neural shock with the usual motor signs of a chronic UMN lesion.
10. Describe how to test and record the range of motion of the joints.

IX. EXAMINATION OF THE SUPERFICIAL REFLEXES (SKIN-MUSCLE REFLEXES)

1. Explain the reason for classification of reflexes into superficial and deep.
2. Recite the superficial reflexes elicited in the Standard NE (**mnemonic hint:** recite them in rostrocaudal order).
3. State the end-point criterion for having properly elicited the plantar reflex.
4. Recite a sentence to prepare the Pt for a plantar stimulus.
5. Demonstrate how to elicit the plantar reflex by stimulation of the sole (Fig. 7-28) and describe the usual movement of the great toe in a normal person.
6. Name the three physiologically significant variables in the stroke used to elicit the plantar reflex.
7. Explain why the Ex applies very slight pressure for the first stimulus to elicit the plantar reflexes.
8. Describe the position of the Pt for eliciting plantar responses.
9. State the dermatome stimulated by Babinski's maneuver and describe the afferent and efferent arcs of the plantar reflex, naming the nerves, spinal cord segments, and muscle groups involved (Figs. 7-29 and 7-31).
10. State the two types of summation required to elicit a plantar response.
11. Describe the lower extremity movements that usually accompany plantar flexion of the great toe after a plantar stimulus in a normal person.
12. Describe ways to investigate whether the plantar response should be judged as a balance between agonist-antagonist muscle contraction or merely an agonist contraction.
13. Describe the response of the great toe to a plantar stimulus in a Pt who has a UMN lesion (Fig. 7-33A). Give two names for it.
14. Describe the additional movements of the lower extremity that usually accompany an extensor plantar response (Fig. 7-33B).
15. When the Pt has an extensor toes sign, describe the timing of the behavior of the great toe in relation to the application and withdrawal of the stimulus.

Learning Objectives for Chapter 7

16. State what tract is interrupted when an extensor toe sign is present.
17. Name several transient pathophysiologic states in which an extensor toe sign or other features of the UMN syndrome may appear without actual anatomic interruption of the pyramidal tract.
18. Describe the response of the toe to plantar stimulation in young infants.
19. State the prognostic implication of absence of a plantar grasp reflex in a young infant.
20. Describe what may happen to the size of the receptive zone for the extensor toe sign after spinal cord transection.
21. Demonstrate several methods in addition to the standard plantar stimulus for eliciting an extensor toe sign (Fig. 7-34). State the common physiologic properties of the stimulus for most of these maneuvers.
22. State several different reasons why a Pt with an undoubted UMN lesion may not show an extensor toe sign.
23. Demonstrate how to palpate the common peroneal nerve (Fig. 7-35).
24. State the nerve that is usually involved and the usual site of the lesion in a Pt with a foot drop.
25. Describe crossed-knee palsy.
26. Demonstrate how to elicit the abdominal and cremasteric reflexes and describe the normal responses (Fig. 7-36).
27. State the physiologic properties shared by the stimulus that produces the abdominal-cremasteric and plantar reflexes.
28. Describe the characteristic changes in the abdominal-cremasteric reflexes in the acute and chronic states of UMN lesions.
29. State some conditions in which absence of the superficial abdominal reflexes does not necessarily implicate UMN interruption.
30. Describe how to elicit the anal wink and bulbocavernosus reflexes and state what level of the spinal cord mediates these reflexes.
31. Show on a stick figure how to record the typical deep and superficial reflex responses in a normal person, a hemiplegic Pt, and a Pt with a chronic lesion at T10 (Fig. 7-37).
32. Describe what would happen to the umbilicus when a supine Pt with a T10-level spinal cord lesion attempts to elevate his head.

X. SUMMARY OF THE STANDARD "TEXTBOOK" SYNDROMES OF UPPER AND LOWER MOTONEURON LESIONS AND THEIR VARIATIONS

1. Recite the clinical signs produced by a slowly evolving or chronic UMN.
2. Contrast the UMN syndrome with the LMN syndrome (Table 7-7).
3. Define so as to differentiate the following clinical terms for syndromes caused by UMN lesions at various sites: hemiplegia, monoplegia, double hemiplegia, spastic diplegia, pseudobulbar palsy, locked-in syndrome, quadriplegia (tetraplegia), and paraplegia.
4. Describe the motor, sensory, and autonomic changes that follow acute spinal cord transection at C1.
5. Describe the effects of spinal shock on the deep and superficial reflexes, both visceral and somatic.

Learning Objectives for Chapter 7

XI. THE THEORY OF DEFICIT AND RELEASE PHENOMENA AFTER LESIONS OF THE MOTOR SYSTEM

1. Define deficit and release phenomena and classify the signs of acute and chronic UMN lesions as one or the other.
2. Apply the concept of deficit and release phenomena to the clinical features of LMN lesions.
3. Apply the concept of deficit and release phenomena to the clinical features of autonomic dysfunction after lesions of the peripheral nervous system (**mnemonic hint:** effect on sweating and vasomotor tone).

XII. INVOLUNTARY MOVEMENT DISORDERS

1. Give an operational definition of voluntary and involuntary movements.
2. Describe some normal involuntary movements or physiologic synkinesias.
3. Describe Bell's phenomenon.
4. Define myoclonic jerks and describe one circumstance in which a myoclonic jerk is normal.
5. Distinguish myoclonic jerks from fasciculations.
6. State which abnormal clinical or EMG findings would distinguish pathologic from benign fasciculations.
7. Define *tremor*.
8. Show how to demonstrate your own physiologic tremor.
9. Describe the clinical characteristics used in the differential diagnosis of tremors.
10. Define the clinical types of tremor and mime them (Fig. 7-38).
11. Describe the clinical characteristics of essential tremor.
12. Differentiate essential palatal tremor from symptomatic palatal tremor (palatal myoclonus) with respect to clinical characteristics and lesion site.
13. Give the clinical characteristics of parkinsonian tremor.
14. List the major neurologic signs in parkinsonism.
15. Describe the effects of parkinsonism on facial expression and speech.
16. Define or describe pill-rolling tremor, lead-pipe rigidity, cogwheeling, akathisia, and oculogyric crisis.
17. Describe the site of the lesion or the system affected for parkinsonian tremor, intention (ataxic) tremor, postural tremor and terminal tremor, or combinations of rest, intention, and postural (rubral) tremor.
18. Describe some of the different applications of the term *myoclonus* and some movement disorders that clinically are difficult to distinguish from myoclonus.
19. Define and mime chorea, athetosis, and dystonia and rank the speed of the movements.
20. Recite the usual sites of the lesion for chorea, athetosis (in cerebral palsy), dystonia, hemiballismus, and terminal, postural, and rubral tremor.
21. Describe one type of focal dystonia.
22. Describe hemiballismus and state the usual site of the lesion.
23. Define a tic and name a syndrome consisting of multiple tics and urgent personality traits.
24. Name the movement disorders often caused by psychotropic drugs.
25. Describe the usual location of involuntary movements in tardive dyskinesias.

Learning Objectives for Chapter 7

26. By applying the basic definitions of deficit and release phenomena, classify the signs of lesions of the basal motor nuclei.
27. Describe some of the motor abnormalities shown by general tests of motor skill such as handwriting, finger-tapping speed, and the Archimedes spiral.
28. Give examples of overactive or driven behavior caused by pathophysiologic imperatives that transcend the Pt's will.
29. Describe the restless-legs syndrome.
30. State how the hyperactivity in the hyperactive child syndrome differs from the standard extrapyramidal hyperkinesias.
31. List several stereotyped mannerisms found in neuropsychiatric disorders such as autism, mental retardation, schizophrenia, and dementia.
32. Describe the effect of pyramidal tract section on voluntary movements and most abnormal involuntary movements of extrapyramidal origin (page 88).
33. Explain why a brief period of observation of a child in the examining room may lead the doctor to erroneously distrust the history given by the mother of a hyperactive child.
34. Discuss the difficulties in deciding which determinants, free will, pathophysiologic imperatives, reflexes, or unconscious motivations, cause any particular behavior.

XIII. SUMMARY OF THE SOMATIC MOTOR SYSTEM EXAMINATION

1. Demonstrate the motor examination (Standard NE, Section VI A to G).

8 Examination for Cerebellar Dysfunction

But how great was his apprehension, when he farther understood, that [the force of parturition] acting upon the very vertex of the head, not only injured the brain itself, or cerebrum—but that it necessarily squeezed and propelled the cerebrum towards the cerebellum, which was the immediate seat of the understanding!—Angels and ministers of grace defend us! Cried my father—can any soul withstand this shock?—No wonder the intellectual web is so rent and tattered as we see it; and that so many of our best heads are no better than a puzzled skein of silk,—all perplexity—all confusion within-side.

—**Laurence Sterne (1713–1768)**

The Life and Opinions of Tristam Shandy, Gentleman

I. FUNCTIONS OF THE CEREBELLUM

A. What the cerebellum does not do

1. Laurence Sterne correctly satirized the speculative neurophysiology of his time, which localized "the immediate seat of the understanding" to the cerebellum. Nevertheless, the cerebellum apparently participates in the regulation of cognition, emotion, and autonomic functions more than generally appreciated (Schmahmann, 2001). Cerebellar lesions can result in the cerebellar cognitive syndrome comprising a constellation of executive, visual spatial, linguistic impairments, and affective dysregulation. A topographical organization has been proposed such that the anterior lobe, parts of medial lobule VI and lobule VIII of the posterior lobe contain the representation of the *sensorimotor cerebellum*; parts of lobule VI and lobule VII of the posterior lobe comprise the *cognitive cerebellum*; and the posterior vermis and the fastigial nucleus are the anatomical substrate for the *limbic cerebellum*. (Stoodley and Schmahmann, 2010)
2. The cerebellum has no clinically evident role in consciousness per se.
3. The cerebellum has no clinically evident role in the conscious appreciation of sensation, despite massive sensory connections. Holmes (1917, 1939) repeatedly stated that standard clinical tests did not reveal sensory deficits in cerebellar patients (Pts).

B. What the cerebellum does do

1. The most explicit function of the cerebellum for clinical testing is its role in coordinating willed muscular contractions. To coordinate means to adjust the rate, range, force, and sequence of willed muscular contractions. In so acting, the cerebellum

belongs to a distributed sensorimotor network for coordination that includes the cerebral cortex, basal motor nuclei, thalamus, and reticular formation (Giron and Koller, 1993).

2. As Hughlings Jackson (1834–1911) stated, "It will not suffice to speak of coordination as a separate 'faculty.' Coordination is the function of the whole and every part of the nervous system." Not the least are the sensory systems. Visual, tactile, and auditory systems send afferents to the cerebellum, but coordination preeminently requires proprioceptive input from joints, muscles, and vestibular system. (See page 404 for a full definition of *proprioception*).
3. To make a movement, the brain must know where the body part starts from to orchestrate the sequence, rate, and force of muscular contractions required to get the part from point A to point B. Musculoskeletal proprioceptors and other senses inform the cerebellum about extremity position and movement, joint angles, and the length of and tension on muscles and joints, i.e., the state of the muscles and skeletomuscular levers at any given instant. From this information, the cerebellum coordinates muscular contractions to produce steady volitional movements and steady volitional postures. Thus, the crucial clinical tests for cerebellar dysfunction expose unsteadiness of volitional movements and unsteadiness of volitionally sustained postures.
4. Now, if you understand the role of the cerebellum, you can answer this question: Could you test a paralyzed or comatose Pt for cerebellar dysfunction? ❒ Yes/ ❒ No. Explain.

☑ No

____

____

A comatose or paralyzed Pt makes no willed movements and maintains no willed postures.

5. Patients with cerebellar lesions make lower scores on neuropsychologic tests and tend to have personality changes, with apathy or disinhibited, socially inappropriate behavior (Karatekin et al., 2000; Malm et al., 1998; Manto and Pandolfo, 2001; Schmahmann and Sherman, 1998). As yet no specific pattern of cognitive or affective dysfunction clearly localizes a lesion to the cerebellum, as do the standard motor tests (Daum and Ackermann, 1997).

BIBLIOGRAPHY · Cerebellum

Schmahmann JD, Sherman JC. The cerebellar cognitive affective syndrome. *Brain*. 1998;121:561–579.

II. ANATOMY OF THE CEREBELLUM

A. The three cerebellar lobes

Nomenclature note: The cerebellum, of all parts of the central nervous system, has too many names for its bumps and crevices. Angevine et al. (1961) listed 24 different nomenclatures. This text uses Larsell's (1972) terms.

1. Larsell divided the cerebellum *transversely* into three lobes and *longitudinally* into three parts, one midline *vermis* uniting two *hemispheres*. Learn Fig. 8-1.
2. In contrast to the schematic depiction of lobes shown in Fig. 8-1, Fig. 8-2 shows the flocculonodular lobe rolled under in its true position. Label the lobes.

B. Cerebellar phylogenesis

1. Phylogeny provides the best understanding of the clinical syndromes of the cerebellum. The cerebellum evolved out of the vestibular nuclei. Its vestibular origin

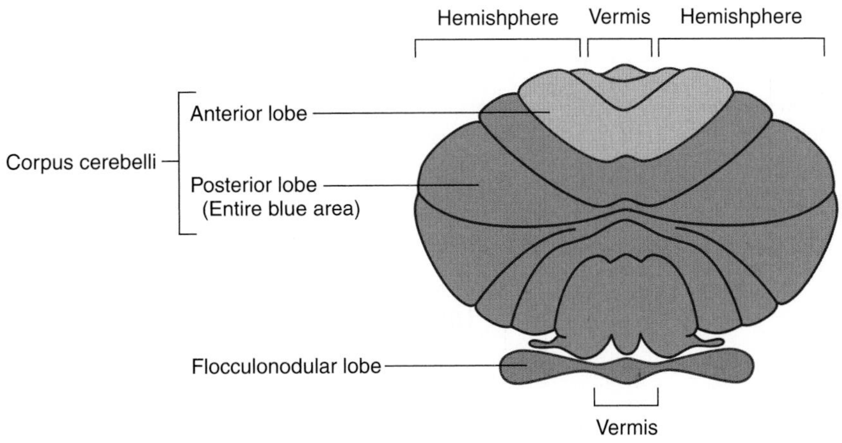

FIGURE 8-1. Schematic dorsal view of the cerebellum (Larsell's nomenclature). In reality, the flocculonodular lobe is rolled under, out of sight, when the cerebellum is viewed dorsally (Fig. 8-2).

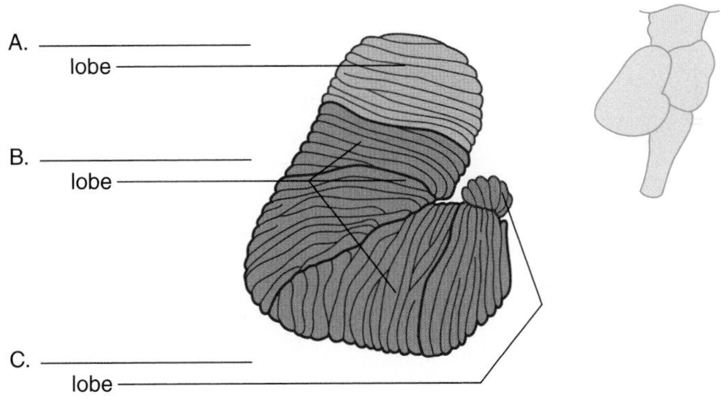

FIGURE 8-2. Right lateral view of the cerebellum. The insert at the right shows the relation of the cerebellum to the brainstem. Label the lobes A to C.

condemns it to straddle forever the vestibular nerves and nuclei, at the pontomedullary junction, and to retain forever its connections with the vestibular system—the law of retained original innervation.

2. Vestibular proprioceptors provide information about the movement of the head and its position in relation to the pull of gravity. Having no limbs, primitive animals require only a small nubbin of cerebellum to coordinate the axial muscles that position the eyes, head, and trunk. This nubbin, the **flocculonodular lobe,** constitutes the **vestibulocerebellum** (or **archicerebellum**).
3. All higher animals retain the vestibulocerebellar connections and their axial functions, but the budding limbs impress new roles on the cerebellum; it must now coordinate axial (trunk) *and* appendicular (limb) muscles. The emergence of the vertical bipedal from the quadripedal posture places particular demands on gait coordination. A second portion of the cerebellum evolves to receive most of the proprioceptive input from limbs and trunk, the **anterior lobe** (the **spinocerebellum** or **paleocerebellum**).
4. The third and newest cerebellar lobe expands in equal measure with the cerebrum, motor cortex, pyramidal tract, pontine basis, and inferior olivary nuclei. The corticopontocerebellar and olivocerebellar pathways send the major inputs to this newest part, the **posterior lobe** (or neocerebellum). The inferior olivary nuclei project topographically to all three cerebellar lobes.
5. To recapitulate: The cerebellum consists of three lobes: the *anterior, posterior,* and *flocculonodular,* based on phylogenesis and the major source of afferent connections. Complete Table 8-1.
6. Lesions of each of the lobes cause different clinical syndromes. From the clinical findings, the examiner (Ex) can predict the location and often the type of lesion (Table 8-3).

Spinocerebellar tracts
Corticopontocerebellar tracts
Vestibulocerebellar tracts
Olivocerebellar tracts

TABLE 8-1 · Some Major Afferent Pathways to the Lobes of the Cerebellum

Cerebellar lobe	Major afferent pathway
Anterior lobe (spinocerebellum)	____________
Posterior lobe (cerebrocerebellum)	____________
Flocculonodular lobe (vestibulocerebellum)	____________
All lobes	____________

C. The three pairs of cerebellar peduncles and their pathways

1. Three pairs of peduncles anchor the cerebellum to the pons, the **superior** (rostral), **middle,** and **inferior** (caudal). These thick stalks convey only and all afferent and efferent cerebellar connections (DeMyer, 1998). Transection of the peduncles allows the cerebellum to fall free from the brainstem (Fig. 8-3).

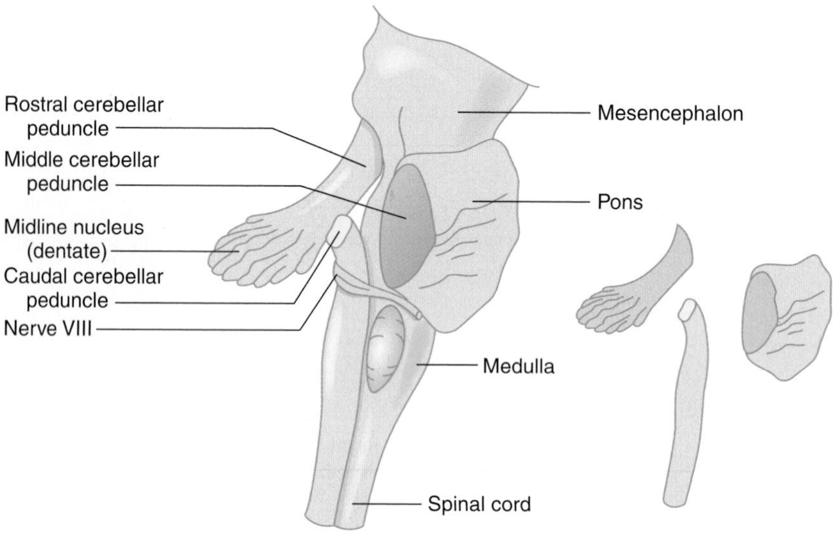

FIGURE 8-3. Right lateral view of the brainstem to show the cerebellar peduncles. The insert at the right is an exploded view of the peduncles.

☑ pons

2. The three pairs of peduncles anchor the cerebellum to only one part of the brainstem, the ❒ mesencephalon/❒ pons/❒ medulla. Therefore, **all cerebellar afferents and efferents must pass through the pons and through one of the peduncles.**
3. The **middle peduncle,** the simplest peduncle in composition, conveys almost exclusively pontocerebellar fibers.

Remember the middLe peduncle by the L mnemonic: Largest, Lateralest, simpLest and phylogenetically Latest: Largest, Lateralist, simpLest, and Latest. Largest by far of the peduncles, it conveys the Largest pathway to the cerebellum; it constitutes the Largest part of the pons (the Largest part of the brainstem); and ends in the Largest lobe of the cerebellum, the posterior lobe; and it is the simpLest peduncle in composition, conveying only one type of fiber, pontocerebellar fibers.

4. The connections of the **inferior cerebellar peduncle** are predicted by its neighbors: the spinocerebellar tracts, medulla, and vestibular nerve. Thus, the inferior peduncle transmits dorsal spinocerebellar, trigeminocerebellar, and olivocerebellar afferents and interchanges afferent and efferent connections with the medullary reticular formation and the vestibular nuclei.

5. The **superior** cerebellar peduncle angles forward and ventrally through the pons and into the midbrain (Fig. 8-3). It contains the major efferent cerebellar pathway, the **brachium conjunctivum,** that aims toward the red nucleus and thalamus. For the priggish neuroanatomist, we note that, the *dorsal* spinocerebellar tract veers directly into the cerebellum via the inferior peduncle, the *ventral* spinocerebellar tract ventures rostrally before entering via the superior peduncle—but the latter fact has no particular clinical value. More importantly, *both* spinocerebellar tracts end in the anterior lobe, especially in the vermis, making the anterior lobe the *spinocerebellum*. These tracts convey proprioceptive information to the anterior lobe from the muscles and joints of the neck, trunk, and extremities.

D. Recapitulation of the cerebellar peduncles

1. In activating muscles for voluntary contractions, the cerebrum communicates with the cerebellum via the corticopontocerebellar pathway, which ends mainly in the ______________ lobe of the cerebellum.

posterior

2. The corticopontocerebellar pathway runs in the ______________ peduncle.

middle

3. The major efferent peduncle, containing the brachium conjunctivum, is the ______________ peduncle.

superior (rostral)

4. Afferents of the olivary, vestibular, and dorsal spinocerebellar systems and cerebellar efferents run through the ______________ peduncle.

inferior (caudal)

5. Recall that the cerebellar lobe that arose out of the vestibular system and retains strong vestibular connections throughout its phylogenetic history is the ______________ lobe.

flocculonodular

6. Of the three cranial nerves (CrNs) attached along the pontomedullary sulcus, the most dorsal one, closest to the inferior peduncle, is CrN ________ and the most ventral one, farthest from the peduncle, is CrN ______________.

VIII; VI. Review Fig. 2-20 if you missed this.

E. Circuits of the cerebellum

1. **Major sources of afferents to the cerebellum arise from the following:**
   a. Spinocerebellar system, via inferior and superior peduncles, to the anterior lobe (paleocerebellum, spinocerebellum).
   b. Corticopontocerebellar system, via middle peduncle, mainly to the posterior lobe (neocerebellum, cerebrocerebellum).
   c. Vestibulocerebellar system, via inferior peduncle, mainly to the flocculonodular lobe (archicerebellum, vestibulocerebellum).
   d. Olivocerebellar system, via inferior peduncle, to all cerebellar lobes.
   e. The afferent fibers send collaterals to the deep cerebellar nuclei on their way to the cerebellar cortex.
2. **Intrinsic cerebellar circuits:** All afferent fibers ascend through the cerebellar white matter to influence ultimately the large Purkinje neurons found ubiquitously throughout the cerebellar cortex. The Purkinje axons afford the only way out of the cerebellar cortex. They descend through the cerebellar white matter, and the vast majority synapse on the deep nuclei of the cerebellum, and a small minority synapse directly on the vestibular nuclei. The deep cerebellar nuclei, the largest of which is the dentate nucleus, sit in the roof of the IV ventricle. Learn Fig. 8-4.

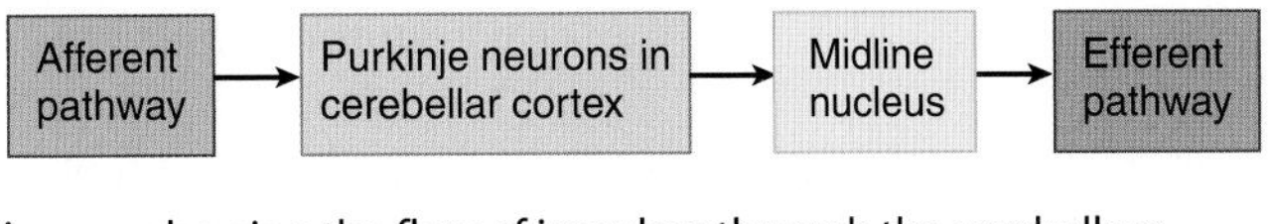

FIGURE 8-4. Diagram showing the flow of impulses through the cerebellum.

3. **Extrinsic cerebellar circuits:** The cortico-ponto-cerebello-thalamo-corticobulbar/corticospinal circuit.

   a. Well, yes, instead of inventing such a word, we could just introduce a law: **Cerebral hemisphere lesions cause contralateral motor signs, whereas cerebellar hemisphere lesions cause ipsilateral signs,** if that's all you want to know. It's more elegant, if more demanding, to learn the actual circuit that underlies the correlation between lesion site and clinical signs (Fig. 8-5). Learning it will cause no harm and has practical value which you can verify at your next opportunity.

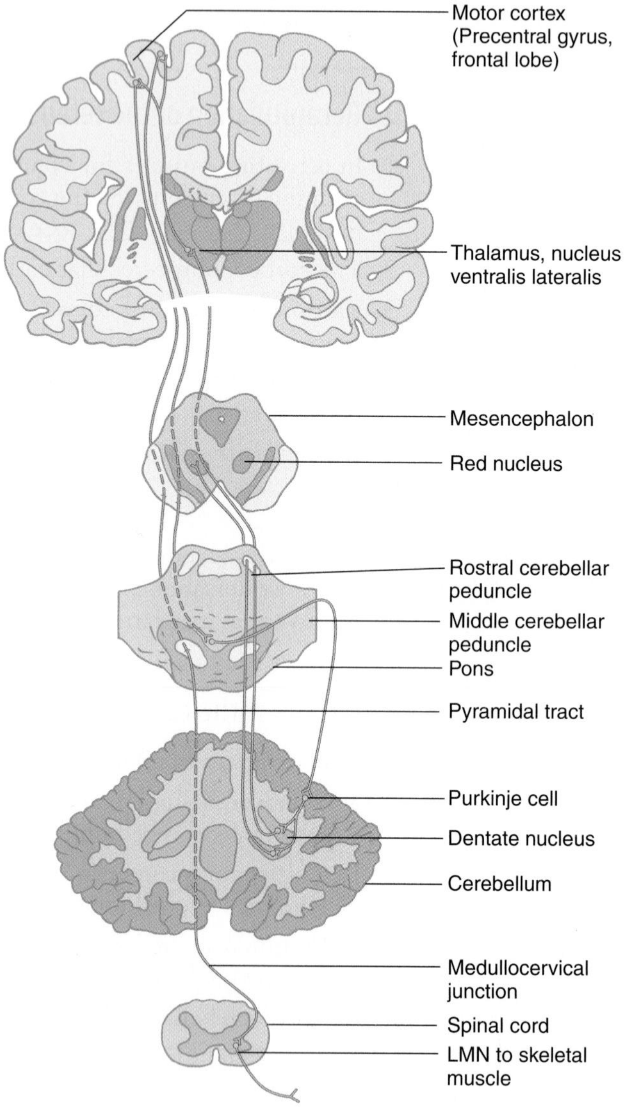

FIGURE 8-5. Diagram of the cerebro-cerebello-cerebral circuit. By this pathway, the cerebellum coordinates volitional movements by feeding back information to the cerebral motor cortex to influence its commands to the lower motoneurons via the pyramidal tract. Start at the motor cortex and trace through the circuit. Notice that the cerebro-cerebello-cerebral circuit double crosses the midline and that the pyramidal crossing brings the influence of one cerebellar hemisphere back to the same side.

   b. **Master Fig. 8-5 this way:**

      i. Learn the labeled structures.

      ii. Start at the motor cortex in the precentral gyrus of the frontal lobe and trace a motor impulse from the motor cortex down to the cerebellar cortex, back to the motor cortex, and down the pyramidal tract.

      iii. Using a colored pencil, draw the circuit on the opposite half of Fig. 8-5. Be sure to include the synapses, marked by Y.

☑ contralateral

c. By means of the single pyramidal decussation, cerebral hemisphere controls volitional movements on the ❒ ipsilateral/❒ contralateral side of the body.

☑ ipsilateral

d. By means of double crossing pathways in conjunction with the pyramidal decussation, one cerebellar hemisphere ultimately coordinates muscular contractions on the ❒ contralateral/❒ ipsilateral side of the body.

☑ ipsilateral. Review the law in 3-a, above.

e. Hence, a lesion of one cerebellar hemisphere causes incoordinated muscular contractions on the ❒ ipsilateral/❒ contralateral side.

III. CLINICAL SIGNS OF CEREBELLAR DYSFUNCTION

A. The keys to detecting cerebellar dysfunction

Four cardinal cerebellar signs consist of **ataxia** (= dystaxia), **tremor (intention tremor and postural)**, and, especially in acute lesions, **hypotonia** and **asthenia.** *Taxis* means "ordered," as in *taxonomy. Ataxia* means "not ordered" or, as applied to the effect of cerebellar lesions, "incoordinated" contractions of muscles during volitional movements or during volitionally sustained postures. Cerebellar signs derive not from weakness or loss of sensation but from loss of the muscular coordination provided by the cerebellum (Lechtenberg, 1993).

As a mnemonic to remember all the clinical manifestations of cerebellar lesions, visualize a drunken person.

Depressants such as alcohol preferentially poison vestibulocerebellar neurons. If you have ever been or seen an inebriated person, you will understand the syndrome immediately. A drunken person cannot coordinate any volitional muscular contractions. Thus, the person sways when standing (when maintaining a volitional posture), reels and missteps when walking, slurs words when talking, and his eyes oscillate when attempting to look at a target. The limbs hang loose and floppy. When a finger approaches a target, such as the nose, it may start to show a tremor as the movement progresses but will then definitely increase as the finger nears the target. If we apply technical terms to these signs, as is the habit of physicians, we can define the cerebellar syndrome as follows:

1. The overall incoordination of intentional muscular contractions is **ataxia** *or* **dystaxia,** although some might prefer **dyssynergia** (Barboi, 2000). A type of sensory ataxia also occurs with peripheral nerve or dorsal column lesions, as in the locomotor ataxia of tabes dorsalis due to syphilis.
2. The tremor of intentionally maintained head or trunk posture or of a limb suspended in front of the body is called **postural, positional** or **static type of action tremor.** (The "action" when holding a volitional posture is the active contraction of the muscles. See Fig. 7-38.) The unsteady oscillations of head and trunk are also called **titubation,** characterized by a low-frequency oscillation of around 3 Hz.
3. The tremor as a limb approaches a target is called **intention, end-point,** or **kinetic tremor.** Classic cerebellar tremor occurs uni or bilaterally depending on the underlying cerebellar disorder and usually has a frequency below 5 Hz.
4. The uncoordinated, slurred speech is called **dysarthria,** like any neurogenic disturbance of voice articulation.
5. The uncoordinated oscillations of the eyes are called **nystagmus.**
6. The loose floppy joints and muscles are called **hypotonia.**
7. The person becomes silly, illogical, disinhibited, and socially inappropriate.
8. List the major clinical signs of cerebellar lesions (**Hint:** start with the head and eyes and work caudally, visualizing a drunken person).

____

____

Nystagmus, dysarthria, dystaxia of posture, arm movement and gait, intention tremor, and hypotonia and personality changes.

☑ rests; ☑ undergoes volitional movement

9. Another common neurogenic tremor, not caused by cerebellar lesions, is the tremor of parkinsonism. This tremor appears when the part ❒ rests/❒ undergoes volitional movement and disappears when the part ❒ rests/❒ undergoes volitional movement.

B. The effect of cerebellar lesions on speech

Dysarthria in cerebellar Pts consists of slowness, slurring of words, and **scanning speech.** In scanning speech, the Pt's voice varies from a low volume to a high volume as if scanning from peak to peak. The Pt fails to meter and modulate the strength of the muscular contractions that produce the speech sounds, thus accentuating the wrong syllables or words, or the Pt may speak too loudly and garrulously. A tremulousness, analogous to postural tremor, also may occur (Ackerman and Ziegler, 1991). Cerebellar lesions seem to affect speech less in children, but they may undergo a peculiar period of mutism after surgery for cerebellar neoplasms (van Mourik et al., 1998).

C. The effects of cerebellar lesions on eye movement

Cerebellar lesions result in nystagmus, dysmetria of saccades, jerky rather than smooth pursuit, slowness in initiating eye movements, and skew deviation (Bogousslavsky and Meienberg, 1987; Glaser, 1999; Pierrot-Deseilligny et al., 1990). Cerebellar nystagmus occurs preeminently during volitional use of the eyes and thus is gaze evoked. Acute unilateral destructive lesions regularly cause a particular gaze-evoked nystagmus with the slow component toward a null or resting point (Holmes, 1917, 1939); see the nystagmus dendrogram in Fig. 5-7.

To test for saccadic dysmetria, have the Pt look straight ahead and place your index fingers in the temporal fields. Ask the Pt to look first at one finger and then the other and then direct the Pt to look rapidly from one to the other several times.

D. Clinical tests for dystaxia of station (stance) and gait

Note: You will learn these tests best if you act them out yourself and perform them on a partner.

1. Symptomatic cerebellar lesions universally impair the gait and stance (the standing posture). Inspect the Pt for swaying when standing, which involves volitional posture, and for dystaxia of gait, which involves volitional foot placement. The unsteady stance and reeling gait of the drunken person need no wordy description. To compensate for unsteadiness of stance and gait, the cerebellar Pt assumes a **broad-based stance** and a **broad-based gait,** just as a toddler does before gaining coordination, or an elderly Pt does after losing some.
2. To challenge the Pt's coordination and overcome the compensatory broad-base, the Ex asks the Pt to stand with the feet together. Similarly, to expose gait incoordination, use a test known to every policeman: ask the Pt to step along a straight line, placing the heel of one foot directly in front of the toe of the other, the so-called **tandem walking.** It is the most sensitive clinical test for gait ataxia (Manto, 2001; Stolze et al., 2002). Now stand up and try tandem walking yourself. You will find that balancing on a narrow base when walking takes no little ability.
3. To judge broad-based gaits, you must know where the heels fall in relation to the midline when a normal person walks. First, just for fun, guess where the medial margins of the heels fall in relation to the midline sagittal plane: ❒ just on the midline/❒ 2.5 cm off/❒ 3 to 5 cm off/❒ more than 5 cm off.

☑ just on the midline

4. Unless the person has huge thighs, the medial margin of the heels falls *exactly* on the line. Verify this the next time you watch someone walk or, just as instructive, note the neat, precise tightrope placement of a dog's hindfeet.

5. Next stretch a string in a straight line or find a straight line on your floor and walk along it with your midline directly above it. Now walk straddling the string by deliberately placing each foot 2 to 3 in. to the side of the midline. Notice that even slight displacement of your heels from the midline will introduce a waddle in your gait. To the original signs of cerebellar dysfunction, we can add a swaying, broad-based stance and gait.

E. Clinical tests for arm dystaxia

1. **Postural tremor and tremor of the arms during the finger-to-nose test**
   a. Ask the Pt to extend the arms straight out in front. Inspect the arms for wavering, indicating incoordination during this volitionally maintained posture, and for frank, rhythmic postural tremor. Having the Pt hold the fingers a little apart in front of the nose, with the arms elevated horizontally, in the bat's wing position, also demonstrates postural instability of the arms or postural tremor (Alusi et al., 2000).
   b. After you have inspected the Pt with the arms held straight out, instruct the Pt to place his index finger on the tip of his nose.
      i. To enlist the Pt's best effort, say, "Move your finger in and place the tip of your finger *exactly* on the tip of your nose. Don't miss!"
      ii. Inspect for dystaxia of the movement in progress or frank tremor that increases as the finger approaches the nose (intention type of kinetic tremor), and whether the Pt fails to precisely place the tip of the finger to the tip of the nose (dysmetria).
      iii. Have the Pt perform this test (and later the heel-to-shin test) three times. If uncertain of the result, have the Pt alternately touch his nose, your finger, and his nose several times.
   c. A tremor of the outstretched hands is called a ______________ tremor.
   d. A tremor that increases as the finger approaches the nose or is reaching a target is called a ______________ tremor.

postural

positional

Intention type of kinetic tremor (called terminal or end-point tremor by some investigators).

2. Cerebellar signs on one side implicate a lesion of the ❐ ipsilateral/❐ contralateral cerebellar hemisphere because of ❐ one/❐ two/❐ three decussations.

☑ ipsilateral; ☑ three (Fig. 8-5)

3. **Dysmetria:** The dystaxic Pt, in seeking a specific end point, such as the nose on the finger-to-nose test, frequently *under*shoots or *over*shoots the target because of failure to control, or *meter,* the muscular contractions that set the distance.
4. **The rapid alternating-movements tests for dystaxia and dysmetria (*dysdiadokokinesia* = dysdiadochokinesia)**
   a. The technical term for dystaxia-dysmetria of rapid alternating, movements, **dysdiadochokinesia,** is a lovely dactylic trimeter. *This* is the *fó*rest priméval: *dys* di á *dó* ko ki *né* si a. This term describes nothing qualitatively different. It means only incoordination of muscular contractions during rapid alternating movements.
   b. The Pt holds out the hands and pronates and supinates them as rapidly as possible. Test the hands separately and together. The dystaxic hand overshoots one time, undershoots the next, and is slower than normal. See Fig. 8-6.
   c. A subtler, superior method is the *thigh-patting test.* Test each hand separately and together. First demonstrate the action to the Pt by lightly slapping your own thigh, alternating first by slapping the palm and then the back of the hand, as rapidly and rhythmically as possible. **Be sure to make an audible sound with each pat.** Instruct the Pt to make actions that *sound* exactly like yours. The Ex sees *and* hears the slow rate and dysrhythmia of the ataxic hand (Fig. 8-7). You can detect the irregular rhythm of the alternating movements much better by sound than by sight.
   d. Here is a challenge to your mastery of this test: If you listen carefully, you will hear a slight but definite difference in the pitch of the sound from

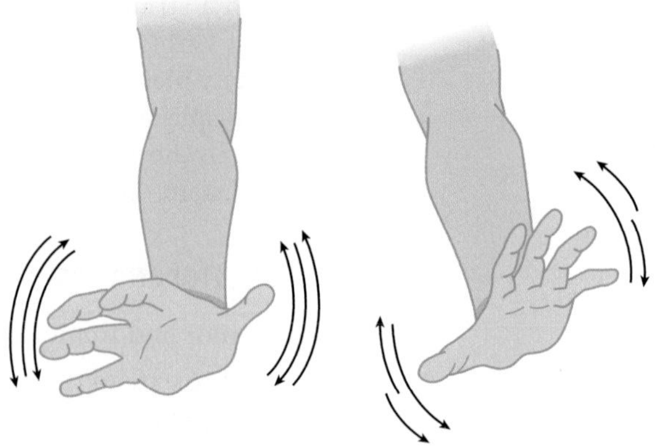

FIGURE 8-6. Pronation and supination test for dystaxia and dysmetria of the hands. Notice the even excursions of the normal right hand and the uneven excursions of the ataxic left hand.

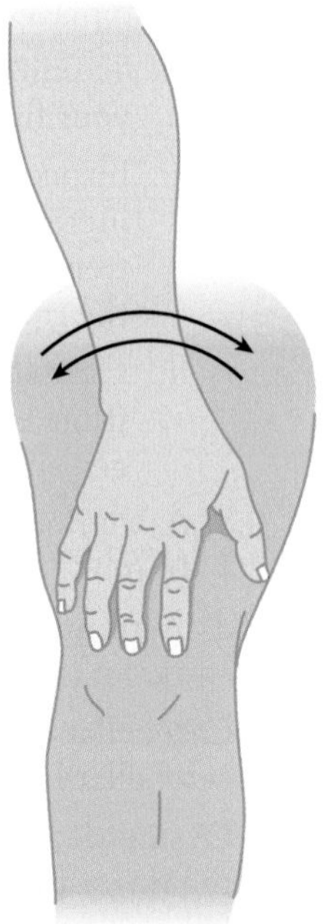

FIGURE 8-7. Thigh-patting test for dystaxia and dysmetria. The cerebellar patient slaps irregularly and turns the hand too much or too little in alternately slapping the front and the back of his hand on his thigh.

slapping the right or left thigh. We don't know the explanation, but the difference is real.

5. **The finger-tapping test:** Listen for dysrhythmia and slowness (Fisher, 1960). See Fig. 7-42.

F. Overshooting and checking tests of the arms

1. The cerebellar Pt has difficulty in maintaining a posture or position against a sudden, unexpected displacement. Have the Pt stand with eyes closed and arms outstretched.
2. Tell the Pt, "I am going to tap your arms. Hold them still. Don't let me budge them." The Ex strikes the back of the Pt's wrist a sharp blow, strong enough to displace the arm. The normal subject's arm returns quickly to its initial position. The cerebellar Pt's arm oscillates back and forth: it *overshoots* several times (Fig. 8-8).

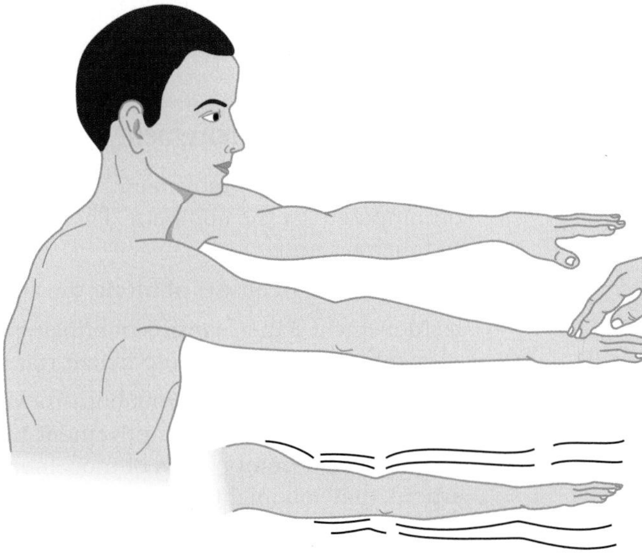

FIGURE 8-8. Wrist-tapping test for abnormal overshooting oscillation after sudden displacement of a part that is maintaining a volitional posture. The thin arrow shows the direction of the examiner's blow, which displaces the part.

3. Holmes (1917) pointed out that cerebellar Pts lack the normal rebound response.
   a. Have the Pt holds the arms extended out front.
   b. Grasp the wrists and ask the Pt to try to hold them in place as you pull down on them. Suddenly release your grip. The normal arm will fly upward a small distance, check and rebound, and quickly resume the resting position. The cerebellar Pt specifically overshoots by flying upward a greater distance and then overshoots the up and down position several times.
   c. Angel (1977) pointed out that neurologists have erroneously called the overshooting phenomenon the rebound sign of Holmes, when in reality the abnormality is failure to check before rebounding. Spastic limbs also rebound excessively.
4. **The *arm-pulling* test also demonstrates overshooting.**
   a. The Ex pulls hard against the Pt's flexed arm. When the Ex suddenly releases the Pt's arm, the cerebellar Pt fails to check the arm's flight (Fig. 8-9).

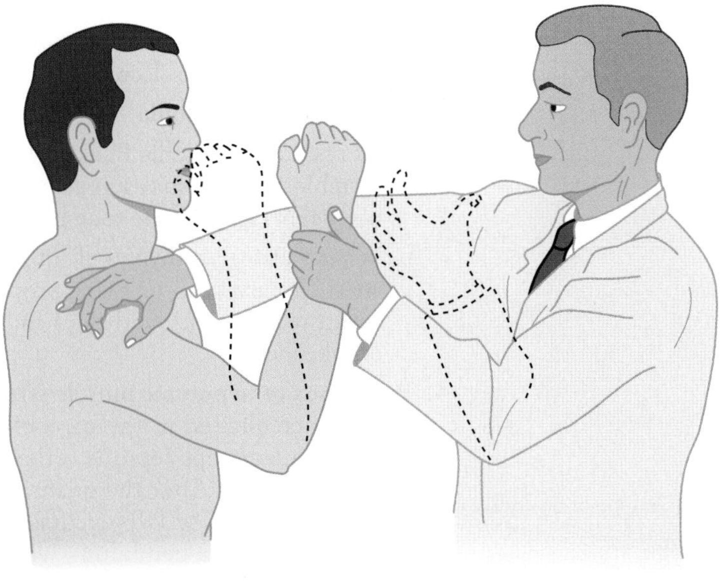

FIGURE 8-9. The arm-pulling test for overshooting. It tests how well the cerebellum functions to check movement and to maintain a given posture after a sudden release of tension on a muscle that is voluntarily contracting.

b. **Precaution:** Notice in Fig. 8-9 how the Ex places an arm to protect the Pt's face in case the Pt's arm fails to check and overshoots.

G. Decomposition of movement

1. In decomposition of movement, the Pt performs a movement as though it were decomposed "by the numbers." The Pt moves the arm from his side in two stages to touch his nose:
   a. Movement 1 consists of lifting the arm to the level of the nose.
   b. Movement 2 then consists of bringing the fingertip to the nose; the two movements produce a long, inefficient trajectory.
2. The normal person performs both movements simultaneously to produce the optimal and most efficient movement trajectory. Gordon Holmes (1876–1965) summarized decomposition of movement among other cerebellar tests in classic articles that you might enjoy reading (1939). You will gain profound insight into the mind of a master clinician at work.

H. Clinical tests for leg dystaxia: the heel-to-shin and heel-tapping tests

1. The **heel-to-shin test** for dystaxia supplements gait testing. Have the Pt supine or sitting. Instruct the Pt to place one heel *precisely* on the opposite knee. Have the Pt hold the heel to the knee for a few seconds and observe for a positional tremor. Then direct the Pt to run the heel in a straight line precisely down the shin. Again emphasize the importance of accuracy in the heel placement and movement.
2. For the **heel-tapping test,** ask the Pt to place one heel over the other shin and to tap the shin with the heel as rapidly as possible on one spot. The cerebellar Pt misses the spot (dysmetria) and taps dysrhythmically (dysdiadochokinesia).
3. Try these tests yourself. Again, such simple tasks offer a considerable challenge. Does your leg waver *at all* as you do the tests?

I. Clinical tests for hypotonia

the muscular resistance the Ex feels when moving the Pt's resting extremity

1. Muscle tone is operationally defined as ______________________________.
2. **Passive movement** discloses the increased range of joint excursions.
3. **Inspection for hypotonia**
   a. At rest, the hypotonic Pt assumes floppy postures and joint positions uncomfortable for a normal subject—rag-doll or dumped-in-a-heap postures. In a normal person, muscle tone helps to limit joint excursions.
   b. When walking, the hypotonic Pt presents a floppy, sagging, loose-jointed appearance. The arms fail to swing properly, the knees may bend backward slightly (genu recurvatum), and the head and trunk bob—a rag-doll gait, as seen in drunkenness.
4. **Pendulous or hypotonic muscle stretch reflexes (MSRs) in cerebellar Pts:** The MSRs, once elicited in the cerebellar Pt, fail to check normally, as best seen with the quadriceps femoris reflex. The Pt sits with the legs swinging freely over a table edge. After the quadriceps MSR is elicited, the leg normally stops swinging after one or two excursions. The cerebellar Pt's leg swings to and fro several times, like a pendulum, without the normal checking of the excursions by muscle tone.
5. Describe how to detect hypotonia in the cerebellar Pt. ______________________________

Passively move the Pt's extremities, inspect for rag-doll postures and a rag-doll gait, and look for pendulous MSRs.

J. Effect of cerebellar lesions on strength and endurance

The cerebellar Pt may experience mild **asthenia,** i.e., weakness, fatigability, and a reluctance to move. Formal strength testing by dynamometry does show some decrease in the maximum force of contraction, particularly in the acute hypotonic phase (Holmes, 1917). The feedback pathway that connects the cerebellar cortex with the cerebral motor cortex (Fig. 8-5) might explain the asthenia. Destruction of the pathway might alter the output of the cerebral motor cortex.

K. Summary of clinical tests for cerebellar dysfunction

1. Review Fig. 8-10, which summarizes the motor tests for cerebellar dysfunction. Act out each test in the dendrogram to ensure that you know how to do it.

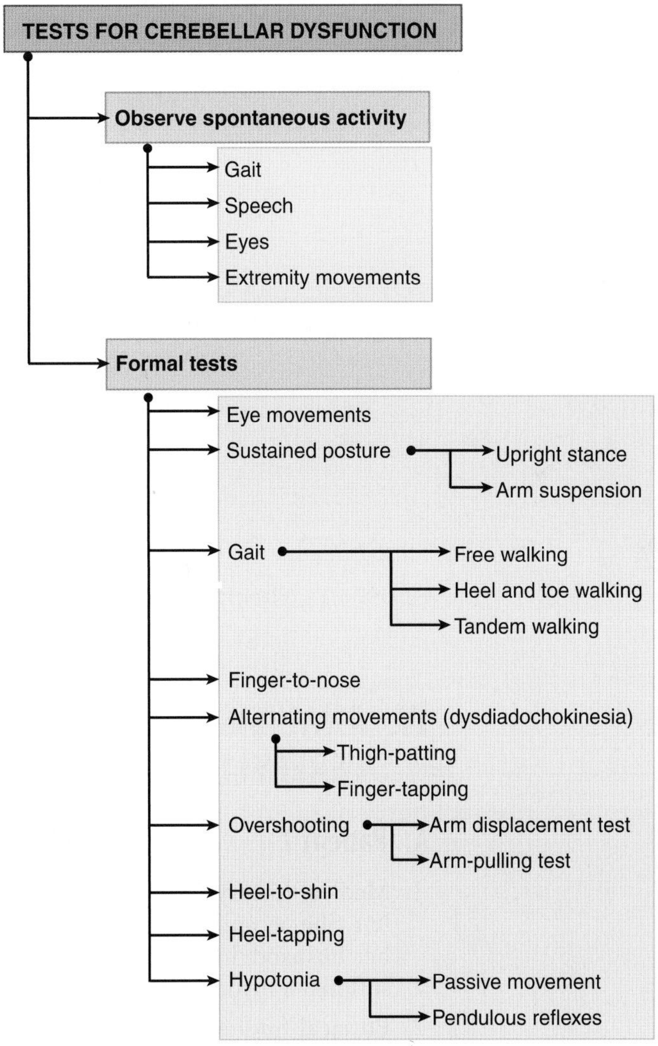

FIGURE 8-10. Dendrogram of motor tests for cerebellar dysfunction.

2. A quantitative battery standardizes the clinical tests for cerebellar dysfunction (Trouillas et al., 1997).

L. Review of circuitry for localization of cerebellar syndromes

Draw the cerebro-ponto-cerebello-dentato-thalamo-cortico-spinal circuit in Fig. 8-11. Compare your drawing with Fig. 8-5.

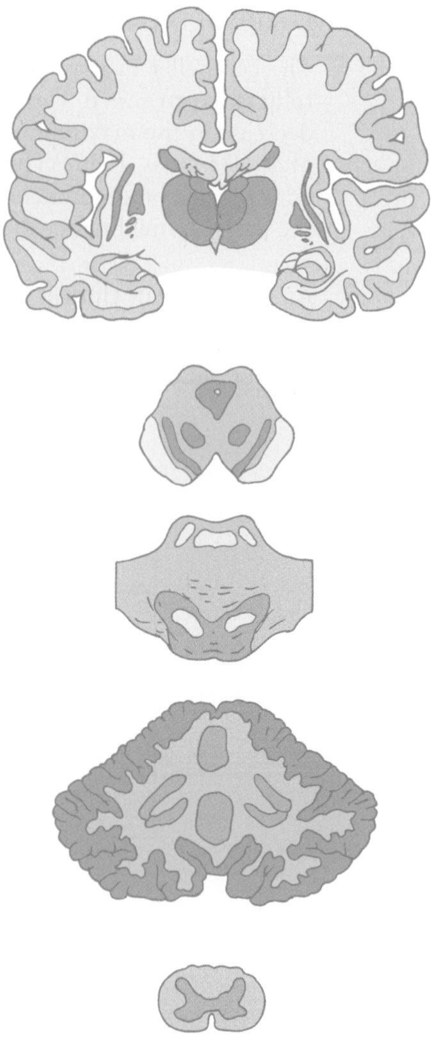

FIGURE 8-11. Blank for drawing the cerebro-cerebello-pyramidal pathway.

IV. ANALYSIS OF PATIENTS AND THE FOUR CEREBELLAR SYNDROMES

A. Patient 1

1. **Medical history:** This 62-year-old woman awakened and, on arising, fell to the left. She became dizzy, vomited, and struggled back into bed. When she called to her husband, he noticed slurred speech. Hypertensive for many years, she had suffered a myocardial infarct at the age of 60.
2. **Physical findings:** The Pt was conscious, cooperative, and intact mentally. She had mild dysarthria. She had a bidirectional nystagmus, with the slow movement toward a null point a little to the right of center. The nystagmus increased when looking to the left. She had slight ptosis of the left eyelid and miosis on the left. The corneal reflex was reduced on the left, and she had hypalgesia on the left side of her face. Pain and temperature discrimination were reduced on the right side of the body and in the right extremities, but the right side of the face was spared. The left side of the palate failed to elevate when she said *Ahhh*. Otherwise, the CrNs functioned normally. She could not walk unless supported. She had somewhat less strength on the left side and definitely less muscle tone. She had severe dystaxia on finger-to-nose and heel-to-knee testing on the left side only. She had left-sided dysdiadochokinesia. Her left arm overshot. Her left quadriceps femoris reflex was pendular. She had flexor plantar responses.

☑ left cerebellar hemisphere

3. **Lesion localization in Pt 1:** Before continuing the text, try to diagnose the location of the lesion. First review the brainstem cross sections in Figs. 2-15 to 2-18. In seeking a single lesion or at least a single pathologic process, first assemble the clinical data that require explanation (Table 8-2). The left-sided dystaxia and other cerebellar signs implicate a lesion of the ☐ vermis/☐ right cerebellar hemisphere/☐ left cerebellar hemisphere.

TABLE 8-2 · Localizing Findings in Patient 1 (Collate with Fig. 10-17)

Clinical sign	Anatomic basis
Left-side ataxia, hypotonia, and mild asthenia	Lesion of the left cerebellar hemisph
Pendular muscle stretch reflexes on the left	Lesion of the left cerebellar hemisphere
Bidirectional nystagmus, increased when looking left (Fig. 5-7)	Lesion of the left cerebellar hemisphere
Left-side ptosis and miosis (Horner's syndrome)	Interruption of descending sympathetic pathway on left
Left-side palatal palsy	Interruption of cranial nerve X intra-axially on the left
Left-side hemifacial hypalgesia	Interruption of the descending root of cranial nerve V on the left
Right-side hypalgesia, sparing face	Interruption of decussated spinothalamictract on the left

Yes. Left cerebellar hemisphere.

4. Review the nystagmus dendrograms (Figs. 5-6 and 5-7) and state whether the Pt's nystagmus helps to localize the lesion and, if so, to where.

---

5. **Noncerebellar findings in Pt 1:** Because lesions limited to the cerebellum do not impair sensation or cause CrN palsies, damage at another site must have caused ptosis, miosis (Horner's syndrome), reduced left corneal reflex palatal palsy, and right-side sensory loss.
6. **Clinicopathologic correlation in Pt 1**
   a. Magnetic resonance imaging (MRI) showed infarction of the lateral aspect of the medulla on the left and of the left cerebellar hemisphere. The lateral wedge of medullary tissue that was infarcted conveys descending autonomic axons and the descending root of CrN V and ascending spinocerebellar tracts (Figs. 2-15 to 2-18, and especially see Fig. 10-23A).
   b. Interruption of the autonomic fibers that descend from the hypothalamus through the medullary tegmentum on their way to the intermediolateral cell column of T1 and T2 accounts for Horner's syndrome.
   c. Interruption of the ipsilateral descending root of CrN V accounts for the reduced the corneal reflex and hemifacial loss of pain and temperature sensation (Fig. 10-2).
   d. Interruption of the crossed, ascending spinothalamic tract that mediates pain and temperature accounts for the loss of pain and temperature on the body and extremities (Figs. 2-28 and 10-23B).
   e. The vertigo and vomiting reflect interruption of the vestibular connections with the medullary reticular formation.
   f. To assign the cerebellar and medullary findings to one cause requires knowledge of the arterial supply of the posterior fossa. One artery, the posterior inferior cerebellar artery (PICA), irrigates the lateral medullary wedge and the overlying cerebellum. Because of the Pt's hypertension, the probable diagnosis is a *PICA syndrome (Wallenberg syndrome)*, i.e., ischemia or frank infarction in the distribution of PICA (the intracranial vertebral artery is primarily occluded). Notice how the history, general physical findings, and knowledge of neuroanatomy, blood supply, and probable pathogenesis converge to make the diagnosis.

g. If we set aside the medullary signs, Pt 1 had the typical **cerebellar hemisphere syndrome** (essentially the posterior lobe syndrome), consisting of the full panoply of cerebellar signs (Table 8-3) *ipsilateral* to the lesion, including a particular type of bidirectional nystagmus. Figure 8-12A shows the unilateral distribution of signs in the cerebellar hemisphere syndrome.

TABLE 8-3 · Four Cerebellar Syndromes That Correlate Lesion Site with the Distribution of Clinical Signs

A	B							C	D
				Dystaxia of					
Distribution of signs	Dysarthria	Arm overshoot	Hypotonia	Arms	Gait and trunk	Legs	Nystagmus	Name of clinical syndrome, based on part of cerebellum affected:	Lobe(s) most affected
1. 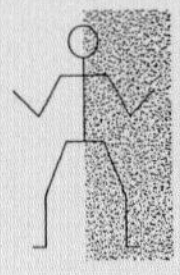	+	+	+	+	+	+	Holmes bidirectional, with null point		
2. 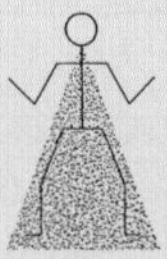	0	±	+	+	+	+	0		
3. 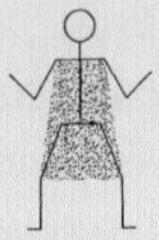	0	0	±	0	0	±	variable		
4. 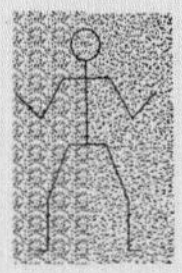	+	+	+	+	+	+	+ (variable type)		

Answers—Table 8-3

C
1. Hemisphere syndrome
2. Rostral vermis syndrome
3. Caudal vermis syndrome
4. Pancerebellar syndrome

D
1. Mainly posterior, variably anterior lobe
2. Anterior lobe
3. Flocculonodular and posterior lobe
4. All lobes

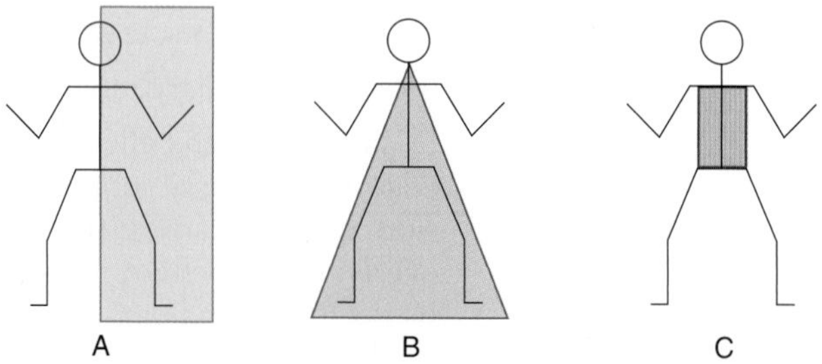

FIGURE 8-12. Distribution of cerebellar signs. (A) Distribution of cerebellar signs in the cerebellar hemisphere syndrome (left hemisphere in this instance). (B) Distribution of signs in the rostral vermis syndrome. (C) Distribution of signs in the caudal vermis syndrome.

Ipsilaterally: cerebellar hemisphere signs, a reduced corneal reflex, facial hypalgesia, Horner's syndrome, and palatal palsy. Contralaterally: loss of pain and temperature sensation on body and extremities sparing the face. See Table 8-2.

h. The cerebellar hemisphere syndrome follows any acute cerebellar hemisphere lesion: infarct, abscess, trauma, hemorrhage, neoplasm, or demyelinating disease.

i. Summarize the neurologic signs of a PICA syndrome. Ipsilaterally:________ ____. Contralaterally: ________ ____.

B. Patient 2

1. **History:** This 48-year-old man had drunk alcohol excessively for 13 years, resulting in numerous hospitalizations for drunkenness, convulsions, and delirium tremens. For 3 years his gait had become increasingly unsteady, to the degree that his family thought he was drunk even when he was sober. He stopped drinking 3 days before the examination.
2. **Physical examination:** The Pt was malnourished and unkempt but sober. He was somewhat disoriented as to time and date. The CrNs functioned normally. He had no nystagmus or dysarthria. Although generally somewhat tremulous, his finger-to-nose, alternating-movements, and overshoot tests of the arms were fairly normal. He had moderate truncal unsteadiness when sitting or standing. He had an unsteady, broad-based gait and could not tandem walk. His heel-to-shin movements were dystaxic. His quadriceps femoris reflexes were pendular. Notice in Fig. 8-13 that the triceps surae MSRs are recorded as ±. Chronic alcoholics often have some degree of peripheral neuropathy.

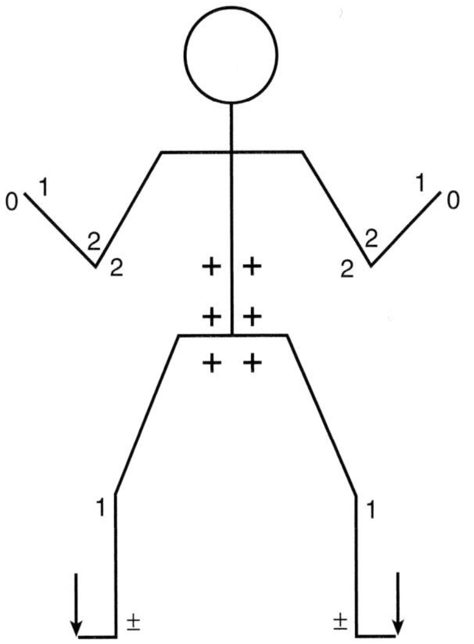

FIGURE 8-13. Reflex stick figure of patient 2.

3. **Course of Pt 2:** Five days after hospitalization, the Pt began to display severe delirium tremens with hyperthermia and convulsions. He died from irreversible hyperthermia. At autopsy, a sagittal cut through cerebellar vermis showed severe atrophy of all the folia of the rostral part. Microscopically the rostral part of the vermis and adjacent anterior lobe cortex showed severe depletion of neurons.
4. **Clinicopathologic correlation in Pt 2**

a. Which panel in Fig. 8-12 shows the distribution of cerebellar signs in Pt 2? ❒ A/❒ B/❒ C.

☑ B

b. The rostral vermis and adjacent cortex belong to which lobe of the cerebellum? ❒ anterior/❒ posterior/❒ flocculonodular.

☑ anterior

c. The rostral part of the vermis receives proprioceptive information from the legs and trunk via the ________________ tracts.

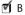

spinocerebellar

d. The clinical picture of classical cerebellar signs in the legs, mild truncal dystaxia, minimal or no arm dystaxia, and absence of dysarthria or nystagmus predicts atrophy limited to the rostral part of the vermis, as shown by Pt 2 (Victor et al., 1959).

e. Patients with anterior cerebellar lobe lesions caused by alcoholism and malnutrition do not show the extensor hypertonus caused by anterior lobe lesions in experimental animals (Ringel and Culbertson, 1988). The gradient of cerebellar signs predicts the lesion location. The signs affect *least* the ❒ CrN musculature/❒ arms/❒ trunk/ ❒ legs and *most* the ❒ CrN musculature/❒ arms/ ❒ trunk/❒ legs.

☑ CrN musculature; ☑ legs

C. Patient 3

1. **History:** This 6-year-old boy had trouble walking for 3 months, with increasing headaches and vomiting. Formerly very active, he no longer ran or played.
2. **Physical examination**

a. CrN examination showed questionable papilledema. He had very faint symmetrical jerk nystagmus in the extreme field of gaze to each side, with the quick component in the direction of gaze. When his eyes were returned slightly toward the midline, the nystagmus disappeared. He walked with a somewhat unsteady gait, but he could not tandem walk. At times he veered to the right, at others to the left. With the boy reclining in bed, formal cerebellar testing showed no definite abnormalities on finger-to-nose or heel-to-knee testing or on the rapid-alternating movements and overshoot tests. However, he had an unsteady trunk in any vertical position—thus when sitting, standing, or walking. In other words, he had predominately an *axial* or *truncal ataxia,* or **titubation.** Sensation was normal. Figure 8-14 shows the reflex pattern.

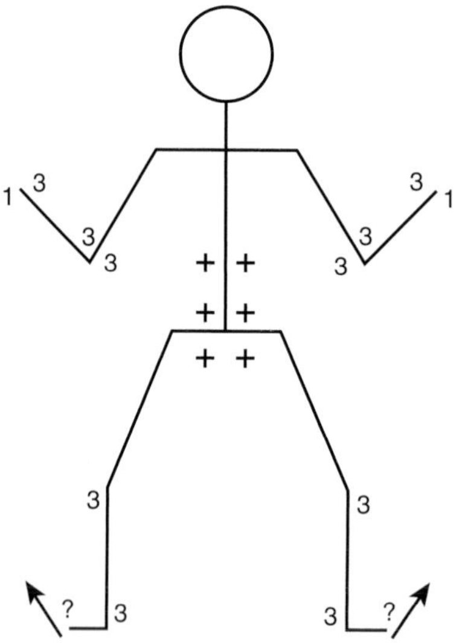

FIGURE 8-14. Reflex stick figure of patient 3.

b. MRI examination showed a posterior fossa tumor occluding the IV ventricle, with enlargement of the aqueduct, III, and lateral ventricles, indicating obstructive hydrocephalus (Figs. 1-25C to 1-25D). Posterior fossa craniotomy disclosed a medulloblastoma involving the flocculonodular lobe and posterior vermis.

3. **Clinicopathologic correlation in Pt 3**

a. From the nystagmus dendrograms, identify the type of nystagmus (Figs. 5-6 and 5-7): ______________________.

pseudonystagmus

b. Pseudonystagmus usually has no pathologic significance and was not clearly related to the neoplasm. The Ex always has to consider whether a finding is new or preexistent and not relevant. The equivocal extensor toe signs and vomiting probably reflect compression of the medulla and the increased intracranial pressure. Because the skull sutures had split, the boy had no florid papilledema, as often occurs from an obstructed IV ventricle.

c. The localizing clinical features in this 6-year-old boy were a nearly pure syndrome of *postural dysequilibrium* or *truncal ataxia* whenever he had to voluntarily maintain an erect posture, either sitting or standing, and severe impairment of tandem walking. However, formal cerebellar tests with the Pt reclining were very nearly normal. It is tempting to suggest that disruption of vestibulocerebellar and cerebellovestibular connections caused the postural disturbance, that he had a *flocculonodular lobe syndrome* or *caudal vermis syndrome* of dystaxia of the axial muscles and severe disturbance of tandem walking (Bastian et al., 1998). But we schematize too much. "The facile gates of hell are too slightly barred" (John Milton, 1608–1674). The large size of the neoplasm and distorted posterior fossa anatomy silence further speculation.

☑ C

d. Which panel in Fig. 8-12 shows the distribution of cerebellar signs in Pt 3? ❐ A/❐ B/❐ C.

D. Summary of the four syndromes of the cerebellum

1. Because the nodule of the flocculonodular lobe is in the caudal part of the vermis, we can contrast the *caudal vermis syndrome* of Pt 3 with the *rostral vermis syndrome* of Pt 2 and the *cerebellar hemisphere syndrome* of Pt 1. Then if we recognize a *pancerebellar syndrome* caused by any agent affecting the entire cerebellum bilaterally, we see that the first step in diagnosing cerebellar lesions is to classify, if possible, the Pt's deficits into one of the four cerebellar syndromes, as follows:

rostral vermis (anterior lobe)

2. Dystaxia predominantly in the legs, sparing the CrN musculature, is the ________________________ cerebellar syndrome.

caudal vermis (flocculonodular lobe)

3. **Dystaxia** or dysequilibrium of stance and gait (axial dystaxia) with little or no extremity dystaxia is the ________________________ cerebellar syndrome.

hemisphere (posterior lobe)

4. Cerebellar signs lateralized to one half of the body is the cerebellar ________________________ syndrome.
5. **Tabular summary of the four cerebellar syndromes:** Study the clinical characteristics listed in Table 8-3, and from these characteristics complete the two right columns.
6. Run down each column in Table 8-3 to discover an important bonus from displaying the data in tabular form. The only column with a strong plus for each of the four cerebellar syndromes is the gait dystaxia column. Gait incoordination is the one ubiquitous cerebellar sign (Bastian, 1998; Stolze et al., 2002) common to all four cerebellar syndromes. The upright posture and gait demand integration of the entire sensory and motor systems by the cerebrum and cerebellum. Hence, gait testing, in particular tandem walking, is the most efficient clinical test for cerebellar dysfunction and many other neurologic deficits.

E. Etiologic implications of the four cerebellar syndromes

1. Earlier I stated that, by identifying the cerebellar syndrome, the Ex could predict the probable lesion. The**rostral vermis syndrome** results from alcoholism and nutritional deficiency. The **caudal vermis syndrome** implies a midline cerebellar neoplasm, usually a medulloblastoma, ependymoma, or astrocytoma. The**cerebellar hemisphere syndrome** comes from an acute destructive lesion, most likely an infarct, hemorrhage, neoplasm, abscess, or trauma. The **pancerebellar syndrome** requires a lesion that affects the entire cerebellum, and, therefore, usually results from vitamin deficiencies (e.g., vitamin E). toxic or metabolic, demyelinating, immune mediated, paraneoplastic, or hereditary (autosomal recessive or autosomal dominant ataxias) or non-hereditary degenerative ataxias (e.g., multiple

system atrophy—cerebellar type). (Klockgether, 2008). Thus, by identifying the cerebellar syndrome, the Ex defines or delimits the diagnostic probabilities, which in turn leads to the most effective diagnostic workup.

2. The pancerebellar syndrome presents the most difficulty in differential diagnosis because the causative agents span the ocean of possibilities from heredofamilial diseases to the toxic effects of drugs. Intermittent pancerebellar signs suggest a metabolic disorder with intermittent flare-ups, disclosed by measuring amino acids and organic acids, or a demyelinating disorder, such as multiple sclerosis. The fairly common vascular lesions that affect the distribution of only one cerebellar artery are relatively easy to diagnose (Amarenco, 1991).
3. **A final warning:** A mass lesion in the cerebellum or posterior fossa is always a danger. It may cause the posterior fossa contents to herniate upward through the tentorial notch or downward through the foramen magnum or directly compress the medullary respiratory center (Chapter 13).

V. SUMMARY OF THE CLINICAL EXAMINATION FOR CEREBELLAR DYSFUNCTION

Rehearsal time again! Can you give the commands, make the observations, and do the tests for cerebellar dysfunction? Work through Fig. 8-10. If you have followed the Standard Neurologic Examination outline, you have already tested muscle tone and elicited the MSRs, which would have disclosed pendular reflexes and hypotonia.

BIBLIOGRAPHY · Cerebellar Dysfunction

Ackerman H, Ziegler W. Cerebellar voice tremor: an acoustic analysis. *J Neurol Neurosurg Psychiatry* 1991;54:74–76.

Alusi SH, Worthington J, Glickman S, et al. Evaluation of three different ways of assessing tremor in multiple sclerosis. *J Neurol Neurosurg Psychiatry* 2000;68:756–760.

Amarenco P. The spectrum of cerebellar infarctions. *Neurology* 1991;41:973–979.

Angel RW. The rebound phenomenon of Gordon Holmes. *Arch Neurol* 1977;34:250.

Angevine J Jr, Mancall E, Yakovlev P. *The Human Cerebellum: An Atlas of Gross Topography in Serial Sections.* Boston, Little, Brown & Co, 1961.

Anthoney TR. *Neuroanatomy and the Neurologic Exam.* Boca Raton, CRC, 1994.

Barboi A. Cerebellar ataxia. *Arch Neurol* 2000;57:1525–1527.

Bastian AJ, Mink JW, Kaufman BA, et al. Posterior vermal split syndrome. *Ann Neurol* 1998;44:601–610.

Bougousslavsky J, Meienberg O. Eye-movement disorders in brainstem and cerebellar stroke. *Arch Neurol* 1987;44:141–148.

Daum I, Ackermann H. Neuropsychological abnormalities in cerebellar syndromes. *Int Rev Neurobiol* 1997;41:455–471.

DeMyer W. *Neuroanatomy,* 2nd ed. Baltimore, Williams & Wilkins, 1998.

Fisher CM. A simple test of coordination in the fingers. *Neurology* 1960;10:745–746.

Giron LT, Koller WC. Anatomic localization of tremor, clinical analysis, pitfalls, and principles. In Lechtenberg R. *Handbook of Cerebellar Diseases.* New York, Marcel Dekker, 1993.

Glaser JS, ed. *Neuro-ophthalmology,* 3rd ed. Philadelphia, Lippincott Williams & Wilkins, 1999.

Holmes G. The cerebellum of man. *Brain* 1939;62:1–30.

Holmes G. The symptoms of acute cerebellar injuries due to gunshot injuries. *Brain* 1917;40:461–535.

Karatekin C, Lazareff JA, Asarnow RF. Relevance of the cerebellar hemispheres for executive functions. *Pediatr Neurol* 2000;22:106–112.

Klockgether T, In: *Therapeutics of Parkinson's Disease and Other Movement Disorders.* Mark Hallet and Werner Poewe (eds.) Wiley-Blackwell 2008; Chapter 27, pp. 407–415.

Larsell O, Jansen J. *The Comparative Anatomy and Histology of the Cerebellum. The Human Cerebellum, Cerebellar Connections, and Cerebellar Cortex*. Minneapolis, University of Minnesota Press, 1972.

Lechtenberg R. Signs and symptoms of cerebellar disease. In Lectenberg R, ed. *Handbook of Cerebellar Diseases.* New York, Marcel Dekker, 1993, Chap. 4, pp. 31–43.

Malm J, Kristensen B, Karlsson T, et al. Cognitive impairment in young adults with infratentorial infarcts. *Neurology* 1998;51:433–440.

Manto MU, Pondolfo M. *The Cerebellum and Its Disorders.* New York, Cambridge University Press, 2001.

Pierrot-Deseilligny C, Amarenco P, Roullet E, et al. Vermal infarct with pursuit eye movement disorders. *J Neurol Neurosurg Psychiatry* 1990;53:519–521.

Ringel RA, Culberson JL. Extensor tone disinhibition from an infarction within the midline anterior cerebellar lobe. *J Neurol Neurosurg Psychiatry* 1988;51:1597–1599.

Schmahmann JD. The role of the cerebellum in affect and psychosis. In Manto MU, Pondolfo M, eds. *The Cerebellum and Its Disorders.* New York, Cambridge University Press, 2001, Chapter 9, pp. 136–153.

Stolze H, Klebe S, Petersen G, et al. Typical features of cerebellar ataxic gait. *J Neurol Neurosurg Psychiatry* 2002;73:310–312.

Stoodley CJ, Schmahmann JD. Evidence for topographic organization in the cerebellum of motor control versus cognitive and affective processing. *Cortex* 2010;46:831–844.

Trouillas P, Takayanagi T, Hallet M, et al. International cooperative ataxia rating scale for pharmacological assessment of the cerebellar syndrome. *J Neurol Sci* 1997;145:205–211.

van Mourik M, Catsman-Berrevoets CE, Yousef-Bak E, et al. Dysarthria in children with cerebellar or brainstem tumors. *Pediatr Neurol* 1998;18:411–414.

Victor M, Adams R, Mancall E. A restricted form of cerebellar degeneration occurring in alcoholic patients. *Arch Neurol* 1959;1:579–688.

VI. AN ESSAY ON TESTING STATION (STANDING) AND GAIT (WALKING)

A. Importance of the station and gait examination

If we had just one chance to make the diagnosis, we would choose the most important single part of the neurologic examination: watching the Pt rise, stand, and walk. First notice how the Pt rises and the steadiness of the vertical posture. Then ask the Pt to walk freely back and forth. As the Pt walks, look for irregular strides, lack of a heel-to-toe foot action, unsteadiness, a wide-based gait, an overplay of involuntary movements, and lack of or excessive arm swinging. Notice whether the Pt turns by stepping around freely or rotates on the spot, en bloc, with tiny steps (see parkinsonian gait and *marche à petit pas,* below). Next, test triceps surae strength and balance by having the Pt walk on the balls of the feet and then on the heels. Next request tandem walking (heel-to-toe down a straight line). Finally, request a deep kneebend. Ask a child to run and hop. Throughout, note how well the Pt comprehends and executes the commands. Retarded, demented, psychotic, and passive-aggressive or oppositional Pts require constant coaxing.

If the Pt rises, stands, and walks completely normally, then, in all probability, the Pt's *motor* system is completely intact. If the Pt's motor system is completely intact, then, in all probability, the *sensory* system is completely intact. If the Pt follows all commands promptly and well, with no confusion or hesitancy, then in all probability the Pt's *mental* state and sensorium are intact. With *motor, sensory,* and *mental* functions intact, then, in all probability, the Pt's nervous system is intact. Of course, you must still complete the entire neurologic examination to confirm these initial inferences. A normal gait requires the integrity of vast circuits of the peripheral and central nervous systems: circuits that underlie the willing of movements and the antigravity, supporting, and righting reflexes; circuits that coordinate the rate, regularity, and force of the muscular contractions; circuits that generate reciprocal limb actions; and circuits that mediate touch, proprioception, and vision. Most disorders of the muscles, nerves, spinal cord, cerebellum, brainstem, basal ganglia, or cerebrum impair the gait and in a characteristic way. Thus, the features of the gait disorder suggest the lesion location and probable cause.

B. Developmental gaits

Gait examination begins with the genetically preprogrammed *automatic* or *reflex stepping* of the neonate. If the Ex holds the neonate vertically, with its feet contacting the bed surface, the infant reflexly lifts its legs alternately and steps. Voluntary trunk control and voluntary standing will later replace automatic stepping, leading to a *cruising gait,* in which the infant takes steps when holding onto a couch or when steadied by a parent. Then, at about 1 year the infant walks freely, with a *toddler's gait,* featured by a broad-base, short, jerky, irregular steps, a semiflexed posture of the arms, and frequent falls (progression by three steps and a plop). After the toddler stage the child develops a normal *mature gait,* with a narrow-based, heel-toe stride, contrabody movement, and reciprocal swinging of the arms (Woollacott et al., 1989). The gait sequence merely reflects a general law of infant development, that **inborn, so-called primitive reflexes or behaviors predate all voluntary actions.** Thus, smiling, chewing, sucking, grasping, breathing, and walking occur reflexly before the brain and its pathways mature to control these actions voluntarily.

C. Neuromuscular gaits

Let us start with the neuromuscular system and work up to cerebral lesions. If you wish to learn the most from this essay, I strongly recommend that you get up and act out the gaits described. First get up and imitate the toddler gait. If an infant has a *clubfoot gait,* the gait depends on which of a variety of valgus or varus deformities exists. With tibial torsion, the infant has an *in-toed* or *pigeon-toed gait.* Many clubfoot deformities correct themselves. Most myopathies (the muscular dystrophies and the polymyositises) weaken the proximal muscles of the shoulders, back, and hips. Because of weak paraspinal muscles, the myopathic Pt shows a characteristic, usually sway-backed, waddle, a *lordotic waddling gait* resembling the *pride of pregnancy gait* of the third trimester. Because of the weak proximal muscles, the myopathic Pt has trouble when getting up on or down from the examining table or when standing up from a sitting or especially a reclining position. In so arising, the myopathic Pt may display **Gower's sign,** the bracing of the arms against the thighs to push the weak trunk erect.

This 4-year-old boy, striding on the balls of his feet, without a definite heel strike has a *toe-walking gait* (Sala et al., 1999). Tight heel cords limit dorsiflexion of the foot to about 90 degrees. Such a gait occurs in Duchenne's muscular dystrophy, in spastic diplegia, and in autistic or other retarded children. But the next toe-walking child moves along jauntily, runs, skips, and hops normally and has none of these serious disorders, merely an idiosyncratic, sometimes familial, gait pattern.

The next Pt's toes do not clear the floor because of paralysis of foot dorsiflexion, causing a *toe-drop* or *foot-drop gait.* In compensation, the Pt jerks the knee high, flipping the foot up into dorsiflexion, and slaps the foot down. With unilateral or bilateral foot-drop gait, the sound of the slapping feet alone permits the Ex to suspect the diagnosis, without even seeing the Pt. Unilateral foot drop suggests a unilateral, perhaps mechanical or compressive, neuropathy of the common peroneal nerve, frequently from a crossed-knee palsy. A *bilateral foot-drop* or *steppage gait* suggests a symmetrical distal peripheral neuropathy of toxic, metabolic, or heredofamilial type, as in alcoholic neuropathy or Charcot-Marie-Tooth progressive peroneal atrophy.

A tibial nerve palsy, in contrast to a peroneal nerve palsy, causes a *heel-drop gait.* The Pt can dorsiflex the foot but not plantar flex it. A complete sciatic palsy causes a *flail-foot gait* in which the Pt can neither dorsiflex nor plantar flex the foot. Now you see why the Ex asks the Pt to walk on the toes *and* the heels. These actions test all the muscles innervated by the sciatic nerve, in addition to proprioception and balance.

D. Sensory gaits

A *tabetic, dorsal column,* or *sensory ataxic gait* resembles a double foot-drop or steppage gait but has its own unique signature. In tabes dorsalis, syphilitic infection causes degeneration of dorsal roots and dorsal columns of the spinal cord. Lacking position sense, the Pt lifts the knees too high and slaps the feet down, placing them irregularly and on a broad base, because of sensory ataxia. The Pt simply does not know where the legs are. When in bed, the Pt literally has to peek under the covers to locate the feet and legs. To compensate for the lack of position sense, the tabetic Pt must use visual cues to stand. Eye closure removes the visual cues that compensate for the absence of position sense. The Pt then sways and falls over, thus failing the Romberg test (Chapter 10), which the cerebellar Pt more or less passes. The steppage gait of dorsal column disease differs from the double foot-drop gait of peroneal palsy by the presence of normal dorsiflexor power, irregular foot placement due to the sensory ataxia, the absence of position and vibration sense in the legs, absence of MSRs, and abnormal Romberg test. The presence of Argyll Robertson pupils and a positive serologic test for syphilis (Table 4-5) separates tabes dorsalis from other dorsal column diseases such as the subacute combined degeneration of pernicious anemia or the spinocerebellar degenerations. The experienced Ex will not confuse any of the gaits in this entire essay with the slow, deliberate, searching steps of the blind Pt, the *blind person's gait.*

The next Pt has a *painful sole* or *hyperesthetic gait.* The Pt sets the foot down gingerly, bears as little weight on it as possible, and limps off the foot as soon as possible while wincing and hunching the shoulders. This feature, the limiting of weight bearing by pain, is the *antalgic gait.* If the pain is unilateral and on the bottom of the ball of the foot, suspect Morton's metatarsalgia, a painful neuroma of an interdigital nerve; if it affects the large toe (podagra), consider gout. If the pain is bilateral, the Pt looks like a person walking barefoot on a hot pavement; suspect hyperesthesia of both soles, common in painful distal peripheral neuropathies, usually metabolic, toxic, or alcoholic or nutritional in origin. When the Pt complains of foot pain, always examine the Pt's shoes—the wear pattern tells a tale in itself—and compare the size and shape of the shoe with the size and shape of the foot and note the heel height.

The next Pt has a *radicular* or *back pain posture* and an *antalgic gait.* The Pt complains of extreme pain radiating into the big toe, caused, in all probability, by a herniated intervertebral disc compressing the L5 nerve root. Coughing, or straight-leg raising causes shooting pain into the foot (pp. 399–404). To rise from a chair, the Pt pushes up with the arms and has a stiff back, with a completely flat lumbar curve. When standing, the Pt does not put weight on the painful leg and gets off of it as soon as possible (*antalgic gait*). The Achilles tendon feels soft to compression by the Ex's thumb, as compared with the weight-bearing leg. When walking, the Pt places little weight on the painful leg and takes stiff, slow, short strides with no heel strike, to avoid painful jarring. Often the Pt's trunk tilts slightly to the side opposite the pain.

Even upper extremity neuropathies may cause a characteristic gait disorder. If the Pt's transverse carpal ligament compresses the median nerve, causing a carpal tunnel syndrome, excruciating pain in the hand typically awakens the Pt at night. Night after night, the Pt gets up and paces the bedroom flipping or shaking the hand in an effort to gain some relief, the *nocturnal flipping-hand gait,* a nearly pathognomonic gait. Autistic and other retarded children show a variety of *flipping-hand gaits* as repetitive, self-stimulating mannerisms.

E. Cerebellar ataxic gaits

Cerebellar lesions cause dystaxia of voluntary movements and of voluntarily maintained postures, hence, a reeling stance and gait. A unilateral cerebellar lesion causes only *ipsi*lateral cerebellar signs, most likely from neoplasm, infarct, or demyelinating disease. After an acute cerebellar lesion, the Pt frequently veers or falls in one direction (*latero*pulsion, *antero*pulsion, or *retro*pulsion). Bilateral cerebellar signs, thus a pancerebellar syndrome, imply a toxic, metabolic, or heredofamilial disorder or multiple sclerosis, if combined with other exacerbating and remitting signs.

Relatively pure dystaxia of the legs and gait, with little or no dystaxia of the arms, and no dysarthria or nystagmus suggest a rostral vermis syndrome, most commonly secondary to alcoholism. The painful peripheral neuropathy of such Pts also may cause an antalgic gait. Relatively pure truncal ataxia suggests a flocculonodular lobe or a caudal vermis lesion, generally a tumor (Bastain et al., 1998; Table 8-3).

F. Spastic gaits

With a *hemiplegic gait,* the Pt circumducts a leg, dragging the toe, placing the ball down without a heel strike, with the ipsilateral arm held in partial flexion or, more rarely, flaccidly at the side. Hemiplegia affects the hand and arm more than the leg and usually causes a closed fist because of flexor spasticity. The lesion is most likely an infarct, tumor, or trauma. The next Pt walks with stiff legs, not clearing the floor with either foot, the exact opposite of the Pt with a high steppage gait. This Pt gives the appearance of wading through water because she must work against the spastic opposition of her own muscles, as if walking in a viscid environment of molasses instead of air. Her knees tend to rub together in a scissoring action. She has a *spastic gait.* If the Pt has a *spastic diplegic gait* from cerebral palsy, she has small, short legs in contrast to normally developed chest, shoulders, and arms. In spastic diplegia, in direct contrast to double hemiplegia, the Pt has severe spasticity in her legs, minimal spasticity in her arms, and little or no deficit in speaking or swallowing (Gage, 1992), whereas the double hemiplegic has pseudobulbar palsy and the arm is weaker than the leg. The cerebral palsy Pt may adduct the legs strongly when walking, causing a *scissors gait.* The knees of some spastic diplegics may remain bent when walking, the *spastic diplegic crouch gait* (Tylkowski and Howell, 1991). The Pt looks as if wading through water or molasses with the knees bent. A pure spastic or *paraplegic gait,* with no sensory deficits, coming on after infancy, suggests a pure corticospinal tract disorder, such as familial spastic paraplegia. If, in addition to spasticity, the disease impairs the dorsal columns or cerebellum, the Pt will have a wider-based unsteady gait and take irregular steps—the *spastic-ataxic gait,* suggesting a spinocerebellar degeneration or multiple sclerosis.

G. Basal motor nuclei gaits

When the Pt with a *choreiform gait* walks, the play of finger and arm movements increases or may even appear clearly for the first time. Random missteps mar the evenness of the strides as the choreiform twitches supervene. Station is characteristically broadbased. A family history of chorea and dementia establishes Huntington's chorea. A history of rheumatic fever, the acute onset of chorea, and a fussy personality signify Sydenham's chorea. When the athetoid Pt walks, the slow writhing movements of fingers and arms tend to increase. A combination of athetosis with moderate spastic diplegia or double hemiplegia, a *spastic-athetoid gait,* usually signifies status marmoratus (*état marbre*) of the basal ganglia and thalamus, secondary to perinatal hypoxia. The Pt's great toe may automatically extend when walking, a so-called *striatal toe.*

Dystonia may first manifest in a child, say of 9 years of age, by an intermittent inturning of one foot that impedes walking, a *dystonic equinovarus gait.* In the later stages, dystonic truncal contortions and tortipelvis may cause the trunk to incline strongly forward. The Pt may take giant uneven strides, exhibiting flexions or rise and fall of the trunk, the dystonic *dromedary gait,* imitating the ungainly gait of a dromedary camel. It looks for all of the world like histrionics, but the Pt has dystonia musculorum deformans, an organic, hereditary disorder. Genetic screening for the DYT gene abnormalities may be useful for patients with early onset dystonia or those with affected relatives. Patients with involuntary movement disorders can sometimes walk backward or dance better than they can walk forward.

This next Pt, with a *parkinsonian gait,* has a tremor at rest that disappears during voluntary movement, a flexed posture, rises and walks slowly with short steps, lacks any arm swing, and turns en bloc like a statue rotating on a pedestal. The Pt does not have a wide-based gait, as in cerebellar disease. If the Ex (after a warning) shoves the parkinsonian Pt, the Pt will move forward or backward on tiny steps of increasing speed and decreasing length, as if chasing the center of gravity, and may fall over, a *festinating gait*. Patients with the *marche à petit pas* often also turn en bloc and festinate. Parkinsonism results from degeneration of the substantia nigra or from neuroleptic medication. *Primary progressive freezing gait* belongs in the Parkinson category but does not respond to levodopa. The Pts freeze when starting to walk and when turning or in response to some stimulus. They show bradykinesia and a masked face. They get progressively worse, begin to fall, exhibit retropulsion, and become wheelchair dependent in about 4 to 5 years (Factor et al., 2002).

H. Cerebral gaits

Gait abnormalities often precede dementia of any type (Verghese et al., 2002). This elderly Pt with the shuffling, short steps, who does not lift the feet far from the floor, has the *marche à petit pas* (the march of small steps; Masdeu et al., 1997; Nutt et al., 1993; Sudarsky, 1990). When the Pt tries to speak, steps cease, leading to the somewhat pejorative, but expressive, colloquialism: "He can't walk and chew gum [in this case walk and talk] at the same time." The aged or demented brain loses the capacity for "dual-tasking" (Haggard et al. 2000). Many of the elderly Pts in a nursing home display this type of gait. It may result from senility (Masdeu et al., 1997), Alzheimer's disease, multi-infarct dementia, or periventricular lesions on MRI (Benson et al., 2002; Whitman et al., 2001).

A glance around a nursing home will disclose many Pts with forward flexion of the head, *head drop* or *head ptosis.* Many times the Pt has lost the sense of verticality: the entire trunk tilts in the chair, and the Pt goes to sleep in the head-dropped, body-tilted posture. The posture may result from neuromuscular disorders that cause weakness of the neck muscles, but it often coexists with dementia, parkinsonism, a forward flexed posture of the entire spine, called *camptocormia* (Umpathi et al., 2002), and usually a disorder of gait.

The next Pt, an elderly woman, has difficulty initiating the sequence of movements to rise, stand, or walk. When lying down, she makes fairly normal leg movements. When trying to rise from the chair, she rocks up and down several times to rise. When commencing to walk, she makes several efforts to move her feet. After these efforts, she appears somewhat puzzled, as if searching for lost motor engrams, or the right button to press to initiate walking. The effort to progress may result only in stepping on the same spot, as if trying to free the feet from thick, sticky mud, the *dancing bear gait.* If she does progress, her feet stick to the floor as if magnetized. Some observers have called the combination of short steps, wide base, and difficulty picking up the feet (magnet sign) a *frontal gait*, an *apraxic gait*, or an *ignition failure gait* (Nutt et al., 1993). Factor et al. (2002) stated that many Pts previously described with such terms may have *primary progressive freezing gait*, but its neuropathologic basis is unknown. Overall, just the presence of a clinically evident gait disorder in the elderly and the rate that it worsens correlate with the risk of death (Wilson et al., 2002).

Some Pts have a syndrome of gait disorder, dementia, and urinary incontinence. They take small steps of reduced velocity and variable stride length, but their feet characteristically turn out (Stolze et al., 2001), a feature unusual in other gait disorders. Formerly called *normal pressure hydrocephalus,* Bret et al. (2002) emphasized that it can also occur in children and prefer the name *chronic hydrocephalus.*

I. Psychiatric gaits

To fully appreciate the *astasia-abasia* (*astasia* = not standing; *abasia* = not walking) of the hysteric Pt, the neophyte physician will have to witness it (Lempert et al., 1991; Keane, 1989). Often the Pt tilts, gyrates, and undulates all over the place, unwittingly proving by not falling during the marvelous demonstration of agility that strength, balance, coordination, and sensation have to be intact. However, do not mistake some of the bizarre involuntary movement disorders, in particular the dromedary gait of dystonia, or some focal seizures for hysteria. Lempert et al. (1991) listed six features of psychogenic gait:

1. Moment-to-moment fluctuation
2. Excessive slowness or hesitation

3. Exaggerated sway on the Romberg test, improved by distraction
4. Postures that waste energy
5. Extremely cautious, restricted steps, like walking on ice
6. Sudden buckling of the knees without falling

To learn how other mental illnesses affect the gait, just watch any group of Pts in a psychiatric hospital as they walk along the hall to the cafeteria. Hardily a single Pt steps out with a perfectly normal gait. This Pt, hopelessly moving along, sighing, shoulders sagging, head down looking at the floor, obviously suffers from depression (Sloman, 1982). The Pt over there wringing her hands and wrinkling her brow has an agitated depression. That unkempt middle-aged man, walking with small irregular, wincing steps placed gingerly on a wide base has spindly arms and legs that contrast with a disproportionate, pregnancy-like fullness of the abdomen. His alcoholism has caused mild shoulder girdle weakness, ascites, a rostral vermis syndrome, and a painful sensory neuropathy with hyperesthetic soles. That young adult Pt with a mild parkinsonian gait is probably a schizophrenic taking large doses of neuroleptic medication. That young woman, gesticulating as if conversing as she walks along, is a schizophrenic, attending to her hallucinations. She is underdosed or her medication has not yet taken hold. That next grim-faced Pt, walking cautiously and peering around suspiciously, suffers from severe paranoid schizophrenia. That child, running helter skelter, bumping into people and objects, giggling inappropriately, has an attention deficit disorder with hyperactivity. The teenager who, of inner necessity, steps on every crack, pats every door, and suddenly halts his progression to whirl around and utter expletives suffers from the disabling compulsions of severe Tourette's syndrome. That aged Pt with silvery white hair, confusion of purpose and direction, and *marche à petit pas* has, as you now know, organic dementia, most likely from senility or Alzheimer's disease. The retarded and autistic children have their gait peculiarities, often characterized by behavioral stereotypies such as hand flapping (Vilensky, 1981). Thus does the gait often disclose the mental and the neurologic status of the Pt.

Gentle reader, if we have overdone the gait examination a little, forgive us. If not quite the whole neurologic examination, nothing else discloses so much so quickly.

BIBLIOGRAPHY · Gait Analysis

Bastain AJ, Mink JW, Kaufman BA, et al. Posterior vermal split syndrome. *Ann Neurol* 1998;44:601–610.

Benson RR, Guttmann CRG, Wei X, et al. Older people with impaired mobility have specific loci of periventricular abnormality on MRI. *Neurology* 2002;58:48–55.

Bret P, Guyotat J, Chazal J. Is normal pressure hydrocephalus a valid concept in 2002? A reappraisal in five questions and proposal for a new designation of the syndrome as "chronic hydrocephalus." *J Neurol Neurosurg Psychiatry* 2002;73:9–12.

Factor SA, Jennings DL, Molho ES, et al. The natural history of the syndrome of primary progressive freezing gait. *Arch of Neurol* 2002;59:1778–1783.

Gage JR. *Gait Analysis in Cerebral Palsy.* New York, Cambridge University Press, 1992.

Haggard P, Cockburn JK, Cock J, et al. Interference between gait and cognitive tasks in a rehabilitating neurologic population. *J Neurol Neurosurg Psychiatry* 2000;69:479–486.

Keane JR. Hysterical gait disorders. *Neurology* 1989;39:586–589.

Lempert S, Brandt S, Dieterich M, et al. How to identify psychogenic disorders of stance and gait. *J Neurol* 1991;238:140–146.

Masdeu JC, Sudarsky L, Wolfson L, eds. *Gait Disorders of Aging.* Baltimore, Lippincott-Raven, 1997.

Nutt JG, Marsden CD, Thompson PD. Human walking and higher-level gait disorders, particularly in the elderly. *Neurology* 1993;43:268–279.

Sala DA, Shulman LH, Kennedy RF, et al. Idiopathic toe-walking: a review. *Dev Med Child Neurol* 1999;41:846–848.

Sloman L, Berridge M, Homatidis S, et al. Gait patterns of depressed patients and normal subjects. *Am J Psychol* 1982;139:94–96.

Stolze H, Kuhtz-Buschbeck JP, Drucke H, et al. Comparative analysis of the gait disorder of normal pressure hydrocephalus and Parkinson's disease. *J Neurol Neurosurg Psychiatry* 2001;70:289–297.

Sudarsky L. Geriatrics: gait disorders in the elderly. *N Engl J Med* 1990; 322:1441–1448.

Swaab Tylkowski CM, Howell VL. Crouch gait in cerebral palsy. *Int Pediatr* 1991;6:153–160.

Umpathi T, Chaudhry V, Cornblath D, et al. Head drop and camptocormia. *J Neurol Neurosurg Psychiatry* 2002;73:1–7.

Verghese J, Lipton RB, Hall CB, et al. Abnormality of gait as a predictor of non-Alzheimer's dementia. *N Engl J Med* 2002;347:1761–1768.

Vilensky JA, Damasio AR, Maurer RG. Gait disturbances in patients with autistic behavior. *Arch Neurol* 1981;38:646–649.

Whitman GT, Tang T, Lin A, et al. A prospective study of cerebral white matter abnormalities in older people with gait dysfunction. *Neurology* 2001;57:990–994.

Wilson RS, Schneider JA, Beckett LA, et al. Progression of gait disorder and rigidity and risk of death in older persons. *Neurology* 2002;58:1815–1819.

Woollacott MH, Connolly K, Shumway-Cook A. *Development of Posture and Gait Across the Life Span*. Columbia, University of South Carolina Press, 1989.

Learning Objectives for Chapter 8

I. THE FUNCTION OF THE CEREBELLUM

1. State as briefly as possible the role of the cerebellum in movement as inferred from clinical observations.
2. Explain the importance of proprioceptive input to the cerebellum.
3. Explain why you cannot test for cerebellar dysfunction in a comatose or paralyzed patient.

II. ANATOMY OF THE CEREBELLUM

1. Name the three lobes of the cerebellum according to Larsell and state the major source of afferent fibers to each one (Table 8-1).
2. Make a schematic dorsal view drawing of the cerebellum showing its division into Larsell's three lobes and into the vermis and hemispheres (Fig. 8-1).
3. State which lobe of the cerebellum anatomically and phylogenetically has the closest relation to the vestibular nerve.
4. Give the phylogenetic name for the three lobes of the cerebellum (Table 8-1).
5. Name the three pairs of peduncles of the cerebellum. State where they attach the cerebellum to the brainstem and their anatomical relation to each other (Fig. 8-3).
6. Recite the "mnemonic of the **L**'s" for the middle cerebellar peduncle.
7. Describe the major afferent and efferent fibers conveyed through each of the three cerebellar peduncles.
8. Describe the general plan of the flow of impulses through the cerebellum, beginning with the afferent pathway (Fig. 8-4).
9. Name the cerebellar neuron that provides the final common pathway out of the cerebellar cortex.
10. Diagram the cortico-cerebello-cortical circuit, beginning with one cerebral motor cortex (Fig. 8-5).
11. Describe the decussations underlying the aphorism: "Cerebral hemisphere lesions cause contralateral motor signs, whereas cerebellar hemisphere lesions cause ipsilateral motor signs."

Learning Objectives for Chapter 8

III. CLINICAL SIGNS OF CEREBELLAR DYSFUNCTION

1. Describe the cardinal signs of cerebellar dysfunction.
2. Describe how visualization of a drunk person aids in remembering the signs of cerebellar dysfunction.
3. Describe or imitate the effects of cerebellar dysfunction on speech.
4. Describe the effects of cerebellar lesions on eye movements.
5. Recite the diagnostic features of the type of nystagmus caused by an acute, large cerebellar hemisphere lesion (Fig. 5-7).
6. Describe the characteristic changes in the gait of a Pt with a cerebellar lesion.
7. Describe where the medial edge of the heels falls when a normal person walks a straight line.
8. Define and demonstrate how to test for postural tremor and intention tremor of the arms.
9. Recite a sentence to get the Pt to perform the finger-to-nose test with maximum effort and accuracy.
10. Define dysmetria and dysdiadochokinesia and describe how to test for them (Figs. 8-6 and 8-7).
11. Describe the advantage that the thigh-patting test for dysdiadochokinesia provides over the free-hand test.
12. Describe how to make the finger-tapping test audible and the information gained.
13. Describe the overshooting (often called rebound) test of the upper extremities (Figs. 8-8 and 8-9) and how to protect the Pt's face during the test.
14. Describe decomposition of movement.
15. Describe the tests for leg dystaxia, in addition to the gait.
16. Describe the clinical manifestations of hypotonia in a Pt with cerebellar dysfunction.
17. Describe in principle the clinical effect of cerebellar lesions on strength and endurance.

IV. ANALYSIS OF PTS AND THE FOUR CEREBELLAR SYNDROMES

1. Describe (or shade on stick figures) the distribution of cerebellar signs in a cerebellar hemisphere lesion, rostral (superior) vermis lesion, caudal (inferior) vermis lesion, and pancerebellar lesions. Relate these syndromes to the cerebellar lobes involved (Table 8-3).
2. Explain why gait testing is the single most important test for cerebellar dysfunction.
3. Describe how the classification of the Pt's cerebellar syndrome into one of the four types, i.e., hemispheric, rostral vermis, caudal vermis, or pancerebellar, suggests the cause or lesion type responsible.

V. SUMMARY OF THE CLINICAL EXAMINATION FOR CEREBELLAR DYSFUNCTION

1. Demonstrate in an orderly sequence how to test a Pt for cerebellar dysfunction. Use Fig. 8-10 as a guide.

VI. AN ESSAY ON TESTING STATION (STANDING) AND GAIT (WALKING)

1. Describe the station and gait examination and what the Ex looks for when a Pt walks.

Learning Objectives for Chapter 8

2. Describe the inferences that the Ex can make about the function of the nervous system if the Pt does all of the station and gait tests perfectly. **Note:** Describe and act out the following features observed in testing station and gait and, where appropriate, describe the pathophysiology or lesion.
3. **Developmental gaits:** Automatic stepping of the newborn, cruising, toddler's gait, and normal mature gait.
4. **Neuromuscular gaits:** Lordotic waddling (myopathic) gait, pride of pregnancy gait, Gower's sign, unilateral and bilateral foot-drop or step-page gait, heel-drop gait, flail-foot gait, and toe-walking gait.
5. **Sensory gaits:** Hyperesthetic gait, radicular pain or antalgic gait, nocturnal flipping-hand gait in an adult and a flipping-hand gait in a retarded child, a sensory ataxia or tabetic gait, and a blind person's gait. Explain why a Pt with degeneration of dorsal columns sways and falls over when closing the eyes (Romberg test) but a Pt with a cerebellar lesion does not.
6. **Cerebellar ataxic gaits:** Describe the four gaits of lesions in different regions of the cerebellum and their etiologic implications (Table 8-3).
7. **Spastic gaits:** Hemiplegic gait, spastic diplegic gait, scissors gait, crouch gait, paraplegic gait, and spastic-ataxic gait.
8. **Basal ganglia gaits:** *Marche à petit pas,* parkinsonian gait, festinating gait, en bloc or pedestal turning, choreiform gait, spastic-athetoid gait, equinovarus dystonic gait, dromedary or tortipelvis dystonic gait.
9. **Cerebral gaits:** *Marche à petit pas,* dancing bear, and the signs of the gait variously named an apraxic gait, frontal gait, ignition failure gait, and progressive primary freezing gait.
10. **Psychiatric gaits:** Astasia-abasia gait of hysteria, gaits of depression and agitated depression, schizophrenic gaits, Tourette's syndrome gait, and hyperactive child gait.

9 Examination of the Special Senses

And there I stood, a man grown, shaking in the sunshine with that old boyish emotion brought back to me by an odour! . . . Often and often have I known this strange rekindling of dead fires. And I have thought how, if our senses were really perfect, we might lose nothing out of our lives: neither sights, nor sounds, nor emotions. . . .

—**Ray Stannard Baker (1870–1946)**

I. THE SENSES

A. Sensation and subjectivity

The possibility for sensation begins when a chemical or physical change stimulates the receptor endings of sensory neurons and alters the flow of impulses in the sensory pathways. The impulses in the sensory pathways then lead to an experience that we call a *sensation*, such as pain, touch, or sight. Nothing is more real to the patient (Pt) than the experience of the sensation, such as pain, nor less real to the observer. Although the Pt can judge the degrees of a sensation, even on scale of 0 to 10 for pain, no one else can verify the sensation or measure it objectively in grams, centimeters, or seconds, the classic units of the physics. Nevertheless, by carefully eliciting the Pt's history, the examiner (Ex) can recognize and diagnose various sensory syndromes, such as migraine or nerve root compression, with about the same degree of certainty as motor syndromes.

B. Classification of sensation

1. Aristotle recognized five primary senses:
   a. Sight
   b. Sound
   c. Smell
   d. Taste
   e. Touch
2. Tradition also recognizes *special* and *general* senses. The special senses are sight, sound, taste, smell, and equilibrium/verticality. The general sensations are the rest. Sensation also can be classified as *somatic* or *visceral*.
3. Charles Sherrington (1857–1952) classified sensation as *exteroception*, *proprioception*, and *interoception*, depending on the origin of the stimulus and the location of the receptor tips of the axons (Sherrington, 1906).

a. **Exteroceptor** axonal tips are located near the external body surfaces. They respond to stimuli that impinge on the body's external surfaces. These stimuli produce sight, sound, smell, taste, and superficial cutaneous sensation. Superficial skin sensations include:
   i. Touch
   ii. Superficial pain
   iii. Temperature
   iv. Itching, tickling, and wetness

b. **Proprioceptor** axonal tips are located beneath body surfaces. They respond to stimuli that originate from receptors deep in the dermis, in muscles, tendons, ligaments, and the vestibular labyrinth. In large part, they record the actions of the body on itself and orientation to the pull of gravity. (See page 404 for a fuller definition of proprioception.) Proprioceptive sensations include:
   i. Position
   ii. Movement
   iii. Vibration
   iv. Pressure, weight, or tension
   v. Deep pain (sometimes included in proprioception)
   vi. Equilibrium and verticality (via vestibular pathways and dorsal columns)

c. **Interoceptor** axonal tips located in the viscera and vessels respond to stimuli that act on the internal surfaces of the viscera or originate in the visceral walls:
   i. Visceral and vascular pain
   ii. Sense of fullness or distention of the viscera

4. Obviously the various sensory classifications overlap and are inconsistent. To obviate memorizing sensory classifications, think systematically and simply sort through your own senses.

Mnemonic for classification of sensation: Start rostrally with the mouth, nose, eyes, ears, skin, and so on over the *exteroceptors* of the body. Then visualize the body in three dimensions, and you will encounter first the deep sensations of the *proprioceptors* and, finally, the *interoceptors.*

C. The concept of sensory modalities

1. No normal person confuses the stench of carrion with a flash of light or a pinprick with a sound. Each unique sensation not resolvable into a more elementary sensation is called a **primary sensory modality.** Ay, but there's the rub: How does one define *unique, resolve,* and *elementary*?
2. **Operations to disclose primary sensory modalities:** Stick yourself with a pin: There, that is pain, one modality. Stroke yourself with a piece of cotton: There, that is touch, another modality.
3. **Operation to disclose multimodal sensations:** Close your eyes and grasp any object, say a quarter, from your pocket or purse. You will recognize it as a metal disc by a combination of touch, texture, weight, size, circularity, and even its slightly cold feel. Thus we can resolve object recognition as a combination of several exteroceptive and proprioceptive modalities. Multimodal sensations include:
   a. Form, size, shape, texture, and weight
   b. Itching, tickling, and wetness

D. Implications of the theory of modality specificity

1. The neurologist constructs the entire sensory examination on modalities because the pathways of the nervous system provide for modality separation. In fact, we

might even define a modality as any sensation that the nervous system represents by a unique pathway, but that requires negative definitions. What is sight? It is that sensation lost after cutting both optic nerves. Each of us has to rely on our private experience to distinguish different modalities.

2. Because unique receptors serve each of the special senses, investigators have sought unique receptors for all modalities. Carried to its extreme, the theory of modality specificity requires unique receptors, unique peripheral axons, unique pathways through the cord, brainstem, and thalamus, and unique cortical receptive areas. Apart from some controversy about the specificity of skin receptors, the theory of modality-specific pathways enables clinicians to localize lesions.
3. By testing all sensations, the Ex tests the integrity of a large volume of neural tissue. Add the volume of tissue assayed by testing motor pathways, and the Ex has tested the integrity of the spinal cord, the brainstem, the cerebellum, and much of the diencephalon and cerebral hemispheres. The more pathways that function normally, the more the Ex can exclude neurologic disease. The more pathways that function abnormally, the more the Ex can predict the size, location, and type of the lesion.

E. Basic principles of sensory physiology

These principles are summarized from the doctrine of specific nerve energies of Johannes Müller (1801–1858):

1. **Sensation is an awareness of the state of nerve impulses in the sensory neural pathways.** We only know the external world by the changes that occur in the state of impulses in our receptor pathways.
2. **Any stimulation of a sensory nerve by any means, electrical, mechanical, or chemical, causes only the type of sensation ordinarily mediated by the nerve.** A blow on the eye causes a sensation of light, not taste.
3. **The same stimulus applied to different sensory organs causes only the sensation appropriate to the organ.** Put a stimulating electrode on the cochlea and you *hear.* Put the same electrode on the skin and you *feel.*

II. SMELL (OLFACTION): CRANIAL NERVE I

A. Olfactory receptor and nerve

1. Learn Figs. 9-1 and 9-2.
2. Mucus covers the olfactory nerve endings. Any odiferous agent must first dissolve in the mucus, which acts as the first censor for smell. Colds or allergic rhinitis impair olfaction by mechanical reduction of airflow and by excessive mucus secretion. *Hyposmia* means partial loss of the sense of smell, and *anosmia* means complete loss.
3. Olfactory impulses travel centrally past the perikarya of the ganglion cells in the nasal mucosa. The ganglion cells are ❒ external to/❒ within/❒ internal to the cribriform plate.

☑ external to (Fig. 9-1)

4. Axons from the olfactory ganglion cells form **olfactory nerve** filaments. The filaments perforate the cribriform plate and attached dura. The olfactory axons then cross the subarachnoid space to synapse on the olfactory bulbs. Organisms may gain access to the subarachnoid space or brain via the olfactory nerve filaments and cause encephalitis.

B. The olfactory stimulus

1. The two cranial nerves (CrNs) that supply sensory fibers to the olfactory epithelium are _____ and _____. Of these, only CrN _____ serves olfaction.

I; V (Fig. 9-2); I

2. As a general law in testing any sensation, the Ex isolates the chosen modality from all other modalities. Otherwise, the Ex does not know which sensory pathway

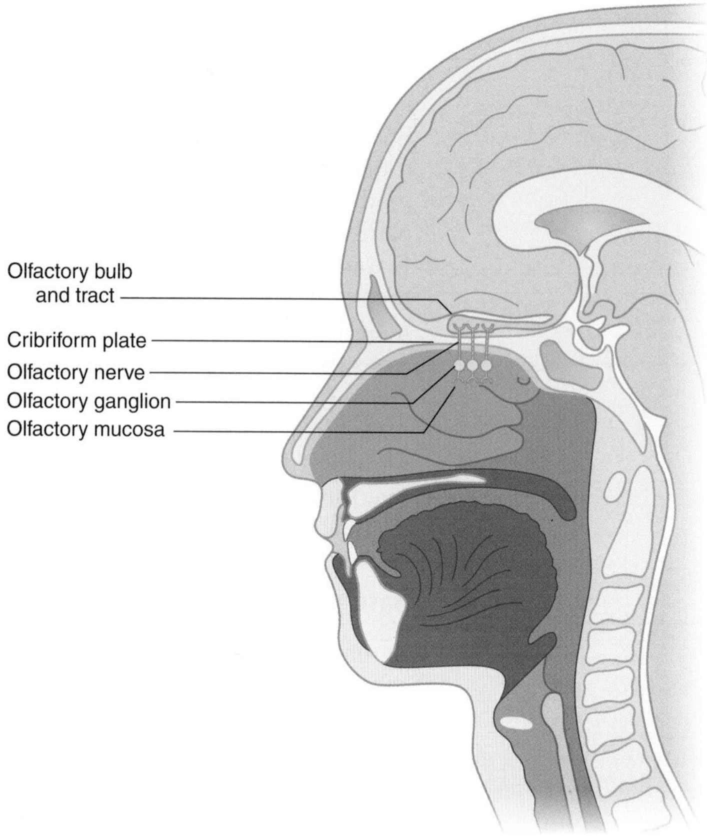

FIGURE 9-1. Sagittal section of head to show olfactory nerve, bulb, and tract.

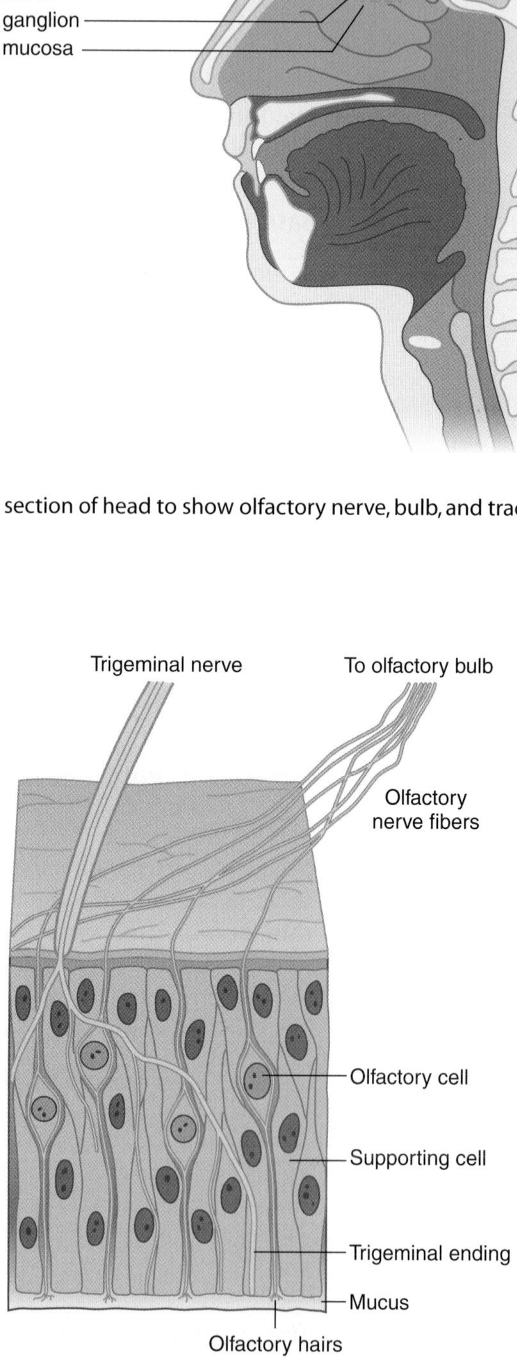

FIGURE 9-2. Microscopic section of olfactory mucosa, showing innervation by cranial nerves I and V. (Reprinted with permission fro Amoore JE, Johnston JW, Rubin M. The stereochemical theory of odor. Sci. Am 1964;210:42–49.)

☑ coffee

☑ opaque
The Ex wishes to test smell, not vision.

caused the response. To test *only* the sense of smell, should the Ex use an irritating substance such as ❒ ammonia or an aromatic substance such as ❒ coffee?

3. Ammonia irritates all receptors of a mucous membrane. Even the conjunctiva reacts to (smells, as it were) ammonia. To test smell, use a vial of coffee grounds. Should the vial be ❒ opaque/❒ transparent? Why?

____

____

4. Other readily available aromatic substances are oil of lemon, orange peel or apple skin, and soap.
5. Although not used in the routine neurologic examination (NE), the University of Pennsylvania Smell Identification Test (available through Sensonics, Inc., Haddonfield, NJ) is a battery for testing olfaction. It tests olfactory memory and discrimination (Doty, 2001; Savic et al., 1997).

C. Technique for testing olfaction

1. Successful sensory testing depends on communication between the Pt and Ex. Say to the Pt, "Close your eyes, sniff, and try to identify this odor."
2. Compress *one* of the Pt's nostrils. Hold the vial in front of the open nostril and ask the Pt to sniff. Wait a moment for the Pt to perceive the odor and then identify it.
3. For the second trial, compress the opposite nostril and this time *do not* present the stimulus. Withholding the stimulus tests the Pt's suggestibility and attentiveness. Incorporate such safeguards in all sensory testing.
4. The third time, present the stimulus to the untested nostril.
5. Other formalized tests of olfaction are widely available, including the Alcohol Sniff Test and the University of Pennsylvania Smell Identification Test (UPSIT) among others.

D. Central olfactory pathways and the concept of a rhinencephalon

1. After receiving the synapses from the primary olfactory axons, the olfactory bulbs send secondary pathways to the adjacent basal frontotemporal junction (basal forebrain). Tertiary pathways then disperse through an array of circuits in the basal forebrain that are not directly accessible to clinical testing but can be imaged (Kareken et al., 2003).
2. Taken together, the olfactory bulbs and tracts and their immediate central connections constitute the **rhinencephalon.** At one evolutionary stage, the cerebrum consisted mostly of rhinencephalon. Ontogenetically and phylogenetically, our own brain retains the primitive rhinencephalic ground plan (Fig. 9-3).

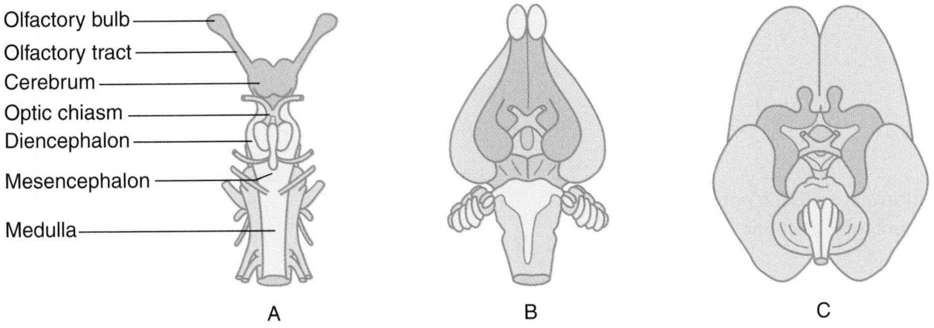

FIGURE 9-3. Ventral views of shark (A), rabbit (B), and fetal human (C) brains. The rhinencephalon (darker tan) comprises most of the shark brain. Notice in the rabbit and human brains that the non-rhinencephalic cortex (unshaded), which began as patches on the cerebral wall of primitive animals, has overgrown to dwarf the rhinencephalon. Nevertheless, the rhinencephalon set its imprint forever on the form and function of the human brain.

3. The sense of smell originally served the two fundamental functions of *feeding* and *mating.* These two visceral drives and their attendant visceral emotions were originally localized in the rhinencephalon before extending to those parts of the forebrain, essentially the limbic lobe, that evolved most directly from the olfactory ground plan. These forebrain derivatives remain the "seats" of emotion and affective experience. Humans no longer exude the natural musks and pheromones, but we assiduously replace them with perfumes and colognes. In any event, smell remains as the most evocative of sensations.
4. ***Déjà vu and déjà pensée:*** The uncus, the medial-most gyrus of the temporal lobe, contains a cortical area for smell. Uncal lesions cause olfactory hallucinations, usually of very disagreeable odors. One of my Pts tore down his bedroom walls because of the conviction that he smelled a dead animal entrapped within them. Each time the odor came powerfully to him, he also experienced a peculiar feeling of familiarity, of something happening that had happened before (just as Baker described). Autopsy showed a metastatic bronchogenic carcinoma in his uncus. The feeling of familiarity, as if something had happened before, is called *déjà vu* (previously or already seen) or *déjà pensée* (previously or already thought). Although we each experience this sense of undue familiarity from time to time, when a Pt reports it in association with an olfactory hallucination, suspect a medial temporal lobe lesion. Get a magnetic resonance imaging (MRI) scan.

E. Olfactory-related consequences of head injuries

1. Head injuries may shear off the delicate olfactory nerve filaments, resulting in anosmia (Doty et al., 1997; Jafek et al., 1989). If the wafer-thin cribriform plate fractures, the meninges may rupture initially or later when the Pt coughs, causing a fistula that allows cerebrospinal fluid (CSF) to gush into the nose. During physiologic fluctuations in intracranial pressure, fluid then refluxes back through the fistula into the subarachnoid space, introducing nasal organisms and causing meningitis or encephalitis. Therefore, consider a CSF fistula in the differential diagnosis of a runny nose (rhinorrhea). Rhinorrhea may occur intermittently and often increases upon bending forward or following the Valsalva maneuver. Suspect such a fistula whenever a Pt, usually one with a history of head injury, has a runny nose and anosmia but does not have a cold or allergic rhinitis (Allen et al., 1972). Persistent CSF fistulas at any level of the neuraxis require surgical closure (Zapalac et al., 2002).
2. To differentiate a CSF leak from nasal mucus or allergic rhinorrhea, test a sample of the fluid for β_2 transferrin (B2Tr) produced in the brain by neuraminidase activity (Warnecke et al., 2004, which is specific for CSF, while results of glucose, total protein content, and chloride are not specific for CSF. To localize the fistula, inspect the nasal cavity with a speculum and endoscopy and proceed through an algorithm that involves high resolution thin sections computed tomography (including paranasal sinus and petrous temporal bones), MRI, MR cisternogram, or radionuclide cisternography (Zapalac et al., 2002; Fig. 9-4).
3. Some nasal complications of a head injury are
   a. Loss of smell, a condition called ________________.
   b. The formation of a fistula between the nasal cavity and the ________________ space.
   c. A potentially lethal complication of such a fistula is ________________.

anosmia; subarachnoid; infection (meningitis, encephalitis)

F. Differential diagnosis of anosmia

1. To analyze anosmia systematically, start at the receptor. What initial barrier must any aromatic agent in the inspired air pass through before it stimulates olfactory receptors? ________________________________

Mucous coating of the olfactory nerve endings.

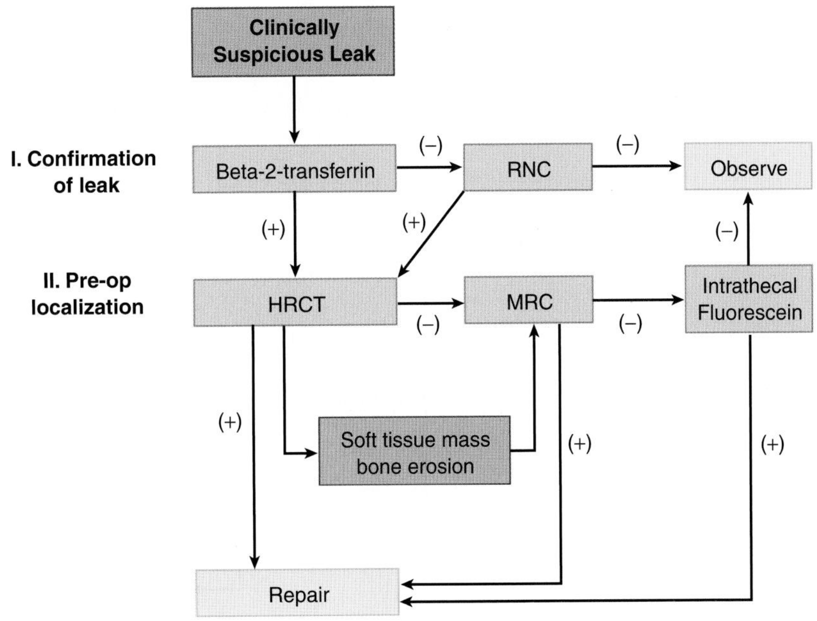

FIGURE 9-4. Diagnostic algorithm for diagnosis and management of suspected skull base cerebrospinal fluid fistulas. HRCT = high-resolution computed tomography; MRC = magnetic resonance cisternography; RNC = radionuclide cisternography. (Reprinted with permission from Zapalac JS, Marple BF, Schwade ND. Skull base cerebrospinal fluid fistulas: a comprehensive diagnostic algorithm. *Otolaryngol Head Neck Surg* 2002;June: 676(6):669–126.)

a. The most frequent causes of anosmia are the common cold, allergic rhinitis, smoking, and head trauma (Hawkes, 2002). Patients with anosmia induced by head trauma have been shown to have reduced serum zinc and increased total serum copper levels (Hirsch, 2009).

b. Olfactory dysfunction may also follow posterior fossa surgery in the sitting position (Ramsbacher et al., 1997), and surgical treatment, either coiling or clipping of intracranial aneurysms (Moman et al., 2009)

c. Sadly, aging diminishes the sensitivity of all sensations—sight, hearing, vibration sense, and so on. Hence, age-related decay of neurons commonly causes hyposmia in the elderly. Hyposmia also occurs in acute viral hepatitis, hypothyroidism, pseudohypoparathyroidism, Wernicke-Korsakoff syndrome, Turner syndrome, Kallman syndrome, Alzheimer's disease, Parkinson's disease (Hirsch, 2009) and perimesencephalic nonaneurysmal subarachnoid hemorrhage (Greebe et al. 2009).

2. Next, consider lesions of the olfactory bulbs and tracts. Although rare, the most significant are meningeal neoplasms—classically, olfactory groove meningiomas—that compress the olfactory bulbs and tracts. The olfactory bulbs and tracts may fail to evaginate (arhinencephaly), resulting in congenital lifelong anosmia (Assouline et al., 1998; DeMyer, 1987).

3. Figure 9-5 reviews the differential diagnosis of anosmia.

4. What is the explanation for nasal drip caused by sneezing or coughing after a head injury?

____

____

The venous system transmits the pressure from coughing or sneezing intracranially, forcing CSF out of a cribriform plate fistula.

5. The Pt with anosmia may complain mainly of loss of taste, because taste and smell are so intimately linked. To appreciate the severe affect of anosmia on the Pt, read Birnberg (1988; taste bibliography).

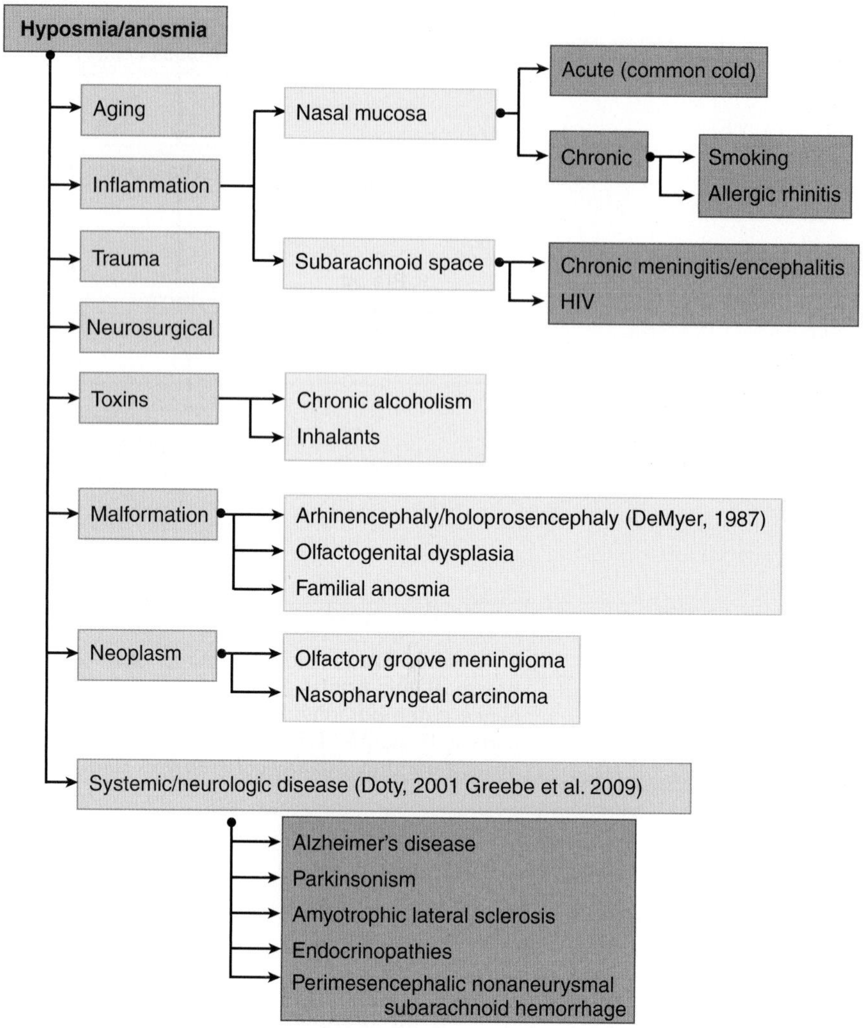

FIGURE 9-5. Dendrogram for the differential diagnosis of hyposmia and anosmia (reference).

BIBLIOGRAPHY · Sensation

Sherrington CS. *The Integrative Action of the Nervous System*. London, Constable & Co Ltd, 1906.

Smell

Allen M Jr, Gammal T, Ihnen, et al. Fistula detection in cerebrospinal fluid leakage. *J Neurol Neurosurg Psychiatry* 1972;35:664–668.

Assouline S, Shevell MI, Zatorre RJ, et al. Children who can't smell the coffee: isolated congenital anosmia. *J Child Neurol* 1998;13:168–172.

Baker RS (David Grayson, pseudonym). *Adventures in Contentment*. New York, Grossett, 1907.

Davidson TM, Murphy C. Rapid clinical evaluation of anosmia. The alcohol sniff test. *Arch Otolaryngol Head Neck Surg* 1997;123:591–594.

DeMyer W. Holoprosencephaly (cyclopia-arhinencephaly). In Vinken PJ, Bruyn GW, Klawans HL, eds. *Malformations. Handbook of Clinical Neurology, vol 6*. Amsterdam, Elsevier Science, 1987, Chapter 13, pp. 225–244.

Doty RL. *Smell Identification Test Administration Manual*. Haddon Heights, NY: Sensonics. 1995.

Doty RL. Olfaction. *Annu Rev Psychol* 2001;52:423–452.

Doty RL, Yousem DM, Pham LT, et al. Olfactory dysfunction in patients with head trauma. *Arch Neurol* 1997;54:1131–1140.

Greebe P, Rinkel GJE, Algra A. Anosmia after perimesencephalic nonaneursmal hemorrhage. *Stroke* 2009;40:2885–2886.

Hawkes C. *Disorders of Smell and Taste*, 2nd ed. Philadelphia, Butterworth-Heineman, 2002.

Hirsch AR. Chemosensory disorders. In Ingrid Kohlstadt, ed. *Food and Nutrition in Disease Management.* Boca Raton, FL: CRS Press.Taylor and Francis Group, 2009, Chapter 3, pp. 43–60.

Jafek BW, Eller PM, Esses BA, et al. Post-traumatic anosmia: ultrastructural correlates. *Arch Neurol* 1989;46:300–306.

Kareken DA, Mosnik DM, Doty RL, et al. Functional anatomy of human odor sensation, discrimination, and identification. *Neuropsychology* 2003 (in press).

Moman MR, Verweij BH, Buwalda J, Rinkel GJL. Anosmia after endovascular and open surgical treatment of intracranial aneurysms. *J Neurosurg* 2009;110(3):482–486.

Ramsbacher J, Brock M, Kombos Th. Permanent postoperative anosmia. A hitherto and described complication following surgery of the posterior cranial fossa in the sitting position. *Acta Neurochirurgica* 1997;139(5):482–483.

Savic I, Bookheimer SY, Fried I, et al. Olfactory bedside test: a simple approach to identify temporo-orbitofrontal dysfunction. *Arch Neurol* 1997;54:162–168.

Warnecke A, Averbeck T, Wurster U, et al. Diagnostic relevance of beta-2 transferrin for the detection of cerebrospinal fluid fistulas. *Arch Otolaryngol Head Neck Surg* 2004;130:1178–1184.

Zapalac JS, Marple BF, Schwade ND. Skull base cerebrospinal fluid fistulas: a comprehensive diagnostic algorithm. *Otolaryngol Head Neck Surg* 2002;126:660–676.

III. TASTE (GUSTATION) AND LOSS OF TASTE (AGEUSIA)

A. Receptors

The epithelium of the tongue and tonsillar pillars contains taste buds (fungiform and circumvallate papillae; Smith and Margolskee, 2001). As in olfaction, the chemical agents that stimulate taste must first dissolve in a liquid, the saliva. Loss of taste is called **ageusia.** Often the Pt who complains of ageusia actually has anosmia, because taste and smell complement each other in producing flavor and full gustatory sensation (Schiffman, 1983a, 1983b). Pathologic changes in taste buds have been found in patients with the syndrome of idiopathic hypogeusia with dysgeusia, hyposmia, and dysosmia. (Henkin et al., 1971). Patients with this syndrome have also been found to have reduced total serum zinc and increased total serum copper levels.

B. Innervation of taste receptors

1. The taste buds of the anterior two-thirds of the tongue are innervated by . . . which CrN was it? Well, if you have forgotten, start at CrN I and sort through them:
   a. CrN _______ smells, and _______ sees.
   b. CrNs _______, _______, and _______ rotate the eyeball.
   c. CrN _______ chews and feels the front of the head.
   d. CrN _______ moves the facial muscles, tears, snots, salivates, and ___________.

I; II

III; IV; VI

V

VII; tastes

2. To test taste, use the anterior two-thirds of the tongue, the area innervated by CrN VII, because of the inconvenience of reaching the taste buds on the posterior third of the tongue and tonsillar pillars. Review Figs. 6-5 and 6-6.

VII; tastes (Should you review the brief description of the CrNs in Tables 2-5 and 2-6?)

3. In contrast to earlier maps, the tongue does not show clinically significant regional differences to salty, sweet, sour, and bitter tastes (Smith and Margolskee, 2001)

C. Review of cranial nerve VII

1. CrN VII attaches to the brainstem at the ______________________ sulcus.

pontomedullary

2. In ventrodorsal order, the CrNs attached to the pontomedullary sulcus are ______________________.

VI, VII, and VIII (Review Fig. 2-20 if you erred.)

3. CrN VII enters the internal auditory meatus in company with CrN ______.

VIII

4. The *primary* neurons for taste occupy the only ganglion on CrN VII, the ______________________ ganglion.

geniculate

5. The name *geniculate ganglion* comes from the knee-like downward bend of CrN VII after it clears the ganglion and heads for the stylomastoid foramen (Figs. 6-5 and 6-6).

D. Central pathways for taste

Lesions of the central taste pathways rarely cause isolated loss of taste. The brainstem pathway ascends ipsilaterally in the tegmentum from the nucleus of the tractus solitarius to the midbrain, where it apparently decussates to terminate in the thalamus (Combarros et al., 2000). Gustatory sensation is probably represented in the insular cortex (island of Reil) and adjacent parietal operculum (area 43 of Brodmann). Irritative lesions in this region may cause gustatory hallucinations (Penfield and Jasper, 1954).

E. Technique of testing for loss of taste (ageusia)

1. **Stimulus:** The stimulus is a salty, sweet, sour, or bitter substance. Table salt, sugar, or quinine are suitable. Conceal the salt or sugar. The Pt who sees a white crystalline substance will almost automatically guess salt or sugar.
2. **Communication with the patient**
   a. Tell the Pt, "I want to place something on your tongue for you to taste. Stick out your tongue and keep it out. When you recognize the taste, hold up your hand."
   b. Place a few crystals of your test material on the right or left half of the tongue and massage these around with the well-moistened cotton tip of an applicator stick. Take care to confine the stimulus to one-half of the tongue. Do not allow the Pt to return the tongue to the mouth because the saliva will diffuse the taste stimulus beyond the area selected for testing. If the tongue is dry, moisten it slightly. Allow 15 to 20 seconds for the substance to dissolve and for the Pt to respond. Some normal subjects will not perceive sugar. Test again with salt.
   c. After the Pt rinses his mouth, test the opposite side of the tongue with the same or a different substance. For routine clinical purposes you need try only one substance to test for ageusia. Although not part of the routine NE, taste can be measured by impregnated paper discs and by galvanic currents.
   d. Test your own sense of taste as described.
   e. The main indications for testing taste are a complaint of loss of appetite, smell, or taste or the presence of a CrN VII palsy. Taste is the only clinically testable sensation mediated by CrN VII. Patients may lose taste or suffer a perversion of taste (**dysgeusia**) because of various medications, systemic illness, cancer, and endocrinopathies (Schiffman, 1983a, 1983b).

F. Clinical value of testing taste in facial palsy

1. **Patient protocol:** A 26-year-old woman awoke one morning with her face "drawn to one side." Examination disclosed that on the left side she could not wrinkle her forehead, close her eye, pull back the corner of her mouth, or wrinkle the skin of her neck. She moved the right side of her face normally. Her complaint of "drawing" of her face was due to the unopposed pull of the intact right-side facial muscles, which pulled her lips to the right when she spoke or smiled (see the Pt in Fig. 6-7). The remainder of the examination was completely normal, including taste sensation and hearing.
2. Analysis of the clinical data will lead to a conclusion as to *where* and *what* the CrN VII lesion is.
   a. In analyzing a motor deficit, consider first its distribution. Does it match a *central* or a pyramidal tract (upper motoneuron) distribution? Does it match a *root* or *peripheral nerve* or *myopathic* distribution?
   b. Which distribution does the motor deficit of the present Pt match? ❒ upper motoneuron/❒ peripheral nerve/❒ myopathic.

☑ peripheral nerve

c. The paralysis involves the muscles of one nerve, CrN ___________.

VII

d. The distribution of the paralysis in the field of one nerve excludes a neuromyal junction disorder or myopathy; these are widespread disorders and not limited to a single nerve.

e. Because interruption of a single nerve explains the paralysis, the disorder consists of a ❒ mononeuropathy/❒ polyneuropathy/❒ myopathy.

☑ mononeuropathy

3. Having identified a mononeuropathy of CrN VII, we have to specify the location of the lesion along the course of the nerve. In analyzing a sensory disturbance or a reflex arc, we invoked the principle of starting at the _____________ to trace along the entire pathway of the nerve impulses.

receptor

4. Where should you start to trace along the course of the impulses in a motor nerve? ________________________________

At the nucleus or cell body of the lower motoneurons.

5. The CrN VII nucleus occupies the ❒ tectum/❒ tegmentum/❒ basis of the ❒ midbrain/❒ pons/❒ medulla.

☑ tegmentum; ☑ pons

6. Because of the close packing of tracts and nuclei, a brainstem lesion would rarely affect just one CrN nucleus. It most likely would involve the neighboring lemniscal, cerebellar, or CrN VIII pathways or neighboring CrNs. In addition to VII, the CrN motor nuclei in the pons are ______________.

V and VI. In Fig. 2-16, notice the relation of the intra-axial course of the axons of VII to the VI nucleus.

7. The Pt had no signs implicating structures in the vicinity of the CrN VII nucleus in the central nervous system (CNS); therefore, the lesion most likely interrupted the nerve ❒ inside/❒ outside the brainstem.

☑ outside

8. After leaving the pontomedullary sulcus of the brainstem and before entering the internal auditory meatus, CrN VII must cross the _________________ space.

subarachnoid

9. The subarachnoid space between the cerebellum and the brainstem is called the **cerebellopontine angle.** A lesion here, such as a neoplasm, would interrupt not only CrN VII, but also CrN ______.

VIII

10. As the neoplasm enlarged, in addition to CrNs VII and VIII, it would affect CrNs _______________________.

V and VI (and possibly IX, X, and XII).

11. Go to Fig. 2-20 to appreciate how a relatively common tumor, an acoustic neuroma, in the cerebellopontine angle can affect additional nerves. Start with your pencil on CrN VIII as the center and shade in a circle about 1 to 1.5 cm in diameter to see how the lesion would encroach on adjacent nerves and the brainstem as it grows.

12. If the lesion occupied the internal auditory meatus or canal, other than CrN VII, which CrN would it affect? _____________________.

VIII

13. If the lesion interrupted the trunk of CrN VII somewhere between its point of exit from the brainstem and the geniculate ganglion, the Pt should have lost _________________ sensation on the anterior two-thirds of the tongue; however, the Pt did *not* have ageusia.

taste (Figs. 6-5 and 6-6)

14. CrN VII innervates one muscle in the middle ear, the ________________ muscle. Contraction of this muscle dampens the vibration of the ossicles, protecting the inner ear from excessively loud sounds. After stapedius muscle paralysis, the Pt experiences ordinary sounds as uncomfortably loud, a symptom called **hyperacusis.**

stapedius

15. Because the Pt retained taste and had no hyperacusis, the CrN VII lesion must be /❒ outside distal to/❒ outside within the middle ear.

☑ distal to

16. If distal to the middle ear, the lesion might be in the facial canal, but a lesion deep within the canal in the temporal bone bars direct clinical examination. If a lesion interrupted CrN VII after its exit from the stylomastoid foramen, the Ex should find pain or swelling in the parotid region, as from an inflammatory or neoplastic mass, but the Pt had no mass or pain in the parotid region.

17. The next link in a motor nerve comes at the terminal tips of its axons, where the axons synapse on the muscles, a region called the ________________ junction.

neuromyal (neuromuscular)

Neuromyal junction lesions, such as myasthenia gravis, or myopathies are diffuse disorders and generally are not confined to a single nerve distribution.

Your line should cross the facial canal distal to the chorda tympani nerve but proximal to the stylomastoid foramen.

18. Explain why the Pt's lesion is not at the neuromyal junction or in the muscle itself.____
19. Make a line across Fig. 6-5 at the most likely site of the Pt's lesion.
20. The Pt had idiopathic facial paralysis (Bell's palsy), a common mononeuropathy of CrN VII. The lesion is usually an inflammation, frequently caused by viruses (several herpes viruses have been implicated, particularly HSV-1) or *Borrelia burgdorferi* (Roberg et al., 1991). The swelling compresses and sometimes completely transects the axons and may occur at various sites along the facial nerve. The Pt recovered good facial function by 6 weeks after onset.
21. This Pt shows how testing taste helps to localize a lesion along the course of CrN VII. Unless the Pt's symptoms and signs implicate taste, smell, or CrN VII, you may omit taste testing; but make the omission by discretion, not carelessness.
22. Read Birnberg's (1988) personal account to appreciate how loss of smell and taste impaired the quality of the Pt's life.

BIBLIOGRAPHY · Taste Testing and Bell's Palsy

Birnberg JR. Living with lack of taste. *Newsweek* 1998; March 21, p 10.

Combarros O, Sanchez-Huan P, Berciano J, et al. Hemiageusia from an ipsilateral multiple sclerosis plaque at the midpontine tegmentum. *J Neurol Neurosurg Psychiatry* 2000;68:795–802.

Henkin RL, Schechter PJ, Hoye R, Mattern CFT. Idiopathic hypogeusia with dysgeusia, hyposmia and dysosmia. *JAMA* 1971;217(4):434–440.

Penfield W, Jasper HH. *Epilepsy and the Functional Anatomy of the Human Brain.* Boston, Little, Brown & Co, 1954.

Roberg M, Ernerudh J, Froberg P. Acute peripheral facial palsy: CSF findings and etiology. *Acta Neurol Scand* 1991;83:55–60.

Schiffman SS. Taste and smell in disease. Part I. *N Engl J Med* 1983a;308:1275–1279.

Schiffman SS. Taste and smell in disease. Part II. *N Engl J Med* 1983b;308:1337–1342.

Smith DV, Margolskee RF. Making sense of taste. *Sci Am* 2001(March):32–39.

IV. HEARING

The specialist told him: "Fine let's leave it at that.
The treatment is done: you're deaf. That's how
It is you have quite lost your hearing."
And he understood only too well, not having heard.

—Tristan Corbiere (1845–1875)

A. Cranial nerve VIII

CrN VIII consists of **cochlear** (auditory) and **vestibular** divisions. Each division has its own specialized receptors, its own bundle within the trunk of VIII, and its own brainstem nuclei and central pathways. The cochlear division mediates hearing only. It detects sound vibrations between 20 and 20,000 cps. By its design, the ear is the most sensitive vibration detector in the human body.

B. Anatomy of the cochlear division of VIII

1. **Receptor for hearing:** The cochlea contains the receptor (the organ of Corti) and the cochlear (spiral) ganglion that originates the cochlear division of VIII (see Fig. 9-6).

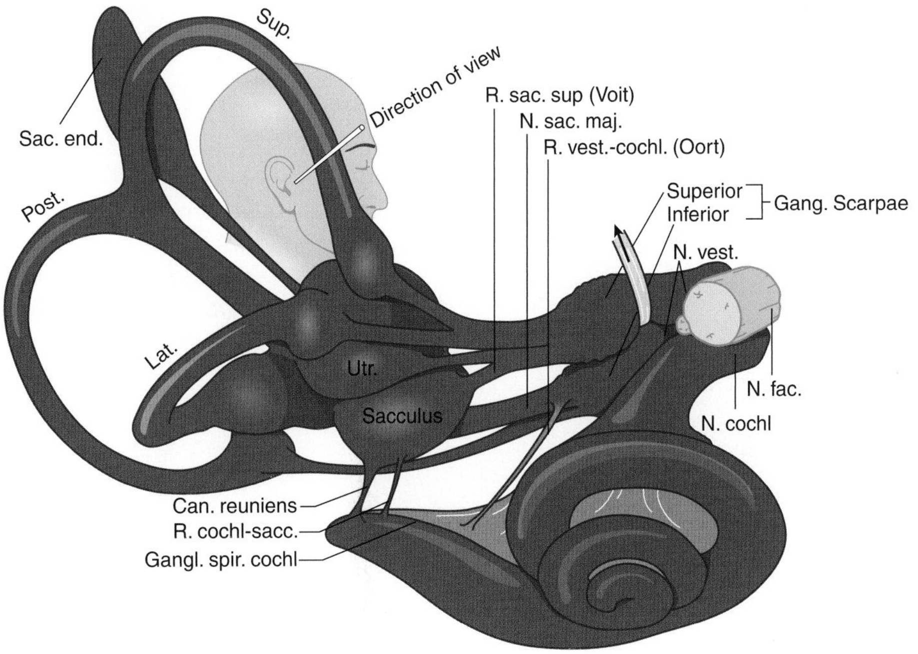

FIGURE 9-6. Drawing of the labyrinth, showing its nerve supply. Notice the intimate relation of the facial nerve (N. fac.) with the vestibular (N. vest.) and cochlear (N. cochl.) divisions of cranial nerve VIII. Lat = lateral semicircular canal; Post = posterior semicircular canal; N = nerve; R = ramus; Sup = superior semicircular canal; Utr = utriculus. (Reprinted with permission from Hardy M. Observations on the innervation of the macula sacculi in man. *Anat Rec* 1934;59:403–418.)

☑ outside primary

2. The cochlear ganglion contains the ❒ outside primary/❒ outside secondary/❒ outside tertiary neurons for hearing.

VII

3. **Peripheral course of the cochlear nerve:** The cochlear and vestibular divisions of VIII run through the internal auditory canal, accompanied by CrN _________________.

pontomedullary

4. CrNs VII and VIII attach to the brainstem at the _________________ sulcus.

5. **Central connections of the cochlear nerve.** Learn Fig. 9-7.

cochlear

a. Upon penetrating the brainstem, the cochlear axons synapse at the _________________ nuclei.

inferior (caudal)

b. These nuclei drape around the _________________ cerebellar peduncle.

☑ secondary

c. In the auditory pathway, the cochlear nuclei contain the ❒ primary/❒ secondary/❒ tertiary neurons.

☑ an auditory nerve

d. In ascending through the brainstem, the auditory pathway disperses about equally ipsilaterally and bilaterally. Therefore, if a Pt has a profound unilateral hearing loss, the lesion most likely would affect ❒ a central pathway/❒ an auditory nerve/❒ the auditory receptive cortex.

lemniscus; inferior colliculus (Fig. 9-6)

e. The name of the auditory pathway that ascends through the brainstem is the lateral _________________, through which axons run to the _________________ colliculus.

medial geniculate

f. From the inferior colliculus, the pathway runs to the _________________ body.

temporal

g. Neurons of the medial geniculate body relay to the superior surface of the _________________ lobe (transverse temporal gyri of Heschl).

☑ No
A unilateral central lesion does not cause unilateral deafness because the brainstem pathways disperse about equally to both hemispheres.

h. Would a unilateral temporal lobe lesion cause complete deafness in either ear? ❒ Yes/❒ No.

Explain.

____.

i. Whenever you test a Pt's hearing, "think through" the auditory pathway, naming the structures en route.

A. Mesencephalon

B. Pons

C. Pontomedullary junction (and superior olivary nucleus)

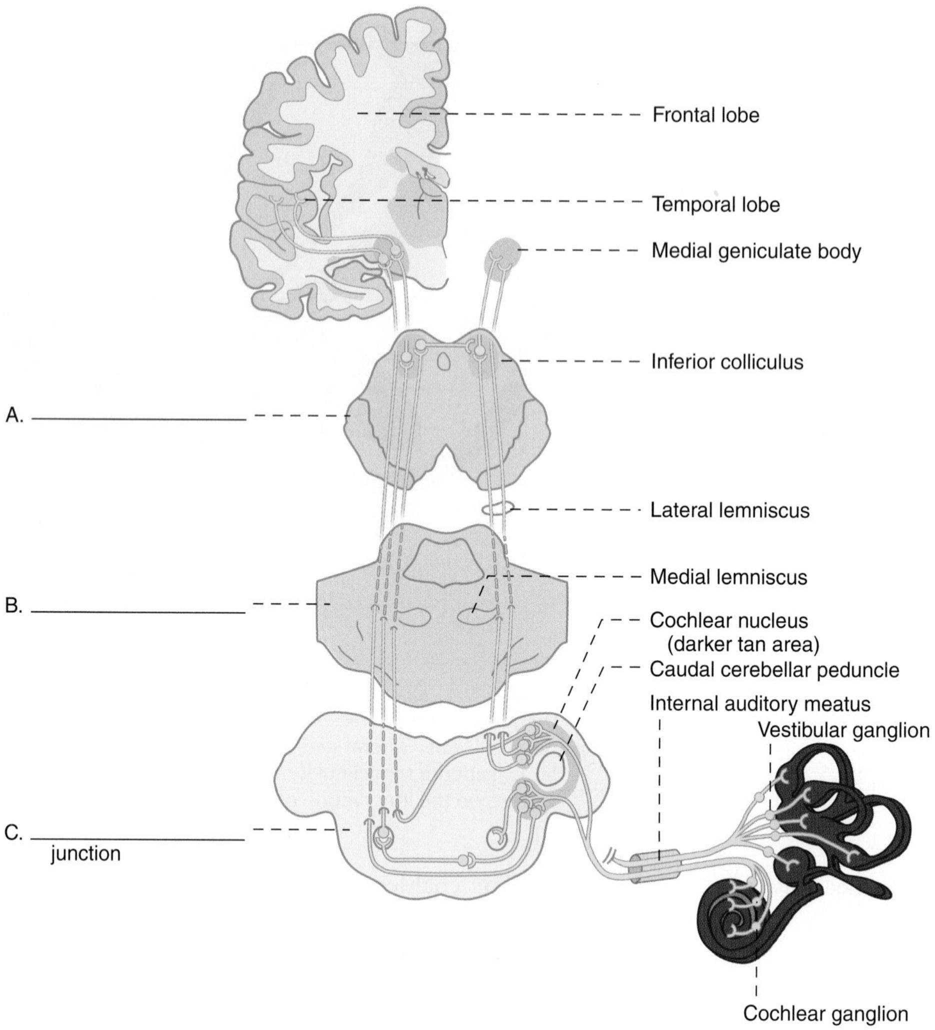

FIGURE 9-7. Diagram of the cochlear (auditory) pathway. On A, B, and C, label the subdivisions of the brainstem.

C. Symptoms and causes of cochlear nerve lesions

The most common symptoms are deafness and tinnitus. **Tinnitus** means a persistent or recurrent hyperacusis usually consisting of a ringing or roaring sound (see Section IV H). The most common causes of impaired hearing and tinnitus are aging (presbyacusis), ototoxic drugs such as aspirin and some antibiotics, viral infections, recurrent otitis media, hereditary cochlear degenerations (Willems, 2000), trauma, and chronic exposure to loud sound.

D. The concept of threshold or sensitivity in testing

In testing olfaction and taste, the Ex merely seeks a *yes* or *no* answer and does not fractionate the strength of the stimulus or test the threshold. For the best test of muscle strength, the Ex requires the Pt to exert the maximum strength. For the best test of a sensory system, the Ex determines not the maximum stimulus it can withstand but the minimum stimulus it can detect; in other words, its sensitivity.

E. Technique for screening hearing

1. **Ask the Pt about hearing deficits:** Can the Pt hear the telephone, normal conversational voice, and whispering? Does the Pt have tinnitus (Lockwood et al., 2002)?
2. **Do otoscopy** to ensure that the external auditory canals are open and that the eardrums are normal. In analyzing hearing deficits, the Ex has to decide whether the Pt has a mechanical impediment to conduction of sound or a nerve lesion.

Otoscopy discloses some obvious mechanical impediments such as damaged eardrums, wax, or foreign bodies in the external auditory canal, but it does not disclose others, such as immobility of the ossicles (otosclerosis). The otologist measures the mechanical conductive ability of the eardrum and ossicles with impedance audiometry and tympanometry (Rapin, 1999).

3. **Rub your fingers together beside one of the Pt's ears and then the other.**
4. **Present a vibrating tuning fork to each ear and ask the Pt to compare the loudness.**
   a. To present the most uniform sound, hold the fork prongs *perpendicular*, not parallel, to the Pt's ear. Forks with a frequency of 512 to 2000 cps match the frequencies most important for speech perception, but they do not vibrate very long. Neurologists compromise by using a fork of 126 or 256 cps (middle C) that also serves to test vibration sense in the digits.
   b. To semi-quantitate the test, move the fork from one ear to the other and ask the Pt to compare the loudness of the sound in the two ears. Also compare the distance from the ear at which you hear the sound with the distance at which the Pt hears it.
5. **Masking the opposite ear:** When the Ex tests one ear, the sound vibrations may travel through air or the skull bone, resulting in detection by the opposite ear, even though the ear directly tested is impaired. To improve test reliability, mask the opposite ear by rubbing the edge of a card along the helix of the ear or rustling your fingers beside it as you present the tuning fork to the other ear. Alternatively, the Ex can insert a stethoscope into the Pt's ears and apply the vibrating tuning fork to the diaphragm. The Ex can then direct the sound to both ears or to one ear by compressing the tubing at the Y of the stethoscope with a hemostat (Arbit, 1977).
6. **The air-bone conduction test of Rinne** compares the efficiency of the conduction of sound vibrations by bone and by air.
   a. Hold a faintly vibrating tuning fork on your mastoid process. Just after the sound disappears, hold the fork beside your ear. Can you hear the sound now? ❐ Yes/❐ No. Normally air conduction is ❐ more/❐ less efficient than bone.

   ☑ Yes; ☑ more
   Sound normally reaches the ear by air conduction.

   b. If you press your fingertip in your ear while holding a tuning fork beside it, you know that that will block the sound. Try this: Place the fork against your mastoid and, as you listen to the sound, press your finger hard into your ear to completely occlude the canal. What happens to the sound? ________________

   It gets louder.

   c. This test shows that, although a mechanical obstruction of the auditory canal causes an ❐ increase/❐ decrease in sound by air conduction, it also causes an apparent ❐ increase/❐ decrease in bone conduction.

   ☑ decrease; ☑ increase

   d. If anything impedes the conduction of sound vibrations through the external auditory canal or ossicles of the middle ear, the Pt has a **conduction** hearing loss. Conversely, reduction of hearing by a lesion of the organ of Corti or of the auditory nerve is called a **neurosensory** loss. Notice that a **conduction** loss of hearing refers to **mechanical** conduction of sound vibrations through the external and middle ear, not to conduction of nerve impulses through CrN VIII. Loss of hearing from a CrN VIII lesion is called a ❐ conduction/❐ neurosensory loss.

   ☑ neurosensory

   e. After application of the tuning fork to the mastoid process, the bone mechanically transmits vibration to the inner ear, bypassing the conduction channels of the external and the middle ear. Bone conduction tests the integrity of the nerve, even though something blocks mechanical conduction of sound vibration through the external auditory canal. Characteristically, neurosensory hearing loss impairs the hearing of high frequencies via air conduction and decreases hearing via bone conduction. Thus, nerve lesions block hearing by air and bone, whereas mechanical lesions block the sounds transmitted through ❐ air/❐ bone.

   ☑ air

f. **Clinical analysis of the air-bone conduction test of Rinne**

1) If a Pt hears better with the fork applied to his mastoid process than with it in the air beside his ear, the best inference is

❒ (a) The Pt is normal.

❒ (b) The Pt must have a lesion of the organ of Corti.

❒ (c) The Pt has a conduction lesion, a mechanical impediment such as wax in the auditory canal, a damaged drum, or immobility of the ossicles.

❒ (d) The Pt has a neurosensory lesion in the organ of Corti or in the auditory nerve.

☑ (c)

2) If the test had shown reduced hearing for air and for bone conduction of sound, the best inference is: ❒ (a)/❒ (b)/❒ (c)/❒ (d).

☑ (d)

7. **The sound-lateralizing test of Weber**

a. For this test, the Ex places a vibrating tuning fork on the middle of the Pt's forehead or the vertex of the skull. Try this test yourself. The sound seems to come from ❒ the right/❒ the left/❒ the center.

☑ the center (if you are normal)

b. Is the sound equally loud in both ears? ❒Yes/❒ No

☑ Yes (if you are normal)

c. With the vibrating fork in place on the vertex of your head, press your fingertip in one ear and then the other. What happens to the sound?

____

It lateralizes to the occluded side.

d. The normal person hears the vertex vibration equally in both ears. If a mechanical impediment blocks sound conduction in one ear, the vertex sound localizes to ❒ the same/❒ the opposite/❒ neither side.

☑ the same

e. If the Pt has an auditory nerve lesion on one side, the vertex vibration sounds loudest on ❒ the same/❒ the opposite/❒ neither side.

☑ the opposite

f. Only a consistent lateralization to one side after several trials is considered significant.

F. Analysis of patients for conduction versus neurosensory hearing loss

1. This Pt showed an increased auditory threshold to finger rustling on the left; the vertex test lateralized to the left, and bone transmission was better than air transmission. These findings most likely indicate:

❒ (a) A normal Pt.

❒ (b) A mechanical impediment, a *conduction* lesion.

❒ (c) An auditory nerve or cochlear lesion, a *neurosensory* lesion.

❒ (d) Temporal lobe lesion.

❒ (e) Insufficient data to reach a conclusion.

☑ (b)

2. This next Pt showed an increased auditory threshold to the tuning fork on the left; bone and air transmissions of sound were reduced on the left, and the vertex test lateralized to the right. Which of the previous inferences applies to this Pt? ❒ (a)/❒ (b)/❒ (c)/❒ (d)/❒ (e).

☑ (c)

G. Testing the auditopalpebral reflex or startle response to sound

While standing just behind the Pt's line of sight, make a loud, unexpected sound such as a hand clap. Observe the Pt for blinking or a startle response. A response indicates an intact auditory pathway. No response means deafness, or that the Pt ignored the stimulus. Use the auditopalpebral reflex to test auditory function in non-cooperative, hysterical, or malingering Pts, infants, and unconscious Pts. Always ask a mother whether her infant shows an alerting response to sound.

H. Auditory tests for cerebral dysfunction

simultaneous (double, bilateral)

1. In testing visual fields, we found that some Pts could not detect visual stimuli from both sides. This test is called ______________________ stimulation.
2. Similarly, the Ex can present simultaneous auditory stimuli, if the previous tests have demonstrated intact auditory pathways (Heilman, 1971). Stand behind the Pt and hold one of your hands beside each of the Pt's ears. Gently rub your fingers together, first on one side and then the other, and have the Pt point to the side from which the stimulus comes. Then rub the fingers of both hands to see whether the Pt identifies the simultaneous stimuli from both sides. Consider only a consistent inattention to sound from one side significant. Repeat the test several times, randomly alternating single and simultaneous stimuli. Patients with large right cerebral hemisphere lesions tend to suppress sound from the left side (see also Chapter 11).
3. The Ex can test sound localization by presenting rustling fingers in the anterior or posterior quadrants of the right and left sides, with the Pt's eyes closed (Klingon and Bontecou, 1966). Chapter 11 describes how to test Pts for auditory aphasia, the inability to understand the symbolic significance of words.

I. Tinnitus

1. **Tinnitus** means an abnormal sound perceived in the ear, unrelated to an outside source. It usually has a buzzing, ringing, roaring, or clicking quality (Marion, 1991). Tinnitus may be continuous or fluctuating and may be perceived in one or both ears.
2. There are two types of tinnitus: *subjective* and *objective.*
   a. **Subjective tinnitus** arises not from real sounds but from some auditory system disorder. It may arise from a disease of the ear such as presbyacusis, cochlear disease, lesions along CrN VIII or central pathways, the auditory cortex, or from drugs such as salicylates, loop diuretics, "mycin" antibiotics, quinine or derivatives, and chemotherapeutic agents such as cysplatin (Lockwood et al., 2002). Tinnitus may be associated with palatal myoclonus (palatal tremor), and with stapedius myoclonus characterized by rapid rhythmic movements of the tympanic membrane. Typewriter tinnitus, an incapacitating unilateral tinnitus, responsive to carbamazepine, has been associated with auditory nerve vascular compression (Levine, 2006).
   b. **Objective tinnitus** is caused by a real sound, audible to the Ex, usually a bruit from an arteriovenous malformation, fistula, or states of high blood flow as in anemia or hyperthyroidism. In these cases, the sound is pulsatile.
3. The Pt with tinnitus requires a thorough head and neck examination, detailed auscultation with gentle pressure on the jugular vein and performance of the Valsalva maneuver to exclude a venous hum (Chapter 1), neuroimaging when appropriate, and laboratory testing for hearing loss, which often accompanies tinnitus (Lockwood et al., 2002). MRA and MRV, or CT angiographic studies, may be needed to look for arterial tortuosity, carotid dissections, fibromuscular dysplasia, aberrancies of the jugular bulb or jugular vein, glomus tumor, carotid aneurysms, or dural arteriovenous fistulas (AVFs).

J. Laboratory tests for auditory dysfunction

1. If the foregoing screening tests suggest loss of hearing, refer the Pt for electronic tests. These may include pure tone audiometry, speech discrimination batteries, recruitment, and the von Bekesy loudness discrimination test. Brainstem auditory evoked responses (BAERs) do not require conscious responses, so you can objectively test the integrity of the auditory pathways in conscious or unconscious Pts, as discussed under Electroneural Diagnosis in Chapter 13.
2. Common causes of delayed speech are deafness and mental retardation. If the child has delayed speech or does not appear to hear, always test thoroughly with bedside and electronic hearing tests.

K. Rehearsal time

Do all of the foregoing hearing tests as outlined in Section V C 3 of the Standard NE.

BIBLIOGRAPHY · Auditory Testing

Arbit E. A sensitive bedside hearing test. *Ann Neurol* 1977;2:250–251.

Heilman K, Pandya DN, Karol EA, et al. Auditory inattention. *Arch Neurol* 1971;24:323–325.

Klingon G, Bontecou D. Localization in auditory space. *Neurology* 1966;16:879–886.

Levine RA. Typewriter tinnitus: a carbamazepine-responsive syndrome related to auditory nerve vascular compression. *ORL J Othorhinolaryngol Relat Spec* 2006;68(1):43–46.

Lockwood AH, Salvi RJ, Burkard RF. Tinnitus. *N Engl J Med* 2002;347:904–910.

Marion MS, Cevette MJ. Tinnitus. *Mayo Clin Proc* 1991;66:614–620.

Rapin I. Hearing impairment. In Swaiman KF, Ashwal S, eds. *Pediatric Neurology*, 3rd ed. St. Louis, Mosby, 1999, Chapter 7, pp. 77–95.

Willems PJ. Genetic causes of hearing loss. *N Engl J Med* 2000;342:1101–1109.

V. THE VESTIBULAR SYSTEM: VERTIGO AND ITS POSTURAL COMPENSATIONS

A. Dizziness and vertigo

1. Among the most common symptoms that plague humankind are headaches, backaches, dizziness, fatigability, and blackout spells.
2. In the Pt's lexicon, dizziness may mean giddiness, light-headedness, unsteadiness, vertigo, spinning, and so on (Baloh, 1998). When the Pt complains of dizziness, ask for a more specific description ("Describe how you feel different when you have the dizziness"). Then echo the Pt's own words to avoid prejudicing the answer. Later ask the Pt to compare the sensation with that produced by a merry-go-round. If strictly defined, vertigo excludes the multitude of less specific symptoms encompassed by dizziness (Evitar, 1999; Rubin and Brookler, 1991). **Vertigo means a specific sense of dysequilibrium as though the person or the world were spinning around or undergoing a swerving or tilting movement** (Baloh and Honrubia, 2001). It is an illusion of movement of self or environment. True vertigo implies a disorder of the vestibular receptors, their nerves, or central connections (Barber, 1974; Brandt et al., 1994; Glasscock et al., 1990). The most frequent causes of peripheral vertigo are benign paroxysmal positioning vertigo (BPPV), Ménière's disease, and vestibular neuritis. Central forms of vertigo are due to lesions involving the neuronal circuitry between the vestibular nuclei and the vestibulo-cerebellum, as well as those involving the vestibular nuclei, the vestibular and ocular motor structures of the brainstem, cerebellum, thalamus, and vestibular cortex (e.g., Wallenberg syndrome, vestibular migraine, cerebellar atrophies).
3. Several afferent avenues contribute to a sense of equilibrium, balance, and verticality: vision, proprioception (vestibular and dorsal column), and cutaneous touch and pressure (Ruge and Bronstein, 1995). Vertigo occurs whenever the major senses provide conflicting information.The vestibular system sends impulses at the rate of 100 impulses per second from each side (Barber, 1974). The brain accustoms itself to the balanced input. With rotation, the input from one side increases and that from the other decreases, thus magnifying the discrepancy between the two sides. The brain interprets the information as movement. If disease causes an imbalance in the vestibular input, the brain interprets it as movement in conflict with other senses that signal no movement (Brandt and Daroff, 1980). A person standing at the top of the Empire State Building or the Grand Canyon who suddenly glances down will feel vertiginous because of the loss of the visual stereoscopy. Even diplopia may cause vertigo or loss of the sense of

balance, because of the mismatch of images from the two eyes. Which image is the person to believe and orient to? When you walk in the dark and put out your hand to touch a wall, you instinctively confirm the role of cutaneous sensation in the sense of balance.

4. **Self-induction of vertigo:** To appreciate how vertigo affects the Pt, try this experiment. Because you may fall, follow the instructions carefully.
   a. Place a penny on the floor about 40 to 50 cm from a bed or a fully cushioned easy chair (to catch you in case you fall).
   b. Stand directly over the penny, with it between your feet and with the receptacle to your *right*.
   c. Flex your neck to stare down at the penny, and while staring at the penny, turn around to your *right* fairly rapidly for six complete turns. At the end of the six turns, stop with your right side toward the receptacle. Then try to stand erect and still and hold your arms straight out. Record these observations.
      i. In which direction do you experience an illusion of movement? ❒to the right/❒ to the left
      ii. Which way do you tend to fall? ❒ to the right/❒ to the left
      iii. Which way do your outstretched arms tend to deviate? ❒ to the right/❒ to the left
   d. Repeat the rotation experiment, but this time rotate to the *left*. The direction of vertigo is to the ❒ right/❒ left, and the direction of falling and arm deviation is to the ❒ right/❒ left.
   e. We can now generalize that, when the person experiences vertigo in one direction, the falling and arm deviation are in the ❒ same/❒ opposite direction.
   f. The vertigo comes from a conflict or mismatch of sensory information (Brandt and Daroff, 1980). When you stop rotating, momentum causes the fluid in the semicircular canals to continue to rotate briefly. The current, deflecting the hair cell receptors of the cristae, signals movement, but the other proprioceptors and vision signal no movement (Brandt and Daroff, 1980). What you have experienced is motion sickness.
   g. During vestibular vertigo, eyelid closure increases postural instability by removing the compensatory information from vision, just as when the Pt has dorsal column disease (Romberg test, pages 410–411). Thus, darkness or deprivation of vision makes Pts with vestibular or dorsal column disease worse, but has little effect on normal persons or Pts with cerebellar ataxia, an important point when taking the history (Barber, 1974).

☑ to the left
Most persons feel as if they were spinning to the left, but some may experience another type of movement.

☑ to the right

☑ to the right

☑ right; left

☑ opposite

B. Symptoms and signs of acute vestibular dysfunction

1. Acute transection of a vestibular nerve causes the full syndrome of vestibular dysfunction (Hotson and Baloh, 1998).
   a. The *symptoms* consist of intense constant vertigo to the opposite side of the lesion, nausea, oscillopsia, and anxiety. The Pt refuses to stand or walk and resists any change in position because it aggravates the symptoms. Nystagmus causes the oscillopsia.
   b. The *signs* consist of falling and past-pointing to the side of the lesion, jerk nystagmus with the slow phase to the side of the lesion, and autonomic dysfunction: vomiting, pallor, sweating, and hypotension. The hypotension does not lead to syncope.
2. Bilateral, symmetrical vestibular disease may produce only unsteadiness of the gait and balance, without the vertigo or autonomic symptoms. Vision and dorsal columns compensate for the loss of vestibular function.
3. CNS or peripheral lesions, such as infarcts, involving the vestibular pathways may cause an ocular tilt reaction with skew deviation of the eyes and tilts of the perceived visual vertical (Brandt and Dieterich, 1994).

C. Physiology of the peripheral vestibular system

1. **Vestibular receptors:** The semicircular canals, utricle and saccule of the vestibular labyrinth of the inner ear, contain the hair cell receptors that initiate vestibular impulses (Fig. 9-7).
2. Each of the three semicircular canals contains an **ampullary crista** that has hair cells sensitive to current flow. The utricle and saccule each contain a **macula** that has otoliths resting on hair cells that are sensitive to inertia and the action of gravity. Head movements and the pull of gravity stimulate the vestibular receptors (Evitar, 1999; Glasscock et al., 1990).
   a. The cristae of the semicircular canals detect fast angular accelerations or rotations of the head in the plane of the canal. Figures 9-8 and 9-9 show the planes of the semicircular canals.

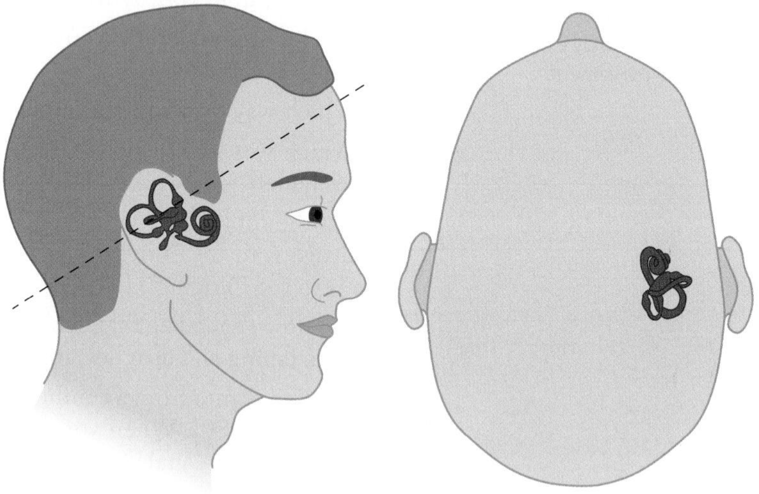

FIGURE 9-8. Orientation of the labyrinth. The size of the labyrinth is exaggerated for clarity of the drawing. (A) Lateral view of the right labyrinth. Notice that the plane (dotted line) of the "horizontal" semicircular canal angles 30 degrees upward from the true horizontal. (B) Superior view of the labyrinth.

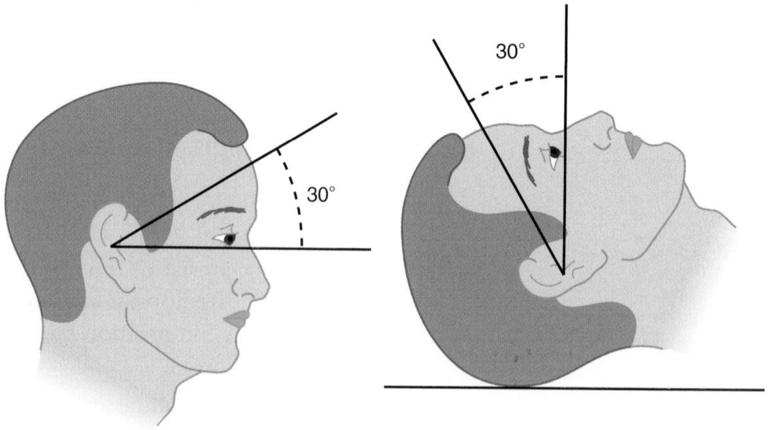

FIGURE 9-9. Inclination of the horizontal canal with the patient erect and supine.

☑ horizontal

   b. In tilting your head downward while spinning around the penny, you placed the *horizontal canal* more truly ❒ horizontal/❒ vertical and therefore in the plane of rotation.
3. The **otoliths** of the **maculae** respond to linear acceleration in the lateral and vertical planes and to slow tilting. They act as "out-of-position" or tilt receptors in

response to gravity and contribute to postural reflexes and a sense of balance and verticality.

4. **In summary, the vestibular receptors initiate three functions:**
   a. They counter-roll the eyes against the direction of head rotation, thus keeping the eyes on the visual target when the head moves; e.g., if the head turns to the right, the vestibular system counter-rolls the eyes to the left.
   b. They detect angular and linear head movements and the inclination of the head with respect to the pull of gravity, which leads to a vertical posture and a sense of balance when the person sits, stands, and walks.
   c. They alter the tone in the antigravity muscles. Through the pathways described next, the vestibular system mediates major postural reflexes, namely the symmetric and asymmetric tonic neck reflexes (Fig. 5-4), head- and trunk-righting reflexes, positive supporting reflexes, Moro's reflex, and decerebrate rigidity (Fig. 12-13).

D. Vestibular pathways

1. The vestibular ganglion occupies the distal end of the internal auditory canal. Hence, the primary vestibular neurons, like the primary cochlear neurons, sit very close to their place of duty (Fig. 9-7). So does the sensory ganglion for CrN ______________.

I

☑ medullopontine (review Fig. 2-21, if necessary)

2. The primary vestibular neurons synapse on the vestibular nuclei at the ☐ cervicomedullary/☐ medullopontine/☐ pontomesencephalic region of the brainstem.

☑ secondary

3. The vestibular nuclei contain the ☐ primary/☐ secondary/☐ tertiary neurons in the vestibular pathway.

4. **The central pathways for the signs of vestibular stimulation**
   a. Pathways from the vestibular nuclei run to the nuclei of CrNs III, IV, and VI. The pathway linking the vestibular system with CrN III, IV, and VI is the ______________________________.

medial longitudinal fasciculus (MLF).

---

   b. These pathways mediate the counter-rolling effect of the vestibular system on eye movement and also mediate nystagmus of vestibular origin.
   c. Extensive connections between the vestibular system and the dorsal motor nucleus of the vagus and the pontomedullary reticular formation mediate the autonomic signs of vestibular dysfunction.
   d. The vestibular nuclei send strong descending pathways to the spinal cord via the MLF and vestibulospinal tracts (Zilstorff-Pederson and Peitersen, 1963). These pathways and reticulospinal pathways coordinate postural reflexes involving the eyes, head, trunk, and limbs, listed in frame V C 4 c. Should you recite these reflexes?

5. **The pathways for the symptoms of vestibular stimulation**
   a. The vestibular nuclei connect to the thalamus by two pathways:
      i. A **ventral** pathway, ventral to the medial lemniscus, passes lateral to the red nucleus and dorsal to the subthalamic nucleus, terminating in the nucleus ventralis posterolateralis, pars oralis (nucleus ventralis intermedius).
      ii. A **dorsal** pathway runs through the lateral lemniscus and brachium of the inferior colliculus to the medial geniculate body, thus paralleling the auditory pathway (Fig. 9-7).
   b. The **vestibular cortex** consists of adjacent areas in the inferior parietal lobe, insula, and superior temporal region. The vestibular cortex is not confined to a discrete strip of striate cortex like other somatic senses. The vestibular cortical regions integrate auditory, visual somatosensory, and vestibular proprioceptive impulses that provide a sense of verticality, balance, and orientation of the body in space (Blanke et al., 2000; Brandt et al., 1994).

6. **Summary:** Vestibular impulses that arrive at the vestibular nuclei can box the compass and disperse to every major subdivision of the CNS: the cerebrum, diencephalon, brainstem, cerebellum, and spinal cord.

vestibulospinal

caudal (inferior)

MLF and in parallel with the auditory pathway

a. If they go *caudally* to the spinal cord, they descend via the MLF and the ______________________ tracts.

b. If they go *dorsally* to the flocculonodular lobe of the cerebellum, they travel via the ____________________ cerebellar peduncle.

c. If they go *rostrally* to nuclei for the ocular muscles, they travel via the ______________________________________.

d. If they go into the reticular formation, the impulses travel through many short circuits of bewildering complexity.

e. If they go to the cortex, they follow a dual pathway to the thalamus and then to areas near the posterior end of the Sylvian fissure, close to the striate cortex of the auditory area.

E. Review of clinical features of acute vestibular dysfunction

Vertigo, nausea, anxiety, oscillopsia, with exacerbation of these symptoms when moving or changing position.

1. Recall that the response to vestibular stimulation is **subjective** and **objective.** List the *subjective* responses, the *symptoms,* by recalling motion sickness.
   ____
   ____

Nystagmus, falling or postural deviation, sweating, pallor, vomiting, and hypotension.

2. List the *objective* responses—the *signs* including somatic and autonomic actions.
   ____
   ____
   ____

F. Physiology of nystagmus from caloric irrigation of the external auditory canals

1. The inertia or flow of fluid within the semicircular canals due to head rotation provides the normal stimulus. Syringing the external auditory canal with warm or cold water induces convection currents in the fluid in the *horizontal* semicircular canal, the closest one. Cooled fluid descends and heated fluid rises. Because of the weak effects of convection, the Ex places the horizontal canal in the vertical plane to add the effect of gravity to the convection currents. Refer to Fig. 9-9 to answer these questions:

30

   a. For a *reclining* Pt, tilt the head ____ degrees forward to get the horizontal canal vertical.

60; ☑ backward

   b. For a *sitting* Pt, tilt the head ___ degrees ❐ forward/❐ backward to get the horizontal canal vertical.

2. **Characteristics of vestibular nystagmus**

☑ jerk

   a. The nystagmus has fast and slow phases. It is therefore a ❐ jerk/❐ pendular nystagmus.

   b. While observing the nystagmus, have the Pt's eyes pursue your finger as you move it from side to side. The nystagmus increases in amplitude when the Pt looks in the direction of the fast component, because the volitional saccade adds to the kickback saccade.

3. **Describing the direction of jerk nystagmus:** Describing the direction of vestibular nystagmus presents a problem. The slow deviation of the eyes is the specific vestibulo-ocular action that initiates the nystagmus. A compensatory saccade then jerks the eyes back toward the midline, centering them for another deviation by the vestibular stimulus. Coma or anatomic interruption of the frontotegmental pathway for saccades may abolish the kickback saccade, even though the deviation phase remains (Beuttner and Zee, 1989). By tradition, the direction of nystagmus is named for the kick-back phase, not for the deviation phase. Understanding that, you can use the well-known **COWS** mnemonic.

COWS mnemonic to recall the expected direction of the fast component of jerk nystagmus induced by caloric stimulation: Cold-Opposite/Warm-Same. **COLD** water irrigation causes the fast phase to the **OPPOSITE** side of the ear irrigated, and **WARM** water to the **SAME** side as the ear irrigated.

4. The term **vestibulo-ocular reflex** (oculocephalic reflex or doll's eye test) means the slow deviation or counter-rolling of the eyes induced by caloric irrigation or by head rotation.

G. Indications for caloric irrigation

Although not part of the Standard NE, consider caloric irrigation if the history or examination indicates dizziness, vertigo, auditory dysfunction, or the recent onset of nystagmus. See Chapter 12 for its use in coma and brain death. Chapter 13 discusses objective recording of nystagmus by electronystagmography (Ruge and Bronstein, 1995). Caloric irrigation becomes reliable in infants after 6 to 8 months of age (Evitar, 1999; Fife et al., 2000).

H. Technique for caloric irrigation

1. **Forewarn and position the Pt:** Because of discomfort, the Ex should warn the Pt about the test, but mentioning the expected symptoms voids the objectivity and validity of the test. Therefore, say this: "I will be rinsing your ear. It's somewhat uncomfortable, but I want you to pay attention to what you feel." Because vertigo may cause the Pt to fall, place the Pt in a sitting or reclining position.
2. **Do otoscopy:** Exclude a mechanical impediment such as wax, otitis, or a perforated eardrum that might allow water into the middle ear, causing pain and infection. Remove excessive wax that may preclude adequate heat conduction.
3. **Place spectacles on the Pt that have strong positive lenses (+10 to 30 diopters, Frenzel lenses).** (You can buy them cheaply in chain stores.) The lenses serve two purposes. They magnify the Pt's eyes, making any nystagmus easier to see, and they impair fixation by blurring vision. Fixation inhibits vestibular-induced nystagmus. Thus, the glasses increase the likelihood of eliciting nystagmus, and make it easier to study if it occurs (Cohen, 1976).
4. **Instruct the Pt to gaze ahead:** Place an emesis basin or a towel next to the Pt's ear to prevent wetting the Pt (and also for emergency service should the Pt vomit).
5. **Irrigate the ear with warm or cold water:** Barber (1974) advocated instilling only 2 mL of ice water through a 14- to 16-gauge needle. Tilt the Pt's head to the opposite side and hold the water in the canal for a timed 20 seconds. After 20 seconds, place the horizontal canal vertical and watch for nystagmus. For a second method, fill a 50-mL syringe with water at a temperature of 7°C above or below the normal 37°C of body temperature (30°C or 44°C). Gently instill the 50 mL of water through a short rubber tube into the external auditory canal over a timed period of 40 seconds (Baloh, 2000; Baloh and Honrubia, 2001). Test both ears because a consistent difference is required for significance. Wait about 5 minutes between each test.
6. **Observe the Pt's responses:** At the end of irrigation, ask the Pt to direct the gaze more or less ahead and hold the arms straight out. Inspect the Pt for the following:
   a. **Nystagmus:** Record the duration and direction.
   b. **Postural deviation and past-pointing:** To test for past-pointing, have the Ex and Pt sit facing each other. Each extends the arms out from the shoulder so that the index fingers of Pt and Ex touch. The Ex instructs the Pt to close the eyes and extend the arm straight up and then bring it back down to touch the

Ex's finger in the original position. Look for the Pt's finger to miss by constantly deviating to one side.

7. **Ask about symptoms:** Ask whether the caloric irrigation reproduced the Pt's usual sensation of movement, and ask about the direction of any vertigo. Patients with vertigo and postural deviations sometimes report confusing directionality, depending on whether they are attending to their vertigo or their body tilt. Normal individuals also respond somewhat variably to caloric irrigation. Some Pts show little or no response from either ear. Determine whether irrigation of the two ears produces any consistent difference. Thus, a strong normal response from the right ear with little or no response from the left indicates a lesion of the vestibular end organ, nerve, or immediate central connections on the left.
8. To gain an enduring sympathy for your vertiginous Pts, submit to caloric irrigation yourself. Get a partner and follow the foregoing instructions. To make all the observations, you may have to irrigate more than once. Use the right ear and ice water and compare your observations with the answers to frames V E 1 and 2.

I. Summary of the results of caloric irrigation

1. If the vertigo goes in one direction, to the right or to the left, the slow deviation phase of the nystagmus, the truncal tilt, arm deviation, and past-pointing go to the *opposite* side.
2. Because the vertigo causes the Pt to feel movement or rotation in one direction, all of the postural deviations can be regarded as reflex compensation for the erroneous information coming from the artificially stimulated horizontal canal. Thus, the Pt compensates for the feeling of moving to the left by leaning and past-pointing to the right. In relation to the vertigo, the Pt compensates by postural deviations that go in the ❒ same/❒ opposite direction.

☑ opposite

J. Summary of vestibular testing

1. The symptoms of vestibular disease are____.

vertigo, nausea, anxiety, oscillopsia, and a resistance to moving around

2. The signs of vestibular disease are____.

nystagmus, postural deviation and falling, vomiting, hypotension, pallor, and sweating

3. What precautions does the Ex take before doing the caloric irrigation test? ____.

Counsel the Pt, do otoscopy, have the Pt sitting or reclining, and protect the Pt against wetting.

4. Describe the nystagmus after irrigating the left ear of a normal person with cold water. ____.

Horizontal jerk nystagmus with the slow phase to the left and rapid phase to the right.

5. In general, the Pt experiences the vestibular-induced vertigo as rotation toward the direction of the ❒ fast/❒ slow component.

☑ fast

6. State the law that relates the postural deviations to the direction of the vertigo. ____.

The posture deviates in the direction opposite to that of the vertigo (as if compensating for it).

7. Now can you put it all together? Figure 9-10 shows a person at the height of a strong vestibular response. Reason out which ear was irrigated with cold water: ❒ right/❒ left.

☑ right

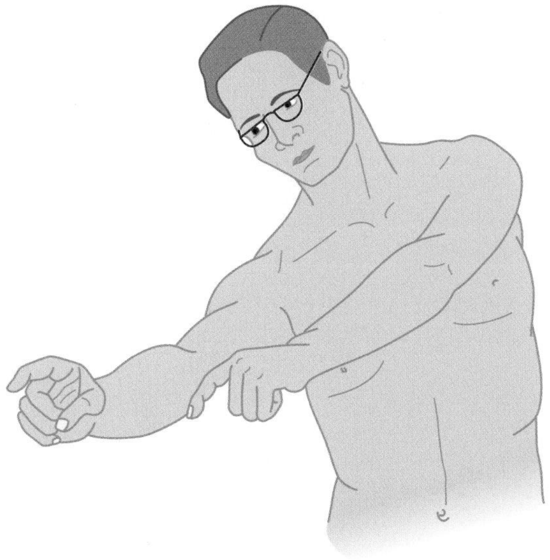

FIGURE 9-10. Postural deviation after one ear was irrigated with cold water. The patient was sitting upright with his head tilted 60 degrees backward during irrigation.

K. Positional vertigo and nystagmus

1. **Introduction:** Whenever a Pt complains of dizziness, the Ex should ask about the effect of changes in posture. Dizziness when first standing up, a phenomenon you have all experienced, suggests orthostatic hypotension. However, disease of the labyrinth or its central connections may cause true vertigo after changes of position, such as turning over in bed (Jannetta et al., 1984; Sharp and Barber, 1992). Positional nystagmus provides an objective sign of organic disease of the labyrinthine system. Free-floating particles in the posterior semicircular canal of the vestibular labyrinth may cause **benign paroxysmal positioning vertigo (BPPV).** Classic BPPV involves the posterior semicircular canal. Bedside maneuvers can move the particles to another location and alleviate the symptoms (Epley, 1992; Furman and Cass, 1999). The episodes of vertigo are typically sudden, last only 10 to 30 seconds and follow turning in bed or changes in position. In contrast, the vertigo of Ménière's disease comes on spontaneously and lasts minutes to hours. Acoustically induced vertigo (Tullio phenomenon), often accompanied by tinnitus, hearing loss, and ear pressure sensitivity, has been mainly attributed to perilymphatic fistula or the superior canal dehiscence syndrome (Tullio, 1929).
2. **Technique to test for positional nystagmus and vertigo (Dix-Hallpike maneuver)**
   a. Occlude visual fixation by Frenzel lenses. Start with the Pt sitting upright near the end of an examining table. Instruct the Pt to look straight ahead during the procedure (Bronstein, 2003). For a trial run, the Ex assists the Pt to drop back down with the head in the midline. After erecting the Pt, drop the Pt back with the head turned 45 to 60 degrees to the right and then to the left. After laying the Pt's head back over the table edge, look for nystagmus for 1 minute before considering the test negative (Fig. 9-11).
   b. After returning the Pt to the erect position, inspect the eyes again for nystagmus. Classic posterior canal BPPV produces geotropic rotatory nystagmus with the involved ear down.
   c. Repeat the procedure with the head turned to the left.
   d. Try fast and slow changes from the initial vertical position.
   e. At the end of any such positional tests, inquire whether the maneuver reproduced the Pt's sensation of dizziness, but do not suggest that it should have.

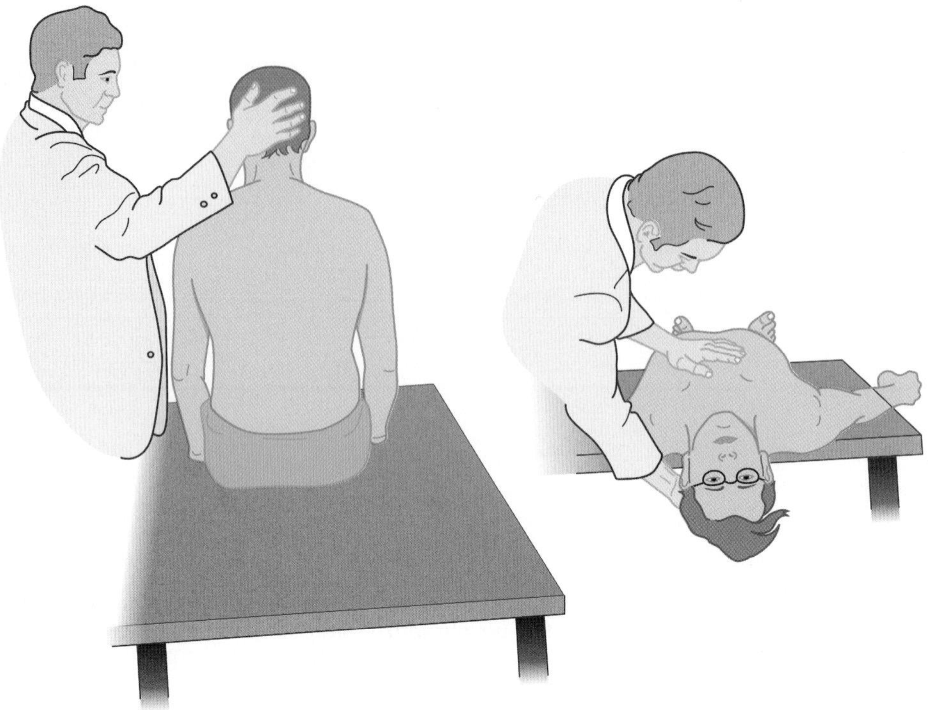

FIGURE 9-11. Method for eliciting positional nystagmus.

f. The Ex may also turn the Pt's head to the sides, or flex and extend it as the Pt sits or reclines. However, any symptoms produced may reflect changes in arterial blood flow through the carotid or vertebral arteries. Even when Pts have a neurologic disorder such as multiple sclerosis, benign paroxysmal positional vertigo, not the underlying disease, may cause the vertigo (Frohman et al., 2000). Hence, the Ex should always consider and test for this possibility.

L. Hyperventilation and dizziness

1. **Indications for hyperventilation:** Hyperventilation causes dizziness and may occur in panic attacks. It may provoke fainting (hyperventilation syncope) and epileptic seizures, in particular petit mal attacks. Hyperventilate the Pt if the history suggests any of these possibilities.
2. **Technique for hyperventilation:** Because the Pt may faint, the Pt sits or semireclines during the test. Ask the Pt to breathe as deeply and quickly as possible for a full 3 minutes by the clock. Throughout the test, keep encouraging the Pt to breathe hard: "Come on now. We are racing up a mountain." At the end, ask how the test made the Pt feel and whether it matched the original symptoms. Be sure to try this test on yourself.
3. **Normal results of hyperventilation:** The Pt feels lightheaded and somewhat faint and may experience tingling in the perioral region and extremities. Carpopedal spasm may also occur.

M. Summary of clinical tests for workup of the dizzy patient

1. See Table 9-1. See also Drachman and Hart (1972), Evitar (1999), and Fife et al. (2000).
2. Frequently the Ex should also order an electroencephalogram and MRI in Pts with dysequilibrium or dizziness (Kerber et al., 1998).

TABLE 9-1 · Clinical Workup of a Patient with Dizziness or vertigo

TESTS FOR VESTIBULAR DYSFUNCTION
Inquire about the circumstances at onset of vertiginous attacks and the necessity of remaining still to avoid vertigo
Inspect the gait and posture for tilting and unsteadiness
Inspect the eyes for nystagmus
Caloric irrigation of the ear
Whirling
Direct whirling of infant
Rotating (Barany) chair
Tilt tests for postural vertigo and nystagmus
Doll's eye maneuver for counter-rolling of the eyes (see Chapter 12)
NON-VESTIBULAR TESTS
Romberg test (increased swaying with vestibular or dorsal column disease, but not with cerebellar disease)
Reclining/standing blood pressure for orthostatic hypotension
Valsalva maneuver
Hyperventilation for 3 min
Carotid sinus stimulation

BIBLIOGRAPHY · Vestibular System, Dizziness, and Vertigo

Baloh RW. Charles Skinner Hallpike and the beginnings of neurotology. *Neurology* 2000;54:2138–2145.

Baloh RW. *Dizziness, Hearing Loss and Tinnitus.* Philadelphia, FA Davis, 1998.

Baloh RW, Honrubia V. *Clinical Neurophysiology of the Vestibular System*. New York, Oxford University Press, 2001.

Barber HO. Diagnostic techniques in vertigo. *J Vertigo* 1974;1:1–16.

Beuttner UW, Zee DS. Vestibular testing in comatose patients. *Arch Neurol* 1989; 46:561–563.

Blanke O, Perrig S, Thut G, et al. Simple and complex vestibular responses induced by electrical cortical stimulation of the parietal cortex in humans. *J Neurol Neurosurg Psychiatry* 2000;69:553–556.

Brandt T, Daroff RB. The multisensory physiological and pathological vertigo syndromes. *Ann Neurol* 1980;7:195–203.

Brandt T, Dieterich M. Vestibular syndromes in the roll plane: topographic diagnosis from brainstem to cortex. *Ann Neurol* 1994;36:337–347.

Brandt T, Dieterich M, Danek A. Vestibular cortex lesions affect the perception of verticality. *Ann Neurol* 1994;35:403–412.

Brandt T, Dieterich M, Strupp M. Vertigo and dizziness—common complaints. London: Springer. 2005.

Bronstein AM. Vestibular reflexes and positional manoevres. *J Neurol Neurosurg Psychiatry* 2003;74:289–293.

Cohen B. Use of Frenzel glasses in diagnosis of lesions of the vestibular system. *J Vertigo* 1976;2:1–10.

Drachman A, Hart C. An approach to the dizzy patient. *Neurology* 1972;22:323–334.

Epley, JM.The canalith repositioning procedure: for the treatment of benign paroxysmal positional vertigo. *Otolaryngol Head Neck Surg* 1992;107:399–404.

Evitar L. Vertigo. In Swaiman KF, Ashwal S, eds. *Pediatric Neurology*, 3rd ed. St. Louis, Mosby, 1999, Chapter 8, pp. 96–103.

Fife TD, Tusa RJ, Furman JM, et al. Assessment: vestibular testing techniques in adults and children: report of the Therapeutics and Technology Assessment Subcommittee of the American Academy of Neurology. *Neurology* 2000;55:1431–1441.

Frohman EM, Zhang H, Dewey RB, et al. Vertigo in MS: utility of positional and particle repositioning maneuvers. *Neurology* 2000;55:1566–1568.

Furman JM, Cass SP. Benign paroxysmal positional vertigo. *N Engl J Med* 1999;341:1590–1596.

Glasscock ME, Cueva RA, Thedinger BA: *Handbook of Vertigo.* New York, Thieme Medical Publishers, 1990.

Hardy M. Observations on the innervation of the macula sacculi in man. *Anat Rec* 1934;59:403–418.

Hotson JF, Baloh RW. Acute vestibular syndrome. *N Engl J Med* 1998;339:680–685.

Jannetta PJ, Moller MB, Moller AR: Disabling positional vertigo. *N Engl J Med* 1984; 310:1700–1706.

Kerber KA, Enrietto JA, Jacobson KM, et al. Disequilibrium in older people. A prospective study. *Neurology* 1998;51:574–580.

Rubin W, Brookler KH. *Dizziness: Etiologic Approach to Management.* New York, Thieme Medical Publishers, 1991.

Ruge P, Bronstein AM. Investigations of disorders of balance. *J Neurol Neurosurg Psychiatry* 1995;59:568–578.

Sharp JA, Barber HO. *The Vestibulo-ocular Reflex and Vertigo.* New York, Raven Press, 1992.

Tullio P. Das *Ohr und die Entstehung der Sprache und Schrift Berlin.* Urban & Schwarzenberg. 1929.

Zilstorff-Pederson K, Peitersen E. Vestibulospinal reflexes. *Arch Otolaryngol* 1963;77:237–242.

Learning Objectives for Chapter 9

I. THE SENSES

1. Enumerate the sensations mediated by exteroceptors, proprioceptors, and interoceptors.
2. Describe how to use your own body to systemically enumerate the special and general senses to avoid formally memorizing them.
3. Define a sensory modality and distinguish between a unimodal and a multimodal sensation.
4. Recite the three principles of sensory physiology as stated in Johannes Müller's doctrine of specific nerve energies.

II. SMELL (OLFACTION): CRANIAL NERVE I

1. On a sagittal diagram of the head, draw the primary olfactory neurons, showing their receptor endings and central synapses (Fig. 9-1).
2. Name the two sensory nerves of the nasal mucosa (Fig. 9-2).
3. Name the bony plate perforated by the olfactory axons.
4. Give the technical term for loss of the sense of smell.
5. Explain why sneezing or coughing may cause a gush of fluid into the nose of a person who has had a head injury.
6. State a potentially lethal complication of a CSF fistula.
7. Name two clinical manifestations of a cribriform plate fracture.
8. Define the rhinencephalon.
9. Explain the evolutionary significance of the rhinencephalon and the original biological importance of the senses of smell and taste (Fig. 9-3).
10. Define *déjà pensée* and *déjà vu.* Explain their clinical significance and localizing value.
11. Name appropriate aromatic substances for testing the sense of smell and explain why to avoid an irritating substance.
12. Demonstrate how to test the sense of smell.
13. Explain how to monitor the Pt's suggestibility and reliability in testing the sense of smell.
14. Describe some common conditions that cause reduction in, or loss of, the sense of smell (Fig. 9-5).
15. Describe how to "think through" the pathway for the sense of smell in analyzing the causes for anosmia.

Learning Objectives for Chapter 9

III. TASTE (GUSTATION) AND LOSS OF TASTE (AGEUSIA)

1. State which CrN innervates the taste buds of the anterior two-thirds of the tongue.
2. Name and locate the ganglion that contains the perikarya of the primary neurons for the sense of taste.
3. State the presumed location of the cortical taste center and contrast it with the presumed cortical center for smell.
4. Name two readily available substances for routine clinical testing of taste.
5. Describe and demonstrate how to test for loss of taste (ageusia).
6. List the muscles, glands, and special sense mediated by CrN VII.
7. Diagram CrN VII and describe the difference in the clinical signs when the nerve is interrupted at various sites along its course (Fig. 6-5).
8. Name the clinical symptom of stapedius muscle paralysis.
9. Describe how taste testing aids in localizing the site of a lesion along the course of CrN VII.
10. Describe some neighborhood signs indicating that a lesion has affected the nucleus or intra-axial course of CrN VII rather than its peripheral or extra-axial course.
11. Discuss the clinical indications for taste testing. Describe the circumstances when you may omit it.

IV. HEARING

1. Trace the auditory pathway from receptor to cerebral cortex, naming the way stations (Fig. 9-7).
2. Explain whether unilateral deafness implicates a lesion of the peripheral nervous system or the CNS.
3. Describe the symptoms of lesions of the cochlear division of CrN VIII.
4. Explain why threshold testing with minimal stimuli provides a better test of sensory systems than the maximal testing used in the strength examination.
5. Describe and demonstrate how to screen a Pt's hearing and how to make the bedside tests semiquantitative.
6. Describe how to mask hearing from the opposite ear when presenting a sound to one ear.
7. Describe and demonstrate how to do the air-bone conduction test of Rinne and state the result in a normal person.
8. Explain the importance of otoscopic inspection of the external auditory canal in interpreting hearing tests.
9. Describe and demonstrate how to do the sound lateralizing test of Weber. Describe the result in a normal person.
10. Describe a simple test on yourself to remember the effect of mechanical impediments to hearing on Weber's sound lateralizing test.
11. Explain the difference between a conductive and a neurosensory hearing loss and describe how to differentiate the two with bedside tests, including tuning fork tests.
12. Deduce the probable type of hearing loss, given various patterns of results from the bedside hearing tests (Section IV F, page 362).
13. Describe how to elicit and interpret the auditopalpebral reflex as a crude test of hearing in an infant or uncooperative patient.
14. Describe how to test the auditory system for inattention to bilateral simultaneous stimuli and for sound localization.

Learning Objectives for Chapter 9

15. Give the name of an electronic test for the integrity of the auditory pathways that does not require a cooperative or even conscious patient.
16. State in principle the kind of information derived from an audiogram and BAER test and give the full name for the BAER acronym.
17. Demonstrate how to do the several bedside tests that screen hearing (see Section V C 3 of the Standard NE).

V. THE VESTIBULAR SYSTEM: VERTIGO AND ITS POSTURAL COMPENSATIONS

1. Define the terms *dizziness* and *vertigo*.
2. Describe the various senses that contribute to the overall sense of balance and equilibrium.
3. State the direction the person will experience postrotatory vertigo after rotating to the *left*.
4. Describe the symptoms and signs that follow acute interruption of the vestibular division of CrN VIII.
5. State the adequate stimulus for the neurons of the semicircular canals (cristae).
6. State in a general way the adequate stimulus for the macula of the utricle and saccule.
7. Enumerate the major normal functions of the vestibular system.
8. Name some postural reflexes mediated through the vestibular system and the spinal pathway that mediates them.
9. Name the brainstem pathway by which axons from the vestibular nuclei reach the nuclei of CrNs III, IV, and VI.
10. Discuss the dispersion of pathways from the vestibular nuclei mentioning, in principle, their destinations.
11. Explain, in terms of the physics involved, why hot or cold water irrigation stimulates the semicircular canals, and how the angle of inclination of the horizontal canal affects the process.
12. Describe how to make the horizontal canal vertical when the Pt is sitting or prone (Fig. 9-9).
13. Describe the type of nystagmus produced by vestibular stimulation and describe the effect of eye movement on it.
14. Describe the convention for naming the direction of a jerk-type nystagmus. State which is the vestibular-induced phase and which is the compensatory or kickback phase and relate this to the COWS mnemonic.
15. State the clinical indications for caloric irrigation, and explain why it is not a necessary part of the routine screening examination.
16. Describe how to prepare the Pt for caloric irrigation, emotionally and physically, and recite the instructions to the Pt before the caloric irrigation test.
17. Explain why the Ex must inspect the external auditory canal before instilling fluid.
18. Explain why the Pt should wear Frenzel (strong positive: +10 to 30 diopters) lenses during caloric irrigation.
19. Describe and demonstrate two alternative caloric irrigation tests. State the water temperature and the amount of water to use.
20. Describe the normal result from cold caloric irrigation of the right ear (Fig. 9-10).
21. Describe when and how to test for positional vertigo and nystagmus (Fig. 9-11).
22. Describe the indications for and how to do the hyperventilation test and the normal result.
23. Recite the battery of bedside tests, vestibular and otherwise, for the workup of the Pt presenting with dizziness or vertigo (Table 9-1).

10 Examination of the General Somatosensory System

Nature, indeed has had a triple end in view in the distribution of nerves: she wished to give sensibility to organs of perception, movement to organs of locomotion, and to all others the faculty of recognizing the experience of injury.

—Galen (A.D. 130–200)

I. INTRODUCTION TO TESTING GENERAL SOMATIC SENSATIONS

A. Special and general senses

The special senses consist of sight, smell, taste, hearing, and equilibrium. The general senses tested in the Standard Neurological Examination (NE) consist of touch, pain, temperature, position, vibration, and stereognosis. Unique receptors and unique central pathways mediate each of the special senses. Some skin receptors and somatosensory pathways serve one general sensory modality, but other receptors in the skin are polymodal.

B. Negative and positive sensory phenomena after lesions of central and peripheral sensory pathways

1. Abnormal or noxious sensations like pain may arise in two ways: from stimulation of receptors or from intrinsic disease of the nerves or central pathways. Disease of afferent nerve fibers centrally or peripherally causes not only negative or **deficit phenomena,** with lack of sensation, as you would expect, but also, paradoxically, may cause **positive phenomena,** with excessive sensation, i.e., pain and tingling (Nashold and Ovelmen-Levitt, 1991).
2. **Nomenclature for deficits in superficial sensation**
   a. *Esthesia* = touch or feeling, so *hypesthesia* = partial loss of touch, and *anesthesia* = total loss. *Anesthesia* is also used to mean lack of pain.
   b. *Therm* = heat, so *thermhypesthesia* = partial loss of temperature sensation, and *thermanesthesia* = total loss.
   c. *Algesia* = pain, so *hypalgesia* = partial loss of pain sensation, and *analgesia* (or anesthesia) = total loss.
3. **Nomenclature for pain and other noxious irritative phenomena after disease of peripheral or central sensory pathways**
   a. **Hyperesthesia, hyperalgesia,** and **hyperthermesthesia** refer to an increased sensitivity to *touch, pain,* and *temperature,* respectively. For example, after a burn

of an area of skin, even slight exposure to heat may cause intense pain, i.e., *hyperthermesthesia*.

b. **Paresthesias** and **dysesthesias** are uncomfortable sensations of numbness, tingling, pins and needles, or burning pain short of neuralgia or causalgia. **Paresthesias** describes such sensations when they accompany a normal external stimulus to the skin. **Dysesthesias** describes their spontaneous occurrence without any obvious external stimulus (Wartenberg, 1953). (Unfortunately some writers reverse the definitions.) You will notice paresthesias and dysesthesias if you study your own sensations when recovering from a local anesthetic for a dental procedure or after having sat too hard on your own sciatic nerve, causing it to "go to sleep."

c. **Hyperpathia** means an extreme overresponse to pain. Hyperpathia associated with a raised pain threshold is called **anesthesia dolorosa.**

d. **Neuralgia** means multiple, very severe, electric shock-like pains that radiate into a specific root or nerve distribution. Examples include trigeminal neuralgia and post-herpetic neuralgia that commonly follow herpetic infection of a dorsal root ganglion (Gilden et al., 1991). The neuralgias may or may not alter the sensory threshold, but they complicate testing because of the intense pain and the presence of trigger points that, if touched, elicit a jolt of pain.

e. **Causalgia,** named by S. Weir Mitchell (1829–1914) but now called **reflex sympathetic dystrophy,** designates an unbearable, burning, relentless hyperesthesia and hyperalgesia that ensue after injury to a peripheral nerve (Low, 1997; Sunderland, 1978). Merely a puff of air or slight movement triggers unbearable pain.

f. **Special irritative or positive sensory disorders of cranial nerves:** See Section II C.

g. **Neurophysiologic mechanisms of such hyperesthesias might include:**

    i. Excessive firing of diseased neurons because of destabilization of their membranes.

    ii. Changes in the sensitivity of receptors or of central conducting mechanisms (Layzer, 2001).

    iii. A discrepancy or imbalance of the sensory information conveyed when disease affects the ratio of impulses delivered by fibers of different diameters.

    iv. Cross talk or short circuiting of impulses in demyelinated axons.

II. GENERAL ANATOMICO-PHYSIOLOGIC PRINCIPLES IN ANALYZING LESIONS OF THE PERIPHERAL NERVOUS SYSTEM

A. Principle 1: The signs and symptoms of peripheral nervous system (PNS) lesions will be expressed in the anatomic distribution of roots, nerve trunks, plexuses, or peripheral nerves

B. Principle 2: The signs and symptoms of PNS lesions depend on the functional types of axons in the nerve: motor (general somatic and visceral efferent, branchial efferent), sensory (general somatic and visceral afferent, special visceral and somatic afferent, or mixed sensorimotor, visceral, and somatic)

C. Principle 3: The signs and symptoms of PNS lesions depend on whether the lesions cause deficit phenomena, irritative phenomena, or both

1. Deficit phenomena after lesions of the somatomotor axons (general somatic efferent, branchial efferent):

a. Paresis or paralysis of individual muscles.
b. Decreased or absent muscle stretch reflexes (MSRs).
c. Denervation atrophy (early and severe).

2. Release phenomena after lesions of somatomotor neurons:
   a. Fasciculations
   b. Fibrillations
3. Autonomic deficit phenomena after lesions of visceromotor neurons (general visceral efferent):
   a. Paralysis and atony of smooth muscle, impairing peristalsis, propulsion, and emptying
   b. Vasomotor paralysis with vasodilation, orthostatic hypotension, and impotence
   c. Anhidrosis
   d. Trophic changes consisting of hair loss, atrophy of skin, and dystrophy of nails
4. Autonomic release phenomena after lesions of the visceral motor neurons (general visceral efferent)
   a. Hyperhidrosis
   b. Vasomotor instability with vasoconstriction and hyperhidrosis, rather than anhidrosis and vasodilation. Often Raynaud's phenomenon
5. Deficit phenomena after lesions of the somatosensory axons (general somatic afferent)
   a. Anesthesia or hypesthesia
   b. Analgesia or hypalgesia
   c. Thermanesthesia or thermhypesthesia
   d. Loss of dorsal column modalities
6. Irritative phenomena after lesions of the somatosensory or special sensory axons or, in some cases, their central pathways
   a. Hyperesthesias: paresthesias and dysesthesias
   b. Hyperalgesia
   c. Hyperthermesthesia
   d. Hyperpathia (anesthesia dolorosa)
   e. Neuralgia
   f. Complex regional pain syndrome Type II (Causalgia)
   g. Symptoms specific to irritation of sensory cranial nerves
      i. Cranial nerve (CrN) I: hyperosmia (usually central in origin)
      ii. CrN II: flashes of light, scintillating scotomas (phosphenes or "seeing stars")
      iii. CrNs V and IX: trigeminal and glossopharyngeal neuralgia
      iv. CrN VII: hypergeusia (increased sense of taste, usually central lesion)
      v. CrN VIII: tinnitus, hyperacusis, diplacusis (auditory division), and vertigo (vestibular division)

D. Principle 4: The sensory nerves function according to the doctrine of specific nerve energies of Johannes Muller (see page 349)

E. Principle 5: To localize lesions of the PNS to a root, plexus, peripheral nerve or branch, detect and list the weak muscles and outline with ink the area of sensory deficit on the patient's (Pt's) skin or on a diagram. Then compare the results with charts of dermatomal, myotomal, and peripheral nerve distributions (Chapter 2)

F. Principle 6: For the localizing analysis, "think along" the course of the PNS nerve fibers, in the direction of the nerve impulse.

1. To analyze a *sensory* disorder in the PNS, commence with the skin and "think along" the PNS from the receptor through the nerve branch or trunk, plexus, and dorsal root into the spinal cord. Continue thinking along the pathway to the primary receptive cortex.
2. To analyze a *motor* disorder, start with the motor cortex and think through the pyramidal tract, ventral motoneuron, ventral root, plexus, nerve trunk, neuromyal junction, and the muscle fiber itself.

G. Principle 7: The size of the nerve fiber and its myelination determine its conduction velocity and relates to its function. Measurement of sensory or motor nerve conduction velocity is often an important adjunct to the clinical examination

1. Peripheral nerves contain unmyelinated and myelinated nerve fibers ranging in diameter from 0.2 to 20 micra (myelin sheath included).
   a. The unmyelinated axons are around 1 micra in diameter (a red blood cell is 7 micra) and conduct at about 1 m/s. They range in size from approximately 0.2 to 0.3 micra to approximately 3 micra.
   b. The myelinated fibers range from 1 to 2 micra to 20 micra in diameter and conduct at rates up to 120 m/s, with a mean near 60 m/s.

$$60 \text{ m/s} \times 60 \text{ s/min} \times 60 \text{ min/h} \times 1/\text{mile } 1609.3 \text{ m} = 216{,}000/1609.3, \text{ or } 134 \text{ miles/h.}$$

2. In general, the larger the fiber diameter, the longer the internodal distance and the faster the conduction. Those fibers conducting faster than 3 m/s are myelinated.
3. The largest nerve fibers innervate joint receptors and muscle fibers.
4. Purely cutaneous peripheral nerves, such as the sural nerve (often chosen for biopsy) or the superficial radial nerve, contain no afferents from joints or muscles and generally have fibers smaller than 12 micra in diameter.
5. In mixed nerves the smallest fibers, generally unmyelinated, are postganglionic sympathetic efferents, visceral afferents, or serve as pain and temperature afferents. The small fibers of purely cutaneous nerves contain only the latter.
6. To classify nerve fibers by size, physiologists use a confusing mixture of three systems: English alphabets (A, B, and C), Greek alphabets (α, β, γ, and δ), and Roman numerals (I to IV) (DeMyer, 1998).

III. GENERAL CLINICAL PRINCIPLES IN TESTING ALL SOMATIC SENSATIONS

A. For the patient

1. To enliven the proceedings, make each test a game or a matter of curiosity: "Let's see how light a touch you can feel." "Let's see whether you can feel the buzz of the tuning fork."
2. Demonstrate and describe the tests. Ask for *yes* or *no* responses, or "Is [stimulus] *one* different from [stimulus] *two*?" a procedure called **forced-choice testing.**
3. Have the Pt close the eyes to avoid visual cues.

B. For the examiner

1. Compare homologous areas of the right and left sides and compare normal areas to any suspected abnormal areas.

2. The skin areas differ greatly in sensitivity. The highly sensitive skin of the face and armpits contrasts with the horny skin of palms and soles. Hairy skin perceives tickling and touch better than glabrous skin. The forehead is the most sensitive area for temperature discrimination. Because cold skin loses sensitivity, ensure a warm skin before testing the Pt.
3. Plan follow-up examinations to recheck any doubtful results.
4. Determine whether sensory deficits match a central pathway, segmental (dermatomal), plexus, or peripheral nerve pattern (Figs. 2-10 and 2-11) or match a nonorganic distribution (Chapter 14).
5. Recognize that the Pt's mental state, legal wrangling, or secondary gain from the illness may drastically alter sensory test results.

BIBLIOGRAPHY · Introduction to Testing General Somatic Sensations

Gilden DH, Dueland AN, Cohrs R, et al. Preherpetic neuralgia. *Neurology* 1991;41: 1215–1218.

Layzer RB. Hot feet: erythromelalgia and related disorders. *J Child Neurol* 2001;16: 199–202.

Low PA, ed. *Clinical Autonomic Disorders. Evaluation and Management*, 2nd ed. Philadelphia, Lippincott-Raven, 1997.

Mitchel SW. *Injuries of Nerves and Their Consequences.* Reprint. New York, Dover Publications, 1965.

Nashold BS, Ovelman-Levitt JO. *Deafferentation Pain Syndromes. Advances in Pain Research and Therapy, Vol 19.* New York, Raven, 1991.

Schwartzman RJ, Erwin KL, Alexander Gm. The nature history of complex regional pain syndrome. *Clin J Pain* 2009;25(4):273–280.

Sunderland S. *Nerves and Nerve Injuries,* 2nd ed. Edinburgh, Churchill-Livingstone, 1978.

Wartenberg R. *Diagnostic Tests in Neurology: A Selection for Office Use.* Chicago, Year Book Publishers, 1953.

IV. EXAMINATION OF SENSORY FUNCTIONS OF CRANIAL NERVE V

A. Functions of the afferents of cranial nerve V

1. **Sensory domain of the trigeminal nerve:** With a single scimitar blow, let us slice the face off from the head, along the line shown in Fig. 10-1, creating the mask of Trigeminus.

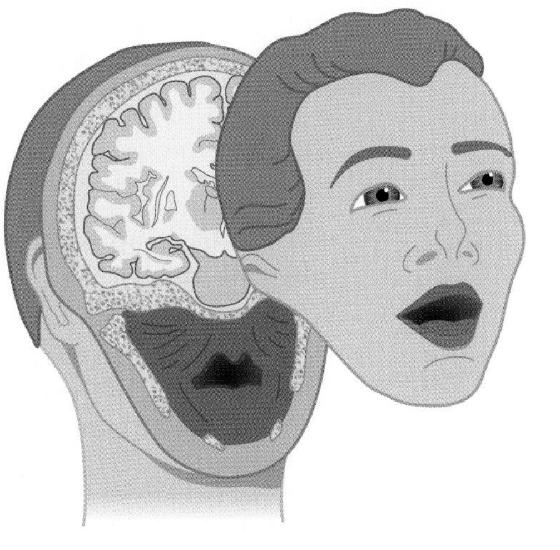

FIGURE 10-1. The mask of Trigeminus. Obtain it by a single slice through the head with a scimitar.

2. **The three dimensions of the mask of Trigeminus**
   a. The mask sliced away by the scimitar is no ordinary Halloween mask. It has three dimensions. It contains all the territory that receives motor and sensory innervations from CrN V: chewing muscles and their proprioceptors, proprioceptors from the eye muscles and general sensation from the facial skin, eyeball and orbit, mucous membranes of the nose, mouth, tongue, and sinuses, the dura mater, and a tad of the external ear.
   b. Of the tissues in the slice, only the cerebrum has no nerve supply. CrN V conveys *no* special sensory fibers. Notice that the cut spares the angle of the mandible, leaving it behind with the head. See the mandibular angle in Fig. 10-2.

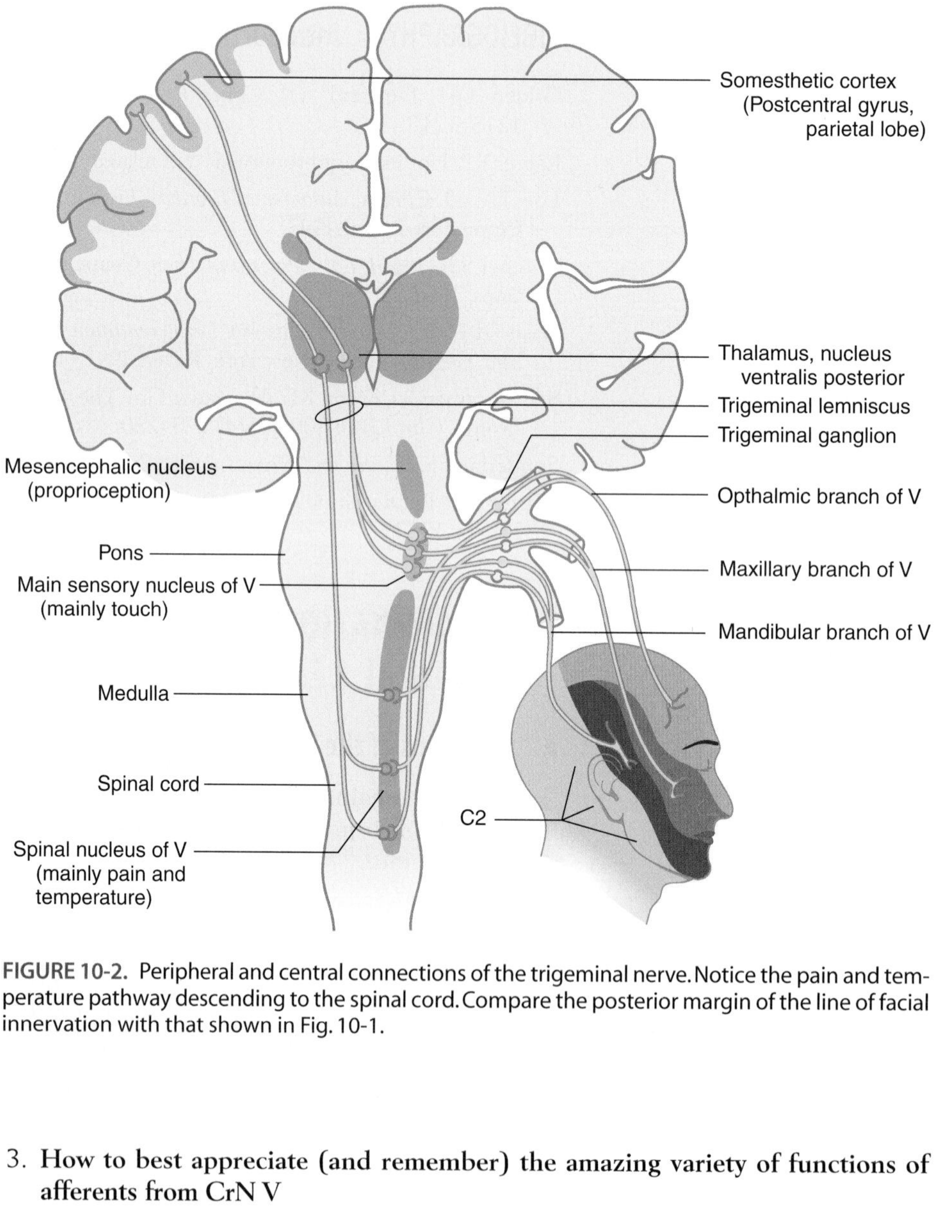

FIGURE 10-2. Peripheral and central connections of the trigeminal nerve. Notice the pain and temperature pathway descending to the spinal cord. Compare the posterior margin of the line of facial innervation with that shown in Fig. 10-1.

3. **How to best appreciate (and remember) the amazing variety of functions of afferents from CrN V**
   a. First, observe a newborn baby: It roots for a nipple, sucks, chews, swallows, searches with its tongue, blinks, cries, and sneezes. Stimuli acting through CrN V initiate all of these reflexes. Then, too, you will understand that the turning of the head toward the stimulus in the rooting reflex depends on the descending root of CrN V that connects with the head-turning muscles of the neck. In fact, the very first cutaneous reflex that the human fetus exhibits is turning of the head in response to stimulation of the upper lip (Hooker, 1969). This behavior appears when the fetus reaches week 8 of gestation, just after the

axons of the root of CrN V have grown down into the cervical region to make this reflex possible. To further understand the descending connections of CrN V, consider the rat, a nocturnal animal with weak eyes, as it feels its way along a totally dark passage. By touching its whiskers against the wall, it gains afferent information to orient the head, neck, and body.

b. Next consider the autonomic responses mediated by CrN V: lacrimation from corneal irritation, rhinorrhea, salivation from mechanical stimulation of the oral mucosa (as opposed to taste), and pupillodilation and bradycardia or tachycardia from facial pain.

c. Then, think of the role of CrN V in sinus pain and toothache, not to mention headache in general. Sensory V is a busy nerve, and that's why it has the largest sensory ganglion in the body.

B. Distribution of the sensory divisions of cranial nerve V

1. From Fig. 10-2 learn the three divisions of the *tri* geminal nerve, their facial skin areas, and central connections.

2. CrN V receives its name *trigeminal* because of its three large sensory divisions, the ________________, ________________, and ________________.

ophthalmic; maxillary; mandibular

3. The three sensory branches funnel into a single root that attaches to the ❒ mesencephalon/❒ pons/❒ medulla.

☑ pons

4. The sensory ganglion of CrN V, the trigeminal (semilunar, gasserian) ganglion, contains the ❒ primary/❒ secondary/❒ tertiary neuron of the sensory pathway from the face.

☑ primary

5. The trigeminal ganglion corresponds to the ________________ ganglia of the spinal nerves.

dorsal root

6. The primary ganglia for the special senses that are very near their end organs belong to CrNs ________________. If you don't recall the answer readily, how should you systematize your approach?

____.

I and VIII

Start at CrN I and sort through them one by one.

7. The trigeminal *nuclei* (*nuclei*, not *ganglia*) contain the ❒ primary/❒ secondary/❒ tertiary neuron of the trigeminal pathway.

☑ secondary

8. Where is the tertiary neuron? ________________.

Thalamus (diencephalon). Review Fig. 10-2 if you missed this.

9. The mesencephalic nucleus of CrN V violates the rule that the primary neuron of a sensory pathway is outside the central nervous system. This nucleus consists of primary neurons within the neuraxis, a unique fact but of no clinical use. The mesencephalic portion of CrN V probably mediates proprioception; the pontine and rostral medullary portion mediates *touch;* and the spinal nucleus mediates *pain* and *temperature* (Humphrey, 1969). Thus, in rostrocaudal order, the functions mediated by the three portions of the sensory nucleus of CrN V are ________________, ________________, and ________________.

proprioception; touch; pain and temperature

10. Taken together, trigeminal sensory fibers and nuclei extend from the rostral part of the cervical region of the spinal cord to the mesencephalon (Fig. 10-2).

C. Technique for testing touch in the area of cranial nerve V

1. **Instruction to the Pt.** Ask the Pt to say *touch* in response to each touch by a wisp of cotton. After the Pt closes the eyes, lightly brush each area of the three sensory divisions of CrN V with a wisp of cotton. Touch alternate areas and sides of the face randomly. Also, change the time between touches to keep the Pt from getting into a rhythm of answering without actually attending to the stimulus.

2. If you used a rigid test object to test for light touch, which principle of sensory testing did you violate?

____

____.

A rigid object causes pressure and touch, violating the rule to test one sensory modality at a time.

Occasionally withhold the stimulus and ask whether the Pt felt something. Recall that in testing smell, the examiner (Ex) also withheld the stimulus at times.

3. After the Pt has responded several times, how would you test the Pt's reliability and attentiveness?

____

____

4. As a rule, if the history indicates a specific area of sensory loss, start sensory testing in a normal area, to give the Pt the experience of the normal sensation. Then start in the middle of the abnormal area and work outward.

D. The corneal reflex

1. **Anatomy of the corneal reflex arc**
   a. The corneal reflex consists of closure of both eyelids in response to touching one cornea. It is entirely distinct from the corneal light reflection described earlier.

ophthalmic

   b. The afferent arc of the corneal reflex travels through the ______________ division of CrN V.

orbicularis oculi; VII

   c. The muscle that closes the eyelid is the ______________ innervated by CrN ______________.

V; VII

   d. The corneal reflex thus tests the integrity of two cranial nerves, (afferent) ______________ and (efferent) ______________.

2. **Technique for the corneal reflex**
   a. Use a free piece of cotton, rolled to a fine point. Do not use cotton attached to a stick (Q tip). Avoid sticks around the eyes. A demented, retarded, or delirious Pt may flinch against the tip of the stick and injure an eye.
   b. Tell the Pt, "I am going to just touch your eyeball very lightly." Instruct the Pt to look to one side and a little up. Gently hold the lids apart to avoid stimulating the eyelashes.
   c. Bring in a wisp of cotton from the lateral side to touch the lateral side of the cornea of the *adducted* eye. **Bring the cotton directly in from the side to avoid entering the field of vision.** That would cause a visually mediated flinch, not a corneal blink reflex. In Fig. 10-3, make an X on the exact spot to stimulate the cornea without entering the Pt's field of vision.

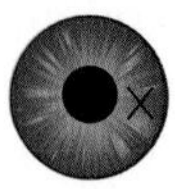

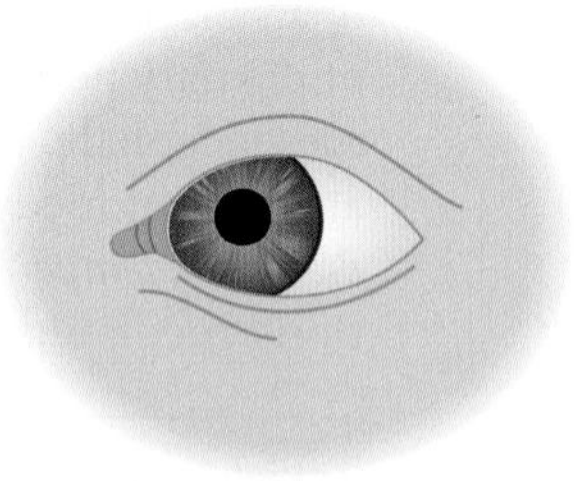

FIGURE 10-3. Blank to mark the site for stimulation of the cornea to elicit the corneal reflex.

3. **Clinical interpretation of the corneal reflex:** Most normal individuals display a corneal reflex. Exceptions include some elderly or postcataract surgery Pts. If no response occurs, do not conclude that the arc from CrN V to VII is interrupted until you have checked for a contact lens. Acute deep hemispheric parietal lesions may abolish the corneal reflex on the contralateral side for hours or days as a deficit or "shock" phenomenon (Ross, 1972). The corneal reflex behaves like other superficial reflexes, the abdominal and cremasteric reflexes, and they all temporarily disappear after an acute upper motoneuron (UMN) lesion. As with the gag reflex, in the absence of symptoms, the Ex may elect to eliminate the corneal reflex from the screening NE.

E. The corneomandibular reflex (von Sölder phenomenon)

Stimulation of one cornea causes contraction of the ipsilateral lateral pterygoid muscle and a twitch of the jaw to the opposite side (Lawton et al., 1963). The jaw twitches *contralaterally* after stimulation of the cornea ipsilateral to a hemispheric lesion. A bilateral reflex may occur in coma, multiple sclerosis, or bilateral hemispheric lesions (Guberman, 1982). It may indicate a UMN lesion more sensitively in amyotrophic lateral sclerosis than other UMN signs. It may also appear in parkinsonism (Okuda, 1999).

F. The glabellar blink reflex

This reflex consists of bilateral contraction of the orbicularis oculi muscles in response to percussion of the glabella with the fingertip or a percussion hammer or to electrical stimulation of the supraorbital branch of the trigeminal nerve. Electrical stimulation during electromyographic (EMG) recording provides an objective, quantitative method of measuring the afferent and efferent arcs of a CrN V to VII reflex. Various lesions of the afferent or efferent arc reduce the blink response. It disappears unilaterally in acute hemiplegia and bilaterally in deep coma (Fine et al., 1992). Usually it fatigues by about 10 taps, but in dementias and parkinsonism (Parkinson's disease, progressive supranuclear palsy, multiple system atrophy) it persists (disinhibited).

G. Technique for testing temperature discrimination

1. **Instruction to the Pt:** State, "I want to see how well you can tell warm from cool. Please close your eyes, and I will place something on your cheek. Tell me whether it is warm or cool."
2. **Tuning fork or finger test:** Apply the metal shaft of a tuning fork to the side of the Pt's cheek for a few seconds and then remove it and apply the side of your little finger to the same spot. Ask the Pt whether each is cool or warm (Fig. 10-4).

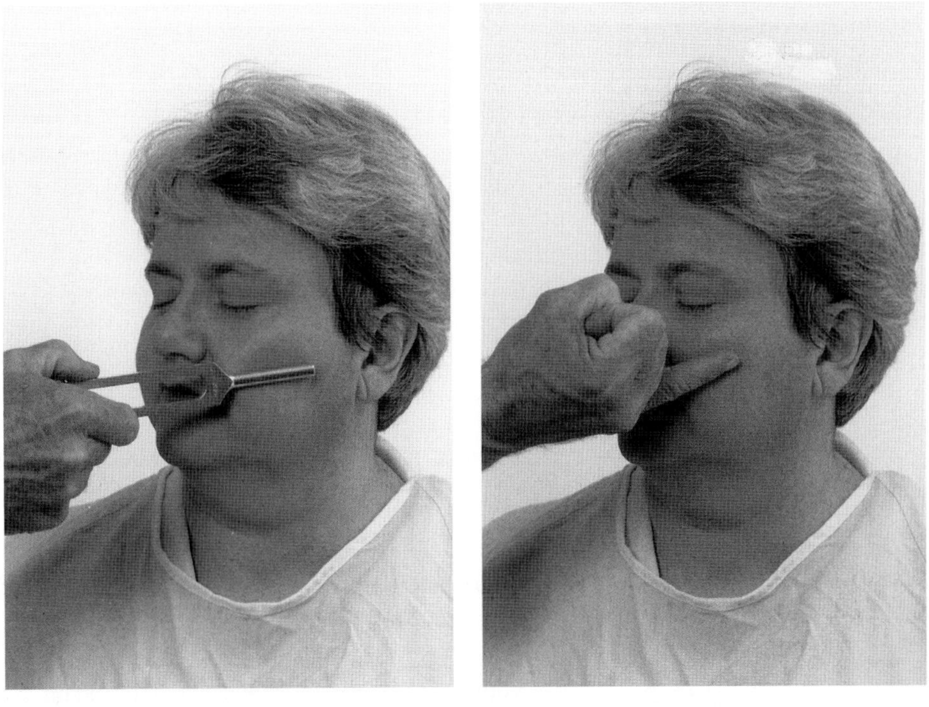

FIGURE 10-4. Randomly touch the tuning fork shaft and your little finger to test temperature discrimination.

a. Use the fork first to establish immediate communication because it will feel colder than the finger. The Pt will attend to the temperature and not to texture or size.

b. Randomly alternate the finger and tuning fork as you proceed over the three trigeminal sensory areas and then over the dorsum of both hands and both feet. Try this test on yourself.

c. To sharpen ambiguous results, say "Which is cooler, number 1 [the tuning fork] or number 2 [the finger]?"

3. **Warm and cold tube test:** Fill one tube with warm water and one with cold. Avoid extremes of temperature. You want to test temperature *discrimination*, not how much heat or cold the Pt can withstand.

4. Because pain and temperature receptors somewhat overlap and share a common pathway in the spinal tract of CrN V and in the trigeminothalamic tract, disease generally affects both modalities. For screening purposes, testing one tests both. Test temperature discrimination first. If the Pt discriminates temperature normally, and the history does not suggest neurologic disease, you do not need to prick every Pt with a pin to test pain. No one relishes a pinprick, especially about the face. If you approach (attack) a young child with a pin first, you will have ended the entire sensory examination. Yet even an intelligent 3- to 4-year-old child will play the temperature game with the tuning fork. By testing temperature sensation, you avoid leaving a trail of pinpricks across the skin, oozing blood, a matter of some importance in this era of acquired immunodeficiency syndrome.

H. Testing pain perception

If the history suggests a sensory disorder, test pain sensation over the face after testing temperature discrimination. See page 391.

I. Differentiation of hysterical from organic loss of facial sensation

1. Draw a line across the head in Fig. 10-5 to show the exact dividing line between the part of the head innervated by CrN V and the cervical dermatomes. Compare it with Fig. 10-2 to see how exact your line is.

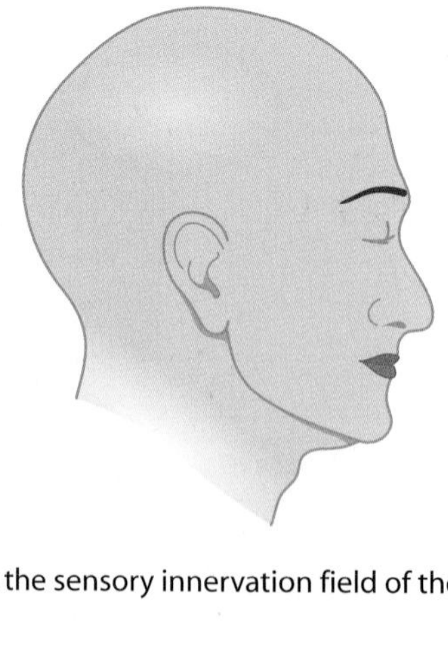

FIGURE 10-5. Blank to draw in the sensory innervation field of the trigeminal nerve.

2. Now shade and label the parts of the face supplied by each of the three major sensory branches of CrN V. Check with Fig. 10-2.

3. Does CrN V innervate the skin over the angle of the mandible? If you included it in your drawing above, check Fig. 10-2 again. You missed a point of importance. Organic sensory loss of facial sensation from trigeminal nerve lesions spares the angle of the mandible, whereas hysterical loss of facial sensation includes it. Review

Figs. 2-10 and 10-2 to recall where CrN V abuts on spinal nerve root C2. Comparison of hysterical with organic sensory losses on the face leads to a useful general law: **In psychogenic illness, Pts lose sensation according to their mental image of the body parts; organic Pts lose sensation according to the wiring diagram of the nervous system.** As another example, in hysteria the loss of sensation in the upper extremity usually cuts off sharply at the wrist, elbow, or shoulder, because that agrees with one's mental image of an arm, but it does not agree with the actual anatomic distribution of peripheral nerves, nerve roots, or their central pathways. See Fig. 14-3.

4. Therefore, in hysterical sensory loss of facial sensation, the angle of the mandible is ❒ spared/❒ affected, whereas in organic loss of affected facial sensation due to a CrN V lesion, the angle of the mandible is ❒ spared/❒ affected.

☑ affected; ☑ spared

J. Analyze this patient

1. This 76-year-old woman complains of severe facial pain, starting 4 months ago and gradually worsening. She describes very brief, shock-like jolts of unbearable pain that runs from the side of her cheek down to the tip of her jaw, on the right side only. She has become irascible and impossible to live with according to her husband. Because eating triggers the pain, she has lost 18 lb. The NE discloses normal motor and sensory functions of the CrNs, except that she will not allow the Ex to test sensation over the right lower jaw because touching the right lower lip triggers excruciating shocks of pain (allodynia).
2. In analyzing a sensory complaint, the Ex must determine its nature and whether its distribution conforms to an anatomic pattern or to the person's mental image of the body and, hence, is psychogenic. The term that best matches the Pt's sensory disorder is (review the descriptors in Section I B 3a to e before answering): ❒ hyperesthesia/❒ hyperalgesia/❒ causalgia/❒ neuralgia.

☑ neuralgia
Although some other terms more or less apply, *neuralgia* is the most specific.

3. Does the location of the sensory disorder match:
   - ❒ a. The distribution of a central pathway?
   - ❒ b. The distribution of a dermatome?
   - ❒ c. The distribution of a peripheral nerve or nerve branch?
   - ❒ d. A nonanatomic distribution that, in combination with the Pt's obvious personality change, indicates a psychogenic disorder?

☑ c

4. Which peripheral nerve area does the Pt's pain correspond to?

____

Mandibular division of CrN V on the right.

5. This Pt had no other abnormalities on the general physical examination or the radiographic examination of the skull with a basilar view to show the foramina of exit of CrN V. She had *trigeminal neuralgia* (tic douloureux), a very typical neuralgia, characterized by repetitive excruciating shocks of pains in one or more of the branches of the trigeminal nerve (Fromm and Sessle, 1991; Rose, 1999). Typically the pain erupts spontaneously and also after touching a "trigger point" on the cheek or the inside of the mouth. It occurs idiopathically with multiple sclerosis (Ferroli and Farina, 2001) and apparently as a result of vascular compression of the root of CrN V by the superior cerebellar artery (Fromm and Sessle, 1991). Medication or surgical treatment may alleviate it (Theodosopoulos et al., 2002). Victor and Ropper (2001) tabulated many other causes of facial pain.

K. Summary of the tests for the sensory functions of the cranial nerves

Get a partner and rehearse Section V, steps C and D, of the Standard NE.

BIBLIOGRAPHY · Examination of Sensory Functions of Cranial Nerve V

Brodsky H, Dat Vuongk, Thomas M et al. Glabellar and palmomental reflexes in parkinsonian disorders. *Neurology* 2004;63:1096–1098.

Ferroli P, Farina L. Linear pontine and trigeminal root lesions and trigeminal neuralgia. *Arch Neurol* 2001;58:1311.

Fine EJ, Sentz L, Soria E. The history of the blink reflex. *Neurology* 1992;42:882.

Fromm GH, Sessle BJ. *Trigeminal Neuralgia: Current Concepts Regarding Pathogenesis and Treatment.* London, Butterworth-Heinemann, 1991.

Galer, BS, Jensen MP. Development and preliminary validation of a pain measure specific to pain: the neuropathic pain scale. *Neurology* 1997;48:332–338.

Guberman A. Clinical significance of the corneomandibular reflex. *Arch Neurol* 1982;39:578–581.

Hooker D. *The Prenatal Origin of Behavior.* New York, Hafner Publishing Co, 1969.

Humphrey T. The central relations of the trigeminal nerve. In Kahn EA, Crosby EA, Schneider RC, Taren JA, eds. *Correlative Neurosurgery,* 2nd ed. Springfield, Charles C Thomas, 1969:477–508.

Lawton SJ, David JN, Mitchell C. The corneomandibular reflex. *Arch Ophthalmol* 1963; 70(1):12–14.

Okuda B, Kodama N, Kawabata K, et al. Corneomandibular reflex in ALS. *Neurology* 1999;52:1699–1701.

Rose FC. Trigeminal neuralgia. *Arch Neurol* 1999;56:1163–1164.

Ross R. Corneal reflex in hemisphere disease. *J Neurol Neurosurg Psychiatry* 1972;35:877–880.

Theodosopoulos PV, Marco E, Applebury C, et al. Predictive model for pain recurrence after posterior fossa surgery for trigeminal neuralgia. *Arch Neurol* 2002;56:1297–1302.

Victor M, Ropper AH. *Adams and Victor's Principles of Neurology.* New York, McGraw-Hill, 2001.

V. EXAMINATION OF SOMATOSENSORY FUNCTIONS OF THE BODY AND EXTREMITIES

A. Testing light touch sensation

1. Test touch over the rest of the body exactly as described for the face. For screening purposes, test only the dorsum of the hands and feet, in addition to the face. The history determines how far to extend the sensory examination. Review Fig. 2-10 to understand why the Ex would move the touch stimulus *up and down* the trunk to discover a dermatomal loss or spinal cord sensory level but *around* the limbs.
2. Quantitative testing of touch and pressure can be done with graded monofilaments (Semmes-Weinstein Esthesiometer, Smith & Nephew Roylan, Inc., Germantown, WI) or hairs (von Frey hairs) of different strengths (Dyck and Thomas, 1993; Perkins et al., 2001; Spreen and Strauss, 1991).
3. Review the anatomy of touch in Fig. 2-28.
   a. Recall that touch impulses ascend to the somesthetic cortex by two spinal pathways: one in the ______________ column of the cord and the other in the ______________ of the cord.
   b. The dorsal column pathway decussates at the ______________ junction, whereas the spinothalamic tract decussates at the ______________.
4. The pathway for touch in the ventrolateral columns most closely resembles the pathway for ☐ pain and temperature/☐ vibration and position sense.
   a. These two tracts, the ventral and lateral spinothalamic tracts, run together as the ______________ lemniscus.
   b. All lemnisci unite in the brainstem to travel to the thalamus as one with the medial lemniscus (DeMyer, 1998). Complete Table 10-1.

Answers (margin): dorsal columns (fasciculi gracilis and cuneatus); ventrolateral column (spinothalamic tract or spinal lemniscus)

cervicomedullary; level of entry of the dorsal root

☑ pain and temperature

spinal

TABLE 10-1 · Origins and Names of the Lemnisci

Site of origin of axons of lemniscus	Name of lemniscus
Trigeminal sensory nuclei	
Cranial nerve VIII nuclei	
Dorsal column nuclei	
Dorsal horn nuclei	

Answers (margin): Trigeminal; Lateral; Medial; Spinal

c. The one sensation that lacks a lemniscus and a specific thalamic relay nucleus is mediated by CrN ___________.

B. Testing temperature sensation from the body and extremities

Proceed exactly as described for the face. Test temperature discrimination first. Use the tuning fork and finger or warm and cold tube tests (Fig. 10-4).

C. Physiology and anatomy of pain

1. **Relation of pain and temperature sensation to types of peripheral axons**
   a. Prick yourself with a pin. After a pinprick you will experience two types of pain: fast and slow. Small myelinated fibers of the A group mediate the first pain, a sharp, bright, localized "fast" pain. This pain is mediated mainly through the classic lateral spinothalamic pain and temperature pathway. Small myelinated axons (IA γ fibers) also mediate cold sensation (Wall and Melzack, 1999; Willis and Coggeshall, 1991; Yarnitsky and Ochoa, 1991).
   b. Unmyelinated C fibers mediate the second type of pain, an afterglow of dull, diffuse, stinging, and burning pain. Diffuse polysynaptic pathways rather than solely the classic spinothalamic pathway likely mediate this pain. This pain connects with the reticular formation and ultimately the limbic system (Casey, 1991; Weiner, 2002). The small, unmyelinated axons (C fibers) also convey warm sensations. In contrast, the largest fibers of the peripheral nerves mediate the so-called dorsal column modalities (Section V).
2. **Clinical classification of pain**
   a. Pain can be classified as **nociceptive** and **neurogenic** (neuropathic).
   b. Pain of **nociceptive** origin is divided into somatic and visceral and arises from some local lesion, such as an invasive carcinoma or trauma that stimulates local pain endings (Victor and Ropper, 2001).
   c. Pain of **neurogenic** origin arises from some form of heightened sensitivity or overactivity from a lesion that affects the peripheral or central nervous system, apart from stimulation of local pain endings. A wide variety of agents, such as a herniated disc, neuropathies, or central lesions, cause neuropathic pain (Bowsher et al., 1998; Casey, 1991). Neurogenic pain may be mediated through the sympathetic nervous system, nonsympathetically mediated or centrally.
   d. The debilitating types of neurogenic pain, i.e., **neuralgias,** such as *trigeminal neuralgia* and *causalgia,* were described in Section I. In these and similar neurogenic pain syndromes such as erythromelalgia, the sensory examination may be difficult or inconclusive (Layzer, 2001). For such Pts, a simple rating scale provides additional insight into the severity and nature of the pain (Galer and Jensen, 1997).
   e. **Referred pain:** The site at which the Pt feels the pain may not correspond to the site of the lesion (Casey, 1991; Hockaday and Whitty, 1967). Thus, cardiac pain is referred down the left arm. In carpal tunnel syndrome, with median nerve compression at the wrist, the Pt may feel pain proximally in the arm and distally in the distribution of the median nerve.
3. **Anatomy of the pain and temperature pathways from the body and extremities**
   a. **Learn Fig. 10-6 and review Fig. 2-28.**
   b. **Draw and verbally trace a nerve impulse for pain and temperature sensation from the skin on the lateral side of the foot to the cerebral cortex.** Start by enumerating the dermatome.

   ____

   ____

   ______________________________.

The S1 dermatome receptor relays to the peripheral branch of dorsal root axon to the central branch to the secondary neuron in the dorsal horn. The secondary axon crosses and ascends in the spinal lemniscus to the tertiary neuron in the nucleus ventralis posterior of the thalamus. The nucleus ventralis posterior relays to somesthetic cortex in the postcentral gyrus of parietal lobe.

4. The pain and temperature axons from the foot, trunk, and hand synapse on secondary neurons at, or within one or two segments of, their level of entry into the spinal cord, but the axons from the face descend through the brainstem to reach their secondary neuron. Review Figs. 10-2 and 10-6.

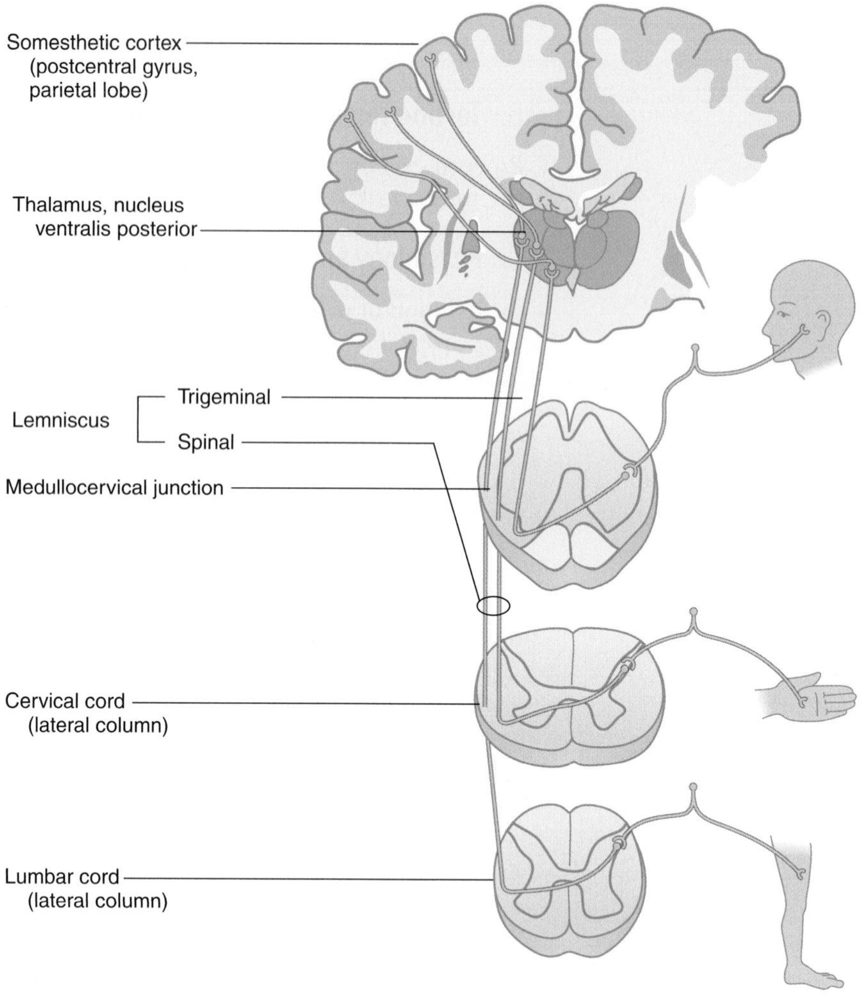

FIGURE 10-6. Pathway for pain and temperature sensation from the periphery to the cerebral cortex. Notice that the sensory axons from the face descend in the descending root of cranial nerve V into the rostral end of the cervical cord.

a. The descent of the axons from the face permits the secondary nucleus that relays pain and temperature sensation to be continuous from the medulla to the last sacral segment. The somatotopic pattern in this continuous long columnar nucleus is *face, neck, arm, trunk, lower extremity,* and *sacral region.* This nucleus, called the **substantia gelatinosa of Rolando,** that relays pain and temperature sensations occupies the tip of the dorsal horn.

b. A surgeon who wanted to abolish only pain and temperature sensation without abolishing touch would make a cut in the ❒ ventrolateral/❒ dorsal column to interrupt the ______________________ tract.

☑ ventrolateral; lateral spinothalamic

c. Neurosurgeons sometimes make such a cut, called a **cordotomy,** in the ventrolateral column of the spinal cord to relieve Pts of intractable pain. Would this cut eliminate touch sensation? ❒ Yes/❒ No. Explain.

____

______________________.

☑ No

Touch impulses reach the thalamus by two pathways, ventral and dorsal columns. Section of only one pathway does not eliminate touch sensation

d. In addition to the foregoing classic spinothalamic pathway (Keele, 1957), a multisynaptic pain pathway ascends from the face, body, and extremities to reach the thalamus and conscious appreciation (Willis and Coggeshall, 1991)

e. Positron emission tomography discloses several cerebral areas that mediate the various affective aspects of pain: the anterior and posterior cingulate and inferior frontal cortices, and periventricular gray matter (Tolle et al., 1999).

D. Testing for pain sensation

1. **Instructions for the Pt:** Show the Pt a straight pin with its sharp and dull ends. Ask the Pt to respond *sharp* or *dull* when you apply the pin. Then have the Pt shut the eyes to prevent visual cues.
2. **Use of the pin:** Alternate touching the Pt with the two ends of the pin randomly to monitor the Pt's attentiveness and reliability. Hold the shaft of the pin lightly between the thumb and the index finger, as if to allow it to slip a little, thus applying the stimulus with the same pressure. Make about three successive pricks for each stimulus because not all individual pricks will hit a pain-sensitive spot. Start with a *normal* area to establish communication, so that the Pt knows what to expect. Test the face and dorsum of the hands and feet. Avoid the horny skin of the palms and soles. Recall the different sensitivities of various skin areas. **Always discard the pin after use.** Never use it again. I don't know how many angels can dance on the point of a pin, but several diseases can: syphilis, infectious hepatitis, and acquired immunodeficiency syndrome, for starters.
3. **Delayed pain and deep pain perception:** If the history and examination suggest a sensory disturbance, proceed as follows to test the extremities, but do not use these tests on the face.
   a. **Testing for delayed pain:** Pinch the dorsum of the Pt's foot briskly between the fingernails of your thumb and index finger. The normal person feels pain almost immediately. A delayed response indicates an abnormality in sensory conduction.
   b. **Testing for deep pain:** Test by squeezing very hard on an Achilles tendon (called **Abadie's sign** when the Pt feels no pain) or a muscle or by compressing very hard over a bony surface. The Pt may feel a delayed pain some seconds after ending the compression. Classic causes of delayed pain or absent deep pain are tabes dorsalis and other diseases that interrupt dorsal roots and dorsal columns.
4. **Location of tender points:** When examining Pts with any acute or chronic pain syndrome, palpate along nerves, muscles, and bony prominences for pain and trigger points. Compress the sites with the ball of the thumb by using firm pressure but short of causing pain in normal persons. Counting the number of tender points assists in the diagnosis of the fibromyalgia syndromes (Goldenberg, 1999).
5. **Pain in neonates and fetuses:** By custom physicians have done procedures such as circumcision on newborn infants without the use of anesthetics, as if the infant felt no pain. Certainly newborns and fetuses show the behaviors associated with pain: crying, agitation, and autonomic responses (Anand et al., 2000). Because infants do react to pain or cold, the Ex can ascertain the sensory level in an infant with a spinal cord transection. Start with the infant quiet. Apply a pin or ice cube to the feet and work up slowly toward the neck. The infant will cry as soon as the stimulus reaches an intact dermatome.
6. **Ancillary methods of investigating pain**
   a. Although available, quantitative or automated methods for testing touch, pain, and temperature are not in routine use (Dyck and Thomas, 1993; Hansson et al., 1991; Meilgaard et al., 1999; Smith et al., 1991; Yarnitsky and Ochoa, 1991). For compression tests to elicit reactions in comatose Pts, see Chapter 12.
   b. Skin biopsies provide an additional method of investigating the integrity of small, unmyelinated nerve fibers (Herrmann et al., 1999; McArthur et al., 1998; Periquet et al., 1999). Sural nerve biopsy likewise aids in categorizing neuropathies (Dyck and Thomas, 1993).
7. Some have remarked that the function of the internist or the surgical consultant is to do the rectal examination (and discover a prostatic carcinoma that has caused the Pt's baffling weight loss and back pain). Physicians habitually neglect the same things, such as the rectal examination, and pain and temperature testing. As a neurologist, my function sometimes is to do the temperature and pain testing that no one else has done, and frequently it pays off.

BIBLIOGRAPHY • Examination of Somatosensory Functions of the Body and Extremities

Anand KJS, Stevens BJ, McGrath PJ. *Pain Neonates,* 2nd ed. *Pain Research and Clinical Management, Vol 10.* New York, Elsevier Science, 2000.

Bateman JE. *Trauma to Nerves in Limbs.* Philadelphia, W.B. Saunders, 1962, p. 79.

Bowsher D, Leijon G, Thuomas K. Central poststroke pain. Correlation of MRI with clinical pain characteristics and sensory abnormalities. *Neurology* 1998;51:1352–1358.

Casey KL, ed. *Pain and Central Nervous System Disease: The Central Pain Syndromes.* New York, Raven, 1991.

DeMyer W. *Neuroanatomy,* 2nd ed. Baltimore, Williams & Wilkins, 1998.

Dyck PJ, Thomas PK, eds. *Peripheral Neuropathy,* 3rd ed. Philadelphia, W.B. Saunders, 1993.

Fisher, CM. Thalamic pure sensory stroke: a pathologic study. *Neurology* 1978;28: 1141–1144.

Galer BS, Jensen MP. Development and preliminary validation of a pain measure specific to neuropathic pain: the neuropathic pain scale. *Neurology* 1997;48:332–338.

Goldenberg D. Fibromyalgia syndrome a decade later. What have we learned? *Arch Intern Med* 1999;159:777–785.

Hansson P, Lindblom U, Lindstrum P. Graded assessment and classification of impaired temperature sensibility in patients with diabetic polyneuropathy. *J Neurol Neurosurg Psychiatry* 1991;54:527.

Herrmann DN, Griffin JW, Hauer P. Epidermal nerve fiber density and sural nerve morphometry in peripheral neuropathies. *Neurology* 1999;53:1634–1640.

Hockaday J, Whitty C. Patterns of referred pain in the normal subject. *Brain* 1967;90: 481–496.

Keele K. *Anatomies of Pain.* Springfield, Charles C Thomas, 1957.

Layzer RB. Hot feet: erythromelalgia and related disorders. *J Child Neurol* 2001;16: 199–202.

McArthur J, Stocks A, Hauer P, et al. Epidermal nerve fiber density. Normative reference range and diagnostic efficiency. *Arch Neurol* 1998;55:1513–1520.

Meilgaard MC, Civille GV, Carr BT. *Sensory Evaluation Techniques,* 3rd ed. Boca Raton, CRC Press, 1999.

Periquet MI, Novak V, Collins MO, et al. Painful sensory neuropathy. Prospective evaluation using skin biopsy. *Neurology* 1999;53:1641–1647.

Perkins BA, Olaleye D, Zinman B, et al. Simple screening tests for peripheral neuropathy in the diabetes clinic. *Diabetes Care* 2001;24:250–256.

Smith SJM, Ali Z, Fowler CJ. Cutaneous thermal thresholds in patients with burning feet. *J Neurol Neurosurg Psychiatry* 1991;4:877–881.

Spreen O, Strauss E. *A Compendium of Neuropsychological Tests.* New York, Oxford University Press, 1991.

Tolle TR, Kaugman T, Siessmeier T, et al. Region-specific encoding of sensory and affective components of pain in the human brain: a positron emission tomography correlation analysis. *Ann Neurol* 1999;45:40–47.

Wall PD, Melzack R, eds. *Textbook of Pain,* 4th ed. Edinburgh, Churchill Livingston, 1999.

Weiner RS, ed. *Pain Management. A Practical Guide for Clinicians.* Boca Raton, CRC Press, 2002.

Willis WD Jr. *The Pain System. The Neural Basis of Nociceptive Transmission in the Mammalian Nervous System. Pain and Headache, Vol 8.* New York, S Karger, 1985.

Willis WD, Coggeshall RE. *Sensory Mechanisms of the Spinal Cord,* 2nd ed. New York, Plenum, 1991.

Yarnitsky D, Ochoa JL. Warm and cold specific somatosensory systems: psychophysical thresholds, reaction times and peripheral conduction velocities. *Brain* 1991;114: 1819–1826.

VI. EXAMINATION TECHNIQUES IN PERIPHERAL NEUROPATHIES

A. Classification of neuropathies

1. Sensory or sensorimotor neuropathies fall into two main types: **diffuse symmetrical polyneuropathies** (Cros, 2001) and **focal neuropathies** or **mononeuritides** (Stewart, 1999). A second major classification consists of **pure sensory, pure motor,** and **combined sensorimotor neuropathies.** The disease may cause an autonomic neuropathy, somatic neuropathy, or combined autonomic-somatic neuropathy.
2. **Diffuse symmetrical polyneuropathies** generally cause sensory disturbances in the distal part of the upper and lower extremities. The Pt has a "stocking and glove" distribution of numbness, tingling, paresthesias, dysesthesias, and pain (Fig. 10-7).

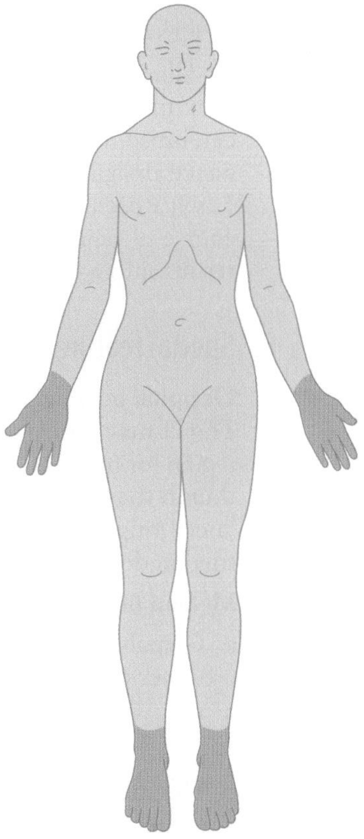

FIGURE 10-7. Areas of sensory loss caused by a diffuse, symmetrical polyneuropathy. The demarcation between affected and unaffected areas fades gradually. Hysterical sensory loss tends to cause sharp margins between the affected and unaffected zones. Compare with Fig. 14-3.

   a. The sensory examination is straightforward. The Ex compares the results of testing pain, temperature, and light touch distally in the extremities with the results of testing proximally. Common causes of polyneuropathies are toxins, drugs, alcoholism, autoimmune disorders, and heredity (Dyck et al., 1996; Victor and Ropper, 2001).
   b. Some symmetrical polyneuropathies cause palpable enlargement of nerve trunks. Inspect and palpate the nerves that cross the posterior triangle of the neck, the ulnar, and the common peroneal nerves. Leprosy also may enlarge peripheral nerves.
   c. Mononeuritis multiplex, such as in diabetes mellitus, may imitate diffuse symmetric neuropathies.

3. **Focal neuropathies or mononeuropathies** generally result from entrapment or mechanical compression (Dawson et al., 1998), but metabolic disorders may predispose to them and may coexist (Stewart, 1999). The entrapment neuropathies often cause extreme pain. The investigation involves a search for trigger factors, often a posture or position, that will elicit or exacerbate the symptoms and for any postures or positions that relieve the discomfort. Compression or percussion over the site of entrapment often will trigger or reproduce the sensory symptoms distal to the entrapment site, a phenomenon called **Tinel's sign** (dysesthesias produced by tapping over the nerve). The phenomenon is equivalent to the pain that radiates down into your little finger when you bang your ulnar nerve at the elbow, called "hitting your crazy bone." Local anesthetic block at the entrapment site abolishes the sensory disturbance and Tinel's sign in the entrapment neuropathies. The text will describe special features of the NE for some of the more common entrapment neuropathies. Granted the importance of corroborative findings on the examination, the diagnosis depends very strongly on the history. Some Pts with entrapment neuropathies by history will not show changes by the clinical or electrophysiologic examination. Most of the entrapment neuropathies respond well to surgical decompression, if conservative therapy fails.
4. Ancillary tests include quantitative sensory testing, EMG and nerve conduction tests, metabolic screening tests, biopsy of sensory nerves or nerve endings in skin, cerebrospinal fluid examination, genetic testing, and sometimes magnetic resonance imaging (MRI) (Dyck et al., 1996; Mendell et al., 2001; Ouvrier et al., 1999; Rosenberg et al., 2001; Andreisek et al., 2006). The Ex can follow the course of neuropathies over long periods by combining clinical and laboratory results into a total neuropathy score (Cornblath et al., 1999).

B. Special features in the examination for entrapment neuropathies

1. **Occipital neuralgia** causes pain radiating from the base of the skull up the occiput. The Pt may notice positions of the head that elicit the pain. Palpate the occipital region for masses, such as lymph nodes. Tap (Tinel's sign) and use the ball of your thumb to compress over the site where the greater occipital nerve exits from the fascial ring, about 2 cm caudolateral to the inion. Local anesthetic block may be tried in doubtful cases.
2. **Median nerve entrapment at the wrist (carpal tunnel syndrome)**
   a. Carpal tunnel syndrome is the most common entrapment neuropathy of the upper extremity.
   b. Review the median nerve motor distribution by the LLOAF/2 mnemonic page 59, and the sensory distribution in Fig. 10-8.
   c. The Pt experiences pain, tingling, and numbness extending from the palmar aspect of the thumb to the radial half of the fourth digit (Rosenbaum and Ohoa, 2002). The symptoms may worsen with the use of the hands, as when driving a car, or may awaken the Pt at night, causing the Pt to pace the floor because of the intense discomfort. The Pt often flaps or flicks the hands to get relief. Women older than 55 years show the peak prevalence. Elevated pressure in the carpal tunnel and resultant ischemia of the median nerve cause the symptoms and signs (Katz and Simmons, 2002).
   d. Inspect the thenar eminence for atrophy. In children with longstanding median nerve lesions, the index finger on the affected side may be smaller (Spinner et al., 1989). Test for loss of strength specifically in the abductor pollicis brevis. The abductor pollicis brevis apparently receives its motor axons exclusively from T1 (Levin, 1999). Thus, testing its strength is one of the few opportunities to test a single motor nerve root. To test it specifically, the Pt must abduct the thumb at an absolute right angle to the plane of the palm. The Ex then matches the Pt's strength with the Ex's own abductor strength (Fig. 10-9).
   e. Test all median nerve sensory modalities in the hand, especially the pad of the index finger. Include two-point discrimination and check for anhidrosis by use

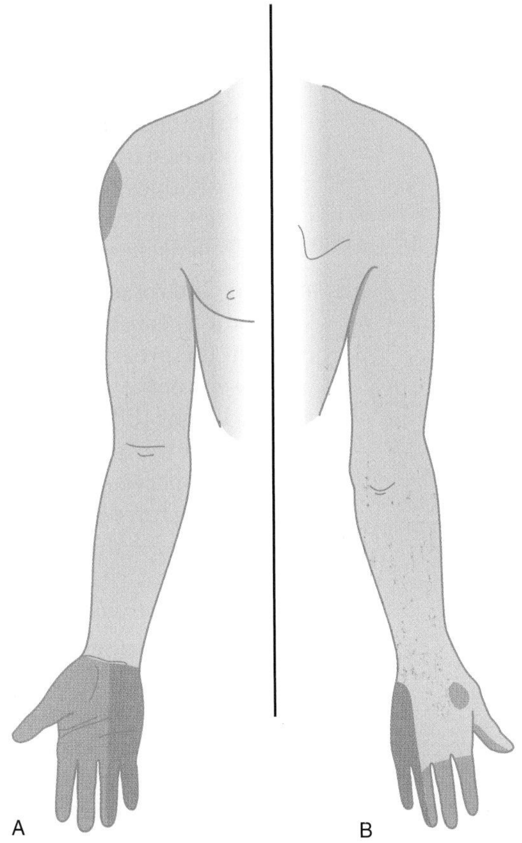

FIGURE 10-8. Sensory distributions of some brachial plexus nerves. (A) Palmar view of the hand: light purple, median nerve; dark purple, ulnar nerve. The light purple over the shoulder indicate the sensory loss after interruption of the axillary (circumflex) nerve (see Fig. 2-11). (B) Dorsal view of the hand: light purple, median nerve; dark purple, ulnar nerve; light purple (near base of thumb), radial nerve.

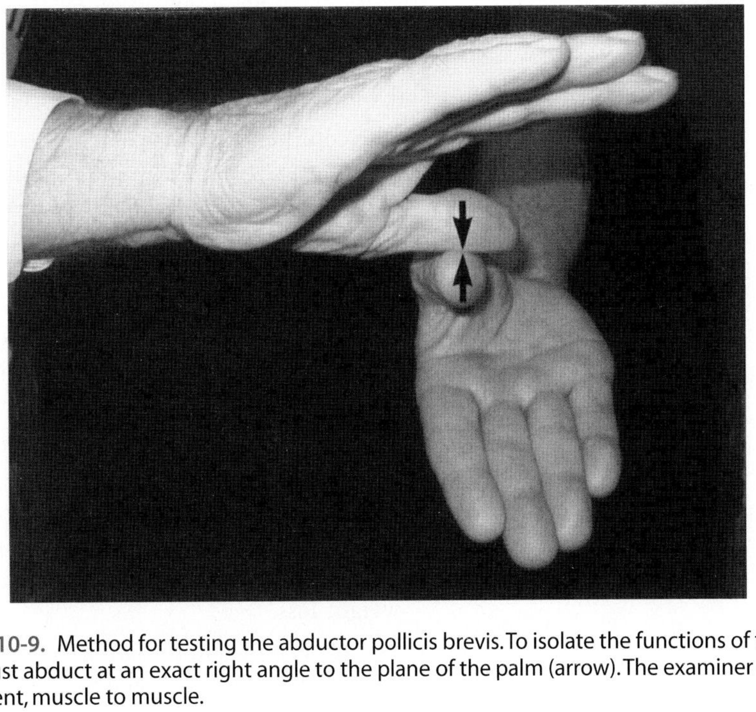

FIGURE 10-9. Method for testing the abductor pollicis brevis. To isolate the functions of the muscle, it must abduct at an exact right angle to the plane of the palm (arrow). The examiner matches the patient, muscle to muscle.

of the ophthalmoscope. **Provocative maneuvers:** Try to elicit *Tinel's sign* by percussing over the median nerve at the wrist (sensitivity ~60%, specificity ~67%) and Phalen's sign by having the Pt flex the hands to a right angle and holding them there for 1 min (sensitivity ~75%, specificity ~47%) by pressing the backs of the hands together (Phalen, 1972).

f. EMG and sensory and motor conduction studies (sensitivity ~85%, specificity ~98%) often prove helpful (Chang et al., 2002), but Pts may experience severe symptoms without diagnostic electrophysiologic changes. False negatives and false positives occur (Padua et al., 1999). MRI, although useful in some Pts, does not replace standard examination techniques (Fleckenstein and Wolfe, 2002; Jablecki et al., 2002; Jarvik et al., 2002).

3. **Anterior interosseus neuropathy(Kiloh-Nevin syndrome):** Anterior interosseus syndrome is caused by entrapment or compression of the anterior interosseus nerve in the proximal part of the forearm (Kiloh & Nevin, 1952). The anterior interosseus nerve, the largest branch of the median nerve, innervates the flexor pollicis longus (FPL), flexor digitorum profundus (FDP) of the index and middle fingers, and the pronator quadratus muscles. Typically patients with anterior interosseus nerve syndrome experience pain in the proximal part of the volar aspect of the forearm and are not able to form an "O" [OK sign] with the thumb and index finger due to involvement of the FPL and radial half of the FDP. A brachial neuritis (Parsonage-Turner syndrome) may mimic the clinical manifestations of an anterior interosseus neuropathy(Parsonage MG et al., 1972).

4. **Ulnar nerve entrapment (the ulnar condyle and cubital tunnel syndromes):** The compression site is at the medial epicondyle of the humerus or the cubital tunnel just distal to the medial epicondyle. The cubital tunnel syndrome is the second most common entrapment neuropathy of the upper extremity. Flexion of the arm may trigger sensation into the little finger (Fig. 10-8). The same diagnostic principles apply as for the median nerve, including matching your *ad* ductor pollicis and your *ab* ductor digiti quinti manus strength directly against the Pt's.

5. **Radial neuropathy:** Wrist drop, the most common presentation of the radial nerve palsy, results from weakness of the extensor carpi radialis longus and extensor carpi ulnaris. It most commonly results from compression of the radial nerve in the spiral groove (Saturday night palsy). Other causes include diabetes, fracture of the humerus, tourniquets, and misplaced injection injuries. Wrist extension weakness may also result from corticospinal lesions.

6. **Lateral femoral cutaneous nerve (meralgia paresthetica):** The Pt experiences sensory disturbances in the anterolateral aspect of the thigh (Fig. 10-10; Williams and Trzil, 1991).

   a. The compression site is where the nerve passes distally under the inguinal ligament. A particular position of the thigh may elicit symptoms. Obesity, pregnancy, diabetes, and a tight belt around the waist, predispose to meralgia paresthetica. Meralgia paresthetica may also develop following surgical procedures (Seror and Seror, 2006)

   b. The nerve is purely sensory. Check for Tinel's sign by percussing and compressing along the lateral third of the inguinal ligament and for symptoms from various positions of the thigh, as in Patrick's sign.

7. **Common peroneal nerve palsy:** The Pt experiences numbness and tingling down the anterolateral aspect of the foot into the dorsum of the foot and has a foot drop (Stewart, 1999). See Fig. 10-10.

   a. The compression site is where the nerve crosses the head of the fibula (Fig. 7-35). Predisposing factors are overt trauma, habitual crossed-kneed sitting posture, lithotomy position, diabetes, knee cast, trauma, and recent weight loss.

   b. Test for loss of skin sensation in a triangular area over the dorsum of the foot (Fig. 10-10) and for weakness of foot and toe dorsiflexion.

8. **Posterior tibial nerve entrapment (tarsal tunnel syndrome):** The Pt feels pain in the lateral aspect of the foot, toes, and sole, particularly when standing or walking, and pain may awaken the Pt at night. The compression site is where the nerve passes under the flexor retinaculum, which runs diagonally anteriorly and upward from the heel (Stewart, 1999).

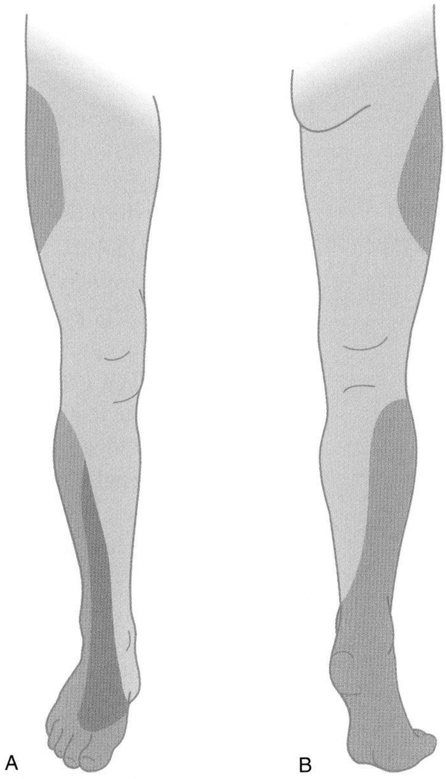

FIGURE 10-10. Distribution of some lumbosacral plexus nerves. (A) Anterior view of the lower extremity: The light purple on the thigh indicate the area of sensory loss caused by interruption of the lateral femoral cutaneous nerve. The light purple below the knee indicate the sensory deficit caused by interruption of the tibial division of the sciatic nerve. The dark purple represents the peroneal division of the sciatic nerve. (B) Posterior view of the leg: The light purple on the thigh represents the distribution of the lateral femoral cutaneous nerve. The light purple below the knee represent the tibial division of the sciatic nerve.

9. **Interdigital nerve entrapment (Morton's metatarsalgia):** The Pt feels pain, numbness, and tingling in the ball of the foot and into toes 3 and 4 or 2 and 3 when walking or wearing shoes that are the least bit tight. The compression site is where the interdigital nerves run along the metatarsal heads, where a neuroma forms. Compression over the neuroma reproduces the sensory symptoms in the toes.

BIBLIOGRAPHY · Examination Techniques in Peripheral Neuropathies

Andreisek G, Crook DW, Burg D, et al. Peripheral neuropathies of the median, radial, and ulnar nerves: MR imaging features. *RadioGraphics* 2006;26:1267–1287.

Chang M-H, Wai S-J, Chiang H-L, et al. Comparison of motor conduction techniques in the diagnosis of carpal tunnel syndrome. *Neurology* 2002;58:1603–1607.

Cornblath DR, Chaudry V, Carter K, et al. Total neuropathy score. Validation and reliability study. *Neurology* 1999;53:1660–1664.

Cros D. Peripheral neuropathy. In Cros D, ed. *A Practical Approach to Diagnosis and Management.* Hagerstown, Lippincott Willliams & Wilkins, 2001.

Dawson DM, Hallett M, Wilbourn AJ. *Entrapment Neuropathies.* Philadelphia, Lippincott-Raven, 2001.

Dyck PJ, Dyck JB, Grant I, et al. Ten steps in characterizing and diagnosing patients with peripheral neuropathy. *Neurology* 1996;47:10–17.

Fleckenstein JL, Wolfe GI. MRI vs EMG. Which has the upper hand in carpal tunnel syndrome. *Neurology* 2002;58:1583–1584.

Jablecki CK, Andray MT, Floeter MK, et al., Practice parameter: electrodiagnostic studies in carpal tunnel syndrome. *Neurology* 2002;58:1589–1592.

Jarvik JG, Yuen E, Hayner DR, et al. MR imaging in a prospective cohort of patients with suspected carpal tunnel syndrome. *Neurology* 2002;58:1597–1602.

Katz JN, Simmons BP. Carpal tunnel syndrome. *N Engl J Med* 2002;346:1807–1812.

Kiloh LG, Nevin S. Isolated neuritis of the anterior interosseus nerve. *Br Med J* 1952;1: 850–851.

Levin KH. Neurologic manifestations of compressive radiculopathy of the first thoracic root. *Neurology* 1999;53:1149–1151.

Mendell JR, Kissel, Cornblath DH. *Diagnosis and Management of Peripheral Nerve Disorders.* New York, Oxford University Press, 2001.

Ouvrier RA, McLeod JG, Pollard JD. *Peripheral Neuropathy in Childhood*, 2nd ed. London, Cambridge University Press, 1999.

Padua L, Padua R, Lo Monaco M, et al. Multiperspective assessment of carpal tunnel syndrome. A multicenter study. *Neurology* 1999;53:1654–1659.

Parsonage MJ, Aldren I, Turner JW. Neuralgic amyotrophy (paralytic brachial neuritis) with special reference to prognosis. Lancet 1957; ii: 209–212Phalen GS. The carpal tunnel syndrome. *Clin Orthop* 1972;83:29–40.

Phalen GS. The carpal tunnel syndrome - clinical evaluation of 598 hands. *Clin Orthop* 1972; (83): 29-40.

Rosenbaum RB, Ochoa JL. *Carpal Tunnel Syndrome and Other Disorders of the Median Nerve*, 2nd ed. Amsterdam, Butterworth-Heinemann, 2002.

Rosenberg NR, Portegeis P, deVisser M, et al. Diagnostic investigation of patients with chronic polyneuropathy: evaluation of clinical guideline. *J Neurol Neurosurg Psychiatry* 2001;71:205–209.

Seror P, Seror R. Meralgia paresthetica: clinical and electrophysiologic diagnosis in 120 cases. Muscle and Nerve. 2006;3395:650–653.

Spinner RJ, Bachman JW, Amadio PC. The many faces of the carpal tunnel syndrome. *Mayo Clin Proc* 1989;64:829–836.

Stewart JD. *Focal Peripheral Neuropathies*, 3rd ed. Baltimore, Lippincott Williams & Wilkins, 1999

Williams PH, Trzil KP. Management of meralgia paresthetica. *Neurosurgery* 1991;74:76–80.

VII. EXAMINATION TECHNIQUES IN LOW BACK PAIN AND PAIN RADIATING DOWN THE LEG: THE SCIATICA SYNDROME

A. The backache syndromes

1. Everyone at one time or another has low back pain, often initiated by a "pop," when lifting or exercising, often recurrent over years or decades. The pain mechanism often remains a mystery, whether muscular, ligamentous, or articular. Despite a thorough workup, the diagnosis often ends up nonspecifically as "lumbosacral strain," if the pain localizes to the back, or "sciatica" if the pain radiates down the leg (Frymoyer, 1988; Rothman and Simeone, 1992; Seimon, 1990).
2. This text focuses on the more specifically neurologic signs of sciatica caused by nerve root compression from a herniated intervertebral disc in the low back.

B. Patient analysis

Off and on for several years, this 34-year-old man has suffered from low back and leg pain. Twelve days ago, when straightening up, he felt a pop in his back. Since then, sharp pain has radiated intermittently into his right foot along its lateral side and into the little toe. Movement or coughing elicits a shock of pain into the leg. He sits rigidly in his chair, with his trunk slightly tilted. When arising, he pushes himself erect with his arms. He stands with most of his weight on his unaffected left leg, holding the knee of the right leg slightly bent. You can confirm the uneven weight distribution by placing your hand around his ankle with your thumb on his Achilles tendon. By squeezing firmly with your thumb, the tendon on the non-weight-bearing leg yields. He stands with his lumbar spine virtually straight, rather than with the normal concavity. Thus simple inspection of how the Pt sits, stands, and walks provides strong objective evidence of the acute back disorder. Palpation of the back discloses paravertebral muscle spasm and mild tenderness. Palpation along the course of the sciatic nerve discloses no tenderness. The triceps surae reflex on the right side is reduced. Plantar flexion is weak on the right, as shown when he tries to rise onto the ball of his right foot, but the action is still too strong for the Ex to overcome by manual opposition. His right calf measures 1.8 cm less than the left. Sensory examination produces uncertain differences between the right and left legs.

C. Localizing the origin of radiating pain

An accurate description of where the pain radiates often identifies the affected nerve or nerve root in a compression syndrome better than the formal examination. Because the Pt has motor and sensory findings, the lesion cannot be limited to one of the small superficial cutaneous nerves of the lateral aspect of the foot. Review Figs. 2-10 and 2-11.

1. If the Pt complains that the pain radiates along the *lateral* side of the foot and into the little toe, you would suspect the involvement of the root to the ___________ dermatome.

S1. Review Figs. 2-10 and 7-29.

2. If the Pt complains of pain radiating toward the *medial* side of the foot or into the great toe, you would suspect the ___________ nerve root.

L5. Review Fig. 2-10, if you erred.

3. What evidence does the history and physical provide that the weakness results from a UMN or lower motoneuron lesion?

____

____

The evidence for a lower motoneuron lesion is weakness confined to one muscle group, atrophy, and a decreased MSR at the ankle (decreased triceps surae reflex). This evidence suggests a lesion confined to the S1 motor root.

4. What would an EMG of the muscles innervated by the S1 nerve root show?

____

Fibrillations, giant motor unit potentials, and possibly fasciculations (Fig. 7-21). In this Pt, the 12-day interval is short for denervation changes to appear, but he has had previous bouts.

5. Notice in Fig. 10-11A that the herniation of a disc at one level (L4 to L5) affects the root of the next level (L5).

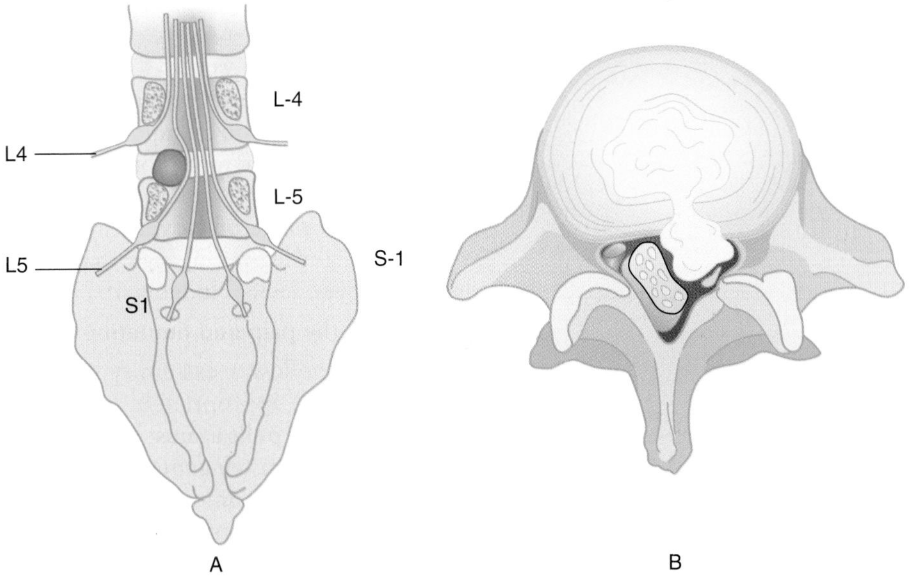

FIGURE 10-11. Intervertebral disc herniation. (A) Dorsal aspect of the lumbosacral spine with the neural arches of the vertebrae and dura mater removed. Nerve roots are labeled on the left, vertebral bodies on the right. Notice how the nerve roots relate to the intervertebral discs and to their point of exit from the vertebral canal. The disc between L4 and L5 has herniated, impinging on nerve root L5. (B) Transverse section of vertebrae L5, as seen from above, showing disc herniation. The dural sac containing the cauda equina remains intact.

D. Leg-raising tests for nerve root compression

Although the foregoing clinical data point to the diagnosis of a nerve root compression syndrome, the leg-raising tests help to confirm it. The tests consist of the **straight-knee** leg-raising test (Lasègue's sign) and the **bent-knee** leg-raising test (Kernig's sign).

1. **Technique of the straight-knee leg-raising test for pain (Laseague's sign)**
   a. The Pt lies supine with the legs relaxed. Grasp the calf or heel of the affected limb and elevate it gently as far as possible, flexing the hip while keeping the knee straight (Fig. 10-12).

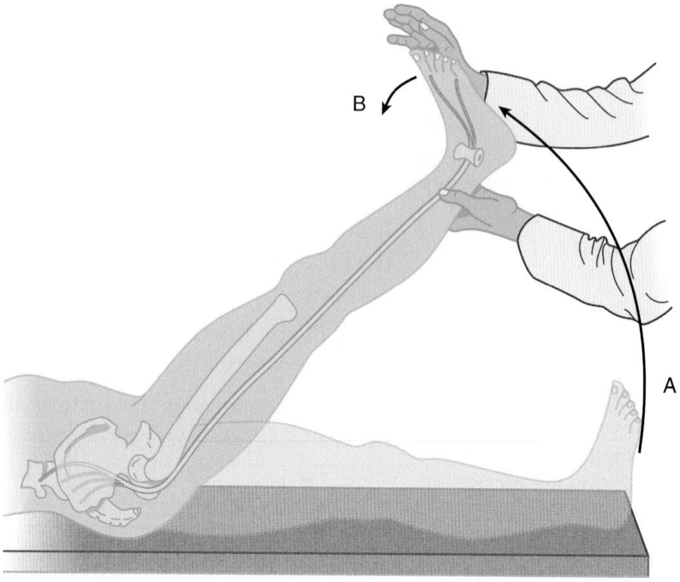

FIGURE 10-12. Straight-knee leg-raising test. (A) The examiner elevates the leg. (B) The examiner then dorsiflexes the foot. Both maneuvers stretch the sciatic nerve and elicit pain if the nerve roots are inflamed, compressed, or imprisoned by a mechanical lesion.

   b. Normally the thigh permits elevation to about 90 degrees. The Pt with nerve root compression winces with pain and flexes the knee at some point less than 90 degrees. Then, if the Ex holds the leg just short of the position of pain, gentle dorsiflexion of the foot produces another twinge of pain, as before, radiating into the foot. The same maneuvers on the unaffected limb may show a nearly normal range of movement without pain or may cause Fajersztajn's crossed, straight leg-raising sign that is nearly pathognomonic of a herniated disc (Frymoyer, 1988; Hudgins, 1977).

2. **Explanation of the pain and limitation of leg elevation**
   a. Elevation of the lower extremity with the knee straight stretches the sciatic nerve. We might appropriately call it the *sciatic nerve stretching test*. As the nerve stretches, it pulls against any impediment to free movement. The resultant pain causes hamstring muscle spasm that arrests farther extension, stretch, and pain. The most common impediment by far is a ruptured intervertebral disc, which impinges on the nerve root (Figs. 10-11A and 10-11B).
   b. Explain what caused the Pt to splint his knee as you reached the end point of excursion in the straight-knee leg-raising test.

   ____

Continued stretch caused nerve root impingement and pain.

   c. When you held the limb just short of maximum permissible elevation, why did dorsiflexion of the foot elicit a twinge of pain?

   ____

Foot dorsiflexion stretched the sciatic nerve more.

   d. We can understand all the postural and movement limitations in this nerve root compression syndrome as protection against pain: the splinting of the back by paravertebral muscle spasm to prevent movement and the limitation of straight leg raising. To test this theory, start with the Pt supine and sit him up, leaving his legs flat against the bed. This action stretches the sciatic nerve. What do you predict that the Pt will do with the affected lower extremity to avoid pain? ____________________.

Flex it

3. **The bent-knee leg-raising test (Kernig's sign):** With the Pt supine as for the straight-knee leg-raising test, keep the knee flexed and flex the limb at the hip. When the thigh reaches the vertical position, gently, *gently* straighten the knee. The Pt will wince with pain, and the reflex hamstring spasm will prevent further straightening of the knee.
4. Xavier et al. (1989) suggested that antidromic activation of peripheral pain receptors, rather than simple mechanical impingement, causes the pain of sciatica.

E. Variations in the sciatica syndrome

1. The typical findings differ in distribution depending on whether the lesion compresses the L5 or S1 root (or both; Table 10-2).

TABLE 10-2 · Differences in Clinical Findings with L_5 and S_1 Nerve Root Compression

Clinical finding	L_5	S_1
Location of back pain and tenderness	Low back pain plus pain in the lateral gluteal region, hip, and posterolateral thigh	Low back pain plus pain in the midgluteal region and posterior thigh
Distribution of radiating pain, paresthesias, dysesthesias, hypalgesia, and hypesthesia	Anterolateral aspect of leg, dorsum of foot and large toe (Fig. 2-10)	Heel extending on the lateral side of sole and foot to the little toe (Fig. 2-10)
Weakness/motor dysfunction	Dorsiflexion of foot and large toe (extensor hallucis longus isan L5 innervated muscle); tendency to stub toe	Plantar flexion, difficulty elevating body weight to stand on ball of foot
Ankle jerk	Present	Reduced or absent
Gait and posture	Antalgic but has more pain when bending back	Antalgic but has more pain when bending forward

2. Within the syndrome of compression of one root, the clinical expression may vary. This Pt may have findings limited to weakness, with little or no pain. In another Pt, pain predominates, with little or no weakness. The next Pt may have well-outlined dermatomal loss on examination, but the next, with equal pain, has no convincing changes on the sensory examination. The findings depend on which motor or sensory axons happen to get compressed. Axons need not be affected equally.
3. In yet another Pt, the pain maximizes in the buttock or hip, imitating hip disease. Such localizations are explained by referral of the pain to sclerotomes and myotomes that come from the L5 and S1 somites. These somites contribute to the pelvic bones, femur, and the associated muscles, and all derivatives retain their innervation from the L5 and S1 roots (Fig. 10-13).
4. Cofactors and comorbidities may confound the diagnosis: anatomic variations in the relation of the nerve roots to the foramina and discs, arthritis, spondylosis, spondylolisthesis, tethered spinal cord or other congenital malformations, diabetes mellitus or other neuropathies, age, occupation, activity level, life style, and secondary gain.

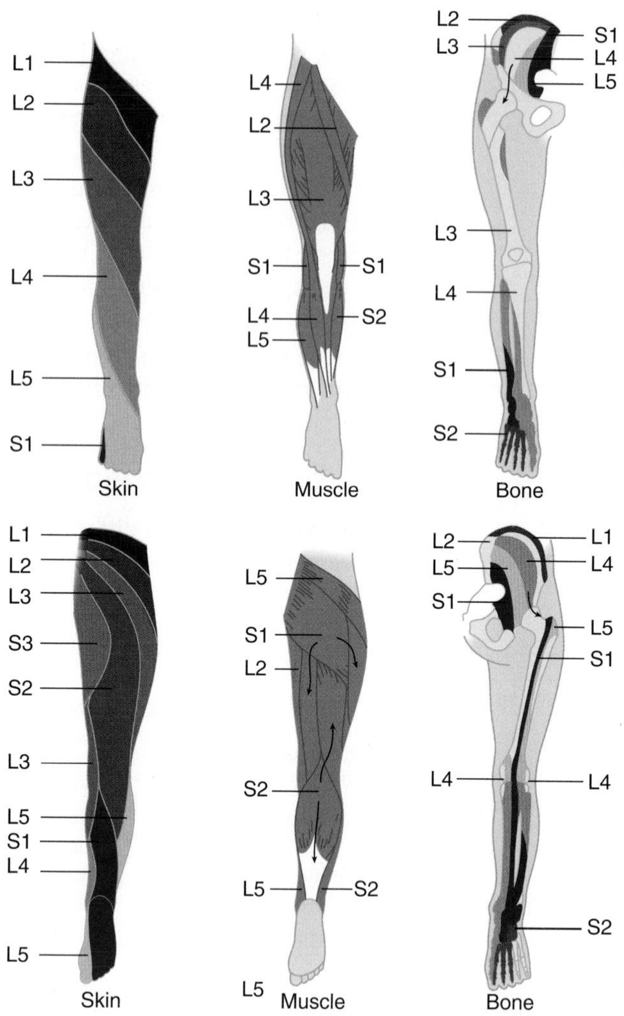

FIGURE 10-13. Distribution of the dermatomes (skin), myotomes (muscles), and sclerotomes (bones) for spinal segments L1 to S3. (Reprinted with permission from Bateman JE. *Trauma to Nerves in Limbs.* Philadelphia, W.B. Saunders, 1962, p. 79.)

F. Summary of the clinical findings in nerve root compression from herniation of an intervertebral disc

1. **Symptoms and signs of disc disease:** motor, sensory, and antalgic posture and gait.
   a. **Motor:** weakness and atrophy in a radicular (myotomal) distribution and reduced triceps surae MSR.
   b. **Sensory:** pain, paresthesias, dysesthesias, numbness in dermatomal distribution. Pain may be local in the back, radicular, referred, or muscle spasm pain.
      i. Pain may be referred to or from viscera. Local radicular and referred pain may coexist.
      ii. Pain may be felt locally in the back, at the level of disc herniation.
      iii. Pain in a radicular (dermatomal sclerotomal/myotomal) distribution (Fig. 10-13).
      iv. Pain over the course of the sciatic nerve (points of Valleix): sciatic notch, retrotrochanteric gutter, posterior surface of thigh, and the head of the fibula.
   c. **Antalgic posture and gait:** pain protective splinting posture, spinal tilt, flattening of the lumbar curve, and a limping gait.
2. **Special features and tests in Pts with suspected disc herniation or radicular compression**

a. Examine the Pt when sitting standing, reclining, and walking.
b. Do the Achilles tendon compression test as an aid in demonstrating less weight-bearing in the affected leg when the Pt stands.
c. Look for sagging gluteal fold in S1 lesions.
d. Compare the circumferences of both legs.
e. Percuss the spine.
f. Palpate for tender points or masses from the costovertebral angle down over lower back, buttock, and along the course of the sciatic nerve.
g. Do the straight-knee leg-raising test, ipsilaterally and contralaterally (Fajersztajn's sign)
h. Test the strength of dorsiflexion and plantar flexion of the foot and the strength of the extensor hallucis longus (L5).
i. Have the Pt bend forward (if possible) as if to touch the floor. The fingertip-to-floor distance should be shorter than 25 cm (Vroomen et al., 2002).

G. Differential diagnosis of low back pain and the sciatica syndrome

1. Disc herniation, lateral or medial: L5 and S1 most frequently.
2. Acute low back strain.
3. Sacroiliac strain: tenderness over the sacroiliac joint pain into the buttocks.
4. Degenerative low back syndrome.
5. Arthritis
6. Myofascial pain, fibromyalgia.
7. Vertebral fractures
8. Spinal Stenosis
9. Spondylolisthesis
10. Facet syndrome
11. Piriformis syndrome
12. Lumbosacral plexus neuritis
13. Coccydynia
14. Osteomyelitis
15. Sacroiliitis
16. Arachnoiditis
17. Carcinoma, pelvic or metastatic
18. Tethered cord or other malformation
19. And, as always, psychosocial factors, pending litigation, secondary gain, etc.

H. Ancillary studies in low back pain and sciatica

1. In view of the numerous causes of low back pain, the sciatic syndrome, and the multiplicity of pain patterns (Jinkins, 1989; Rothman and Simeone, 1992; Seimon, 1990), additional studies may be required to establish the correct diagnosis. These include EMG, somatosensory evoked potentials, plain radiographs, myelography, computed tomography, MRI, and sometimes nuclide scan. None of these is routine and must be judiciously selected, depending on the overall results of a complete history and physical examination (Deen, 1996; Deyo and Weinstein, 2001).
2. Treatment has shifted from bed rest to early mobilization. Manipulative methods of treatment appear to offer no benefit over nonmanipulative methods (Hsieh, 2002).

I. Radicular pain in the neck and arms

1. The causes of local or radiating pain in the neck and shoulders overlap with the causes of low back pain and require a similar workup (McNab and McCulloch, 1994; Nachemson and Jonsson, 2000; Victor and Ropper; 2001).

2. An additional sign to seek with cervical lesions, whether from midline disc herniation, intrinsic neoplasm, or multiple sclerosis, is **Lhermitte's head flexion sign.** Sharp flexion of the head by the Pt causes an electric shocklike sensation of pain or "pins and needles" in the body and extremities. Stretch of the neural tissue at the site of the lesion of the cord apparently causes the sensation. See Fig. 12-23.

BIBLIOGRAPHY · Examination Techniques in Low Back Pain and Pain Radiating Down the Leg: The Sciatica Syndrome

Deen HG. Diagnosis and management of lumbar disk disease. *Mayo Clin Proc* 1996;71: 283–287.

Deyo RA, Weinstein JN. Low back pain. *N Engl J Med* 2001;344:363–370.

Frank AO, DeSouza LH, McAuley JH, et al. A cross sectional survey of the clinical and psychological features of low back pain and consequent work handicap: use of the Quebec Task Force Classification. *Int J Clin Pract* 2000; 54 (10): 639–644 (Medline).

Frymoyer JW. Back pain and sciatica. *N Engl J Med* 1988;318:291–300.

Hsieh CY. Effectiveness of four conservative treatments for subacute low back pain. *Spine* 2002;27:1142–1148.

Hudgins WR. The cross-straight leg raising test. *N Engl J Med* 1977;297:1127.

Jinkins JR. Pathoanatomic basis of pain in lumbar disc extrusion. *MRI Decisions* 1989; Nov/Dec:28–33.

McNab I, McCulloch J. *Neck Ache and Shoulder Pain.* Baltimore, Williams & Wilkins, 1994.

Nachemson AL, Jonsson E. *Neck and Back Pain.* Baltimore, Lippincott Williams & Wilkens, 2000.

Papadopoulos EC, Kahn SN. Piriformis syndrome and low back pain: a new classification and review of the literature. *Orthop Clin North Am* 2004;35(1):65–71.

Rothman RH, Simeone FA. *The Spine,* 3rd ed. Philadelphia, Saunders, 1992.

Seimon LP. *Low Back Pain. Clinical Diagnosis and Management,* 2nd ed. New York, Demos, 1990.

Victor M, Ropper AH. *Adams and Victor's Principles of Neurology.* New York, McGraw-Hill, 2001.

Vrooman PCAJ, de Kron MCTFM, Wilmink JT, et al. Diagnostic value of history and physical examination in patients suspected of lumbosacral nerve root compression. *J Neurol Neurosurg Psychiatry* 2002;72:630–634.

Xavier AV, McDanal J, Kissin J. Mechanism of pain caused by nerve-root tension test in patients with sciatica. *Neurology* 1989;39:601–602.

VIII. EXAMINATION OF THE DORSAL COLUMN, DISCRIMINATIVE OR DEEP MODALITIES: PROPRIOCEPTION, POSITION SENSE, VIBRATION, AND DIRECTION OF MOVEMENT

A. Definition of proprioception

Sherrington's term *proprioception* comes from *proprius* (one's own as in *property,* and *capio* = to *take* or *capture;* literally, to take or capture one's own). The term refers to the capturing, by receptors within the depth of one's own body, of the movements of one's own body parts. The body parts that move consist of one's own muscles and joints, i.e., the skeletomuscular apparatus, and one's vestibular fluid and otoliths. **Formally defined, proprioception is the sense of movement, of position, and of skeletomuscular tension provided by deep mechanical receptors in muscles, joints, connective tissue, and the vestibular system.** Along with vision and touch, it provides a sense of equilibrium or verticality.

We arrived earlier at the notion that the field of reception which extends through the depth of each segment is differentiated from the surface field by two main characters. One of these was that while many agents which act on the body surface are excluded from the deep field as stimuli, an agency which does act there is mass, with all its mechanical consequences, such as weight, mechanical inertia, etc., giving rise to pressures, strains, etc., and that the receptors of this field are adapted for these as stimuli. The other character of the stimulations in this field we held to be that the stimuli are given in much greater measure than in the surface field of reception, by actions of the organism itself, especially by mass movements of its parts .... In many forms of animals, e.g., in vertebrates, there lies in one of the leading segments a receptor-organ (the labyrinth) derived from the extero-ceptive field of the remaining segments. This receptive organ, like those of the proprio-ceptive field, is adapted to mechanical stimuli. It consists of two selective parts, both endowed with low receptive threshold and with refined selective differentiation. One part, the otolith organ, is adapted to react to changes in the incidence and degree of pressure exerted on its nerve-endings by a little weight of higher specific gravity than the fluid otherwise filling the organ. The other part, the semicircular canals, reacts to minute mass movements of fluid contained within it. These two parts constitute the labyrinth .... This system as a whole may be embraced within the one term "proprio-ceptive."

—Charles Sherrington (1859–1952)

B. Neuroanatomy of skeletomuscular proprioception

Compare your answers with Fig. 10-6.

1. Review the pathway through the dorsal columns in Fig. 10-14.

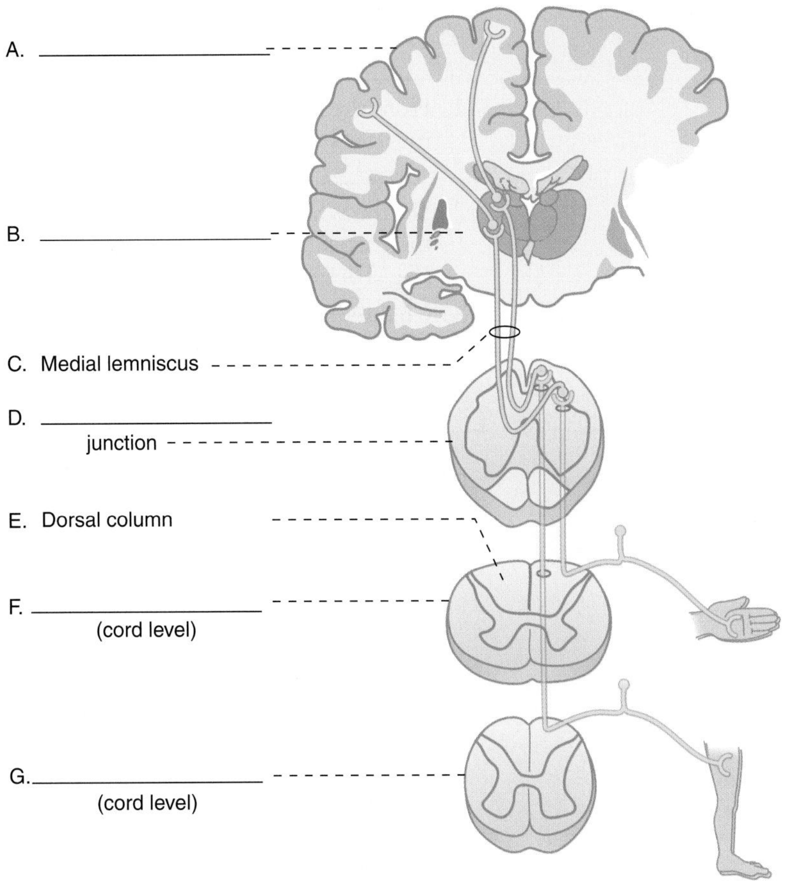

FIGURE 10-14. Pathway for dorsal column modalities from the periphery to the cerebral cortex. Complete labels A to G and compare with Fig. 10-6.

dorsal root ganglia

cochlear (spiral); vestibular

☑ primary

☑ medial to

At the medullocervical junction.

medial lemniscus

ventralis posterior

postcentral; parietal

2. A variety of receptors in the connective tissue of joints and tendons mediates proprioception. The muscle spindles would, a priori, seem ideal to mediate a sense of movement, yet no relevant pathway to the somesthetic cortex is known. The primary skeletomuscular proprioceptive neurons, like all primary somatic sensory neurons, occupy ____________________.
3. CrN VIII has two ganglia that are homologous to dorsal root ganglia, the ____________ ganglion and the ____________ ganglion.
4. The axons ascending in the dorsal columns arise from ❒ primary/❒ secondary/ ❒ tertiary neurons.
5. Figure 10-13 shows that the processes of dorsal root ganglion cells extend from the toe to the dorsal column nuclei, the remarkable distance of 170 cm in man, the astonishing distance of 450 cm in a giraffe, and the incredible distance of 2000 cm in the blue whale.
6. The axons from the foot ascend ❒ lateral to/❒ intermingled with/❒ medial to those from the arm.
7. **Nomenclature note:** Anatomists call the **leg dorsal column** the fasciculus gracilis or column of Goll and the **arm dorsal column** the fasciculus cuneatus or column of Burdach. I prefer the terms *arm dorsal column* and *leg dorsal column* rather than *fasciculus gracilis* and *cuneatus*, which you will forget 2 days after you lay aside the text. The sensory homunculus in the dorsal columns is a headless man sitting with his rump on the dorsal median septum. The head gets added to the homunculus as the trigeminal lemniscus joins the medial lemniscus (DeMyer 1998). Review Fig. 2-12D.
8. At what level of the neuraxis is the secondary neuron of the dorsal column pathway? ____________________.
9. The decussating axons are secondary axons conveying impulses to the thalamus, impulses destined to affect consciousness. In the brainstem they form a tract named the ____________________.
10. The medial lemniscus terminates in a thalamic nucleus called the nucleus ____________.
11. From the nucleus ventralis posterior, the pathway for the dorsal column modalities goes to the somesthetic cortex in the ____________ gyrus of the ____________ lobe.
12. Try the whole thing at once. Wiggle your toe and think through the pathway to the cortex by which you know your toe has wiggled. Can you draw the pathway (Fig. 10-14)?
13. Chapter 9 describes the anatomy of the other component of the proprioceptive system, the vestibular system.

C. The general concept of the dorsal column, discriminative, or deep modalities

1. The dorsal columns mediate many sensations besides position and movement. In general, these sensations depend on receptors deeply placed in the dermis and the connective tissue of the joints, tendons, and muscles. These deep receptors are attuned, as Sherrington said, to mass, inertia, pressure, and movement. Because distance is inherent in the concept of movement, we have the ingredients of classic Newtonian mechanics. The proprioceptive or proprioceptive-related discriminatory sensations mediated by the dorsal columns are
   a. Sense of position or posture
   b. Sense of movement of joints and body (kinesthesia) and of something moving on the skin
   c. Vibration (pallesthesia)
   d. Two-point discrimination
   e. Sense of pressure

   f. Texture
   g. Touch localization (topognosia)
   h. Sense of weight (baresthesia)
   i. Sense of numbers or letters written on the skin (graphesthesia)
   j. Sense of form (stereognosis)

2. The following considerations rationalize the association of these sensations as basically mechanical stimuli:
   a. Vibration is easy to associate with proprioception as mediated by mechanical receptors. Recall that the cochlea, a receptor exquisitely specialized for detecting vibration, developed as the phylogenetic kin of the vestibular apparatus, a receptor exquisitely specialized for detecting the movement of fluids and otoliths. Vibration sense is merely the detection of fast changes in the pressure on and position of a minute portion of tissue, the eardrum being the most specialized example.
   b. The amount of pull on the joint and connective tissue proprioceptors leads to a sense of weight.
   c. To a large extent, discriminative touch, such as texture, depends on minute variations in the pressure on any area of skin. You feel texture best by moving an object across your skin or across your fingernail, causing almost a slow vibration sense. Discrimination of characters written on the skin demands first of all the perception of the path traced by an object pressing on the skin (a sense of movement), followed by comparison of the pattern with memory traces. Touch itself involves some mechanical displacement, i.e., some pressure. Two-point discrimination is the distance between two pressure points. Localization of a touch stimulus depends on comparing the location of a touch stimulus with the mental image of the body parts. It is essentially the problem of distance. In contrast with all these mechanical deformations of skin or joints that cause sensations conveyed by dorsal columns, an object that does not directly touch you, such as the sun 93,000,000 miles away, can burn you and cause pain. Ventrolateral, not dorsal, column pathways mediate these temperature and pain sensations.

D. Technique for testing digital position sense

1. **Instruction to the Pt**
   a. With one hand, support the Pt's hand or foot and ask the Pt to remain completely relaxed. With the other hand, grasp the digit by its side and wiggle it up and down, stopping randomly in one direction or the other. Separate the digit being tested so that you do not touch other digits (Fig. 10-15).

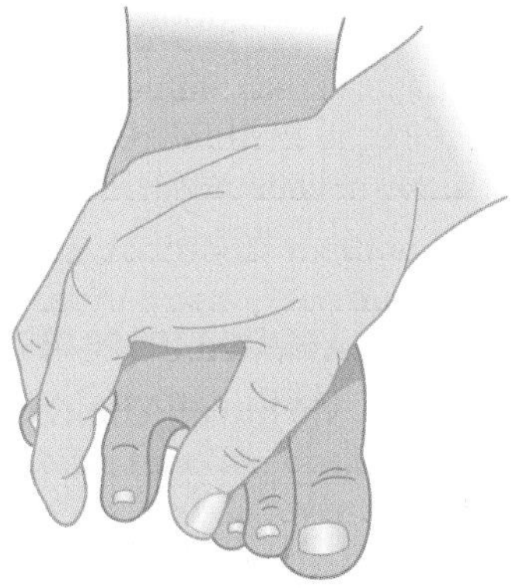

FIGURE 10-15. Method of separating the digits to test position sense in the fourth toe. With his other hand the examiner grasps the toe on the sides and randomly moves it up or down and asks the patient to respond to each new position.

b. While the Pt watches, stop the digit at one position or the other and instruct the Pt to report whether the finger is *up* or *down*. This step communicates what the Ex expects of the Pt. Then, for the actual testing, the Pt closes the eyes. In addition, instruct the Pt *not* to move the digits at all. The digits should remain totally passive. Tell the Pt, "Let me do all of the moving." Test the digits of all four extremities.

c. Take care not to apply different pressures or use a different tone of voice on the up or down movement. The Pt may attend to the wrong stimulus.

2. **Use of the fourth digit in testing position sense**

a. When testing position sense, the novice instinctively grasps the thumb, index finger, or large toe; but using digit 4 presents the greatest challenge to and therefore the best test of position sense. Not infrequently in early central nervous system disease, such as in degenerative diseases of the dorsal columns, you can demonstrate definite loss of position sense in the fourth digit when it is preserved in the other digits. Figure 10-16 shows why.

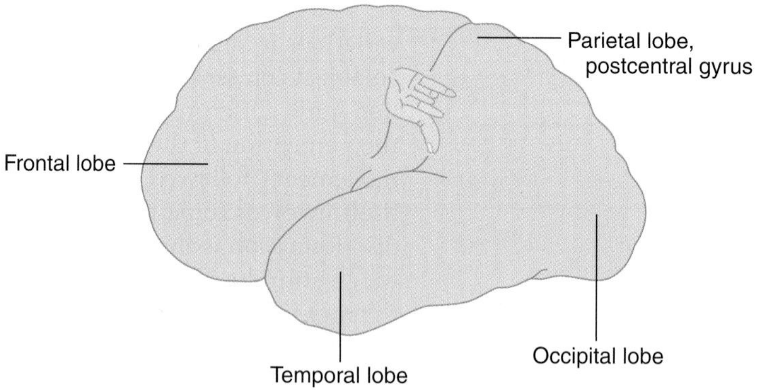

FIGURE 10-16. Lateral view of the left cerebral hemisphere. The right hand is projected onto the left postcentral gyrus to show the relative area devoted to each digit. The face projects to the area immediately inferior to the hand, the trunk, and leg superior, as in the precentral motor cortex (see Fig. 2-2C).

b. The first, second, and fifth digits of the hands and feet have the richest innervation and the largest cortical representation. Therefore, interrupting position sense of these digits requires a relatively large lesion. Practice using digit 4 of the hand and foot (Fig. 10-15).

c. When initial testing suggests loss of position sense, always test several digits several times. After understanding the test, the Pt should reply promptly and make no, *no* errors. Occasionally, the Pt will become bored or carelessly state one direction while meaning the other. A delay in responding means lack of attention or genuine loss of position sense. Immediate repetition and inquiry will disclose whether the error implies carelessness or disease.

3. If position sense is normal distally, it will be normal proximally. If abnormal at the digits, work proximally to test it at the wrist or ankle to establish the severity of the loss.

E. Position sense testing, probability theory, and *yes* or *no* forced-choice sensory tests

1. Patients with defective position sense often give an answer because they know a reply is expected, and they try to please the Ex. The Ex who does not understand probability theory may misinterpret the responses of the Pt with mild or even complete position sense loss or the malingering Pt who deliberately gives wrong answers.

☑ 50%

2. Even with *no* position sense at all, what percentage of the time would the Pt guess the correct direction when a digit is randomly placed up or down? ❒ 0%/❒ 25%/❒ 50%/❒ 75%.

3. The situation exactly duplicates trying to call heads or tails in flipping a coin. The guesser wins 50% of the time on average.

0

4. Next consider impaired but not absent position sense. The Pt responds correctly, sometimes because of chance and sometimes because of correct perception of the position. The novice Ex may erroneously conclude that the Pt is unreliable, because he misses one time and then gives several correct responses. If you are satisfied that the Pt has not simply made a careless error, recall the rule that says the normal person makes _______________% errors.

One method is to give three alternatives, *up, down,* and *straight.* Start by wiggling the finger up and down and then stop *up, down,* or in the *neutral* position; or you can move the digit medially or laterally.

5. The next problem is how to reduce the probability of getting the correct answer by chance. How can you accomplish this?

____

_________________________________.

three

6. By giving three alternatives instead of two, you reduce the chance of guessing the correct answer from one in two to one in _______________.

0 $(1/2)^3$ = one in eight

7. Ordinarily, *two*-alternative testing is easier and faster than *three*-alternative testing and is as reliable. Probability theory sets the minimum number of trials that should be made in a *two*-alternative testing of position sense. As in flipping a coin, you will expect to call heads or tails correctly about one-half the time; the mathematical notation is $(1/2)^1$. When you try to call the coin twice in a row, the probability of being right is $(1/2)^2$, or one in four. The probability of calling three in a row would be $(1/2)^3$, or one in _______________.

☑ doubles

8. Each time you try to stretch your luck one more time, the denominator ❒ halves/❒ doubles/❒ triples/❒ quadruples. Soon the odds against chance are very great.

five trials: $(1/2)^5 = 1/32$, which is less than the needed 1/20 and therefore makes chance unlikely.

9. In testing position sense, the problem is where to cut off the trials to have confidence that the Pt has not succeeded by chance alone, when in fact the Pt has no position sense. Statisticians agree that when the probability of an event is 1 in 20 or less, chance is an unlikely explanation. Thus, in testing position sense, where chance has a 50% success rate, the smallest number of trials the Pt must get right to make chance success unlikely is _______________.

50

10. Some mental Pts reply exactly the opposite to each up or down position, ipso facto proving intact position sense. Even with no position sense, a Pt just guessing gets _______________% right by chance.

11. **Final admonition:** In previous sensory tests, we implicitly relied on statistical concepts. If we offer coffee as a smell stimulus to anosmic Pts, some will reply because they expect to smell something. The question then becomes, How many Pts with anosmia will report coffee when they smell nothing? Because the probability of reporting coffee is less than 1 in 20, chance is an unlikely explanation for a correct answer. The same consideration holds for taste. In testing pain, we have to consider probability and the fact that some pinpricks do not stimulate pain endings. Hence, the Pt may report no pain on a particular prick, even though you stuck him. Moreover, pain thresholds differ considerably from Pt to Pt and from age to age. These facts lead to a general observation: as a teacher I find that medical students and residents often report that the history or the sensory examination "was unreliable." What that generally means is that the student failed to communicate adequately with the Pt to derive the historical information or produce the test results that the Pt was actually capable of. Usually such a Pt has a different culture, diction, syntax, and dialect than the student. Nothing tests the skill of the Ex more than the sensory examination. Make a successful sensory examination a matter of personal pride. By practicing sensory testing on yourself and many other subjects, you will appreciate the variables and avoid coming to erroneous conclusions about the Pt's reliability.

F. Clinical testing of position sense by the swaying (Romberg) test

1. **Technique and instructions to the Pt:** Ask the Pt to stand with the feet together. Note whether the Pt sways. Then ask the Pt to close the eyes, and note whether the swaying increases. Stand behind the Pt with arms held up ready to catch the Pt, but do not touch the Pt.
2. **Results of Romberg swaying test**
   a. *Normal subjects* will sway minimally with the eyes closed but not fall. Stand up and try this test yourself. Stand on both feet and then on one foot.
   b. Patients with acute **unilateral vestibular disease** tend to sway to the side of the lesion, but the nervous system compensates in chronic vestibulocerebellar disease, unilateral or bilateral (Lanska and Goetz, 2000). Many Pts with vestibular disease perform well on the Romberg test (Hotson and Baloh, 1998).
   c. Patients with **dorsal column lesions,** such as tabes dorsalis, sway much more with eyes closed and may fall unless supported. They do not compensate with time. Patients with severe sensory polyneuropathies also sway more with eyes closed. Swaying is never the sole sign of peripheral nerve or dorsal column lesions. It provides an auxiliary test for pathways tested more directly and specifically by digital position sense, vibration, directional scratch test, and stereognosis.
   d. Patients with **hysteria** cause the most difficulty in interpreting the swaying test. Hysterical Pts often gyrate wildly but usually do not fall, thus proving that they have intact balance.
      i. The Ex often can divert the hysterical Pt into performing well on the swaying test. At some time later in the examination, have the Pt stand with the feet together, arms straight out in front, and eyes open. Ask the Pt to continue alternately touching his nose with his right and left index fingers. While the Pt concentrates on repeating the finger-to-nose action, ask the Pt to close the eyes. Usually the Pt, now engrossed in the finger-to-nose task, will automatically maintain the posture without swaying.
      ii. Hysteria never manifests solely by a positive swaying test. It is only one shadow in a pattern of psychiatric findings.
3. **Interpreting the Romberg swaying test**
   a. Students often mistakenly consider the swaying test as a test of cerebellar function, but the cerebellum does not depend on vision to do its job of coordinating. An analysis of the three operations of the test will explain how to interpret it.
      i. *Operation 1* requires the Pt to stand with the feet together, thus narrowing the base and increasing the stress on balance.
      ii. *Operation 2* requires the Pt to close the eyes, thus removing visual clues for balance.
      iii. *Operation 3* requires the Ex to judge whether the Pt sways more with eyes open or eyes closed.
   b. Hence, we compare the degree of swaying when the Pt stands with heels together and eyes open with the degree of swaying with the eyes closed. This is an ❐ operational/❐ interpretational definition.

      ☑ operational
   c. We interpret the test as showing that the removal of vision places the burden of afferent information for balance on the dorsal column proprioceptive system. We believe this because loss of dorsal column modalities, as in tabes dorsalis, causes the most severe swaying with eyes closed. Normally, a distributed sensorimotor complex, consisting of the proprioceptive system (including the vestibular apparatus, dorsal columns, and cerebellum), visual system, thalamus, basal ganglia, pyramidal tracts, and parietal lobes, maintains the standing posture and verticality.
   d. Why do you ask the Pt to close the eyes for the swaying test? ____.

      To deprive the Pt of visual cues for balance and to place the afferent responsibility on the dorsal column proprioceptive system tandem walking

e. Which part of the gait examination uses the principle of narrowing the base, thus increasing the stress on balance? ________________________.

G. Cerebellar versus sensory dystaxia

1. Earlier we stated that the cerebellum could coordinate muscular contractions only if it received the proper proprioceptive information. Loss of proprioceptive afferents via dorsal roots and dorsal columns results in sensory dystaxia that has to be distinguished from cerebellar dystaxia.
2. In theory, we might expect dystaxia from lesions of the corticopontine pathways. In practice, ataxia from corticopontine pathway lesions is unusual, although a controversial form of ataxic hemiplegia has been advocated and questioned (Landau, 1988).
3. Romberg's test shows that vision can substitute for proprioception. Hence, in distinguishing sensory from cerebellar dystaxia, have the Pt perform with eyes open and then closed. Which type of dystaxia, sensory or cerebellar, would distinctly worsen with the Pt's eyes closed? ❒ sensory/❒ cerebellar. Explain.

____

____.

☑ sensory
Because visual guidance substitutes for proprioceptive guidance, eye closure increases sensory dystaxia much more than cerebellar.

4. The differentiation of cerebellar from sensory dystaxia comes from the pattern of cerebellar signs and the pattern of sensory and reflex findings. Complete Table 10-3.

TABLE 10-3 · Differentiation of Sensory and Cerebellar Dystaxia*

Clinical finding	Sensory dystaxia	Cerebellar dystaxia
Loss of vibration and position sense		
Areflexia		
Nystagmus		
Hypotonia		
Dystaxia much worse with eyes closed		
Overshooting on release		

*Place a plus sign in the appropriate column or columns.

Sensory	Cerebellar
+	
+	
	+
+	+
+	
	+

H. Testing for loss of vibration sense (pallanesthesia)

1. **Preparation of the Pt:** As usual, start with the Pt's eyes open and show the Pt what you will do, but do the test with the Pt's eyes closed.
2. **Test procedure:** Hold a tuning fork (128 or 256 cps) by the round shaft and strike the tines a crisp blow against the ulnar side of your palm to set the fork vibrating. Apply the free end of the shaft to the Pt's fingernails and toenails or just proximal to the nail bed. If you press upward with the index finger pad of your free hand against the Pt's finger pad, you can feel the fork nearly as long as the Pt can.
3. **Inquire:** "Do you feel the buzz?" If the Pt fails to feel vibration at the nails for as long as you can, apply the fork to proximal bony prominences: ulnar styloid process or distal radius and internal malleolus or shin.
4. **Reliability monitoring in testing for pallanesthesia**
   a. How would you monitor the Pt's attentiveness and reliability in this test?

   ____

   ____.

   Sometimes apply the tuning fork when it is not vibrating.

   b. To monitor reliability, strike the tines to set them vibrating. Although the Pt's eyes are closed, the Pt hears the strike and expects to feel vibration; instead, squeeze the vibrating tines immediately *after* striking the fork, stopping its vibration before applying the fork to the Pt. Strike your fork and squeeze its ends to familiarize yourself with the action. Thus, sometimes when you apply the fork, it is vibrating but not at other times.

5. **Interpretation of vibration testing**
    a. Aging increases the threshold to vibration and reduces the sensitivity. Normally the hands feel vibration better than the feet at all ages (Calne and Pallis, 1966; Martina et al., 1998).
    b. At spinal levels, dorsal column pathways mediate vibration, but some evidence suggests that the pathway may also travel in the dorsal part of the lateral columns (Willis and Coggeshall, 1991). Interruption of the pathway from the peripheral receptors up through the thalamus reduces vibratory perception. Suprathalamic lesions more or less spare vibration (Roland and Nielsen, 1980).
    c. Of the quantitative tests of vibration, the Reidel-Seiffer tuning fork is the most practical for routine use (Dimitrakoudis and Bril, 2002; Martina et al., 1998; Merkies et al., 2000).

I. Alternative efficient tests for dorsal column dysfunction

1. **Directional scratch test**
    a. Draw two transverse lines 2 cm apart across the distal shin and the dorsum of the hand.
    b. Using your finger tip, the tip of a tongue blade broken longitudinally, or the butt of the tuning fork, make a 2-cm-long stroke between the two lines, randomly alternating between a proximal (up) and distal (down) direction.
    c. Ask the Pt to state whether the object moved *up* or *down*. Start with two practice trials with the Pt's eyes open to establish communication. Then, with the Pt's eyes closed, make 10 trials in random *up* or *down* directions. The normal person gets all 10 correct. If the Pt errs, increase the distance to 5 cm and then to 10 cm to get a quantitative estimate of the deficit. Hankey and Edis (1989) claimed this test is superior to the standard tests of position and vibration, and that it correlates well with abnormal evoked responses (Motoi et al., 1992).
2. **Two-point discrimination**
    a. **Test items:** Use a calipers or a device called a Disccriminator. A paper clip bent to free the ends substitutes for a formal device.
    b. **Technique:** Start with the device wider than the expected distance to establish communication and gain the Pt's cooperation. Randomly alternate touching one or two points of the calipers. The Ex may use the static method in which the two points remain in place or the moving test in which the calipers are moved a slight distance.
    c. The Pt should discriminate two points at a distance: 2 to 4 mm on the fingertips, 4 to 6 mm on the dorsum of the fingers, 8 to 12 mm on the palm, and 20 to 30 mm on the dorsum of the hand (Meilgaard et al., 1999; Richards et al., 1998). Children older than 7 years can respond reliably (Cope and Anthony, 1992). Two-point discrimination decreases somewhat with aging, but is equal between the sexes.
    d. Peripheral nerve, central pathway, and parietal lobe lesions impair two-point discrimination. Although an excellent test (Krumlinde-Sundholm and Eliasson, 2002), it takes too much time for the screening NE.
3. **Stereognosis:** *stereo* = form, *gnosis* = knowing. Test form knowing by presenting objects of different shapes for recognition: a square or rectangular block, pyramid, cone, or marble. See the distinction between stereognosis and tactile agnosia in Section IX.

J. Review of somatosensory pathways

1. Practice testing yourself and a companion with a cotton wisp, a pin, and a tuning fork for temperature (Fig. 10-4) and vibration sense and then do the directional scratch test and test position sense. As you test each modality, "think through" the pathway to the cerebral cortex. You must, in particular, review the location

of the secondary neuron and the level of the decussation. To prove that you can "think through" these pathways, draw them (Figs. 10-6 and 10-14).

2. Cortical lesions may somewhat impair the simple modalities of touch, pain, and temperature sensation but less than infracortical lesions of the pathways (Adams and Burke, 1989). Some appreciation of these modalities may occur at thalamic or infracortical levels. Unilateral suprathalamic lesions do not increase the vibration threshold (Roland and Nielsen, 1980).

BIBLIOGRAPHY · Examination of the Dorsal Column or Deep Modalities

Adams RW, Burke D. Deficits of thermal sensation in patients with unilateral cerebral lesions. *Electroencephalogr Clin Neurophysiol* 1989;73:443–452.

Calne D, Pallis C. Vibratory sense: a critical review. *Brain* 1966;89:723–746.

Cope EB, Anthony JH. Normal values for the two-point test. *Pediatr Neurol* 1992;8: 251–254.

Dimitrakoudis D, Bril V. Comparison of sensory testing on different toe surfaces: implications for screening. *Neurology* 2002;59:611–613.

Hankey GJ, Edis RH. The utility of testing tactile perception of direction of scratch as a sensitive clinical sign of posterior column dysfunction in spinal cord disorders. *J Neurol Neurosurg Psychiatry* 1989;52:395–402.

Hotson JF, Baloh RW. Acute vestibular syndrome. *N Engl J Med* 1998;339:680–685.

Krumlinde-Sundholm L, Eliasson A. Comparing tests of tactile sensibility: aspects relevant to testing children with spastic hemiplegia. *Dev Med Child Neurol* 2002;44: 604–612.

Landau W. Neuromythology, part III: ataxic hemiparesis: special deluxe stroke or standard brand? *Neurology* 1988;38:1799–1801.

Lanska DJ, Goetz CG. Romberg's sign. Development, adoption, and adaptation in the 19th century. *Neurology* 2000;55:1201–1206.

Martina ISJ, van Konigsveld R, Schmitz PIM, et al. Measuring vibration threshold with a graduated tuning fork in normal aging and in patients with polyneuropathy. *J Neurol Neurosurg Psychiatry* 1998;65:743–747.

Meilgaard MC, Civille GC, Carr T. *Sensory Evaluation Techniques,* 3rd ed. Boca Raton, CRC Press, 1999.

Merkies ISJ, Schmitz PIM, van der MechÈ FGA, et al. Reliability and responsiveness of a graduated tuning fork in immune mediated polyneuropathies. *J Neurol Neurosurg Psychiatry* 2000;68:669–671.

Motoi M, Matsumoto H, Kaneshige Y, Chiba S. A reappraisal of "direction of scratch" test: using somatosensory evoked potentials and vibration perception. *J Neurol Neurosurg Psychiatry* 1992;55:509–510.

Richards PM, Persinger MS, Michel RN. Ontogeny of two-point discrimination for fingers and toes in children (ages 7–15). *Percept Motor Skills* 1998;86:1259–1262.

Roland PE, Nielsen VK. Vibratory thresholds in the hands. *Arch Neurol* 1980;37:775–779.

Sherrington C. *The Integrative Action of the Nervous System*. Reprint. New Haven, Yale University Press, 1952.

Willis WD, Coggeshall RE. *Sensory Mechanisms of the Spinal Cord,* 2nd ed. New York, Plenum, 1991.

IX. EXAMINATION FOR ASTEREOGNOSIS AND TACTILE AGNOSIA

A. The concept of agnosia

1. We can regard sensations as requiring two stages of cortical activity. The first stage occurs in the primary cortical receptive areas as they register the sensory impulses that shuttle in from the thalamic relay nuclei. For the next stage, the brain has to elaborate the meaning or significance of the cascade of sensory impulses. The brain matches these impulses with stored memories and integrates them into the

value system of the individual to adjudicate their significance and to know whether to act on them or ignore them. For example, to recognize a dime placed in your hand in the dark, you have to recognize its distinct form, its weight, its size and texture, its metallic nature, and its symbolic significance as money.

2. The parietal lobe mediates these subsequent, discriminative aspects of somatic sensations, such functions as stereognosis, graphesthesia, two-point discrimination, and position sense (Bassetti et al., 1993): The part of the parietal lobe adjacent to the primary sensory cortex of the post-central gyrus acts as the association area for "knowing" the symbolic significance or meaning of sensations. The association areas for sight and sound occupy the zones adjacent to their primary sensory receptive areas in the occipital and temporal lobes. These zones meet and become confluent at the parieto-occipito-temporal junction, a region called the **posterior parasylvian area.** The anterior part of this area also integrates vestibular sensation with the other senses. See Fig. 10-17.

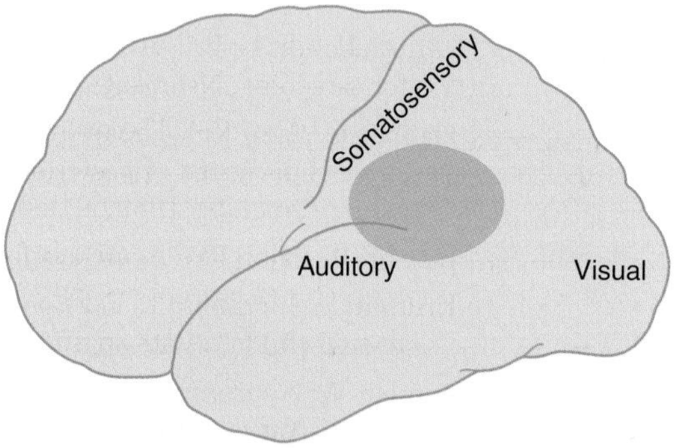

FIGURE 10-17. Lateral view of the left cerebral hemisphere. The dots indicate the posterior parasylvian area. Notice the bordering somatosensory, auditory, and visual receptive areas.

B. The gnosias, the nomenclature of knowing

1. Clinicians have devised a sensory nomenclature based on the theory that the ultimate meaning of afferent stimuli depends on an association cortex (Critchley, 1966). The sensations that require a high degree of cortical integration, i.e., that require a great deal of knowing, we call **gnosias.** The terms *knowledge* and *gnosia* are etymologically related: *diagnosis* literally means *through* or *thorough* knowing (*dia* = through as in *dia* r-rhea; *gnosis* = know). *Prognosis* means knowing beforehand (*pro* = before; *gnosis* = knowing).

2. The three-dimensional sense of form is called stereo ________________.

gnosis

3. Sense of localization of a skin stimulus is topo________________.

gnosia (*topo* = place)

4. The *graphic* sense of numbers or letters written on the skin is ________________.

graphognosia

5. Sense of awareness of a bodily defect is named by using the root *nosos* for disease. Hence, *nosology* is the science of disease classification, and the sense of awareness of disease is ________________.

nosognosia

6. Give the medical meanings of these roots:

a. *Stereo-* means ________________.

b. *Topo-* means ________________.

c. *Grapho-* means ________________.

d. *Noso-* means ________________.

form (three-dimensional)
place
writing
disease

C. The agnosias, the terms for not knowing

1. The negating prefix to designate lack of or absence of is __________ before a vowel or __________ before a consonant. Hence, *agnosia* literally means ________________.

an; a; not knowing

2. To designate a *gnostic* defect secondary to a lesion in the association cortex or its circuitry, we negate the term for the normal sensation:
   a. Loss of form sense is called ________________ognosis.
   b. Loss of cutaneous localization is called ________________ognosia.
   c. Loss of graphic sense is called ________________ognosia.
   d. Loss of disease awareness is called ________________ognosia.

astere

atop

agraph

anos

D. Is the lesion in the sensory pathway or the association circuit

1. Lesions may interfere with the knowing of sensory stimuli in two ways: by interrupting the sensory pathways from receptor to primary sensory cortex or by interrupting the association cortex or its circuits with the thalamus and hippocampal formation.
   a. If the lesion destroys the receptor, the sensory pathway through nerve or neuraxis, or the primary receptive cortex, the impulses cannot reach the association cortex for interpretation. The Pt does not know because the association cortex does not receive sensory information. We return to one of Müller's laws: all we know of the external world is a change of state in the impulses in one of our afferent pathways (see page 349).
   b. If the lesion destroys the association cortex or its circuits with the thalamus or hippocampal formation, the Pt does not know because of inability to appreciate the significance or meaning of the impulses that reach the primary cortex.
2. After transection of a peripheral nerve or the spinal cord, the complete loss of sensation is called *anesthesia*. If sensation is merely reduced, it is called __________esthesia.

hypesthesia

3. Similarly, complete lack of pain sensation is called __________algesia, reduced pain sensation is called __________algesia, and excessive pain sensation is called __________algesia.

analgesia; hypalgesia; hyperalgesia

4. Loss of sense of form because of interruption of the pathway between the receptor and the primary sensory cortex is called *stereoanesthesia*. Loss of sense of form because of a lesion of the association cortex is called __________.

astereognosis

5. Loss of hearing because of interruption of CrN VIII is ❒ deafness/❒ auditory agnosia.

❒ deafness

6. What would *auditory agnosia* mean?
   ____
   ____

Inability to understand the meaning of words or sounds because of a defect in the auditory association cortex.

7. If a lesion in the optic pathways or calcarine cortex causes hemianopsia, the Pt has ❒ blindness/❒ visual agnosia in that field of vision.

☑ blindness

8. Explain why we say the Pt in frame 7 is blind, rather than having visual agnosia.
   ____
   ____
   ____

Because the lesion affects the optic pathway or calcarine cortex, not the association cortex, the primary impulses for vision cannot get to the visual association cortex for interpretation. It is improper to diagnose agnosia, if impulses fail to reach the association cortex.

E. Testing for astereognosis and tactile object agnosia

1. **Definition**
   a. *Stereognosis* as commonly used means object recognition through touch. Some tests also use vision.
   b. **Distinction between stereognosis and tactile agnosia:** Caselli (1991) separated tactile gnosia, or full recognition of objects placed in the hand, from simple form perception, such as distinguishing a cone from a pyramid, which he called *stereognosis.* Although lesions of the postcentral gyrus of the parietal lobe may cause astereognosis and tactile object agnosia (Takeda et al., 2000), functional MRI studies show that the cerebral circuitry for tactile object recognition

involves not only the parietal lobe but also the visual association cortex and, surprisingly, the frontal polar cortex (Deibert et al., 1999).

2. **Technique to test for astereognosis and tactile agnosia**
   a. **Test items:** Use a series of common objects known to the Pt, such as keys, safety pins, paper clips, buttons, and coins, such as a penny, dime, nickel, and quarter. The penny and dime are especially hard to distinguish, and the normal person may miss occasionally.
   b. With the Pt's eyes closed, place various common objects that the Pt has not seen in the Pt's hand. Test each hand separately. Instruct the Pt to feel the object and identify it.
   c. Lack of dexterity, as with the spastic or paralyzed hand, reduces the Pt's ability to recognize objects (Krumlinde-Sundholm and Eliasson, 2002). If the Pt's hand is paralyzed, the Ex may move the item over the fingers to substitute for the Pt's active finger movement.

☑ left

3. If you place the object in the Pt's right hand, you are testing the ❒ left/❒ right parietal lobe.

stereoanesthesia

4. If the Pt has lost the sense of form because of a lesion in the periphery, spinal cord, brainstem, or thalamus, the term *astereognosis* is incorrect. The correct term is stereo____________.

☑ association circuitry

5. The term *agnosia* correctly applies only if the lesion is in the ❒ nerve/❒ spinal cord/❒ brainstem/❒ thalamus/❒ association circuitry.

BIBLIOGRAPHY · Examination for Astereognosis and Tactile Agnosia

Bassetti C, Bogousslavsky J, Regli F. Sensory syndromes in parietal stroke. *Neurology* 1993;43:1942–1949.

Caselli RJ. Rediscovering tactile agnosia. *Mayo Clin Proc* 1991;66:129–142.

Critchley M. *The Parietal Lobes.* New York, Hafner Publishing, 1966.

Deibert E, Kraut M, Kremen S, et al. Neural pathways in tactile object recognition. *Neurology* 1999;52:1413–1417.

Krumlinde-Sundholm L, Eliasson A. Comparing tests of tactile sensibility: aspects relevant to testing children with spastic hemiplegia. *Dev Med Child Neurol* 2002;44:604–612.

Takeda K, Shozawa Y, Sonoo M, et al. The rostrocaudal gradient for somatosensory perception in the human postcentral gyrus. *J Neurol Neurosurg Psychiatry* 2000;69:692–693.

X. REVIEW OF SOMATOSENSORY DISTRIBUTIONS

A. Figure 10-18 summarizes distributions of sensory symptoms

B. Note: This section distinguishes tongue-tip neuroanatomy that you need to be able to recite as you analyze the patient and fingertip neuroanatomy that you look up as needed

1. **Dermatomal distributions:** Review Fig. 2-10 and recite the mnemonic for remembering dermatomal distributions. Start with the "hooded cape" and end with **L5** and **S1** and the **coccygeal bull's eye.**
2. **Peripheral nerve distributions:** Review Fig. 2-11.

a. For focal or mononeuropathies, recall the trigeminal, ulnar/median (Fig. 10-9), lateral femoral cutaneous (Fig. 1-10), and common peroneal distributions and then use Fig. 2-11 to look up the other nerves. Distinguishing symptoms of some dermatomal and some peripheral nerve distributions is often difficult.

b. For symmetrical polyneuropathies, recall the "stocking and glove" distribution (Fig. 10-7).

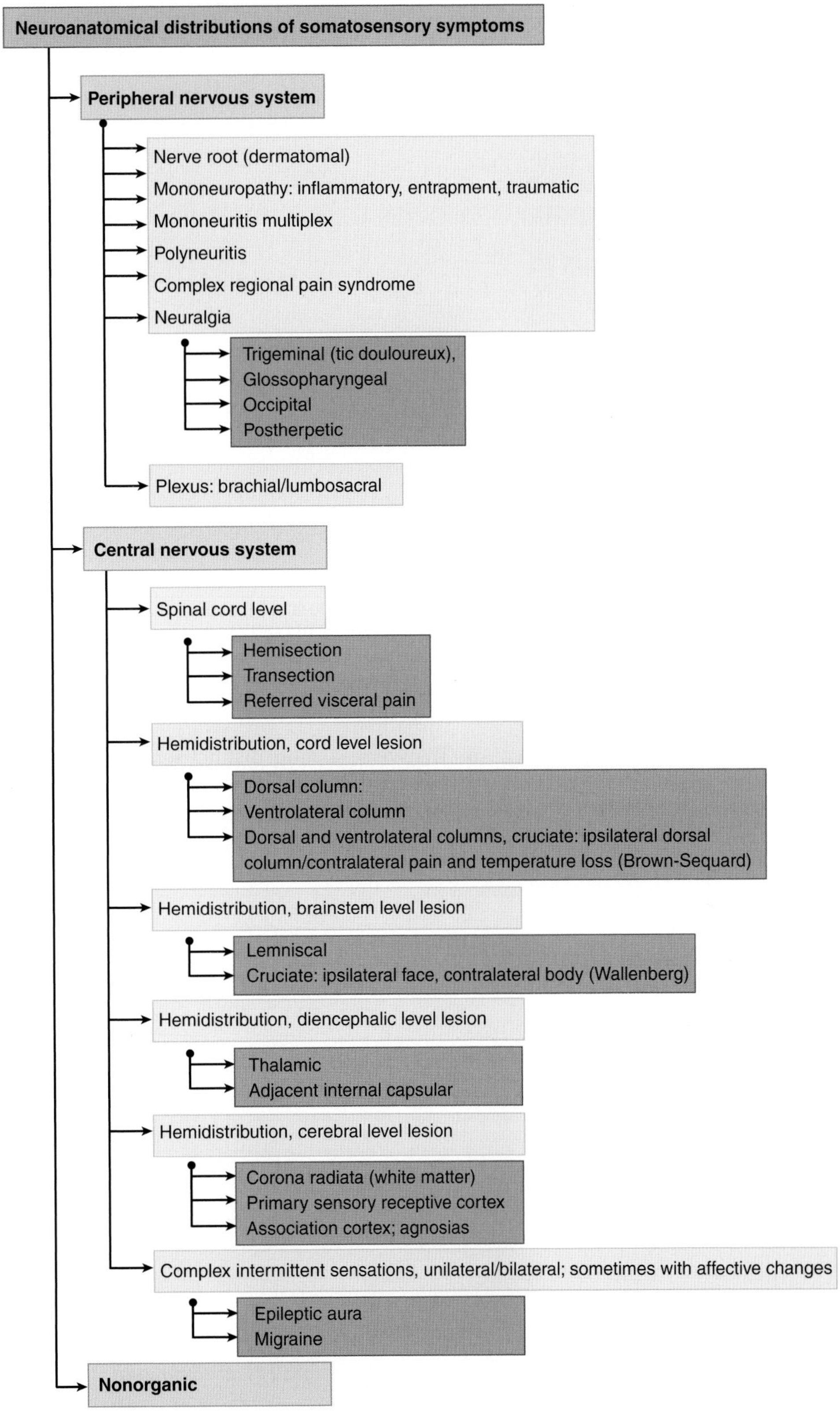

FIGURE 10-18. Neuroanatomic distributions of somatosensory symptoms (reference).

3. **Plexus distributions:** Use the motor, sensory, and segmental distribution tables and figures in Chapter 2 to look up the information as needed (fingertip neuroanatomy).
4. **Spinal cord distributions**
   a. Conus medullaris distribution (Fig. 10-19)

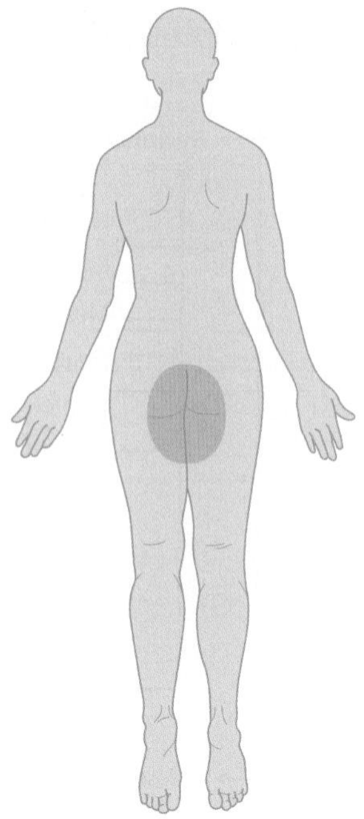

FIGURE 10-19. Sacral loss of sensation caused by a lesion of the distal or sacral part of the spinal cord (the conus medullaris and cauda equina). The conus gives rise to the cauda equina, the lumbosacral roots that descend from the conus to exit through the intervertebral foramina.

b. Transverse section: distinct sensory level with loss of all somatosensory sensation caudal to the lesion or with sacral sparing (Fig. 10-20).

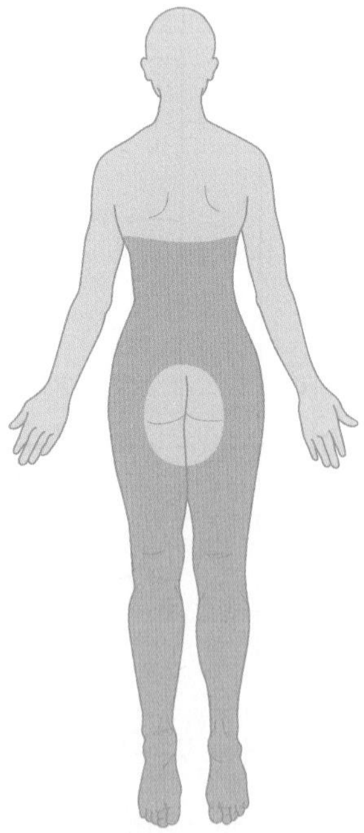

FIGURE 10-20. A transverse lesion at the midthoracic level causes sensory loss caudal to the lesion. Because the ascending fibers from the sacral area occupy the extreme periphery of the cord, the lesion may spare these fibers, a phenomenon called *sacral sparing* (white round area).

c. Hemisection of the right or left half of the spinal cord (Brown-Sequard syndrome; Figs. 10-21A and 10-21B; Aminoff, 1993).

d. Syringomyelia distribution (Figs. 10-22A and 10-22B).

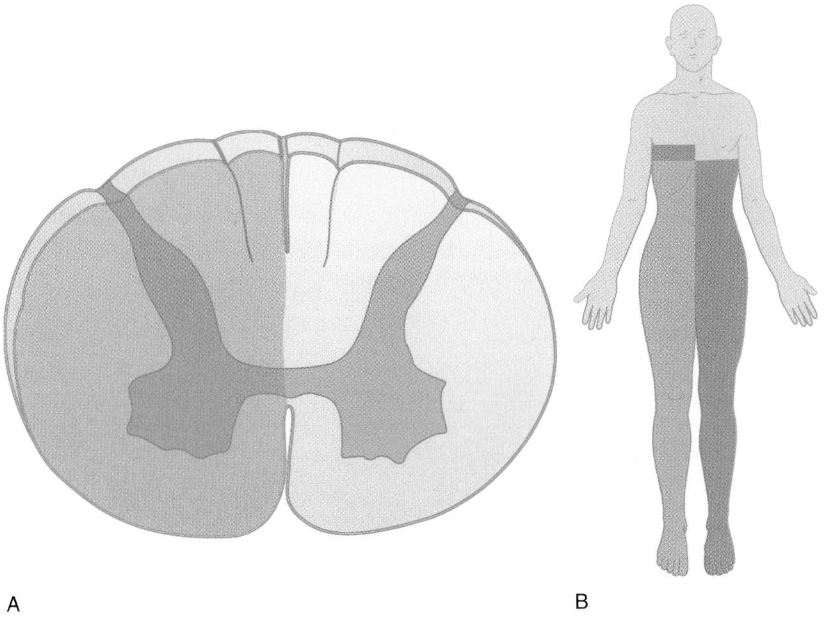

FIGURE 10-21. Sensory loss in the Brown-Sequard syndrome of hemisection of the spinal cord in the upper thoracic region. (A) Draw in the corticospinal tract and spinothalamic tract on the side of the lesion (light and dark purple) and compare with Fig. 2-12. (B) The transverse band of dark purple represents the sensory deficit at the level of the lesion from interruption of the dorsal root. The light purple indicates the ipsilateral loss of deep modalities from interruption of the dorsal columns and the ipsilateral leg paralysis from interruption of the corticospinal tract. The dark purple represents the loss of pain and temperature sensation in the contralateral side of the body and leg from interruption of the spinothalamic tract, which has crossed.

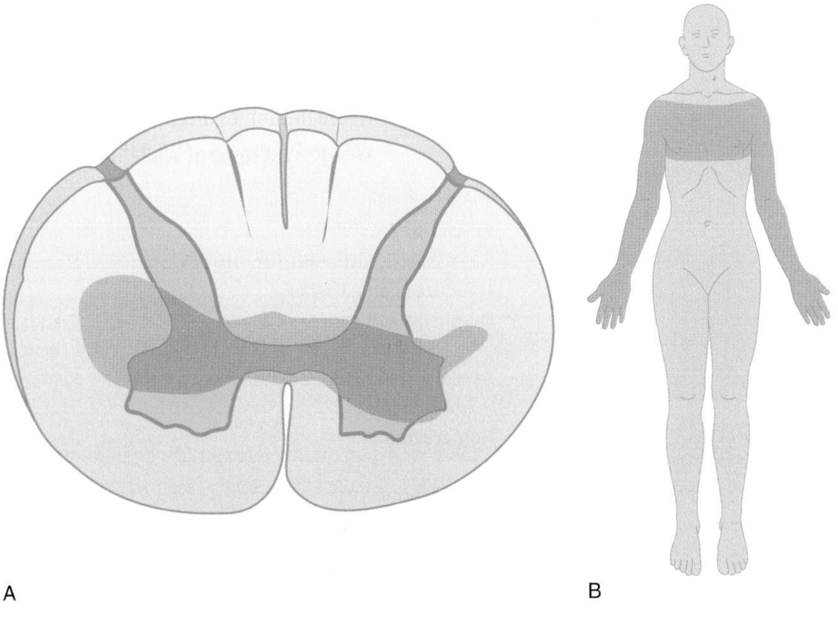

FIGURE 10-22. Pattern of sensory loss with syringomyelia. (A) A syrinx, a cavitating lesion of the cord, interrupts the pain and temperature axons that cross the midline to ascend in the spinothalamic tract. (B) With a syrinx extending from C4 to T5, the patient loses pain and temperature sensation in the light purple region. The lesion does not interrupt the pain and temperature pathways from the trunk and leg because these pathways run in the periphery of the spinal cord (Fig. 2-12).

5. **Lateral medullary wedge syndrome of Wallenberg):** Ipsilateral face/contralateral body and extremities. See Fig. 10-23A and 10-23B and Table 10-4.
6. **Hemisensory distribution:** Medial lemniscus/thalamic/internal capsule/cortical/ distributions (Fig. 10-24).

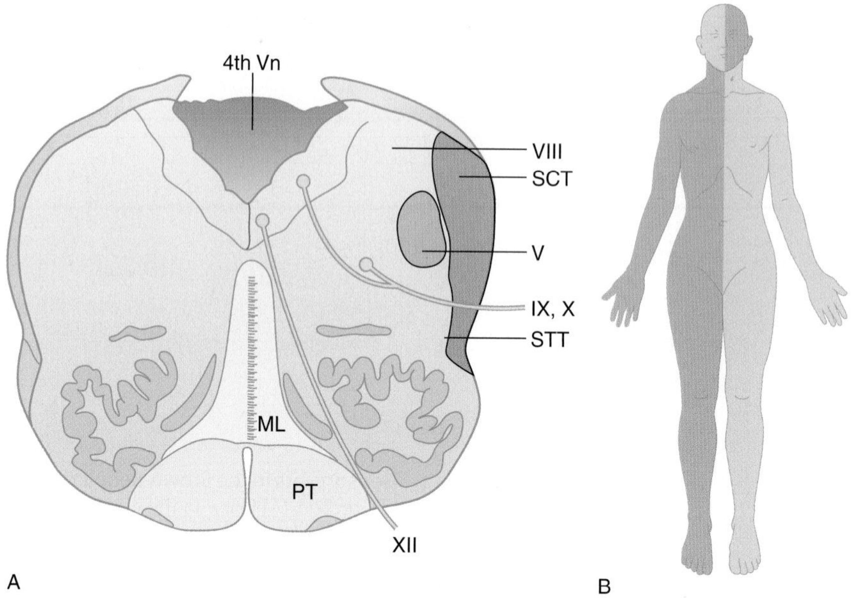

FIGURE 10-23. Cruciate areas of sensory loss with medullary lesions. (A) Transverse section of the medulla showing the lesion site (outlined structure) for Wallenberg's lateral medullary wedge syndrome, usually due to occlusion of the posterior inferior cerebellar artery. (B) Interruption of the descending root of cranial nerve V causes ipsilateral loss of pain and temperature on the face. Interruption of the STT causes contralateral loss of pain and temperature sensation. See Table 10-4 for the remainder of the syndrome. ML = medial lemniscus; PT = pyramidal tract; SCT = spinocerebellar tracts; STT = spinothalamic tract; Vn = ventricle; V = descending nucleus and root of cranial nerve V; VIII = vestibular nuclei; IX, X = nucleus ambiguus for cranial nerves IX and X; XII = cranial nerve XII.

TABLE 10-4 · Neuroanatomic Correlation of Symptoms and Signs of the Lateral Medullary Wedge Syndrome of Wallenberg*

Symptom or sign	Structure involved
Ipsilateral	
Facial pain, dysesthesia or anesthesia, reduced corneal reflex	Descending root of CrN V
Dysphagia and dysarthria	CrNs IX and X or nucleus ambiguus; paralysis of palatal elevation; pharyngeal constrictors, and vocal cord
Ataxia, dysmetria, intention tremor, or hypotonia	Spinocerebellar tracts and cerebellar hemisphere
Horner syndrome	Descending sympathetic tract in lateral reticular formation
Contralateral	
Loss of pain and temperature	Lateral spinothalamic tract
Nonlateralized Symptoms	
Nausea, vomiting, vertigo, and hiccoughing	Reticular formation and vestibular nuclei

*Also see Fig. 10-23 and review Section IV A of Chapter 8.
ABBREVIATION: CrN = cranial nerve.

BIBLIOGRAPHY · Review of Somatosensory Symptom Distributions

Aminoff MJ. Sensory modulation and the spinal cord. *Ann Neurol* 1993;34:511–512.

Kim JS, Lee JH, Lee MC. Patterns of sensory dysfunction in lateral medullary infarction. *Neurology* 1997;49:1557–1563.

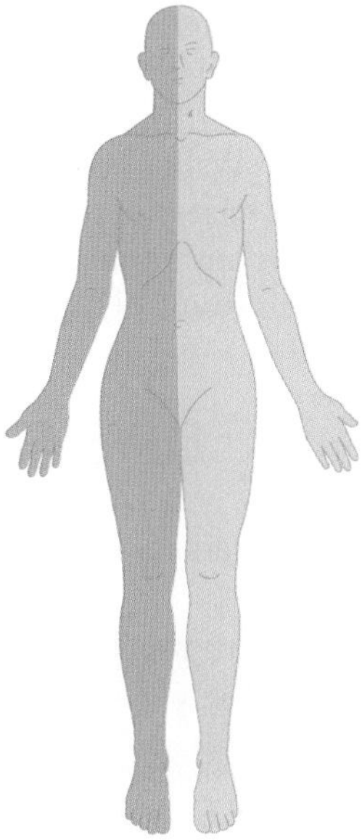

FIGURE 10-24. Hemisensory loss due to interruption of sensory pathways through the medial lemniscus-thalamo-cortical pathway. Hysteria also can cause hemisensory loss. Chapter 14 discusses the differentiation from organic anesthesia.

XI. STEPS IN THE CLINICAL ANALYSIS OF A SENSORY DISORDER

A. Inquire whether the symptom is intermittent or constant.

B. Ask the Pt to delineate the area of pain or sensory change. If intelligent, observant, and nonpsychiatric, the Pt will map it out as well or better than the Ex can with pin and cotton, and much more quickly.

C. **Inquire about any factors or maneuvers that exacerbate or relieve the symptom.** Have the Pt demonstrate any postures or maneuvers that alter the symptom. Ask the Pt's opinion as to the cause for the complaint. Frequently the answer discloses fears of cancer or some other dreaded malady. You can then plan how to discuss the differential diagnosis effectively, and Pts appreciate your interest in their observations and opinions.

D. **Before each test, establish communication.** State clearly what you expect. Don't equivocate but don't suggest responses. Ask for *yes* or *no* responses, or "Is [stimulus] 1 different from [stimulus] 2?"

E. **Isolate the modality for testing from other sensory modalities.** Do most sensory tests with the Pt's eyes closed.

F. **Monitor the suggestibility and attentiveness of the Pt by sometimes withholding the stimulus and asking whether the Pt perceived something.**

G. **Draw the area of the deficit on the Pt or on a diagram.** Delineate the borders only as sharply as the results warrant. Repeat the examination on another day to test the reproducibility of the deficit. When satisfied with the accuracy of the drawing, place it in the Pt's chart.

H. **Think through the anatomic pathway for the modality.** Know the location of the secondary sensory neuron and therefore the site of decussation of the pathway.

I. **Try to match the distribution of the Pt's sensory findings with the neuroanatomic distribution of the sensory pathways.** As always in diagnosis, the clinician has to decide whether the finding is **organic, nonorganic,** or **mixed organic/nonorganic.**

J. **Make a decision on the probable diagnosis and cause for the symptom** (Fig. 10-24).

K. **Final warning:** Although the classic findings of lesions at various sites enable localization of most organic diseases, variations within the compass of the classic syndromes is frequent. The Pt may feel the discomfort of the carpal tunnel syndrome in the forearm, not just the hand. The Pt with Brown-Sequard cord hemisection syndrome often has ipsilateral hyperesthesias. The Pt with Wallenberg's lateral medullary wedge syndrome may not show the classic cruciate sensory pattern. See Kim et al. (1997) and Aminoff (1993) in the previous bibliography. The Pt's mental state and motives may drastically change the result of sensory testing.

XII. SUMMARY OF SOMATIC SENSORY TESTING

Rehearse Section VII, steps A and B, of the Standard NE.

Learning Objectives for Chapter 10

I. INTRODUCTION TO TESTING GENERAL SOMATIC SENSATIONS

1. List the special senses and the general senses tested in the Standard NE.
2. Recite and define the words used to describe deficient or excessive senses of touch, pain, and temperature.
3. Give examples of paresthesias and dysesthesias experienced by everyone.
4. Define hyperpathia, neuralgia, and complex regional pain syndrome Type I and II (reflex sympathetic dystrophy and causalgia).
5. Discuss some neurophysiologic theories to explain the positive or irritative sensations caused by lesions that affect sensory fibers.

II. GENERAL ANATOMICO-PHYSIOLOGIC PRINCIPLES IN ANALYZING LESIONS OF THE PERIPHERAL NERVOUS SYSTEM

1. Recite the deficit and irritative or release phenomena found clinically after disease of somatomotor axons.
2. List the deficit and irritative or release phenomena after interruption of visceromotor axons.
3. List and define several irritative phenomena after disease of somatosensory axons.
4. Describe irritative phenomena after disease of the main sensory components of CrNs I, II, V, and VII.
5. State where to start the "thinking through" process in trying to localize lesions along the course of motor and sensory pathways.
6. In a general way, relate axon size to function in the PNS.

III. GENERAL CLINICAL PRINCIPLES IN TESTING ALL SOMATIC SENSATIONS

1. Explain how to reduce the tedium and enliven the process of sensory testing.
2. Explain the process known as *forced-choice testing* of sensation.
3. Describe differences in sensitivity to stimuli, in particular touch, in different areas of skin.
4. Describe the distributional patterns that organic diseases of the PNS usually match.

IV. EXAMINATION OF SENSORY FUNCTIONS OF CRANIAL NERVE V

1. Explain how the concept of a three-dimensional "mask of Trigeminus" enables you to recall the posterior border of the innervation field of CrN V on the surface skin and deep structures (teeth, oral cavity, nasal passages, and sinuses).
2. Describe the range of functions mediated by CrN V. (**Mnemonic:** Recite the facial, feeding, and respiratory-related reflexes and certain facial and oral autonomic reflexes of a newborn infant.)

Learning Objectives for Chapter 10

3. Draw a lateral view of the face to show the area of distribution of the three major sensory divisions of the CrN V and name the three branches (Fig. 10-2).
4. Draw a dorsal view of the brainstem and show the three subdivisions of the trigeminal sensory nucleus.
5. Diagram the sensory pathway that connects the sensory nuclei of CrN V with the thalamus (Fig. 10-2).
6. Explain the unique anatomic and functional features of the mesencephalic nucleus of CrN V.
7. Describe and demonstrate how to test touch over the trigeminal area.
8. Explain how to monitor the Pt's attentiveness and suggestibility while testing skin sensation.
9. Explain why, if you suspect a numb area from the Pt's history, you should begin sensory testing with a normal area and then work from the numb area out to the normal area.
10. Describe and demonstrate how to test the corneal reflex.
11. Name the cranial nerves that mediate the corneal reflex.
12. Describe the corneomandibular and glabellar blink reflexes.
13. Explain why you should use subtle rather than obvious differences in testing temperature sensation.
14. Describe and demonstrate how to test for temperature discrimination by the tuning fork versus finger test and the warm and cool tube test.
15. Explain why you should usually test for temperature discrimination before testing for pain, especially in a child.
16. Explain the clinical importance of recognizing that the sensory innervation field of CrN V spares the skin over the mandibular angle.
17. Explain, in principle, how the pattern of sensory loss found during the examination distinguishes organic from hysterical loss of sensation, and describe the usual pattern of hysterical loss of sensation in the arm.
18. Describe the clinical characteristics of trigeminal neuralgia.

V. EXAMINATION OF SOMATOSENSORY FUNCTIONS OF THE BODY AND THE EXTREMITIES

1. Explain why, in testing for a dermatomal loss of sensation or spinal cord sensory level, the Ex moves the stimulus *up* and *down* the trunk but *around* the limbs (Fig. 2-10).
2. State the location of the nerve cell body for the primary, secondary, and tertiary neurons in the pathways for pain and temperature, touch, and dorsal column modalities (Fig. 2-28).
3. Describe the pathways by which touch reaches conscious appreciation from the body and extremities.
4. Explain the importance of knowing the location of the secondary neuron in the somatic sensory pathways.
5. Define a lemniscus and name the lemnisci (Table 10-1).
6. Define the spinal lemniscus.
7. On a generalized cross section of the brainstem, locate the lemnisci (Fig. 2-14).
8. Name the one sensation that does not, in fact or theory, have a specific thalamic relay nucleus. (In answering this question, recall how to use your own body to systematically enumerate the senses.)
9. Describe the two types of pain in terms of time of response to a pinprick and relate these to the kind of peripheral nerve fiber that conducts each type of pain.

Learning Objectives for Chapter 10

10. Define referred pain and give an example.
11. Distinguish between nociceptive pain and neurogenic pain.
12. Diagram the pathway for pain and temperature sensation from the trunk and extremities to the cerebral cortex (Fig. 10-6).
13. Explain how the pain and temperature pathway from the face resembles and differs from the pathway for the rest of the body (Figs. 10-2 and 10-6).
14. Describe the order of representation of the entire face and body in the pain and temperature nucleus (substantia gelatinosa of Rolando) and state the location of that nucleus.
15. Describe a neurosurgical operation on the spinal cord that would abolish pain and temperature sensation but would not abolish touch or cause motor disturbances.
16. Describe the type of pin to use to test pain sensation and how to hold it to ensure a uniform stimulus for the pinpricks.
17. Explain why you make multiple pinpricks at each site rather than single pricks in testing pain sensation.
18. Explain why you should test temperature and pain sensation on the dorsum of the hands and feet rather than on the palms and soles.
19. Explain why you should always discard a pin after using it to test pain sensation.
20. Describe how to test for delayed pain and deep pain.
21. State the evidence suggesting that a neonate or possibly even a fetus might feel pain.
22. Describe how to test sensation to accurately and reliably determine the level of a spinal cord transection in a newborn or young infant.
23. State the type of biopsies that aid in investigating disease of small nerve fibers.

VI. EXAMINATION TECHNIQUES IN PERIPHERAL NEUROPATHIES

1. Describe the typical distribution of sensory loss in polyneuropathies.
2. State which nerves to palpate to identify hypertrophic neuropathy.
3. Describe Tinel's "tapping the nerve" sign.
4. Describe ancillary procedures commonly used in the differential diagnosis of polyneuropathies.
5. Describe occipital neuralgia.
6. Describe the distribution of the sensory deficit in the carpal tunnel syndrome.
7. Recite the LLOAF/2 mnemonic for the muscles innervated by the median nerve.
8. Name the most important muscle to test in the carpal tunnel syndrome and demonstrate how to test it.
9. Demonstrate Phalen's sign.
10. State the usual site of entrapment of the ulnar nerve.
11. Name two muscles in the hand that can be readily tested for weakness from an ulnar neuropathy.
12. Describe the distribution of the sensory disturbance in entrapment of the lateral femoral cutaneous nerve.
13. Contrast the sensory and motor deficits from entrapment of the common peroneal nerve and the posterior tibial nerve.
14. Describe the site of the lesion and distribution of the pain in Morton's metatarsalgia.

Learning Objectives for Chapter 10

VII. EXAMINATION TECHNIQUES IN LOW BACK PAIN AND PAIN RADIATING DOWN THE LEG: THE SCIATICA SYNDROME

1. Contrast the clinical findings on the NE of a Pt with an acute compression of the L5 nerve root with compression of the S1 root from intervertebral disc herniation. (**Hint:** Cover the L5 and S1 columns in Table 10-2 and recite the findings.)
2. Describe how to do the sciatic nerve stretching tests and the biomechanics involved.
3. In a nonpsychiatric Pt, what is generally the best way to identify the distribution of radicular pain?
4. Explain how an EMG can help localize the myotome affected in root compression syndromes.
5. In the straight-knee leg-raising test, explain why, when the Ex stops just short of eliciting pain and then manually dorsiflexes the Pt's foot, pain is produced.
6. Describe the results and significance when the straight-knee leg-raising test on one side produces radicular pain in the other leg.
7. Explain why the distribution of pain from L5 or S1 may affect the buttock, hip, or thigh as much as or more than radiating down into the foot.
8. Describe several methods of examining the back and leg of a Pt with the sciatica syndrome in addition to the standard testing of sensation, strength, and MSRs (Section VII F 2).
9. Show how to test the one muscle usually exclusively innervated by L5.
10. List a number of disorders or comorbidities involved in the differential diagnosis of sciatica.
11. Describe ancillary studies often required in the differential diagnosis of sciatica.

VIII. EXAMINATION OF THE DORSAL COLUMN, DISCRIMINATIVE OR DEEP MODALITIES: PROPRIOCEPTION, POSITION SENSE, VIBRATION, AND DIRECTION OF MOVEMENT

1. Define proprioceptive sensation.
2. Explain how the etymology of the word *proprioception* applies to its use in neurology.
3. Summarize the reasoning that led Sherrington to recognize a proprioceptive system.
4. Diagram the skeletomuscular proprioceptive pathway from the foot and hand (Fig. 10-14).
5. Describe the location of the second-order neuron in the dorsal column proprioceptive pathway from the extremities. State where its axon decussates and the name of the pathway it takes to the thalamus.
6. Diagram the sensory homunculus in the dorsal columns and give the technical terms for the fasciculi of the dorsal columns (the arm dorsal column and the leg dorsal column; Fig. 2-12D).
7. Contrast the nature of the stimuli received by deep and superficial receptors.
8. Discuss the relation between the concepts of the mechanoreceptors (dorsal column modalities) and classic Newtonian physics.
9. Describe and demonstrate how to test for position sense in the digits.
10. Explain why testing digits 3 or 4 provides a greater challenge to the Pt's position sense than digits 1, 2, or 5 and why, if you find normal position sense in digits 3 and 4, you do not have to test other digits or proximal joints in the routine screening NE (Fig. 10-16).

Learning Objectives for Chapter 10

11. State which joints you examine next to determine the severity of the loss, if the Pt has no position sense in digits 3 and 4 in the hands or feet.
12. Discuss whether a normal person who is attending to the stimulus will make any errors in digit position.
13. State the probability that a Pt who has no position sense will correctly guess the *up* or *down* position of the digit.
14. Describe the methods of making position sense testing more challenging than simple *up* or *down* alternatives.
15. In *up* or *down* position sense testing, state the minimum number of trials necessary to make success by chance improbable.
16. Discuss the clinical interpretation when the Pt consistently gives the wrong or exactly opposite answer to the *up* or *down* position of the digit.
17. Discuss the reason the sensory examination requires such a high degree of skill on the part of the Ex.
18. Discuss some reasons inexperienced Exs may misinterpret the Pt's response to sensory testing as unreliable.
19. Recite the instructions the Ex gives the Pt for the swaying (Romberg) test.
20. Give an operational description of the Romberg test.
21. Give an interpretational description of the Romberg test.
22. State the critical sensory pathway for maintaining the upright posture with the eyes closed.
23. Explain why you ask the Pt to stand with the feet together for the Romberg test.
24. Describe how to divert the hysterical patient into performing well in the Romberg test.
25. Describe the effect of closing the eyes on cerebellar and sensory dystaxia.
26. Describe how to differentiate sensory from cerebellar ataxia (Table 10-3).
27. Describe the result of the swaying test in a normal person, in a hysteric, in Pts with lesions of the cerebellum or dorsal column, and in Pts with vertigo.
28. Describe and demonstrate how to test for vibration sense.
29. Explain how to monitor the Pt's attentiveness and reliability in testing vibration sense.
30. Describe the directional scratch test for dorsal column dysfunction.
31. Review the pathways for conscious perception of touch, temperature and pain, position, and vibration.
32. Demonstrate how to test for two-point discrimination.
33. Compare the relative impairment of the foregoing sensations by lesions of the PNS or central pathways up to the somesthetic cortex.

IX. EXAMINATION FOR ASTEREOGNOSIS AND TACTILE AGNOSIAS

1. Describe the role of the primary sensory cortex and the association cortex in the recognition of objects and form.
2. Make a lateral drawing of a cerebral hemisphere. Shade the posterior parasylvian area and indicate the location of the primary sensory cortices (Fig. 10-17).
3. Define *gnosia* as used in neurology and give examples of gnosia by using the following roots: *stereo-*, *topo-*, *grapho-*, and *noso-*.
4. Distinguish between *stereoanesthesia* and *astereognosis.*
5. Distinguish between *deafness* and *auditory agnosia* and between *blindness* and *visual agnosia* and explain what these terms imply about the location of the lesion along the course of the sensory pathways.

Learning Objectives for Chapter 10

6. Distinguish between *astereognosis* and *tactile agnosia.*
7. Describe the items used and how to test for tactile agnosia.

X. REVIEW OF SOMATOSENSORY DISTRIBUTIONS

1. Recite the mnemonic for remembering dermatomal distributions (see page 62).
2. Diagram the sensory distributions of the trigeminal, median, ulnar, lateral femoral cutaneous, and common peroneal nerves (Fig. 2-11).
3. Describe the sensory findings in the Brown-Sequard cord hemisection syndrome (Fig. 10-21).
4. Describe the sensory loss in the cervical syringomyelia syndrome (Fig. 10-22).
5. Describe the sensory findings in Wallenberg's lateral medullary wedge syndrome (Fig. 10-23).
6. Recite the nonsensory symptoms and signs of Wallenberg's syndrome (Table 10-4).
7. Describe the distribution of sensory loss after interruption of the somatosensory pathway through the upper brainstem to the primary somatosensory cortex of the postcentral gyrus (Fig. 10-24).

XI. STEPS IN THE CLINICAL ANALYSIS OF A SENSORY COMPLAINT

1. Enumerate the steps in the clinical analysis of a sensory complaint and describe the distributions implicating an organic sensory abnormality (Fig. 10-13).
2. Rehearse Section VII of the Standard NE.

11 The Patient's Mental Status and Higher Cerebral Functions

As not only the disease interested the physician, but he was strongly moved to look into the character and qualities of the patient. . . . He deemed it essential, it would seem, to know the man, before attempting to do him good.

—Nathaniel Hawthorne (1804–1864)

I. THE MENTAL STATUS EXAMINATION: A NONPROGRAMMED INTERLUDE

A How to derive the mental status information

1. Most of the data for judging the patient's (Pt's) mental status emerge as a natural consequence of the questions posed during the standard medical history, which this text does not cover. Although you do the basic Neurologic Examination (NE) by a set routine, you should probe the Pt's mental status unobtrusively and flexibly. If you blurt out questions obviously designed to test the mental status, such as, "Do you hear voices?" the Pt may respond with annoyance, sullen silence, or outright anger. Nevertheless, just such a question, introduced at the proper time, encourages the disclosure of distressing thoughts. The Pt then may describe the voice that repeats, "You have a duty to kill your family." Because your personal characteristics and interview techniques condition what the Pt can and will disclose, you must remain flexible, empathetic, and nonjudgmental. This is the first point: **the interview technique is everything.**
2. By monitoring the Pt's responses, you determine which questions to use and how far to pursue any particular line of inquiry. As long as the Pt talks productively, continue the line of inquiry. If the Pt changes the subject or becomes evasive, flustered, or silent, you have pressed too hard. The Pt isn't ready to talk about that. Try another tack. A mentally ill Pt may permit a full NE but completely resist inquiries obviously designed to disclose thoughts. Patients will talk about whatever problems and anxieties occupy their thoughts, if they can tolerate the thought and its communication. This is the second point: **Pts will disclose their mental state, particularly their worries and concerns, if you provide a free opportunity.** Nathaniel Hawthorne (1804–1864) marvelously described the correct interview technique in *The Scarlet Letter:*

So [Dr.] Roger Chillingworth—the man of skill, the kind and friendly physician—strove to go deep into his patient's bosom, delving among his principles, prying into his recollections, and probing everything with a cautious touch, like a treasure-seeker in a dark cavern. Few secrets can escape an investigator, who has opportunity and license to undertake such a quest, and skill to follow it up. A man burdened with a secret should especially avoid the intimacy of his physician. If the latter possess native sagacity, and a nameless something more—let us call it intuition; **if he show no intrusive egotism, nor disagreeably prominent characteristics of his own;** if he have the power, which must be born with him, to bring his mind into such affinity with his patients' that this last shall unawares have spoken what he imagines himself only to have thought; **if such revelations received without tumult, and acknowledged not so often by an uttered sympathy as by silence, an inarticulate breath, and here or there a word, to indicate that all is understood;** if to these qualifications of a confidant be joined the advantages afforded by his recognized character as a physician—then, at some inevitable moment will the soul of the sufferer be dissolved, and flow forth in a dark, but transparent stream, bringing all its mysteries into the daylight [emphasis added].

3. We have highlighted the two most important statements. With these in mind, you may find it useful to reread Chapter 1, Section I E.

B. Categories of the mental status examination

1. The examiner (Ex) must know and explore each category of the mental status examination (Arciniegas and Beresford, 2001; Strub and Black, 2000). Learn Table 11-1.

TABLE 11-1 · Outline of Mental Status Examination

I. General behavior and appearance	Is the patient normal, hyperactive, agitated, quiet, immobile? Is the patient neat or slovenly? Do the clothes match the patient's age, peers, sex, and background?
II. Stream of talk	Does the patient converse normally? Is the speech rapid, incessant, under great pressure, or is it slow and lacking in spontaneity and prosody? Is the patient discursive, tangential, and unable to reach the conversational goal?
III. Mood and affective responses	Is the patient euphoric, agitated, giggling, silent, weeping, or angry? Is the mood appropriate? Is the patient emotionally labile?
IV. Content of thought	Does the patient have illusions, hallucinations or delusions, and misinterpretations? Does the patient suffer delusions of persecution and surveillance by malicious persons or forces? Is the patient preoccupied with bodily complaints, fears of cancer or heart disease, or other phobias?
V. Intellectual capacity	Is the patient bright, average, dull, or obviously demented or mentally retarded?
VI. Sensorium	A. Consciousness B. Attention span C. Orientation for time, place, and person D. Memory, recent and remote E. Fund of information F. Insight, judgment, and planning G. Calculation

2. Because much of the mental status examination belongs to the psychiatric history, this text focuses on the **sensorium** because:
   a. Sensorial testing uses questions that require more or less objective answers for passing or failing, e.g., either you know what day it is, or you don't know what day it is.
   b. Sensorial deficits are sensitive to organic impairment of the brain.

C. The nature of the sensorium

I think; therefore I am.

—René Descartes (1596–1650)

The sensorium is that place where you are aware that you are aware.

1. We all intuitively recognize our awareness of ourselves and our environment. Without consciousness, no other categories of the sensorium are tenable or testable. But consciousness requires a content. At any moment we are conscious of objects, the state of our bladder, the time of day, our feelings, etc. We call our awareness the **sensorium.**
2. Functions of the sensorium:
   a. Registers current internal and external contingencies.
   b. Relates current internal and external stimuli to our memories and to our future hopes and desires.
   c. Invests the streams of afferent stimuli with emotion, determines their significance, and assigns priority that results in neglect or attention.
   d. Proposes various actions and their consequences.
   e. Directs the motor system in the actual behaviors that achieve personal survival and satisfaction.
   f. Allows us to experience life as a conscious process with a past, present, and future and to respond appropriately (Fig. 11-1).

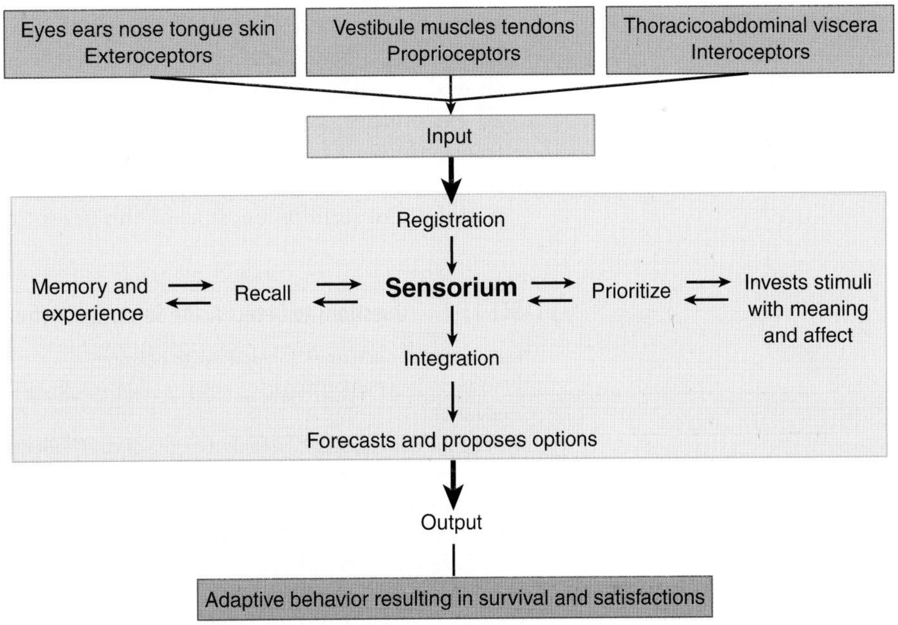

FIGURE 11-1. Diagram of the sensorium as an input-output system.

3. **Examples of sensorial responses to internal or external contingencies**
   a. **Internal contingencies:** Anxiety about academics: "Maybe I better study tonight." Hunger: "Maybe I better eat something."
   b. **External contingencies:** Fire: "I better get away from here." Meeting another person: "Mmmm I'd like to know that person better" or "Mmmm, I should avoid that person."
   c. The sensorium is ever vigilant and somewhat suspicious in order to avoid harm and gain advantage.

D. The sensorium commune: the common sense of all human kind

1. **The ancients recognized that every person who is sound of mind has a *sensorium commune*,** a sense in common of:
   a. **Who** they are, their role, and station in life: parent, child, student.
   b. **Where** they are: at home, school, hospital, the bathroom.
   c. **When** it is: It's noon. It's today, a particular date. Yesterday has passed. Tomorrow will come. It's winter, not spring, summer, or fall.
   d. **What** is happening: It's snowing. The house is on fire. A dog is barking.
   e. **How** the wise and prudent person should behave: Thus, we have the common sense to come in out of the snow, to get out of a burning house, and to yell at the dog to stop yapping, because we all sense these circumstances as dangers or nuisances.
2. **What is uncommon sense (unshared sense)?**
   a. The uncommon senses or perceptions that we don't share are our personal political, religious, and moral beliefs, e.g., there is a God/there is no God.
   b. Hence, we avoid specific questions about these topics and most of all avoid debating them in the medical setting because they generate argument, not medical data. Questions on such topics lack quantifiable, objective end points that test the organic condition of the brain, as do questions about the sensorium.

E. Testing for acute dysfunction of the sensorium after a concussion

1. **Patient analysis:** A blow to the head has rendered a 21-year-old athlete unconscious for 2 minutes. As the Ex reaches the player, who still lies on the playing field, consciousness appears to have returned. The Ex's quick neurologic appraisal shows normal breathing, pupils, eye movements, and spontaneous movements of all extremities. These findings exclude a major catastrophe such as spinal cord transection or a large cerebral lesion. To quickly, but effectively, evaluate the athlete's sensorium, the Ex asks a series of **who, where, when,** and **what** questions, posing them *seriatim* because of the urgent circumstances (Table 11-2).

TABLE 11-2 · Questions to Detect Acute Sensorial Dysfunction After a Head Injury

"Hello, what is your name?" (orientation to person)
"Who am I?" (orientation to person and your role as a physician: an athlete should know the team physician)
"What is the day and date?" "What is the time of day?" (orientation to time)
"Where are we?" (orientation to place: practice field or stadium)
"What has just happened to you?" or "What was the last play?" (current events and recent memory)
"What team are you playing?" (current events and recent memory)
"What is the score of the game?" (current events and recent memory)
"Can you repeat the months of the year backward?" (comprehension and attention span)
"Can you remember these three items?" Recite an item such as *table,* a *color,* and an *address* and ask the patient to repeat them after a few minutes. (recent memory)
Ask about pain, blurred or double vision, tinnitus, dizziness, and numbness or tingling. (Checks current neurologic symptoms)
Complete a Standard Neurologic Examination

2. By correctly answering all questions, the athlete demonstrates the first four sensorial functions: consciousness; attention span; orientation for time, person, and place; and recent memory (Table 11-1).
3. Asking the Pt to learn three unrelated items, a color, an address, and an object, and then repeat them after 5 minutes adds another useful test, as does spelling the word *world* backward or reciting the months backward (McCrea et al., 1998).

4. The Ex then asks about neurologic symptoms such as blurred vision, double vision, numbness, and so forth and completes a Standard NE.
5. **As an exercise, try to select from Table 11-2 the single most, symbolic, generic question that best tests the athlete's sensorium if you were limited to one question.**
   a. We submit, "What is the score of the game?" as the best question, although you may feel differently.
   b. Basically the sensorial tests determine whether the person knows the score, or in street-talk expressing the same thing when meeting someone, we say, "Hey man, what's coming down?" "What's happening?" Asking "What's the score?" subsumes all of these statements that invite newly met persons to display their sensorium.
6. Here is a marvelous, true anecdote of a mother who brought her 8-year-old child into the Emergency Room for examination after a hard fall on concrete had caused severe scalp bleeding:
   a. When asked whether the fall had stunned the child. The mother said: "Oh no. I knew she wasn't stunned 'cause I asked her who was she and who was I and where was she and what had just happened to her, and she knew all that."
   b. The Ex said: "Those are certainly the right questions. Where did you learn that?" She said: "Why? anybody knows that." In other words, she posed her perfectly scripted questions from an intuitive appreciation of "common sense" as a test of brain function, the matching of one brain's perceptions against those of another's.
7. **Operation of the sensorium in animals:** Just for fun, analyze two dogs meeting. Each exploits all of its exteroceptors to maximize information—eyeing, sniffing, nuzzling, licking, whining, growling, ruffling fur, and stalking about—in a primal exploration of each other's sensorium as reflected in behavior. Then comes the dog's decision concerning the best behavior for survival and satisfaction: flee, fight, or copulate.

F. Testing for chronic dysfunction of the sensorium in the brain-impaired or demented patient

The principle is the same as in acute concussion but the form of the questions differs. Avoid machine-gunning the Pt with a series of simplistic questions: "What is your name? Where are you? What is the day, date, and week? Do you hear voices? Who is the president? Can you remember an item, a color, and an address?" If you ask questions that crudely, the Pt, especially if somewhat demented or mentally ill, will quickly realize that you are probing their mental status. Often they will reply (not a little piqued): "What's the matter, Doc; do you think I'm crazy?" The Ex ultimately must derive answers to the questions in Table 11-3, but derive them artfully in the natural course of the interview. The Pt should experience it all as an ordinary conversation, not as an inquisition.

G. An operational definition of the sensorium

These deliberations allow us to hazard an operational definition: **The sensorium consists of those brain functions tested by a standard set of questions that elicit more or less objective answers about the person's past, present, and future.**

For clinical purposes, we judge "objectivity" and "normality" by matching the Pt's answers against the answers that standard persons with common sense would make.

H. Where does the sensorium reside within the body

1. The sensorium cannot be in the limbs and other parts of the body. Their destruction does not alter the sensorium. The two historical contenders for the site have been the heart and the brain.
2. Many ancient savants and scholars located the sensorium in the heart (Keele, 1957: Gross, 2009). After all, the heart races when you are frightened, and when the heart stops, the sensorium stops.

TABLE 11-3 · Questions to Detect Chronic Sensorial Dysfunction in Dementia

Area of sensorium tested	Questions
Orientation to person, time, and place; recent and remote memory; consciousness of self and environment	"What is your name?" "How old are you?" "When is your birthday?" "What is your address?" "What kind of work do you do?" "Do you have a spouse/children?" "What are their names/ages/occupations/addresses?" "Where are they now?"
Orientation to time and recent memory	"Do you happen to know the time of day?" "Have you had to wait long to see me?" "What is the day/date/month/year?" "What is the season/weather?" "What did you do yesterday?"
Doctor/patient role: judgment and insight as to presence of illness or need for medical attention	"What have you come to see me about?" or "Do you feel any need for medical help?"
Judgment and planning	"What are your plans for the future?" or "How long do you expect to be off work?"
Recent memory, fund of information and attention span	"What do you think of. . . ." (mention a recent item in the news). "How has your memory been?" "Are you worried about it?" "Suppose we test it. Can you name the last several presidents?" "See whether you can remember. . . ." (name an item, e.g., a table, a color, and an address)
Calculation and attention span	"Subtract 7 from 100, then take off seven more and continue subtracting 7's." "Spell *world*" (or other word) backward, forward, or by alphabetical sequence of the letters.

a. The ancient Egyptians seemed to favor the heart because in their embalming practices they always preserved the heart in a canopic jar or by returning it to the thorax, but they discarded the brain.

b. Aristotle, a Greek (384–322 b.c.), advocated the heart. In his *De Partibus Animalum*, he asserted:

> For the heart is the first of all the parts to be formed; and no sooner is it formed than it contains blood. Moreover the motions of pleasure and pain, and generally of all sensations plainly have their source in the heart and find in it their ultimate termination.

3. But dissenters throughout time raised their voices. Hippocrates (5th century b.c.) said:

> And men should know that from nothing else but from the brain came joys, delights, laughter and jests, and sorrows, griefs, despondency and lamentations. And by this, in especial manner, we acquire wisdom and knowledge, and see and hear and know what are foul and what are fair, what sweet and what unsavory.

4. Aristotle's view of the heart as the site of life and consciousness has persisted in our popular culture, and until the 1960s persisted also in medicine in the very definition of death.
   a. In our vernacular, the heart remains the site of consciousness and emotion.
      i. We say that a person with no feeling or compassion has no heart. Or the person may be faint-hearted or lion-hearted.
      ii. We still speak of love as an affair of the heart, and the heart remains the Valentine's Day symbol of love. (Can we ever change our vocabulary from

sweetheart to "sweetbrain" and declare, "I love you with all of my brain," rather than, "I love you with all of my heart"?)

b. The Aristotelian view, even though acknowledged as wrong, determined the very definition of death into the 1960s. Medically and legally, death was defined as irreversible cessation of the heartbeat and breathing. We still record the time of death as when the heart stops, even though the brain died long before.

I. Where does the sensorium reside within the brain

1. Indisputable evidence from clinicopathologic studies clearly places the sensorium in the brain. No contrary evidence exists, now that the critical and decisive experiment, heart transplantation, has once and for all excluded the heart as the site of the sensorium.
2. Although not localizing as specifically as sensorimotor functions, certain parts of the sensorium appear to localize to particular brain regions.
   a. Consciousness and attention span to some degree co-localize through the ascending reticular activating system.
   b. Recent memory and orientation to person, time, and place are impaired after lesions of the medial temporal lobes and the closely related hippocampal-fornix-mamillary body circuit and basal forebrain (Fig. 11-10), but diffuse cortical or white matter lesions also impair these functions.
   c. Calculation has a nodal point in the left angular gyrus region.
   d. Insight, judgment, and planning are in large measure executive functions of the frontal lobes.
3. Functional brain imaging undoubtedly will localize sensorial functions, affective states, and thought processes better than the clinicopathologic correlation studies of the past.
4. To end the preliminaries poetically, we may regard the sensorium as the place of knowing, that place where we know what we see, hear, and feel; or, ironically in Aristotelian terms, it's where the heart is, where we have our perceptions, feelings, and priorities.

J. The sensorium and sensory deprivation

The notion that the sensorium knits all of the individual sensory impressions into a stream of consciousness anticipated modern studies in sensory deprivation. A person confined to a stimulus-free, totally dark, totally soundproof, constant-temperature chamber devoid of environmental fluctuations and human contact finds that the sensorium weakens. Boredom alternates with fright. The thoughts become loose and detached, and hallucinations follow. Continued isolation causes complete disintegration. The sensorium requires incessant change—the interplay of light and dark, sound and silence, pain and pleasure—to function. The philosophic ideal of pure thought, free from the fetters of the flesh and its environment, is therefore exposed as a fraud. The sensorium functions not floating free as a cloud but with respect to the ever-changing stream of internal and external stimuli. Thus, you behave differently in a classroom than in a swimming pool, and you survive in both.

K. Detailed examination of the sensorium

1. **Consciousness:** Because you obviously cannot respond consciously when asleep, the sensorium is a property of the waking state. For the moment, we define consciousness intuitively as *awareness of self and environment.* (Chapter 12 discusses operational tests of consciousness.) Does the Pt make responses that prove awareness of self and environment?
2. **Attention span:** After consciousness comes attentiveness, the attention span of the individual. Can the Pt attend to stimuli long enough to comprehend and respond to them, or attend to a task long enough to complete it? For a simple,

effective test, ask the Pt to recite the months backward or spell the word *world* backward (McCrea et al., 1998).

3. **Orientation:** If conscious and attentive, does the Pt comprehend **who** and **where** he or she is and **when** it is? This orientation as to person, place, and time requires ongoing sensory impressions. Have you ever awakened from a deep sleep momentarily disoriented as to the day, the hour, or even where you were? If so, you had to process different afferent stimuli, until all of the pieces of the puzzle suddenly fell into place. Judge the Pt's orientation:
   a. As to **person:** Does the Pt recognize him- or herself and his or her role, the other people present, and their roles?
   b. As to **place:** Does the Pt recognize that he or she is in a clinic or hospital, its name, and the name of the city and state?
   c. As to **time:** Can the Pt recite the time of day, day of the week, the month, and the year?
4. **Memory:** Orientation, attention span, and memory intertwine inextricably. Screen for memory this way:
   a. Note how well the Pt recalls and relates the events of the medical history.
   b. Inquire, "Does your memory work all right?" Or more bluntly, "Do you have trouble with your memory?" If you suspect a memory disturbance, say to the Pt, "Suppose we try out your memory?" Ask the Pt to name the presidents backward from the present one. Although also requiring a long attention span, this task requires more attention and memory than reciting the months backward.
   c. Next provide the Pt with an **address,** a **color,** and an **object** to remember, three nonsense items that have no special relation: *5330 Broadway, orange,* and *table.* Have the Pt repeat the items to ensure that they have registered. Then, at the end of the NE, ask the Pt to recite them.
   d. Determine whether the Pt differs in the ability to recall recent or remote events. Can the Pt remember what he or she ate for breakfast? Recent memory suffers most in aging or brain diseases in general. To easily remember this difference, recall that grandfather cannot remember where he just laid his glasses, but he can wax eloquently about the events of long ago.
5. **Fund of information:** The oriented, attentive Pt with a good memory knows what's happening in the world. Ask about current activities or events. If unable to discuss current activities and events, the Pt has organic brain disease, cultural deprivation, or is so withdrawn as to need psychiatric care.
6. **Insight, judgment, and planning:** Simply ask what the Pt plans to do. Do the proffered goals and plans match the Pt's physical and mental capabilities? The quadriplegic Pt who expects to work as a carpenter or the individual with a borderline IQ who expects to become a chemist lacks insight, judgment, and planning. Does the Pt recognize the illness and its implications?
7. **Calculation:** Test calculation by asking whether the Pt can balance a checkbook, make change, do formal paper-and-pencil calculations, and subtract 7's serially from 100.

L. Affective responses

Besides being conscious, attentive, and oriented, having a good memory, a fund of information, insight, judgment, and planning, the standard person reacts emotionally to ongoing events. Imagine your reaction to a hand grenade thrown onto your table or merely to a cockroach. Your alarm or aversion differs in the two cases. Affective responses should have the appropriate *quality* and *quantity.*

1. Assay affective responses not by blunt questions, but by comparing the observed with the expected reactions. What affect would you expect as a Pt discusses her paralyzed arm? What affect would you expect if the Pt complains that the "apparatus" plots to kill him? A blunted, bland, or indifferent affect occurs most commonly with hysteria, schizophrenia, and bifrontal lobe lesions.

2. If you have cause to cry or laugh, how much provocation does it take to make you start and how much time does it take you to get over it? If the Pt cries for 15 seconds and then starts to laugh when you ask him to tell you a funny story, the Pt has affective *lability*, the opposite of affective *blunting*. Affective lability, on-and-off laughing and crying, commonly accompanies bilateral upper motoneuron (UMN) disease, as we have seen in pseudobulbar palsy and diffuse brain diseases.

M. Perceptual distortions: illusions, hallucinations, and delusions

1. **Illusions:** Everyone has experienced the illusion of water shimmering on a hot highway on a summer's day. The water is an *illusion*. **An illusion is a false sensory perception based on natural stimulation of a sensory receptor.** The healthy person recognizes the illusory nature of such an experience, but the sick person may not.
2. **Hallucinations:** Observe that sweating, tremulous man cowering on the bed, screaming about dogs and snakes in the corner of his room. Or observe this calm woman with an expressionless face who tells you in a flat voice that she hears God's voice ordering her to drown her baby. Both Pts display characteristic hallucinations: the man has delirium tremens, and the woman schizophrenia. Before an epileptic seizure, many Pts experience visual, auditory, or somatic hallucinations. **An hallucination is a false sensory perception not based on natural stimulation of a sensory receptor.** The mentally ill Pt usually does not recognize the hallucination as a false representation of reality, whereas the Pt with epilepsy does.

   Hypnagogic and hypnopompic hallucinations are not true hallucinations. A hypnagogic hallucination represents wakeful dreaming while falling asleep, while a hypnopompic hallucination represents wakeful dreaming immediately after waking up.
3. **Delusions:** This Pt, eyeing a nurse carrying a tray into the room, says to you *sotto voce*, "There is one of them now. She's trying to poison me." You err in responding to this remark if you try to reason with him that she has merely come to take his temperature. Somehow, his psychic economy needs to misperceive the nurse as a conspirator, and all the reason in the world will not dispel his belief. **A delusion is a false belief that reason cannot dispel.**
4. Literary geniuses frequently depict illusions, hallucinations, and delusions. Try to identify these perceptual distortions (and get re-accustomed to the programming that follows in the next section):

   a. Here, Macbeth muses alone after murdering Duncan:

   Is this a dagger which I see before me,
   The handle toward my hand? Come, let me clutch thee:
   I have thee not, and yet I see thee still.
   Are thou not, fatal vision, sensible
   To feeling as to sight? Or art thou but
   A dagger of the mind, a false creation,
   Proceeding from the heat-oppressed brain?…
   Mine eyes are made the fools o'th'other senses.
   Or else worth all the rest: I see thee still.…

   —William Shakespeare (1564–1616)

☑ hallucination
a false sensory perception not based on natural stimulation of a sensory receptor

   b. This exemplifies ❒ an illusion/❒ an hallucination/❒ a delusion, which is defined as____
____.

   c. Here is a passage from Gérard De Nerval's poem *The Dark Blot:*

He who has gazed against the sun everywhere he looks thereafter, palpitating on the air before his eyes, a smudge that will not go away.

☑ illusion

a false sensory perception based on natural stimulation of a sensory receptor

d. This exemplifies ❒ an illusion/❒ a hallucination/❒ a delusion which is defined as ____.

e. Here, lawyer Porfiry Petrovitch, in Fyodor Dostoyevsky's *Crime and Punishment*, discusses a client:

"Yes, in our legal practice there was a case almost exactly similar, a case of morbid psychology," Porfiry went on quickly. "A man confessed to murder and how he kept it up! It was a regular hallucination; he brought forward facts, he imposed upon every one and why? He had been partly, but only partly, unintentionally the cause of a murder and when he knew that he had given the murderers the opportunity, he sank into dejection, it got on his mind and turned his brain, he began imagining things, and he persuaded himself that he was the murderer. But at last the High Court of Appeals went into it and the poor fellow was acquitted and put under proper care."

☑ No

☑ delusion

A delusion is a false belief that reason cannot dispel.

i. Was lawyer Petrovitch correct in stating that his client suffered from "a regular hallucination"? ❒ Yes/❒ No.

ii. Is the client's mental aberration ❒ an illusion/❒ a delusion?

iii. Define a delusion.

____

Editorial Note: Although lawyer Petrovitch mistakenly stated that his client had hallucinations rather than delusions, his legal instinct was right. Even a harsh, oppressive society like czarist Russia recognized that a confession does not establish guilt, because delusions may cause people to confess to crimes they did not commit. Moreover, if the police concentrate too much on obtaining confessions (often by physical and mental duress), they may not concentrate enough on obtaining conclusive, objective evidence of the real perpetrator. This magnificent insight against self-incrimination, reflected in our Fifth Amendment, protects persons against their own mental quirks and against overzealous prosecution.

5. **Localizing significance of hallucinations:** Although hallucinations may accompany a variety of mental illnesses or diffuse metabolic diseases, repetitively experienced hallucinations may indicate a lesion of the appropriate sensory cortex. A lesion in the occipital cortex might cause hallucinations of vision; in the uncus, of smell; and in the postcentral gyrus, of somatic sensation. Such hallucinations often constitute part of the aura, or forewarning, of an epileptic seizure produced by a focal epileptic discharge in one of these areas.

BIBLIOGRAPHY · The Mental Status

Arciniegas DB, Beresford TB. *Neuropsychiatry.* New York, Cambridge University Press, 2001.

Gross CG. A Hole in the head. More Tales in the History of Neuroscience. The MIT Press. Cambridge, Massachusetts, London, England, 2009.

Keele K. Anatomics of pain. Springfield, IL, Charles C. Thomas, 1957.

McCrea M, Kelly JP, Randolph C, et al. Standardized assessment of concussion (SAC): on site mental status evaluation of the athlete. *J Head Trauma Rehabil* 1998;13:27–35.

Strub RL, Black FW. *The Mental Status Examination in Neurology,* 4th ed. Philadelphia, FA Davis, 2000.

II. AGNOSIA, APRAXIA, AND APHASIA

I translate into ordinary words the Latin of their corrupt preachers, whereby it is revealed as humbug.

—**Bertolt Brecht (1898–1956)**

A. Introduction to agnosia, apraxia, and aphasia

Fate foredooms every medical student to address the deficits signified by these three mystifying Greek terms. Despite the fascinating subject, the name-plagued literature on agnosia, apraxia, and aphasia discourages even the hardiest scholar. Aphasiologists, in particular, are a contentious lot. Each one, compulsively it seems, must disagree with the methods, concepts, and nomenclature of their predecessors. Philosophy and polysyllabic words prevail, resulting in considerable humbug, hence, the quote from Brecht. For salvation, we shun the rhetoric and simply ask: By what operations do we discover the signified deficits?

B. Agnosia

1. **Review of agnosia:** A*gnosia* means literally *not knowing.* A root of a word when attached to *-agnosia* or *-ognosia* then specifies what the Pt does not know. As a review from Chapter 10, list some common agnosias tested in the Standard NE.

   ____

   ____

Astereognosia, agraphognosia, atopognosia, anosognosia, and tactile agnosia.

2. **General definition of agnosia:** Knowing the operations that disclose agnosia (e.g., give the Pt certain stimuli to identify) justifies a general definition. **Agnosia is the inability to understand the meaning, import, or symbolic significance of ordinary sensory stimuli even though the sensory pathways and sensorium are relatively intact.** Learn this definition. Agnosias affect various modalities, visual, auditory, or tactile. The Pt may fail to recognize stimuli in one modality but then recognize them in another.
3. An optimal definition not only states what something is but what it is not and the conditions necessary to diagnose it. The necessary conditions to diagnose agnosia are
   a. The Pt's sensory pathways are relatively intact.
   b. The Pt's sensorium and mental status are relatively intact.
   c. The Pt previously understood the symbolic significance of the stimulus, i.e., was familiar with it.
   d. An organic cerebral lesion causes the deficit.
4. These conditions exclude Pts with interrupted sensory pathways, mental retardation, overt dementia, and functional mental illnesses such as hysteria and negativism.
5. Agnosias beyond the scope of this text include **associative** visual agnosia (modality-specific inability to recognize and name previously known objects or their pictures or to demonstrate their use), **apperceptive** visual agnosia (impaired perception of patterns and inability to recognize shapes; Giannakopoulos, 1999), and **color** agnosias.

C. Agraphognosia (agraphesthesia)

1. **Technique for testing:** With the Pt's eyes closed, trace letters or numbers between 1 and 10 on the skin of the palm or fingertips. Use any blunt tip, such as the cap end of a ballpoint pen.
   a. Normal educated persons rarely miss the traced figures, but a normal person unpracticed in numbers may sometimes err.
   b. In testing for agraphognosia in the left hand, you test the ❒ right/❒ left ______________ lobe of the brain.

☑ right; parietal

graphanesthesia

2. For a Pt unable to recognize letters written on the skin and whose lesion had destroyed sensory pathways, the correct term would be ________________.
3. The same pathway from the periphery to the somatosensory cortex that detects the direction of movement of a stimulus across the skin also mediates graphognosia (Bender et al., 1982).

D. Prosopagnosia

1. **Prosopagnosia** means the inability to recognize faces in person or in photos.
2. **Technique to test for prosopagnosia:** The Ex asks someone known to the Pt to enter the room. The Pt cannot recognize the person's face but does recognize the individual immediately by the voice sound when the person speaks. When looking at a facial photo of family or a well-known celebrity, the Pt can see the face and can even describe the parts but fails to recognize who the person is. It probably should be noted that this syndrome is not just limited to recognizing human faces, but to recognizing items with specific historical significance within a class of objects. As such, patients with prosopagnosia also have trouble identifying their car among a series of cars, their own clothing, etc.
3. The lesion usually occupies the inferomedial temporo-occipital region, irrigated by cortical branches of the posterior cerebral artery (Damasio and Damasio, 1989; Hudson and Grace, 2000; Tranel and Damasio, 1996). The lesion is usually bilateral, but if unilateral, it is usually right-sided (Wada and Yamamoto, 2000). Lesions in this region also cause an acquired type of color agnosia (achromatopsia or chromatagnosia).

E. Technique to test for agnosias of the body scheme: autotopagnosia (asomatognosia)

1. **The concept of a body scheme:** One's brain knows one's anatomic parts, boundaries, and postures as a grand gestalt called the **body scheme** or **somatognosia** (Castle and Phillips, 2002; Coslett et al., 2002; Miller et al., 2001). Even a puppy knows its parts and separates self from nonself. The normal body scheme, such as finger localization (finger gnosia) and right-left orientation, only becomes formally testable in 4- to 6-year-old children and thus illustrates a definite developmental timetable (Reed, 1967).
2. Neuropsychiatric disorders may cause body scheme delusions (Castle and Phillips, 2002). In anorexia nervosa, the person perceives herself as too fat, no matter how emaciated she actually becomes. A person may erroneously perceive normal body parts, such as the nose, breasts, or, in transsexuals, the genitalia, as misshapen.
3. Several terms express the concept of *somatognosia* or its antonym *somatagnosia*. **Topagnosia** is the inability to localize skin stimuli. **Autotopagnosia** means the inability to locate, identify, and orient one's body parts, i.e., body scheme agnosia.
4. **Technique to test for two autotopagnosias: tactile finger agnosia and right-left disorientation**
   a. For identifying the fingers, assign the numbers 1 to 5 to the digits of each of the Pt's hands, beginning with the thumb, or use names. Then, with the Pt's eyes closed, randomly touch a digit on the right or left hand and ask the Pt to identify the finger by number or name and whether it is the right or left hand (Reitan and Wolfson, 1993).
      i. If the Pt seems to have right-left disorientation, give further commands such as, "Touch your right hand to your left ear," to verify the deficit.
      ii. To further explore right-left disorientation, ask the Pt to point out your own right and left hands and digits by number or name.
      iii. The lesion usually occupies the region of the left angular gyrus (posterior parasylvian area). See Gerstmann's syndrome, Section IIIO.
   b. Also test the Pt for autotopagnosia by placing a part in one position and asking the Pt to duplicate the position with the opposite extremity, with the

eyes closed. For example, elevate the Pt's arm to a position on one side and ask the Pt to hold it there and to duplicate the position with the opposite extremity.

F. Left-side hemispatial inattention

1. Patients with right parietal lesions often fail to attend to the entire left half of space. Evidence for this unilateral neglect comes from observing that the Pt ignores persons, objects, or any stimuli from the affected side, fails to dress that side, and fails to eat the food from that half of the plate. Such Pts, at least early after an acute lesion, often have anosognosia (see Section G).
2. **Technique to test for left-side hemispatial inattention**
   a. Ask the Pt to draw a cross or any symmetrical figure such as a bicycle wheel with spokes or the face of a clock. The Pt will draw the right half of the figure accurately but make mistakes in completing the drawing on the opposite side (Fig. 11-4; Critchley, 1953; Stone et al., 1991).
   b. The line bisection test demonstrates left-side inattention better than drawing a clock face (Ishiai et al., 1993). Draw a straight line 20 cm long across a sheet of paper and ask the Pt to make a pencil mark exactly in the center. The Pt with a right parietal lobe lesion makes the mark considerably to the right of the true center because of neglect of the left half of space (Tegner and Levander, 1991).

G. Anosognosia

1. **Definition:** Josef Babinski (1857–1932) introduced *anosognosia* to describe a Pt who had a left hemiplegia and left-side sensory loss but who was unaware of his neurologic deficits. Some authors now use *anosognosia* generically for lack of awareness of any bodily defect. Although highly characteristic on the left side after right parietal lesions, it can affect the right side after left parietal lesions, particularly in the acute phase of the lesion (Stone et al., 1991).
2. **Technique to test for anosognosia**
   a. The Ex, noting a left hemiplegia, asks the Pt whether anything is wrong with the side. The Pt replies *No.* If the Ex asks whether the Pt can move the left arm, the Pt will reply *Yes* despite complete hemiplegia (Levine et al., 1991).
   b. The most dramatic test for anosognosia is this: Stand on the left side of the Pt's bed and place the Pt's hemiplegic arm on the bed alongside the Pt. Lay your own left arm across the Pt's waist. Ask the Pt to reach over and pick up his own left hand. He will grope across his abdomen, grasp your hand, and hold it triumphantly aloft, never realizing the error.

H. Inattention to double simultaneous cutaneous stimuli

1. Synonyms include *sensory suppression*, *sensory extinction*, and *sensory inattention*. As with agnosias, the sensory pathways from the periphery to and including the primary sensory cortex must be intact, making the phenomenon a test of association cortex. Inattention to bilateral double stimuli occurs with vision (Chapter 3, Section I B 2), hearing (Chapter 8, Section IV H), and touch.
2. **Technique to test for tactile inattention to simultaneous bilateral stimuli (double simultaneous stimulation)**
   a. Inform the Pt that you may touch one or both sides. With the Pt's eyes closed and using light pressure, brush one or simultaneously both cheeks randomly with the tips of your index finger or wisps of cotton.
   b. The Pt reports whatever is felt and should perceive one or both stimuli. Similarly test the dorsum of the hands and then the feet.
   c. If the Pt reports only one stimulus after the Ex has applied simultaneous stimuli, the Ex again states, "I may be touching you in more than one place. Don't let me fool you." Then alternate, randomly touching only one or both sides,

until you determine whether the Pt consistently does or does not feel bilateral simultaneous stimuli.

d. Inattention to simultaneous bilateral stimuli is most prominent after right parietal lobe lesions, in which case the Pt fails to attend to the stimulus on the left (Bender, 1952; Critchley, 1966; Meador et al., 1998; Weinstein and Friedland, 1977). Occasionally, with left parietal lesions, the Pt will not attend to the right side on simultaneous stimulation. After simultaneous stimulation of both sides, the Pt with a right parietal lesion *inattends* to stimuli from the ❒ right/❒ left side.

☑ left

3. **Technique to test for inattention to simultaneous unilateral stimuli**

a. On one side, simultaneously touch the face and hand several times, and then the foot and hand and face and foot. The person normally reports both stimuli. Parietal lobe lesions impair recognition of both stimuli.

b. Learning-disabled children without gross structural lesions of the brain often suppress double stimulation on one side. Usually the Pt feels the face or foot stimulus and suppresses the hand stimulus.

I. Review of localization of agnosias and loss of discriminative sensory modalities

1. Recite the definition of agnosia and the qualifying requirements.
2. Agnosias generally signify lesions of the association areas that extend from the primary sensory receptive areas or of the thalamocortical circuits of the association areas. The cortex works by thalamocortical and corticothalamic feedback circuits. The association nuclei of the thalamus project to the association areas of the cortex, just as the sensory nuclei of the thalamus project to the respective sensory cortices. The thalamic projections to primary sensory cortex run courses different from those for the association pathways and can be preserved when lesions interrupt the association circuitry. Interruption of a feedback circuit at any point may cause defects similar to lesions of only the cortical component of the circuit. Thus thalamic lesions may cause hemineglect, some agnosias, and aphasia (Bruyn, 1989). In these instances, the sensory pathways are at least partly preserved, as the definition requires.
3. Although right parietal lesions most commonly cause contralateral hemiinattention, lesions of either parietal lobe regularly cause loss of discriminative modalities contralaterally, such as astereognosis, agraphognosia, atopagnosia, and loss of two point discrimination (Fig. 11-9). The primary modalities of touch, pain and temperature, and vibration remain more or less intact with cortical lesions. Lesions of infracortical pathways or in the periphery more commonly significantly impair these modalities.
4. For autotopagnosias such as finger agnosia and right-left disorientation, the relevant association area is the left posterior parasylvian area. In this case, a unilateral lesion causes bilateral deficits of the body scheme. Lesions of the left posterior parasylvian area cause, in addition to bilateral finger agnosia and right-left disorientation, dyscalculia and dysgraphia (see Gerstmann's syndrome).
5. In summary, lesions of *either* parietal lobe may cause contralateral loss of astereognosis and other discriminative modalities, but hemispatial inattention and anosognosia are more common with ❒ right/❒ left parietal lobe lesions.
6. In contrast, finger agnosia and right-left disorientation are more common with ❒ right/❒ left posterior parasylvian lesions.

☑ right

☑ left

BIBLIOGRAPHY · Agnosia

Bender M. *Disorders in Perception, with Particular Reference to the Phenomena of Extinction and Displacement.* Springfield, Charles C Thomas, 1952.

Bender M, Stacy C, Cohen J. Agraphesthesia: a disorder of directional cutaneous kinesthesia or a disorientation in cutaneous space. *J Neurol Sci* 1982;53:531–555.

Bruyn RPM. Thalamic aphasia: a conceptual critique. *J Neurol* 1989;236:21–25.

Castle DJ, Phillips Ka. *Disorders of Body Image.* Petersfield, United Kingdom, Wrightson Biomedical, 2002.

Coslett HB, Saffran EM, Schwoebel J. Knowledge of the human body. A distinct semantic domain. *Neurology* 2002;59:357–363.

Critchley M. *The parietal lobes*. London, Edward Arnold & Co,1953.

Damasio H, Damasio AR. *Lesion Analysis in Neuropsychology.* New York, Oxford University Press, 1989.

Hudson AJ, Grace GM. Misidentification syndromes related to face specific area in the fusiform gyrus. *J Neurol Neurosurg Psychiatry* 2000;69:645–648.

Ishiai S, Sugishita M, Ichikawa T, et al. Clock-drawing test and unilateral spatial neglect. *Neurology* 1993;43:106–110.

Levine DN, Calvanio R, Rinn WE: The pathogenesis of anosognosia for hemiplegia. *Neurology* 1991;41:1770–1780.

Meador KJ, Ray PG, Day L, et al. Physiology of somatosensory perception. Cerebral lateralization and extinction. *Neurology* 1998;51:721–727.

Miller BL, Seeley WW, Mychak P, et al. Neuroanatomy of the self. Evidence from patients with frontotemporal dementia. *Neurology* 2001;57:817–821.

Reed J. Lateralized finger agnosia and reading achievement at ages 6 and 10. *Child Dev* 1967;38:213–220.

Reitan RM, Wolfson D. *The Halstead-Reitan Neuropsychological Test Battery. Theory and Clinical Interpretation,* 2nd ed. Tucson, Neuropsychology Press, 1993.

Stone SP, Wilson B, Wroot A, et al. The assessment of visuo-spatial neglect after acute stroke. *J Neurol Neurosurg Psychiatry* 1991;54:345–350.

Tegner R, Levander M. The influence of stimulus properties on visual neglect. *J Neurol Neurosurg Psychiatry* 1991;54:882–887.

Tranel D, Damasio AR. Agnosias and apraxias. In Bradley WG, Daroff R, Fenichel GM, Marsden CD, eds. *Neurology in Clinical Practice. Principles of Diagnosis and Management,* 2nd ed. Boston, Butterworth Heinemann, 1996, Chapter 16, pp. 119–130.

Wada Y, Yamamoto T. Selective impairment of facial recognition due to a haematoma restricted to the right fusiform and lateral occipital region. *J Neurol Neurosurg Psychiatry* 2000;71:254–257.

Weinstein EA, Friedland RP, eds. *Hemi-attention Syndromes and Hemisphere Specialization. Advances in Neurology, Vol 18.* New York, Raven, 1977.

J. Apraxia

1. **Definition of apraxia:** The ability to execute a voluntary act is called **praxia** (*praxis* = action, as in *practice*). By negating *praxia*, the ability to act, we describe *apraxia*, the inability to act. **Apraxia means the inability to perform a voluntary act even though the motor system, sensory system, and mental status are relatively intact.** Learn this definition.
2. **Formal criteria to distinguish apraxia from other motor defects**
   a. The Pt's motor system is sufficiently intact to execute the act.
   b. The Pt's sensorium is sufficiently intact to understand the act.
   c. The Pt comprehends and attempts to cooperate.
   d. The Pt's previous skills were sufficient to perform the act.
   e. The Pt has an organic cerebral lesion as the cause of the deficit.
   f. In summary, the Pt must comprehend the act, cooperate in attempting it, and have a motor system sufficiently intact to execute the act. These requisites exclude Pts with paralysis or functional mental illnesses, such as hysteria or negativism, profound dementia, and mental retardation, to whom *apraxia* is not meant to apply.
   g. If the definition and conditions for diagnosing apraxia causes the strange feeling of repeating a previous experience (the déjà vu of anterior temporal lobe lesions), we are on the right track. Review frame II B 2 that defines agnosia.
3. **Distinction between apraxia and other motor deficits:** Apraxic Pts are often unaware of their deficits and may do an act automatically that they cannot do on command. For example, apraxic Pts may fail to stick out their tongue and lick

their lips on command but may then lick their lips automatically. The Pt may fail to make a fist when asked in close the fingers but may automatically grasp an object, such as a spoon.

a. With pyramidal lesions, the paralysis precludes doing the act voluntarily or automatically, thus violating a necessary condition that the motor system be fairly intact. The paralyzed Pt may also have apraxia, but the paralysis prevents its recognition.

b. The Pt with a cerebellar lesion retains the ability to perform an act but cannot perform it smoothly.

c. With basal motor nuclei lesions, involuntary movements or rigidity impede down the act, but the sequence of the act remains possible.

K. Technique to test for common apraxias

1. The Ex tests for apraxia almost inadvertently in giving routine commands such as: "Stick out your tongue." "Make a fist." "Walk across the room." These commands disclose tongue, hand, and gait apraxias, respectively.
2. For formal testing, the Ex makes special verbal requests and, if that fails, demonstrates acts for the Pt to pantomime.
3. **Face-tongue (bucco-facial) apraxia:** Ask the Pt to protrude the tongue and move it up, down, right, and left and lick the lips. Ask the Pt to act as if blowing out a match or sucking on a straw. If verbal instruction fails, try miming.
4. **Arm (ideomotor) apraxia:** More complicated apraxias such as ideomotor apraxia require sequential actions. Ask the Pt to demonstrate a sequence: how to use silverware, thread a needle, strike a match and light a candle, and use a key to lock and unlock a lock, or use scissors or other tool. The Ex may provide the actual materials or tools or may have the Pt imitate gestures and hand positions (Heilman and Valenstein, 1979; O'Hare et al., 1999).
5. **Constructional apraxia:** Ask the Pt to copy geometric figures (a cross, interlocking pentagons, or clock face) or construct them out of matchsticks.
6. **Dressing apraxia:** Watch the Pt try to get dressed. The apraxic Pt cannot orient the clothes to put them on and gets the shoes on the wrong foot. Usually this is associated with right parietal lesions and is part of the neglect syndrome.
7. **Gait apraxia (Bruns ataxia):** Ask the Pt to rise and walk.
8. **Writing and speaking apraxia (aphasia):** Explained in the next section.
9. **Global apraxia in children:** The child lags in motor skills such as chewing, swallowing, dressing, tying shoelaces, buttoning, and the use of cutting tools such as a knife and fork and scissors.

L. Patient analysis for identification of constructional and dressing apraxia

1. **Medical history:** A 67-year-old right-handed salesman with a college education had noticed dizziness, fatigue, and blurring of vision for 3 months. Three weeks before hospitalization, he began to have right frontal headaches. For 1 week, he had noticed weakness and slight numbness of his left extremities. Although he appeared dull and apathetic and did arithmetic poorly, his sensorium was otherwise intact.
2. **Motor examination:** The Pt could walk, but movements on the entire left side were moderately weak, except for normal frontalis and orbicularis oculi strength. He had no atrophy, tremor, dystaxia, or involuntary movements. Manipulation of the Pt's left extremities showed an initial catch followed by yielding of the part. Figure 11-2 shows the reflex pattern.

☑ upper motoneuron

a. His facial weakness was ☐ upper motoneuron/☐ lower motoneuron.

clasp-knife spasticity

b. Manipulation of the Pt's left extremities showed a type of hypertonus called ________________.

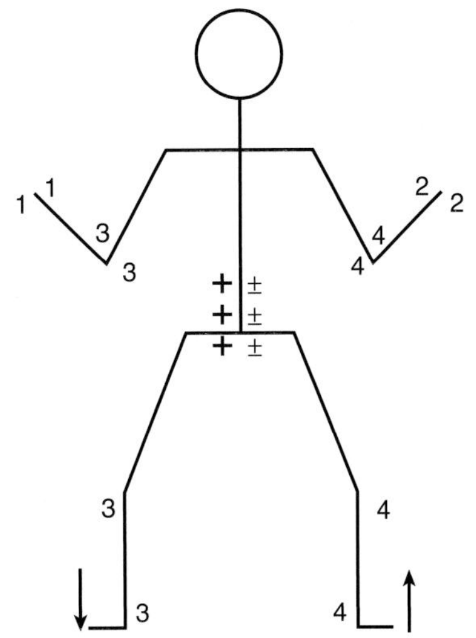

FIGURE 11-2. Reflex figurine of the patient.

spastic, hyperreflexic left hemiparesis with extensor toe sign, and reduced left-side abdominal and cremasteric reflexes

c. Integrate the total information from the physical examination and Fig. 11-2 to summarize the motor deficits and reflex changes detected thus far:

____

____.

3. **Sensory examination**

inattention or sensory suppression

a. Although the Pt could feel light touch on either side, perhaps less well on the left, he consistently failed to report a left-side stimulus when the Ex simultaneously touched both of the Pt's hands. He failed to report left-side stimuli when simultaneous sound stimuli were presented. This type of sensory deficit is called sensory _______________.

b. On the line bisection test, the Pt made the mark to the right of the true center.

astereognosis or tactile agnosia

c. The Pt recognized coins or a safety pin by vision or when placed in the right hand, but not in the left. The left-side deficit is called _______________.

agraphognosia

d. He had difficulty recognizing numbers traced on the left palm, a defect called _______________.

incomplete left homonymous hemianopsia

e. The visual field defect shown in Fig. 11-3 is called

____.

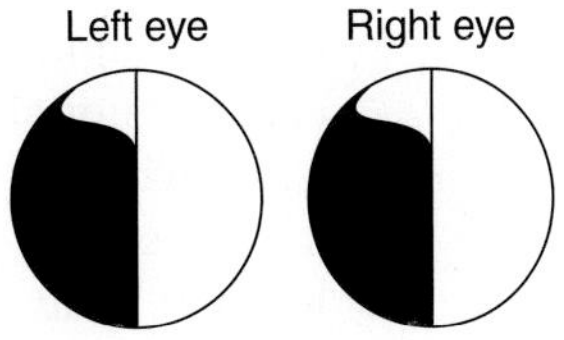

FIGURE 11-3. Visual fields of the patient.

☑ No

f. Would the Pt perceive simultaneous stimuli presented in the upper part of the left visual field and the temporal half of the right visual field? ❐ Yes/ ❐ No.

☑ No
The Pt had a left incomplete homonymous hemianopsia, which means blindness in the left visual field. His lesion had to interrupt the optic pathway to the visual cortex. Because the lesion interrupted the modality pathway or the defect does not qualify as agnosia.

g. Could you correctly say that the Pt had visual agnosia for the entire left half of space? ❐ Yes/❐ No. Explain.

____

____

4. **Testing for constructional apraxia**

a. As part of the test battery (to be described), the Pt named and tried to copy several geometric figures. Study his efforts in Fig. 11-4.

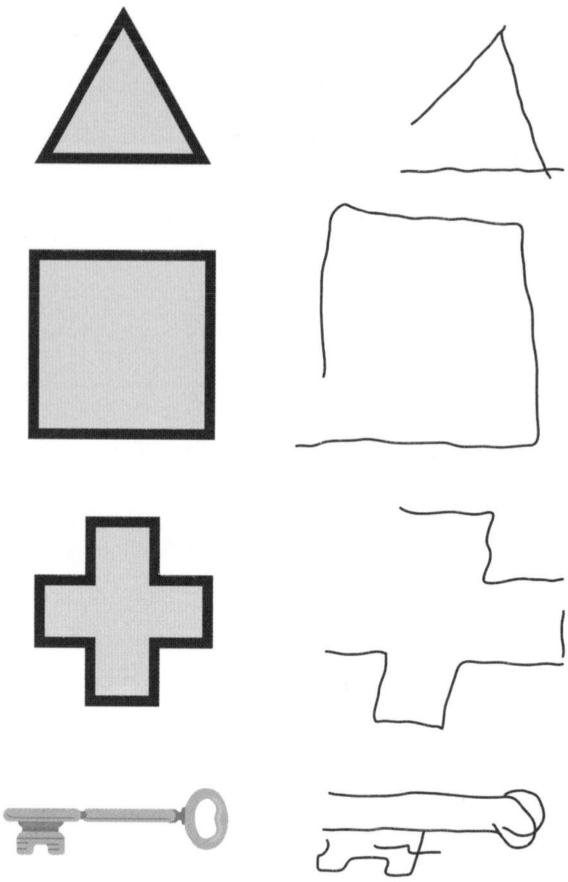

FIGURE 11-4. Stimulus figures for patient to name and copy. In the right-hand column are the attempts of the patient to copy the figures after he had named them correctly.

☑ left

b. In each instance, the Pt failed to complete the ❒ right/❒ left side of the figure. To appreciate the limitation of the defect to the left side, draw a vertical line to divide each of the Pt's figures exactly into right and left halves.

c. This Pt, a college graduate, failed to complete a simple voluntary act such as copying geometric figures. Yet he understood the task and had normal motility of his right hand. At first thought, you might suspect that his left hemianopsia caused the difficulty, but experience shows that Pts with only hemianopsia complete such figures. Because the present Pt met all of the criteria for apraxia, his deficit in the construction of geometric figures is called **constructional apraxia.** He also could not construct figures from match sticks. In Pts with left hemisphere lesions, the type of constructional apraxia for drawing or copying involves the gestalt of the figure, or both sides, rather than the left half, as in the Pt just described.

5. **Testing for dressing apraxia:** At the end of the NE, the Ex handed the Pt his pajama top. Ordinarily, if the Pt is disabled, the Ex helps the Pt dress. Watching this Pt dress constituted an essential part of the NE. He repeatedly fumbled the garment while trying put it on, demonstrating **dressing apraxia.**

6. **Localizing significance of dressing apraxia and left-side constructional apraxia**

☑ sensory inattention;
☑ anosognosia

a. Dressing apraxia and constructional apraxia, in which the Pt fails to complete the left side of figures, occur most frequently with a right posterior parietal lesion (Critchley, 1969; Joynt and Goldstein, 1975; Weinstein and Friedland, 1977). Check the finding(s) that would most likely accompany a right posterior parietal lesion: ❒ sensory inattention/❒ anosognosia/❒ bilateral finger agnosia/❒ right-left disorientation.

b. Ideomotor apraxias occur with lesions of the language-dominant hemisphere, almost always the left (Heilman et al., 2000; Meador et al., 1999). Usually the

Pt with ideomotor apraxia also has aphasia (Papagno et al., 1993). Both hands are usually affected, although the lesion is unilateral.

7. **Summary of the Pt's clinical deficits**
   a. **Motor:** Mild spastic, hyperreflexic left hemiparesis with an extensor toe sign. Severe constructional and dressing apraxia.
   b. **Sensory:** Slight left hemihypesthesia and hemihypalgesia, left-side astereognosis, left-side tactile and auditory inattention, and incomplete left homonymous hemianopia.
8. **Localizing significance of the Pt's neurologic signs:** How to "think circuitry."
   a. This Pt's hemiparesis implicates involvement of the ________________ tract.

pyramidal

   b. To cause the hemiparesis, the pyramidal lesion would have to involve some level between the motor cortex and the upper cervical cord. What *motor* finding locates the pyramidal tract lesion at or rostral to the pons?

   ____

   ____

UMN facial palsy from interruption of corticobulbar fibers that activate the lower part of the face.

   c. The agnosia and apraxia implicate a lesion at the level of the ❒ brainstem/ ❒ sensorimotor cortex/❒ association cortex or its intracerebral connections.

☑ association cortex or its intracerebral connections

   d. The particular types of agnosia and apraxia implicate a lesion of the ❒ right/ ❒ left/❒ both cerebral hemisphere(s), mainly in the ❒ frontal/❒ parietal/ ❒ occipital/❒ temporal region.

☑ right; ☑ parietal

9. **The principle of parsimony:** Although a brainstem lesion might account for the Pt's left hemiparesis and mild hemihypesthesia, his apraxia and agnosia require a lesion of the dorsolateral cerebral wall in the parietal region. Thus, although we might postulate separate lesions at the levels of the brainstem and cerebral wall, we now invoke a most important principle in diagnosis, the *principle of parsimony*. Called *Occam's razor* (William of Occam, 1280–1349), this principle requires us to seek the simplest explanation: a single lesion and a single diagnosis. In other words, we seek the simplest, the most *parsimonious*, explanation. Thus, if a single lesion caused the hemiparesis, hemihypesthesia, and agnosia-apraxia, it involves the ❒ spinal cord/❒ brainstem/❒ dorsolateral cerebral wall.

☑ dorsolateral cerebral wall

   a. The hemianopsia indicates a lesion at some level along the visual pathway. Review the visual pathway in Fig. 3-4 and the course of the optic radiation through the lateral cerebral wall in Figs. 3-5 and 3-6. Hemianopia implicates a lesion:

      ❒ (1) In the retina or optic nerve

      ❒ (2) In the anterior part of the temporal lobe

      ❒ (3) Between the optic chiasm and the visual cortex of the calcarine fissure

☑ (3)

   b. Applying the principle of parsimony, could the previously postulated lesion of the dorsolateral cerebral wall in the parietal lobe also interrupt the optic pathway? If so, where? ❒ Yes/❒ No. Explain.

   ____

   ____

☑ Yes
The geniculocalcarine tract runs through the deep white matter of the parietotemporal region. See Fig. 3-5A.

   c. The preservation of a bit of the superior visual field indicates that the most inferior axons of the geniculocalcarine tract are intact. The lesion that causes the partial hemianopia involves the superior part of the geniculocalcarine tract, which runs through the parietal lobe and adjacent temporal and occipital lobes (Fig. 3-5A).
   d. In addition to the agnostic-apraxic and visual field deficits, implicating the posterior inferior parietal area, the slight hemihypalgesia and hemihypesthesia implicate the primary somesthetic receptive region of the ________________ gyrus of the ❒ right/❒ left ________________ lobe.

postcentral; ☑ right; parietal

   e. The mild left hemiparesis implicates the motor area located in the right ________________ gyrus.

precentral

   f. The left-side auditory inattention implicates the auditory association area in the ❒ anterior/❒ posterior part of the ❒ right/❒ left temporoparietal region.

☑ posterior; ☑ right

g. Shade Fig. 11-5 to show the presumed extent of the lesion. Use dark shading for the regions that have produced the severest or most complete deficits and lighter shading for the regions responsible for the lesser deficits. Frame L 7, earlier, summarizes the deficits that require a localizing explanation.

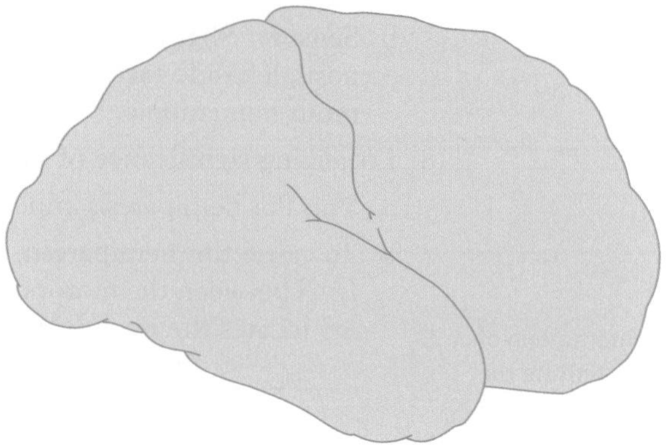

FIGURE 11-5. Blank of right cerebral hemisphere to be shaded to show the presumed location of the patient's lesion.

10. **Neuropathologic considerations**

a. By causing edema and compressing vessels, focal lesions may impair the function of surrounding brain tissue. The severest signs usually reflect the site of maximum tissue damage and, therefore, best predict the lesion site. The Pt's severest defects, the hemianopia and dressing and constructional apraxia, suggest maximum damage to the right posterior parasylvian area, with less involvement of the sensorimotor cortex of the paracentral region.

b. Radiographic examination showed a mass in the predicted right parieto-occipital region. Craniotomy and biopsy disclosed a large, expanding neoplasm, a glioblastoma multiforme, causing pressure on the surrounding brain. The surgeon removed the right occipital lobe, providing internal decompression. Postoperatively, the left hemiparesis disappeared, suggesting that pressure and edema from the neoplasm had caused it, rather than direct extension of the neoplasm to the paracentral area (Fig. 11-6).

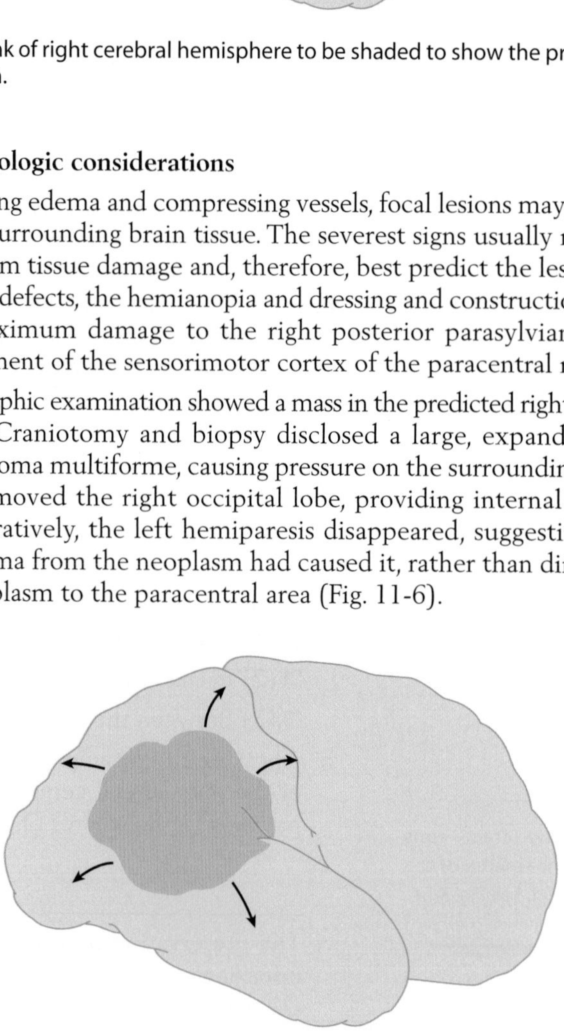

FIGURE 11-6. Lateral view of the right cerebral hemisphere to show the actual location of the patient's lesion, as determined at autopsy examination. The arrows indicate the surrounding edema of the hemisphere, which led to clinical signs such as hemiparesis, implicating damage to tissue beyond the immediate confines of the neoplasm.

c. Ordinarily, a Pt with a lesion in the right posterior parasylvian area might also have anosognosia. The Pt failed to show it before the operation, but afterward he failed to recognize that he had a left hemianopia. Anosognosia occurs more commonly with large, acute lesions, such as infarcts, than when lesions evolve relatively slowly, as with neoplasms.

BIBLIOGRAPHY · Apraxia

See end of Aphasia section.

III. APHASIA: AGNOSIA AND APRAXIA OF LANGUAGE

A. Survey of the levels and types of speech disturbance

1. Communicative speech consists of words arranged according to the rules of grammar and syntax and invested with prosody. Many factors—culture, thought disorders such as schizophrenia, neuroses, and structural lesions of the brain—alter the communicative content and emotional connotation of speech.
2. We may now distinguish four levels of disturbed speech production: **dysphonia, dysarthria, dysprosody,** and **dysphasia.** At the lowest level, **dysphonia** consists of a disturbance in, or a lack of, the production of sounds in the larynx. **Dysarthria** means a disorder in articulating speech sounds. Then come the **dysprosodies** that consist of scanning speech (cerebellar), plateau speech (basal motor nuclei/parkinsonian), and stuttering, cluttering, and absence of emotional inflections (cerebral). At the highest level, **dysphasia** means a disturbance in the understanding or expression of words as symbols for communication. Review (or if you wish, write out) the definitions of these terms and check your definitions against the ones given in Section III of the Standard NE.
3. One end of the neuropsychiatric spectrum of speech disorders consists of little or no speech, called **mutism** or **aphonia.** Varieties of mutism include deaf mutism, elective mutism, psychogenic mutism, autism and other retardation syndromes, catatonia, depression, postictal state, and cerebellar mutism following posterior fossa surgery. (Gordon, 2001). Akinetic mutism or bradylalia may follow bilateral lesions of the thalamus, basal motor nuclei, or upper brainstem. Absence of speech or delayed speech in a child always raises the question of mental retardation, autism, or deafness.
4. The other end of the speech spectrum consists of too much speech, logorrhea (pressure of speech or an increase in the amount and rate of speech, as seen in mania), fluent aphasia, cluttering, echolalia, vocal tics, and finally the compulsive talker, the conversational narcissist who never has a silent thought and articulates every bit of trivia that comes to mind.

B. Definition of aphasia

1. Literally, *a* = lack of, and *phasis* = speech. **Aphasia means the inability to understand or express words as symbols for communication, even though the primary sensorimotor pathways to receive and express language and the mental status are relatively intact.** Learn this definition. The definition excludes language disturbances caused by functional mental illness, global retardation, dementia, blindness, deafness, stuttering, or neuromuscular disease.
2. The purist would reserve *aphasia* for total loss of language, and *dysphasia* for partial loss, but clinicians use the prefixes *a-* and *dys-* interchangeably.

C. The four avenues for communication by language

1. A moment's introspection discloses four major avenues of language. We express language by *speaking* or *writing,* and we receive it by *reading* or *listening.* Thus, we *speak/write* and *listen/read*. Additional modes of communication include Morse code, Braille, sign language, facial expression, pantomime, not to mention "body language" and the information conveyed by clothing, tattoos, hair style, and makeup.
2. Some Pts with brain lesions, although neither deaf nor blind, fail to understand the meaning of spoken or written words. The general term for failure of a mentally intact Pt with intact sensory pathways to understand the meaning of a stimulus is

agnosia

______________. Because of the special significance of language for human communication, we designate agnosia for spoken or written words as **receptive** or **sensory aphasia.**

apraxia

3. Some Pts with brain lesions produce the wrong syllables, wrong words, or even no words when attempting to speak or write. The general term for failure of a mentally intact, nonparalyzed Pt to execute such voluntary acts is ______________.
4. We call apraxia for writing or speaking **expressive** or **motor aphasia.**

reading; listening; writing; speaking

5. Recite the four ordinary avenues for receiving and expressing language: ______________, ______________, ______________, and ______________.

D. Volitional, propositional, or declarative speech versus automatic or exclamatory speech

1. Some speech, **exclamatory speech,** communicates the emotional state of the moment, rather than ideas. On stubbing a toe, we automatically exclaim, "Ouch!" Exclamations, particularly expletives, erupt spontaneously, unwilled, without deliberation or forethought, although we can also produce them volitionally. Patients with Tourette's syndrome may produce involuntary exclamations as vocal tics.
2. In contrast, we communicate ideas by volitional **declarations** or **propositions.** The sentence may consist of a simple declaration, "The fire engine is red," or a distinct proposition, "Fire engines ought to be red." A proposition states something for analysis that *was, is,* or *could* be. A proposition is preeminently volitional, planned, and often crafty. **Aphasics lose declarative and propositional speech but tend to retain some exclamatory speech.** Thus, after struggling but completely failing to produce a propositional statement, the aphasic Pt sighs in anger and exclaims spontaneously and with perfect clarity, "Oh damn, I can't." Yet when asked to repeat the automatically uttered sentence, the Pt fails again because it now has become propositional or volitional speech. In analogy, recall that in pseudobulbar palsy, the Pt loses volitional movements but retains or even shows exaggerated, automatic laughing or crying. These facts demonstrate that the brain uses different circuits for volitional behavior, as contrasted to emotional or more automatic behavior (Bookheimer et al., 2000). In general, aphasics also retain humming and singing better than spoken language.

E. Clinical testing for aphasia

1. **Detecting aphasia during the history:** Aphasia testing begins with the history. You will readily detect gross defects in language reception or expression. The mildly aphasic Pt produces less than the expected amount of written and spoken language. Although the Pt's conversation remains goal directed, the Pt fails to hit the nail on the head with crisp, logical statements. The speech may degenerate to circumlocutions, platitudes, and clichés dredged more from memory than composed of volitional, novel, or artful word combinations. Less commonly, the aphasic Pt becomes wordy, as if by preempting the conversation, the Pt can prevent the other person from saying something that the Pt cannot understand, or the Pt may show a gratuitous redundancy in searching for *le mot juste* (just the right word). The clues to dysphasia are as follows:
   a. Searching for words, pauses, and hesitations.
   b. Substitution of the wrong words or phonemes.
   c. Poverty of speech or the converse, excessive production of sounds that resemble words but fail to communicate.
   d. Puzzlement and hesitations in response to ordinary statements made in the course of conversation.
   e. Loss of intonation and prosody.

f. Frequent dysarthria.

g. Irritation or distress at the inability to communicate.

2. **Usual operational steps in examining the Pt for aphasia**

   a. During the give and take of the history, listen for word choice, in particular word substitutions, a searching for words, articulation, hesitations, prosody, and the quantity of speech.

   b. Test ability of the Pt to repeat words spoken by the Ex.

   c. Test word comprehension by questions and commands.

   d. Show the Pt common objects to name.

   e. Have the Pt write a sentence to dictation.

   f. Have the Pt read and interpret a sentence, a paragraph, or symbols.

3. **Formal aphasia screening tests:** The Ex uses a formal and comprehensive battery (e.g., Boston Diagnostic Aphasia Examination, Western Aphasia Battery) to test the Pt's ability to read, write, name things, repeat words and sentences, and copy them to dictation and to follow written and verbal commands. The indication for the test battery is a suspicion raised during the history or NE of a brain lesion (Damasio, 1992).

F. General classification of aphasia

1. **Expressive and receptive aphasia:** Traditionally, neurologists have classified aphasia as **receptive, expressive,** or **mixed expressive-receptive aphasia,** also called **global aphasia.** Most Pts have mixed expressive and receptive language deficits, with at least some impairment of all four avenues of language. In judging relative loss of receptive and expressive language, recall that the active expression of language requires more effort than receiving it. Therefore, aphasics typically comprehend language better than they express it, just as children do as they learn to talk.

2. **Fluent and nonfluent aphasia:** Many researchers classify aphasia as *fluent* or *nonfluent*, depending on the amount of speech sounds produced and combine these terms with the traditional expressive-receptive scheme (Goodglass, 1993; Table 11-4).

TABLE 11-4 · Classification of the Aphasias

Type of aphasia	Fluency	Understands	Repetition	Naming	Lesion location
Broca's	Poor; effortful	Good	Poor	Poor	Left posterior inferior frontal operculum (Fig. 11-7A)
Wernicke's	Good; fluent sounds but "word salad"	Poor	Poor	Poor	Posterior parasylvian, temporal operculum (Figs. 11-7F and 11-7C)
Conduction	Good; poor articulation	Good	Poor	Poor	Posterior parasylvian (Figs. 11-7C and 11-7B–11-7E)
Transcortical motor	Poor	Good	Good	May be normal	Frontally (Fig. 11-7A) and superiorly, extending inward to striatum
Transcortical sensory	Good	Poor	Good	Usually normal	Parietal, temporal (Fig. 11-7C) involving the thalamocortical circuit
Global	None or scanty; or expletives only	Very poor	Very poor	Very poor	Entire parasylvian area (Figs. 11-7A–11-7F)

SOURCE: Data from Damasio AR. Aphasia. *N Engl J Med* 1992;326:531–539.

G. General localization of lesions causing aphasia

1. **Localization to the left hemisphere**

   a. The lesion that causes aphasia occupies the left cerebral hemisphere in almost all right-handed and most left-handed Pts. Therefore, we designate the left hemisphere as usually dominant for language. Operationally, in designating a hemisphere as dominant for language, we mean that a lesion of that hemisphere will result in aphasia, that physiologic tests, such as cortical stimulation (Penfield and Roberts, 1959), electrocorticography, and that functional scans will document activation of one or more zones of the left hemisphere during language tasks. Functional magnetic resonance imaging studies have indicated that 96% of right-handers are left hemisphere dominant, 76% of left-handers are left hemisphere dominant, and 10% of left-handers are right hemisphere dominant, at least for silent word generation (Pujol et al., 1999).

b. Normal hemispheres are anatomically asymmetric, with the left hemisphere larger than the right, particularly the **planum temporale.** The planum is a submerged area between the transverse temporal gyri (the primary auditory sensory cortex) and the posterior end of the sylvian fissure.

c. **Localization within the dominant hemisphere:** The lesion usually involves the parasylvian region of the left hemisphere (Fig. 11-7).

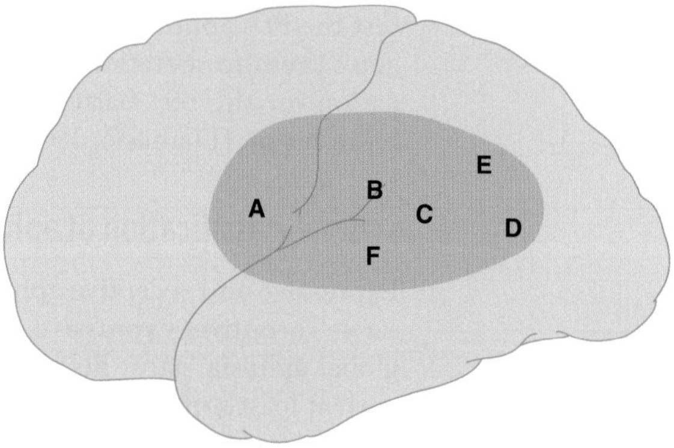

FIGURE 11-7. Lateral view of the left cerebral hemisphere to show the expected lesion sites in aphasic patients.

d. The lesion may extend into the subjacent deep white matter and into the caudate-putamen or the thalamus, thus interrupting the connections of the parasylvian cortex with the deep nuclear masses (Bruyn, 1989; Damasio, 1992; Kreisler et al., 2000; Mega and Alexander, 1994). Uncommonly, mostly in left-handers, the lesion occupies the homologous regions of the right hemisphere.

e. The clinical features of the aphasia fairly well predict the site of the lesion within the aphasiogenic zone depicted in Fig. 11-7. The lesions that cause expressive aphasia are more forward, toward the anterior inferior frontal region, and the lesions causing receptive aphasia are more posterior, toward the parieto-occipito-temporal junction (posterior parasylvian area; Brazis et al., 2001).

H. Broca's aphasia (motor aphasia, or nonfluent aphasia

1. **Clinical features**

a. The nonfluent aphasic Pt speaks telegraphically, sparsely, and slowly—hence, the term *nonfluent* (Mohr et al., 1978). The Pt has difficulty in word finding and naming. The Pt may use some nouns and verbs but omits the small connecting words, conjunctions such as *but*, *or*, and *and*, and articles such as *a*, *an*, or *the*, and prepositions. The Pt says, "I go house," instead of "I go to the house." In fact, as an excellent test sentence, ask the Pt to repeat "No *if*'s, *and*'s, *but*'s, *for*'s, or *or*'s."

b. The Pt fails to make associations, such as naming the makes of automobiles or naming a number of objects that are red.

c. The Pts with Broca's aphasia fails to inflect and modulate the normal rhythms of speech and thus displays one form of **dysprosody.**

d. The Pt with Broca's aphasia also has difficulty writing, suggesting that the posterior inferior part of the frontal lobe mediates speaking and writing.

e. Importantly, the Pt retains the ability to audit language and to read, but lacks the ability to repeat sentences.

2. **Lesion site for Broca's aphasia:** The lesion occupies the anterior part of the aphasic zone, in the posterior inferior part of the frontal lobe (Broca's area, site A in Fig. 11-7). This region abuts on the classic motor area, in harmony with the predominantly motor function of this region. Because of the inverted homunculus in the motor strip, the speech area abuts on the face area of the primary motor cortex. Thus, a right-side upper motoneuron facial palsy, if not a frank right hemiplegia, frequently accompanies Broca's aphasia.

I. Wernicke's aphasia (receptive aphasia, fluent aphasia)

1. **Clinical features:** In direct contrast to Broca's aphasia, the fluent aphasic produces plentiful but garbled sounds, perhaps best described as a "word salad" or "word potpourri." The substitution of erroneous words or parts of words and phonemes (paraphasia) robs the speech of meaning. Even so, the jargon may retain prosody, rhythm, and inflection, thus sounding like speech but deficient in meaning. Thus, the term **fluent aphasia,** implying fluent communication is almost an oxymoron. Children also may have fluent aphasia.
2. Patients with fluent aphasia lose the ability to audit their own words and the words of others and often fail to realize the severity of their deficit in expression. They cannot use their auditory feedback to monitor or correct their own errors in word production. To appreciate the experience of a Pt with medication-induced Wernicke's aphasia, read Lazar et al. (2000).
3. **Lesion site for receptive aphasia:** The lesion occupies the region around the posterior end of the Sylvian fissure at the parieto-occipito-temporal confluence, in the auditory and visual word association area (sites B, C, and F of Fig. 11-7). Thus, the lesion affects the aphasic zone more posteriorly and temporally than in expressive aphasia.
4. **The arcuate fasciculus (Wernicke's arc)** curves in a U-shape from the temporal lobe around to the posterior inferior frontal region, connecting Wernicke's area (F of Fig. 11-7) with Broca's (A of Fig. 11-7) (Pearce, 2000).

J. Dyslexia and alexia (word agnosia and word blindness)

1. **Clinical features: Dyslexia** means agnosia for the meaning of written words despite adequate intelligence and exposure to conventional methods of instruction. Hence, the Pt cannot read. Depending on the time of onset, dyslexia can be classified as **congenital** or **acquired.** In contrast, some children—normal, learning disabled, autistic, or retarded—have **hyperlexia** (Mehegan and Dreifuss, 1972). They may read prematurely at very young ages but fail to comprehend what they read.
2. **Clinical examination for dyslexia**
   a. If the Pt is a child, review the history for accompanying language and behavioral problems: delay in acquiring speech; difficulty in naming letters; letter reversals such as *d* for *b;* and abnormal sequencing such as *was* for *saw* (Shaywitz and Shaywitz, 1999) The child often has attention deficits and the inability to organize, plan, and carry out actions such as completing homework assignments.
   b. The Ex should test for the ability to recognize individual letters, small words, and long words and the ability to sound out long words, to read phrases, sentences, and paragraphs, and to explain them.
   c. Test for the ability to copy sentences from print and from dictation. Even though the Pt can write a dictated sentence, he cannot then read it.
   d. Test for the elements of Gerstmann's syndrome (Section III-O)
   e. Test for other visual agnosias such as the inability to name colors.
3. **Lesion site for dyslexia**
   a. In **congenital** dyslexia, the Pt usually has no gross lesion but may show microdysgenesia of the cortex. Functional studies agree with the pathoanatomic studies in locating the critical area in the parieto-occipito-temporal confluence, centering on the angular gyrus (Shaywitz and Shaywitz, 1999). Dyscalculia often accompanies dyslexia.

b. In **acquired** dyslexia, the lesion usually occupies the posterior end of the aphasic zone (sites D and E in Fig. 11-7) or somewhat more posteriorly. The lesion damages the word association cortex of the parieto-occipito-temporal confluence or disconnects it from afferents that arrive from the corpus callosum or from the lingual gyrus of the occipital lobe and fusiform gyri of the temporal lobe (Greenblatt, 1977). Benson (1977) described a type of dyslexia after lesions of the dominant frontal lobe that may be associated with Broca's aphasia.

K. Auditory agnosia (word deafness)

The Pt with relatively pure auditory aphasia fails to understand spoken words but can read, write, and speak. The lesion occupies the posterior part of the left superior temporal gyrus (site F in Fig. 11-7), next to the primary auditory receptive area in the transverse gyri, in the floor of the Sylvian fissure. Temporal lobe lesions cause other auditory agnosias such as interpreting the meaning of diverse sounds other than language.

L. Global aphasia

1. **Clinical features:** The Pt has expressive and receptive dysphasia that may eliminate all receptive and expressive communication by words. Initially after the lesion, the Pt may be entirely mute. Any speech retained is mainly exclamatory or severely telegraphic.
2. **Lesion site:** In global aphasia, the lesion destroys most of the left parasylvian cortex (sites A to F, entire shaded area in Fig. 11-7) or its connections with the caudate-putamen or thalamus. Because the middle cerebral artery exclusively irrigates the entire parasylvian cortex and most of the striatum, aphasia commonly results from infarction in its territory. Shade this zone in Fig. 11-8.

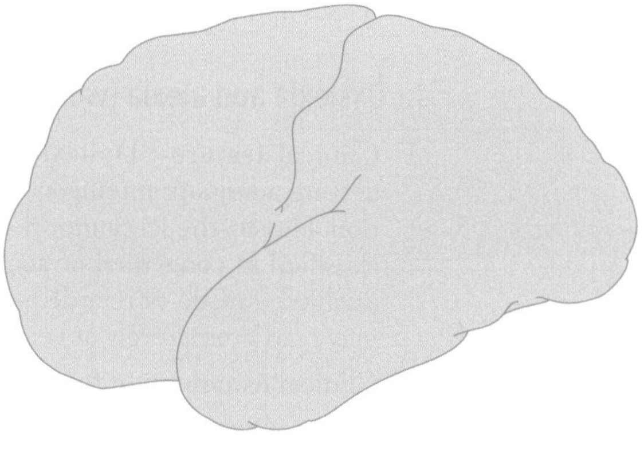

Check your drawing against Fig. 11-7.

FIGURE 11-8. Blank of the left cerebral hemisphere. Shade it to show the expected lesion site in the aphasic patient.

M. Review of the neurologic findings associated with the types of aphasia

1. The neurologic deficits that accompany aphasia will depend on the location of the lesion within the aphasic zone, but they follow a definite logic, if you understand the location of the motor area and the separate primary receptive cortices for vision and hearing (Fig. 2-2C).
2. A lesion in the **anterior** part of the parasylvian zone may extend into the motor area, whereas a more posterior lesion may extend into the optic radiation (geniculocalcarine tract). Review Fig. 3-5, if necessary.
3. The Pt with nonfluent Broca's aphasia would more likely have ❒ hemiparesis/ ❒ hemianopsia/❒ right-left confusion, because the lesion is located ______________________________.

☑ hemiparesis

anteriorly in the aphasic zone next to the motor area

☑ hemianopsia

posteriorly in the aphasic zone, overlying the geniculocalcarine tract

4. The fluent aphasic would more likely have ❐ hemiparesis/❐ hemianopsia/❐ anosognosia, because the lesion is located____.

☑ fluent
Because the lesion is more posterior, toward the auditory and visual word association region.

5. Which type of aphasic would most likely have a severe receptive aphasia: the ❐ fluent/❐ nonfluent. Explain. ____

N. Role of the right hemisphere in language

1. The **left** cerebral hemisphere invests words with their meaning or semantic content as symbols for communication. The right hemisphere can do so only to a limited extent, after the brain reaches developmental maturity. The right hemisphere has to deliver the language stimuli it receives to the left hemisphere via the corpus callosum for interpretation and motor expression (Greenblatt, 1977).
2. Ross (1981) proposed that the parasylvian zone of the **right** hemisphere invests speech with the intonations, melody, pauses, and phrasing, the **prosody** that adds emotion to speech. Lesions in the right parasylvian zone or its subcortical connections impair the Pt's ability to invest his own speech with its emotional coloring and to interpret the emotional meaning or emotional gestures of others.
   a. In analogy to aphasia, the Pt whose speech lacks emotional inflection has **expressive dysprosody.**
   b. The Pt who cannot differentiate the emotional inflections of language spoken by others has **receptive dysprosody,** or the Pt may have **global dysprosody** (Ross, 1981).
   c. Subsequent studies have not fully supported this theory, but prosody comes from some site or sites in the cerebrum (Van Lanker and Breitenstein, 2000).
3. **Testing for dysprosody**
   a. To detect *expressive dysprosody,* listen for flat emotionless speech during the medical history and ask the Pt to say a test phrase while investing it with different emotional inflections. To appreciate the power of prosody in communication, try this exercise: say, "Would you come here," out loud, saying it as softly and seductively as possible, and then as angrily as possible. Play with this phase as a thespian might, to discover how many different emotions it can convey.
   b. To detect *receptive dysprosody,* say a test phrase in different emotional inflections, and ask the Pt to interpret the emotion conveyed. Tape recordings can provide standardized phrases.
4. **Differential diagnosis:** A flat expressionless speech can also occur with various other neuropsychiatric disorders: depression, dementia, Broca's aphasia, and diseases of the thalamus or basal motor nuclei, such as parkinsonism.
5. Expressive dysprosody would qualify as a form of ❐ apraxia/❐ agnosia, whereas receptive dysprosody would qualify as ❐ apraxia/❐ agnosia.

☑ apraxia; ☑ agnosia

O. Gerstmann's syndrome

1. **Clinical features:** The core signs of Gerstmann's syndrome consist of **dysgraphia, dyscalculia, finger agnosia,** and **right-left disorientation,** but most Pts also have some degree of aphasia or dyslexia. The Pt often has dysgraphia for spontaneous writing but can copy. Children normally go through a developmental Gerstmann's syndrome (Gordon, 1992; O'Hare et al., 1991), but it may also persist as part of an overall learning disability (Suresh and Sebastian, 2000).
2. **Lesion site:** Although a lesion of the left angular gyrus, at the parieto-occipito-temporal junction (site E in Fig. 11-10), may cause the four core components of Gerstmann's syndrome, one or all of the components can occur with lesions of more distant sites (Heimberger et al., 1964). Even though the lesion is unilateral, the finger agnosia and right-left disorientation affect both sides of the body, thus representing bilateral autotopagnosia.

3. List the four signs of Gerstmann's syndrome.

____
____

Dysgraphia, dyscalculia, finger agnosia, and right-left disorientation.

P. Focal and asymmetrical cortical degeneration syndromes

Although the various agnosias and apraxias characteristically result from focal lesions such as infarcts and neoplasms, sometimes diffuse cortical degenerative diseases may affect lobes or parts of lobes. The Pt has, for example, aphasia as the leading component of the disease, if it focuses on the left parasylvian area. Overall, the Pt later becomes demented, but the focal signs may predominate, at least in the early stages (Casselli, 1995).

Q. Review of the definitions of agnosia, apraxia, and aphasia

Now that you know the operational methods to test for these disorders, give general interpretational definitions of the following:

1. Agnosia:

____
______________________________.

See frame II B 2, page 439.

2. Apraxia:

____
______________________________.

See frame II J1, page 443.

3. Aphasia:

____
______________________________.

See frame III B, page 449.

4. The requisites to distinguish agnosia from other disturbances of sensation, comprehension, or perception are

____
____
______________________________.

See frame II B 3, page 439.

5. The requisites necessary to distinguish apraxia from other disorders of execution are

____
____
______________________________.

See frame II J 2, page 443.

BIBLIOGRAPHY · Aphasia: Agnosia and Apraxia of Language

Arciniegas DB, Beresford TB. *Neuropsychiatry.* New York, Cambridge University Press, 2001.

Benson D. The third alexia. *Arch Neurol* 1977;34:327–331.

Bookheimer SU, Zeffiro TA, Blaxton Ta. Activation of language cortex with automatic speech tasks. *Neurology* 2000;55:1151–1157.

Brazis PW, Masdeau JC, Biller J. *Localization in Clinical Neurology,* 5th ed. Philadelphia, Lippincott Williams Wilkins, 2001.

Bruyn RPM. Thalamic aphasia: a conceptual critique. *J Neurol* 1989;236:21–25.

Casseli RJ. Focal and asymmetric cortical degeneration syndromes. *Neurologist* 1995;1:1–19.

Critchley M. *Developmental Dyslexia.* London, William Heinemann Medical Books, 1964.

Critchley M. *The Parietal Lobes.* New York, Hafner Publishing, 1969.

Damasio AR. Aphasia. *N Engl J Med* 1992;326:531–539.

Freedman M, Leach L, Kaplan E, et al. *Clock Drawing: A Neuropsychological Assessment.* New York, Oxford University Press, 1994.

Giannakopoulos P, Gold G, Duc M, et al. Neuroanatomic correlates of visual agnosia in Alzheimer's disease. A clinicopathologic study. *Neurology* 1999;52:71–77.

Goodglass H. *Understanding Aphasia.* San Diego, Academic Press, 1993.

Goodglass H, Kaplan E, Barresi B. Boston Diagnostic Aphasia Examination. 3rd ed. (Edition (BDAE-3). Pro-Ed 2000.

Gordon N. Children with developmental dyscalculia. *Dev Med Child Neurol* 1992;34: 459–463.

Gordon N. Mutism: elective or selective and acquired. *Brain Development* 2001;23:83–87.

Greenblatt SH. Neurosurgery and the anatomy of reading. A practical review. *Neurosurgery* 1977;1:6–15.

Grigoletto F, Zappala G, Anderson DW. Norms for the Mini-Mental State Examination in a healthy population. *Neurology* 1999;53:315–320.

Heilman KM, Meador KJ, Loring DW. Hemispheric asymmetries of limb-kinetic apraxia. A loss of deftness. *Neurology* 2000;55:523–526.

Heilman KM, Valenstein E. *Clinical Neuropsychology.* New York, Oxford University Press, 1979.

Heimberger R, DeMyer W, Reitan R. Implications of Gerstmann's syndrome. *J Neurol Neurosurg Psychiatry* 1964;27:52–57.

Joynt RJ, Goldstein MN. Minor cerebral hemisphere. In Friedlander WJ, ed. *Advances in Neurology, Vol 7.* New York, Raven, 1975, pp. 147–183.

Kreisler A, Godefroy O, Delmaire C, et al. The anatomy of aphasia revisited. *Neurology* 2000;54:1117–1123.

Lazar RM, Marshall RS, Prell GD. The experience of Wernicke's aphasia. *Neurology* 2000;55:1222–1224.

Meador KJ, Loring DW, Lee K, et al. Cerebral lateralization. Relationship of language and ideomotor praxis. *Neurology* 1999;53:2028–2031.

Mega MS, Alexander MP. Subcortical aphasia: the core profile of capsulostriatal infarction. *Neurology* 1994;44:1824–1829.

Mehegan H, Dreifuss F. Hyperlexia. *Neurology* 1972;22:1105–1111.

Mohr JP, Pessin MS, Finkelstein S, et al. Broca aphasia: pathologic and clinical. *Neurology* 1978;28:311–324.

O'Hare AE, Brown JK, Aitken K. Dyscalculia in children. *Dev Med Child Neurol* 1991;33:356–361.

O'Hare A, Gorzkowska J, Elton R. Development of an instrument to measure manual praxis. *Dev Med Child Neurol* 1999;41:597–607.

Papagno C, Sala SD, Basso A. Ideomotor apraxia without aphasia and aphasia without apraxia: the anatomical support for a double dissociation. *J Neurol Neurosurg Psychiatry* 1993;56:286–289.

Pearce JMS. Aphasia and Wernicke's arc. *J Neurol Neurosurg Psychiatry* 2000;70:699.

Penfield W, Roberts L. *Speech and Brain Mechanisms.* Princeton, Princeton University Press, 1959.

Pujol J, Deus J, Losilla JM, et al. Cerebral lateralization of language in normal left-handed people studied by fMRI. Neurology 1999;52:1038–1043.

Ross ED. The aprosodias. *Arch Neurol* 1981;38:561–569.

Shaywitz SE, Shaywitz BA. Dyslexia. In Swaiman KF, Ashwal S, eds. *Pediatric Neurology,* 3rd ed. St. Louis, Mosby, 1999, Chapter 33, pp. 576–584.

Shewan CM, Kertesz A. Reliability and validity characteristics of the Western Aphasia Battery (WAB). *J Speech Hearing Disorders* 1980;45:308–324.

Suresh PA, Sebastian S. Developmental Gerstmann's syndrome: a distinct clinical entity of learning disabilities. *Pediatr Neurol* 2000;22:267–278.

Van Lanker D, Breitenstein C. Emotional dysprosody and similar dysfunctions. In Bogousslavsky J, Cummings JL, eds. *Behavior and Mood Disorders in Focal Brain Lesions.* Cambridge, Cambridge University Press, 2000, Chapter 12, pp. 327–368.

Weinstein EA, Friedland RP, eds. *Hemi-inattention Syndromes and Hemisphere Specialization. Advances in Neurology, Vol 10.* New York, Raven, 1977.

IV. A RESUMÉ OF CEREBRAL LOCALIZATION

A. Review of the lobes of the cerebrum

Celsus, in approximately A.D. 25, remarked, "... nor can a diseased portion of the body be treated by one who does not know what that part is." If you cannot draw the lobes of the brain and define their boundaries, review Fig. 2-2.

B. The concept of localization and clinicopathologic correlation

1. Localization of the sites of lesions that cause specified signs and symptoms and the localization of functions are not the same. We do not worry ourselves with localizing functions if we recall the operational steps for localizing lesions: Give a test, executing it and judging the results according to a standard procedure. Then correlate the results with the sites of brain lesions in a series of Pts. Just because an Ex can localize a lesion from the deficit of function does not mean the function has been localized; localizing the function in this circumstance indulges in the sin of circular reasoning:

   Sequence 1
   Child: "Daddy, why do things fall to the ground?"
   Daddy: "Why, that's simple, because there is gravity."

   Sequence 2
   Child: "Daddy, why do you say there is gravity?"
   Daddy: Why, that's simple, because things fall to the ground."

2. Localization by the clinicopathologic method led to the construction of Fig. 11-9 which correlates signs and symptoms with lesion site.

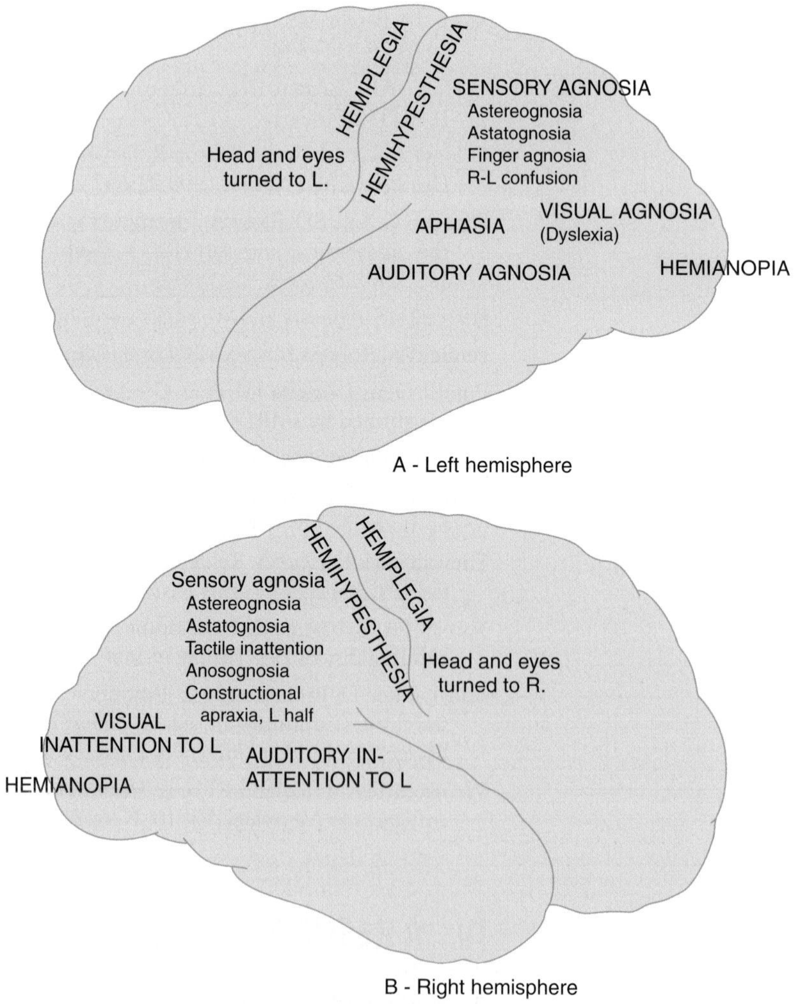

FIGURE 11-9. Summary of the signs and symptoms caused by focal destructive lesions in the right or left cerebral hemisphere. (A) Lateral view of left cerebral hemisphere. (B) Lateral view of the right cerebral hemisphere. Note that some signs, such as hemiplegia, appear after lesions of either hemisphere, but that other signs depend on which hemisphere contains the lesion.

3. Functional brain imaging shows that mental functions involve many more areas of the brain, probably including the cerebellum, than deduced from clinicopathologic correlation (Mazziotta et al., 2000). Thus the sites or localizations established by clinicopathologic correlation remain valid but should be viewed as nodal points in distributed networks rather than as autonomous sites that solely mediate the functions operationally determined at the bedside.
4. **Localization of memory:** Although diffuse disease of the gray or white matter of the cerebrum impairs memory, bilateral lesions restricted to the medial temporal lobe or diencephalon and basal forebrain can cause a relatively pure memory loss called the **pure amnestic syndrome.** The Pts lack recent memory but retain their previous IQ and have no other frank neurologic signs (Victor and Ropper, 2001; Fig. 11-10).

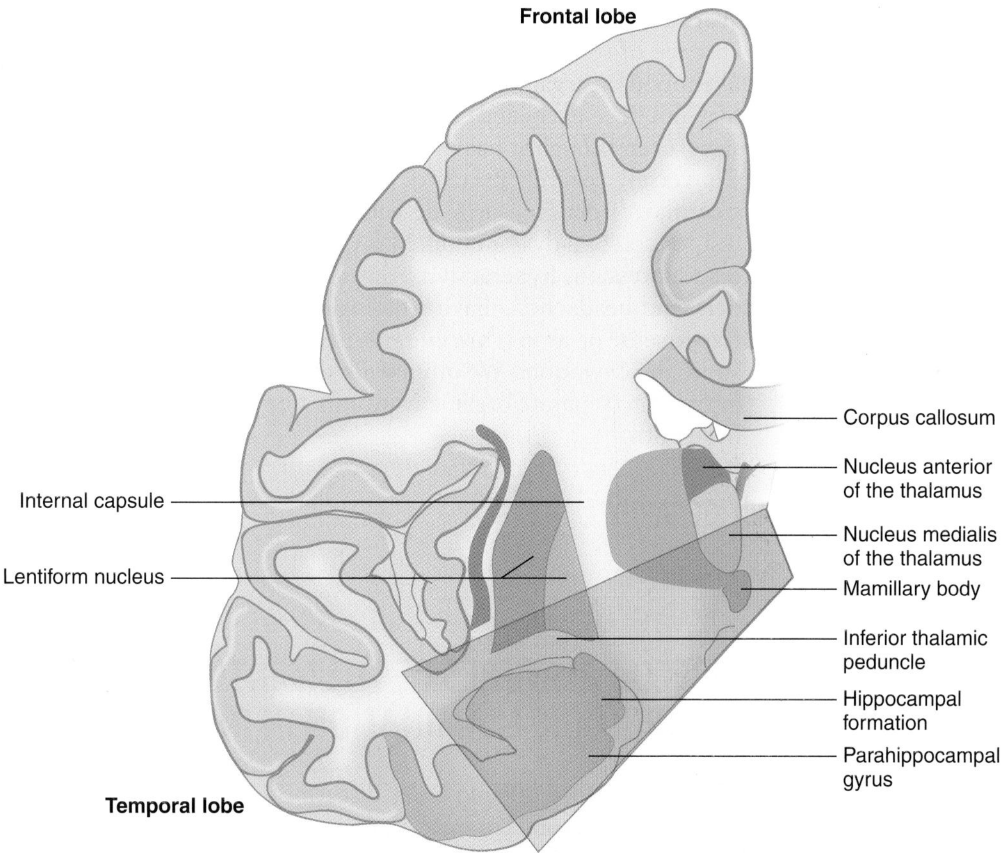

FIGURE 11-10. Coronal section of a cerebral hemisphere showing the region that, when damaged bilaterally, causes loss of recent memory. (Reproduced with permission from Horel Ja. The neuroanatomy of amnesia: A critique of the hippocampal memory hypothesis, *Brain* 1978;101:403–445.)

C. Diagnostic value of agnosia, apraxia, and deficits of the sensorium in the functional-organic dichotomy

1. At the end of each history and NE, the Ex has to make a dichotomy between probable organic disease and probable functional (psychogenic) disease for guidance in selecting diagnostic tests and management.
2. If you realize that a large percentage of Pts has functional disorders, you will realize the importance of making the first dichotomy in diagnosis correctly.

3. In essence, the Ex must recite this catechism:
   a. Does the Pt have a lesion (biochemical or anatomic)?
   b. Where is the lesion?
   c. What is the lesion?
   d. What critical diagnostic procedures are required?
4. If the Pt has frank neurologic signs, such as hemiplegia or hemianopsia, agnosia, or apraxia, the first diagnostic dichotomy is easy: the Pt has ❒ organic/❒ functional disease.

☑ organic

5. Most functional diseases spare most of the sensorium. Therefore, the average neurotic or mildly psychotic Pt has no sensorial defect. Brain lesions may impair memory, orientation, and consciousness—sensorial functions—without causing more obvious neurologic signs. Therefore, sensorial defects themselves may indicate organic disease. Disordered memory, orientation, or consciousness in a mentally disturbed Pt most likely indicates ❒ organic/❒ functional disease.

☑ organic

6. Preservation of memory, orientation, or consciousness in a mentally disturbed Pt most likely indicates ❒ organic/❒ functional disease.

☑ functional

7. **Warning:** Although useful, the organic-functional dichotomy is artificial. The absence of sensorial defects or frank neurologic signs, although reducing the likelihood of organic brain lesions, never guarantees their absence. The lesion may not have exceeded the safety factor of the tissue to cause frank neurologic signs, even though it has produced changes recognized by the Pt or associates. Conversely, severely psychotic Pts with severe schizophrenia or severe depression may display sensorial defects and perform poorly on the Halstead-Reitan test for cerebral dysfunction. Many so-called functional disorders—schizophrenia, depression, hyperactivity, anorexia nervosa, bulimia, obesity, sleep disorders, and headaches—have a biological basis but no identifiable lesions in the classic sense or, as in schizophrenia, subtle measurement are required to demonstrate the deviations. We often walk the fine edge between triumph and diaster in trying to separate organic from functional disease, and, of course, the Pt may have both.

BIBLIOGRAPHY

See bibliography of next section.

V. SPECIAL FEATURES OF THE MENTAL STATUS AND NEUROLOGIC EXAMINATION IN DEMENTIA AND AGING

Patients with diffuse organic brain disease of different types present with certain common symptoms and common signs of mental dysfunction, called **dementia,** such as disorientation in time and memory loss (*Diagnostic and Statistical Manual of Mental Disorders*, 4th ed.; Cummings and Benson, 1992; Victor and Roper, 2001). However, focal lesions can also cause changes in overall behavior and mood and some features of dementia (Bogousslavsky and Cumnings, 2000). The Pt, often unaware of the loss of mental abilities, is usually brought in because of a concerned family. Family members often express these changes as "Grandmother just does not act like herself any more."

A. Bedside screening tests for cognitive deficits in dementia

1. **The problems**
   a. Extensive test batteries sensitive to dementia and brain lesions require training, equipment, and time. Standard IQ tests, such as the Stanford-Binet and Wechsler, strongly reflect environmental influences and education and are

relatively insensitive to early dementia and many focal brain lesions. For example, Pts with amnestic and confabulatory syndromes with no recent memory or who have had prefrontal lobotomies score normally on IQ tests, whereas culturally deprived or illiterate persons with normal brains score poorly.

b. Investigators have extracted items from the larger batteries for shorter tests for dementia, to follow the course of demented Pts through trials of drug treatments, and for the differential diagnosis of dementias (Lopez et al., 1999). The race is on; in fact, a cottage industry exists to find reliable tests for dementia that require little time. Most popular is the Mini-Mental State Examination (MMSE) available from Psychologic Assessment Resources Inc. (www.parinc.com), which takes 10 minutes plus, but it has shrunken to a Micro-MMSE that takes 1.5 to 3 minutes. The Memory Impairment Scale takes only 4 minutes. A three-step spelling of *world* (forward, backward, and in the alphabetical order of the letters—thus *dlorw*) is touted to be about as good but takes only 1 minute (Leopold and Borson, 1997). See Table 11-5 for categories of cognition evaluated with these tests.

TABLE 11-5 · Categories of Cognition Tested in Mental Status Examination

Orientation	Ask patient to state where they are; for example, city, state, hospital Ask patient to state day of the week, month, year
Attention	Ask patient to count backwards from 100 by 7. Stop after 5 correct answers.
Registration	Name three objects (for example, pen, bed, nose); then ask patient to repeat the three objects
Complex Tasks	Give the patient a three-step command, such as: "get your coat, put it on the chair, and come sit down."
Naming	Ask patient to name two objects visible in the room by pointing and saying, "what is this?"
Repetition	Ask the patient to repeat a sentence
Recall	Ask patient to recall the three objects they were given above
Reading	Write the phrase, "close your eyes," and show it to the patient, saying please do what the card says
Writing	Ask the patient to write a simple sentence
Copying	Ask the patient to copy overlapping shapes

In the Mini-Mental State Examination (MMSE), the categories of cognition are assessed and scored with one point being given for each correct answer.

c. Another screening test that may be more sensitive at detecting mild cognitive impairment is the Montreal Cognitive Assessment (MOCA) (Nasreddine et al., 2005).

d. Matching the proliferation of instant cognitive tests are symptom checklists. All you have to do is have a clerk, the Pt, or parents fill out a check list, add up the score, and, presto, you can diagnose autism, attention-deficit/hyperactivity disorder, depression, dementia, delirium, etc.—instant and painless diagnosis.

e. The astute clinician learns a great deal by observing the Pt's reactions and behavior and interacting with the Pt during the test. You accomplish much more than getting a numerical score. The test becomes part of the interaction that leads to knowing the Pt's real problems and circumstances. If you don't have the time to devote to the task, don't even pretend to evaluate the Pt's mental status. Decisions about driving, schooling, living arrangements, wills, and money management require the most careful clinical judgment.

f. The two critical problems in the mental status evaluation are

   i. Early detection of the mild cognitive impairment that heralds the onset of most gradually evolving dementias (Bennett, 2002).

   ii. Differentiation of the causes of dementia, most importantly, separating the treatable from the nontreatable, for which the "instant" tests are of no value.

2. **The solution**

   a. Learn to use the appropriate mental status questions for screening the sensorium (Table 11-3).

   b. Familiarize yourself with and use one of the numerous quick screening tests (Albert and Knoefel, 1994; Bennett, 2002; Houx et al., 2002; Petersen, et al., 2001; Table 11-4), Of the brief screening tests, the MMSE of Folstein is the most popular and has norms for children (Besson and Labbé, 1997; Ouvrier et al., 1999) and adults (Dufouil et al., 2000; Grigoletto et al., 1999), but it is strongly biased by education (Doraiswamy and Kaiser, 2000; Grigoletto et al., 1999). Solomon et al. (1998) devised a brief battery for office use in the diagnosis of Alzheimer's disease that answers some of the criticisms of the MMSE. Most normal, well-educated younger persons make no errors and score the full 30 allowable on the MMSE, but the scores for normal persons decline strikingly with age (after 60 to 65 years), education level, and sex (Grigoletto et al., 1999; Fig. 11-11).

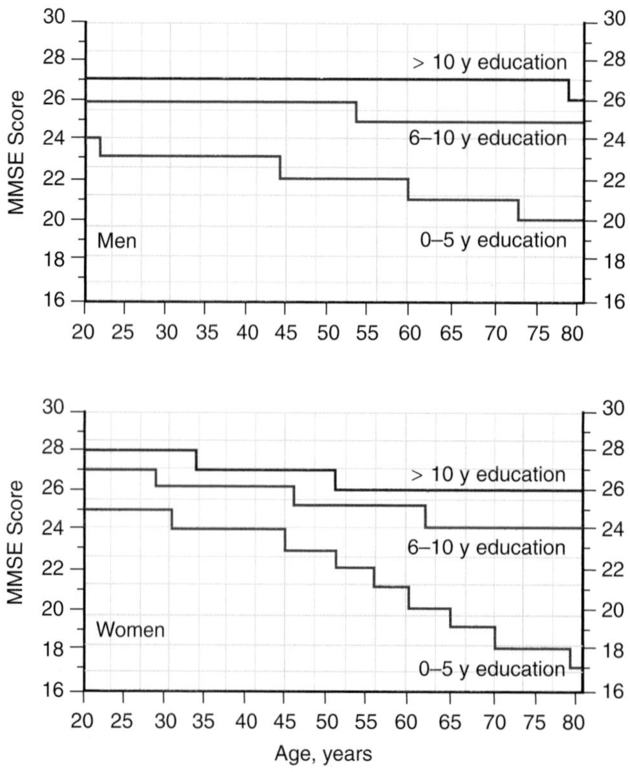

FIGURE 11-11. Fifth percentile norms for the Mini-Mental State Examination. (Reproduced by permission from Grigoletto F, Zappala G, Anderson DW. Norms for the Mini-Mental State Examination in a healthy population. *Neurology* 1999;53:315–320.)

c. The Ex must fully recognize the limitations in interpreting any neuropsychological tests. Validity rests on the assumption that the Pt has cooperated fully, did his or her best, and belongs to the culture on which the test was standardized.

d. Then decide whether to order a full-scale neuropsychologic battery (Green, 2000). When in doubt, refer the Pt to a specialized dementia center.

B. Additional methods of assessing the demented patient

1. Several researchers list the methods to diagnose and evaluate the physical, cognitive, and emotional status of Pt with dementia. The major thrust is to separate treatable dementias, such as syphilis and Wilson's hepatolenticular degeneration, from the untreatable and to determine prognosis (Camicioli and Wild, 1997b; Chui and Zhang, 1997; Clark and Trojanowski 2000; Knopman et al., 2001; Petersen et al., 2001; Fig. 11-12).
2. Applegate et al. (1990) listed several scales for the clinician to assess daily living activities in aging and depression as part of the overall neurologic evaluation.

C. Clinical findings that differentiate aphasia from dementia or other forms of mental illness

Patients with global aphasia cannot respond to the standard questions for testing the sensorium and fail the mental status tests. The clinical features that distinguish aphasics from demented Pts are

1. Retention of personal habits and hygiene.
2. Sense appropriate times for daily activities and attends to daily tasks of living.
3. Continent of urine and feces.
4. Socially appropriate behavior.
5. Can often identify the correct word or answer if the Ex recites a list of alternatives that contain it.

D. Primitive reflexes in aging and dementia

Sometimes the convolutions [gyri] are simply reduced in volume, at other times they are puckered; in other cases there is induration. The patient lives a life of mere excito-motory and nutritive kind. The cerebral functions are obliterated. The true spinal and ganglionic functions remain alone. There is much for the physiologist to investigate in this singular return to a sort of infantile existence.

—Marshall Hall (1790–1857)

1. **The theory of primitive reflexes:** At term the infant's preprogrammed primitive reflexes, such as breathing and sucking, determine its behavior (O'Doherty, 1986). As the infant's cortex matures, it comes to dominate or inhibit the primitive inborn behaviors. Then, with aging or dementia, the cortex loses neurons, thus disinhibiting the primitive reflexes and allowing them to reappear in the brain-impaired adult (Huff et al., 1987; Jenkyn et al., 1977; Rao, 2000).
2. **The flexion attitude or posture**

   a. The infant emerges at term in an attitude of universal flexion, the so-called *fetal posture,* with the head flexed on the chest, the chest flexed on the pelvis, and the arms and legs flexed on the body. Yakovlev (1954) interpreted this posture as a "grasp reflex of the body upon the body." The flexion attitude dominates in the normal newborn to the point that the infant cannot completely extend its knees and elbows, nor can the Ex by passive manipulation.

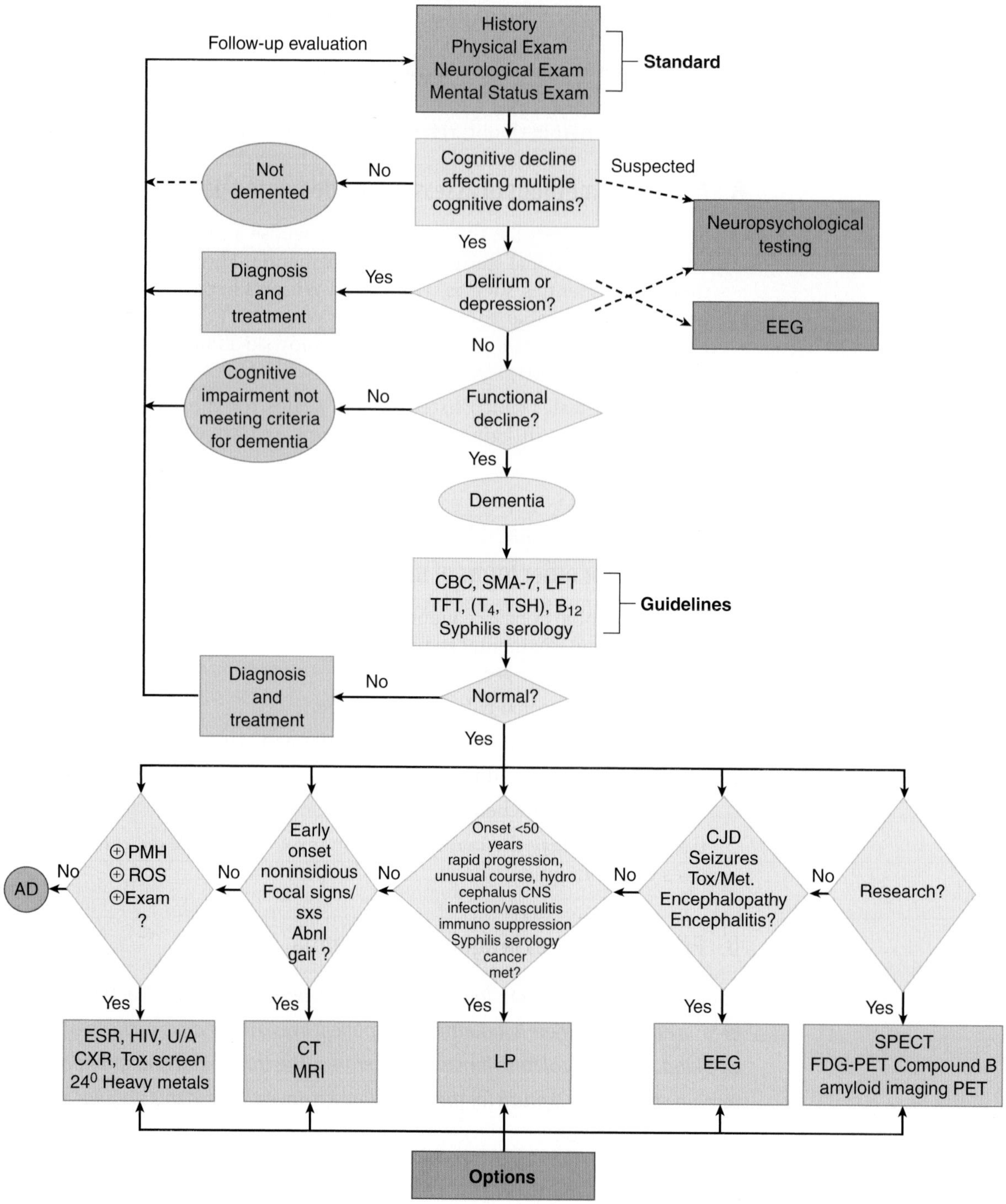

FIGURE 11-12. Algorithm for the diagnosis and evaluation of dementia. CJD = Creutzfeldt-Jacob disease; LFT = liver function tests; TFT = thyroid function tests. (Slightly modified and reproduced with permission from Chui H, Zhang Q. Evaluation of dementia: a systematic study of the usefulness of the American Academy of Neurology's Practice Parameters. *Neurology* 1997;49:925–935.)

b. During the first year, as the cerebral cortex matures, the normal infant unfolds from this flexion attitude, unfolding from itself and unfolding in defiance of gravity, to reach an erect posture and to extend the limbs from the trunk and free them for action.

c. In advanced dementia, as the cerebral cortex degenerates, the flexed fetal posture reemerges. The Pt again folds up on himself and again succumbs to gravity. Shakespeare spoke of this life cycle of flexion, vertical posture, and flexion as twice an infant, once an adult (Fig. 11-13).

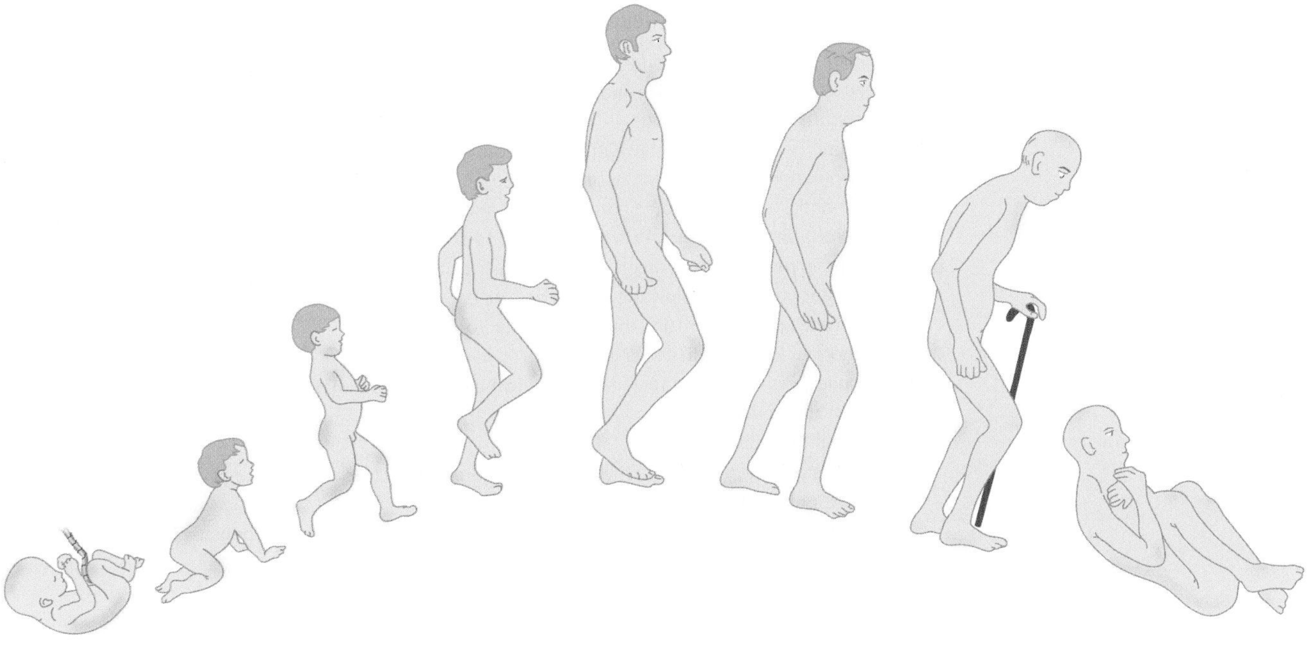

FIGURE 11-13. The cycle from flexion to verticality to flexion during the lifespan of the individual: twice an infant, once an adult. (After Yakovlev P. Paraplegia in flexion of cerebral origin. *J Neuropathol Exp Neurol* 1954;3:267–296.)

3. **Significance of primitive reflexes:** The primitive reflexes, although generally nonlocalizing as to lesion site, do reflect diffuse brain dysfunction, but do not strictly correlate with dementia (Huff et al., 1987; Jenkyn et al., 1977; Jenkyn and Reeves, 1981; Koller et al., 1982; Owen and Mulley, 2002; Rao, 2000; Tweedy et al., 1982). See Table 11-6.

E. Clinical features of diffuse brain disease, dementia, and aging

1. **Alterations in mentation and behavior caused by diffuse brain disease:** The Pt exhibits:
   a. Poor planning, judgment, and decision-making, with poverty of thought and action, negativism, childishness, and loss of flexibility.
   b. Loss of interest in current events with circumscription of activities, hypochondriasis, and self-preoccupation.
   c. Forgetfulness, with recent memory worse than remote memory—"living in the past."
   d. A state of *abulia* (*a* = lack of; *boule* = will; therefore, lack of will). The Pt exhibits an overall inertia about making decisions and taking actions. Part of the conservatism of aging and dementia is this pervasive inertia in making decisions and acting on them. Abulia also characterizes the impairment of executive function with large bifrontal lobe lesions (Dubois et al., 2000). The Pt seems apathetic, lacks spontaneity, motivation, interest, and the energy to initiate and persevere in completing tasks. The Pt speak sparsely, slowly, and shows long delays in responding, making no attempt to expand a conversation or to play with ideas. In a phrase, the Pt's battery has run down.
2. **Alterations in affect**
   a. Depression with mixture of apathy, irritability, and often complaints of undue fatigability. Less frequently, aggression or mania.
   b. Anxiety and worry over trivial matters.
   c. Emotional lability (pseudobulbar affect) or emotional blunting. Mood swings with mania or depression.

TABLE 11-6 · Nonlocalizing Neurologic Signs in Diffuse Organic Brain Dysfunction

1. *Range of eye movement and smooth pursuit.* Instruct Pt to hold head still and follow Ex's finger through extremes of horizontal gaze and vertical gaze. Hold a transparent ruler in front of the cornea to measure range of deviation.
   Normal: Eyes move smoothly, without nystagmus, 7 mm upward and 10 mm in other directions.
   Abnormal: Irregular, hesitant, or saccadic smooth pursuit. Upward gaze usually most limited. Upward gaze and lateral gaze should equal at least 5 and 7 mm, respectively.
2. *Lateral gaze impersistence.* Pt holds head still and deviates the eyes as far as possible to the left to maintain persistent fixation on a point on the wall for a timed 30-s period. Instruct the Pt to blink, if necessary, but not to allow the eyes to deviate back to the middle.
   Normal: Pt persists in maintaining fixation for 30 s.
   Abnormal: Pt unable to persist for 30 s.
3. *Tongue impersistence.* Instruct Pt to protrude the tongue in the midline as far as possible for a timed 30-s period.
   Normal: Pt persists for 30 s.
   Abnormal: Pts with involuntary movement syndromes, such as chorea, invariably fail, as often do demented Pts or Pts with a short attention span.
4. *Glabellar blink.* Pt looks at a point across room. Ex stands at sides and brings index finger down from above the forehead and taps the glabella rapidly 10 times.
   Normal: Reflex closure of eyelids inhibited after several taps; lids remain open.
   Abnormal: Continuous reflex blinking of upper or lower lid or both, with or without lid closure (disinhibition). Some normal individuals may continue to blink.
5. *Snout reflex.* The Pt closes his eyes. The Ex taps the philtrum several times at a medium rate, or the Ex may press the tip of a test tube firmly (not so as to cause pain) against the philtrum, compressing the upper lip against the gum.
   Normal: No response.
   Abnormal: Puckering or pursing of the lips
6. *Suck reflex.* The Pt closes the eyes. Using the rounded tip of a test tube, the Ex strokes the Pt's lips from the center of the crevice to the sides.
   Normal: Sucking response in young infant. Thereafter, no response.
   Abnormal: Any pursing or sucking motion of lips in Pt older than early infancy. Failure of young infant to suck.
7. *Nuchocephalic reflex.* Pt stands relaxed with eyes lightly closed. The Ex tells the Pt to relax and let the body and arms be loose and floppy. The Ex briskly turns the Pt's shoulders 1/8 to 1/4 turn to the right and to the left several times, stopping randomly with shoulders turned in one direction or another.
   Normal: Head reflexly turns in the direction of the shoulder movement after about a 0.5-s lag to realign straight ahead with the new shoulder position. (Exclude cervical spondylosis before trying the test.)
   Abnormal: Head holds original position and does not turn to align with the new position of the shoulders. (The reflex is "disinhibited.")
8. *Grasp reflex.* Ex uses index and middle finger to stroke the Pt's palm from the hypothenar eminence toward the junction of the Pt's thumb and index finger.
   Normal: Present in early infancy but not thereafter.
   Abnormal: The Pt grasps the Ex's fingers. Forced groping may ensue, in which the Pt maintains the grasp and moves the hand wherever the Ex moves the hand, or the Pt may involuntarily grope for an for an object presented to vision.
9. *Palmomental reflex.* The Ex instructs the Pt to relax. Pt sits or reclines. Break a wooden tongue blade transversely and use the serrated margin to stroke proximodistally along the Pt's thenar eminence on the right and left hands (Owen and Mulley, 2002).
   Normal: No contraction of mentalis muscle, but the reflex occurs in most Pts if the stimulus is very strong (Koller et al., 1982).
   Abnormal: Readily elicited ipsilateral and sometimes bilateral mentalis contraction.
10. *Arm-dropping test.* Ex instructs the Pt: "Relax your arms completely. Let me do all of the work."
    Ex grasps Pt's arm by wrist, elevates it, and lets it drop. The Ex catches the Pt's arm with the other hand to avoid injury. This test is most successful when done after the nuchocephalic test, which gives the Pt experience in what a totally floppy arm feels like.
    Normal: Free fall of the arm.
    Abnormal: Failure to let the arm drop freely. Occasionally, a normal subject cannot relax to allow free fall of the arm.
11. *Leg-dropping test.* Repeat as for arm dropping. The Pt sits with the legs dangling over a table edge. The Ex grasps the ankle, extends the leg, and allows it to drop.
12. *Paratonia* (Gegenhalten). Ex grasps Pt's wrist and passively moves the Pt's arms in various directions.
    Normal: Free, nonoppositional response.
    Abnormal: More or less continuous opposition to movement in any direction, which may give in and then resume. Must differentiate from parkinsonian rigidity.

ABBREVIATIONS: Ex = examiner; Pt = patient.

3. **Alterations in vegetative function and personal hygiene**
   a. Sudden or premature aging in facial appearance and posture. The Pt who looks 80 years old usually is not that old, or, if you look 80 at 70, you aren't likely to make it to 80.
   b. Slovenly personal appearance, often with bladder and bowel incontinence.
   c. Decreased appetite, usually with weight loss.
   d. Disordered sleep cycle, often with nocturnal disorientation.
   e. Decrease in sexual activity and interest or, less commonly, hypersexuality or inappropriate sexuality.

F. Neurologic signs in diffuse brain disease, aging, and dementia

1. **Alterations in speech**
   a. Dysarthria
   b. Poverty of speech and associations, circumlocutions, aphasia-like word searching and anomia.
   c. Monotonous or plateau speech, lacking in prosody.
   d. Perseveration and echolalia.
2. **Alterations in gait** (Camicioli et al., 1997a; Joseph and Young, 1992; see the gait essay at the end of Chapter 8).
   a. Unsteadiness, broad base, and falling (Tinetti, 2003).
   b. Shortening of stride length; *marche à petit pas.*
   c. Gait apraxia.
   d. Loss of verticality with retropulsion or anteropulsion and festination.
3. **Alterations in overall motor function**
   a. Bradykinesia, poverty, and slowness of all volitional movements.
   b. Increasing flexion posture.
   c. Rigidity, either lead-pipe rigidity or paratonic rigidity (Gegenhalten).
   d. Facial immobility.
   e. Deterioration of handwriting: dysgraphia and micrographia. Inspect samples of the Pt's signature over several years (using old checks, etc.).
   f. Involuntary movements: orolingual hyperkinesias and mild resting or action tremors.
   g. Disinhibition and emergence of primitive reflexes (Table 11-6).
   h. Disordered motor functions in subcortical dementia: Alzheimer's disease causes predominantly cortical degeneration. Extrapyramidal signs are frequent such as rigidity and bradykinesia, but usually not prominent (Lopez et al., 1997). The so-called subcortical dementias affect basal motor nuclei and the rostral brainstem as much as or more than the cortex. Such Pts, as with Huntington's chorea, thalamic degeneration, parkinsonism, or Wilson's hepatolenticular degeneration, present with early or conspicuous extrapyramidal signs in addition to dementia (Cummings and Benson, 1992). Separation on purely clinical grounds of cortical and subcortical dementia remains questionable, but the "cortical" dementias feature aphasia and apraxia over the subcortical (Victor and Ropper, 2001).
4. **Alterations in muscle stretch reflexes:** All muscle stretch reflexes are brisk (including jaw jerk) except for reduced or absent triceps surae (due to mild distal senile peripheral neuropathy).
5. **Alterations in visual function**
   a. Reduction in vision: often has cataracts or macular degeneration.
   b. The pupils become miotic and, in the very elderly, may fail to react to light and in accommodation (Jenkyn and Reeves, 1981).
   c. Poor fixation and smooth pursuit, with limited upward gaze.

6. **Alterations in sensation**
   a. Anosmia common in Alzheimer's disease.
   b. Reduced deep modalities, such as vibratory sensation in feet.
   c. Presbyacusis.

G. Clinical distinctions between dementia, delirium, and mania

1. Dementia is a chronic, more or less permanent change in mentation, often insidious in onset, and often progressive. Delirium, although clinically similar to dementia, is transient. Delirium tremens is the classical example.
2. The delirious Pt has temporary but global disorders of cognition and attention, an altered level of conscious but not coma (although it may precede or alternate with coma), increased or decreased activity, amnesia and disorientation, often with hallucinations and delusions, and a disturbed sleep cycle with the delirium worsening or only appearing at night (Lipowski, 1989).
3. The manic Pt shows grandiosity, exaggerated self-esteem and sense of power and invincibility, pressure of speech, distractibility, insomnia, flight of ideas, and pleasure-seeking or goal-seeking despite consequences, but the Pt retains memory and orientation to person, time, and place.

BIBLIOGRAPHY · Special Features of the Mental Status and Neurologic Examination in Aging and Dementia

Albert M, Knoefel J. *Clinical Neurology of Aging,* 2nd ed. New York, Oxford University Press, 1994.

American Psychiatric Association. *Diagnostic and Statistical Manual of Mental Disorders,* 4th ed. Washington, DC, American Psychiatric Association, 1994.

Applegate JP, Blass JP, Williams TP. Instruments for the functional assessment of older patients. *N Engl J Med* 1990;322:1207–1214.

Bennett DA, Wilson RS, Schneider, JA, et al. Natural history of mild cognitive impairment in older persons. *Neurology* 2002;59:198–205.

Besson PS, Labbé EE. Use of the modified Mini-Mental State Examination with children. *J Child Neurol* 1997;12:455–460.

Bogousslavsky J, Cummings JL, eds. *Behavior and Mood Disorders in Focal Brain Lesions.* New York, Cambridge University Press, 2000.

Camicioli R, Panzer V, Kaye J. Balance in the elderly. Posturography and clinical assessment. *Arch Neurol* 1997a;54:976–981.

Camicioli R, Wild K. Assessment of the elderly with dementia. In Herndon R, ed. *Handbook of Neurologic Rating Scales.* New York, Demos Vermande, 1997b, Chap. 6, pp. 125–141.

Chui H, Zhang Q. Evaluation of dementia: a systematic study of the usefulness of the American Academy of Neurology's Practice Parameters. *Neurology* 1997;49: 925–935.

Clark CM, Trojanowski JQ, eds. *Neurodegenerative Dementias.* New York, McGraw-Hill, 2000.

Cummings JL, Benson DF. *Dementia: A Clinical Approach.* Stoneham, Butterworth-Heinemann, 1992.

Doraiswamy PM, Kaiser L. Variability of the mini-mental state examination in dementia. *Neurology* 2000;54:1538–1539.

Dubois B, Slachevsky A, Litvan I, et al. The FAB. A frontal assessment battery at bedside. *Neurology* 2000;55:1621–1626.

Dufouil C, Clayton D, Brayne C, et al. Population norms for the MMSE in the very old. Estimates based on longitudinal data. *Neurology* 2000;55:1609–1613.

Green J. *Neuropsychological Evaluation of the Older Adult.* San Diego, Academic Press, 2000.

Grigoletto F, Zappalà G, Anderson D. Norms for the Mini-Mental State Examination in a healthy population. *Neurology* 1999;53:315–320.

Horel Ja. The neuroanatomy of memory. *Brain* 1978;101:403–445.

Houx PJ, Shepherd J, Blauw G-J, et al. Testing cognitive function in elderly populations: the PROSPER study. *J Neurol Neurosurg Psychiatry* 2002;73:385–389.

Huff FJ, Boller F, Luccelli F, et al. The neurologic examination in patients with probable Alzheimer's disease. *Arch Neurol* 1987;44:929–933.

Jenkyn LR, Reeves AG. Neurologic signs in uncomplicated aging (senescence). *Semin Neurol* 1981;1:21–30.

Jenkyn LR, Walsh DB, Culber CM, et al: Clinical signs in diffuse cerebral dysfunction. *J Neurol Neurosurg Psychiatry* 1977;40:956–966.

Joseph AB, Young RR. *Movement Disorders in Neurology and Neuropsychiatry.* Cambridge, Blackwell, 1992.

Klelin SK, Masur D, Farveer K, et al. Fluent aphasia in children: definition and natural history. *J Child Neurol* 1992;7:50–59.

Knopman DS, DeKosky ST, Cummings JL, et al. Practice parameter: diagnosis of dementia (an evidence based review). Report of the Quality Standards Subcommittee of the American Academy of Neurology. *Neurology* 2001;56:1143–1153.

Koller WC, Glatt S, Wilson RS, et al. Primitive reflexes and cognitive function in the elderly. *Ann Neurol* 1982;12:302–304.

Leopold NA, Borson AJ. An alphabetical "World." A new version of an old test. *Neurology* 1997;49:1521–1524.

Lipowski J. Delirium in the elderly patient. *N Engl J Med* 1989;320:578–582.

Lopez OL, Litvan I, Catt KE, et al. Accuracy of four clinical diagnostic criteria for the diagnosis of neurodegenerative dementias. *Neurology* 1999;53:1292–1299.

Lopez OL, Wisnieski SR, Becker JT, et al. Extrapyramidal signs in patients with probable Alzheimer's disease. *Arch Neurol* 1997;54:969–974.

Lopresti BJ, Klunk WE, Mathis CA, et al. Simplified Quantification of Pittsburgh Compound B Amyloid Imaging PET Studies: A Comparative Analysis. Journal of Nuclear Medicine 2005;46(12):1959–1972.

Mazziotta JC, Toga AW, Frackowiak RSJ, eds. *Brain Mapping: The Disorders.* San Diego, Academic Press, 2000.

Nasreddine ZS, Phillips NA, Bedirian V, et al. The Montreal Cognitive Assessment, MoCA: A Brief Screening Tool for Mild Cognitive Impairment. *J Am Geriatr Soc* 2005;53:695–699.

O'Doherty N. *Neurologic Examination of the Newborn.* Lancaster, MTP Press, 1986.

Owen G, Mulley GP. The palmomental reflex: a useful clinical sign? *J Neurol Neurosurg Psychiatry* 2002;73:113–115.

Ouvrier R, Hendy J, Bornholt L, et al. SYSTEMS: School-Years Screening Test for the Evaluation of Mental Status. *J Child Neurol* 1999;14:772–780.

Petersen RC, Stevens JC, Ganguli M, et al. Practice parameter: early detection of dementia: mild cognitive impairment (an evidence based review). Report of the Quality Standards Subcommittee of the American Academy of Neurology. *Neurology* 2001;56:1133–1142.

Rao R. Frontal release signs in older people with peripheral vascular disease. *J Neurol Neurosurg Psychiatry* 2000;68:105–106.

Solomon PR, Hirschoff A, Kelly B et al. A 7 Minute Neurocognitive Screening Battery Highly Sensitive to Alzheimer's Disease. *Arch Neurol.* 1998;55:349–355.

Strub RL, Black FW. *The Mental Status Examination in Neurology*, 2nd ed. Philadelphia, FA Davis, 2000.

Tinetti ME. Preventing falls in elderly persons. *N Engl J Med* 2003;348:42–49.

Tweedy J, Reding M, Garcia C, et al. Significance of cortical disinhibition signs. *Neurology* 1982;32:169–173.

Victor M, Ropper AM. *Adams and Victor's Principles of Neurology*, 7th ed. New York, McGraw-Hill, 2001.

Yakovlev P. Paraplegia in flexion of cerebral origin. *J Neuropathol Exp Neurol* 1954;3:267–296.

VI. REVIEW OF CLINICAL TESTS FOR CEREBRAL DYSFUNCTION

A. Rehearsal time again

Define the sensorium, state the seven areas of the sensorium, and give an example of a question designed to test each of the areas.

B. **Distinguish between an illusion, a hallucination, and a delusion.**

C. **Define agnosia, aphasia, and apraxia, and describe tests for each.**

D. **With a partner, practice how to elicit the nonlocalizing signs of cerebral dysfunction (refer to Table 11-6 for guidance).**

Learning Objectives for Chapter 11

I. THE MENTAL STATUS EXAMINATION

1. Describe how to monitor the appropriateness of any particular line of inquiry in the mental status examination and describe some of the adverse responses Pts make when the Ex makes a mistake in technique.
2. Explain the need for flexibility in collecting the data for the mental status examination and the need for a specific outline to arrange it.
3. Write down the outline for the mental status examination (Table 11-1).
4. Give an interpretational definition of the sensorium commune.
5. Describe how the *who, where, when,* and *what* questions illustrate the concept of the sensorium.
6. Explain why the Ex avoids discussing personal attitudes to social, political, and religious questions in evaluating the sensorium.
7. Recite the actual questions to test whether a person who had just received a head injury had regained full sensorial function (Table 11-2).
8. Explain why the Ex should not, except in emergencies, ask the questions that screen the sensorium in serial order.
9. Recite an operational definition of the sensorium.
10. Describe in historical perspective the concept of a common sensorium (*sensorium commune*) and its localization in the brain.
11. Describe what happens to the sensorium in total sensory deprivation.
12. List the seven areas of the sensorium (Table 11-1, item VI) and give examples of questions designed to test each area (Table 11-3).
13. Describe how to test orientation to time, person, and place.
14. Describe a three-item test to test a Pt's memory.
15. Describe what is meant by a *blunted* or a *labile* affect.
16. Define and give an example of an *illusion,* a *delusion,* and an *hallucination.*
17. Discuss the localizing significance of hallucinations produced by organic disease.

II. AGNOSIA, APRAXIA, AND APHASIA

1. Describe several types of agnosia and give a general definition of agnosia.
2. Recite the qualifications that separate agnosia from other disturbances of sensory reception.
3. Demonstrate how to test for agraphognosia.
4. Describe how to test for prosopagnosia.
5. Discuss the concept of a body scheme or autotopognosia (somatognosia).
6. Give some examples of distortion of the body scheme by Pts with neuropsychiatric disorders.
7. Demonstrate how to test for finger agnosia and right-left disorientation and the localizing significance of the deficits.
8. Describe how to test for left-side hemispatial inattention.
9. State the original definition of anosognosia and describe how to test for it.

Learning Objectives for Chapter 11

10. Describe how to test for tactile inattention to double simultaneous stimulation (tactile suppression) and its localizing significance.
11. Demonstrate how to test for inattention to double simultaneous auditory and visual stimuli.
12. Review the concept of the primary and association cortex and explain why deep lesions, such as in the thalamus, may cause signs and symptoms similar to cortical lesions.
13. Discuss the difference in the effect of cortical lesions on the discriminative sensations and the primary sensations such as pain and touch.
14. Define apraxia.
15. Recite the qualifications that separate apraxia from other disturbances of execution.
16. Describe or demonstrate how to test for tongue apraxia, ideomotor apraxia, constructional apraxia, and dressing apraxia.
17. Describe the difference in the constructional apraxia for drawings shown by Pts with left parasylvian as contrasted to right parasylvian area lesions.
18. Explain how the principle of parsimony (Occam's razor) applies to localizing a neurologic lesion.
19. Explain how a mass lesion such as a neoplasm may produce signs or symptoms of impairment of neural tissue beyond the actual border of the lesion.

III. APHASIA: AGNOSIA AND APRAXIA OF LANGUAGE

1. Define so as to differentiate dysphonia, dysarthria, dysprosody, and dysphasia.
2. Describe several types or causes for mutism.
3. Describe several causes of excessive speech production.
4. Define aphasia.
5. Name the two avenues by which the normal person receives language and the two for expressing it. Describe how to test these four avenues of language.
6. Explain the difference between emotional or expletive speech and volitional or propositional speech.
7. Describe several features of aphasia that may be evident when taking a history.
8. Describe the clinical difference between fluent and nonfluent aphasia and the differences in speech output.
9. Explain how to determine the dominant hemisphere for language operationally.
10. State which hemisphere is language dominant in most persons, whether right- or left-handed.
11. Make a lateral drawing of a cerebral hemisphere and shade the usual location within the dominant hemisphere of the lesions that cause aphasia (Fig. 11-7). Recite the name for this area.
12. Distinguish in general between expressiveor non-fluent aphasia, receptive dysphasia, dyslexia, auditory agnosia, mixed aphasia, and global aphasia.
13. Describe where, within the aphasic zone, a lesion would most likely produce: relatively pure expressive or nonfluent Broca's aphasia; Wernicke's aphasia; dyslexia; combinations of fluent aphasia, auditory aphasia, dysgraphia, and dyslexia; and global aphasia (Fig. 11-7).
14. Describe which type of aphasia would most likely be associated with each of the following: the inability to write; UMN facial palsy/hemiparesis; and hemianopia.
15. Describe the location of Wernicke's arcuate fasciculus and the regions it connects.
16. Define dyslexia.
17. Describe neurologic and learning problems often found with congenital dyslexia.

Learning Objectives for Chapter 11

18. State the usual site of the lesion for dyslexia (word agnosia).
19. Describe the function postulated for the right hemisphere in language and how to test that function.
20. List several causes for a flat expressionless type of dysprosody.
21. Recite the components of Gerstmann's syndrome and state the expected site of the lesion.

IV. A RESUMÉ OF CEREBRAL LOCALIZATION

1. Draw lateral and medial views of the cerebral hemispheres and demarcate the lobes (Fig. 2-2).
2. Contrast in principle the effect of a lesion of the posterior parasylvian region of the left cerebral hemisphere with a similar lesion on the right (Fig. 11-9).
3. Describe the general location of the lesion that would selectively impair recent memory, giving a pure amnestic syndrome (Fig. 11-10).
4. Recite the questions of the catechism that the Ex must address in analyzing the presence or absence of a lesion and in making the distinction between organic and psychogenic illnesses.
5. Explain how to use testing of the sensorium and the nonlocalizing signs of diffuse cerebral dysfunction (Table 11-6) to differentiate functional from organic mental illness in Pts who do not have frank localizing signs on the Standard NE.
6. Discuss the pitfalls in trying to dichotomize disease into functional and organic types.

V. SPECIAL FEATURES OF THE MENTAL STATUS AND NEUROLOGIC EXAMINATION IN DEMENTIA AND AGING

1. Describe the invaluable additional information beyond a test score number that the Ex gains in personally administering certain neuropsychological tests.
2. Describe typical alterations in intellectual, affective, and vegetative functions in dementia and aging.
3. List several treatable dementias.
4. Describe the meaning of *twice an infant, once an adult* (Fig. 11-13).
5. Describe the clinical distinctions between a Pt with global aphasia and one with dementia.
6. Explain the concept of primitive reflexes as related to dementia and aging.
7. Describe the technique and normal result of testing for motor impersistence, glabellar blink, snouting and sucking reflexes, grasp reflex, palmomental reflex, arm- and leg-dropping tests, and paratonia (Table 11-6).
8. Describe some typical changes in overall mentation in diffuse brain disease.
9. Define abulia.
10. Describe common alterations in affect in dementia.
11. Describe alterations in vegetative function and personal hygiene.
12. Describe typical alterations in speech in dementia.
13. Describe typical alterations in gait and overall motor function in "cortical dementia."
14. Name the signs of motor dysfunction suggesting dementia with "subcortical lesions."
15. Name a muscle stretch reflex typically reduced in aged individuals and explain.
16. Describe the changes disclosed by the NE in smell, hearing, vision, and pupillary responses in aging and dementia.
17. State which direction of eye movement is usually most impaired in diffuse cortical disease.
18. Distinguish between dementia and delirium.
19. Describe the clinical features of mania.

12 Examination of the Patient Who Has a Disorder of Consciousness

I may speak alike to you and my own conscious heart.

—Percy Bysshe Shelley (1792–1822)

I. EVALUATION OF CONSCIOUSNESS

A. Two definitions of consciousness: intuitive and operational

1. Intuitively, we define consciousness as the awareness of self and environment. Or, more introspectively, we define consciousness as the awareness of our sensorium.
2. Operationally, physicians determine consciousness by practical steps.

B. Operations that establish consciousness

Physicians customarily employ inspection, verbal stimuli, and, if necessary, pain to determine the patient's (Pt's) awareness of self and environment.

1. **Inspection:** Does the Pt appear to adapt appropriately to the ongoing visual, auditory, and tactile stimuli of the ordinary environment?
2. **Verbal stimuli:** Does the Pt respond appropriately to inquiries and requests?
3. **Pain:** Does the Pt respond appropriately to pain?
4. For proof of conscious awareness, the Pt must have a receptor and its sensory pathway intact enough to receive stimuli and deliver those stimuli to the cerebrum. Then the Pt must have a motor pathway, neuromuscular junction, and an effector intact enough to produce a volitional behavior, verbal or nonverbal, that depends on consciousness. The examiner (Ex) cannot determine consciousness by clinical tests in a curarized Pt on the intensive care unit, a Pt with severe complete Guillain-Barré, or a Pt with bilateral complete hemiplegia, who lacks an intact effector system. See, however, the locked-in syndrome, pages 41-42.

C. Pathologic alterations in the level of consciousness

1. Disease may alter consciousness by causing various stages of **delirium** or **coma**.
2. **Delirium (acute confusional state): Delirium** means an acute, transient confusional state characterized by global impairment of the sensorium. The Pt shows

disorientation, amnesia, misperceptions, hallucinations, (often vivid) delusions, brief attention span, disconnected thoughts, irrational or incoherent mutterings, and abnormally decreased or increased psychomotor activity (agitation). Rating scales enable a quantitative assessment (Trzepacz et al., 2002). In a phrase, the Pt is "out of his head." The sleep and wake periods fail. Any such state of excessive neuronal activity may eventually cause tremors and convulsions (*Diagnostic and Statistical Manual of Mental Disorders,* 4th ed., 1994; Lipowski, 1989; Victor and Ropper, 2001). The delirious Pts then return to their previous mental state, or delirium may precede coma. Demented Pts may have periods of superimposed delirium. In aged and demented persons, delirium occurs most commonly at night. The causes of delirium include intracranial hemorrhage, infection, sleep deprivation, various drugs or withdrawal from drugs, toxic or metabolic states, and fever. Withdrawal from alcohol or other depressant drugs causes **delirium tremens,** the classic example of delirium with excitement and often seizures (Chapter 11).

3. Coma (from the Greek word *Koma* meaning *deep sleep*) is sustained pathologic unconsciousness resulting from dysfunction of the ascending reticular activating system (ARAS) in the brainstem tegmentum or both cerebral hemispheres. Comatose patients cannot be aroused and their eyes remain closed (The Multi-Society Task Force on PVS, 1994).
4. Depression of consciousness may evolve through several stages or come on abruptly.
5. Recite the minimum neuroanatomic connections necessary for a valid bedside appraisal of consciousness.

____

____

Receptor, receptor pathway to the cerebrum, motor pathway through the central nervous system (CNS) and into the peripheral nervous system, across the neuromuscular junction, and the effector itself.

D. The Glasgow Coma Scale (GCS) for tracking the level of depressed consciousness

1. A grading scale forces the Ex to observe systematically and accurately. The necessity to grade a response, as in eliciting muscle stretch reflexes (MSRs), makes you observe better than if you do not face such a reckoning.

Depend on it, sir, when a man knows he is to be hanged in a fortnight, it concentrates his mind wonderfully.

—**Samuel Johnson (1709–1874)**

2. For the Glasgow Coma Scale (total score 3 to 15), the Ex periodically grades eye opening from 1 to 4, the best verbal response from 1 to 5, and the best motor response to pain from 1 to 6 (Teasdale et al., 1978). The trend lines derived from these simple tests readily disclose deterioration or improvement. In Fig. 12-1, the trend lines document a declining level of consciousness in a Pt with cerebral edema. After the Pt receives intravenous mannitol, a hyperosmolar agent that reduces edema, the trend lines document the abrupt improvement.
3. Like the Apgar score, the total score for the three categories provides a prognosis (Bates, 1991; Evans et al., 1976; Teasdale et al., 1978). A GCS score from 3 to 8 implies a poor prognosis (Levin et al., 1991). The GCS should report the total score as well as the individual scores for each of the three items of the scale. Valuable as these scales are, some interexaminer variability occurs (Newton et al., 1995; Wiese, 2003).
4. In some intensive care unit Pts with the eyes swollen shut and who are sedated and intubated, the GCS is difficult to apply. Besides, the GCS is insensitive to brainstem function (lack of assessment of pupillary size and reactivity). Thus, modifications of the GCS and new proposals for more reliable coma scales have

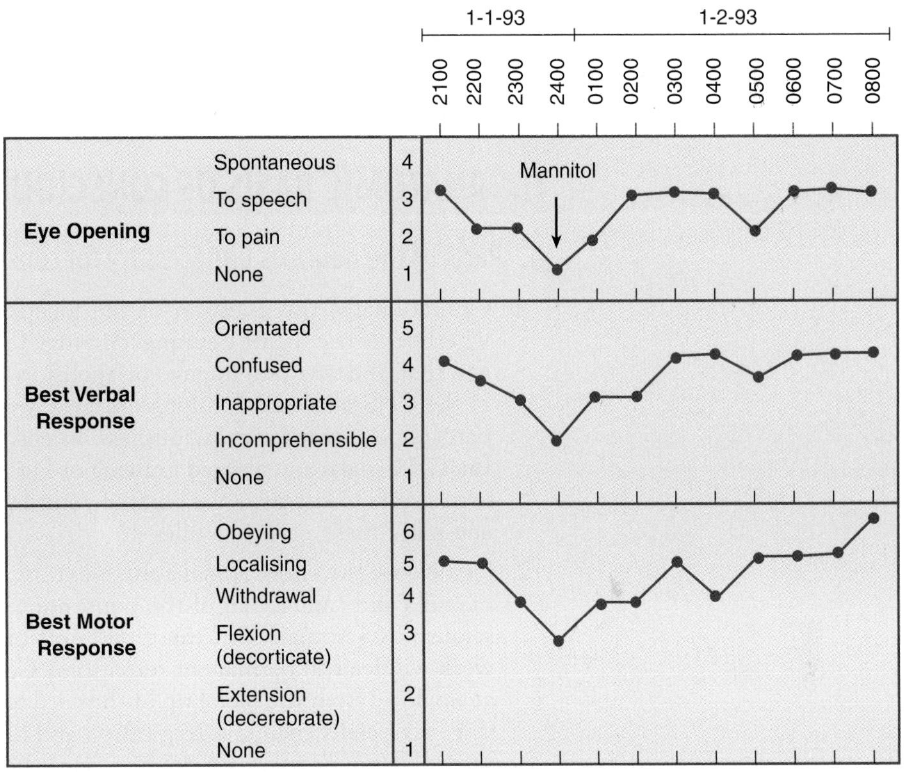

FIGURE 12-1. The Glasgow Coma Scale (GCS). Notice the declining level of consciousness until after mannitol treatment, which reduces brain edema.

TABLE 12-1 · Full Outline of UnResponsiveness (FOUR) Scale

Eye Response
- 4 = eyelids open or opened, tracking, or blinking to command
- 3 = eyelids open but not tracking
- 2 = eyelids closed but open to loud voice
- 1 = eyelids closed but open to pain
- 0 = eyelids remain closed with pain

Motor Response
- 4 = thumbs-up, fist, or peace sign
- 3 = localizing to pain
- 2 = flexion response to pain
- 1 = extension response to pain
- 0 = no response to pain or generalized myoclonus status

Brainstem Reflexes
- 4 = pupil and corneal reflexes present
- 3 = one pupil wide and fixed
- 2 = pupil or corneal reflexes absent
- 1 = pupil and corneal reflexes absent
- 0 = absent pupil, corneal, and cough reflex

Respiration
- 4 = not intubated, regular breathing pattern
- 3 = not intubated, Cheyne-Stokes breathing pattern
- 2 = not intubated, irregular breathing
- 1 = breathes above ventilator rate
- 0 = breathes at ventilator rate or apnea

source: Wijdicks et al., 2005.

since been proposed but not universally accepted. The Full Outline of UnResponsiveness (FOUR) score scale (Table 12-1; Wijdicks et al., 2005), proposed as an alternative to the GCS's, a new scale for improved assessment of coma. The scale has been validated in different settings, and it consists of four components (Eye Response, Motor Response, Brainstem Reflexes, and Respiratory Pattern. The total score is 0 to16, and each component has a maximal score of 4.

II. ANATOMIC BASIS OF CONSCIOUSNESS

A. Parts of the neuraxis unnecessary for consciousness

1. Operationally, the question of the location of consciousness boils down to whether we can locate neuronal circuitry that must be active for consciousness and that, if destroyed, impairs or abolishes consciousness. To identify the parts of the CNS necessary for consciousness, we will first cut away and discard the parts *un*necessary for consciousness. To ensure that you know the gross parts of the CNS, make an enlarged drawing of Fig. 2-1 on a loose sheet of paper. Then use scissors to cut away the parts of your drawing, as described next in the text, and place these parts in a pile.
2. First excise the entire spinal cord. Next excise the cerebellum. Then excise the medulla and caudal half of the pons: none of these parts is necessary for consciousness. (Actually cut these parts off of your drawing. This seeming busy work will lead to permanent retention.) Complete transection of the neuraxis at any level from the sacral tip of the cord to the midpons spares consciousness, if we artificially maintain respiration and blood pressure. The pile of parts discarded as unnecessary for consciousness now contains the entire spinal cord, medulla, caudal half of the pons, and the cerebellum. Next, however, complete transection of the brainstem in the upper pons will temporarily abolish consciousness, whereas complete midbrain transection will permanently abolish consciousness.
3. Next, instead of *complete* transections of the pons and midbrain, let us make *partial* transections to determine what must remain to support consciousness. To appreciate the partial cuts, review the cross-sectional anatomy of the brainstem by drawing the generalized cross section of the brainstem (Figs. 2-13 and 2-14). Actually cut the parts off of your drawing as called for in the text.
4. We find that complete transection or even removal of the entire basis of the midbrain or pons bilaterally does not abolish consciousness. If we start with a completely intact nervous system, bilateral destruction of the basis of pons or midbrain spares vertical eye movements but causes complete paralysis of all other volitional movements (Chapter 5). The Pt retains full sensation and full consciousness but can communicate that consciousness by the only available effector mechanism, the vertical eye movements (see the locked-in syndrome). Now snip off the brainstem basis bilaterally and place it on the discard heap.
5. After transecting the basis, we can insert the knife blade a little deeper to transect the medial and lateral lemnisci. The Pt loses the sensations mediated by these pathways, but consciousness remains. Next transect the tectum. Consciousness remains. Next, core out the cranial nerve motor nuclei. Consciousness remains. Thus, from your cross-sectional drawing of the brainstem, cut away the tectum, lemnisci, and cranial nerve nuclei and add them to the discard heap.
6. Now transection of the tegmentum bilaterally between the midpons and rostral midbrain abruptly abolishes consciousness. For consciousness, the midbrain and rostral half of the pontine tegmentum must remain intact (Reznick, 1983) and in continuity with the cerebrum and the diencephalon. Except for the rostral half of the pontomesencephalic tegmentum, we have discarded all other parts of the neuraxis caudal to the diencephalon.
7. From your original drawing, you now have left in your hand a cerebrum in continuity with the diencephalon and pontomesencephalic tegmentum. Now we will determine the role of the remaining parts of the CNS in consciousness

by transecting the diencephalon and basal ganglia at successively more rostral levels. We must insert the knife from the bottom of the cerebrum to transect these gray masses bilaterally without damaging the surrounding white matter or cortex. Bilateral transection of the diencephalon permanently and irreversibly abolishes consciousness. As we extend more rostrally into the basal ganglia, the evidence becomes a little less secure because of the lack of pure lesions in human disease; however, early in the history of surgery on the basal ganglia and diencephalon to treat involuntary movement syndromes, neurosurgeons learned not to make bilateral lesions because of the impairment of mentation, consciousness, and speech. Tentatively, we can state that acute bilateral destruction of the globus pallidus and striatum abolishes consciousness—at least, if the lesion extends, as it usually does, a little into the neighboring diencephalon or septal region, or into the neighboring medial hemispheric wall (Freemon, 1971). Thus, we find that bilateral lesions at any level, from the pontomesencephalic tegmentum up through the diencephalon and basal ganglia to the medial hemispheric wall, abolish consciousness (Figs. 12-2 and 12-3).

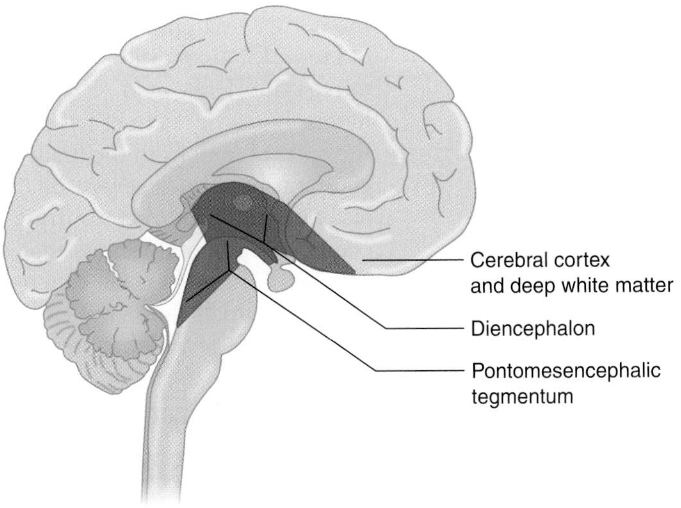

FIGURE 12-2. Sagittal section of the brain. The stippling shows the part of the pontomesencephalic tegmentum, diencephalon, and basal forebrain in which bilateral lesions abolish consciousness.

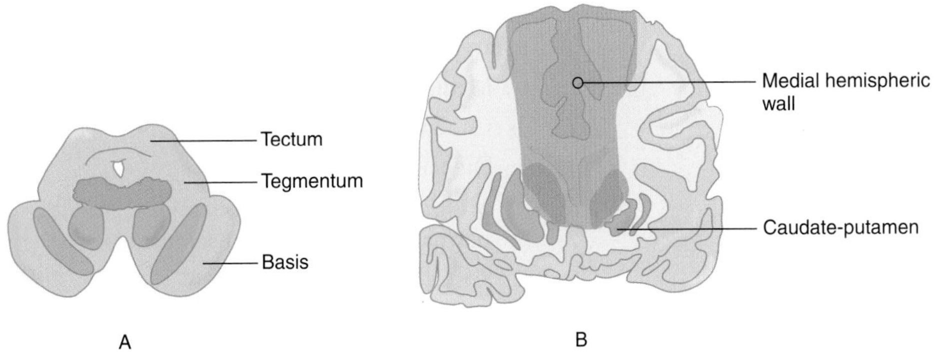

FIGURE 12-3. Coronal sections of the midbrain (A) and the cerebrum (B) at the level of the caudate nuclei. The shaded area shows the sites and comparative sizes of lesions that abolish consciousness.

8. Notice in Figs. 12-2 and 12-3 that, because the lesions involve structures rostral to the midbrain, in particular the basal ganglia and medial hemispheric wall, they must become increasingly larger than those required in the pontomesencephalic tegmentum and diencephalon.
9. The next anatomic region consists of the deep white matter surrounding the diencephalon and basal ganglia, which conveys axonal circuits between those neuronal masses and the cortical neurons. If we destroy the deep white matter of one hemisphere, scrape off all of its cerebral cortex, or remove the white matter and cortex by a hemispherectomy, the Pt can retain consciousness. (However, large acute lesions of a hemisphere temporarily impair consciousness. Curiously, left hemisphere lesions impair consciousness about twice as often as right hemisphere lesions [Albert et al., 1978].) Actually trace a hemisphere from Fig. 12-2, cut it out, and add it to the discard heap. The discard heap of the gross parts unnecessary for consciousness thus includes.

____

____

The spinal cord, medulla, caudal pons, cerebellum, entire basis and tectum of the pons and midbrain, the lemnisci and cranial nerve nuclei, and either one of the two cerebral hemispheres.

10. Although one of the two cerebral hemispheres is dispensable, we cannot dispense with both. We can discard any pair of the frontal, parietal, occipital, and temporal lobes. We profoundly alter personality and sensorimotor functions, but consciousness per se remains. But if we remove too much of the cerebrum bilaterally, scrape the cerebral cortex off *both* hemispheres, or destroy much or all of the cortex by hypoxia or hypoglycemia, we produce an **apallic syndrome,** an old term for a condition that is now considered equivalent to a persistent vegetative state (Dalle et al., 1977). If we suck out the deep white matter from both hemispheres, or if the Pt has a severe demyelinating disease, thus disconnecting the cortical shell from the brainstem and diencephalon, the Pt permanently loses consciousness. Such severe, bilateral destructive decorticating or demyelinating lesions stand in direct contrast to the tiny, confined, bilateral pontomesencephalic tegmental lesions that exquisitely and selectively abolish consciousness, with little effect on functions mediated through other pathways. Review Fig. 12-3, which shows the location in the midbrain tegmentum of the smallest, most discrete lesion that will permanently abolish consciousness.

B. Summary of the parts of the neuraxis necessary and unnecessary for consciousness

1. The previous observations show that full consciousness requires the pontomesencephalic tegmentum of at least one-half of the brainstem and the ipsilateral diencephalon and some of the ipsilateral cerebral hemisphere. This may, just may, constitute the minimal amount of brain required to function as a person. Although a necessary condition for consciousness, an intact pontomesencephalic tegmentum alone is not a sufficient condition or at least not sufficient to provide operational evidence of consciousness. That requires, in addition, a cerebral hemisphere or most of a hemisphere with an output pathway to some effector to produce behavioral responses that signify consciousness. What is not expendable bilaterally without profoundly affecting or abolishing consciousness is
   a. Medial hemispheric wall down to and including basal forebrain
   b. Caudate-putamen (striatum)
   c. Diencephalon
   d. Midbrain tegmentum: Bilateral tegmental lesions of small size completely and permanently abolish consciousness
   e. Rostral pontine tegmentum
2. To justify your having learned the structures unnecessary for consciousness, note this supreme fact: If your Pt has a lesion confined to one of these structures and is or becomes unconscious, something else has caused the unconsciousness. The usual cause is that the lesion has herniated or shifted the brain to compress the structures indispensable for consciousness. Without medical or surgical

intervention, the Pt will die. Section III discusses these brain herniations and their clinical recognition.

C. To prove your knowledge of the neuroanatomic basis of consciousness

1. Enumerate the parts of the neuraxis that we can discard without abolishing consciousness.

____

____.

Spinal cord, medulla, and caudal half of the pons (but we must support breathing and blood pressure); cerebellum; tectum; basis; lemnisci; cranial nerve (CrN) nuclei of the brainstem; any pair of the four cerebral lobes or one cerebral hemisphere (and maybe a little of the other hemisphere).

2. Enumerate the various sites of lesions within the neuraxis that will abolish consciousness. Assume artificial support of breathing and blood pressure to ensure that the neural lesion causes loss of consciousness, not hypoxia or ischemia.

____

____.

Make the lesions bilaterally at any level from the rostral pontine midbrain tegmentum, diencephalon, basal ganglia, or medial hemispheric wall, including the basal forebrain region. Alternatively, destroy bilaterally the cerebral cortex or the deep white matter.

3. State where to put the smallest lesion that will most selectively abolish consciousness.

____

____.

Place the lesion bilaterally in the midbrain tegmentum (Fig. 12-3A).

D. Operational demonstration of the pathways for consciousness

1. Insert a *stimulating* electrode into the midbrain reticular formation of an animal.
2. Apply *recording* electrodes over the scalp. The record obtained from the scalp electrodes is called an **electroencephalogram** (EEG).
3. After the animal goes to sleep, stimulate the reticular formation and observe:
   a. That the animal opens its eyes and looks around.
   b. That the EEG shows a distinct change in the electrical activity of the brain (Fig. 12-4).

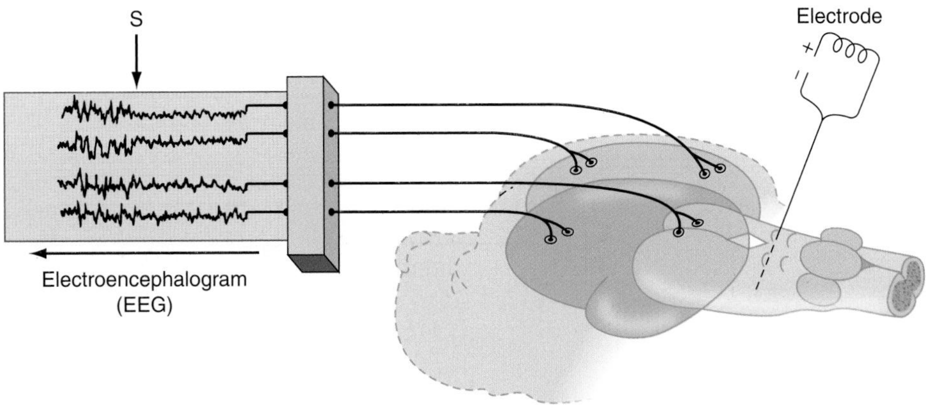

FIGURE 12-4. A sleeping animal with an electrode inserted into the midbrain reticular formation is hooked to an EEG machine. Stimulation of the electrode causes an abrupt awakening. *S* marks the point of stimulation during the EEG recording. Notice the abrupt change in the entire EEG from the high-amplitude slow waves of sleep to the low-amplitude fast activity of the waking state. EEG = electroencephalography.

4. After having awakened the animal with a stimulus to the reticular formation, the experimenter can greatly increase the current to make an electrolytic lesion around the tip of the electrode. The animal will lapse into unconsciousness.
5. Similar stimulation of the midline and intralaminar nuclei of the thalamus will produce an alerting response. Bilateral destruction abolishes consciousness.

6. **Interpretation of the experiment:** Demonstration of a nonspecific ascending pathway.
   a. The initial stimulation through the electrode was like throwing on a master switch: The entire cortex lit up. Because the entire cortex responded, we say that a **diffuse** or **nonspecific** ascending pathway has been stimulated. Because these impulses run through the thalamus, we conclude that the experiment demonstrates an ascending reticulo-thalamo-cortical pathway. We call this entire pathway the **ascending reticular activating system** (ARAS). Although the physiologic evidence points to a thalamocortical projection of the ARAS, the actual axons have yet to be fully demonstrated. The axons of some of the chemically specified reticular formation nuclei that belong to the ARAS bypass the thalamic nuclei.
   b. Notice that the operational definition of the ARAS depends on two lines of evidence: Stimulation of the system ❏ heightens/❏ decreases consciousness, whereas destruction ❏ heightens/❏ decreases consciousness.

☑ heightens; ☑ decreases

7. Give an operational definition of the ARAS based on the effects of stimulation or destruction.____
____.

The ARAS consists of the neuronal groups in the pontomesencephalic tegmentum and diencephalon that increase consciousness when stimulated and decrease it when destroyed.

E. Demonstration of specific thalamocortical pathways

1. The thalamocortical pathways of the sensory nuclei have a very specific, point-to-point relation to the cerebral cortex, in contrast to the ARAS, which projects diffusely or nonspecifically. To demonstrate this contrasting, specific system, do the following:
   a. Insert a *stimulating* electrode into one of the sensory relay nuclei of the thalamus.
   b. Apply *recording* electrodes over the cortical receptive area of the nucleus. In Fig. 12-5, the *stimulating* electrode is inserted into the nucleus ventralis posterior, and the *recording* electrodes are placed over the somesthetic receptive area in the postcentral gyrus. Study Fig. 12-5.

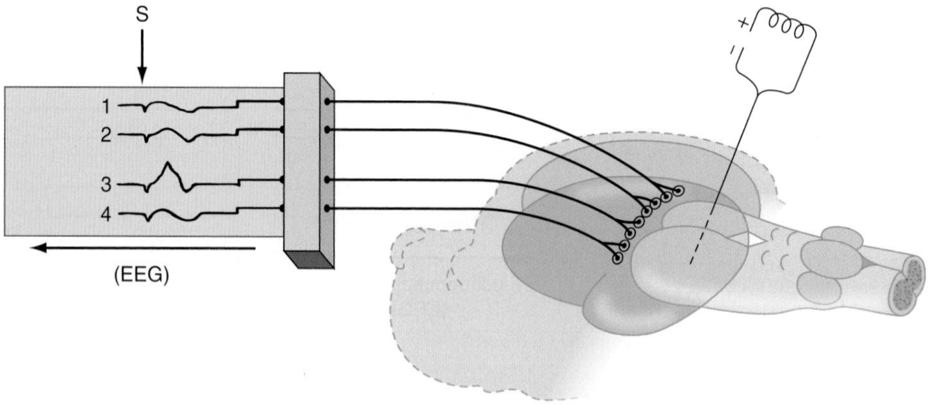

FIGURE 12-5. An electrode stimulated after insertion into one specific site in a thalamic somatosensory relay nucleus causes only one specific point of cortical excitation, in lead 3 of the electroencephalogram, rather than a generalized response as in Fig. 12-4.

2. The specific systems are so specific that stimulation of minute retinal areas, stimulation of the cochlea by discrete sound frequencies, or stimulation of the skin of the individual digits evokes a response in a tiny, specific cortical sensory area. Review the specific thalamic sensory relay nuclei and their cortical projection areas in Table 12-2.
3. The ❏ specific/❏ nonspecific pathways of the ARAS mediate the general state of consciousness, whereas the ❏ specific/❏ nonspecific thalamocortical pathways mediate consciousness of particular sensory events.

☑ nonspecific; ☑ specific

lateral geniculate body; occipital
medial geniculate body; temporal
nucleus ventralis posterior; parietal

TABLE 12-2 · Specific Sensory Relay Nuclei of the Thalamus

Modality	Thalamic nucleus	Cortical receptive area
Vision		Calcarine cortex in ______ lobe
Hearing		Superior temporal gyrus in ______ lobe
Somatic sensation		Postcentral gyrus in ______ lobe

BIBLIOGRAPHY · Consciousness

Albert ML, Silverberg R, Reches A, et al. Cerebral dominance for consciousness. *Arch Neurol* 1978;33:453–454.

Bates D. Defining prognosis in medical coma. *J Neurol Neurosurg Psychiatry* 1991;54:569–571.

Dalle OG, Gerstenbrand F, Lucking CF, et al. The apallic syndrome, Berlin. Germany. Springer-Verlag. 1977.

Evans BM. Patterns of arousal in comatose patients. *J Neurol Neurosurg Psychiatry* 1976;39:392–402.

Freemon FR. Akinetic mutism and bilateral anterior cerebral artery occlusion. *J Neurol Neurosurg Psychiatry* 1971;34:693–698.

Iyer VN, Mandrekar JN, Danielson RD, et al. Validity of the FOUR score coma scale in the medical intensive care unit. Mayo Clin Proc. 2009; 84 (8): 694–701.

Levin HS, Williams DH, Eisenberg HM. Serial MRI and neurobehavioral findings after mild to moderate closed head injury. *J Neurol Neurosurg Psychiatry* 1991;55:255–262.

Lipowski ZJ. Delirium in the elderly patient. *N Engl J Med* 1989;52:578–582.

Newton CRJC, Kirkham FJ, Johnston B. Inter-observer agreement of the assessment of coma scales and brainstem signs in non-traumatic coma. *Dev Med Child Neurol* 1995;37:807–813.

Posner JB, Saper CB, Schiff ND, et al. Plum and Posner's Diagnosis of Stupor and Coma. Oxford University Press, 2007.

Plum F, Posner J. The Diagnosis of Stupor and Coma, 3rd ed. Philadelphia, FA Davis, 1980.

Reznick M. Neuropathology of seven cases of locked-in syndrome. *J Med Sci* 1983;60:67–68.

Stead LG, Wijdicks EFM, Bhagra A, et al. Validation of a new coma scale, the FOUR Score, in the Emergency Department. Neurocritical Care. 2008; 10 (1); 50–54.

Teasdale G. Jennett B. assessment of coma and impaired consciousness. A practical scale. Lancet 1974; 2: 81–84.

Teasdale G, Knill-Jones R, van der Sande J. Observer variability in assessing impaired consciousness and coma. *J Neurol Neurosurg Psychiatry* 1978;41:603–610.

The Multi-Society Task Force on PVS. Medical Aspects of the Persistent Vegetative State—First of Two Parts. N Engl J Med1 1994; 330: 1499–1508.

Trzepacz PT, Meagher DJ, Wise MG. Neuropsychiatric aspects of delirium. In Yudofsky SC, Hales RE, eds. *Textbook of Neuropsychiatry and Clinical Neuroscience,* 4th ed. Washington, DC, American Psychiatric Publishing, 2002, Chap. 14, pp. 525–564.

Victor M, Ropper AM. *Adams and Victor's Principles of Neurology*, 7th ed. New York, McGraw-Hill, 2001.

Wiese MF. British Hospitals and different versions of the Glasgow Coma Scale; telephone survey. BMJ 2003-; 327 (418) 782–783.

Wijdicks EFM, Bamlet WR, Maramattom BV, et al. Validation of a new coma scale. The FOUR Score. Ann Neurol.2005; 58: 585–593.

III. INTERNAL HERNIATIONS OF THE BRAIN: EFFECT ON CONSCIOUSNESS, NEUROLOGIC FUNCTION, AND VASCULAR SYSTEM

A. Causes and consequences of internal herniations

The most common causes of internal herniations of the brain are cerebral contusions, hematomas, abscesses, neoplasms, and cerebral edema. The mass effect of these lesions increases the intracranial pressure and causes internal shifts or herniations of the brain that compress the normal tissue, in particular the diencephalon and brainstem (Cuneo et al., 1979; Davis and Robertson, 1991; Posner et al., 2007; Sunderland, 1958). This compression impairs consciousness and the life-sustaining functions of breathing, blood pressure control, and temperature regulation. Herniations also compress cerebral arteries, resulting in infarctions.

B. Anatomy of the intracranial partitions and compartments

To understand how space-occupying lesions act to cause coma or kill Pts, learn Figs. 12-6 to 12-8, and complete the subsequent exercises.

falx; tentorium

1. The cranial cavity is divided by tough, dural partitions called the ________________ cerebri and the ________________ cerebelli.

falx cerebri

2. The dural partition that divides the supratentorial space into right and left halves is the ________________.

temporo-occipital

3. The tentorium cerebelli forms a tent over the cerebellar hemispheres by inserting itself between the cerebellar hemispheres below and the ________________ lobes above.

notch (opening)

4. The space between the free, medial edges of the tentorial halves is called the tentorial ________________.

vermis

5. The part of the cerebellum that protrudes through the tentorial notch is the superior tip of the ________________.

☑ mesencephalon

6. The tentorial notch surrounds the ☐ pons/☐ mesencephalon/☐ diencephalon.
7. In Figs. 12-6 and 12-7 notice that:

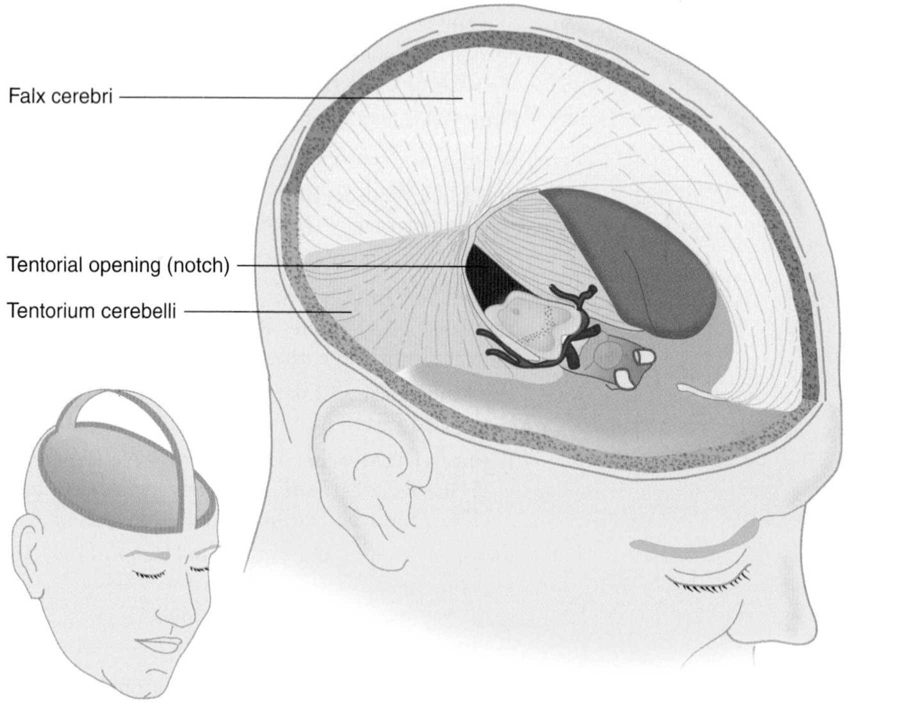

FIGURE 12-6. Basket-handle dissection of the skull and removal of the cerebral hemispheres. Notice that the falx cerebri and tentorium cerebelli, folds of the dura mater, partition the intracranial space. The mesencephalon was transected and left in situ in the tentorial opening. The posterior cerebral arteries course along the ventral edge of the midbrain and extend laterally to cross the free edge of the tentorium to reach the temporo-occipital portions of the cerebrum. Locate the III nerves issuing from under the posterior cerebral artery. See also Fig. 12-7.

   a. The transected brainstem remains in situ after removal of the cerebral hemispheres and diencephalon. Notice that the posterior cerebral artery passes over the free edge of the tentorial notch to reach the temporo-occipital portions of the cerebrum.

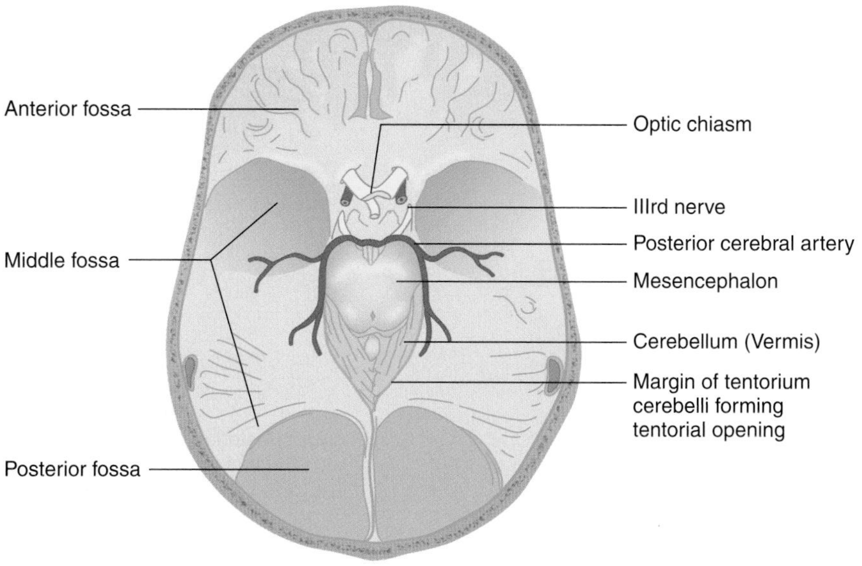

FIGURE 12-7. Base of the skull after removal of the basket handle and its attached falx cerebri. The mesencephalon remains *in situ,* as in Fig. 12-6. Notice the IIIrd nerve traveling under the PCA = Notice that the cerebellar vermis occupies the apex of the tentorial opening. The posterior fossa is under the tentorium. PCA posterior cerebral artery. (Redrawn with permission from Plum F, Posner J. *The Diagnosis of Stupor and Coma,* 3rd ed. Philadelphia, FA Davis, 1980.)

b. CrN III issues from the mesencephalon and passes *under* the posterior cerebral artery.

C. Responses of the fluid pools of the intracranial space to increased pressure

1. Water comprises 75% of the brain. Water is physically incompressible and biologically relatively immobile, although in cerebral edema it may increase the brain volume by 20% to 30%. This relatively immobile brain water contrasts with the two rapidly mobile liquid pools of the intracranial space, the **intravascular blood** and the **cerebrospinal fluid** (CSF). If brain tissue swells, what will happen to the lumen of the veins and capillaries? ________________

It will collapse.

2. After studying Figs. 12-8 and 12-9, describe what pressure does to the ventricles, sulci, and subarachnoid spaces of a swollen hemisphere. ________________

Collapses or displaces them.

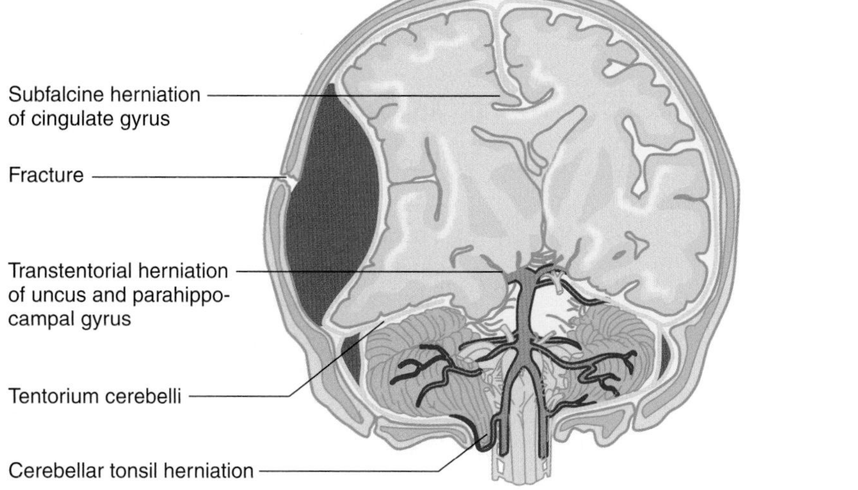

FIGURE 12-8. Coronal section of the head; ventral view of the brainstem and cerebrum. A large epidural hematoma has shifted the brain from right to left. Notice the herniation of the right uncus over the tentorial edge. Follow along the vertebral and basilar arteries to their terminal branches, the posterior cerebral arteries. Notice how the posterior cerebral artery on the right impinges on the IIIrd nerve. (Redrawn with permission from Netter F. *Ciba Symp* 1966;18, Plate XI.)

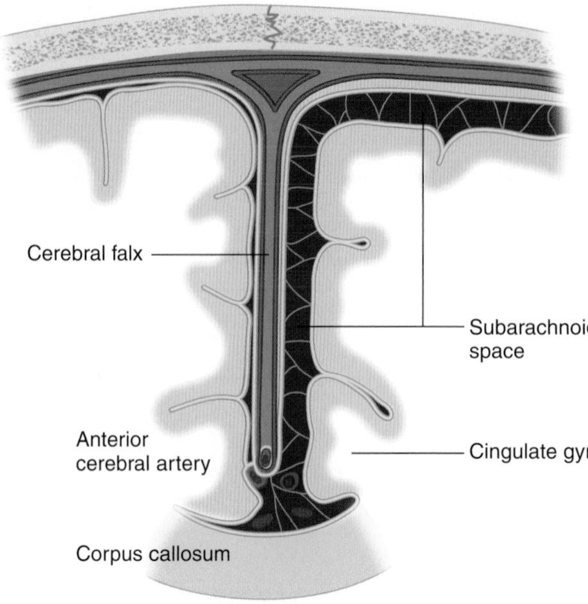

FIGURE 12-9. Coronal section through the falx and adjacent portions of the cerebrum along the interhemispheric fissure. Notice that the swollen hemisphere (reader's left) has collapsed the subarachnoid space and that the cingulate gyrus has begun to herniate under the free, inferior edge of the falx, impinging on the anterior cerebral artery.

CSF and intravascular blood

3. Thus, the first compensation for increased pressure is a reduction in the two rapidly mobile intracranial fluid pools, the ________________________.

bulging fontanels, split sutures, and increased occipitofrontal circumference (Chapter 1).

4. The infant has additional ways to compensate for increased intracranial pressure, manifested by the following physical signs: ____ ________________________.

puberty (10 to 12 years; Chapter 1)

5. As the skull matures, it no longer yields to increased intracranial pressure. If you find split sutures on a skull radiograph of an 18-year-old Pt, the increased pressure must have started before the age of ________________.

medially under the falx or downward over the edge of the tentorial notch

6. If the hemispheric swelling exceeds the compensatory mechanisms in an infant or adult, the affected tissue can only respond by herniating. Study Fig. 12-8 and state the only *two* places the shifting hemisphere can go ____________ ________________________________.

subfalcial (the *x* becomes *c*)

7. Because part of the swollen hemisphere has shifted *under* the falx cerebri, this shift is called ________________ herniation.

D. Anatomy of transfalcine herniation

cingulate

1. The part of the hemisphere that shifts under the falx is called the ________________ gyrus.
2. The anterior cerebral arteries run parallel to the free edge of the falx. When the cingulate gyrus herniates, it may compress the artery against the free edge of the falx, causing infarction of the medial hemispheric wall dorsal to the corpus callosum (Fig. 12-9).

☑ leg

3. In view of the representation of body parts in the motor cortex on the medial aspect of a hemisphere (Fig. 2-2C), this infarction would cause upper motoneuron (UMN) paralysis of the ❒ leg/❒ arm/❒ face/❒ leg, arm, and face.

E. Anatomy of transtentorial herniation of the cerebrum

1. With a space-occupying lesion in one hemicranium, the bony wall of the calvarium prevents herniation or decompression outward. The cerebral hemisphere can herniate only *medially* or *downward* (Fig. 12-8).

a. The dural membrane that opposes *medial* shift of the cerebrum is the ____________________.

falx cerebri

b. The dural membrane that opposes *downward* shift of the cerebrum is the ____________________.

tentorium cerebelli

2. *Trans* means *over* or *across*, hence, *trans* continental. The shifting of a swollen hemisphere *across* the free edge of the tentorium cerebelli is called ____________________tentorial herniation.

transtentorial

3. Hence, the two internal herniations of a swollen hemisphere are ____________________ herniation and ____________________ herniation.

transtentorial; transfalcine

4. The parts that undergo transtentorial herniation are the medial parts of the temporal lobe, namely the ____________________ and ____________________ gyrus.

uncus; parahippocampal (see Figs. 12-8 and 12-9, if you missed)

5. Fig. 12-10 shows a brain removed at autopsy. Fill in the labels and, in the blanks below, describe what is wrong.
____.

The left uncus and parahippocampal gyrus have herniated across the tentorial notch, thus compressing CrN III and the midbrain.

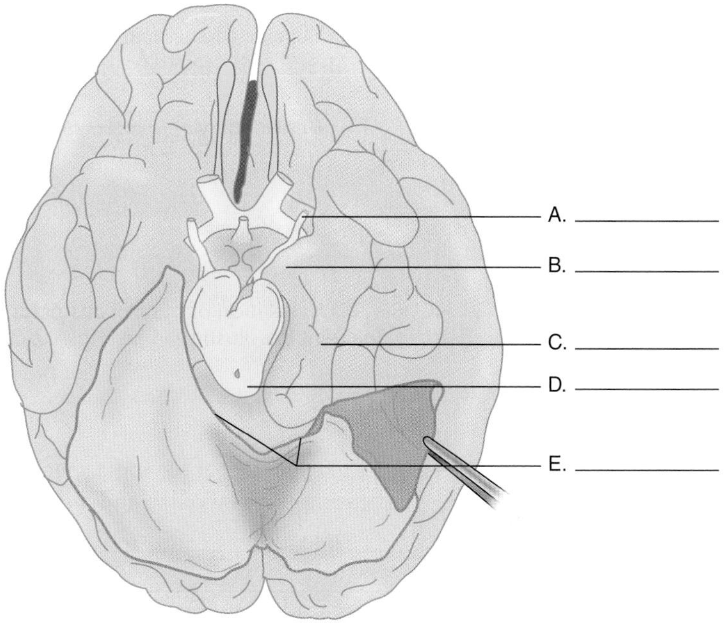

A. CrN III
B. Uncus
C. Parahippocampal gyrus
D. Midbrain
E. Free edge of tentorium (tentorial notch)

FIGURE 12-10. Ventral view of the cerebrum with the tentorium cerebelli reflected on the left side. Complete the blanks on the right side. (Redrawn with permission from Peele T. *The Neuroanatomic Basis for Clinical Neurology,* 2nd ed. New York, McGraw-Hill, 1961.)

6. In coursing from the basilar artery to the cerebrum, the posterior cerebral artery crosses the free edge of the falx, where the herniation may compress it (Figs. 12-6 and 12-7 and Table 12-5). This artery irrigates the medial part of the temporo-occipital region and the occipital pole. Infarction of this region, particularly on the right, would cause two ophthalmologic disorders, ____________________ and ____________________ (Keane, 1980, Alexia with agraphia has also been rarely observed as a result from compression of left posterior cerebral artery by transtentorial herniation [Kirschner et al., 1982]).

contralateral homonymous hemianopsia; prosopagnosia

F. Effect of transtentorial and subfalcine herniation on consciousness

Because subfalcine and transtentorial herniations compress the medial hemispheric wall, diencephalon, and mesencephalon, they interfere with the ARAS and alter the Pt's level of consciousness. Medial shift of the brain alone may impair consciousness (Fisher, 1995; Inao et al., 2001; Pullicino et al., 1997; Ropper, 1993) but, if combined with transtentorial herniation, compresses the brainstem and may kill the Pt.

G. Effect of transtentorial herniation on cranial nerve III

constrict

1. As transtentorial herniation increases, the uncus displaces the posterior cerebral artery and CrN III. CrN III contains parasympathetic fibers that, when stimulated, cause the pupil to _______________.

Increases

The unopposed tonic action of the pupillodilator muscle (sympathetic) enlarges the pupil. The dilated pupil of transtentorial (uncal) herniation is known as Hutchinson pupil.

2. After compression of CrN III, what happens to the pupillary size? Explain.

____

____

3. Because the pupilloconstrictor fibers occupy the superomedial part of CrN III, the caudally displaced posterior cerebral artery impinges on them first when the temporal lobe herniates (Fig. 12-11).

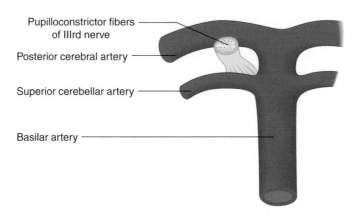

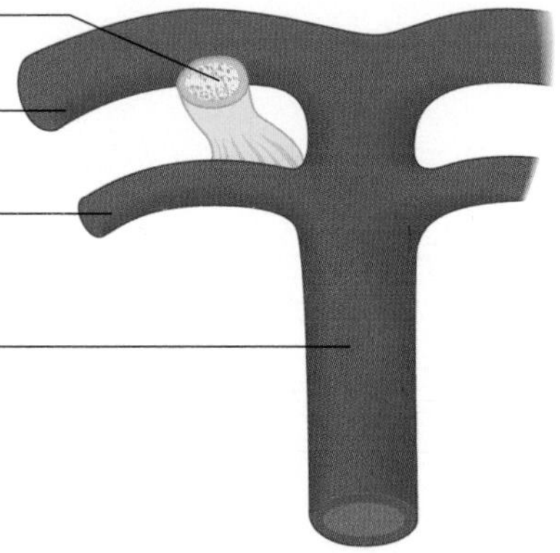

FIGURE 12-11. Relation of pupilloconstrictor fibers of cranial nerve III to the posterior cerebral artery. To orient this illustration, see Figs. 12-6 and 12-8.

Transtentorial herniation, brainstem compression, and death.

4. In a Pt suspected of having a space-occupying intracranial lesion, what would an increasing pupillary size and a decreasing level of consciousness imply?

____

____

5. As transtentorial herniation advances, both III nerves may crease to function. Both pupils become *dilated* and *fixed*, no longer responding to light. Before dilating, the opposite pupil may go through a phase of mild constriction (Forbes et al., 1965; Ropper, 1990). Whereas a unilateral dilated and fixed pupil announces danger requiring prompt or even heroic intervention, bilateral dilated and fixed pupils from brainstem compression are almost synonymous with death without prompt neurosurgical intervention (Clusmann et al., 2001).

H. Effect of transtentorial herniation on motor function

☑ left-sided

1. Consider a Pt with a large acute right hemisphere lesion. It would cause a ☐ left-sided/☐ right-sided hemiplegia.
2. As the herniating right hemisphere compresses the mesencephalon, the left basis gets pushed against the opposite free edge of the tentorium on the left side, indenting the basis (Kernohan-Woltman notch). Notice in Fig. 12-7 the close relation of the basis mesencephali to the tentorial edges, affording virtually no safety factor.

right; ☑ ipsilateral

3. After compression of the *left* basis, the UMN fibers cannot transmit impulses. The Pt now shows a _______________-sided hemiplegia in addition to the original left-sided hemiplegia. The new hemiplegia is ☐ ipsilateral/☐ contralateral to the right hemisphere lesion.

☑ same

4. Such an ipsilateral hemiplegia is called a **paradoxical hemiplegia** because it is on the ❒ same/❒ opposite side as the hemispheric lesion. Sometimes the paradoxical hemiplegia appears first, constituting a false localizing sign of the side of brain herniation.

Decrease or disappear.

5. Hence, if a Pt started out with a large right hemispheric lesion and left hemiplegia and then had a right hemiplegia, the Pt has double hemiplegia. If the double hemiplegia evolves very rapidly, the Pt might display cerebral shock. What would happen to the MSRs and tone? _______________.
6. Thus, depending on the rapidity of evolution of the lesion, the MSRs and tone may change from time to time and from side to side.
7. Recite the neurologic findings in transtentorial herniation with respect to the IIIrd nerve, the ARAS, and the pyramidal tracts in the basic mesencephali. Check the preceding frames to be sure that you have recited the effects correctly.
8. The Kernohan-Woltman notch/paradoxical hemiplegia sequence can be regarded as a *contrecoup* condition because it is on the opposite side of the inciting hemispheric lesion; but in acute head injury a *coup* type of displacement may similarly nick the midbrain *ipsilaterally* (Saeki et al., 2000).

I. Bilateral transtentorial herniation

1. Many pathologic conditions cause **bilateral** transtentorial herniation. The lesion may consist of cerebral edema from trauma, encephalitis, or metabolic disorders such as uremia and hepatic coma. Of the structural lesions, head injuries, subdural hematomas, hydrocephalus, multiple metastatic neoplasms or abscesses, and intracranial hemorrhage lead the list. If both hemispheres swell, the unci and parahippocampal gyri of both sides try to squeeze down through the tentorial notch. The ring of swollen tissue acts exactly like a ligature around the midbrain.
2. The *coup de grace* to the Pt with transtentorial herniation, bilateral or unilateral, is mesencephalic and pontine hemorrhage secondary to the herniation (Friede and Roessmann, 1966; Hassler, 1967). The stretching and compression of the brainstem vessels stops the blood flow. The vessel walls rupture. The consequent brainstem hemorrhage is usually the terminal event that causes the Pt to die (Fig. 12-12).

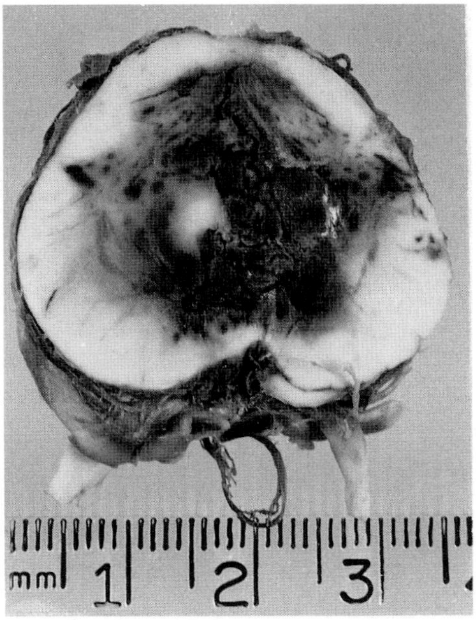

FIGURE 12-12. Transverse section of the mesencephalon showing hemorrhages secondary to transtentorial herniation. The IIIrd nerves are seen exiting ventrally. The caudal displacement of the brainstem by the herniating cerebrum stretches and compresses the brainstem vessels until they rupture, killing the patient.

J. Decerebrate rigidity, a postural syndrome of midbrain lesions

1. **Description of the decerebrate posture:** Extensive midbrain lesions, intrinsic or from unilateral or bilateral transtentorial herniation, disconnect the cerebrum and diencephalon from the rest of the brainstem, i.e., decerebrate the individual. The "decerebration" can, in fact, be toxic-metabolic rather than anatomic. Along with the IIIrd nerve signs, double hemiplegia, and loss of consciousness, the Pt may show a diagnostic postural syndrome called **decerebrate rigidity** (gamma rigidity). Study Fig. 12-13 and assume the decerebrate posture yourself. Can you maintain it easily?

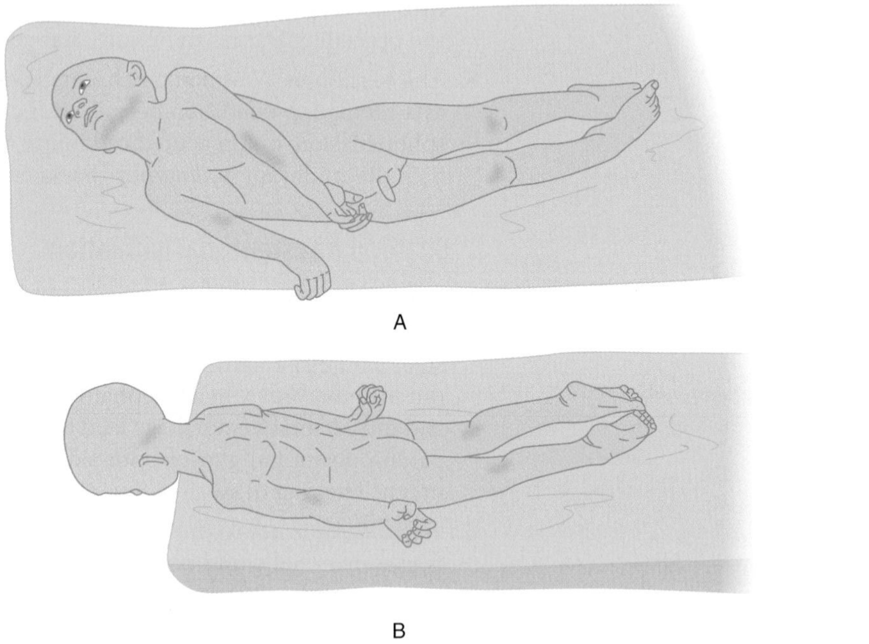

FIGURE 12-13. Decerebrate posture in an unconscious Pt. (A) Patient placed on his side. (B) Patient placed with his head over the edge of the table to show the rigid extension of his neck. (Redrawn with permission from Penfield W, Jasper H. *Epilepsy and the Functional Anatomy of the Human Brain.* Boston, Little, Brown & Co., 1954).

2. After carefully inspecting the head, jaw, trunk, and limb postures of the Pt, cover Fig. 12-13 and test your powers of observation by completing Table 12-3.

☑ closed
☑ extended
☑ extended
☑ extended
☑ flexed
☑ flexed
☑ extended
☑ plantar flexed
☑ plantar flexed

TABLE 12-3 · Posture in Decerebrate Rigidity

The mouth is ☐open/☐closed.
The head is ☐extended/☐flexed.
The trunk is ☐extended/☐flexed.
The arms are ☐extended/☐flexed (and pronated).
The wrists are ☐extended/☐flexed.
The fingers are ☐extended/☐flexed.
The legs are ☐extended/☐flexed.
The feet are ☐extended/☐plantar flexed.
The toes are ☐plantar flexed/☐dorsiflexed.

3. **Muscle tone in decerebrate rigidity:** Testing of the muscle tone of the Pt shown in Fig. 12-13 would disclose rigid extension of the extremities and spine, but if you once bend the part, it will yield like a clasp knife. Hence, the tonic disturbance seems to combine features of spasticity and rigidity.

☑ extended
☑ flexed
☑ internally

4. **Descriptive definition of decerebrate rigidity:** The Pt displays an involuntary posture with the:
   a. Proximal joints (spine, shoulders, hips, elbows, and knees) rigidly ❒ extended/❒ flexed.
   b. Distal joints (wrists/ankles, fingers/toes) rigidly ❒ extended/❒ flexed.
   c. Forearms and legs ❒ internally/❒ externally rotated.
5. **Pathophysiologic explanation of the decerebrate posture:** As a prelude to interpreting the decerebrate posture, review the strength of the muscle actions listed in Table 12-4. Actually test a normal subject to complete the table.

TABLE 12-4 · Comparative Strength of Postural Deviation in Decerebrate Rigidity

Action	Stronger than	Weaker than	Opposing action
Jaw closure is	❒	❒	Jaw opening
Head extension is	❒	❒	Head flexion
Trunk extension is	❒	❒	Trunk flexion
Arm extension is	❒	❒	Arm flexion
Forearm pronation, arm extended is	❒	❒	Supination
Wrist flexion is	❒	❒	Wrist extension
Finger flexion is	❒	❒	Finger extension
Leg extension is	❒	❒	Leg flexion
Inversion of foot is	❒	❒	Eversion
Ankle flexion is	❒	❒	Ankle extension
Toe flexion is	❒	❒	Toe extension

   a. After completing Table 12-4, you can conclude that the direction of pull of the strongest muscles determines the posture of the spine and extremities assumed by the decerebrate Pt.
   b. Figure 12-14 shows the posture of a quadruped with decerebrate rigidity. A quadruped with decerebrate rigidity will stand, if set on its feet. Review also Fig. 7-2.

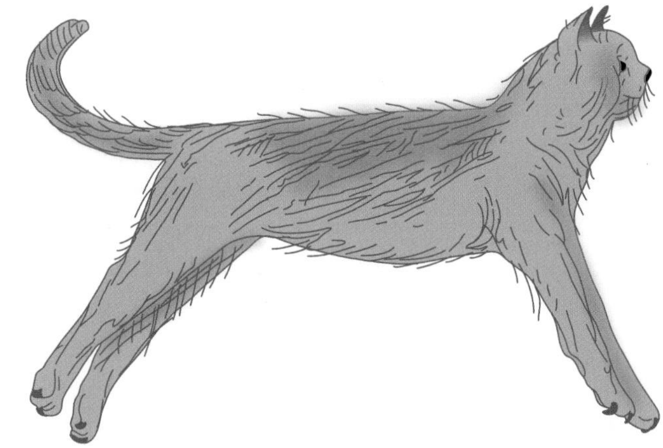

FIGURE 12-14. Decerebrate posture in the cat. (Reproduced with permission from Pollock L, Davis L. The reflex activities of a decerebrate animal. *J Comp Neurol* 1930;50:377–411.)

   c. The extended head, tail, and extremities and the closed jaw of the quadruped indicate that the muscles that acting to cause the decerebrate posture support a quadruped animal's posture against collapse due to the pull of gravity. These same muscles cause it to leap and locomote in defiance of gravity. Hence, we interpret decerebrate rigidity as that posture maintained by excessive contraction

☑ quadruped (Review Table 12-3 and Fig. 7-2, if you missed.)

of the antigravity muscles of the quadruped. In general, the strongest muscles of humans are the true antigravity muscles of a ❑quadruped/❑biped.

Transect or compress the midbrain.

d. Describe how you could produce the decerebrate posture in an experimental animal.______________________

If you tested carefully, you should have checked the Stronger Than column every time.

6. **Role of the vestibular system in decerebrate rigidity:** After decerebration by midbrain transection interrupts the impulses descending from the cerebrum, the vestibular system becomes overactive, causing it to overstimulate or drive the powerful antigravity muscles.

Decerebrate rigidity is a new behavior, released by interruption of descending pathways.

a. Explain whether you should classify the decerebrate posture as a deficit or a release phenomenon.______________________

____

See next frame.

b. Describe a surgical experiment or series of experiments to prove that the drive for the decerebrate posture comes from the vestibular system. Think carefully.

____

______________________.

c. Like any release phenomenon, decerebrate rigidity not only requires a lesion to release it but also an intact neural mechanism to produce, drive, and perpetuate it. The term "decerebrate rigidity" was first used by Sherrington (1898) after an intercollicular transection (between the red nuclei and the vestibular nuclei) in animal studies. Sherrington showed that destruction of the vestibular system abolishes the decerebrate posture. Apparently the activity that drives the decerebrate posture arises in the vestibular system and is conveyed to the spinal cord by the vestibulospinal tracts. Dorsal or ventral root transection also abolishes it.

midbrain; vestibular system, vestibulospinal tract, and dorsal and ventral roots

d. For decerebrate rigidity to appear, the critical neural structure transected or compressed is the ______________. The critical neural structures that must remain intact are the ______________________.

The decerebrate posture consists of the rigid extension of the neck, trunk, arms, and legs with wrist pronation and wrist and finger flexion, and ankle and toe flexion with internal rotation of the feet.

7. **Give a succinct clinical description of the decerebrate posture.** Be sure to separate observation from interpretation.______________________

____

It is a release of the antigravity posture of the quadruped, maintained by the vestibulospinal system and dorsal root afferents, after actual mesencephalic lesions or after toxic and metabolic states that functionally decerebrate the Pt.

8. **Give the pathophysiologic interpretation of decerebrate rigidity.**

____

____

9. Some unconscious Pts show decerebrate posturing only in response to pain. To elicit the posture, press the ball of your thumb or a knuckle hard for several seconds against the Pt's sternum.

10. Despite the relatively poor prognosis, rarely Pts with decerebrate rigidity remain conscious (Halsey and Downie, 1966) and rarely recover (Brandler and Selverstone, 1970; Damasceno, 1991; Kao et al., 2006).

K. Decorticate versus decerebrate posture

1. The decerebrate posture differs from chronic hemiplegia (after the state of cerebral shock or diaschisis in acute hemiplegia has passed). Compare Figs. 12-13 and 12-15.

The hemiplegic Pt holds the arm flexed rather than extended at the elbow. Otherwise, the wrist and finger postures and the leg posture resemble it.

2. Describe the major difference in the posture of the arm in decerebrate rigidity versus hemiplegia.

____

____

L. Respiratory and autonomic effects of brainstem lesions and transtentorial herniation

1. The unconscious Pt may display strong inspiratory stridor because of collapse of the oropharyngeal muscles. Simply place your fingers behind the ramus of the mandible and pull the mandible forward. The Pt will immediately breathe more freely. Positioning the head to the side or placing an oropharyngeal airway then solves the problem.

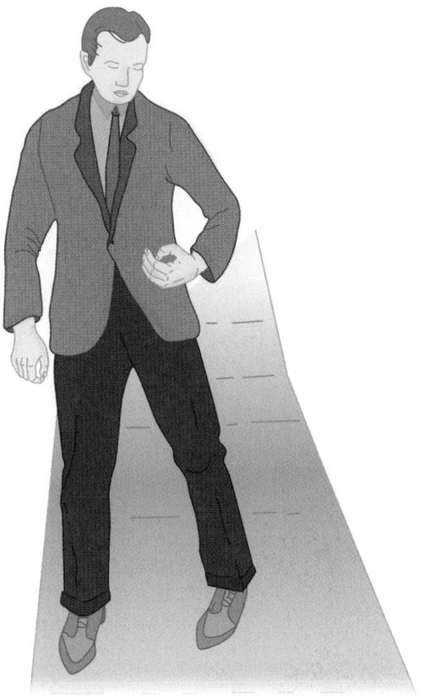

FIGURE 12-15. Posture in an adult with chronic hemiplegia. Compare the arm position with that shown in Fig. 12-13.

2. Lesions at various levels from the cerebrum to the upper cervical cord cause characteristic respiratory dysrhythmias. Figure 12-16 depicts some of the dysrhythmias, but it depicts their localizations more schematically than the data warrant.

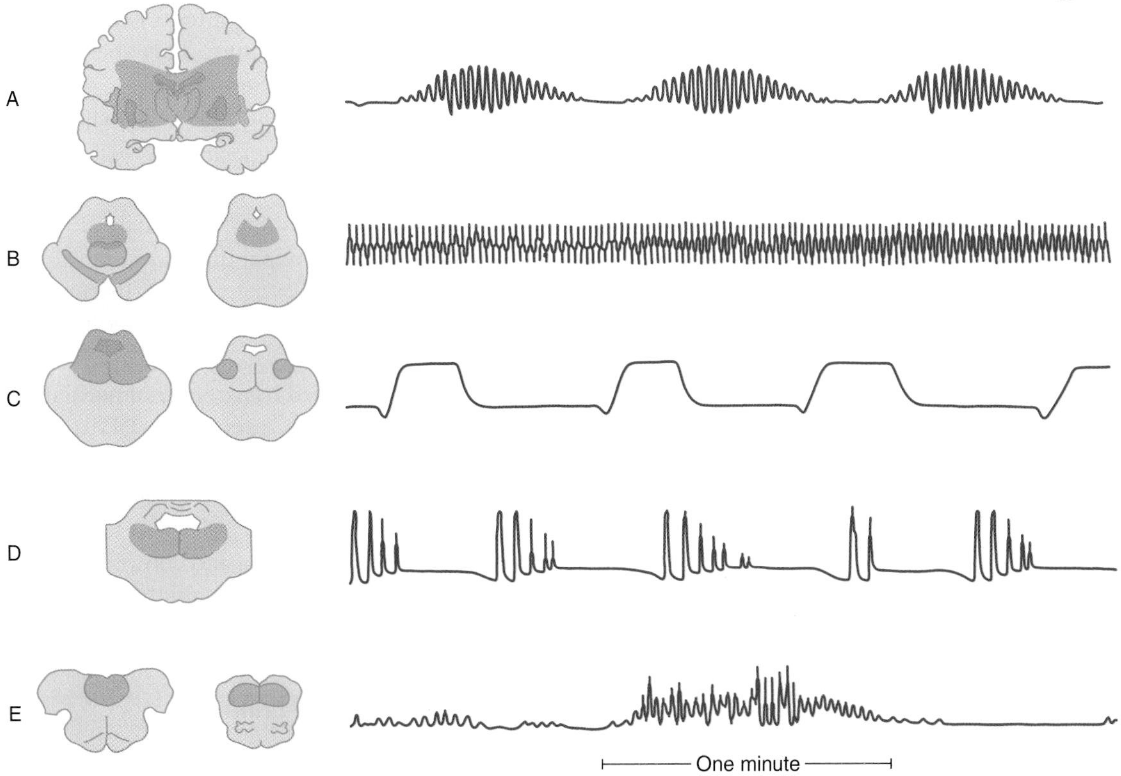

FIGURE 12-16. Correlation of intra-axial brainstem lesions at successive levels, with the type of respiratory dysrhythmia caused. (A) Cheyne-Stokes respiration. (B) Central neurogenic hyperventilation. (C) Apneustic breathing. (D) Cluster breathing. (E) Ataxic breathing. (Redrawn from Plum F, Posner J. *The Diagnosis of Stupor and Coma*, 3rd ed. Philadelphia, FA Davis, 1980.)

3. Transtentorial herniation, by external compression, caudal displacement, and kinking of the brainstem, causes a "wave of failure" to pass caudally from diencephalon to medulla. The Pt passes in succession through the various respiratory dysrhythmias shown in Fig. 12-16 that reflect the effects of lesion at various rostrocaudal levels. One type of dysrhythmia seen with intrinsic brainstem lesions but not with transtentorial herniation is apneustic breathing (Fig. 12-16C; Plum and Posner, 1980).
4. Among many other dysrhythmias not specific as to lesion site or cause are **Biot's** and **Kussmaul's.**
   a. Kussmaul's breathing is characterized by "air hunger," with deep regular sighing respiration (increase tidal volume), whether the rate is slow, normal, or fast. Kussmaul respiration suggests the presence of metabolic acidosis, and is the result of stimulation of the brainstem respiratory centers by the low blood pH. It occurs with metabolic disorders, such as diabetic acidosis and uremia, exogenous acids (e.g., intoxication with salicylates methanol, or ethylene glycol), and other severe systemic illnesses.
   b. Biot's breathing resembles Cheyne-Stokes breathing (Fig. 12-16A) by consisting of periods of apnea that alternate irregularly with series of breaths, but the four to five breaths have equal length and terminate abruptly rather than fading in and out.
5. The effect of transtentorial herniation or other brainstem lesions on blood pressure and pulse varies. Although hypertension or hypotension and tachycardia or bradycardia may occur, typically increased intracranial pressure causes a *slowing* of the pulse rate and an *increasing* blood pressure (Cushing's phenomenon). Many factors, such as the ventilatory efficiency, may alter this formula. Thus, the Ex must expect changes in the vital signs and monitor them carefully.

M. Transforaminal herniation

1. **Anatomy of transforaminal herniation:** The diffusely swollen, herniating brain may impose the death penalty by a mechanism other than transtentorial herniation. As increased pressure pushes the intracranial contents caudally, the cerebellum and medulla herniate into the foramen magnum. This aperture is designed to accommodate only the cervicomedullary junction.
   a. Because the caudalmost part of the cerebellum, the cerebellar *tonsils,* is the part of the cerebellum to herniate, this lesion is called **tonsillar** or **transforaminal herniation.** See the herniated right cerebellar tonsil shown in Fig. 12-8.
   b. Transforaminal herniation may result from expanding *supra* tentorial lesions or from expanding *infra*tentorial lesions, such as a cerebellar hemorrhage or neoplasm. Chapter 13 describes the danger of transforaminal herniation after lumbar puncture.
   c. Infratentorial masses also may cause **upward transtentorial herniation,** causing midbrain compression and midbrain signs (Cuneo et al., 1979).
2. **The clinical syndrome of transforaminal herniation:** The clinical syndrome mimics transection of the neuraxis at the medullocervical junction level. The Pt becomes quadriplegic and totally apneic (Table 12-5). The total apnea results from the quadriplegia that stops volitional breathing and compression of the reticulospinal tracts that stops automatic breathing. No respiratory drive reaches the lower motoneurons (LMNs). Review Fig. 6-17.

N. Summary of the internal herniations of the brain

1. Name the three common internal herniations of the brain.

   ____

   Subfalcine, transtentorial, and transforaminal.

2. Name the parts of the brain that herniate in transtentorial herniation and in transforaminal herniation. ______________________________

   ____

   Parahippocampal gyrus and uncus in transtentorial herniation; cerebellar tonsils and medulla in transforaminal herniation.

TABLE 12-5 · Summary of Vascular Complications and Clinical Signs of Internal Herniations of the Brain

Type of herniation	Vascular complications	Clinical signs
Subfalcine herniation medially of the cingulate gyrus	Compression of anterior cerebral artery under free edge of the falx, causing infarction of medial hemispheric wall and motor area for the leg (Figs. 2-2C and 12-9)	Obtundation, disorientation, monoparesis of contralateral lower extremity
Transtentorial herniation downward and medially of the uncus and parahippocampal gyrus	Compression of posterior cerebral artery against free edge of tentorium (Figs. 12-6 and 12-7); brainstem hemorrhages (Fig. 12-12) The anterior choroidal and posterior communicating arteries may be displaced inferomedially in severe cases	Increasing loss of consciousness, pupillodilation; and IIIrd nerve palsy; hemianopsia
Transtentorial herniation upward of the cerebellar vermis and midbrain	Compression of superior cerebellar artery by free edge of tentorium and compression of midbrain and brainstem vessels	Increasing obtundation, pretectal/rostral midbrain syndrome (Table 5-2), IIIrd nerve palsy
Transforaminal herniation downward of the cerebellar tonsils and medulla oblongata	Infarction of the cervicomedullary junction and rostral 1–2 segments of spinal cord from compression of ventral and posterior spinal arteries that arise inside the foramen magnum from the vertebral and posterior inferior cerebellar arteries; hemorrhagic necrosis of the cerebellar tonsils	Neck stiffness or head tilt. Apnea and quadriparesis from compression of the medullocervical junction

By causing brainstem compression that impairs vital functions such as breathing, pulse rate, and blood pressure, and ultimately by causing brainstem hemorrhage.

3. State, in principle, how brain herniations kill the Pt.

____

☑ No
Clinical tests for cerebellar dysfunction require conscious responses by the Pt.

4. Could you test for cerebellar function in a comatose Pt? ❒ Yes/❒ No. Explain.

____

See next frame.

5. If a comatose Pt removed from a wrecked car shows distinct decerebrate rigidity in the upper extremities and the lower extremities are totally flaccid, what would be the best clinical conclusion? Think circuitry to figure out and explain the answer.

____.

6. The Pt may have suffered spinal cord transection and a brain injury, a not uncommon association. In this case, a single lesion does not explain the clinical picture, but a single cause, trauma, does. Sometimes however, even with an intact spinal cord, only the arms will show decerebrate posturing. Hence, the action of the legs proves that the cord is intact, but the absence does not. Extremely rarely, posturing of the arms resembling decerebrate rigidity occurs as a spinal reflex (Saposnik et al., 2000; Brain Death bibliography).

O. Brain herniations: a clinical summation and critique

1. Table 12-5 summarizes the internal herniations. Cover the text in columns 2 and 3 and recite the text by using the headings in column 1 as a prompt.
2. When any modern gladiator, a boxer, a football player, or a race driver, dies after a head injury, in sacrifice to our appetite for brutality, you can surmise that the mechanism of death was brain edema and herniation (Jordan, 1992; Unterharnscheidt, 2003). If we, as a people, do not value above all else the preciousness and fragility of life, one might suppose that we would, at least, value and protect the brain, which gives us the means to seek advantages. For the brain functions not, as you might have supposed, as an organ of intelligence, but, as Szent-Györgyi said, as an advantage-seeking organ. The television hero stunned by a head injury who, without lingering effects, immediately returns to chasing the bad guys represents an egregious error in medical management because it trivializes head injury. Getting "dinged" is sports slang to minimize a possible life-taking event. **Any person**

stunned or unconscious from a blow to the head requires rest and careful medical observation. You must presume that any Pt with any head injury may have a life-threatening epidural or subdural hematoma—albeit initially inapparent. Whether to send home the Pt who has had a seemingly trivial blow to the head or to hospitalize for observation is one of the most difficult of all medical decisions. You must deal with prediction, the most difficult of all the arts. Remember that the specter of death is looking over your shoulder.

Life is short, the art long, opportunity fleeing, experience treacherous, judgment difficult.

—Hippocrates (4th Century B.C.), Aphorisms, Section 1.

3. To carefully monitor every Pt who has a potential brain herniation, record the mental status and all signs: vital signs, such as blood pressure and pulse, and physical signs, such as the pupillary diameters in millimeters. Record the presence or absence of venous pulsations (Jacks and Miller, 2003). The goal always is to intervene early to prevent herniations. Given a Pt with a head injury and left hemiparesis who is initially conscious, outline the sequence of events that will predict transtentorial herniation and list the sequence of events to death:
   a. Consciousness: ______________________.
   b. Extremity movement and posture: ______________________.
   c. Pupillary changes: ______________________.
   d. Respiration changes: ______________________
   e. Pulse and blood pressure: ______________________.

See the next frame for the answers.

4. Answers to frame 3
   a. May have some excitement or delirium and then pathologic sleep, stupor, semicoma, and coma.
   b. Left hemiparesis may worsen to hemiplegia, and right hemiparesis appears and leads to double hemiplegia, often followed by decerebrate rigidity and then complete flaccidity just preceding death as the brainstem becomes more and more damaged.
   c. The right and then the left pupil become dilated and fixed. Both eyes become immobile.
   d. Cheyne-Stokes, central neurogenic hyperventilation, cluster breathing, ataxic or Biot's respiration, and total apnea.
   e. Pulse and blood pressure may fluctuate, but there is a tendency for blood pressure to increase with decreasing pulse rate (Cushing's phenomenon).
   f. Hemorrhage into the brainstem, secondary to stretching of the brainstem vessels.
5. The time to help has essentially passed when the Pt shows the full signs of brain herniation, with deep coma, bilateral pupillodilation, and decerebrate rigidity. At that point, many Pts are irretrievable. The Ex must have recognized the Pt's increased pressure and potential for herniation and called for neurologic help (Clusmann et al., 2001). If the physicians can relieve the pressure early, the Pt recovers; if not, the Pt dies. That is the importance of understanding the mechanisms and clinical signs described here.

BIBLIOGRAPHY · Internal Herniations of the Brain: Effect on Consciousness, Neurologic Function, and Vascular System

Brandler SJ, Selverstone B. Recovery from decerebration. *Brain* 1970;93:381–392.

Clusmann H, Schaller C, Schramm J. Fixed and dilated pupils after trauma, stroke, and previous intracranial surgery: management and outcome. *J Neurol Neurosurg Psychiatry* 2001;71:175–181.

Cuneo RA, Caronna JJ, Pitts L, et al. Upward transtentorial herniation. Seven cases and literature review. *Arch Neurol* 1979;36(10):618–623.

Damasceno BP. Decerebrate rigidity with preserved cognition and gait: a possible role of anoxic-ischemic brain damage. *Int J Neurosci* 1991;58:283–287 (Medline).

RL Davis and DM Robertson, Editors, *Textbook of Neuropathology*. 2nd Edition. Williams and Wilkins, Baltimore 1991.

Fisher CM. Brain herniation: a revision of classical concepts. *Can J Neurol Sci* 1995;22:83–91.

Forbes H, Norris JR, Fawcett J. A sign of intracranial mass with impending uncal herniation. *Arch Neurol* 1965;12(4):381–386.

Friede R, Roessmann U. The pathogenesis of secondary midbrain hemorrhages. *Neurology* 1966;16:1210–1216.

Halsey J, Downie A. Decerebrate rigidity with preservation of consciousness. *J Neurol Neurosurg Psychiatry* 1966;29:350–355.

Hassler O. Arterial pattern of human brainstem: normal appearance and deformation in expanding supratentorial conditions. *Neurology* 1967;17:368–375.

Inao S, Kawai T, Kabeya R, et al. Relation between brain displacement and local cerebral blood flow in patients with chronic subdural haematoma. *J Neurol Neurosurg Psychiatry* 2001;71:741–746.

Jordan B. *Medical Aspects of Boxing*. Boca Raton, CRC Press, 1992.

Kao CD, Guo WY, Chen JT, et al. MR findings of decerebrate rigidity with preservation of consciousness. *AJNR* 2006;27:1074–1075.

Keane JR. Blindness following tentorial herniation. *Ann Neurol* 1980;8:186–190.

Kirschner HS, Staller J, Webb W, et al. Transtentorial herniation with posterior cerebral artery territory infarction. A new mechanism of the syndrome of alexia without agraphia. *Stroke* 1982;13:243–246.

Plum F, Posner J. *The Diagnosis of Stupor and Coma*, 3rd ed. Philadelphia, FA Davis, 1980.

Pollock L, Davis L. The reflex activities of a decerebrate animal. *J Comp Neurol* 1930;50:377–411.

Pullicino, PM, Alexandrov AV, Shelton JA, et al. Mass effect and death from severe acute stroke. *Neurology* 1997;49:1090–1095.

Ropper AH, ed. *Neurological and Neurosurgical Intensive Care*, 3rd ed. New York, Raven Press, 1993.

Ropper AH. The opposite pupil in herniation. *Neurology* 1990;40:1707–1709.

Saeki N, Higuchi Y, Sunami K, et al. Selective hemihypaesthesia due to tentorial coup injury against the dorsolateral midbrain: potential cause of sensory impairment after closed head injury. *J Neurol Neurosurg Psychiatry* 2000;69:117–118.

Sherrington CS. Decerebrate rigidity and reflex coordination of movements. *J Physiol* 1898; 22:319–322.

Sunderland S. The tentorial notch and complications produced by herniations of the brain through that aperture. *Br J Surg* 1958;45:422–438.

Unterharnscheidt F. About boxing: review of historical and medical aspects. *Texas Rep Biol Med* 1970;28:421–425.

Unterharnscheidt F, Unterharnscheidt JT, eds. *Boxing Med Aspects.* San Diego, Academic Press, 2003.

Walker A. The syndromes of the tentorial notch. *J Nerv Ment Dis* 1963;136:118–129.

IV. INITIAL NEUROLOGIC EXAMINATION OF THE UNCONSCIOUS PATIENT

A. Introduction

1. For the most difficult diagnostic challenge of all, we would ask you to evaluate a Pt brought in comatose off the street, with no history available. Review the Neurologic Examination of the Unconscious Patient on page XXV, at the front of the text. Recite the **ABCDEE** mnemonic, the **5H** mnemonic for enemies of the brain (hint: start with **H**ypoxia), and review the differential diagnostic dendrogram. At your leisure, read Fisher (1995) and Posner et al. (2007) for masterful descriptions of the neurologic examination (NE) of the unconscious Pt.
2. In trying to determine whether the putatively unconscious Pt is arousable, the inexperienced Ex seems instinctively to want to move the Pt's head from side to side, shake a limb, or jar the gurney. Avoid these maneuvers until you can be sure that the Pt doesn't have a broken neck or a broken arm.

3. The seemingly unresponsive Pt may have a toxic or metabolic state, an anatomic lesion, trauma, or a mental illness. The Ex has to determine immediately whether the Pt has an anatomic lesion or a metabolic or toxic disorder that threaten life (Fig. NE-3). **Asymmetric neurologic signs, such as a hemiparesis or a cranial nerve palsy, provide the best evidence of an anatomic lesion as the cause for the coma.** The mental disorders get sorted out in the course of the evaluation for life-threatening disorders. Mental illnesses include hysteria, malingering, and psychosis with catatonia (catatonia consists of catalepsy or waxy flexibility, negativism, mutism, and bizarre posturing).

B. Inspection of the comatose patient

1. If the Pt can breathe adequately, so can the Ex. The Ex has at least a little time for contemplation. Proceed to look for what is "good" and favorable and what is "bad" and evil. Anything that works normally, i.e., breathing and pupillary light reflexes, is good. What does not work at all is evil. Therefore, we extract a "cosmic law" about the NE of the unconscious Pt. **Whatever behavior the Pt shows, a pupil constricting or a limb moving, establishes the integrity of some neuroanatomic circuit and the function of some intact neurophysiologic mechanism.**
2. If the Pt fails to make any responses, the Ex has to decide whether this results from anatomic interruption of central neuroanatomic circuits, the depth of the coma, or total effector paralysis, as in severe Guillain-Barré syndrome or the Pt curarized for management on a respirator.

C. "Good" behaviors disclosed by the four-glance, instant screening neurologic examination of the acutely unconscious patient

Given a Pt who is unconscious (but not comatose, with no reflexes or behavior at all), the Ex can complete a preliminary but surprisingly adequate four-glance survey of the Pt's neuroanatomic circuits. The value of the observations depends on your ability to "think circuitry" and the implications of the behavior observed.

1. **Normal breathing and oropharyngeal reflexes:** Breathing and related reflexes, such as coughing, swallowing, hiccuping, or yawning, establish that CrNs IX, X, and XII, the pontomedullary reticular formation, and cervical and thoracic levels of the spinal cord are intact and cannot be the site of a lesion (Fig. 6-17).
2. **Blinking or tonic closure of the eyelids:** CrNs V and VII work.
3. **Random slow conjugate drifts of the eyes to the sides:** CrNs III, IV, and VI and the frontopontine pathway that drives eye movements are intact (Fig. 2-30). Together with the integrity of CrNs V and VII, the entire pontine tegmentum is intact, because the nucleus of CrN V is in the *rostral* part of the pontine tegmentum, the nuclei of CrNs VI and VII are in the *caudal* part, and the medial longitudinal fasciculus extends the *entire length*. Given the drifts of the eyes, the same considerations prove that the midbrain is intact: the nucleus of CrN III is in the rostral midbrain tegmentum, that of CrN IV is in the caudal, and the medial longitudinal fasciculus (MLF) extends the entire length.
4. **Random spontaneous, particularly semi-purposive symmetrical movements of all four extremities:** Both pyramidal tracts, from the motor cortex to the sacral level of the spinal cord, work (Fig. 2-27). At this point, the Ex knows that the entire length of the neuraxis, from the cerebral cortex to the tip of the spinal cord, is more or less intact. If after the four glances, you then find intact pupillary, corneal, vestibular, and auditopalpebral reflexes, further demonstrating the functional integrity of the midbrain, pons, medulla, and their cranial nerves, you have completed a cerebral cortex to sacral cord screening NE that virtually excludes a large anatomic lesion as the cause for the unconscious episode.
5. In addition to random or semi-purposive movements, the unconscious Pt may show myokymia and a variety of mutterings, shivers, shudders, twitches, and myoclonias difficult to classify, in addition to more patterned movements of choreiform, athetoid, or dystonic type; or aimless picking at the bedclothes, a sign

called **carphologia.** These actions are of uncertain localizing or prognostic import but generally require intact pyramidal tracts.

Mnemonic: Start examining the unconscious Pt with this four-glance inspection for four almost alliterative behaviors, **breathing/eyelids closing/eyeballs drifting/ extremities roving,** and recite the circuitry involved.

6. In the differential diagnosis of coma, recall that active pulsations of the retinal veins almost exclude the presence of increased intracranial pressure. In fact, spontaneous venous pulsations disappear when the intracranial pressure as measured by lumbar tap exceeds 190 mm of water (Levin, 1978). The presence of pulsations means more than their absence, because some normal persons do not show pulsations (Jacks and Miller, 2003). To best visualize venous pulsations requires direct ophthalmoscopy.
7. During this quick inspection, you may encounter more or less diagnostic odors of alcohol, fetor hepaticus, diabetic ketosis, or lung gangrene. The odor of alcohol does not establish it as the cause for the coma; perhaps the Pt has a subdural or epidural hematoma.
8. Also during the preliminary stage, note the Pt's body temperature; hyperthermia and hypothermia suggest different categories of diagnosis.

D. "Bad" behaviors disclosed by inspection of the unconscious patient

1. Worst of all is no behavior whatsoever: flaccid eyelids and no pupillary responses; no eye drifts (in deep coma and brain death, the eyes return to and remain fixed in the neutral position); no breathing; no spontaneous movements; a totally flaccid, dumped-in-a-heap posture; and no response to any stimulus. At this point the Ex does not know whether the absence of behavior results from destructive lesions, with neural shock or brain death, widespread LMN paralysis, or merely the depth of the coma, e.g., as in a massive overdose of barbiturates.
2. Next worst is a sustained or driven posture: sustained deviation of the head and eyes or decerebrate rigidity.
   a. Focal seizures may cause deviation of the head and eyes. In the absence of convulsions, you would expect a destructive lesion in the conjugate gaze center in the posterior frontal region of the ❒ ipsilateral/❒ contralateral hemisphere or in the ❒ ipsilateral/❒ contralateral half of the pons.
   b. List which CrN(s) would most likely be paralyzed by a large lesion affecting the region of the pontine conjugate lateral gaze center.________________________
3. **Prognostically bad findings:** No prognostic formula unerringly predicts death, but Pts who fail to recover corneal and pupillary light reflexes within 24 hours of the onset of coma generally die. Similarly, Pts who have an acute head injury and who lack pupillary and vestibulo-ocular reflexes generally die. Prognostic scales have an error rate of 5% to 20% when applied to nontraumatic coma and require judicious interpretation to avoid premature termination of life support (Bates, 1991). The Ex should remain vigilant to the possibility of treatable metabolic derangements (e.g., hypermagnesemia) mimicking herniation syndromes with fixed and dilated pupils (Rizzo et al., 1993)

☑ ipsilateral; ☑ contralateral (Review Figs. 5-1 and 5-3 if you missed.)

VI and VII (Fig. 5-1)

E. Detecting hemiplegia in the unconscious patient

1. **Inspection:** The acute, severe anatomic lesions that cause unconsciousness or the hemiplegia that follows focal seizures (Todd's paralysis) usually cause flaccid hemiplegia (cerebral shock). Look for unilateral asymmetry of movement, posture, muscle tone, and most importantly, unilateral flaccidity of the extremities. Unless deeply comatose, the unconscious Pt with intact pyramidal tracts moves all four extremities spontaneously or more or less purposively in response to pain. A tip-off posture of flaccid hemiplegia is that the leg rests in external rotation, with the foot turned out. Hemiplegia and a broken hip are the two most common

reasons for this posture. Flaccidity on one side and absence of spontaneous or pain-induced movements identify acute hemiplegia. The face and extremities on the intact side continue to show some muscle tone.

2. **Flaccidity of the cheek:** When the unconscious hemiplegic Pt inhales, the cheek on one side sucks in; when the Pt exhales, that cheek puffs out. It will be on the ❒ hemiplegic/❒ nonhemiplegic side. Explain.

☑ hemiplegic
Flaccid paralysis involves the buccinator and other facial muscles on the hemiplegic side. Therefore, the flaccid cheek on the hemiplegic side sucks in with inspiration and puffs out with expiration. The tone in the facial muscles on the other side holds the cheek in place.

____

____

3. **The eyelid-release test**

   a. Review of facial motor innervation

      i. Diagram the UMN and LMN innervations of the right side of the face in Fig. 12-17. Check it against Fig. 6-3.

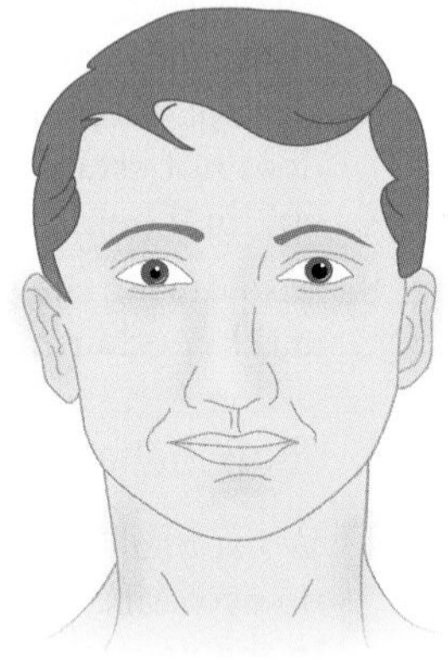

FIGURE 12-17. Blank to draw in the upper motoneuron innervation of the VIIth nerve nucleus and the lower motoneuron innervation of the face.

      ii. Recall that the LMNs for the orbicularis oculi muscle may receive innervation by many crossed and uncrossed UMNs. Hence, in acute hemiplegia, after sudden interruption of UMNs, the eyelid may also show flaccidity and weakness. The eyelid-release test demonstrates this, because even in the unconscious (but not completely comatose) Pt, the eyelids remain closed because of tonic innervation, i.e., by a positive drive.

   b. **Procedure for eyelid-release test:** Gently pull both eyelids up with your two thumbs and then release them simultaneously (Fig. 12-18).

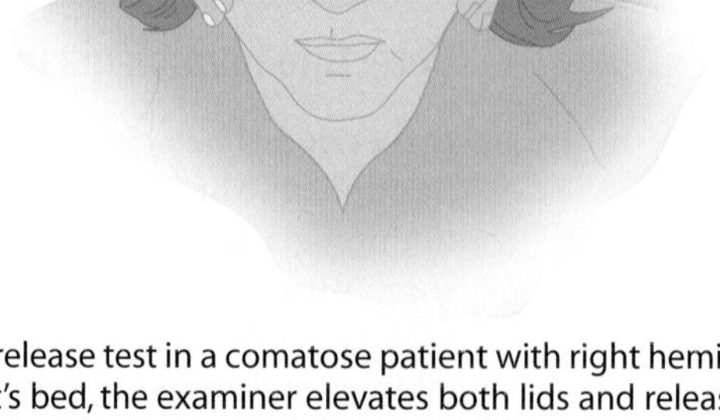

FIGURE 12-18. Eyelid-release test in a comatose patient with right hemiplegia. While standing at the head of the patient's bed, the examiner elevates both lids and releases them simultaneously. The lid of the hemiplegic side closes slowly because of flaccidity of its orbicularis oculi muscle, whereas the lid of the normal side closes briskly because of tonus in its orbicularis oculi muscle.

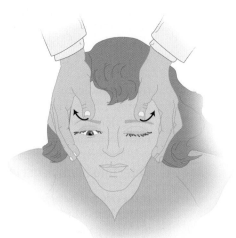

The orbicularis oculi muscle of the normal side is not paralyzed and retains muscle tone.

c. **Results:** The eyelid of the hemiplegic side glides down slowly, whereas the opposite lid closes rapidly. In fact, it almost snaps shut, unless the Pt is deeply comatose. Why does the eyelid on the nonhemiplegic side close faster? ____

d. Rarely, the eyelids of the unconscious Pt will remain open and unblinking (Keane, 1975).

4. **The limb-dropping tests:** The limb-dropping tests demonstrate flaccid paralysis of the extremities.

a. **The wrist-dropping test:** Grasp both of the Pt's forearms just proximal to the wrist. Hold the forearms vertical, as shown in Fig. 12-19. The flaccid hemiplegic wrist drops at right angles, whereas the nonhemiplegic wrist, having some tone, remains to some degree vertical.

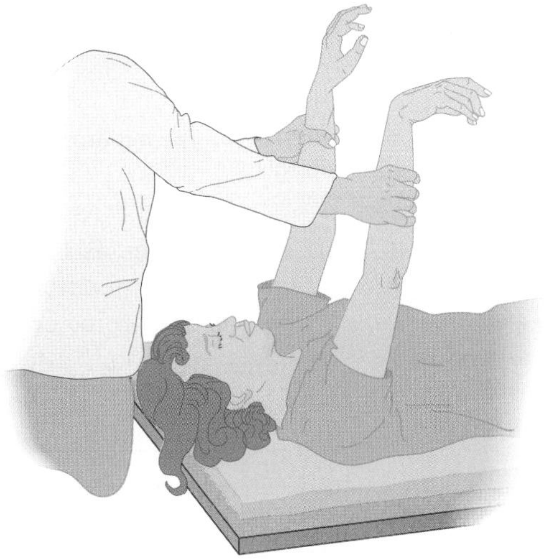

FIGURE 12-19. The wrist-dropping test for flaccid hemiplegia in a comatose patient with right hemiplegia.

b. **The arm-dropping test:** Grasp both forearms, as in the wrist-dropping test, and release them simultaneously. The hemiplegic arm drops limply, whereas the normal arm glides or floats down (Fig. 12-20). Lift the arm only a few inches and cushion its drop. Beware of ulnar nerve injury.

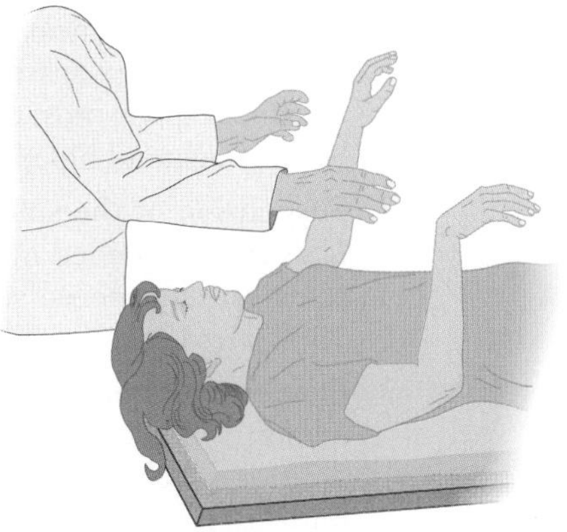

FIGURE 12-20. The arm-dropping test for flaccid hemiplegia in a comatose patient with right hemiplegia.

c. **The leg-dropping test:** Crook the Pt's knees on your arm. Extend one leg first and drop it, and do the same with the other (Fig. 12-21). The Ex can both see and hear the difference as the flaccid hemiplegic leg drops more rapidly to strike the bed.

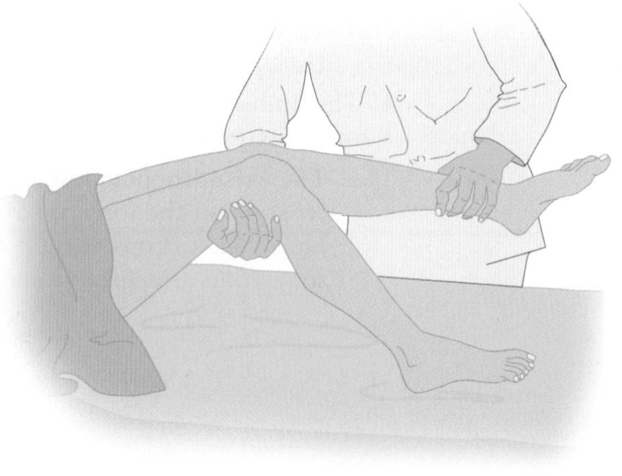

FIGURE 12-21. The leg-dropping test for flaccid hemiplegia in a comatose patient with right hemiplegia.

Inspect for asymmetry of movement and puffing out of one cheek. Test for asymmetry of muscle tone by manipulation of the extremities and by the eyelid closure and extremity-dropping tests.

d. The dropping tests depend on the principle of asymmetry of muscle tone. For correct interpretation, the nonhemiplegic side must have some muscle tone. Hence, deep coma or LMN paralysis invalidates the tests.

5. Summarize the methods of detecting acute flaccid hemiplegia in an unconscious Pt.____

F. Resistance to movement: paratonia (Gegenhalten)

1. The paratonic Pt may resist movement of a part of the body in any direction. It occurs in conscious and unconscious Pts. It is as if the Pt divines every movement you impose and automatically counteracts it.
2. Paratonia, like any resistance dependent on muscular contraction, does not occur on the side of acute flaccid hemiplegia or in the deeply comatose Pt when all tone is lost. The novice often misidentifies the nonhemiplegic side as hemiplegic because of mistaking paratonia for the increased tone of a UMN lesion.

G. Resistance to movement: nuchal rigidity and meningeal irritation signs

1. **Definition of nuchal rigidity:** The term *nucha* refers to the back of the neck. **Nuchal rigidity** means that neither the Pt nor the Ex can flex the Pt's head because of reflex spasm of the nuchal (extensor) muscles. Irritation of the subarachnoid space, most commonly by inflammation (encephalitis or meningitis) or by subarachnoid blood, causes nuchal rigidity.
2. **Suspension of the spinal cord:** The spinal cord is buoyed by the surrounding CSF and suspended in position by its attachment to the medulla, by its nerve roots, and by special suspensory ligaments, the **denticulate ligaments** (Emery, 1967; Fig. 12-22).
3. **Biomechanics of neck flexion and extension:** By understanding the mechanics involved in eliciting nuchal muscle spasm, you get a bonus: You learn how to position a Pt who has suffered a vertebral fracture and how to interpret Lhermitte's sign. Study Figs. 12-23 and 12-24.

   a. Line A-A' in Fig. 12-23 impales the neuraxis. It simulates a lever with the fulcrum at the top of the vertebral column. Thus, flexion of the head causes ❒ relaxation/❒ stretching of the spinal cord.

☑ stretching

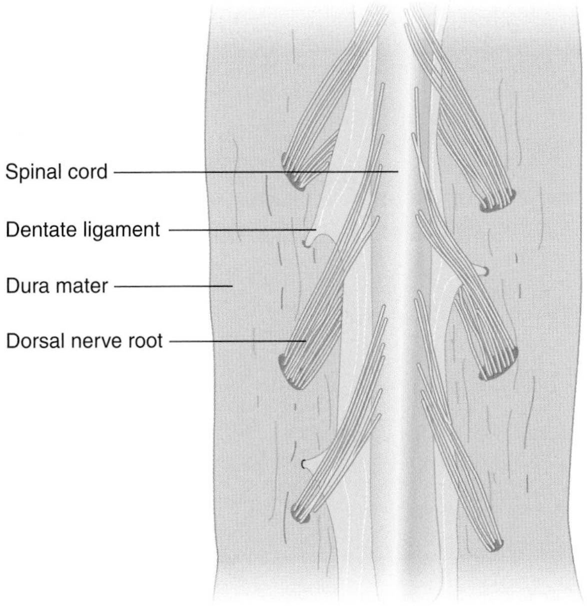

FIGURE 12-22. Dorsal view of the spinal cord, with the dura split open. Notice the dentate (denticulate) ligaments that suspend the spinal cord.

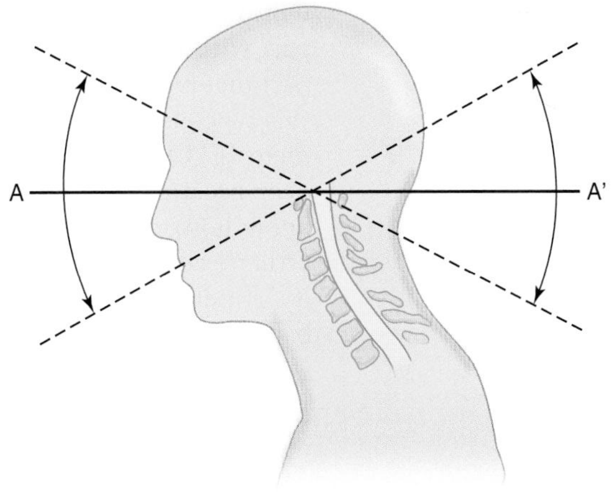

FIGURE 12-23. Sagittal section of the head to show the effect of head extension and flexion in stretching and relaxing the spinal cord. Imagine a steel rod driven through the head (A-A'). It acts as a lever with the fulcrum over the body of the first cervical vertebra.

b. During neck flexion and extension, movement occurs not only between the skull and first cervical vertebra but also between all other cervical vertebrae. The neck does not bend as though hinged at one point: It bends in a curve, like a sapling. The interrupted lines in Figs. 12-24A and 12-24B show the actual changes in vertebral angulation with flexion and extension and the accompanying changes in tension on the nerve roots and spinal cord (Breig, 1978; Goel and Weinstein, 1989).

4. **The mechanism of spasm of the nuchal (extensor) muscles: The pain-spasm-pain cycle**

   a. During the range of movement from neck extension to flexion, the cord and roots change from a relaxed accordion-like wrinkling to a stretched condition

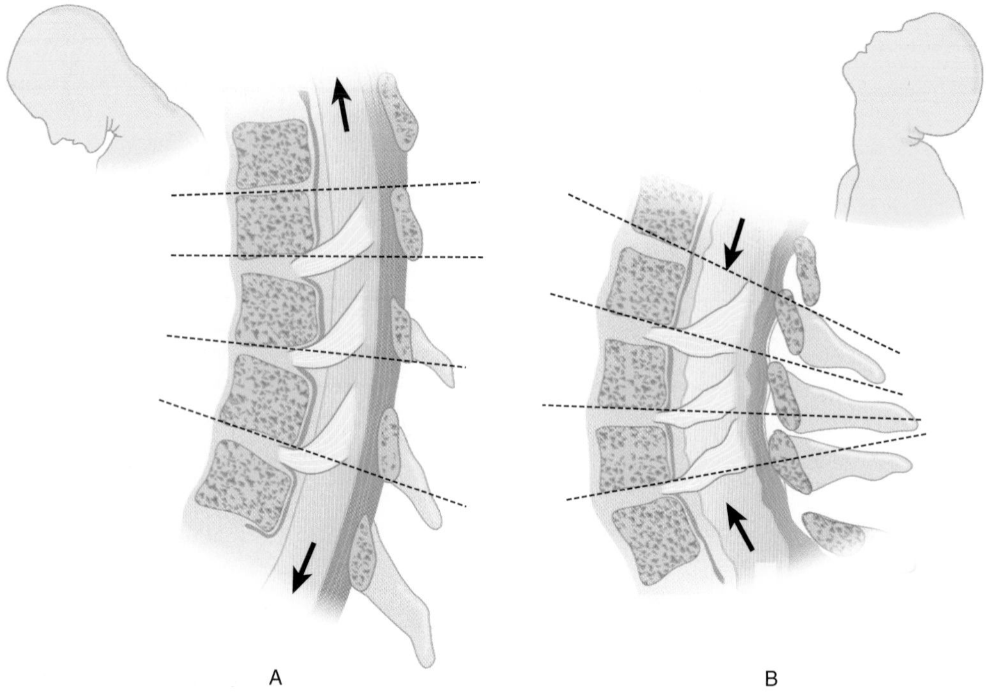

FIGURE 12-24. Sagittal sections through the cervical spinal cord and vertebrae. (A) Head flexion. (B) Head extension. Notice that the spinal cord and nerve roots are stretched and lengthened in A and relaxed and pleated in B.

(Fig. 12-24; Breig, 1978). When, however, roots, meninges, and cord are inflamed and swollen, the ordinarily innocuous act of flexing the head puts tension on the inflamed structures. It's like pressing on a boil. As long as the part with the boil remains still, it does not hurt. However, movement of the part that places tension on the swollen tissues causes intense pain. Any pain of this type elicits immediate muscle spasm, which prohibits the painful movement (O'Connell, 1946; Wartenberg, 1950). If you have ever tried to take a deep breath when you had a "stitch" in your side from a pleuritic rub, you will know how effectively pain inhibits the muscular contraction that causes it. Other examples of pain-avoiding muscle spasm are the abdominal wall rigidity of peritonitis and back rigidity from a lumbar sprain, i.e., a "crick in the back."

b. With inflamed meninges, the position that causes pain from tension on the cord and nerve roots is neck ❒ extension/❒ flexion.

☑ flexion

H. Technique to test for nuchal rigidity

1. With the Pt supine and relaxed, place your hand under the Pt's occiput and gently attempt to flex the neck. Normally, it bends freely. If the Pt has nuchal rigidity, the neck resists flexion and the Pt winces with pain. If nuchal rigidity is severe, you can lift up the Pt's head and trunk as if the spine were a rigid rod or as if the Pt were a statue (Fig. 12-25A).
2. Because true nuchal rigidity indicates meningeal irritation, the Ex must distinguish it from other forms of cervical rigidity. With true nuchal rigidity, the neck resists only flexion. The neck moves freely through rotation and extension, because these movements do not stretch meninges, spinal cord, and nerve roots. To demonstrate that rigidity affects only the nuchal muscles, do the following two things:
   a. Place your hand on the Pt's forehead. Passively roll the Pt's head from side to side to demonstrate free head rotation despite resistance to flexion (Fig. 12-25B).
   b. Then lift the Pt's shoulders to let the head fall backward, testing for freedom of extension (Fig. 12-25C).

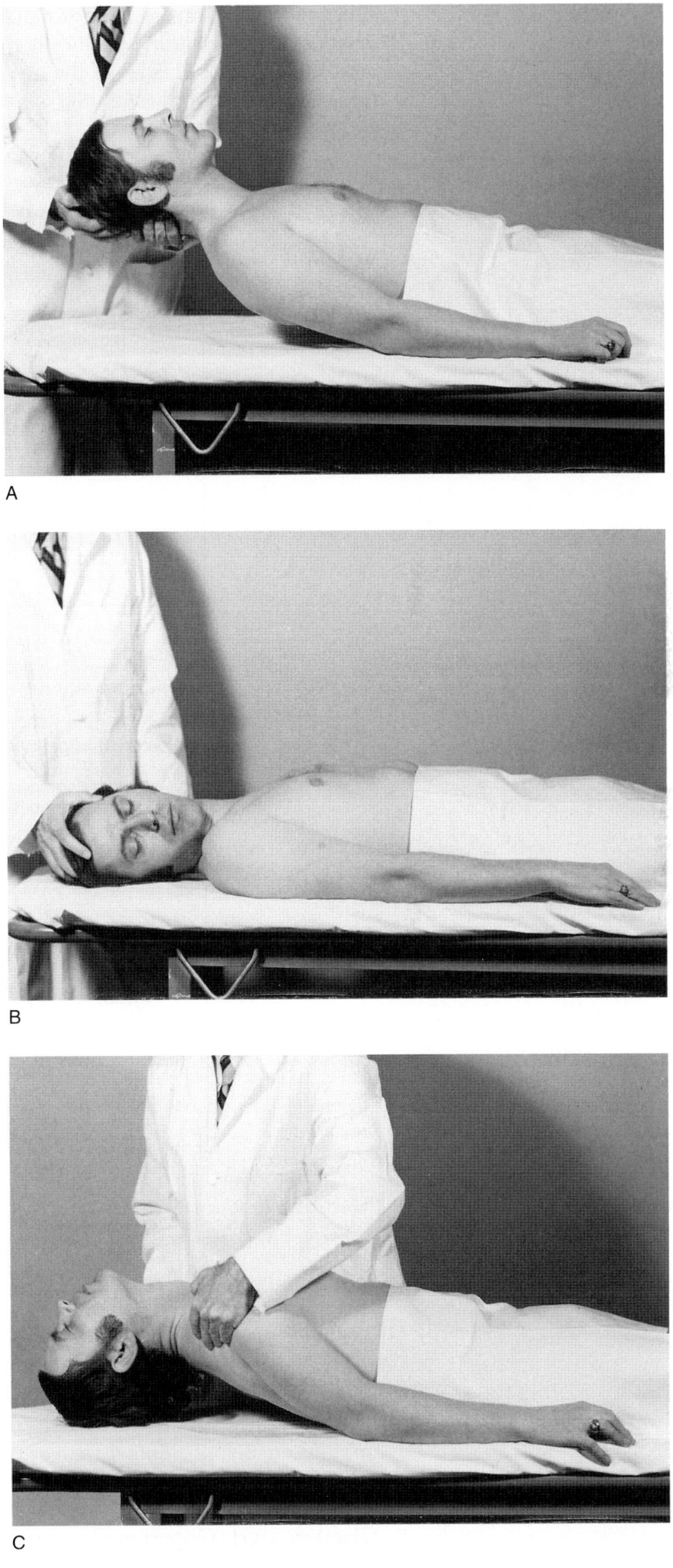

FIGURE 12-25. Diagnosis of pure nuchal rigidity, indicative of meningeal irritation. (A) The neck strongly resists flexion, often to the degree that the examiner can actually pick up the patient's head and spine like a statue. (B) The neck rotates freely despite extreme nuchal rigidity that resists flexion. (C) The head falls back freely when the examiner lifts the patient's shoulders.

☑ back (nape)

c. **Cervical rigidity** means any resistance to neck movement in any direction. In contrast, **nuchal rigidity** specifically means resistance to neck flexion, i.e., rigidity of the ❒ back/❒ front of the neck. Figure 12-26 lists some of the numerous causes of cervical rigidity.

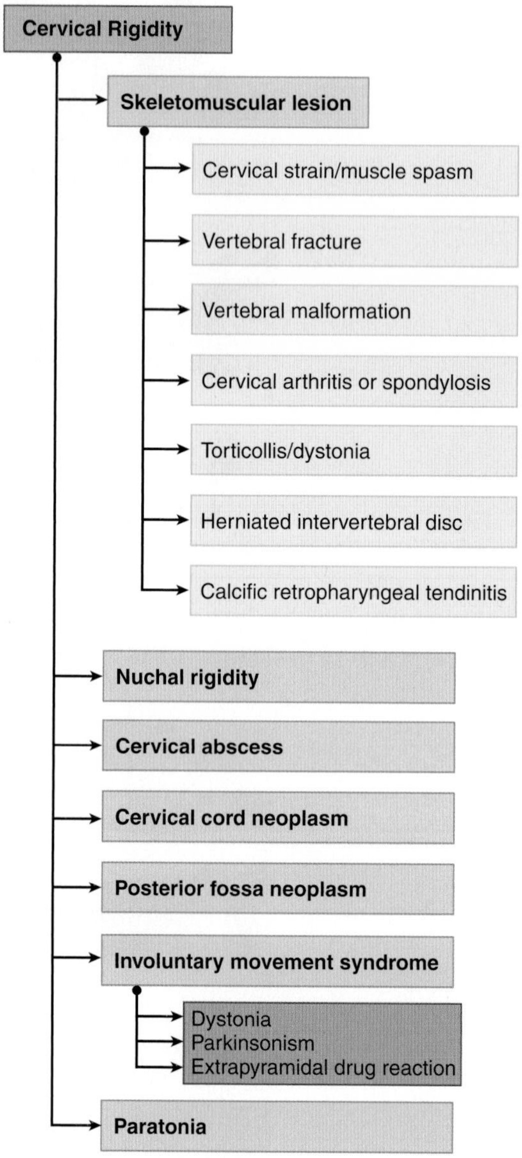

FIGURE 12-26. Dendrogram for causes of cervical rigidity (reference).

I. Neck manipulation and spinal cord injury (Fig. 12-27)

1. **Contraindications to neck manipulation:** Study Fig. 12-27, which shows a fracture dislocation of the cervical vertebrae but can represent any mass lesion, such as a tumor or herniation of an intervertebral disc, that compresses the cervical cord.
   a. Head flexion would place tension on the swollen spinal cord. The cord will impinge on any intruding mass. For this reason, do not test for nuchal rigidity in a Pt suspected of a cervical cord lesion. Always suspect that any Pt unconscious from trauma has a cervical fracture and obtain cervical spine films (Trunkey, 1991; Gisbert et al., 1989). Be cautious about any neck manipulation in any comatose Pt, particularly a neonate, because the pain-protective reflexes may not be active.
   b. In addition to cervical cord injury, neck manipulation may compress the vertebral artery (Fig. 12-34) and cause vertebrobasilar stroke (Garg et al., 1993, Williams and Biller, 2003) or cause vascular insufficiency of the cord (Linssen et al., 1990). This complication may follow chiropractic manipulation.

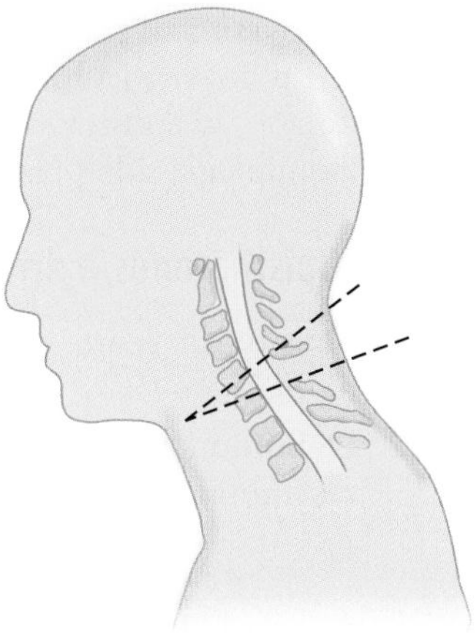

FIGURE 12-27. Fracture and dislocation of C5 on C6. The displaced vertebrae have impinged on the contused and swollen cord.

2. **Positioning of a Pt with known or suspected cervical cord injury:** Your natural tendencies urge you to place an injured Pt supine with the head flexed on a pillow, exactly the wrong position. In a suspected cervical cord injury, splint and transport the Pt with the neck in a position to reduce tension on the cord—in other words, in a neutral or slightly ______________ position.

extended

3. **Lhermitte's sign after neck flexion:** Neck flexion in the alert Pt may cause a shocklike sensation extending from the neck to the feet. Coughing, sneezing, or straining may elicit the same sensation. The explanation is mechanical stretch of the cord in the presence of a cervical cord lesion causing irritation of the sensory pathways. It is common in multiple sclerosis (Gutrecht, 1989).

J. Review of nuchal rigidity

1. In nuchal rigidity, the neck moves freely in all directions except for ______________.

flexion

2. State the maneuvers to show that a Pt with resistance to neck flexion has nuchal, and only nuchal, rigidity.

____
______________________.

With the Pt supine, roll the Pt's head from side to side and lift the shoulders to allow the head to drop back, thus showing free movement in all directions except flexion.

3. Then, and only then, is it a reliable sign of an irritative process in the ______________ space, the two most common causes of which are ______________.

subarachnoid; meningitis and subarachnoid hemorrhage

4. If the head of the Pt with decreased consciousness resists movement in all directions, and the extremities do likewise, then the Pt has the generalized hypertonia called ______________.

paratonia

K. Confirmatory signs of meningeal irritation: Brudzinski's and Kernig's signs

1. **Brudzinski's sign:** When testing for nuchal rigidity, watch for adduction and flexion of the legs (Brudzinski's sign) as you attempt to flex the head (Wartenberg, 1950). Why would the Pt's knees flex?

____
____

Flexion of the neck places tension on the entire cord and roots (review nerve root stretching tests, Fig. 10-12, if you missed this question). Flexion of the legs reduces stretch on nerve roots.

2. **Leg-raising tests:** With the Pt supine, do the **bent-knee** and **straight-knee leg-raising tests** of Kernig and Lasègue (Fig. 10-7). Meningeal irritation causes the Pt to resist leg movement in both cases.

L. Absence of meningeal irritation signs in the presence of meningeal irritation

The usual meningeal irritation signs may fail to occur in five circumstances: infancy, senility, coma, with peripheral neuromuscular paralysis, and after acute interruption of the pyramidal tracts. The proof of inflammation or subarachnoid hemorrhage in these Pts requires a lumbar tap (Chapter 13). In addition, meningeal leg signs may fail to appear on the side of a hemiplegia. Unilateral absence may aid in identifying the hemiplegic side (Thorner, 1948).

M. Opisthotonos, a driven posture

1. First of all, learn to pronounce the word correctly: *ah-piss-THAH-tonos,* not *oh-PISS-tho-tonos.*
2. **Definition: Opisthotonos** means a bowed-backward, or hyperextended, position resembling a "wrestler's bridge" (Fig. 12-28).

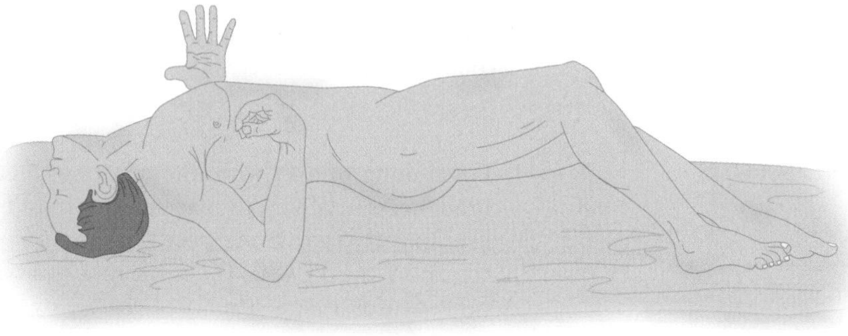

FIGURE 12-28. Severe opisthotonos. (Redrawn with permission from Dorland WAN: *Dorland's Illustrated Medical Dictionary,* 25th edition. Philadelphia, W.B. Saunders, 1974)

3. **Causes:** Opisthotonos results from overcontraction of the immensely powerful extensor muscles of the spine. It occurs with meningeal irritation, decerebrate rigidity, tetanus, and strychnine intoxication, hence, from several different pathophysiologic mechanisms. It may also occur with exposure to centrally acting dopamine receptor blocking agents, and in somatoform disorders and catatonic schizophrenia, conditions without demonstrable lesions (Fig. 12-29).
   a. In meningeal irritation, opisthotonos results from spasm of the powerful extensor muscles that splint the neck and back against flexion, which causes pain. We can regard it as a pain-protective reflex posture in these cases.
   b. In decerebrate rigidity, the opisthotonic posture results from the hypertonus of the quadrupedal antigravity muscles driven by the vestibular system after an anatomic midbrain lesion or a metabolic lesion that has inactivated or disconnected the cerebrum from the brainstem.
   c. In tetanus and strychnine intoxication, MSR and LMN excitability increase tremendously. All skeletal muscles become extremely hypertonic. Tetanus toxin, in addition to its central excitatory effects, has a contractile action on muscles, causing them to remain cramped even after transection of their nerves (Dastur et al., 1977). When all muscles contract maximally, the strongest muscles dictate the posture by overpowering their weaker antagonists. However, in tetanus in particular, local factors based on variability in the excitability of the LMN pools and the direct cramping action of the toxin may alter the strongest muscle law. Thus, as shown in Fig. 12-28, the arm flexors may overcome their stronger antagonists, the extensors. To appreciate what the opisthotonic Pt suffers, lie down supine, extend your neck and legs into the wrestler's bridge position, clench your teeth (lock-jaw), and contract every muscle in your body as hard as you can for 1 minute.
4. **In summary,** opisthotonos results from at least three different pathogenic mechanisms.
   a. In decerebrate rigidity:

hypertonus of antigravity muscles

____.

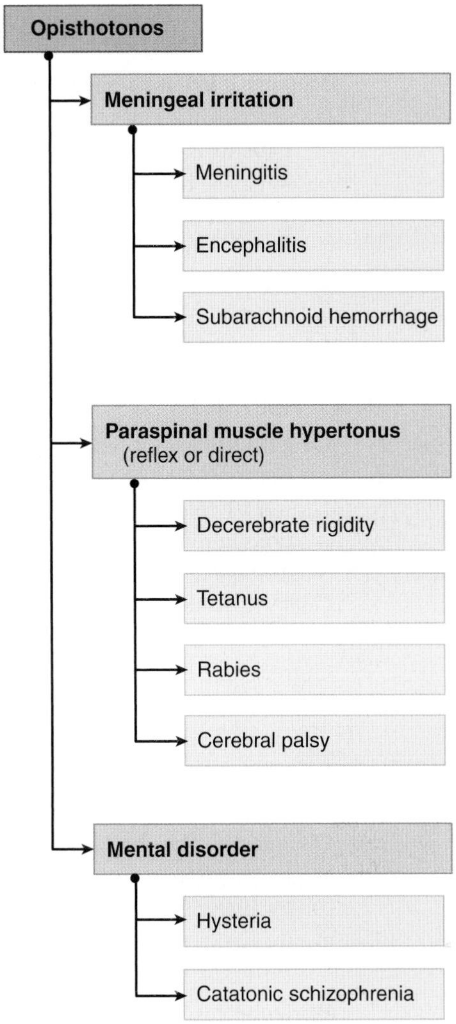

FIGURE 12-29. Dendrogram for causes of opisthotonus (reference).

reflex pain-protective extensor spasms

increased reflex and muscular irritability

b. In meningeal irritation: ______________________________.

c. In strychnine or tetanus intoxication: ______________________________.

BIBLIOGRAPHY · Neurologic Examination of the Unconscious Patient

Emery JL. Kinking of the medulla in children with acute cerebral oedema and hydrocephalus and its relationship to the dentate ligaments. *J Neurol Neurosurg Psychiatry* 30:267–275, 1967.

Fisher CM. The neurological examination of the comatose patient. *Acta Neurol Scand* 1969;45(suppl 36):1–56.

Jacks AS, Miller NR. Spontaneous retinal venous pulsation: aetiology and significance. *J Neurol Neurosur Psychiatry* 2003;74:7–9.

Keane JR. Spastic eyelids. Failure of levator inhibition in unconscious states. *Arch Neurol* 1975;32:695–698.

Levin BE. The clinical significance of spontaneous pulsations of the retinal vein. *Arch Neurol* 1978;35:37–40.

Plum F, Posner J. *The Diagnosis of Stupor and Coma,* 3rd ed. Philadelphia, FA Davis, 1980.

Posner JB, Saper CB, Schiff ND, et al. *Plum and Posner's Diagnosis of Stupor and Coma,* 4th ed. Oxford, England. University Press 2007.

Rizzo MA, Fisher M, Lock JP. Hypermagnesemic pseudocoma. *Arch Int Med* 1993;153(9): 1130–1132.

Wijdicks EFM, Bamlet WR, Maramattom BV, et al. Validation of a New Coma Scale: the FOUR score. *Ann Neurol* 2005;58:585–593.

Meningeal Irritation Signs: Nuchal Rigidity and Opisthotonos

Anastasopoulous D, Maurer C, Nasiosti G, Mergner T. Neck rigidity in Parkinson's disease patients is related to incomplete expression of reflexive head stabilization. *Exp Neurol* 2009;217(2):336–346.

Breig A. *Adverse Mechanical Tension in the Central Nervous System: An Analysis of Cause and Effect*. New York, Wiley, 1978.

Dastur FD, Shahani WR, Dastoor DH, et al. Cephalic tetanus: demonstration of a dual lesion. *J Neurol Neurosurg Psychiatry* 1977;40:782–786.

Emery J. Kinking of the medulla in children with acute cerebral oedema and hydro-cephalus and its relationship to the dentate ligaments. *J Neurol Neurosurg Psychiatry* 1967;30:267–275.

Garg B, Ottinger CJ, Smith RR, et al. Strokes in children due to vertebral artery trauma. *Neurology* 1993;43:2555–2558.

Gisbert VL, Hollerman JJ, New AL. Incidence and diagnosis of C7-T1 fractures and subluxations in multiple trauma patients: evaluation of the advanced trauma life support guidelines. *Surgery* 1989;106:702–708.

Goel VK, Weinstein JN. *Biomechanics of the Spine: Clinical and Surgical Perspective*. Boca Raton, CRC Press, 1989.

Gutrecht JA. Lehrmitte's sign: from observation to eponym. *Arch Neurol* 1989;46:557–558.

Hunderfund ANL, Robertston CE, Bell ML, et al. Calcific retropharyngeal tendinitis. Unusual cause of neck pain with nuchal rigidity. *Neurology* 2008;71(10):778.

Linssen WHJP, Praamstra P, Fons JM, et al. Vascular insufficiency of the cervical cord due to hyperextension of the spine. *Pediatr Neurol* 1990;6:123–125.

O'Connell J. The clinical signs of meningeal irritation. *Brain* 1946;69:9–21.

Thorner J. Modification of meningeal signs by concomitant hemiparesis. *Arch Neurol Psychiatry* 1948;59:485–495.

Trunkey D. Initial treatment of patients with extensive trauma. *N Engl J Med* 1991;324:1259–1263.

Wartenberg R. The signs of Brudzinski and Kernig. *J Pediatr* 1950;37:679–684.

Williams LS, Biller J. Vertebrobasilar dissection and cervical spine manipulation. A complex pain in the neck. *Neurology* 2003;60(9):1048–1049.

V. SENSORY TESTING OF UNCONSCIOUS PATIENTS

A. First principles

1. **Necessity for effector integrity:** Bedside testing of sensation in the unconscious Pt requires eliciting motor responses. Three conditions may reduce or block the motor response: LMN paralysis, UMN paralysis with cerebral shock, and simply the depth of coma. If no response occurs, then the Ex does not know whether the afferent or efferent limb of the arc has failed. To bypass the necessity for intact effectors, the Ex can assess the integrity of sensory pathways by electronically recording evoked responses to somatosensory, visual, and auditory stimuli (Chapter 13).
2. **Follow a rostrocaudal routine:** As with an alert Pt, the Ex adopts a rostrocaudal routine to test the sensory systems. Start with the rostralmost CrNs and proceed caudally over the body. Skip CrN I.

B. Testing the pupillary light reflex and cranial nerves II and III

1. Test pupillary reaction to light with a flashlight. If the pupils do not seem to react, darken the room completely and then suddenly turn on the overhead light while watching the pupils through a magnifying glass.
2. Measure and record the size of the pupils in millimeters. Use an actual scale of dots (Fig. 12-30).

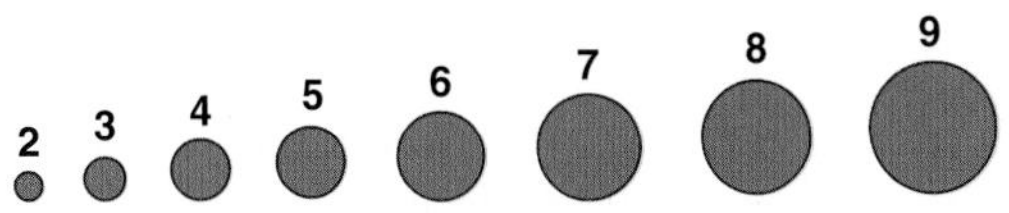

FIGURE 12-30. Scale in millimeters for measuring pupillary size.

3. Many factors can alter pupillary size (Table 12-6). Always consider the possibility that the Pt has taken a drug that can alter pupillary size.

TABLE 12-6 · Pupillary Findings in the Unconscious Patient

Size and reactions	Toxic-metabolic agents	Anatomic lesions
Widely dilated, nonreactive	Strong cholinergic blocker or sympathomimetic drugs	Midbrain failure or bilateral CrN III lesions
Widely dilated but reactive	Mild anticholinergics in some OTC sleeping and cold medications; adrenergic vasopressors	May mean early midbrain failure
Midposition or mildly dilated (4–6 mm) and sluggish or nonreactive	Glutethimide (Doriden)	May mean both sympathetic and parasympathetic paralysis: Adie's syndrome
Pupilloconstriction	Sleep, anoxia, uremia; glaucoma drugs or other parasympathomimetics	Interruption of descending sympathetic pathway
Pinpoint but reactive if bright light used	Opiates	Massive pontine lesion, often a hemorrhage, that disrupts descending sympathetic pathways

ABBREVIATIONS: CrN = cranial nerve; OTC = over the counter.

4. The pupillary light reflex involves CrNs II (afferent) and III (efferent) simultaneously. In Fig. 12-31, draw the pupilloconstrictor reflex pathway. Start, as usual, at the receptor and trace through the pathway.

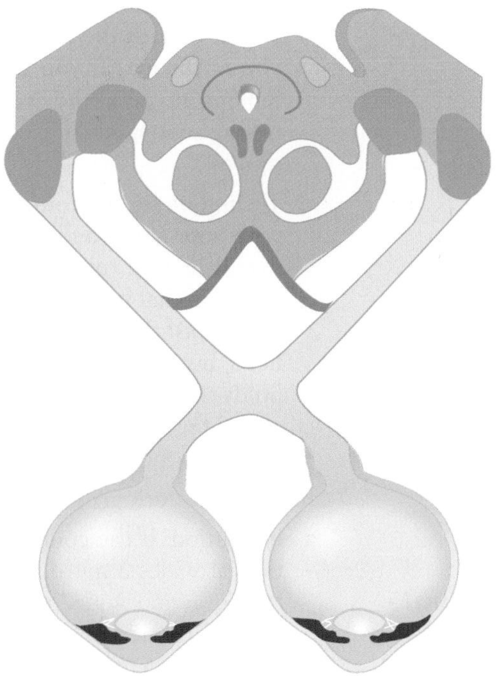

FIGURE 12-31. Blank to draw the pathway of the pupilloconstrictor reflex. Start with a retinal neuron. Check your drawing against Fig. 4-30, page 159.

C. Technique for testing sensory function of cranial nerve V

1. **Corneal reflex (V afferent, VII efferent):** Test with a wisp of cotton, as in the conscious Pt.
2. **Supraorbital compression test for reflex of CrNs V to VIII**
   a. Press your thumbnail strongly into the Pt's eyebrow over the superciliary notch, the exit site of the ophthalmic division of CrN V. Locate your own notch by pressing the ball of your thumb from medial to lateral along your eyebrow. Then press your fingernail in until you feel pain.
   b. With an intact pons and CrNs V and VII, the unconscious Pt responds with an *ipsilateral* facial grimace with eyelid closure. Hence, the Ex can test each half of the face separately. In the comatose Pt with acute hemiplegia, the grimace would be absent or weaker on the ❒ hemiplegic/❒ nonhemiplegic side. Explain. ____

   ☑ hemiplegic
   After acute UMN lesions, the excitability of reflexes is temporarily reduced during the phase known as **cerebral shock.**

   c. If the Ex suddenly and unexpectedly flicks the closed eyelashes of the Pt in feigned coma, the Pt often shows an exaggerated response with grimacing and head retraction. This is practically never seen in organic coma (Wiggs, 1973).

D. Testing hearing: the auditory division of cranial nerve VIII (auditopalpebral reflex)

Test by a sudden sound, such as a clap or clanging metal pans together, and observe the Pt for a startle response.

E. Testing the vestibular division of cranial nerve VIII

Two tests, **caloric irrigation** and the **counter-rolling test,** elicit a **vestibulo-ocular reflex** that causes conjugate deviation of the eyes. The receptors for the tests are essentially the cupulae of the semicircular canals, but the cristae and neck proprioceptors may add somewhat to the response (Buettner and Zee, 1989). The vestibular nuclei relay the vestibular impulses through the MLF to activate CrNs VI and III.

1. **The counter-rolling test for the vestibulo-ocular reflex (doll's eye test or oculocephalic reflex)**
   a. **Principle of the test:** If you have an old-fashioned doll, hold it up in front of you. If you tilt the doll's head *down,* the eyes will turn *up* to remain looking at you in the eye. If you tilt the doll's head *up,* the eyes rotate *down* to remain looking at you in the eye. Counterweights behind the eyes cause this counter-rolling action, which essentially keeps eyes on the visual target when the head moves.
   b. **Technique for the counter-rolling test:** Hold the Pt's head in a neutral position with your hands and briskly rotate it to the *right* and *left* and *up* and *down,* and stop it in each rotated position. For example, rotate the head to the right and stop it in that position. During the initial rotation to the right, the eyes *counter-roll against* the direction of head turning, thus turning to the left relative to the head, but actually the eyes simply maintain their original position. As the Ex holds the head in the rotated position, the eyes quickly turn and align straight ahead for the new head position. Failure of the eyes to counter-roll indicates failure of the vestibulo-ocular reflex.
2. **Review of caloric irrigation**
   a. **Indication:** If the counter-rolling test fails, do caloric irrigation. Caloric irrigation provides a more powerful stimulus than head turning, but the counter-rolling action added to caloric irrigation is more effective than either alone (Fisher, 1969).
   b. **Precaution:** What precaution must you take before injecting water into the external auditory meatus? ______________________.

   Inspect it, remove wax, and inspect for otitis or a perforated eardrum. The Pt's coma might have come from extension of a middle-ear infection into the brain.

c. **Technique for caloric irrigation:** Review the technique for caloric irrigation from Chapter 9. Give details of position, equipment, and water temperature.

____

Flex the supine Pt's head 30 degrees. Irrigate the auditory canals with 100 mL of water at 30°C over a period of 40 seconds or with 5 mL of ice water and tilt Pt's head to opposite side for 20 seconds (Chapter 9).

d. **Normal response to cold caloric irrigation:** The Pt shows nystagmus featured by slow deviation of the eye *ipsilaterally* and quick, saccadic jerks that restore the eyes to the primary position. As the coma deepens, the frontopontine pathway fails and the saccades disappear, but the vestibular deviation remains. In yet deeper coma, the deviation lessens until no response is obtained at all, even though the pathways remain anatomically intact.

e. If the Pt shows no response, you have to "think circuitry" to locate the reason for the failure:

   i. Start with the nature of the stimulus. The stimulus may have been inadequate. Try colder water and irrigate longer.
   ii. The Pt's labyrinths are inexcitable or CrNs VIII are interrupted.
   iii. The vestibular nuclei or MLF are interrupted by an extensive tegmental lesion.
   iv. The peripheral nerves to the ocular muscles are interrupted, or neuromuscular transmission has failed.
   v. The Pt may be in a stage of profound coma or may be brain dead. Obviously, any response provides more useful information than no response.

f. **Significance:** Normal pupillary reactions to light and full normal conjugate counter-rolling of the eyes in response to the vestibulo-ocular stimuli virtually exclude an anatomic lesion of the pontomesencephalic tegmentum as the cause for the unconsciousness. The Pt has a supratentorial lesion or metabolic-toxic coma. Fixed eyeballs, and thus no vestibulo-ocular reflex, with normally reactive pupils, suggest depressant drugs, generally barbiturates.

3. Summarize three methods used to investigate the comatose Pt for the integrity of the MLF in its course through the tegmental core of the brainstem.

____

Inspect for random horizontal drifts and do the caloric irrigation and the counter-rolling tests.

4. Which method should you choose to test the MLF in a Pt unconscious from head trauma? ❒ caloric irrigation/❒ counter-rolling test. Explain.

____

☑ caloric irrigation

Do not manipulate the neck in a Pt with suspected head trauma because of the possibility of a cervical fracture.

5. An alternative to caloric irrigation is galvanic stimulation of the labyrinth (Toglia et al., 1981).

F. Cranial nerves IX and X

Spontaneous swallowing or groaning constitutes a sufficient test. Actually eliciting the gag reflex may induce vomiting and aspiration of stomach contents into the lungs. However, see the brain death protocol, page 607.

G. Techniques for eliciting responses to noxious stimuli: cold and pain

1. To test the somatic pathways in unconscious Pts, use stimuli that a conscious Pt would perceive as noxious or painful. First, make a decision whether to use cold or pain. Cold is often the more appropriate stimulus for infants and children (especially when the parents are looking on) and for partly conscious Pts.
2. **Technique to test for response to cold:** Apply an ice cube to the Pt's face, hands, and feet. If there is no response, apply it to armpits, abdomen, or inner thighs (actions that will get your attention quickly).
3. **Techniques to test for pain responses**

a. **Mandibular test for pain response:** Place your fingers on the temporomandibular joints and press (Wijdicks, 1996) or place your fingers behind the ramus of the mandible and compress the tips against the bone, as if to pull the mandible forward. This provides a very strong pain stimulus. Try it on yourself and a partner.

b. **Knuckle rub tests for pain response:** Make a fist and press or rub your knuckles strongly against the Pt's sternum. Observe for an arousal response with eye opening or decerebrate posturing.

c. **Nail compression tests for pain:** Test for localized pain responses by stimulating each extremity separately. Pinch the Pt's fingernails or toenails hard, or press them with the rubber tip of a pencil. To ensure a painful stimulus, the Ex must apply the pinch correctly. Grasp your left thumbnail between the tip of the right thumbnail and index finger and pinch it hard. You may or may not feel much pain. Next grasp your left thumbnail by placing the center of the tip of the right thumb over the margin of the left thumbnail where it attaches to the flesh, and this time squeeze and torque, or twist, the left nail, as though trying to screw on a bottle cap. Try the technique with other fingers. With practice you can learn to torque only the fingernail, not the entire digit, which may injure the Pt's finger joints.

d. **Skin pinch test for pain response:** As an alternative pain stimulus, try pinching the Pt's skin between your thumb tip and index finger. In this era of acquired immunodeficiency syndrome and infectious hepatitis, avoid pinpricks. They often leave a trail of dots of blood. Also do not use your fingernails, except to compress the supraorbital nerve, where the eyebrow provides protection, or you may leave visible wounds. Try the various ways of testing facial and body pain on yourself to learn the proper strength of stimulus to use.

4. Do not overdo pain testing in the Pt suspected of feigned coma. The Pt may have a steely resolve not to respond. Sudden, unexpected stimuli, such as flicking a closed eyelid, are more likely to elicit a response than extremely strong ones (Wiggs, 1973).
5. Record the result of pain testing in the Glasgow Coma Scale. In general, the arm responses are more informative than the leg responses because a purely spinal reflex can cause flexion of the leg in a Pt with a transected cord or in the brain-dead Pt whose spinal cord remains intact.
6. Review the mandibular, sternal rub, nail, and skin pinch tests for responses to pain in the comatose Pt.

BIBLIOGRAPHY · Sensory Testing of Unconscious Patients

Buettner UW, Zee DS. Vestibular testing in comatose patients. *Arch Neurol* 1989;46:561–563.

Fisher CM. The neurological examination of the comatose patient. *Acta Neurol Scand* 1969;45(suppl 36):1–56.

Toglia JU, Adam RU, Steward G. Galvanic vestibular tests in the assessment of coma and brain death. *Ann Neurol* 1981;9:294–295.

Wijdicks EF. The Diagnosis of Brain Death. *N Eng J Med*. 2001;344:1215–1221.

Wiggs JW. Detection of feigned coma. *N Engl J Med* 1973;289:379.

VI. FACTORS THAT COMPOUND AND COMPLICATE THE NEUROLOGIC EXAMINATION OF THE UNCONSCIOUS PATIENT

A. The muscle stretch reflexes and toe signs

The MSRs and toe signs that prove so valuable in the alert Pt take a secondary role in coma. You may find decreased, equal, or increased MSRs or no MSRs depending on cerebral shock and the depth of the coma. Even when the MSRs are unequal, you may not know whether one side is pathologically depressed or the other pathologically active. Depression of consciousness for any reason, even deep sleep in some individuals, may cause bilateral extensor toe signs. Thus, in coma, neither the presence nor the absence of the typical UMN signs have the significance that they do in the alert Pt.

B. Preexisting neurologic signs

Preexisting conditions may confuse the diagnosis. Is a given finding preexistent or new? The apparent unconsciousness may be the result of petit mal or psychomotor status epilepticus; the failure to react to sound may represent preexisting deafness; the immobile eye with the nonreactive pupil may be a glass eye; the Pt may have congenital ptosis or anisocoria; the pupils may react sluggishly; the MSRs may be absent because of Adie's syndrome (Table 4-5); the hemiplegia may be a postictal paralysis after a focal seizure (Todd's paralysis); or the Pt may have had a preexisting hemiplegia or other neurologic signs before the coma. Mild diffuse atrophy, brisk MSRs, and spasticity, particularly of the fingers, suggest a preexisting hemiplegia. Photographs and family members can document preexisting illness.

C. How to address the unconscious patient: the law of respect

Because of the difficulties in judging the level of consciousness, the Ex must never, never, make flippant or pejorative remarks at the bedside of a presumably unconscious or anesthetized Pt or discuss prognosis or management controversies. Anesthetized or unconscious Pts often hear and remember more than expected (Baier and Schomaker, 1990; Cheek, 1960). Always assume that the Pt hears and understands everything said at the bedside. The physician, ward personnel, and family should address the Pt by name and talk to the Pt as if he were conscious (LaPuma et al., 1988). Although such stimulation may or may not speed recovery (Pierce et al., 1990), addressing unconscious Pts by name and avoiding thoughtless comments causes no harm and does affirm the Pt's status as a human being rather than as just a carcass.

BIBLIOGRAPHY · How to Address the Unconscious Patient

Baier S, Schomaker MS. *Bed Number Ten: A Patient's View of Long Term Care.* Boca Raton, CRC Press, 1990.

Cheek DB. What does the surgically anesthetized patient hear? *Rocky Mtn Med J* 1960;57:49–53.

LaPuma J, Schiedermayer DL, Gulyas AE, et al. Talking to comatose patients. *Arch Neurol* 1988;45:20–22.

Pierce JP, Lyle DM, Quine S, et al. The effectiveness of coma arousal intervention. *Brain Inj* 1990;4:191–197.

VII. THE NEUROLOGIC EXAMINATION IN THE LOCKED-IN SYNDROME (DE-EFFERENTED STATE)

You survive, but you survive with what is so aptly known as "locked-in syndrome". Paralyzed from head to toe, the patient, his mind intact, is imprisoned inside his own body, unable to speak or move. In my case, blinking my left eyelid is my only means of communication.

—Jean-Dominique Bauby
The Diving Bell and The Butterfly

A. Clinical features

1. Bilateral extensive lesions—infarction, trauma, demyelination, or neoplasm—may destroy both pyramidal tracts in the basis pontis or midbrain (Chia, 1991; Feldman, 1971; Reznick, 1983; Turazzi and Bricolo, 1977). The Pt suffers complete bilateral hemiplegia, anarthria, aphagia, and incontinence. The Pt retains full consciousness and sensation because the lesion spares the tegmentum and its contained reticular formation and lemnisci. Breathing continues automatically, but the only volitional movements remaining are vertical eye movements and sometimes blinking. The pathways for these actions enter the pretectum and tectum rostral to the lesion. Usually the lesion interrupts the pathways to the conjugate lateral gaze center in the pons, causing paralysis of volitional horizontal eye movements (Nordgren et al., 1971; Fig. 2-30). The Pt, although conscious, may display decerebrate posturing to stimuli (Feldman, 1971; Nordgren, 1971).
2. The Ex can communicate with the Pt and establish consciousness by the only volitional effector mechanism remaining, the eye movements, by using upward movements for *yes* and downward for *no*. Otherwise, the Pt's consciousness, deprived of any efferent pathways to other effectors, remains "locked-in." In rare instances when the lesion destroys the pyramidal tracts at the midbrain level, the Pt may also retain volitional blinking and horizontal eye movements (Chia, 1991).
3. If unrecognized by the Ex, the locked-in state condemns the Pt to the cruelest of existences. Perfectly conscious and in possession of all senses and faculties, the Pt cannot avoid even the most trifling annoyances. The Pt cannot adjust a heel to relieve pressure, scratch an itch, flick a fly from the face, or voluntarily swallow to relieve a flooded pharynx. Although thought and emotion remain as powerful as ever, the Pt cannot utter the faintest whisper or write a single letter. Even the total helplessness is not the worst of it, if others make unintended but dehumanizing remarks at the bedside, as if the Pt were a non-person. Moreover, because a Pt may pass through the locked-in state during recovery from coma, the Ex must always anticipate the return of sentiency and monitor for it daily by meticulous NEs.

BIBLIOGRAPHY · The Locked-in Syndrome

Bauby JD. *The Diving Bell and the Butterfly*. Random House, 1997.

Chia L-G. Locked-in syndrome with bilateral ventral midbrain infarcts. *Neurology* 1991;41: 445–446.

Feldman MH. Physiological observations in a chronic case of "locked-in" syndrome. *Neurology* 1971;21:459–478.

Nordren RE, Markesbery WR, Fukuda K, et al. Seven cases of cerebromedullospinal disconnection: the "locked-in" syndrome. *Neurology* 1971;21:1140–1148.

Reznick M. Neuropathology in seven cases of locked-in syndrome. *J Neurol Sci* 1983;60: 67–78.

VIII. THE NEUROLOGIC EXAMINATION IN THE PERSISTENT VEGETATIVE STATE

A. Definition

Jennett and Plum (1972) defined the persistent vegetative state (PVS) as a persistent state after coma, characterized by eye opening and "a return of wakefulness accompanied by an apparent total lack of cognitive function." In essence, the Pt, appears awake but remains unaware of self and environment. Awareness is abolished but arousal from sleep persists, thus implying the separation of these two functions.

1. **Persistent** emphasizes that the PVS has already lasted for some time, 4 weeks at a minimum, and implies that the Pt may remain that way for an extended period.
2. **Vegetative** emphasizes the assumption that the Pt, devoid of mind or volitional actions, retains only autonomic, vegetative, or reflex functions (Munsat et al., 1989).

3. Some states such as the *akinetic mutism* of Hugh Cairns (1941, 1952), the decorticate or *apallic state* of Kretchsmer (Dalle et al., 1977), and the *coma vigile* of the French resemble, or are synonymous with, the PVS, but sometimes coma vigile is identified with the locked-in syndrome (Victor and Ropper, 2001).

B. Neuropathology of the persistent vegetative state

1. The most common causes of the PVS are severe hypoxia, head trauma, or massive infarction, resulting in permanent bilateral diffuse damage, usually at multiple levels from the rostral brainstem through diencephalon, basal ganglia, deep white matter, and cerebral cortex (Adams et al., 2000; Jennett, 2002; Kinney and Samuels, 1994). After such a catastrophe, the stage of eyes-closed unconsciousness usually lasts no more than a month. Then the Pt will enter the stage of eyes-open unconsciousness, the so-called PVS.
2. Patients with progressive cerebral degenerative diseases may also end in a vegetative state, and some infants with severe brain malformations meet the criteria (Multi-Society Task Force, 1994). Estimates place the number of PVS Pts in the United States as between 10,000 and 25,000 adults and 4000 and 10,000 children (Multi-Society Task Force, 1994).

C. Clinical features of the persistent vegetative state (Jennett, 2002)

1. The Pts cannot sit, stand, walk, or talk. The Pts remain mute and completely devoid of any verbal or nonverbal communication or of any purposeful or adaptive behavior that offers operational proof of consciousness or volition.
2. PVS Pts are akinetic or hypokinetic. Although the Pt may display more or less severe paralysis, spasticity, rigidity, or paratonia and sometimes hypotonia, the akinesia is out of proportion to and not directly caused by a UMN syndrome. The Pt cannot do any self-help tasks such as dressing or feeding.
3. PVS Pts exhibit apparent sleep and wake cycles. They open their eyes during the day or sometimes in response to putatively painful stimuli.
4. PVS Pts may blink, move their eyes spontaneously, and may fixate and pursue to some degree. They do not actively fixate and selectively move the eyes from target to target, which would imply consciousness. Vestibulo-ocular reflexes generally remain.
5. PVS Pts flex their limbs in response to pain but show no purposive or adaptive avoidance. They fail to orient actively or adaptively to light, sound, or touch but may startle reflexively in response to these stimuli.
6. PVS Pts retain many autonomic and somatic reflexes. They are incontinent for urine and feces but generally support their own blood pressure and breathe automatically.
7. PVS Pts show many of the primitive reflexes reviewed in Table 11-6: grasping, sucking, automatic yawning, and chewing, but not purposeful chewing and swallowing. They may show cyclic automatic chewing movements unrelated to feeding. Feeding is by tube or gastrostomy. Some Pts display the spontaneous crying or laughing of pseudobulbar palsy (Higashi et al., 1977).

D. The minimally conscious state

Some Pts fall somewhere beyond a true PVS but are far from fully conscious (Table 12-8; Giacino et al., 2002). They show inconsistent but at least some discernible behavioral signs suggestive of consciousness. This diagnostic category remains in need of further study before full acceptance (Bernat, 2002; Coleman, 2002).

E. Prognosis for survival and recovery from the persistent vegetative state

1. Survival time in the PVS has increased with improvement in overall management (Strauss et al., 1999). Children have a greater potential for survival than adults (Kreil et al., 1993). Operational proof of consciousness has returned to some Pts who have been in the PVS for as long as 18 to 36 months (Arts et al., 1985; Higashi et al., 1981; Rosenberg, 1977) and anecdotally after more than a decade.

Seen in this light, the PVS may represent a phase, after coma, preceding the return of consciousness. For these reasons, the Ex must periodically repeat the NE in all Pts with altered consciousness and must not hastily dismiss the Pt as a "vegetable" or too quickly terminate support. The critical question is how long do we wait on a Pt in the PVS to recover consciousness before giving up? As a final confounding factor, even though a person in the PVS or minimally conscious state had previously given directives about life support, further reflection may change the Pt's mind. Patients who wanted to die under one circumstance may later change their minds and want to live (Patterson, 1993).

2. The Pt in the "minimally conscious state" further complicates matters (Wijdicks, 2006). The burden of decision challenges the *epistemology* of the NE, but we have had no better way. Magnetic resonance imaging spectroscopy of the thalamus, a crucial neuronal station in the neuroanatomy of consciousness, shows differences in Pts who recovered from the PVA as contrasted to those who remained in that state (Uzan et al., 2003). In any event the burden does not rest on the Pt to prove "worthiness," consciousness, and the existence of personhood but on the neurologic evaluation to refute these attributes. If all this uncertainty about our ability—yours and mine—to judge consciousness worries you, you have the right attitude. Conversely, if the PVS exemplifies the failure of the NE to provide an absolute solution, the brain death protocol (next section) fully demonstrates the validity and power of the NE. Most neurologists agree that the diagnosis of brain death is straightforward, reliable, and uncontroversial.

BIBLIOGRAPHY · The Neurologic Examination in the Persistent Vegetative State

Adams JH, Graham DI, Jennett B. The neuropathology of the vegetative state after an acute brain insult. *Brain* 2000;123:1327–1338.

Arts W, van Dongen H, Van Hof-van Duin J, et al. Unexpected improvement after prolonged post-traumatic vegetative state. *J Neurol Neurosurg Psychiatry* 1985;48:1300–1303.

Bernat JL. Questions remaining about the minimally conscious state. *Neurology* 2002;58: 337–338.

Cairns H. Disturbances of consciousness with lesions of the brainstem and diencephalon. *Brain* 1952;75:109–146.

Cairns H, Oldfield R, Pennybacker JB, et al. Akinetic mutism with an epidermoid cyst of the third ventricle. *Brain* 1941;64:273–290.

Coleman D. The minimally conscious state: definition and diagnostic criteria. *Neurology* 2002;58:506.

Dalle Ore G, Gerstenbrand F, Lucking CH, et al, editors. *The Apallic Syndrome*. New York, Springer-Verlag, 1977.

Giacino JT, Ashwal S, Childs N, et al. The minimally conscious state. Definition and diagnostic criteria. *Neurology* 2002;58:349–353.

Higashi K, Hatano M, Abiko S, et al. Five-year follow-up study of patients with persistent vegetative state. *J Neurol Neurosurg Psychiatry* 1981;44:552–554.

Jennett B. *The Vegetative State. Medical Facts, Ethical and Legal Dilemmas.* New York, Cambridge University Press, 2002.

Kinney HC, Samuels MA. Neuropathology of the persistent vegetative state. A review. *J Neuropath Exp Neurol* 1994;53:548–558.

Kriel RL, Krach LE, Jones-Saete C. Outcome of children with prolonged unconsciousness and vegetative states. *Pediatr Neurol* 1993;9:362–368.

Multi-Society Task Force. Medical aspects of the persistent vegetative state. Part 1. *N Engl J Med* 1994;330:1499–1508.

Multi-Society Task Force. Medical aspects of the persistent vegetative state. Part 2. *N Engl J Med* 1994;330:1572–1579.

Munsat TL, Stuart WH, Cranford RE. Guidelines on the vegetative state: commentary on the American Academy of Neurology statement. *Neurology* 1989;39:123–124.

Patterson DR, Miller-Perrin C, McCormick TR, et al. When life support is questioned early in the care of patients with cervical level quadriplegia. *N Engl J Med* 1993;328:506–509.

3. These ancillary procedures prove useful if something prevents a full, adequate NE, such as severe burns of the face and head or traumatic destruction of facial parts. A radionuclide scan or EEG may be added to conclude the BDP after only one NE to facilitate organ transplantation rather than waiting for a prolonged period for a second clinical examination (Schneider and Ashwal, 1999).
4. The time of death is recorded as the time at which the Ex reaches a diagnosis of brain death.

J. Rationale for confirmatory tests and for involving more than one physician in the brain-death protocol

Involvement of at least three different physicians—the attending physician, the neurologist, and the radiologist or electroencephalographer—to diagnose brain death increases the probability that at least one of them will be honest, competent, and incorruptible. Then, if a pathologist does an autopsy, a fourth physician ensures the validity of the diagnosis. The pathologist by gross and microscopic examination can determine whether the brain had died many hours before removal, as distinguished from a brain subjected to prompt fixation shortly after death (Walker, 1985). The involved physicians do *not* meet as a committee and do not vote on whether the Pt's brain is dead. They all ascertain independently of each other that brain-death criteria have been met, according to the techniques that each knows and thoroughly understands. With these safeguards, the diagnosis of brain death then becomes as infallible as humanly possible, and the process is protected from fraud, incompetence, or as a shield for murder.

K. Brain-death protocol in infants and children

Because of presumably greater resistance to hypoxia, the BDP for infants, in particular premature infants, is somewhat more conservative than for older Pts (Kohrman and Spivak, 1990; Schneider and Ashwal, 1999).

L. Pitfalls and precautions in the diagnosis of brain death by the neurologic examination

1. The two greatest pitfalls in the diagnosis of brain death are hypothermia and an overdose of depressant drugs. Rarely, a nonbarbiturate drug may cause abolition of brainstem reflexes (Richard et al., 1998; Rizzo et al., 1993) as may toxic levels of aminoglycosides, anticholinergics, neuromuscular blocking agents, severe Guillain-Barré syndrome (Hassan and Mumford, 1991). In severe pharmacologic depression or hypothermia, the NE may show no brain function, and the EEG may be isoelectric, *yet the Pt may recover completely*. Radionuclide scans or direct angiography will still demonstrate cerebral blood flow in these Pts who show no clinical or electrical evidence of brain function, but whose brains remain alive. And consider this scenario: a murderer who wanted to make a Pt appear brain dead could administer atropine to block pupillary and cardioinhibitory responses and curarize the Pt to block skeletomuscular responses. Such a Pt would have no effector responses and meet brain-death criteria on the purely clinical examination, but the EEG would demonstrate electrical activity and the radionuclide scan would demonstrate cerebral blood flow.
2. True decerebrate or decorticate posturing are inconsistent with the diagnosis of brain death. Some purely spinal reflexes remain in a large percentage of brain-dead Pts. The mechanism that caused brain death, such as cerebral edema or transforaminal herniation, may leave the spinal cord intact, whereas hypoxia-induced brain death may cause the cord to die also. With an intact cord, the Pt may show finger jerks, whole arm posturing, triple flexion, MSRs, and, extremely rarely, movements of the arms resembling decerebrate rigidity triggered by stimuli below the neck but not the face (Marti-Fabregas et al., 2000; Saposnik et al., 2000). Most dramatic of all is the "Lazarus sign" in which the arms flex and

adduct, crossing the hands in front of the chest. The possibility of such ghastly movements that to the layman are totally mystifying and impossible to understand is one of the many reasons I always ask the family to remain in the waiting room during the examination.

3. By informing the family on a day-to-day basis of the Pt's condition and prognosis, the physician encourages a rational response to the BDP. The family must understand that the purpose of the BDP is to recognize and verify beyond doubt that the person has already died and that continued support of the remaining organs is futile. Otherwise the family may misperceive termination of support as an effort to save money for an insurance company or the hospital, to provide organs for transplantation, or to commit euthanasia or genocide.
4. When all criteria for brain death have been rigidly fulfilled with respect to the NE and the appropriate ancillary studies (EEG and blood flow) have been correctly performed, the possibility for a mistake is virtually nil in Pts with mature brains. Because of different reactions of the immature and immature brains, the timing of the tests and some criteria for the BDP differ for infants (Schneider and Ashwal, 1999).

M. Permission for organ donation

Most physicians agree that no one on the organ transplant team should approach the family before completion of the BDP, because of the obvious conflict of interest. I think it best in general that the attending physician or neurologist raise this question after completion of the BDP and then introduce the representative from the transplant team.

N. Tabular summary of the neurologic examination of patients in coma, the persistent vegetative state, minimally conscious state, and locked-in syndrome (Table 12-8)

BIBLIOGRAPHY · The Neurologic Examination in the Diagnosis of Brain Death

American Academy of Neurology. Practice parameters for determining brain death in adults (summary statement). *Neurology* 1995;45:1012–1014.

Facco E, Liviero MC, Munari M, et al. Short latency evoked potentials: new criteria for brain death. *J Neurol Neurosurg Psychiatry* 1990;53(4):351–353.

Goudreau, Jl, Wijdicks EFM, Emery SF. Complications during apnea testing in the determination of brain death: predisposing factors. *Neurology* 2000;55:1045–1048.

Gutmann DH, Marino PL. An alternative apnea test for the evaluation of brain death. *Ann Neurol* 1991;30:852–853.

Hassan T, Mumford C. Guillain-Barré syndrome mistaken for brain death. *Postgrad Med J* 1991;67:280–281.

Kohrman MH, Spivak BS. Brain death in infants: sensitivity and specificity of current criteria. *Pediatr Neurol* 1990;6:47–50.

Marks SG, Zisfein J. Apneic oxygenation in apnea tests for brain death: a controlled trial. *Arch Neurol* 1990;47:1066–1068.

Marti-Fabregas J, Lopez-Navidad A, Caballero F, et al. Decerebrate-like posturing with mechanical ventilation in brain death. *Neurology* 2000;54:244–227.

Plum F, Posner J. *Diagnosis of Stupor and Coma*, 3rd ed. Philadelphia, FA Davis, 1980.

Richard IH, Lapointe M, Wax P, et al. Non-barbiturate, drug induced reversible loss of brainstem reflexes. *Neurology* 1998;51:639–640.

Ringel RA, Riggs, JE, Brick JF. Reversible coma with prolonged absence of pupillary and brainstem reflexes: an unusual response to a hypoxic-ischemia event in MS. *Neurology* 1988;38:1275–1277.

TABLE 12-8 · **Neurologic Examination in Brain Death, Coma, PVS, Minimally Conscious State, and Locked-in Syndrome**

	Consciousness	Communication	Emotion	Sleep-wake cycles	Auditory function	Visual function	Breathing	Motor function	EEG	Prognosis
BRAIN DEATH	None	None	None	None	None	None	None	None or only spinal reflexes	Isoelectric (no activity)	Dead
COMA	None	None	None	None	None	None	Minimal or none	None in deep coma	Polymorphic delta	Depends on cause
PERSISTENT VEGETATIVE STATE	No operational evidence of consciousness	None	No operational evidence of emotional experience	Present	None, or startle or brief orientation to sounds*	None to minimal visual orientation*	Adequate automatic breathing	Withdraws from noxious stimuli*; no volitional movements	Polymorphic delta, theta, or slow alpha rhythm	Worsens with time in PVS; rarely, consciousness returns
MINIMALLY CONSCIOUS STATE	Intermittent, incomplete, unsustained	Minimal contingent vocalization; no speech as such	Some reactive smiling or crying (pseudobulbar?)	Present	Orients to sound; cannot follow commands	Some fixation and following	Adequate automatic breathing	Some posturing, localizes pain	Delta, theta, or alpha	Worsens with time
LOCKED-IN SYNDROME	Fully conscious	Only by vertical eye movements or blinking	Experiences full range	Present	Responds with eye movements	Normal vision	Adequate automatic breathing	Double hemiplegia	May be normal	Poor for motor recovery

*Presumed to be reflex only, not volitional.

ABBREVIATIONS: EEG = electroencephalography; PVS = persistent vegetative state.

Rizzo MA, Fisher M, Lock JP. Hypermagnesemic pseudo coma. *Arch Int Med* 1993;153(9): 1130–1132.

Saposnik G, Bueri JA, Maurino J, et al. Spontaneous reflex movements in brain death. *Neurology* 2000;54:221–223.

Schneider S, Ashwal S. Determination of brain death in infants and children. In Swaiman KE, Ashwal S, eds. *Pediatric Neurology: Principles and Practice,* 3rd ed. St. Louis, Mosby, 1999, Chapter 62, pp. 969–980.

Walker AD. *Cerebral Death,* 3rd ed. Baltimore, Urban and Schwarzenberger, 1985.

Wijdicks EFM. The diagnosis of brain death. *N Engl J Med* 2001a;344:1215–1221.

Wijdicks EFM, ed. *Brain Death.* Hagerston, Lippincott Williams & Wilkins, 2001b.

Wijdicks EFM. Brain death worldwide. Accepted fact but no global consensus in diagnostic criteria. *Neurology* 2002;58:20–25.

Zuckier L, Kolano J. Radionuclide studies in the determination of brain death. Criteria, Concepts, and Controversies. *Seminars in Nuclear Medicine* 2008;38(4);262–273.

X. THE NEUROLOGIC EXAMINATION IN INTERMITTENT DISTURBANCES OF CONSCIOUSNESS: SYNCOPE, SEIZURES, AND BLACKOUT SPELLS

A. Definition

Syncope means a sudden, brief lapse of consciousness, with loss of postural tone and spontaneous recovery, but not caused by epilepsy. Lay people call it *fainting, falling out,* or *blacking-out*. The medical investigation focuses on what precedes or triggers the syncope, either emotional factors or pathophysiologic events. The incidence of organic syncope increases dramatically after the age of 70 years and almost doubles for Pts with cardiovascular disease. The sex incidence remains about equal (Soteriades et al., 2002). Figure 12-33 shows a classification of syncope.

B. Pathophysiologic mechanisms of syncope

Whether triggered by emotional or organic causes, the final event that causes loss of consciousness is cerebral ischemia induced by several factors (Grubb and Olshansky, 1997).

1. Vagal inhibition of the heart, causing bradycardia or asystole.
2. Loss of vasoconstrictor tone by sympathetic inhibition or insufficiency, causing hypotension. Sympathetic and parasympathetic discharges occur in syncope (Shen and Gersh, 1997).
3. Hydraulic or hypovolemic decreases in cerebral blood flow. The causes may be pooling of blood in the large veins, intrinsic heart disease with inadequate output, or occlusive vascular disease.
4. Cardiac dysrhythmias.

C. The medical history in syncope or any intermittent disorder such as headaches or seizures.

1. **The three-phase description:** For all intermittent clinical events, syncope, headaches, pain, and epilepsy divide the inquiry into **preictal events,** the **ictus** itself, and the **postictal events** or recovery period. Question family members who have seen an attack and view videos, if possible. Most important, learn the mode of onset. **The clue to the cause comes from how the attack starts, not how it ends.**
2. **Preictal phase**

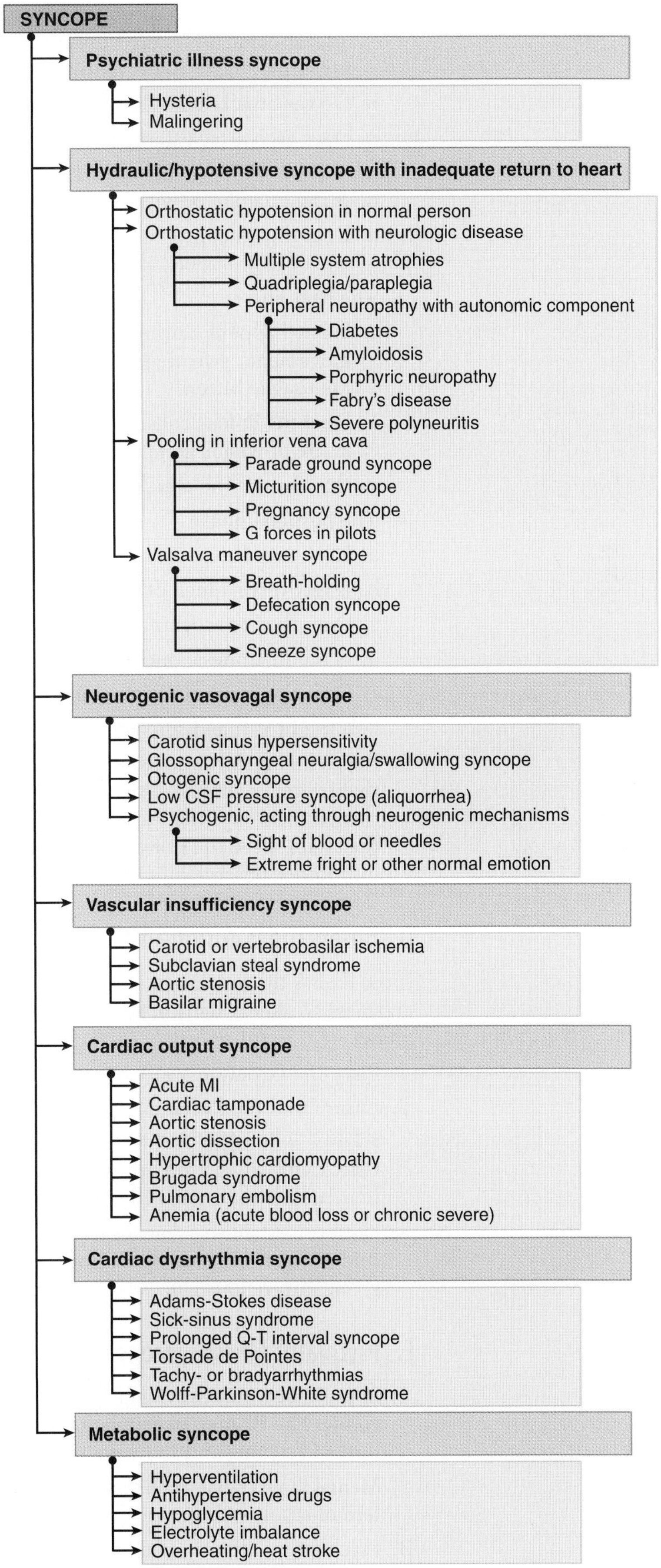

FIGURE 12-33. Dendrogram for causes of syncope (reference only).

a. What symptoms, posture, activities, and social circumstances prevail when the attacks come on? Is the Pt standing, sitting, moving, changing position, coughing, urinating, or hyperventilating?

b. Do the attacks all follow a pattern?

c. Does each attack start the same way? Ask the Pt: "What is the first change or warning of an attack?"

d. Is the Pt alone or with people, and, if with people, which ones?

e. Does the syncope evolve immediately or over minutes with premonitory feelings of fear, anxiety, impending doom, dizziness, and nausea?

3. **The ictal phase**

a. What happens during the attack: changes in breathing, falling, convulsive movements, sweating, pallor, cyanosis, and incontinence? Is the Pt injured? Is the tongue bitten?

b. Does the Pt lose consciousness? Ask: "Can you talk during the attack? Are you aware of what's going on?"

c. How long is the attack?

4. **The postictal phase**

a. How does the ictus end?

b. Is recovery sudden or gradual?

c. Does the Pt recognize that an ictus has occurred?

d. Is the Pt amnesic or disoriented?

e. Does the Pt regularly sleep afterward?

f. Is the Pt stiff and sore after an attack?

5. **Reproducing the circumstances of the attack:** Try to reproduce the circumstances that trigger an attack. If the Pt reports that a posture, such as head turning, elicits an attack, have the Pt turn the head. If hyperventilation or coughing precedes the attack, have the Pt hyperventilate or cough. If the Pt faints in the presence of his mother, observe him in the presence of his mother.

D. Observations during an attack

If the Ex has the fortune to witness an attack, have the Pt describe the symptoms—dizziness, weakness, nausea, flashing lights, etc. Protect the Pt during the unconscious phase.

1. Place the Pt flat on a soft surface.
2. Ensure that the Pt has an open airway. Turn the Pt's head to the side to prevent aspiration in case of vomiting.
3. Check vital signs, blood pressure, pulse, respiratory rate, pupillary size and reaction, muscle tone, and reflexes.
4. Until you establish a diagnosis, draw a blood sample for hypoglycemia or hypocalcemia whenever you observe any attack that alters consciousness and consider giving intravenous glucose.

E. Psychiatric illness syncope (Fig. 12-33)

1. In psychiatric illness syncope, the Pt usually has a conversion disorder or is malingering. The Pt may experience weakness, sweating, nausea, abdominal discomfort, and sighing and show pallor at the onset, or it may be instantaneous.
2. Mental illness never manifests solely by syncope. It is only one shadow in the pattern of emotional turmoil (Leis et al., 1992).
3. Psychogenic attacks usually occur in the presence of people emotionally entangled with the Pt. At the end of the NE, call in the family to see how the family and Pt interact. The Pt may faint on the spot, thus clinching the diagnosis. Organic syncope is not "socially dependent."

4. If Pts fall during the ictus, they usually do not hurt themselves or become incontinent. As in hysterical swaying on the Romberg test, the Pt may conveniently fall into the observer's arms. In organic attacks, the fall often injures the Pt, but this distinction is by no means absolute.
5. Preceding an attack, some Pts hyperventilate. Always ask about changes in breathing and any associated symptoms (Hoefnagels et al., 1991) and do the hyperventilation test (pages 371–372). The test and an EEG are particularly important in the differential diagnosis of epilepsy (Stephenson, 2002).

F. Mechanical/hypovolemic syncope from inadequate return of blood to the heart (Fig. 12-33)

1. **Orthostatic syncope (orthostatic hypotension)**
   a. Upon suddenly rising from a sitting or reclining position, the Pt feels giddy or may faint. The blood pressure has dropped rather than automatically adjusting to the erect position. Everyone experiences this phenomenon to some degree.
   b. Take the blood pressure and pulse rate with the Pt reclining and upright. Normal young persons display an acceleration of the pulse by 5 to 25 beats and a drop in systolic blood pressure of no more than 25 mmHg and an increase of up to 10 mmHg in the diastolic pressure (Arnold et al., 1991). In association with symptoms, a consistent drop below 90 mmHg in systolic pressure establishes orthostatic hypotension. The elderly show a lower blood pressure on standing than young persons. A tilt table test refines the analysis of orthostatic hypotension, and the Valsalva maneuver may provide further evidence of autonomic insufficiency (Almquist et al., 1989; Chen et al., 1989). Ask about medications that might cause hypotension.
2. **Parade-ground syncope:** If a person stands still for a period of time, as a soldier on a parade ground, blood pools in the inferior vena cava and in the lower extremities. After the person faints and becomes horizontal, blood returns to the circulation, allowing prompt recovery.
3. **Micturition syncope:** During urination, particularly with a very full bladder, the Pt faints (Lyle, 1961). The release of a large volume of urine from the bladder and the sudden relaxation of the abdominal wall drops abdominal pressure. Venous blood pools in the tributaries of the inferior vena cava, thus curtailing venous return to the heart. Also, cardioinhibitory reflexes may arise from the bladder. Similarly, the drop in abdominal pressure may cause syncope after rapid removal of ascitic fluid from the abdomen. Cardiac inhibition or vasodilation from loss of sympathetic vasoconstrictor tone may add to the mechanical effects in reducing cerebral blood flow.
4. **Pregnancy syncope:** When the pregnant woman lies on her back, the gravid uterus compresses the inferior vena.
5. **Breath-holding spells**
   a. The most common syncope in children 6 to 48 months of age evolves through a stereotyped tetrad (DeMyer, 2002). The child may have literally dozens of these spells. Learn this tetrad.
      i. Provocation by anger or frustration
      ii. Expiratory apnea and cyanosis
      iii. Unconsciousness and opisthotonic rigidity
      iv. Stupor and somnolence
   b. Notice that part (1) is the preictal stage, (2) and (3) are the ictus, and (4) is the postictal stage. The history is all important in establishing the triggering emotional event before each spell. The NE is normal. The mechanism may involve the compression of the vena cava by the prolonged forced expiration and vasovagal reflexes. The uncommon pallid type of breath-holding spell is more likely vasovagal (Shore and Painter, 2002).

6. **Cough (ptussive) syncope:** The Pt, usually one with lung disease, has syncope after prolonged coughing. The syncope may result from a vagal reflex or from the Valsalva effect, both of which reduce the return of blood via the vena cava. In some cases, coughing or sneezing may precipitate syncope in Pts with the Chiari malformation (Corbett et al., 1976; Weig et al., 1991) or other posterior fossa lesions or with neck masses.
7. **Stretch syncope:** The Pt faints when extending the head while stretching. The syncope may result from a combination of the Valsalva maneuver, vasovagal mechanisms, and positional occlusion of the vertebral artery (Fig. 12-34; Pelekanos et al., 1990; Sturzenegger et al., 1995).

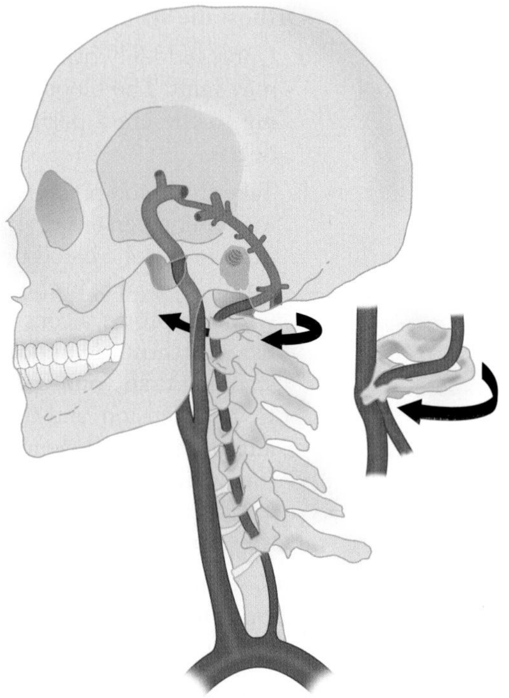

FIGURE 12-34. Diagram to show how turning of the head may kink or compress the carotid or vertebral arteries, thereby interfering with blood flow to the brain.

G. Neurogenic (vasovagal) syncope

1. Either a physical stimulus, such as coughing or head turning, or an emotional event, such as the sight of blood, triggers the syncope. In either case, the syncope has a pathophysiologic basis in bradycardia/hypotension acting through vasovagal mechanisms that inhibit the heart and vascular tone (Arnold et al., 1991). Cholinergic stimulation predominates, producing sweating, increased peristalsis, salivation, and bradycardia.
2. Syncope triggered by an emotional stimulus such as the sight of blood, a needle prick, or bad news may be called **psychogenic vasovagal syncope.** The interpretation and definition of this category, often called *vasovagal syncope,* differs from investigator to investigator (Landau and Nelson, 1996; Nahm and Freeman, 2001). Because these responses happen in otherwise normal persons, psychogenic vasovagal syncope, as defined here, differs from psychiatric illness syncope per se (Fig. 12-33).

H. Neurogenic vasovagal syncope, reflexogenic type, from swallowing, ear stimulation, or carotid sinus

1. **Swallowing or glossopharyngeal syncope:** The Pt faints when swallowing or in association with spontaneous pain in the ear and throat (glossopharyngeal neuralgia, analogous to trigeminal neuralgia).

2. **Otogenic syncope:** The Pt faints after stimulation of the external auditory canal, as during the insertion of an otoscope, or as a result of ear disease. Because the auditory canal and drum originate from the branchial arches, they receive sensory twigs from the branchial arch nerves, including CrNs IX and X. Thus, stimulation of the external auditory canal or drum may directly stimulate CrN IX or X afferents.
3. **Reflexogenic syncope from carotid sinus hypersensitivity**
   a. **Pathophysiology:** Increased BP stimulates baroreceptors in the carotid sinus that compensate by causing vasodilation or cardiac inhibition. Hypersensitivity of the reflex causes syncope.
      i. The carotid sinus is innervated by CrN ________.

IX

      ii. Cardiac inhibition is a parasympathetic reflex with the efferent arc through CrN ____________.

X

      iii. If carotid sinus hypersensitivity causes syncope by bradycardia/asystole, it is **cardioinhibitory syncope** (70%–75% of cases).
      iv. If carotid sinus hypersensitivity causes syncope from inhibition of sympathetic vasoconstrictor tone, it is **vasodepressor syncope** (5%–10% of cases).
      v. A third, controversial type of carotid sinus syncope is the **cerebral type** in which neither the pulse nor the blood pressure changes radically (Reese et al., 1962).
      vi. A paradoxical reflex may inhibit the sympathetic outflow rather than causing the expected vasoconstriction and tachycardia. It may worsen hypotension from hemorrhagic shock and during isoproterenol infusion (Almquist et al., 1989).

   b. **Complete** Table 12-9.

TABLE 12-9 · Mechanisms of Carotid Sinus Syncope

Type of carotid sinus syncope	Mechanisms of syncope
Vasodepressor	
Cardioinhibitory	
Cerebral	

Decreased sympathetic vasoconstrictor tone
Reflex asystole or bradycardia
Unknown

   c. **Role of head turning and neck manipulation in syncope**
      i. A Pt with a hypersensitive carotid sinus or with swollen lymph nodes may faint when turning the head because of inadvertent mechanical stimulation of the carotid sinus.
      ii. Head turning also may cause syncope by temporarily occluding a carotid or vertebral artery. In a normal young person, occlusion of a major cerebral artery may cause no symptoms or signs. In elderly, hypertensive, or arteriosclerotic Pts with occlusive arterial disease, the other arteries may fail to supply the brain adequately after occlusion of one (Fig. 12-34).
      iii. Chiropractic neck manipulation may cause death or severe neurologic disability from vertebrobasilar infarction.
   d. **Indications for the carotid sinus massage test**
      i. A Pt with syncope precipitated by head turning or who has enlarged cervical lymph nodes.
      ii. A Pt with lapses of consciousness for whom the history, physical examination, and other tests disclose no cause.
   e. **Contraindications to the carotid sinus massage test for carotid sinus sensitivity**
      i. Do not perform carotid sinus massage if patient has had an MI, stroke or transient ischemic attack in the previous three months.
      ii. History of ventricular fibrillation, ventricular tachycardia, or carotid bruits, are relative contraindications.

f. **Technique for the carotid sinus massage test**

i. The technique for the carotid sinus massage has not been standardized. Some authors use carotid Doppler ultrasound to guide carotid sinus massage, and do not perform the maneuver if there is = 70% carotid artery stenosis.

ii. Complete the general physical and NE, including palpating the neck for nodes and listening over the head and neck for bruits. Monitor the Pt by electrocardiography (ECG) and preferably also EEG.

iii. Place the Pt sitting upright in a chair. A standing Pt may fall during the test or, if recumbent, may not have sufficient hypotension to faint, even though the Pt has a hypersensitive carotid sinus.

iv. Have the Pt repeat whatever head maneuver or position results in syncope.

v. The Ex must use a control test for suggestibility to exclude psychogenic syncope. State that you will rub the Pt's neck, but do not suggest the outcome. Select any point on the neck away from the carotid sinuses and massage gently for 5 to 15 seconds. Fainting suggests psychogenic syncope.

vi. Locate the carotid sinus by gently palpating the carotid bifurcation. Press your fingers gently backward, just below the angle of the mandible and anterior to the sternocleidomastoid muscle. Record the blood pressure and pulse. Massage the carotid bulb with very gentle pressure for 5 to 15 seconds and again record the blood pressure and pulse. After 5 minutes, massage the other carotid bulb.

vii. In normal subjects, the pulse slows by about 15% (Arnold et al., 1991). Asystole lasting more than 3 s or a drop of more than 50 mmHg in the systolic blood pressure indicates carotid sinus hypersensitivity. (Fujimura et al., 1989).

viii. Carotid sinus hypersensitivity can be treated by surgical denervation of the sinus or by parasympathetic blocking agents.

g. Name two mechanisms by which head turning can cause loss of consciousness.

____

____

Stimulation of a hypersensitive carotid sinus or occlusion of a major cerebral artery.

h. What is the position of the Pt for the carotid sinus massage test? ❒ sitting/ ❒ standing/❒ reclining. Explain.

____

____

☑ sitting
If standing, the Pt may fall. If reclining, the Pt may not faint, even with a hypersensitive carotid sinus.

i. Similar considerations apply to the vasovagal reflex that follows ocular compression (Shore and Painter, 2002; Stephenson, 1990).

I. Vascular occlusive syncope

1. **Carotid or vertebrobasilar transient ischemic attacks:** Complete a thorough neurovascular examination. See Chapter 1, Section V B and Fig. 12-34.
2. **Subclavian steal syndrome:** The Pt has stenosis, or occlusion, of the left subclavian artery proximal to the origin of the left vertebral artery. The Pt may have a bruit over the supraclavicular fossa and sometimes a thrill. The blood pressure in the left arm is reduced. Exercise of the left arm "steals" blood from the vertebral system, resulting in dizziness, blurred vision, long tract and cranial nerve, and other brainstem signs, including syncope (Fig. 12-35). Subclavian steal syndrome from Takayasu arteritis may rarely present with syncope.

J. Cardiac dysrhythmia syncope

This type of syncope results from a faulty impulse generation or transmission in the heart (Fujimura et al., 1989). Of special importance, look for Adams-Stokes atrioventricular block and for the prolonged QT interval syndrome, because its treatment prevents death. Syncope frequently requires an intensive cardiac and cardiovascular workup.

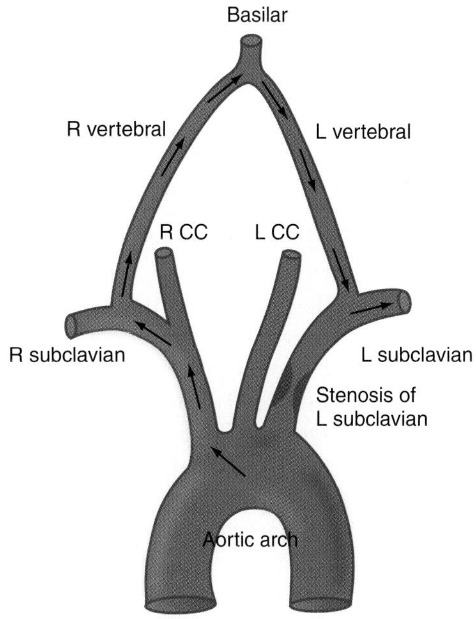

FIGURE 12-35. Diagram of the path of blood in the subclavian steal syndrome. Stenosis of the left subclavian artery reduces the pressure in the left subclavian artery, causing it to "steal" blood from the vertebral system (arrows). L = left; LCC = left common carotid artery; R = right; RCC = right common carotid artery.

K. Epilepsy versus syncope

1. The most common differential diagnosis in syncope is epilepsy. Careful history and an epileptiform EEG generally distinguish epilepsy from syncope (Table 12-10).

TABLE 12-10 · Comparison of Neurologic Findings in Vasovagal/Hydraulic Hypotensive Syncope, Epilepsy, and Psychiatric Illness Syncopes

	Vasovagal and hydraulic/ hypotensive syncope	Epilepsy	Psychiatric illness syncope
Age of onset	Rare in infants	Any age	Adolescents/young adults (not in children)
Sex	About the same	About the same	Female > male
Emotional instability	Not correlated	Not correlated	Always present
Trigger factors	Standing after reclining, standing motionless, head postures, Valsalva maneuver	Flashing lights, drug/ alcohol withdrawal, hyperventilation, metabolic imbalance	Presence of significant persons; emotionally trying events
Preictal symptoms	Weakness, dizziness, blurred vision, chest pain, sweating, abdominal discomfort	Frequent aura, varying from hallucinations to abdominal discomfort	Histrionic gestures and postures
Length	Seconds to minutes	Seconds to minutes	Brief to prolonged
Autonomic signs	Pallor, tachycardia, sweating	Cyanosis, flushing	None
Blood pressure during attack	Decreased	Increased in motor seizures	Normal
Heart rate during episode	Slow and forceful or rapid	Rapid	Normal
Incontinence	Rare	Often	Never
Injury during attack	Rare	Frequent: bruises, tongue biting	Almost never
Postictal phase	Prompt recovery with amnesia for duration of unconsciousness	Confusion, retrograde/ anterograde amnesia, sore muscles, hemiparesis, drowsiness	May or may not have amnesia
EEG during attack	Diffuse slowing	Epileptiform discharges	Normal
EEG between attacks	Normal	Abnormal usually	Normal

ABBREVIATION: EEG = electroencephalography.

2. Because cerebral ischemia disrupts brain metabolism, the Pt not only may faint but also may have a convulsion—an epileptic seizure—as part of an attack of syncope or breath-holding.

L. Subsequent workup of syncope when the initial evaluation fails to establish a diagnosis

The diagnosis of a single episode of syncope involves very different considerations from recurrent episodes of syncope. Syncope on exertion raises the question of cardiac output insufficiency. If the history and physical examination fail to establish the trigger factor for syncope, proceed with ECG and EEG or combined EEG, ECG, and video monitoring, or 24-hour ambulatory monitoring (Grubb and Olshansky, 1997; Low, 1997; Stephenson, 2002). Kapoor et al. (2000) recommended ECG for most syncope Pts, but first be sure that you have exploited all the bedside tests. A tilt table test is indicated if the clinical findings suggest neurogenic vasovagal syncope. Occasionally, magnetic resonance imaging examination will disclose an unsuspected lesion, particularly of the posterior fossa, such as a Chiari type I malformation that causes the syncope (Weig et al., 1991). Despite a full workup, many Pts with blackout spells will remain undiagnosed after the initial evaluation (Kapoor et al., 1983; Soteriades et al., 2002). Above all, follow the Pt. The number of Pts with no diagnosis will drop as the follow-up visits continue.

BIBLIOGRAPHY · Syncope

Almquist A, Goldenberg IF, Milstein S, et al. Provocation of bradycardia and hypotension by isoproterenol and upright posture in patients with unexplained syncope. *N Engl J Med* 1989;320:346–351.

Arnold RW, Dyer JA, Gould AB, et al. Sensitivity to vasovagal maneuvers in normal children and adults. *Mayo Clin Proc* 1991;66:797–804.

Chen MY, Goldenberg AB, Milstein S, et al. Cardiac electrophysiologic and hemodynamic correlates of neurally mediated syncope. *Am J Cardiol* 1989;63:66–72.

Corbett JJ, Butler AB, Kaufman B. "Sneeze syncope" basilar invagination and Arnold-Chiari type I malformation. *J Neurol Neurosurg Psychiatry* 1976;39:381–384.

DeMyer W. Breath-holding spells. In Maria BL, ed. *Current Management in Child Neurology*. London, BC Decker, 2002, Chapter 25, pp. 321–323.

Fujimura O, Yee R, Klein GJ, et al. The diagnostic sensitivity of electrophysiologic testing in patients with syncope caused by transient bradycardia. *N Engl J Med* 1989;321:1703–1706.

Grubb BP, Olshansky B. *Syncope: Mechanisms and Management*. Armon, Futura Publishing, 1997.

Hoefnagels WAJ, Padberg GW, Overweg J, et al. Syncope or seizure? The diagnostic value of the EEG and hyperventilation test in transient loss of consciousness. *J Neurol Neurosurg Psychiatry* 1991;4:953–954.

Kapoor W, Karpf M, Wieland S, et al. A prospective evaluation and follow-up of patients with syncope. *N Eng J Med* 1983;309:197–204.

Kapoor WN. Syncope. *N Engl J Med* 2000;343:1856–1861.

Kaufman H, Saadia D, Voustianiouk A. Midodrine in neurally mediated syncope: a double-blind, randomized, crossover study. *Ann Neurol* 2002;52:342–345.

Landau WM, Nelson DA. Clinical neuromythology XV. Feinting science: neurocardiogenic syncope and collateral vasovagal confusion. *Neurology* 1996;46:609–618.

Leis AA, Ross MA, Summers AK. Psychogenic seizures: ictal characteristics and diagnostic pitfalls. *Neurology* 1992;42:94–99.

Lempert T, Bauer M, Schmidt D. Syncope: a videometric analysis of 56 episodes of transient cerebral hypoxia. *Ann Neurol* 1994;36:233–237.

Low P, ed. *Clinical Autonomic Disorders*. Philadelphia, Lippincott-Raven, 1997.

Lyle C, Monroe JT, Flinn DE, et al. Micturition syncope. Report of 24 cases. *N Engl J Med* 1961;265:982–986.

Nahm F, Freeman R. Vasovagal syncope. The contributions of Sir William Gowers and Sir Thomas Lewis. *Arch Neurol* 2001;58:509–511.

Pelekanos JT, Dooley JM, Camfield PR, et al. Stretch syncope in adolescence. *Neurology* 1990;40:705–708.

Reese C, Green J, Elliott F. The cerebral form of carotid sinus hypersensitivity. *Neurology* 1962;12:492–494.

Shen W, Gersh BJ. Fainting: approch to management. In Low PA, ed. *Clinical Autonomic Disorders*, 2nd ed. Philadelphia, Lippincott-Raven, 1997, Chapter 48, pp. 649–680.

Shore PM, Painter M. Adolescent asystolic syncope. *J Child Neurol* 2002;17:395–397.

Soteriades ES, Evans JC, Larson MG, et al. Incidence and prognosis of syncope. *N Engl J Med* 2002;347:878–885.

Stephenson JBP. Fainting and syncope. In Maria BL, ed. *Current Management in Child Neurology*. London, BC Decker, 2002, Chapter 56, pp. 345–351.

Sturzenegger M, Newell DW, Douville CM, et al. Transcranial Doppler and angiographic findings in adolescent stretch syncope. *J Neurol Neurosurg Psychiatry* 1995;58:367–370.

Toole JF. *Cerebrovascular Disorders*, 5th ed. Baltimore, Lippincott Williams & Wilkins, 1999.

Weig SG, Buckthal PE, Choi SK, et al. Recurrent syncope as the presenting symptom of Arnold-Chiari malformation. *Neurology* 1991;41:1673–1674.

Learning Objectives for Chapter 12

I. EVALUATION OF CONSCIOUSNESS

1. Give a succinct, general (interpretational) definition of consciousness.
2. Describe the standard bedside operations to test for consciousness.
3. Describe the advantages of a quantitative scale for numerical grading of consciousness (Fig. 12-1).
4. Recite the three responses graded for the Glasgow Coma Scale.

II. ANATOMIC BASIS OF CONSCIOUSNESS

1. Recite the parts of the CNS that can be excised without abolishing consciousness (assuming artificial support of breathing and blood pressure).
2. Recite the parts of the CNS required for consciousness.
3. Recite the sites of lesions that abolish consciousness and state where to place the smallest lesion that will most selectively abolish consciousness.
4. Name the neuronal system that mediates alerting and consciousness and describe as precisely as possible its location and components.
5. Describe how to demonstrate the ARAS in an experimental animal, based on stimulation or lesion placement (Figs. 12-4 and 12-5).
6. Describe the difference in the EEG response to stimulation of the ARAS and a specific thalamic sensory relay nucleus.

III. INTERNAL HERNIATIONS OF THE BRAIN

1. Give some examples of space-occupying intracranial lesions that may result in herniation of the brain.
2. Name the large, tough dural membranes that separate the intracranial space into compartments (Figs. 12-6 to 12-10).
3. Make a drawing of the skull base (with the calvarium removed) to show the tentorium and the transected mesencephalon, posterior cerebral artery, and III nerves in situ after removal of the cerebral hemispheres (Figs. 12-6 and 12-7).
4. Draw the outline of the tentorial opening (incisura tentorii cerebelli) and state which parts of the brain occupy the tentorial notch.
5. Name the parts of the brain separated by the tentorium cerebelli (Fig. 12-8).
6. Explain in terms of its consistency and water content why the brain readily herniates out of its normal position.
7. State the two fluids that respond or readjust most readily to shifts or compression of the brain.

Learning Objectives for Chapter 12

8. State the only two places a herniating cerebral hemisphere can go and give the names of these two types of internal brain herniation.
9. Describe the effect of subfalcine herniation on the anterior cerebral artery and the resultant clinical signs (Table 12-7).
10. State which parts of the cerebrum herniate in transtentorial herniation.
11. Name the major artery and nerve encountered by the herniating medial edge (uncus and parahippocampal gyrus) of the temporal lobe (transtentorial herniation; Figs. 12-8 and 12-8).
12. Describe the clinical effects of transtentorial herniation on consciousness.
13. Describe the effect of transtentorial herniation on pupillary size.
14. Make a drawing showing the location of the pupilloconstrictor fibers in the III nerve and the relation of the III nerve to its adjacent arteries (Fig. 12-11).
15. Describe the clinical significance of an alteration of consciousness and increasing pupillary size in a Pt who may have a supratentorial lesion.
16. Describe the pupillary changes as transtentorial herniation advances.
17. State the clinical implications of dilated, fixed pupils in an unconscious patient (who has no pharmacologic reason for dilated pupils).
18. Explain how transtentorial herniation can give rise to an ipsilateral or paradoxical hemiplegia (**Hint:** The Kernohan-Woltman notch).
19. Describe and explain the changes in UMN signs that may evolve during transtentorial herniation.
20. Describe the terminal pathologic event in the brainstem of the Pt with transtentorial herniation (Fig. 12-12).
21. Assume the decerebrate posture and describe how it affects the position of the jaws, neck, trunk, arms, wrists, hands, legs, and feet (Fig. 12-13 and Table 12-3).
22. Describe the body's posture when it assumes the position dictated by the pull of its strongest muscles.
23. State the site of the anatomic lesion that causes decerebrate rigidity.
24. Discuss the neurophysiologic explanation for the decerebrate posture. State where the drive that maintains the decerebrate posture is thought to originate.
25. Describe the disturbance in muscle tone seen in the decerebrate state.
26. Explain whether to classify the decerebrate state as a *release* or a *deficit* phenomenon.
27. Contrast the posture of the arm in the decerebrate and decorticate (hemiplegic) postures (Fig. 12-15).
28. Describe how to elicit decerebrate posturing in an unconscious Pt.
29. Describe the characteristic respiratory dysrhythmias that result from brainstem lesions and state the location of the responsible lesion (Fig. 12-16).
30. Describe the typical effect of increased intracranial pressure on pulse and blood pressure (Cushing's phenomenon).
31. Define and describe transforaminal herniation of the brain and explain how it may kill the patient (Table 12-5).
32. Give an orderly description of the signs of transtentorial herniation as related to:
    a. Consciousness
    b. Motor signs in the extremities
    c. Pupillary and IIIrd nerve signs
    d. Respiration
    e. Pulse and blood pressure

Learning Objectives for Chapter 12

33. Name the common internal herniations of the brain. Name the parts of the brain that herniate in each instance and the vascular complications (Table 12-5).
34. Describe, in principle, how brain herniations kill the Pt.

IV. INITIAL NEUROLOGIC EXAMINATION OF THE UNCONSCIOUS PATIENT

1. Recite the **AABCDEE** mnemonic that reminds the Ex of the priorities in first approaching an unconscious Pt.
2. Recite the **H** mnemonic for the five enemies of the brain in coma (**Hint:** Start with **H**ypoxia).
3. Enumerate some causes for coma that the Ex can discover by smelling the Pt's breath.
4. Describe the type of findings on the NE that best help to differentiate anatomic from toxic-metabolic causes of coma.
5. Describe the positive, favorable motor findings apparent immediately on inspection that suggest an anatomically intact nervous system in an unconscious but not comatose Pt (the four-glance NE).
6. Explain how to conclude whether an unconscious Pt has an intact pyramidal tract and the importance of this observation for identifying an anatomic lesion.
7. Describe the immediate findings that suggest a poor prognosis for the unconscious Pt.
8. Describe the series of observations and maneuvers that detect acute hemiplegia in the unconscious Pt (Figs. 12-18 to 12-21).
9. Explain the significance of paratonia on the opposite side from a flaccid hemiplegia in an acutely unconscious Pt.
10. Define the term *nucha* and state the clinical significance of *nuchal rigidity*.
11. Name and describe the ligaments that tether the spinal cord to the dura (Fig. 12-22).
12. Describe how extension and flexion of the head affect the tension on the spinal cord and nerve roots (Figs. 12-23 and 12-24).
13. Explain the pathophysiology of nuchal rigidity in response to meningeal irritation.
14. Describe the maneuvers to separate pure nuchal rigidity from other forms of a stiff neck (Fig. 12-25A to 12-25C).
15. Describe how to position the head of a Pt who may have suffered a neck injury before moving or transporting the Pt. State which position to avoid and why.
16. State a catastrophic result of excessive or forceful neck manipulation in a Pt with a mass lesion in the cervical vertebral canal.
17. Describe Lhermitte's sign of a cervical cord lesion.
18. Describe and name the leg signs of meningeal irritation.
19. List three circumstances in which a Pt with meningeal irritation may fail to show the classic meningeal irritation signs.
20. Pronounce *opisthotonos* correctly and describe the opisthotonic posture (Fig. 12-28).
21. Enumerate several conditions that cause the opisthotonic posture (Fig. 12-29).
22. Describe at least two different basic pathophysiologic mechanisms that cause opisthotonos.

V. SENSORY TESTING OF UNCONSCIOUS PATIENTS

1. State the only bedside method for determining the integrity of CrN II in an unconscious Pt.

Learning Objectives for Chapter 12

2. Describe the conditions and technique for examining the pupils in an unconscious Pt.
3. State which class of pharmacologic agents must be excluded for valid testing of the pupillary light reflex.
4. Describe two different tests for the integrity of the afferent arc of CrN V in the unconscious Pt.
5. Describe how the facial muscles of an unconscious Pt with an acute, completely flaccid hemiplegia respond to an ipsilateral or contralateral corneal stimulus or supraorbital compression.
6. Describe how to test the integrity of the auditory division of CrN VIII in an unconscious Pt.
7. Describe how to test the integrity of the vestibular division of CrN VIII in an unconscious Pt.
8. Demonstrate how to do the doll's eye, or counter-rolling, test in an unconscious Pt.
9. Explain the anatomic significance of intact vestibulo-ocular reflexes in the unconscious Pt.
10. State the normal response to caloric irrigation in an unconscious Pt.
11. State which phase of caloric-induced nystagmus disappears first in the unconscious Pt.
12. Describe a possible danger in eliciting the gag reflex in an unconscious Pt.
13. Discuss circumstances in which it is preferable to start with cold rather than pain as the noxious stimulus.
14. Describe and demonstrate three different ways of inflicting pain in examining an unconscious Pt.
15. Describe some drawbacks to using pinprick to elicit pain.

VI. FACTORS THAT COMPOUND AND COMPLICATE THE NEUROLOGIC EXAMINATION OF THE UNCONSCIOUS PATIENT

1. Describe how the MSRs in unconscious Pts may differ from normal and explain why their interpretation is more difficult than in the alert Pt.
2. Describe the effect of decreased levels of consciousness on the plantar responses.
3. State whether the Ex can elicit MSRs or a plantar reflex in a deeply comatose Pt.
4. Describe several preexisting neurologic findings that confound the NE of the comatose Pt.
5. Discuss the question of addressing the Pt assumed to be unconscious and discuss the conversational content appropriate for the Pt's bedside.

VII. THE NEUROLOGIC EXAMINATION IN THE LOCKED-IN SYNDROME (DE-EFFERENTED STATE)

1. Define the *locked-in state* and explain the meaning of the term.
2. State which volitional movements the Pt in the locked-in state retains.

VIII. THE NEUROLOGIC EXAMINATION IN THE PERSISTENT VEGETATIVE STATE

1. Define the PVS.
2. Describe the location and types of lesions that lead to the PVS.
3. Describe some differences between the comatose Pt and the PVS Pt.
4. Describe some of the behaviors seen in the PVS that are not regarded as volitional and indicative of consciousness.

Learning Objectives for Chapter 12

5. Discuss the factors that affect how long the Pt in the PVS should receive life support.
6. Discuss the limitations of the NE or any other method of determining lack of consciousness.

IX. THE NEUROLOGIC EXAMINATION IN THE DIAGNOSIS OF BRAIN DEATH: THE BRAIN-DEATH PROTOCOL

1. Recite the traditional definition of death until about 1960.
2. State what two major advances in medical technology led to a redefinition of death as brain death.
3. Explain the difference between the process of terminating support after the diagnosis of brain death and terminating support for euthanasia.
4. State the three fundamental ways of demonstrating functions of a living brain but that are always absent in a dead brain.
5. From Table 12-7, describe how to do the NE for the BDP.
6. Describe ancillary diagnostic procedures that supplement the NE in determining brain death.
7. Explain why apnea testing is the last step in the BDP.
8. Describe variations in opinions as to what to include in the BDP beyond the indispensable NE.
9. Describe the results of an EEG and blood flow studies of a brain-dead Pt.
10. Discuss whether to involve more than one physician in the BDP.
11. State some conditions in which the NE may fail to elicit any responses, but the brain remains alive.
12. Describe some spinal reflexes that may remain in a brain-dead Pt.
13. Name the two most important pitfalls that must be avoided for a valid determination of brain death.
14. Explain why the criteria for the BDP differ somewhat for infants.
15. Describe the main clinical differences between brain death, coma, persistent vegetative state, minimally conscious state, and locked-in syndrome. Cover the text of Table 12-8 and work through the columns and rows.

X. THE NEUROLOGIOC EXAMINATION IN INTERMITTENT DISTURBANCES OF CONSCIOUSNESS: SYNCOPE, SEIZURES, AND BLACKOUT SPELLS

1. Define *syncope*.
2. Outline the major categories for the classification of syncope (Fig. 12-32).
3. Describe several pathophysiologic mechanisms that may result in syncope.
4. State the single most important historical information to diagnose the cause of syncope.
5. Describe the three phases in the description of syncope.
6. State the most important observations the Ex should make in witnessing an attack of syncope and describe how to protect the Pt.
7. State what blood test should always be considered when the Ex witnesses any unexplained episode of altered consciousness.
8. Describe the most common change in breathing that precedes psychogenic syncope and describe how to test for it (pages 371–372).
9. Describe several types of hydraulic/hypotensive syncope.
10. Define orthostatic hypotension and describe how to test for it.

Learning Objectives for Chapter 12

11. State two types of cardiac dysrhythmia that may lead to syncope.
12. State the normal limits for changes in blood pressure and pulse in testing for orthostatic syncope (orthostatic hypotension).
13. Describe the sequence of parade-ground and micturition syncope.
14. Describe the mechanism of syncope in the late stages of pregnancy.
15. Describe the clinical features of the most common nontraumatic, nonepileptic cause of loss of consciousness in young children between 6 and 48 months of age and the findings, if any, on the NE.
16. Describe the pathogenic mechanism(s) involved in swallowing, coughing, and otogenic syncope.
17. Describe the cholinergic signs that occur during vasovagal syncope.
18. Distinguish between psychiatric illness syncope and psychogenic vasovagal syncope.
19. Describe the afferent and efferent pathways in swallowing and otogenic syncope.
20. Explain how head turning can trigger syncope (Fig. 12-34).
21. Describe three types of carotid sinus syncope.
22. List the contraindications for the carotid sinus massage test.
23. Describe and demonstrate how to test for a hyperactive carotid sinus.
24. Describe the course of blood and the diagnostic physical findings in a Pt with the subclavian steal syndrome (Fig. 12-35).
25. Contrast the important distinctions between vasovagal syncope, epilepsy, and psychiatric illness syncope. Cover the text in Table 12-10 and work through the rows and columns.
26. State the ancillary neurodiagnostic procedures that the Ex should consider when the initial history and NE fail to disclose the cause for syncope.

13 Ancillary Neurodiagnostic Procedures—Lumbar Puncture and Neuroimaging

We have instruments of precision in increasing numbers with which we and our hospital assistants at untold expense make tests and take observations, the vast majority of which are but supplementary to, and as nothing compared with, the careful study of the patient by a keen observer using his eyes and ears and fingers and a few simple aids.

—**Harvey Cushing (1869–1939)**

I. ARRAY OF NEURODIAGNOSTIC PROCEDURES

After completing the history and neurologic examination (NE) and proposing a tentative diagnosis, the examiner (Ex) has to decide whether further studies are required. Table 13-1 reviews the array of standard diagnostic tests. The goal is to choose the one or two safest, least invasive, and most economical procedures that will *best* confirm or refute the tentative diagnosis. Do not order every conceivable test to cover every diagnostic possibility. Go for the jugular. If you fail initially to secure the diagnosis, select successive tests in a logical order. In this section we will discuss the clinical use of lumbar puncture and neuro-imaging studies.

II. THE CEREBROSPINAL FLUID EXAMINATION

A. Location, origin, and circulation of the cerebrospinal fluid

1. Examination of the cerebrospinal fluid (CSF) dates to Heinrich Quincke who introduced spinal puncture in 1891 for the treatment of hydrocephalus.
2. **Location of the CSF:** The CSF occupies the ventricles and subarachnoid spaces. The total volume of CSF is about 150 mL. The subarachnoid space separates the arachnoid membrane from the pia mater. In addition to the CSF, the subarachnoid space contains the blood vessels that enter or leave the central nervous system (CNS).
3. **Formation of the CSF**
   a. The CSF is formed by:
      i. The choroid plexuses of the lateral, III, and IV ventricles.
      ii. Water produced by oxidative metabolism.

TABLE 13-1 · Ancillary Neurodiagnostic Procedures

A. Neuroradiologic imaging
   1. Plain films
   2. CT (enhanced and unenhanced)
   3. MRI (enhanced and unenhanced)
   4. Angiography: MRA, direct injection, CTA, Doppler sonography
   5. Cranial ultrasonography
   6. Radionuclide scanning: PET, SPECT

B. Electroneurodiagnosis
   1. Electroencephalography (EEG)
   2. Electromyography (EMG)
   3. Nerve conduction velocity (NCV)
   4. Evoked responses: visual, auditory, and somatosensory
   5. Audiogram

C. Punctures
   1. Subarachnoid (LP or cisternal) for CSF
   2. Subdural for blood, pus, or fluid
   3. Ventricular for blood or CSF
   4. Stereotaxic for lesion biopsy

D. Blood biochemistry
   1. Complete metabolic profile
   2. Toxicology screen
   3. Quantitative amino acids and organic acids
   4. Serum enzymes
   5. Long-chain fatty acids, cholesterol, cholestanol
   6. Serum ceruloplasmin
   7. B_{12} and folic acid
   8. Lysosomal enzymes
   9. Collagen vascular screen
   10. Disease-specific tests for inborn errors of metabolism
   11. Hypercoagulable screen
   12. Protein fractionation

E. Neuro-ophthalmology
   1. Visual acuity
   2. Visual fields, central and peripheral
   3. Ophthalmoscopy direct and indirect, slit-lamp inspection of media and fundus
   4. Visual evoked response (VER)
   5. Electroretinogram (ERG)
   6. Electronystagmography

F. Urinalysis
   1. Routine including specific gravity
   2. Screen for inborn errors of metabolism
   3. Toxicology screen
   4. Catecholamines

G. Neuropsychological tests
   1. Developmental
   2. IQ
   3. Achievement
   4. Neuropsychological battery
   5. Personality profile

H. Biopsy
   1. Muscle
   2. Nerve
   3. Skin
   4. Brain

I. Microbiologic tests
   1. Serologic
   2. Culture of microorganisms
   3. Immunologic screen, T and B cells, blood titers, γ-globulin
   4. Polymerase chain reaction

J. Genetic tests
   1. Karyotype
   2. Genotype

ABBREVIATIONS: CSF = cerebrospinal fluid; CT = computed tomography; CTA = Cranial computed tomography angiography; LP = lumbar puncture; MRA = magnetic resonance angiography; MRI = magnetic resonance imaging; PET = positron emission tomography; SPECT = single-photon emission computed tomography.

iii. An ultrafiltrate through the blood-brain barrier of the cerebral capillaries (Fishman, 1992; May et al., 1990).

b. The rate of production is 0.3 to 0.4 mL/min, or about 500 mL/day.

4. **Circulation of the CSF**

a. The CSF exits the ventricles by flowing out of the foramina into the IV ventricle, the Lateral foramina of Luschka and the Median foramen of Magendie. The ependyma lining the ventricles absorb some CSF (Rando and Fishman, 1992). Learn Fig. 13-1.

b. After exiting from the foramina of the IV ventricle, the CSF enters the subarachnoid space. It may then percolate *downward* around the spinal cord or *upward* over the cerebral hemispheres to the superior sagittal sinus.

i. Pacchionian granulations that extend from the subarachnoid space into the lumen of the sinus allow absorption of the CSF into the venous blood (Fig. 13-2).

ii. At the spinal level, drainage takes place at the root sleeves, where the pia and arachnoid fuse with the connective tissue of the spinal nerves.

5. Trace a drop of CSF from the temporal horn of the lateral ventricle to its absorption into the blood.

____

Temporal horn, trigone (atrium), anterior horn, interventricular foramen, III ventricle, aqueduct, IV ventricle, subarachnoid space, and Pacchionian granulations or root sleeves. Some absorbs through the ependymal lining.

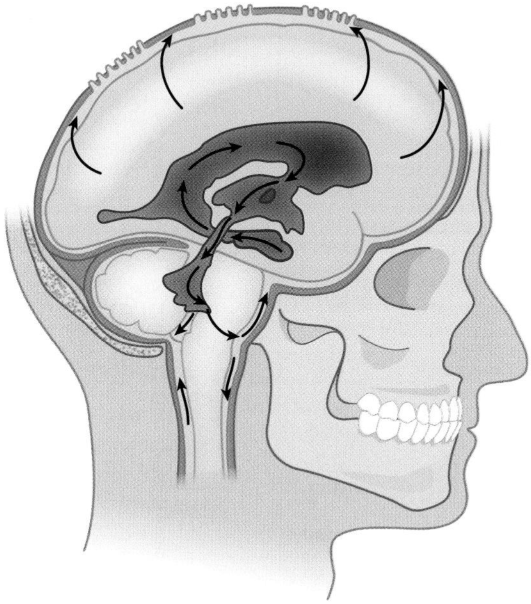

FIGURE 13-1. Lateral view of the ventricular system and CSF circulation. Beginning in the temporal horn, trace a drop of CSF through the III ventricle, aqueduct, out the IV ventricle, into the subarachnoid space, and up over the convexity of the hemisphere to the Pacchionian granulations along the superior sagittal sinus. CSF = cerebrospinal fluid.

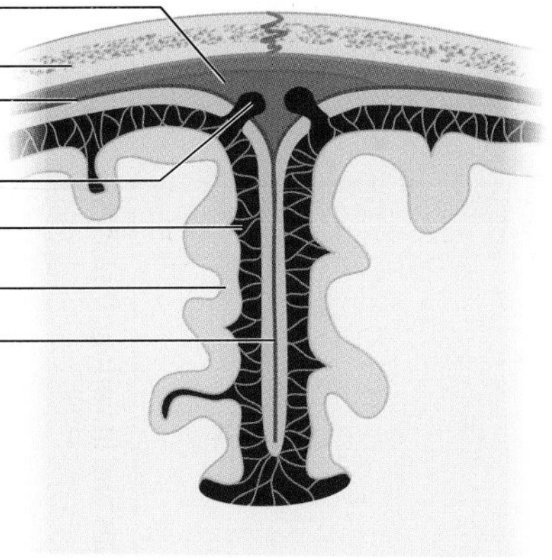

FIGURE 13-2. Coronal section through the cerebral falx to show the Pacchionian granulations projecting directly into the superior sagittal sinus. The CSF passes through the granulations into the venous blood of the sinus. CSF = cerebrospinal fluid.

B. Functions of the cerebrospinal fluid

1. The CSF in the subarachnoid space provides a flotation layer around the brain and spinal cord that cushions them from trauma.
2. The CSF permits circulation of metabolites and electrolytes, neurotransmitters, peptide hormones, antibodies, leukocytes, and various other normal and abnormal cells.
3. The CSF aids in regulating the pH and electrolyte balance of the extracellular space of the CNS.

C. Composition of the cerebrospinal fluid

The CSF is a sparkling clear salt solution containing a few white blood cells (WBCs), proteins, sugar, traces of enzymes, neurohumors, neurotransmitters, and other metabolites (Fishman, 1992). The cell count, sugar, and protein levels change with age. See the top rows of Table 13-2 and Fig. 13-3.

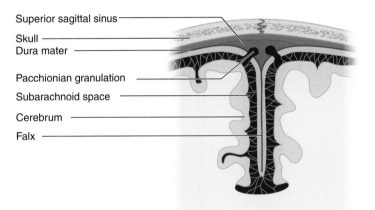

TABLE 13-2 · Typical Cerebrospinal Fluid Profiles in Normal Individuals and in Various Diseases

			Cytology				Chemistry	
	Color	Pressure	Cells/mm^3	Cell type	Stained smear, culture	Glucose % of blood sugar	Total protein	Special tests
Normal young infant	Sparkling clear	10–100 mm H_2O	<15	Mononuclear	No bacteria	≈ 66% of blood	20–170 mg %	Normal
Normal adult	Sparkling clear	80–180 mm H_2O	<5	Mononuclear	No bacteria	≈ 66% of blood	10–40 mg %	Normal
Meningitis acute bacterial	Cloudy	↑	500–1000	Polymorphonuclear	Bacteria present	<50% of blood	↑	Antibody batteries
Tuberculous	Cloudy, xanthochromic	N or ↑	10–500	Mostly mononuclear	Bacteria present	<50% of blood	↑	PCR, culture
Fungal	Cloudy, xanthochromic	N or ↑	<500	Mostly mononuclear	Fungi present	<50% of blood	↑	Staining, some immunologic tests, culture
Encephalitis	Clear to faintly cloudy	N or ↑	<500	Mononuclear after first hours	Negative stain; culture may be positive	N	N to moderate ↑	Serology, PCR, immunoassays, culture
Subarachnoid hemorrhage	Erythrochromic or xanthochromic	N or ↑	100's–1000's	RBCs	Negative	N	Varies with amount of blood	Detection of ferritin
Demyelinating diseases	Sparkling clear	N	N or slight ↑	Mononuclear, plasma cells	Negative	N	N to slight ↑	Increased γ-globulin
Neoplasm	Sparkling clear or xanthochromic if protein ↑	N to ↑	N or slight ↑	Neoplastic cells sometimes present	Negative	N	N to slight ↑	N or nondiagnostic

ABBREVIATIONS: N = normal; PCR = polymerase chain reaction; RBCs = red blood cells.

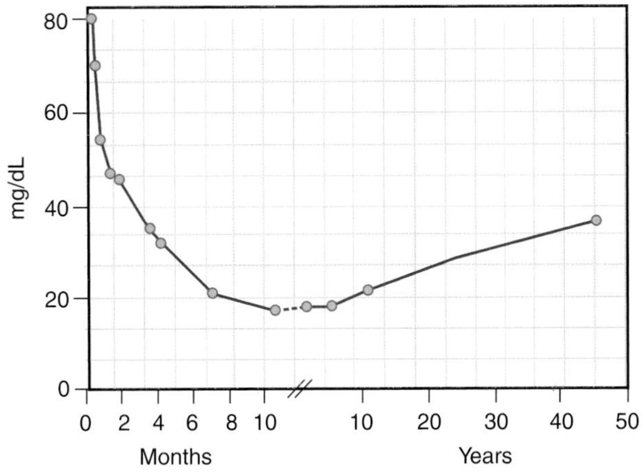

FIGURE 13-3. Age-related changes in the average total protein content of the cerebrospinal fluid. (Modified from Widell S: On the cerebrospinal fluid in normal children and in patients with acute abacterial meningo-encephalitis, *Acta Paediatr Nov*; 47(6):711–713, 1958.)

D. Normal pressure of the cerebrospinal fluid

Measure the pressure of the CSF by attaching a manometer to a needle inserted into the subarachnoid space (Fig. 13-4A). The normal CSF pressure depends on the patient's (Pt's) age (Table 13-2): 10 to 100 mm of water for young infants, 80 to 180 mm of water for normal mature individuals, and up to 250 mm of water for grossly obese individuals, perhaps because of increased intra-abdominal pressure. Diseases may increase or decrease intracranial pressure. Increased intracranial pressure is by far the most common problem.

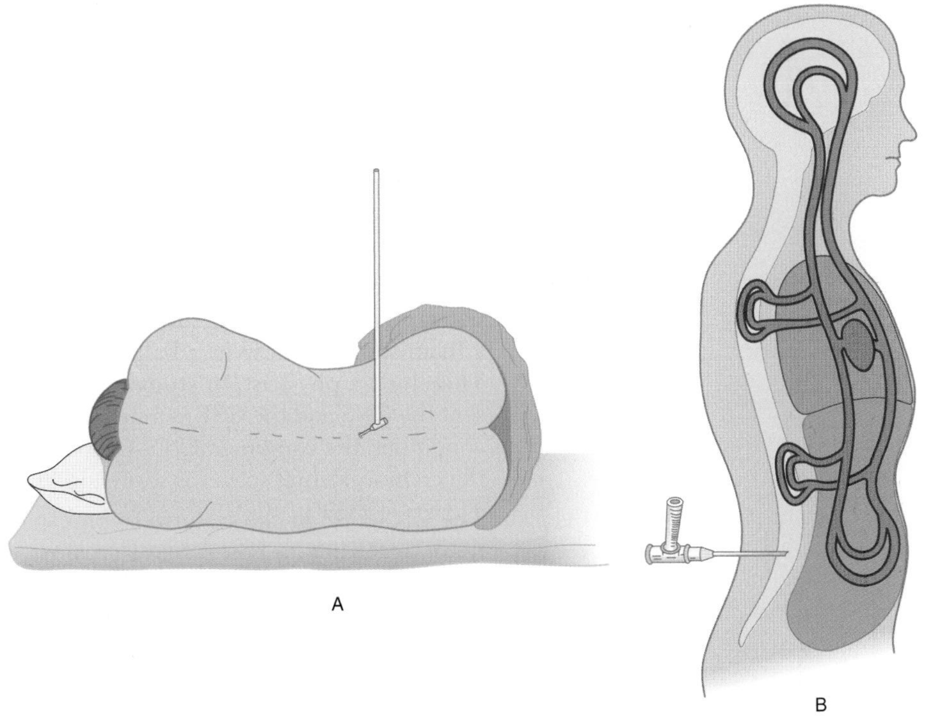

FIGURE 13-4. (A) Patient in left lateral position with legs and back flexed. A manometer is attached to a needle inserted into the subarachnoid space. (B) Top view of patient diagrammatically representing the continuity of vessels inside and outside the craniovertebral cavity.

E. Increased intracranial pressure

1. **Symptoms of increased intracranial pressure:** Symptoms consist of headaches, nausea and vomiting, dizziness, transient blurring of vision or blindness (transient obscurations of vision), and mild obtundation. Mothers of children who have

shunts to treat increased pressure often can tell by overall changes in the child's behavior that the shunt is blocked or malfunctioning.

2. **Signs of increased intracranial pressure**
   a. Increased pressure in infants causes a bulging fontanel, split sutures, and an increasing occipitofrontal circumference that moves successively upward on the percentile lines of an occipitofrontal circumference chart (Fig. 1-23).
   b. In older Pts, papilledema occurs and often a VI nerve palsy develops as a consequence of compression of the nerve during its long intracranial course.
3. **Causes of increased intracranial pressure**
   a. **Expanding lesions** within the craniovertebral space, such as hematomas, neoplasms, abscesses, and brain edema. Rarely, increased production of CSF may cause increased pressure.
   b. **Prolonged status epilepticus** *or* hypoxia, which causes brain edema.
   c. **Metabolic encephalopathies:** Hepatic, uremic, Reye's syndrome, pseudotumor cerebri (idiopathic intracranial hypertension), and endocrinopathies.
   d. **CNS infections:** Meningitis and encephalopathies may incite extreme edema and increased pressure.
   e. **Obstructive lesions** that impede the flow of CSF from the ventricles to the subarachnoid space and through the Pacchionian granulations. The most common sites of blockage are
      i. The **interventricular foramen of Monro,** usually by a neoplasm.
      ii. The **cerebral aqueduct,** usually by congenital atresia or stenosis, inflammatory adhesions, or neoplastic compression.
      iii. The **IV ventricle and its outlets,** usually by posterior fossa neoplasms, inflammatory adhesions or failure of outlets to perforate, as in the Dandy-Walker malformation.
      iv. The **subarachnoid space,** usually by adhesions after meningitis or subarachnoid hemorrhage.
      v. The **Pacchionian granulations,** because of clogging of the granulations (and root sleeves) by blood or extremely high CSF protein.
      vi. The **intracranial venous sinuses,** because of thrombosis.
4. **Increased intracranial pressure and Pascal's law**
   a. Physically, the CSF is essentially water and the CNS is about 80% water. Students who have handled only the stiff, formalin-fixed brain of the cadaver do not appreciate the supple softness of the living brain. Its compliancy resembles a foam sponge pillow or a balloon (the pia-arachnoid) filled with molasses. Therefore, a physicist, in studying intracranial hydrodynamics, might represent the CNS and the CSF as a single homogeneous fluid. To duplicate biologic conditions, the combined CNS-CSF model includes the vascular space within the craniovertebral space, as shown in Fig. 13-4B.
   b. The CNS-CSF in the craniovertebral space is itself incompressible, like any fluid. According to Pascal's law, pressure exerted on a fluid in a closed container is transmitted equally in all directions. The pressure transmission is independent of the size or shape of the container. Therefore, pressure in the lumbar CSF reflects the intracranial pressure, although biological factors alter the simple expression of Pascal's law.
   c. As intracranial pressure increases, it displaces CSF and the intravascular blood (Fig. 12-9). If these compensations fail, any further increase in pressure causes the brain to herniate down through the foramen magnum, the only place it can go, the only way out of the brain case (Chapter 12).

F. Low cerebrospinal fluid (CSF) volume (pressure)syndrome

1. **Symptoms and signs:** The Pt experiences orthostatic headache, vertigo, tinnitus, nausea, and vomiting, especially when rising from a reclining to a vertical position,

and may faint. The symptoms could occur because of loss of flotation, allowing the cerebrum to sag onto the brainstem. A variety of connective tissue disorders have been associated with the development of this syndrome (Schievink, 2006).

2. **Causes of low CSF pressure**
   a. Medical procedures that pierce the meninges and establish a CSF leak include lumbar puncture and neurosurgical operations.
   b. Basal skull fractures that create fistulae in the nose or middle ear, causing CSF rhinorrhea or otorrhea.
   c. Severe dehydration.
   d. Leakage along nerve roots (Rando and Fishman, 1992).
   e. Idiopathic aliquorrhea (Rando and Fishman, 1992).

G. Indications for lumbar puncture (spinal puncture or spinal tap)

1. To identify infections of the CSF. Repeated lumbar punctures (LPs) serve to monitor the effect of treatment.
2. To identify subarachnoid bleeding.
3. To identify neoplastic invasion or seeding of the subarachnoid space by gliomas, carcinomas, or leukemias and lymphomas.
4. To measure and fractionate CSF proteins in suspected immunologic diseases, especially multiple sclerosis, and for the differential diagnosis of some neuropathies, such as Guillain-Barré syndrome (albuminocytologic dissociation).
5. To measure pH, electrolytes, enzymes, neurotransmitters, and trace constituents in the diagnosis of the genetic/metabolic encephalopathies (Hyland and Arnold, 1999).
6. To introduce chemotherapeutic or antibacterial agents or anesthetics.
7. To introduce contrast agents for myelography or radionuclides for study of CSF flow dynamics and to locate leaks.
8. To measure for increased CSF in patients with possible pseudotumor cerebri (idiopathic intracranial hypertension). In such cases, imaging studies have excluded a mass lesion that would cause herniation. An LP is also required to document low CSF pressure in low-pressure syndromes.

H. Contraindications to a lumbar puncture

1. **Infection of the lumbar skin** or deeper tissues through which the needle must pass.
2. **Coagulopathies:** Spinal subarachnoid hemorrhage or spinal subdural hematomas may follow an LP in these Pts (Masdeu et al., 1979). Diseases, such as hemophilia and thrombocytopenia, or anticoagulant therapy represent relative rather than absolute contraindications.
3. **Cervical cord lesions:** Removal of CSF from the lumbar region may cause the cord to shift against the lesion, resulting in quadriplegia, apnea, and death.
4. **Increased intracranial pressure** from a suspected or known intracranial mass lesion.
   a. If the history, NE, or ophthalmoscopic examination suggest a mass lesion or increased intracranial pressure, an LP generally should not be done. The presence of distinct venous pulsations virtually excludes increased intracranial pressure. Nearly 90% of normal persons show pulsations if both eyes are carefully examined (Levin, 1978). The absence of venous pulsations does not establish increased pressure because some normal Pts do not show such pulsations.
   b. The most common mass lesions that cause brain herniation include neoplasms, hematomas, abscesses, cerebral edema, and massive cerebral or cerebellar hemispheric infarction or hemorrhage. Of 22 Pts with brain abscess, five showed evidence of herniation within 2 hours of an LP (Samson and Clark, 1973). Do not perform LPs in Pts with brain abscess. The diagnosis depends on radiographic imaging findings.

c. Posterior fossa lesions, which may cause transforaminal herniation, also pose a great threat. Signs of impending transforaminal herniation include a stiff neck, hiccups. irregular breathing, apnea, hypotension, and quadriparesis (Hartmann et al., 1994). Note also that posterior fossa masses may cause upward herniation out of the posterior fossa, thereby compressing the midbrain. **If the clinical findings raise any question of a mass lesion that may cause transtentorial or transforaminal or upward herniation, always order computed tomography (CT) or, better, magnetic resonance imaging (MRI) before doing an LP.** The radiographic examination may clinch the diagnosis and render the LP useless and potentially harmful.

d. Sometimes clinical exigencies will call for an LP even in the presence of increased pressure, to identify or exclude a specifically treatable disorder. Conditions with possible increased pressure that may require an LP include suspected meningitis or encephalitis and pseudotumor cerebri. Then the Ex has to weigh the indications against the contraindications (Fishman, 1992). In these cases, consider pretreating the Pt with mannitol and hyperventilation to reduce intracranial pressure before the LP.

e. In the management of increased pressure from acute head injuries and other emergencies and coma, neurosurgeons implant a pressure transducer within the skull for continuous monitoring of the results of treatment.

I. Complications of a lumbar puncture

1. **Transtentorial or transforaminal herniation of the brain,** causing death.
2. **Back pain** at the puncture site.
3. **Bleeding:** Epidural, subdural, or subarachnoid; a so-called bloody tap (Masdeu et al., 1979). A spinal hematoma may produce progressive radicular pain and sphincter disturbances. Most neurologic sequelae seem to relate to inadvertent insertion of the needle at too high a level (Hamandi et al., 2002).
4. **Headache and post-LP low CSF volume (pressure) syndrome:** See Section F. Most Pts have some backache and approximately 10% have headache after an LP. Low CSF pressure from CSF leakage presumably causes post-LP headache.
   a. The headache begins a day or two after the LP, is often throbbing, mainly occurs in the upright position, is worsened by coughing or straining, and improves when the Pt reclines. The Pt may have a stiff neck, nausea and vomiting (Kuntz et al., 1992).
   b. Most post-LP headaches resolve spontaneously. Bed rest (none, 2 to 8 hours, or up to 48 hours), forcing fluids, or intravenous caffeine are of questionable benefit in helping to prevent post-LP headaches (Roos, 2003a).
   c. Refractory headaches respond to an epidural injection of 15 to 20 mL of autologous blood at the puncture site (Sencakova et al., 2001), presumably because it seals the puncture wound.
5. **Double vision**, which usually results from unilateral or bilateral cranial nerve VI palsies is usually self-limited.
6. **Iatrogenic infection:** very rare.
7. **Implantation of epidermoid tumors in the lumbosacral canal:** a very rare complication.
8. In summary, the three most dangerous circumstances for an LP are increased intracranial pressure, a mass lesion capable of producing herniation, and a high cervical cord lesion.

J. Preparation for a lumbar puncture

1. Always get an MRI or CT scan whenever the Pt has the new onset of overt neurologic signs and symptoms, an altered consciousness, or seizures.
2. Always get an MRI if the Pt might have a compressive spinal cord lesion.

3. Ensure that the radiographs are competently read, particularly with respect to ventricular size, presence of absence of sulci and cisterns, and the absence of a posterior fossa lesion. MRI is usually superior to CT, except for emergency screening for large mass lesions, edema, or recent bleeding.
4. Review the history and medical record for a bleeding tendency. The platelet count should exceed 50,000 and the international normalized ratio (INR) should be less than 1.5.
5. Decide whether to send a simultaneous blood sample for comparison with the CSF with respect to chemistry and rising antibody titers.
6. **Psychological preparation of the Pt for an LP:** Everyone dreads needles, particularly a stab in the back. Every layperson, it seems, knows of someone who had one of "those taps" and afterward had a permanent backache or never walked again. Of course, that conclusion has reversed cause and effect: the LP was done because of the disability, but litigious Pts today blame the doctor, not the disease. The Ex must ensure that the indications are valid and that the Pt understands the reasons for the procedure. Because an LP counts as surgery, have the Pt sign a consent form listing complications such as backache, headache, infection, and bleeding.

K. Technique for lumbar puncture

1. **Positioning of the Pt for an LP**
   a. The Pt assumes the lateral recumbent position with the head, spine, and extremities flexed (the fetal position; Fig. 13-4A). A pillow under the head keeps it aligned with the spine. In the trunk-flexed position, the distance between the dorsal processes and lamina of adjacent vertebrae ❐ increases/❐ decreases.
   b. Cooperative and not acutely ill Pts may sit with the spine flexed. However, in this position, the measurement of the intraspinal pressure is unreliable. If the pressure reading is important (e.g., in a patient with possible pseudotumor cerebri), the lateral recumbent position is preferred.

☑ increases
Spinal flexion thus increases the target area for the needle. Review Fig. 12-24 if you erred.

2. **Needle insertion and manometry for measuring CSF pressure**
   a. Clean the lower lumbar area with Betadine or 70% alcohol and apply a sterile drape.
   b. Select the vertebral interspace, between L3 and L4, between L4 and L5, or between L5 and S1, by palpation or by lining up the vertebral inter-space with the top of the iliac crests, which is at the interspace between L3 and L4. Insertion of the needle rostral to that level may damage the distal tip of the spinal cord, which usually ends at L2 (Fishman, 1992).
   c. Depending on the Pt, anesthetize the insertion point with 1% lidocaine.
   d. Insert a 20- to 22-gauge needle, with its stylet in place, into the inter-space between the dorsal processes of the vertebrae at the selected level. Angle the needle slightly cephalad to parallel the slant of the dorsal spines of the vertebrae (Fig. 12-24). Insert the needle until a slight "pop" is felt as the needle pierces the dura and enters the subarachnoid space. The larger the bore of the needle, the easier it is to reach the subarachnoid space, but the greater the leakage of fluid after withdrawal of the needle.
      i. Insert the needle with the bevel of the needle turned *parallel* to the long axis of the spine (Roos, 2003b). The bevel then is thought to more cleanly separate rather than transect the longitudinal fibers of the dura, thus reducing post-LP leakage of CSF. A problem with the theory is that dural fibers run in a variety of directions, not just longitudinally.
      ii. To reduce post-LP leakage and post-LP headaches, Whitacre or Sprotte dull-tipped needles have been advocated to replace the standard sharp-tipped Quincke needle (Strupp et al., 2001). These needles have a blunt tip alleged to separate rather than cut the dural fibers. The needles drain CSF through an oval opening on the lateral aspect of the shaft, just proximal to the blunt tip, rather than through the tip itself (Evans et al., 2000).

iii. Before insertion of a blunt-tipped needle, the Ex uses a sharp-tipped "introducer" needle to cut a path about two-thirds of the way in.

e. After feeling the initial pop, the Ex withdraws the stylet. A drop of CSF should appear at the hub of the three-way stopcock on the LP needle. Attach a manometer and allow the fluid level to stabilize in the manometer. Record the opening pressure. At the end of the procedure, record the closing pressure.

f. If the history or ophthalmoscopic examination raises a concern about increased pressure, proceed this way. Insert a needle through the skin but stop it just short of the subarachnoid space. Remove the stylet and attach a manometer. With the manometer in place and with a fingertip blocking the open bore at the top of the manometer, advance the needle into the subarachnoid space and allow the fluid to fill the manometer gradually. Otherwise, the Ex may insert the needle with its regular stylet in place, withdraw it, and quickly attach a three-way stopcock and manometer.

g. For premature and young infants, use a standard butterfly needle (Greensher et al., 1971). The Ex should limit the depth of any needle puncture to 2.5 cm in these infants.

3. **Fluctuations in the meniscus in the manometer**

a. The meniscus of CSF in the manometer will fluctuate around some mean value, e.g., 120 mm of water (Fig. 13-5).

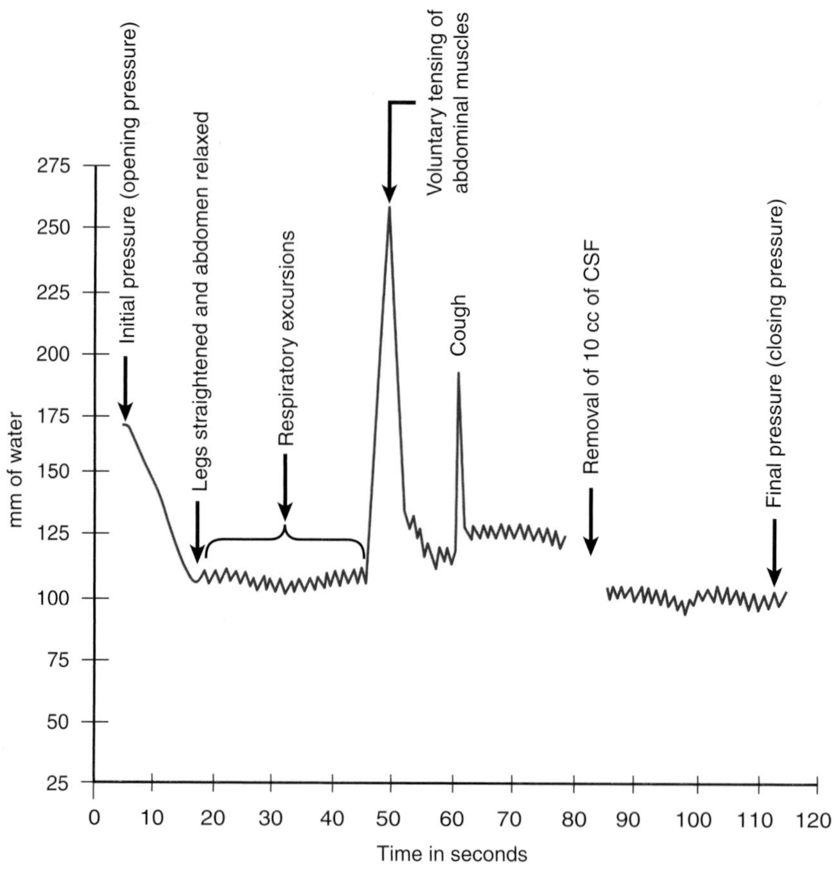

FIGURE 13-5. Graph of cerebrospinal fluid pressure, as measured by manometry. Starting at the left, read through the legends just above the arrows.

☑ decreases
The intrathoracic pressure decreases with inspiration. Inspiration sucks blood from the CNS veins and the CNSCSF pressure drops. Breathing causes rhythmic excursions of the manometer meniscus at the rate of 16 per minute, as shown in Fig. 13-5.

b. **Causes for fluctuations:** As shown in Fig. 13-4B, the intracranial and intraspinal veins communicate directly with the extracranial and extravertebral veins. Because these communications lack valves, the extracranial veins transmit any change in their pressure directly into the craniovertebral space, in particular the changes in intrathoracic and intra-abdominal pressure. When a person inhales air, the CNS-CSF pressure ☐ increases/☐ decreases/☐ does not change.

☑ increase
The intervertebral veins reflect the increased intra-abdominal pressure backward into the craniovertebral space, thus reducing the outflow of blood from the CNS. Because the arterial input continues, the CNS-CSF pressure increases.

c. Contraction of the abdominal muscles would ❒ increase/❒ decrease the intracranial pressure. Explain.

____

______________________________________.

d. The pulse causes smaller excursions of the meniscus (not shown in Fig. 13-5 because of their small amplitude). Because the arterial walls absorb much of the arterial pressure, the CNS-CSF pressure most closely reflects the capillary and venous pressures.

L. Clinical evaluation of increased pressure as registered by manometry

☑ high

1. Assume that the opening pressure in the manometer is 240 mm of water, which is ❒ normal/❒ low/❒ high.
2. Two explanations exist:
   a. The intrinsic CNS-CSF pressure is too high.
   b. The pressure reflects factors extrinsic to the craniovertebral space.
3. An LP always makes the Pt anxious and causes increased tension in the skeletal muscles. What, then, is a simple extrinsic cause for increased CNSCSF pressure? ______________________________.

Abdominal muscle, tension

☑ high

4. Encourage the Pt to relax the flexed position and to take a few deep breaths. In the Pt with the opening pressure of 240 mm of water, these maneuvers dropped the pressure to 210 mm of water. This value is ❒ normal/❒ low/❒ high.
5. The flexed posture has caused the Pt to flex the head on the chest, and it may have bent somewhat to the side while resting on the pillow. Because flexion or turning of the head may compress the jugular veins, the Ex straightened the Pt's head and readjusted it on the pillow. These maneuvers failed to drop the pressure below 200 mm of water, indicating that the Pt had slightly increased intrinsic intracranial pressure.
6. If an expanding intracranial lesion raises the CNS-CSF pressure, visualize what might happen after removal of CSF from the lumbar region (Fig. 13-6).

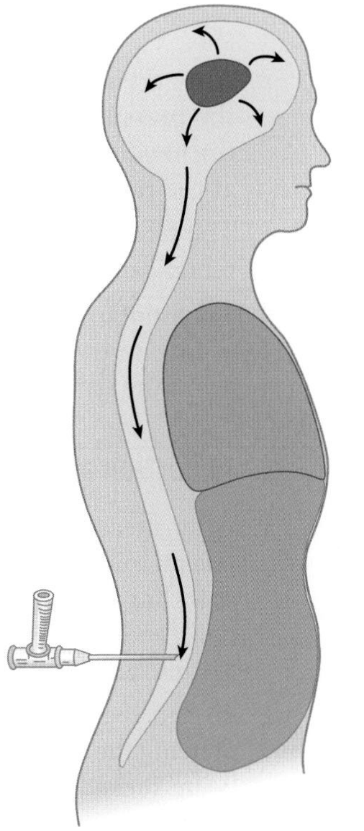

FIGURE 13-6. Depiction of an expanding intracranial lesion (oval black mass) causing increased intracranial pressure. The pressure exerts itself equally in all directions. Escape of cerebrospinal fluid through a lumbar needle allows the intracranial contents to flow (herniate) toward the region of lowered pressure.

7. Increased intracranial pressure may have caused impending herniation of the brain. The system may be delicately balanced, with the uncus and parahippocampal gyrus poised ready to plunge over the edge of the tentorium, or the cerebellar tonsils may be ready to herniate through the foramen magnum. These two potentially fatal herniations are called ________________ and ______________ herniation.

transtentorial; transforaminal

8. Withdrawal of fluid from the lumbar region will allow the brain to flow down toward the point of low pressure, according to Pascal's law. The potential herniation is converted to actual herniation. The Pt will ______________!

die

9. If, after careful measurement, the Ex concludes that the Pt truly has intrinsic increased intracranial pressure, what is the next step? ☐ Withdraw fluid rapidly./☐ Withdraw fluid cautiously./☐ Withdraw the needle immediately!

☑ Withdraw the needle immediately! The small amount of fluid in the manometer suffices for a cell count or to see blood in the CSF, which is often the most important information needed.

10. Describe the safe maneuvers used to exclude extrinsic factors as the cause for high spinal fluid pressure fluid.____

Have the Pt straighten the legs slightly and take several deep breaths. Extend the Pt's head and reposition it on the pillow.

M. Cessation of cerebrospinal fluid flow

1. Frequently, the flow of fluid starts but stops. Very rarely, transforaminal herniation, like a plug in a drain, blocks the transmission of intracranial pressure after a small amount of CSF has drained out. In this case, the Pt shows dramatic signs of apnea and quadriplegia. Most commonly, the cause is far more benign: Something has blocked the needle (Table 13-3).

TABLE 13-3 · Common Causes for Cessation of Cerebrospinal Fluid Flow and Their Remedies

Cause	Remedy
Blood clot in the needle lumen	Replace stylet to ream out the needle
Nerve root has fallen over the bevel of the needle	Rotate the shaft of the needle
Displacement of the tip of the needle from the subarachnoid space or incomplete penetration	If you think the needle tip is too deep, withdraw it slightly; if too shallow, insert it farther

2. After trying the maneuvers in Table 13-3, reattach the manometer to measure the pressure again. If the system is open from the subarachnoid space through the needle to the manometer, the manometer meniscus should show excursions at the rate of 16 per minute, caused by ______________.

breathing

3. The CSF may also stop flowing through the needle if a lesion occludes the vertebral canal.
4. **What not to do if CSF stops flowing through the needle:** Exasperation may tempt the Ex to try to suck CSF out with a syringe. If at this point you do not understand the dangers, this text has totally failed.

N. Collection and appearance of the cerebrospinal fluid

1. After measuring the opening pressure, collect 10 to 15 mL of CSF by allowing several milliliters to drip into each of three or four tubes. The normal fluid appears sparkling clear in all tubes. Inspect all tubes for *cloudiness*, *redness* (erythrochromia), and *yellowness* (xanthochromia). The attending physician, not the laboratory technician, bears the responsibility for proper inspection of CSF after collection.
2. To end the LP, measure the closing pressure and replace the stylet before withdrawing the needle. Replacing the stylet is thought to keep arachnoid strands from being sucked through the dural puncture site, which might prolong CSF leakage.

O. Cloudiness of the cerebrospinal fluid

1. Cloudiness usually means an increased number of WBCs in the CSF. Rarely, numerous bacteria cause cloudiness. Normally, the CSF contains five or fewer

WBCs per mm^3. **More than 300 polymorphonuclear WBCs/mm^3** or more than **400 to 500/mm^3 of lymphocytes or monocytes will cause detectable cloudiness, if the Ex inspects the CSF properly.** Obvious cloudiness occurs with counts of 600 to 800 WBCs/mm^3.

2. To detect minimal cloudiness with counts in the range of several hundred WBCs per cubic millimeter, do the following:
   a. Obtain an exact duplicate of the tube used to collect the CSF and add the same amount of water as is in the CSF tube. The duplicate tube must have the same translucency, color, and refractive index as the CSF tube.
   b. Hold the duplicate and CSF tubes side-by-side against a white sheet of paper, against a dark background, and then against a light source. Use daylight, if at all possible. Compare the CSF with the water by looking through the sides of the tubes, as in using a colorimeter. The direct, side-by-side comparison enables the Ex to detect very subtle cloudiness or color changes.
   c. In bright sunlight, even mild CSF pleocytosis with WBCs or red blood cells (RBCs) can cause the Tyndall effect, a snowy iridescence.
   d. Students may suppose that this is all unnecessary because the CSF goes to the laboratory for the "official" examination and cell count anyway, so why bother? Well, the careful physician inspects the CSF personally and does the cell count on the spot, before the cells have undergone the autolysis that commences in an hour, and to gain the information quickly and reliably. In the second place, personal inspection checks the accuracy of the laboratory, a check that unfortunately is necessary. If the laboratory reports 20 WBCs/mm^3 after the Ex has seen a cloudy fluid, the laboratory must be wrong. If the Pt has meningitis, you must avoid an error on this critical point.

P. Bloody taps, erythrochromia, and xanthochromia

1. RBCs get into the CSF at one of two times in relation to the tap:
   a. From *preexisting* bleeding caused by a ruptured blood vessel or other CNS lesion.
   b. From *inadvertent* bleeding caused by the needle puncture, a "traumatic" or "bloody tap."
2. Frank bleeding causes a red CSF, called **erythrochromia.** It takes an RBC count of 100 to 300/mL to cause erythrochromia. Normally the RBC count in the CSF is ___________.

zero

3. In contrast to *erythrochromia,* a yellowish CSF is called **xanthochromia.**
4. **Differentiation of preexisting bleeding from a bloody tap:** A traumatic tap is generally inconsequential, whereas preexisting bleeding may foretell a life-threatening lesion. Three tests distinguish the two sources of RBCs, the **four-tube test, centrifugation for xanthochromia,** and **cytologic demonstration of erythrophagocytosis** by monocytes.
   a. **The four-tube test:** Compare the redness of the successive tubes. Blood that enters the CSF before the tap will have mixed freely with the CSF. All tubes display the same color and will have the same cell count. Blood from a traumatic tap tends to clear in successive tubes.
   b. **Centrifugation for xanthochromia:** If the tubes are uniform in color, centrifuge one to deposit the RBCs on the bottom and compare the supernatant fluid with a control tube, as described above. If the CSF is completely colorless, the RBCs entered the CSF recently, either less than 2 to 4 hours ago or from the tap itself. Discoloration of the super-natant fluid means that the RBCs entered more than 2 to 4 hours before and have undergone lysis. Free hemoglobin in solution causes the xanthochromia. If the bleeding occurred days before the tap, degradation products of hemoglobin, methemoglobin, and bilirubin cause the color. Because RBCs undergo crenation in the CSF, crenation does not signify preexisting blood.
   c. **Erythrophagocytosis:** Cytologic examination proves preexisting bleeding by demonstrating phagocytosed RBCs in macrophages, but it takes many hours to days to develop.

5. **Correction of the WBC for blood contamination:** Subtract 1 WBC/mm^3 for each 700 RBCs/mm^3. The remainder approximates the true CSF WBC count.

Q. Cerebrospinal fluid xanthochromia

1. **Xanthochromia** means a yellowish discoloration of the CSF detected by controlled comparison of the CSF sample with water. The most common causes are free hemoglobin, oxyhemoglobin, methemoglobin, bilirubin, and high protein (usually > 200 mg/dL. Less likely causes of xanthochromia include jaundice secondary to liver disease or hemolytic disease in the newborn, diet high in carotenes, and rifampin therapy (Fishman, 1992). Distinguish the possibilities this way:
   a. Xanthochromia from very high protein will clot quickly when the CSF stands in the tube (Froin's syndrome). With protein values above 150 mg/mL, CSF may look slightly yellow because of albumin-bound bilirubin that does not come from blood. Or if bleeding causes more than 150,000 RBCs/mL, the amount of serum may tinge the CSF.
   b. Dip a hemoglobin test tape into the CSF to identify hemoglobin. An Ictotest reagent tablet identifies bilirubin. Neither reagent reacts if only protein is present.
2. The final arbiter is spectrophotometry, which can distinguish the successive degradation products of red cell lysis: oxyhemoglobin, methemoglobin, and bilirubin. Spectroscopy can be positive even with xanthochromia too faint for detection by the unaided eye.

R. Laboratory examination of the cerebrospinal fluid

1. The routine tests include cell count and cell identification, sugar, total protein, protein fractionation, and the Venereal Disease Research Laboratory test for syphilis. Chloride determination has little value with the routine specimen.
2. Successful exploitation of the CSF depends on careful planning. Molecular biology advances so rapidly that the Ex almost has to consult the literature for the best tests to apply to each new CSF sample. For example, the CSF level of hypocretin in narcolepsy (Mignot et al., 2002), the measurement of CSF tau and CSF-Aβ42 in Alzheimer's disease (Andreasen et al., 2001; Riemenschneider et al., 2002), the identification of ferritin indicating activation of phagocytosis by microglia as an index of intracranial bleeding (Thompson, 1995), the identification of transferrin protein to detect a CSF fistula in rhinorrhea (page 352), and the increase in prolactin (Aydln et al., 2002) in CSF from seizures, and the reduced levels of homovanillic acid, biopterin, and neopterin in dopa-responsive dystonia (Nygaard, 1993), now qualify as diagnostic tests. The vast array of possibilities places even more value on the clinical findings to guide the selection of tests for the particular Pt. See Fig. 13-7.
3. **Glucose content of CSF**
   a. The CSF glucose normally is about 66% of the blood glucose or higher in preterm or term infants. The CSF glucose concentration lags some hours behind changes in the blood glucose. In general, the Ex should determine the blood glucose at the time of the LP for comparison. A 50-mL bolus of 50% glucose IV will equilibrate with the CSF in 30 min to several hours. When feasible, do the LP in the morning to allow for overnight equilibration of blood and CSF levels.
   b. High CSF glucose reflects high blood values.
   c. Low CSF glucose implies diffuse meningeal disease, usually because of increased because WBCs or neoplastic seeding. The usual causes include:
      i. Acute bacterial meningitis, tuberculous meningitis, and fungal meningitis.
      ii. Herpes simplex encephalitis (but not typically with most viral infections).
      iii. Neoplastic seeding of the CSF with lymphoma or acute leukemias or carcinomatosis of the meninges.

EXAMINATION OF CSF

- **Pressure**
  - Direct manometry during lumbar puncture
  - Surgically implanted intracranial transducer
- **Gross appearance**
  - Normal: sparkling clear (compare with control tube)
  - Abnormal:
    - Cloudy
    - Erythrochromia or xanthochromia
      - High protein
      - Hemoglobin/oxyhemoglobin
      - Methemoglobin
      - Bilirubin
    - Three tube test
    - Centrifugation
  - Spectroscopy to define pigment
  - Test tapes for hemoglobin, bilirubin, glucose, and protein
- **Microscopic examination of cell contect**
  - WBC count: normal <5/mm^3
  - RBC count: normal 0
  - Differential cell count: Normal: 75% lymphocytes, 24% monocytes; no RBCs polymorphonuclear leukocytes, plasma cells or eosinophils
  - Cytospin or sedimentation cytology: identifies types of WBCs and neoplastic cells
  - Immunohistochemical battery for identification of neooplastic cells
- **Chemistries**
  - Glucose (66% of blood sugar) do concomitant blood sugar
  - Protein analysis: do concomitant serum analysis
    - Total protein, varies with age, neonates to <170 mg%, adults to <45 mg%
    - Electrophoresis, isoelectric focusing, immunoglobulin fractionation, IgG index, oligoclonal bands. Do concomitant serum
    - Myelin basic protein: increased in myelinoclastic diseases
  - Amino acids, neurotransmitters, and trace metabolites depending on clincial clues:
    - Glutamine: hepatic encephalopathy
    - Lactate: mitochondrial encephalopathy; CSF lactate ≥ 4.0 mmol/L raises possibility of bacterial meningitis
    - Prolactin: seizure marker
    - Ferritin: intracranial bleeding
    - Catecholamines
    - Biomarkers for incipient Alzheimer's disease
- **Microbiology/immunology**
  - Stain: gram, India ink, Diff-quick, Wright-Giemsa, Papanicolaou, and Romanowsky
  - Culture: aerobic and anaerobic bacteria, fungi, viruses, TB
  - Serologic testing
    - VDRL
    - Blood and CSF titers for viruses
  - Viral screen
    - Immunoassays: ELISA becoming method of choice
    - Nucleic acid hybridization by Southern (DNA) and Northern (RNA) Blot
    - PCR
  - Bacterial antigen screening battery for acute bacterial meningitis
  - Cryptococcal surface antigen

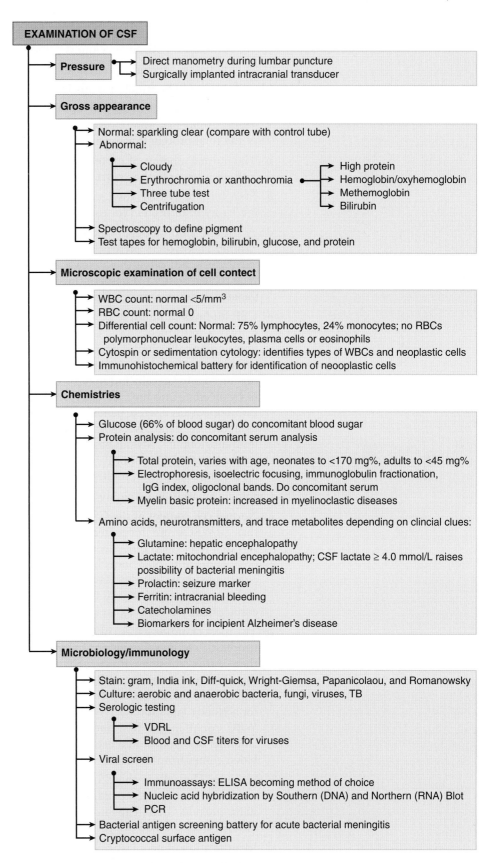

FIGURE 13-7. Dendrogram showing methods for examining the cerebrospinal fluid (reference). CSF = cerebrospinal fluid; ELISA = enzyme-linked immunosorbent assay; IgG = immunoglobulin G; PCR = polymerase chain reaction; RBC = red blood cell; TB = tuberculosis; VDRL = Venereal Disease Research Laboratory test; WBC = white blood cell.

iv. Systemic causes of hypoglycemia, including prolonged insulin shock.

v. Sometimes with subarachnoid hemorrhage.

vi. Idiopathic aglycorrachia (Fraser, 1991).

4. **Identification of abnormal proteins in the CSF**

a. The total protein is measured and the proteins are fractionated (Thompson, 1995). Abnormal immunoglobulins can be detected even without elevation of the total protein (Swaiman, 1999).

b. The normal amount of protein varies with the Pt's age (Fig. 13-3). The total protein is lower in the ventricular and cisternal CSF than in the lumbar CSF.

c. Even for bloody CSF, the Ex can estimate the total CSF protein by subtracting 1 mg/dL of protein for each 1000 RBCs/mm^3.

d. A striking albuminocytologic dissociation occurs in the Guillain-Barré syndrome. The protein increases to several 100 mg/dL without corresponding pleocytosis, but often the increase in protein or the peak does not occur for days to weeks after the onset of the illness. The CSF below a block in the spinal canal also shows a strong albuminocytologic dissociation.

e. **CSF findings in multiple sclerosis and other immunopathies:** The CSF may display a mild pleocytosis. Cytologic examination reveals plasma cells and immunologically altered lymphocytes. The CSF contains increased γ-globulin, mainly immunoglobulin G (IgG), and an increased CSF IgG index. IgG is manufactured intrathecally but may enter through a disrupted blood-brain barrier or by bleeding into the CSF. Agarose electrophoresis demonstrates oligoclonal gammopathy as discrete bands, whereas normal CSF immunoglobulins migrate as a diffuse band. Isoelectric focusing shows heavy and light chains of immunoglobulins. Myelin basic protein is frequently increased in all demyelinating diseases. The clinical findings, CSF profile, and MRI findings together certify the diagnosis of multiple sclerosis (Swaimann, 1999).

5. **Cytologic analysis and staining**

a. **Normal cell content of the CSF:** The normal total CSF WBC counts are fewer than 20 WBCs/mm^3 for preterm infants to neonates, fewer than 15 WBCs/mm^3 at 4 to 8 weeks, and generally no more than 5 WBCs/mm^3 in older infants, children, and adults. Newborns have about 60% polymorphonuclear cells, but in older individuals lymphocytes make up 75% of the total and monocytes 25% make up the rest. Normally CSF contains no polymorphonuclear leukocytes, eosinophiles, plasma cells, and RBCs, but it may rarely contain ependymal cells.

b. The most common causes of CSF pleocytosis are meningitis, encephalitis, and neoplastic seeding. Convulsions alone can cause a slight pleocytosis that may then cause confusion with encephalitis (Clark, 1985; Edwards et al., 1983). If the cell count exceeds 5 WBCs/mm^3, the cells should be smeared on a slide and stained for organisms. To estimate the total WBC count to compensate for a bloody tap, subtract 1 WBC/mm^3 for each 700 RBCs. Also compare the WBC count in the first and last of the four tubes collected. Decreasing amounts of blood should cause a decreased cell count in the last tube, if the blood comes from the tap. Preexisting blood is evenly mixed.

c. **Staining:** The cells in the CSF are concentrated by centrifugation or by sedimentation methods. Depending on the diseases suspected clinically, the cell stains include Gram, Papanicolaou, Romanowsky, and WrightGiemsa stains, the Diff-quik methods, or India ink for fungi (Bigner, 1992).

d. **Identification of neoplastic cells in the CSF:** Neoplastic cells in the CSF arise from seeding by intrinsic gliomas, blood dyscrasias, or metastatic carcinoma. An immunohistochemistry panel aids in differentiating the various types of neoplastic cells (Bigner, 1992). In acute encephalitis, the activated lymphocytes require differentiation from neoplastic cells. The neoplastic cells of lymphomas and acute leukemia commonly invade the CSF, but chronic leukemias uncommonly do so. Immunophenotyping helps distinguish lymphomas, which are usually monoclonal B cells.

i. The most common carcinomas that seed the subarachnoid space arise from the breast, lung, and skin (melanoma).

ii. The common gliomas that seed the CSF are medulloblastoma, pineoblastoma, retinoblastoma, and neuroblastoma. The glial cells stain with antibodies to glial fibrillary acid protein.

S. Cerebrospinal profiles in acute bacterial meningitis and viral meningoencephalitis

1. **CSF in acute bacterial meningitis:** Polymorphonuclear pleocytosis with more than 100 to 500 WBCs/mm^3, increased pressure, decreased glucose, and increased protein (Table 13-2). Brief pretreatment with antibiotics does not reduce the cell count but does reduce the demonstration of the organism by stain or culture.
2. **CSF in viral meningitis:** Lymphocytic pleocytosis, normal glucose, slightly too moderately increased protein, and increased pressure (Table 13-2). The most common causes are enteroviruses, herpes viruses, and human immunodeficiency virus (HIV; Johnson, 1998; Roos, 1997).

T. Identification of infectious agents in the cerebrospinal fluid

1. Molecular biology has greatly improved the diagnosis of meningitis and encephalitis. Previously, the diagnosis depended mainly on the Gram stain, India ink, culture, and antibody titers. These remain as staples, but the newer techniques prove particularly valuable when pretreatment with antibiotics prevent demonstration of microorganisms by stain or culture. Many serologic tests depend on matching serum and CSF titers and estimating the rate of production of antibodies and their passage through the blood-brain barrier (Roos, 1997). Newer techniques include:
   a. The polymerase chain reaction (PCR) for nucleic acids of most common viruses and bacteria.
   b. Improved test batteries for virus-specific antibodies.
   c. Counterimmune electrophoreses and latex particle agglutination tests for antigens of common bacterial meningitides such as *Haemophilus influenzae* type B, *Neisseria meningitidis, Streptococcus pneumoniae* and other streptococci, and *Escherichia coli* (screening panel for acute meningitides).
   d. The limulus amebocyte lysate assay for gram-negative endotoxins and gram-negative meningitis.
2. **Herpes simplex:** Identified by PCR (Kennedy and Chaudhuri, 2002). The detection of this virus, with its predilection for the temporal lobe, is extremely important because of the potential for treatment with acyclovir.
3. **Enteroviruses:** Identified by viral culture or reverse transcriptase PCR.
4. **Arthropod borne viruses:** The diagnosis depends on a fourfold or greater increase in virus-specific IgG between acute and convalescent sera or by identification of virus-specific IgM in CSF or serum.
5. **HIV:** Identified by PCR. HIV is recoverable from the CSF in all stages of infection, even before any clinical signs of acquired immunodeficiency syndrome and in the absence of virus recovery from the blood. The neurologic complications span the gamut: dementia, aseptic meningitis, myelopathy, polyneuropathy, secondary opportunistic meningitides, and vasculitis (Harrison and MacArthur, 1995; Sharer, 1992).
6. **Epstein-Barr (infectious mononucleosis):** Quantitative PCR level for the virus (Weinberg et al., 2002).
7. **Syphilis:** Identified by a positive Venereal Disease Research Laboratory (VDRL) test which is highly specific but only 30% to 70% sensitive for neurosyphilis (Castro et al., 2008). The CSF fluorescent antibody absorption test (FTA-ABS) is more sensitive but not specific as false positives are common (Marra et al., 1995).

8. ***Cryptococcus:*** The most frequent fungal infection of the CSF is detected by India ink staining, culture, and latex agglutination tests.
9. ***Borrelia burgdorferi* (Lyme disease):** Detected by the Western blot test.
10. ***Tuberculous meningitis:*** Detected by staining, culture, PCR, and nucleic acid amplification (Pai et al., 2003).

U. Summary of the cerebrospinal fluid examination

1. Review Table 13-2 for the CSF changes in various disorders, but do not memorize the information.
2. Describe the differences in the pressure, cell count, and protein values during maturation from preterm infants to adults.

See Table 13-2 and Fig. 13-3.

____

BIBLIOGRAPHY · The Cerebrospinal Fluid Examination

Andreasen N, Minthon L, Davidsson P, et al. Evaluation of CSF-tau and CSFA 42 as diagnostic markers for Alzheimer disease in clinical practice. *Arch Neurol* 2001;58: 373–379.

Aydln GB, Köse G, Değerliyurt A, et al. Prolactin levels in cerebrospinal fluid of patients with infantile spasms. *Pediatr Neurol* 2002;27:267–270.

Bigner SH. Cerebrospinal fluid (CSF) cytology: current status and diagnostic applications. *J Neuropathol Exp Neurol* 1992;51:235–245.

Blennow K, Hampel H. CSF markers for incipient Alzheimer's disease. The Lancet Neurology 2003; 2: 605–613.

Castro R. Prieto ES, da Luz Martins Pereira F. Nontreponemal tests in the diagnosis of neurosyphilis: an evaluation of the Venereal Disease Research Laboratory (VDRL) and the Rapid Plasma Reagin (RPR) tests. *J Clin Lab Anal* 2008;22(4):257–261.

Edwards R, Schmidley GW, Simon RP. How often does a CSF pleocytosis follow generalized convulsions? *Ann Neurol* 1983;13:460–461.

Evans RW, Armon C, Frohman EM, et al. Assessment: prevention of post-lumbar puncture headaches. Report of the Therapeutics and Technology Assessment Subcommittee of the American Academy of Neurology. *Neurology* 2000;55:909–914.

Fishman RA. *Cerebrospinal Fluid in Diseases of the Nervous System*. Philadelphia, WB Saunders, 1992.

Fraser JL. Persistent lumbar aglycorrachia of unknown cause. *Neurology* 1991;41:1323–1324.

Greensher J, Mofenson HC, Borofsky LG, et al. Lumbar puncture in the neonate: a simplified technique. *J Pediatr* 1971;78:1034–1035.

Hamandi K, Mottershead J, Lewis T, et al. Irreversible damage to the spinal cord following spinal anesthesia. *Neurology* 2002;59:624–626.

Harrison, MJ, McArthur JC, eds. *AIDS and Neurology*. New York, Churchill Livingstone, 1995.

Hartmann A, Stingele R, Schnitzer, M. General treatment strategies for elevated Intracerebral pressure, in Hanley DF, Einhaupl KM, Bleck TP, et al., (eds). *Neural Critical Care*, Berlin, Springer-Verlag, 1994.

Hasbun R, Abrahams J, Jekel J, et al. Computed tomography of the head before lumbar puncture in adults with suspected meningitis. *N Engl J Med* 2001;345:1727–1733.

Hyland K, Arnold LA. Value of lumbar puncture in the diagnosis of genetic metabolic encephalopathies. *J Child Neurol* 1999;14(suppl 1):S9–S15.

Johnson RT. *Viral Infections of the Nervous System*, 2nd ed. Baltimore, Lippincott Williams & Wilkins, 1998.

Kennedy PDE, Chaudhuri A. Herpes simplex encephalitis. *J Neurol Neurosurg Psychiatry* 2002;73:237–238.

Kuntz KM, Kokmen E, Stevens JC, et al. Post lumbar puncture headache: experience in 501 consecutive procedures. *Neurology* 1992;42:1884–1887.

Leib SL, Boscacci R, Gratzl O, et al. Predictive value of cerebrospinal fluid (CSF) lactate level versus CSF/blood glucose ratio for the diagnosis of bacterial meningitis following neurosurgery. *Clinc Infect Dis* 1999;29(1):69–74.

Levin BE. The clinical significance of spontaneous pulsations of the retinal vein. *Arch Neurol* 1978;35:37–40.

Marra CM, Critchlow CW, Hook EW, et al. Cerebrospinal fluid treponemal antibodies in untreated early syphilis. *Arch Neurol* 1995;52(1):68–72.

Masdeu JC, Breuer AC, Schoene WC. Spinal subarachnoid hematomas: clue to a source of bleeding in traumatic lumbar puncture. *Neurology* 1979;29:872–876.

May C, Kaye JR, Atack MB, et al. Cerebrospinal fluid production is reduced in healthy aging. *Neurology* 1990;40:500–502.

Mignot E, Lammers GJ, Ripley B, et al. The role of cerebrospinal fluid hypocretin measurement in the diagnosis of narcolepsy and other hypersomnias. *Arch Neurol* 2002;59:1553–1562.

Nygaard TG. Dopa-responsive dystonia. Delineation of the clinical syndrome and clues to pathogenesis. *Adv Neurol* 1993;60:577–585.

Pai M, Flores LL, Pai N, et al. Diagnostic accuracy of nucleic acid amplification tests for tuberculous meningitis: a systematic review and meta-analysis. *Lancet Infect Dis* 2003;3(10):633–643.

Quincke H. *Über hydrocephalus. Verhandlungen des Congresses für innere Medizin, Vol 10.* Wiesbaden, JF Bergman, 1891, p. 321.

Rando TA, Fishman RA. Spontaneous intracranial hypotension: report of two cases and review of the literature. *Neurology* 1992;42:481–487.

Recommendations for test performance and interpretation from the Second National Conference on Serologic Diagnosis of Lyme Disease. *MMWR Morb Mortal Wkly Rep*1995;44(31):590–591.

Riemenschneider M, Lautenschlager N, Wagenpfeil S, et al. Cerebrospinal Tau and β-amyloid 43 proteins identify Alzheimer Disease in subjects with mild cognitive impairment. *Arch Neurol* 2002;59:1729–1734.

Roos KL, ed. *Central Nervous System Infectious Diseases and Therapy.* New York, Marcel Dekker, 1997.

Roos KL. Lumbar puncture. *Semin Neurol* 2003a; 23(1):105–114.

Roos KL. Cerebrospinal fluid. In Joynt RJ, Griggs RC, eds. *Baker's Clinical Neurology.* Baltimore, Lippincott Williams & Wilkins, 2003b.

Samson DS, Clark K. A current review of brain abscess. *Am J Med* 1973;54:201–210.

Sencakova D, Mokri B, McClelland RL. The efficacy of epidural blood patch in spontaneous CSF leaks. *Neurology* 2001;57:1921–1923.

Sharer LR. Pathology of HIV-1 infection of the central nervous system. *J Neuropathol Exp Neurol* 1992;51:3–11.

Shievink WI. Spontaneous spinal cerebrospinal fluid leaks and intracranial hypotension. *JAMA* 2006; 295:2286–2296

Strupp M, Schueler O, Straube A, et al. "Atraumatic" Sprotte needle reduces the incidence of post-lumbar puncture headaches. *Neurology* 2001;57:2310–2312.

Swaiman KF. Spinal fluid examination. In Swaiman KF, Ashwal S, eds. *Pediatric Neurology,* 3rd ed. St. Louis, CV Mosby, 1999, Chapter 10, pp. 115–121.

Thompson EJ. Cerebrospinal fluid. *J Neurol Neurosurg Psychiatry* 1995;59:349–357.

Van Der Meulen J. Cerebrospinal fluid xanthochromia: an objective index. *Neurology* 1966;16:170–178.

Weinberg A, Shaobing L, Palmer M, et al. Quantitative CSF PCR in Ebstein-Barr virus infection of the central nervous system. *Ann Neurol* 2002;52:543–548.

Whiteley W, Al-Shahi R, Wardlow CP, et al. CSF opening pressure: reference interval and the effect of body mass index. *Neurology* 2006;67:1690–1691.

III. NEURORADIOLOGY

A. Plain skull and spine radiographs

1. **Structures visualized by plain films**
   a. Plain skull films show bone, teeth, and air-filled cavities including the nasopharynx. The films show the contours of bone, its thickness, density, vascular markings, foramina, orbits, and the state of the sutures. Plain films show calcifications,

normal, as in the pineal body, and in calcified lesions. Plain films do not show the ventricles and subarachnoid spaces, brain parenchyma or its lesions (unless calcified), or normal blood vessels.

b. Bony lesions shown include hyperostoses, erosions, fractures, and synostosis.

c. Plain spine films show vertebral contours, malformations, fractures, and the intervertebral disc spaces.

2. **Indications for plain skull or vertebral radiographs**

a. In most instances, you should bypass plain films in favor of CT or MRI, which visualize CNS parenchyma and its lesions, the CSF spaces, and vessels, thus providing far more information.

b. Plain skull films quickly and inexpensively screen for infection in the sinuses and mastoids by showing mucosal thickening, clouding, and fluid levels. Skull films are also useful in the evaluation of shunt integrity in previously shunted patients with hydrocephalus. Order lateral, Waters, and Towne views to visualize all of the sinuses and the mastoid air cells. Sinus-dedicated CT is currently the best method of sinus visualization but it is far more expensive. Plain films serve little purpose if MRI or CT is required, because these procedures also show sinus disease.

c. Vertebral radiographs aid in screening for malformation syndromes involving bone, for spondylosis, and for cervical fractures and dislocations in unconscious Pts with acute head injuries.

d. Surveys of the skull, ribs, and long bones by plain radiographs identify previous fractures in battered infants.

3. **Risk of plain radiographs:** Minimal radiation.

B. Computerized axial tomography

1. **Structures visualized:** CT serves many of the previously listed indications for plain radiographs, but, in addition to showing bone and air filled cavities, it shows brain parenchyma and many parenchymal lesions, calcifications, and the CSF spaces. These structures appear as black or shades of gray, depending on their ability to absorb radiation (Table 13-4 and Figs. 13-8A to 13-8C). Intravenous injection of iodinated contrast material demonstrates the larger brain vessels.

TABLE 13-4 · Gray Scale for Structures and Fluids in Radiographs

	Normal gray matter	Normal white matter	CSF spaces	Bone	Air-filled cavities	Usual lesions
Plain films	Not seen	Not seen	Not seen	White	Black	Seen if calcified
CT	Light gray	Intermediate gray	Black	White	Black	Bright
T1-MRI	Intermediate gray	Light gray	Black	—	Black	Dark (fat bright)
T2-MRI	Light gray	Very dark	Bright	—	Black	Bright
FLAIR	Gray	Medium gray	Black	—	Black	Bright
DWI	Light gray	Medium gray	Dark	—	—	Bright

ABBREVIATIONS: CSF = cerebrospinal fluid; CT = computed tomography; DWI = diffusion weighted imaging; FLAIR = fluid attenuating inversion recovery; T1-MRI = T1-weighted magnetic resonance imaging; T2-MRI = T2-weighted magnetic resonance imaging.

2. **Indications for CT**

a. For most Pts requiring an imaging procedure, order an MRI. Substitute CT for MRI if the Pt has magnetic metal in the body, certain electronic devices (e.g., pacemaker). (Greenspan and Montesanno, 1993).

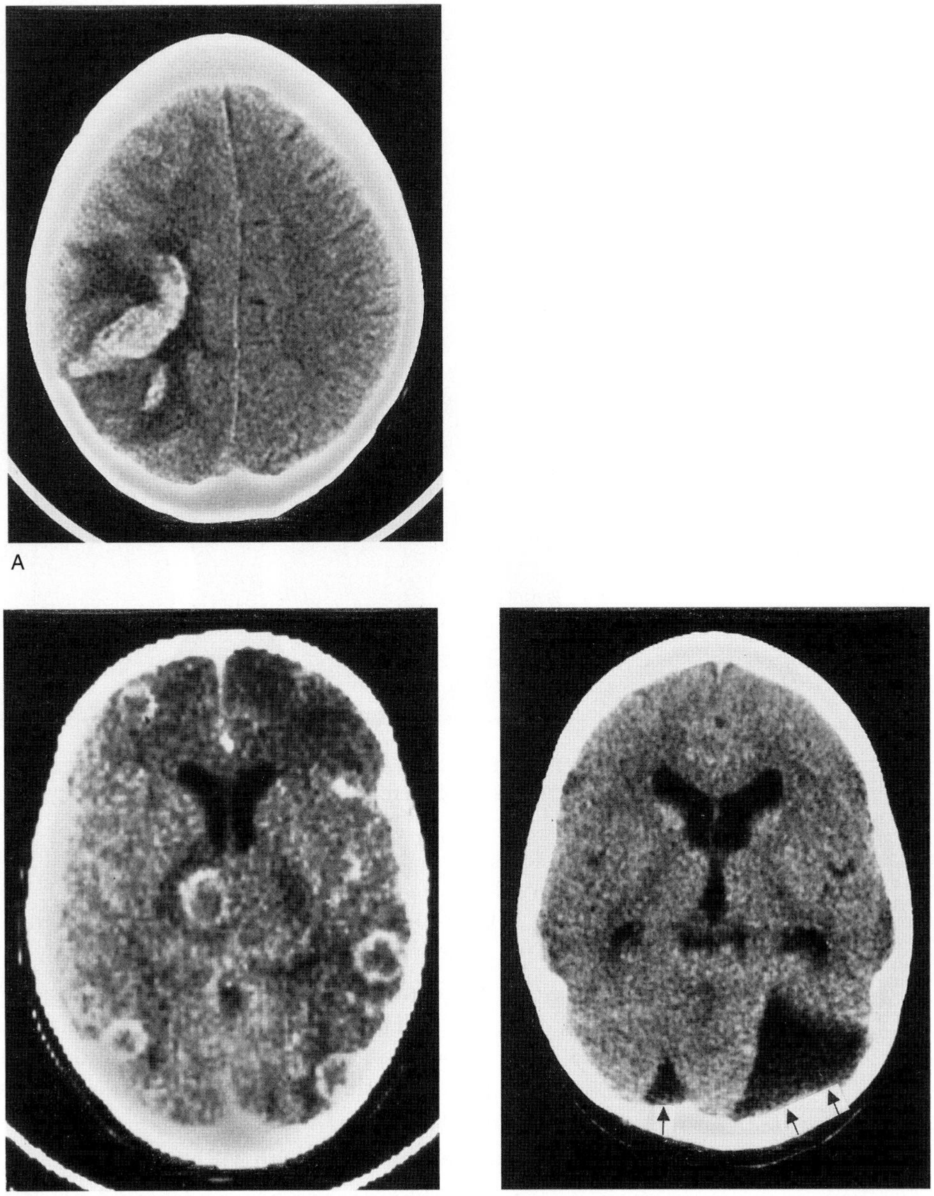

A B C

FIGURE 13-8. (A) CT scan, horizontal section at a high level of the cerebrum, above the ventricles, shows a recent hemorrhage in the left parieto-occipital region. Edema causes the dark zone around the hemorrhage. (B) CT scan, horizontal section of the cerebrum, shows contrast-enhanced white rings of vascularity around multiple abscess cavities. (C) CT scan, horizontal section of the brain, shows congenital arachnoid cyst of the posterior fossa (two arrows). It has displaced the cerebellum and caused slight ventricular enlargement from obstructive hydrocephalus. The single arrow (to the reader's left) points to the displaced cisterna magna cerebelli. CSF = cerebrospinal fluid; CT = computed tomography.

b. Substitute CT for MRI when time is critical, as in the diagnosis of acute intracranial bleeding from a head injury or when you have to identify or exclude quickly a lesion requiring surgical intervention. CT often shows intracranial bleeding better than MRI.

c. CT suffices to follow the changes in ventricular size after shunt operations for hydrocephalus.

d. CT shows normal intracranial calcification and calcified lesions (Fig. 13-9).

e. CT can visualize the skull and sutures in three dimensions, enabling surgeons to better plan the correction of craniofacial malformations and some facial injuries.

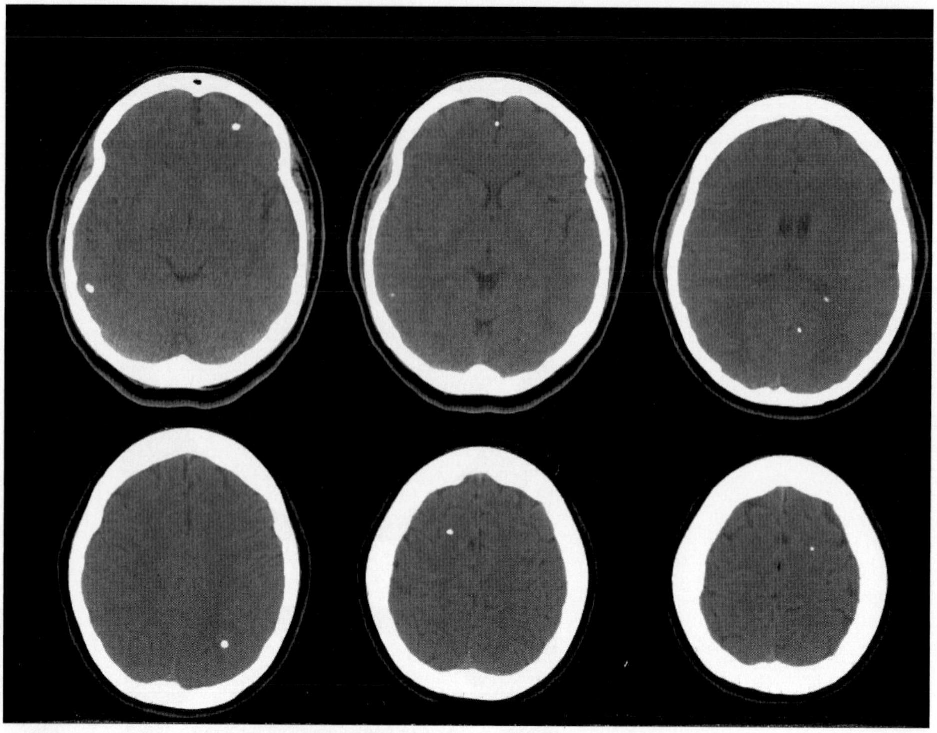

FIGURE 13-9. Axial non-contrast computed tomography (CT) of the brain shows multiple calcifications in a patient with neurocysticercosis. (Courtesy of Jordan Rosenblum, MD.)

f. CT can be obtained more conveniently than MRI for imaging of deeply comatose intensive care Pts or determination of brain death.

g. **Angiography with CT:** Iodinated contrast material injected into a peripheral vein will display blood vessels and enhance many lesions that have abnormal blood vessels or blood-brain barrier disruption (Fig. 13-8B). CT angiography provides a three-dimensional view of the vessels of the brain and neck (Mazziotta, 2000).

3. **Comparison of CT with MRI**

a. CT is cheaper and more widely available. Its wider availability, shorter scanning time, and lower cost make it suitable as a substitute for MRI in some cases., It shows calcifications, whereas MRI does not.

b. CT poorly visualizes lesions of the posterior fossa or base of the skull because the dense petrous bone degrades the image.

4. **Risk of CT:** Some uncooperative Pts and infants require sedation. Some Pts may have allergic reactions to injected contrast material containing iodine. The fluid load from IV contrast may be of danger to a patient with renal impairment.

C. Magnetic resonance imaging of the head and spine

1. **The superiority of MRI to CT:** MRI exploits the paramagnetic signals from the protons and does not expose the Pt to radiation. Because of its vastly superior specificity and sensitivity, MRI is the procedure of choice for imaging the brain and spinal cord (Modic et al., 1993; Osborn, 1994), with the few exceptions listed above. Radiographs show the normal anatomy and lesions of the CNS as black or on a gray scale. See Figs. 13-10 and 13-11A to 13-11E and Table 13-4.

2. The number and variety of imaging procedures, far from replacing the history and NE, places an even greater premium on the clinical findings to enable the Ex to select the appropriate procedures that are safe, decisive, and as economical as possible. The more focused the clinical information, the better the clinician can "go for the jugular" in selecting the one or two best tests.

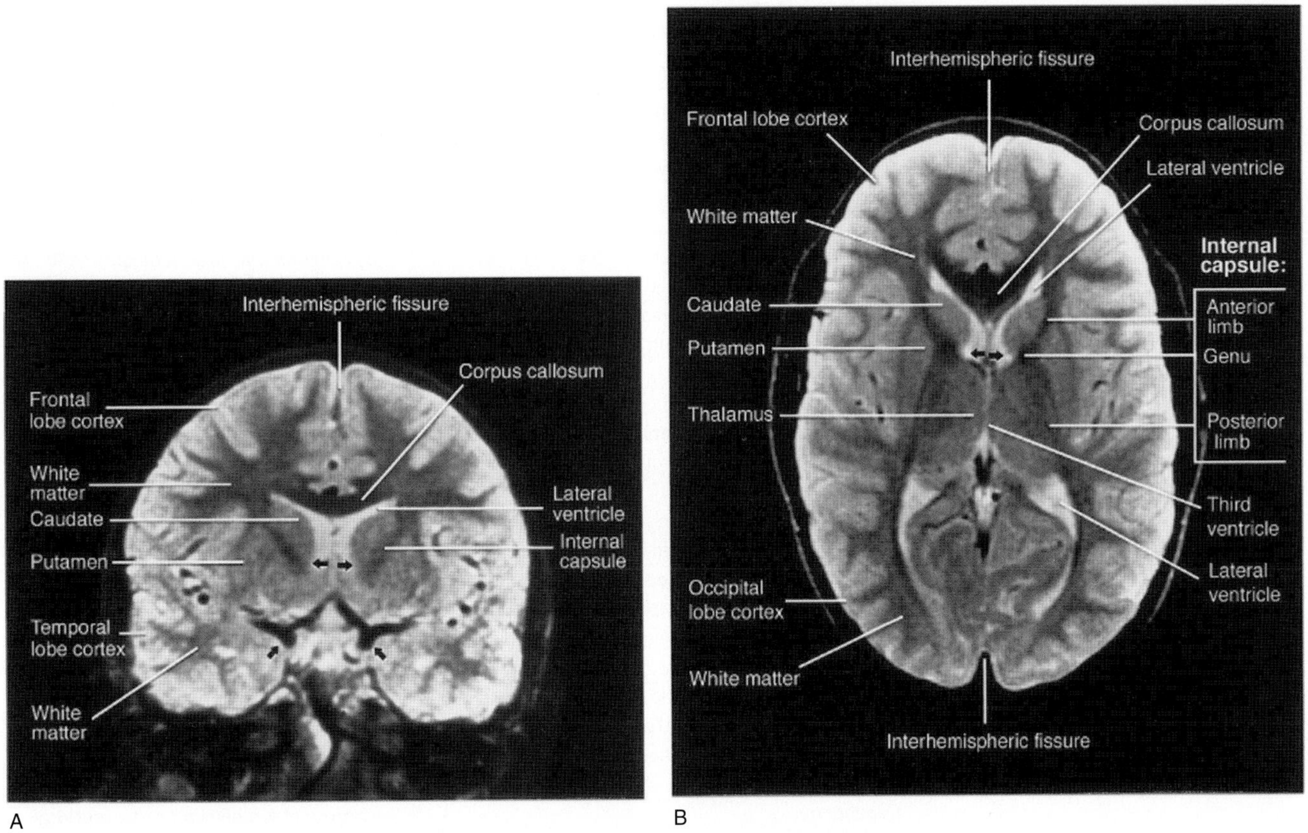

FIGURE 13-10. (A) Coronal section, T2-weighted image, at the level of the genu of the internal capsule. The upper arrows point to the genu of the internal capsule at the foramen of Monro. The two foramina of Monro lead from the lateral ventricles into the III ventricle. The lower arrows show the *Y* of the internal carotid artery (shown as a black flow void) as it bifurcates into the middle and anterior cerebral arteries. (B) Horizontal section, T2-weighted image, at the level of the genu of the internal capsule. The arrows point to the genu of the internal capsule at the foramen of Monro.

3. **Types of MRI procedures:** Table 13-5 (Atlas, 1995; Osborn, 1994; Orrison, 2000).
   a. "Standard" MRI
      i. T1-weighted imaging
      ii. T2-weighted imaging
   b. Diffusion weighted imaging
   c. Perfusion weighted imaging
   d. MRA
   e. Functional MRI (fMRI).
   f. Magnetic resonance spectroscopy (MRS).
4. **Indications for MRI**
   a. History or NE that raises the suspicion of an extra-axial or parenchymal lesion of the CNS or surrounding tissues (Yock, 2002).
   b. Suspected cerebrovascular disease: infarction (Fig. 13-11A), hemorrhage, aneurysms, and arteriovenous malformations.
      i. MRA demonstrates the intracranial and neck vessels, in lieu of invasive angiography. Various imaging techniques taken together, as listed in C 3 a to 3 f, define the necrotic core of an infarct that cannot recover, the penumbra of ischemic but recoverable tissue, the age of the lesion, and the time that blood has been in the tissue (Baldoli et al., 2002; Choi et al., 2000; Davis et al., 2003; Schlaug et al., 1999).
      ii. MRA and other angiographic techniques aid in determining the site of occlusion of the vessels and provide insight as to the mechanism of the infarct (Osborn, 1994; Fig. 13-12).

TABLE 13-5 · MRI Techniques for Brain Imaging and Their Application

Procedure	Principle	Application
Standard T1 and T2 MRI	Exploits paramagnetic properties of protons, most of which are in extracellular space	Shows normal anatomy of parenchyma and CSF spaces and most lesions; vessels appear as flow voids or bright with injection of contrast material
Diffusion weighted imaging (DWI)	Measures changes in diffusion; diffusion means thermally driven Brownian movement; decreased diffusion shows bright signal	Detects fluid shifts caused by membrane dysfunction (cytotoxic edema); in early stroke, it shows bright areas within minutes; conventional MRI takes hours; shows response to thrombolytic therapy; delineates neoplasms, abscesses, trauma and demyelination; some tumors usually dark
Diffusion tensor imaging (DTI)	Maps anisotropic and isotropic diffusion	Identifies some white matter lesions missed on standard MRI and further characterizes others; can trace CNS tracts, normal or degenerating
Perfusion weighted imaging (PWI)	Injected gadolinium discloses regional differences in blood flow by paramagnetic changes in neighboring molecules; areas of low blood flow appear black	Identifies sites of abnormal blood flow; DWI shows the core infarct, and perfusion MR defines the sites of potentially reversible damage; used to localize and grade brain tumors and in measuring response to treatment
Functional MRI (fMRI) = BOLD = *B*lood *O*xygen *L*evel *D*ependent	Shows regional blood flow in relation to changes in deoxyhemoglobin level	Shows sites of increased or decreased blood flow dependent on functional activity or lesions; used in presurgical mapping of sensorimotor cortex and localization of speech, memory, and other mental and sensorimotor functions; EEG can be time locked to trigger fMRI during epileptogenic discharges to localize the site
Fluid Attentuation inversion recovery (FLAIR)	Images resemble T2 films but the signal from CSF is suppressed, making it dark rather than bright	Especially shows lesions adjacent to CSF spaces, such as periventricular leukomalacia and other parenchymal lesions; shows mesial temporal sclerosis in temporal lobe epilepsy

ABBREVIATIONS: CSF cerebrospinal fluid; EEG electroencephogram; MRI magnetic resonance imaging.

iii. Autopsy examination (Kelly et al., 2001) and agreement between MRI techniques confirm the accuracy of the MRI procedures in cerebrovascular disease (Lansberg et al., 2000; Neumann-Hafelin et al., 2000).

c. Suspected demyelinating disease of adults or children (Fig. 13-11B).

d. Neoplasia: primary or metastatic (Fig. 13-11C).

e. Craniospinal trauma (Fig. 13-11D).

f. Dementia (Fig. 13-11E).

g. Acute infections: meningitis, encephalitis, and abscesses (Fig. 13-8B).

h. Investigation of the developmental level of the brain (Thatcher et al., 1996), neuropsychiatric disorders in adults and children (Garreau, 1998), and developmental retardation as related to microcephaly, macro-cephaly, hydrocephaly, cerebral palsy, anoxic encephalopathy, and malformations (Barkovich, 2000).

i. Investigation of the cause of seizures and the origin of epileptogenic activity.

j. Acute or new onset headaches, in particular "thunderclap" headaches that may signify subarachnoid hemorrhage (CT is also useful in detecting acute subarachnoid hemorrhage).

k. MRI can estimate the age of intracerebral hemorrhage by changes in paramagnetic properties of the decomposition products from oxyhemoglobin through deoxyhemoglobin, methemoglobin, transferrin, and hemosiderin (Osborn, 1994).

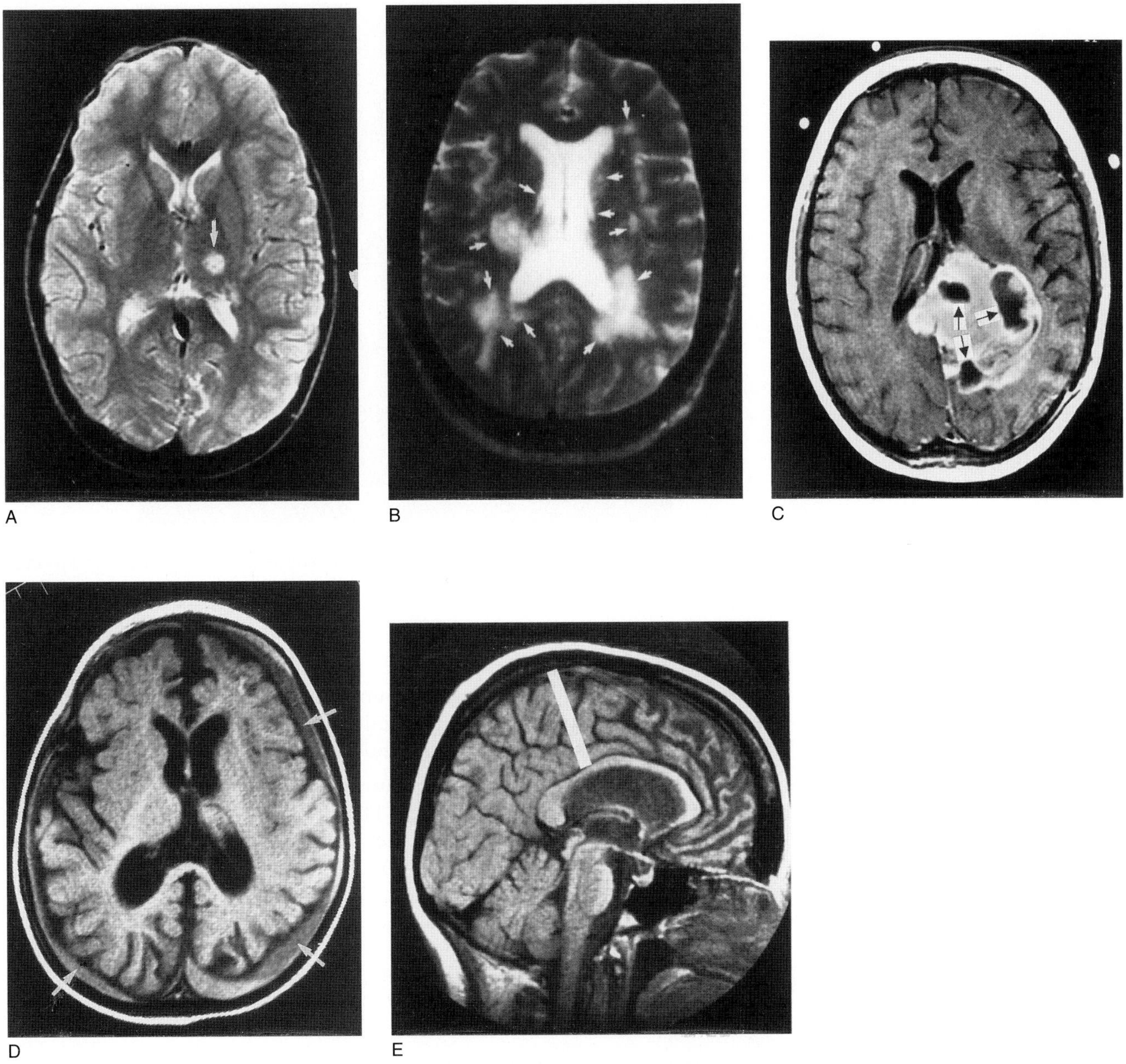

FIGURE 13-11. Montage of lesions demonstrated by MRI. The left side of the patient's brain is to the reader's right. All horizontal scans are mounted with the frontal lobes up. (A) MRI, horizontal T2-weighted section of the brain, shows a subacute infarct (arrow) in the left thalamus. (B) MRI, horizontal T2-weighted section of the cerebrum, shows multiple areas of periventricular demyelination (arrows) in multiple sclerosis. (C) MRI, horizontal T1-weighted section of brain, gadolinium enhanced, shows an astrocytoma with cystic cavities (arrows). The tumor is bright, and the fluid-filled cysts and CSF are black in T1-weighted images, in contrast to bright areas in T2-weighted images. (D) MRI, horizontal T1-weighted section of the brain, shows bilateral subdural hematomas (arrows) and atrophic cerebrum with enlarged ventricles and subarachnoid spaces. The patient, a battered child, had received multiple head injuries. (E) MRI, sagittal T1-weighted section of the brain. The medial wall of the hemisphere shows severe atrophy of the frontal lobe gyri, with extreme widening of the sulci. Notice the normal size of the gyri and sulci in the parts of the cerebrum posterior to the white marker. The patient has a form of dementia called *Pick's disease.* MRI = magnetic resonance imaging.

5. **Enhancement with gadolinium:** Gadolinium is a magnetic metallic element of the rare earth group (atomic weight = 157.25). The IV injection of gadolinium shows the blood vessels and sites of increased blood-brain barrier permeability, as in infarcts, neoplasms, and demyelinating lesions (Fig. 13-11C) or contusions. If you are selecting the right Pts for MRI, those with reasonably strong clinical

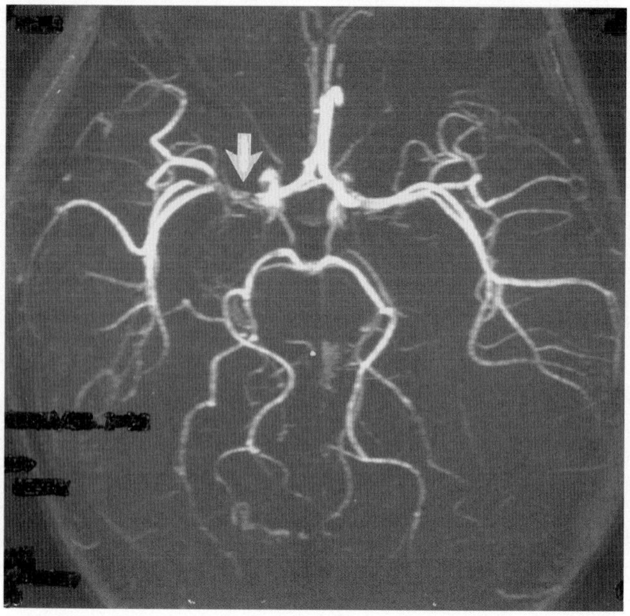

FIGURE 13-12. Magnetic resonance angiogram. The arrow shows the site of embolic occlusion of the right middle cerebral artery.

evidence of a neurologic lesion, gadolinium enhancement is generally indicated (Elster, 1993). Even if normal, a gadolinium scan provides valuable evidence against highly aggressive or destructive lesions.

6. **Risks of MRI:** MRI per se causes no known adverse biological effects, but the strong magnetic field precludes MRI for Pts with certain paramagnetic implants and certain electronic devices. Some Pts get claustrophobia when inserted into the MRI tube. Uncooperative Pts and infants require sedation or anesthesia to prevent movement during an MRI scan. Avoid gadolinium in pregnant women and Pts with a history of allergic reactions. Also always check renal function before giving gadolinium as rarely this agent has been linked with occurrence of nephrogenic systemic fibrosis (NSF) also known as nephrogenic fibrosing dermopathy (NFD). (Marckmann et al., 2006)

D. Computed tomography and magnetic resonance myelography

Visualization of the spinal cord and vertebral lesions by CT or MRI has reduced the need for direct injection of contrast material into the subarachnoid space via an LP (Atlas, 1995; Greenspan and Montesonno, 1993; Modic et al., 1993). Myelography is still needed when MR is contraindicated, when searching for certain CSF leaks, or when artifacts from spinal fusion devices preclude adequate visualization of the spinal cord.

E. Diffusion weighted imaging (diffusion weighted magnetic resonance imaging)

This technique shows cytotoxic edema as bright areas. In acute infarction it visualizes the lesion sooner than with conventional MRI or CT, and it supplements standard MRI in many other disorders that cause anatomic lesions. Perfusion weighted imaging adds additional information about blood flow and blood-brain barrier disruption (Tables 13-4 and 13-5). Diffusion tensor imaging shows normal and degenerating CNS tracts (Ciccarelli et al., 2001; Werring et al., 2000).

F. Magnetic resonance spectroscopy

1. Standard MRI displays anatomy by using the signals from water protons. MRS displays metabolites by using signals from nonwater protons or phosphorus. (Proton

MRS = PMRS = ^{1}H-MRS; phosphorous MRS = ^{31}P-MRS.) By using voxels of 1 to 2 cm^2, proton MRS displays spectral peaks for the metabolites involved in the mitochondrial electron-transport chain, oxidative phosphorylation, Krebs cycle, aerobic glycolysis, and anaerobic metabolism (Fig. 13-13).

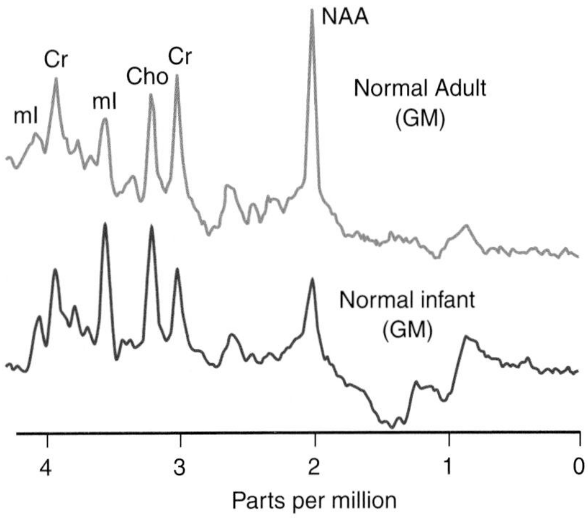

FIGURE 13-13. Magnetic resonance spectroscopy of the gray matter. Notice the higher NAA peak in the adult GM, indicating further neuronal development. Cho = choline; Cr = creatine; GM = gray matter; ml = myo-inositol; NAA = *N*-acetyl aspartate. (Adapted with permission from Danielsen ER, Ross B. *Magnetic Resonance Spectroscopy Diagnosis of Neurological Diseases.* New York, Marcel Dekker, 1999.)

2. The major resonances charted are from **lactate, *N*-acetyl aspartate, glutamine, creatine, choline,** and **myo-inositol** (Fig. 13-13).
   a. **Lactate** is an end product of glycolysis. It does not show a distinct peak in normal persons but increases in anaerobic metabolism and marks sites of tissue damage. Lactate peaks:
      i. In the acutely ischemic or necrotic tissue, when oxidative metabolism fails.
      ii. In tissue infiltrated by inflammatory cells. The lactate in ischemic tissue may come from the infiltrating macrophages.
      iii. In mitochondrial encephalopathies.
      iv. In fluid-filled cysts.
   b. ***N*-acetylaspartate** (NAA) is a marker of neuronal density and viability. NAA is an amino acid of unknown function located almost exclusively in mature perikarya and their processes, including axons. Its presence reflects neuronal density in the gray matter and axonal integrity in the white matter. Its decrease reflects neuronal destruction, as in degenerative diseases, infarction, and glial tumors. NAA appears as early as 16 weeks in the fetal cortex, increases rapidly, and reaches the adult level by around 16 years.
   c. **Creatine** is distributed fairly uniformly and serves as an internal standard for comparison of other metabolites. It occurs alone or as phosphocreatine. It increases in some lesions, such as tumors. Neuronal loss causes a decrease in the NAA-to-creatine ratio because the creatine is considered the basis for comparison of spectral peaks.
   d. **Choline** (Cho) levels reflect free choline and phosphoryl and glucophosphoryl choline of the phospholipids of cell membranes. Membrane disruption, as in acute demyelination, releases phospholipids and increases choline levels. Brain tumors have a high Cho level because of increased cellular density.
   e. **Myo-inositol** serves as a marker of astrocytes, where it is found almost exclusively.
3. **Clinical application of MRS** (Danielsen and Ross, 1999; Rudkin and Arnold, 1999).

a. **Cerebrovascular disease:** Decreases of NAA and increases of lactate in the ischemic zone allows estimation of the distribution and severity of neuronal damage.

b. **Epilepsy:** Localizes epileptogenic foci by elevated lactate during seizure discharge and by decreased NAA levels in the focus.

c. **Multiple sclerosis:** Decreased NAA shows axonal damage in plaques and in adjacent tissue in chronic multiple sclerosis. Increased Cho indicates demyelination in plaques.

d. **HIV:** NAA decreases and Cho increases before clinical signs and changes on standard MRI.

e. **Brain tumors:** Aids in differentiating histologic type of tumor and in guiding stereotaxic biopsy.

f. **Neurodegenerative diseases:** Spectroscopy shows neuronal loss in numerous degenerative diseases including amyotrophic lateral sclerosis, parkinsonism, and Parkinson plus syndromes, Huntington's chorea, and various metabolic disorders.

g. **Inborn errors of metabolism:** Currently, MRS lacks the sensitivity to detect the primary defect in most cases but can document the neuronal and axonal loss, demyelination, and lactate level. Future technical improvements undoubtedly will make MRS more valuable in these diseases.

BIBLIOGRAPHY · Computed Tomography, Magnetic Resonance Imaging, and Magnetic Resonance Spectroscopy

Atlas SW. *Magnetic Resonance Imaging of the Brain and Spine,* 2nd ed. New York, Raven, 1995.

Baldoli C, Righini A, Parrazini C. Demonstration of acute ischemic lesions in the fetal brain by diffusion magnetic resonance imaging. *Ann Neurol* 2002;52:243–246.

Barkovich JA. *Pediatric Neuroimaging,* 3rd ed. Philadelphia, Lippincott Williams & Wilkins, 2000.

Choi SH, Na DL, Chung CS, et al. Diffusion-weighted MRI in vascular dementia. *Neurology* 2000;54:83–89.

Ciccarelli O, Werring DJ, Wheeler-Kingshott CAM, et al. Investigation of MS normal-appearing brain using diffusion tensor MRI with clinical correlations. *Neurology* 2001;56:926–934.

Danielsen ER, Ross B. *Magnetic Resonance Spectroscopy Diagnosis of Neurological Diseases.* New York, Marcel Dekker, 1999.

Davis S, Fisher M, Warach S, eds. *Magnetic Resonance Imaging in Stroke.* New York, Cambridge University Press, 2003.

Elster AD. Is gadolinium required for routine cranial MR imaging? An update. *MRI Decisions* 1993; September/October.

Garreau B, ed. *Neuroimaging in Child Neuropsychiatric Disorders.* Heidelberg, Springer-Verlag, 1998.

Gilman S. Imaging of the brain. *N Engl J Med* 1998;338:812–820, 889–896.

Greenberg JO, ed. *Neuroimaging,* 2nd ed. New York, McGraw-Hill, 1999.

Greenspan A, Montesanno P. *Imaging of the Spine in Clinical Practice.* St Louis, Mosby, 1993.

Kelly PJ, Hedley-Whyte ET, Primavera J, et al. Diffusion MRI in ischemic stroke compared to pathologically verified infarction. *Neurology* 2001;56:914–920.

Krings T, Schreckenberger M, Rohde V, at al. Metabolic and electrophysiological validation of functional MRI. *J Neurol Neurosurg Psychiatry* 2001;71:762–771.

Lansberg MG, Norbash AM, Marks MP, et al. Advantages of adding diffusion-weighted magnetic resonance imaging to conventional magnetic resonance imaging for evaluating acute stroke. *Arch Neurol* 2000;57:1311–1316.

Marckmann P, Skov L, Rossen K, et al. Nephrogenic systemic fibrosis: suspected causative role of gadodiamide used for contrast-enhanced magnetic resonance imaging. *J Am Soc Nephrol* 2006;17(9):2359–2362 (Medline).

Mazziotta JC. Imaging: window on the brain. *Arch Neurol* 2000;57:1413–1421.

Modic MT, Masaryk TJ, Ross JS. *Magnetic Resonance Imaging of the Spine.* St Louis, Mosby, 1993.

Neumann-Hafelin T, Moseley ME, Albers GW. New magnetic resonance imaging methods for cerebrovascular disease: emerging clinical applications. *Ann Neurol* 2000;47:559–570.

Orrison W, ed. *Neuroimaging.* Philadelphia, WB Saunders, 2000.

Osborn AG. *Diagnostic Neuroradiology.* St Louis, Mosby, 1994.

Osborn AG. *Diagnostic Cerebral Angiography,* 2nd ed. Philadelphia, Lippincott Williams & Wilkins, 1999.

Rudkin TM, Arnold DL. Proton magnetic resonance spectroscopy for the diagnosis and management of cerebral disorders. *Arch Neurol* 1999;56:919–926.

Schlaug G, Benfield A, Baird AE, et al. The ischemic penumbra operationally defined by diffusion and perfusion MRI. *Neurology* 1999;53:1528–1537.

Thatcher RW, Lyon GR, Rumsey J, et al. *Developmental Neuroimaging.* San Diego, Academic Press, 1996.

Werring, DJ, Toosy AT, Clark CA, et al. Diffusion tensor imaging can detect and quantify corticospinal tract degeneration after stroke. *J Neurol Neurosurg Psychiatry* 2000;69:269–272.

Yock DH. *Magnetic Resonance Imaging of CNS Diseases. A Teaching File,* 2nd ed. St Louis, Mosby, 2002.

G. Introduction to dynamic techniques for localization of functions and lesions in the brain

1. **Functional localization** means detecting sites of brain function involved in the performance of specified mental, motor, and sensory processes. Examples of localized mental process include word generation and reactions to anxiety or pain. Localized motor actions include finger tapping or tongue movement. Rather than mapping the brain as a mosaic of isolated areas, the newer functional methods demonstrate distributed systems or linked areas, including the cerebellum. These methods extend the localization doctrines derived from classic clinicopathologic correlations at autopsy and from static radiographic films (Frank and Pavlakis, 2001). Functional techniques fall into two large groups: *radiographic* and *electromagnetic.*
2. The functional *radiographic* techniques demonstrate focal differences in metabolism and cerebral blood flow that depend on neuronal activity (Orrison, 2000). Radiographic techniques for recording focal variations in blood flow include fMRI, positron emission tomography (PET), and single-photon emission computed tomography (SPECT). MRS will evolve to include more and more functional applications.
3. The functional *electromagnetic* techniques depend on the fact that masses of neurons produce recordable electrical potentials and recordable differences in magnetic field. Electroencephalography (EEG) noninvasively records electrical potentials from masses of neurons from scalp electrodes. Electrocorticography records from electrodes placed directly on the cortex or electrodes can also be inserted into the depths of the brain. Various sensory stimuli applied to receptors or sensory pathways evoke recordable electrical potentials from farther along the pathway or at the cortical receptive areas (Section IV). Magnetoencephalography involves recording magnetic fields produced by the electrical potentials from masses of active neurons.
4. Most of the functional techniques for studying brain lesions and localization of functions are also applied to the analysis of normal and abnormal development of the brain (Thatcher et al., 1996). The supplement to the December 2002 issue of the *Journal of Cell Biology,* pages 1 to 248, thoroughly reviews all aspects of molecular imaging.

H. Functional magnetic resonance imaging

When active neurons at a site increase the local metabolic rate and blood flow, the increased blood flow more than meets O_2 demand, paradoxically causing the deoxyhemoglobin level to fall. Deoxyhemoglobin reduces the magnetic signal from neighboring water molecules (Buxton, 2002; Pritchard and Cummings, 1997). Functional MRI exploits this difference as a measure of increased flow and increased neuronal activity. The focal increases in cortical blood flow occur within seconds when the brain engages in specified mental, motor, or sensory processes. More commonly used as a research tool, fMRI is beginning to have clinical application (Table 13-5).

I. Radionuclide scanning

1. Radionuclide scans use injected or inhaled radioactive substances detected by external scanning. The substances are administered by breathing, IV injection, or injection into the subarachnoid space, as for detecting a CSF fistula.
2. The two methods most widely used are SPECT and PET (Diksic and Rega, 1991; Gjedde et al., 2000).
   a. SPECT typically uses technetium, a gamma emitter. It is relatively cheap and widely available.
   b. PET uses a positron-emitting isotope of C, O, or F, typically fluorodeoxyglucose. Fluorodeoxyglucose is metabolized only to the first step, phosphorylation. Because it does not proceed down the metabolic path, it accumulates in the tissue for measurement. The technique is expensive and requires access to a cyclotron. PET scanning is more expensive than SPECT, but the cost has been decreasing due to greater availability of the isotope. PET scanning now plays an important part in the clinical management of many cancers (Fig. 13-14). Although of great research value, PET scanning is not a routine clinical procedure.

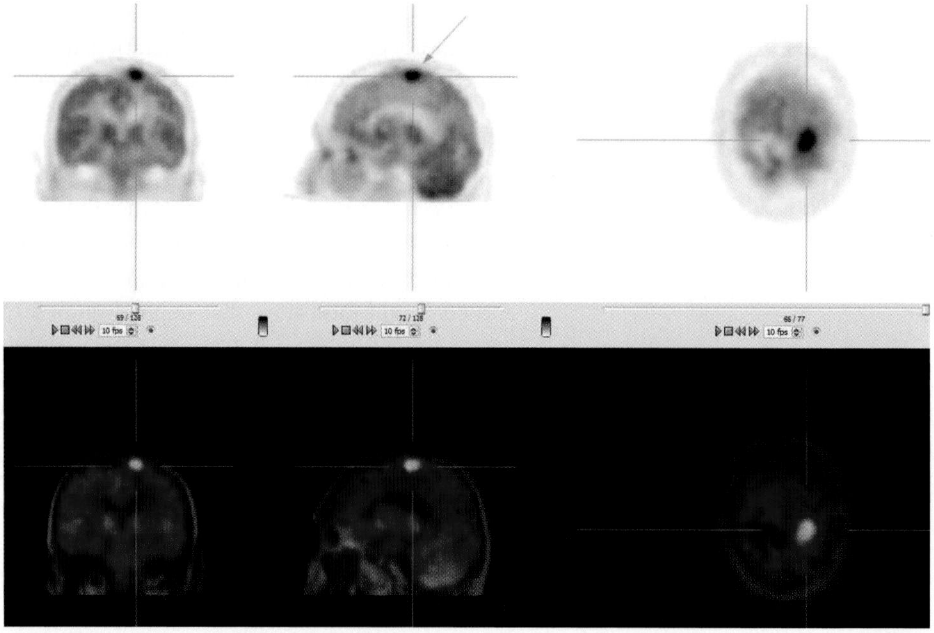

FIGURE 13-14. F-18 FDG PET images (top) demonstrate a focus of hypermetabolic activity near the vertex of the skull (arrow) just to the left of the midline. Fusion imaging with a recent MRI study (bottom) is useful to more precisely localize the focus. The finding is consistent with recurrent glioblastoma in this patient. (Courtesy of Robert H. Wagner, MD.)

3. Radionuclide scans show blood flow through the various regions of the brain. When using fluorodeoxyglucose as the radioactive signal, PET shows sites of glucose use. By combining other chemicals such as neurotransmitters with radioactive isotopes, a wide range of metabolic activity can be investigated.
4. **Clinical applications**
   a. Studying the dynamics of glucose metabolism or other metabolites.
   b. Studying blood flow, whether hyperperfusion or hypoperfusion.
   c. Determining the absence of cerebral blood flow in the diagnosis of brain death (SPECT).
   d. Studying the dynamics of CSF flow (Fig. 13-15) and detecting fistulae (SPECT).

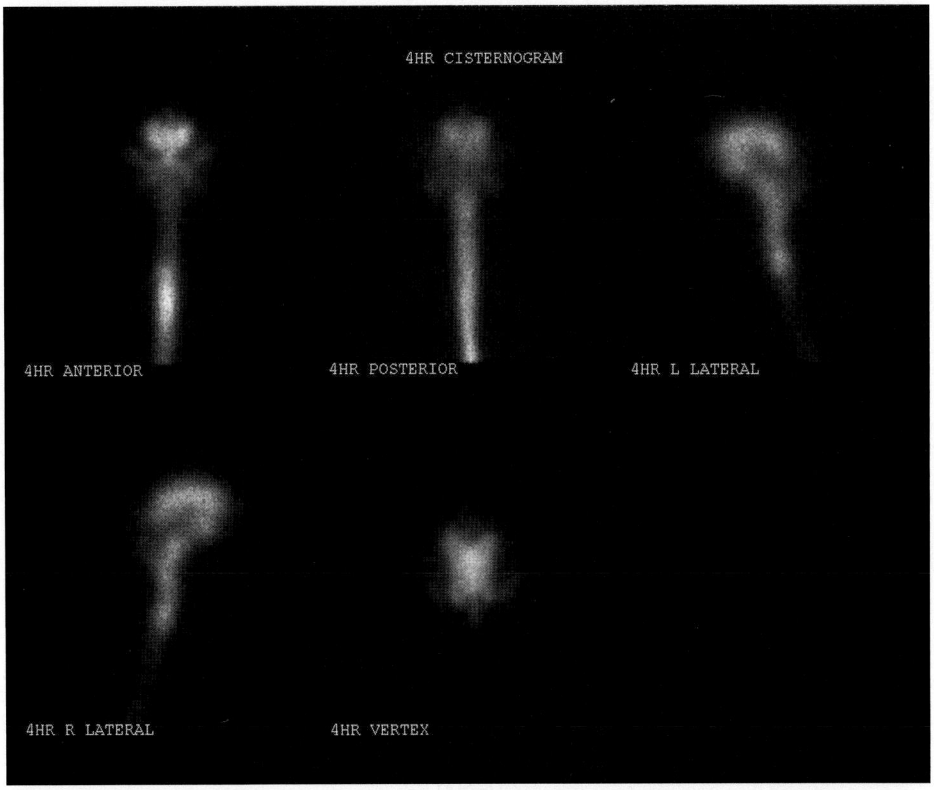

A

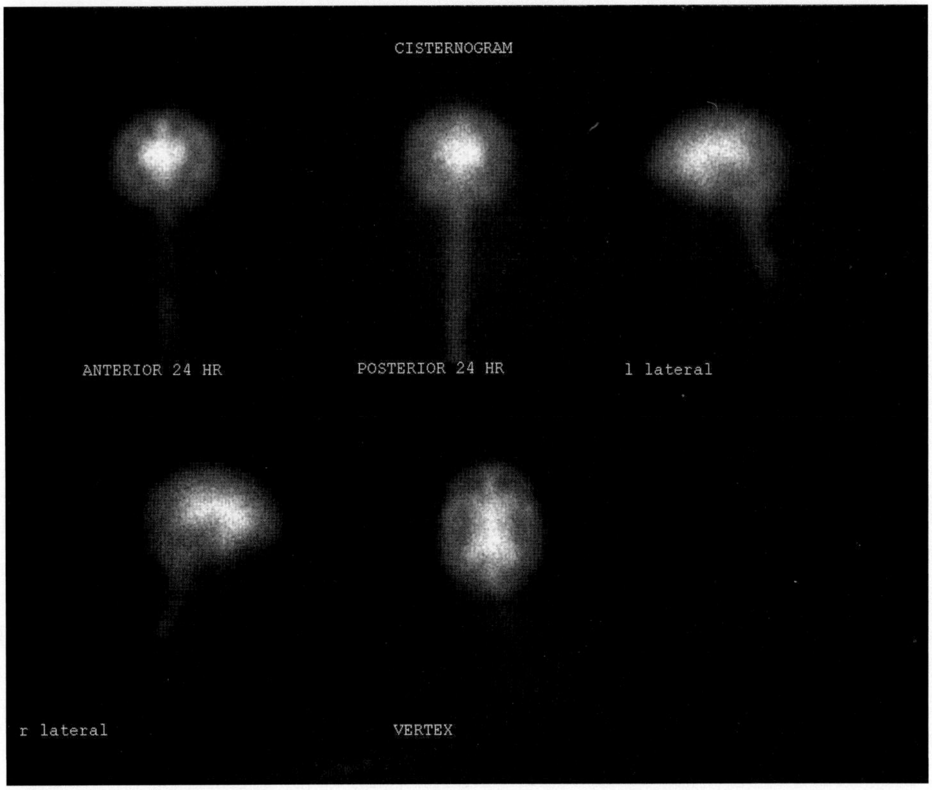

B

FIGURE 13-15. Cisternography. The 4-hour images (figure 1) demonstrate early visualization of the lateral ventricles. Delayed images at 24 hours (figure 2) and at 48 hours demonstrate persistence of activity in the ventricles consistent with the diagnosis of normal pressure hydrocephalus. (Courtesy of Robert H. Wagner, MD)

e. Localizing an active epileptogenic focus before surgical removal (SPECT and PET).

f. Localizing brain activity during specified mental tasks, sensory stimuli, or motor actions (PET).

g. Analysis of neuropsychiatric disorders of adults and children (O'Tuama et al., 1999).

BIBLIOGRAPHY · Functional Imaging and Radionuclide Scanning

Buxton, RB. *Introduction to Functional Magnetic Resonance Imaging: Principles and Techniques.* New York, Cambridge University Press, 2002.

Diksic M, Rega RC. *Radiopharmaceuticals and Brain Pathophysiology Studied with PET and SPECT.* Boca Raton, CRC Press, 1991.

Frank Y, Pavlakis SG. Brain imaging in neurobehavioral disorders. *Pediatr Neurol* 2001;25: 278–287.

Gjedde A, Hansen SB, Knudsen GM, et al., eds. *Physiological Imaging of the Brain with PET.* San Diego, Academic Press, 2000.

Mazziotta JC, Toga AW, Frackowiak RSJ. *Brain Mapping: The Disorders.* New York, Cambridge University Press, 2000.

O'Tuama LA, Dickstein DP, Neeper R, et al. Functional brain imaging in neuropsychiatric disorders of childhood. *J Child Neurol* 1999;14:207–221.

Pritchard JW, Cummings JL. The insistent call from functional MRI. *Neurology* 1997;48: 797–800.

Thatcher RW, Lyon GR, Rumsey J, et al. *Developmental Neuroimaging.* San Diego, Academic Press, 1996.

J. Angiography of the central nervous system: arteriography and venography

1. **Definition: Angiography** means the radiographic visualization of the course, distribution, and caliber of blood vessels (Huber, 1982). The process differs from methods for detecting regional differences in blood flow by functional imaging or Doppler ultrasound.
2. **Methods for demonstrating CNS vessels**
   a. CT shows vessels, albeit crudely, after IV injection of iodinated compounds. 3D reconstructions from CT demonstrates the vessels in three dimensions.
   b. Standard MRI films show blood vessels as flow voids (Fig. 13-11A). An IV injection of gadolinium increases the visibility of the vessels.
   c. MRA shows the vessels satisfactorily, but not as well as with injection of contrast agents by catheterization (Fig. 13-12). Improvements in MRA have reduced the need for, and may ultimately eliminate, direct injection angiography.
   d. Direct injection angiography of iodinated contrast material into an intra-arterial catheter demonstrates the arteries and veins best of all the methods.
   e. Doppler ultrasound studies demonstrate blood flow in the neck and some intracranial vessels but do not produce angiograms.
3. **Indications for invasive angiography (as a supplement to MRA)**
   a. Demonstration of degrees of narrowing of vessels in the neck and intracranial arteries (e.g., CNS vasculitis).
   b. Investigation of subarachnoid hemorrhage and demonstration of aneurysms and arteriovenous malformations of the brain and spinal cord (Djindjian, 1970).
   c. Preoperative planning of surgical procedures that may involve or displace vessels.
4. **Risk of invasive angiography:** Arterial thrombosis, embolization, dissection, and allergic reactions to the contrast medium. Because the kidneys excrete the contrast material, renal failure may preclude contrast angiography (this is a relative contraindication as limited angiography may still be possible), but MRA without contrast is still safe.

BIBLIOGRAPHY · Angiography

Djindjian R. *Angiography of the Spinal Cord.* Baltimore, University Park Press, 1970.

Huber P. *Krayenbuhl/Yasargil Cerebral Angiography,* 2nd ed. Stuttgart, Georg Thieme Verlag, 1982.

Newton TH, Potts DG, eds. *Radiology of the Skull and Brain, Vols 1–3.* St. Louis: CV Mosby, 1974.

Osborn AG. *Diagnostic Cerebral Angiography,* 2nd ed. Philadelphia, Lippincott Williams & Wilkins, 1999.

Learning Objectives for Chapter 13

I. ARRAY OF NEURODIAGNOSTIC PROCEDURES

State the principles that govern the selection of laboratory tests.

II. THE CEREBROSPINAL FLUID EXAMINATION

1. Describe the location of the CSF.
2. Trace a drop of CSF from its origin to its absorption (Fig. 13-1).
3. Draw a lateral projection of the ventricular system.
4. List the functions of the CSF.
5. Describe the changes in the total CSF protein level with age (Fig. 13-3)
6. Describe the composition of normal CSF (Table 13-2).
7. Contrast the normal pressure of the CSF in infants and adults.
8. Describe the signs and symptoms of increased intracranial pressure in infants and older Pts.
9. Describe, in principle, the causes for increased CSF pressure.
10. Recite the usual sites of obstruction of the CSF and name some of the types of lesions that cause obstruction.
11. State Pascal's law of distribution of pressure in an enclosed container.
12. Describe the signs and symptoms and some causes of low CSF pressure.
13. List several common indications for an LP.
14. List and explain the most important contraindications for an LP.
15. Describe some situations in which the Ex may elect to do an LP despite increased pressure.
16. Describe the complications of an LP.
17. Describe the post-LP headache syndrome and its presumed cause.
18. Review the suggestions for prevention and management of the post-LP headache.
19. Describe the treatment for prolonged post-LP headache.
20. Discuss the Pt's apprehensions with regard to an LP.
21. Describe how to position a Pt for an LP and why that position is chosen (Fig. 13-4).
22. Describe the levels of the vertebral column to choose for an LP.
23. Describe how to angle and align the bevel of the needle for an LP.
24. Describe how to measure the CSF pressure and state the normal range.
25. State the precautions the Ex takes in measuring the CSF pressure when the history or clinical examination raise the possibility of increased pressure.
26. State what causes the normal fluctuations in the level of the CSF meniscus in the manometer (Fig. 13-5).
27. State, in principle, the relation between the CSF pressure and the pressure in the extracranial veins.

Learning Objectives for Chapter 13

28. Describe the changes in CSF pressure with inspiration and expiration and explain why these changes occur.
29. State whether the intracranial and CSF pressure is most closely related to the arterial or capillary and venous pressure.
30. State the mechanism by which an anxious Pt's abdominal muscle tension may increase the opening CSF pressure.
31. Describe how to induce the anxious Pt to relax the abdominal muscles.
32. Explain how neck flexion may increase the CSF pressure.
33. Summarize the actions or instructions the Ex uses to exclude extrinsic causes for a high opening CSF pressure.
34. Describe how an LP can cause the death of a Pt with intrinsically increased intracranial pressure.
35. State what actions to take if the opening CSF pressure remains increased after having completed the usual maneuvers to exclude extrinsic causes for increased pressure.
36. Enumerate the causes and describe what to do if the flow of CSF stops or the manometer excursions cease (Table 13-3).
37. Describe the clinical signs of transforaminal herniation (Chapter 12).
38. Describe how to determine whether the CSF and manometer system is patent..
39. Explain why the Ex generally should not aspirate CSF with a syringe, if the flow suddenly stops.
40. Explain the rationale for collecting CSF in three different tubes.
41. Describe the gross appearance of normal CSF.
42. Describe the usual pathologic alterations in the gross appearance of the CSF.
43. Describe the proper way to inspect a sample of CSF for changes in gross appearance.
44. State how many RBCs or WBCs must be present to alter the gross appearance of the CSF.
45. State the usual cause for cloudiness of the CSF.
46. Explain how to interpret the situation if the Ex has seen a cloudy CSF and the laboratory reports a count of less than 200 WBCs/mm^3.
47. Explain why the Ex cannot delegate the immediate inspection of the CSF to the laboratory.
48. Distinguish between erythrochromia of the CSF and xanthochromia.
49. Define what is meant by a *traumatic* or *bloody tap.*
50. Describe the methods for distinguishing a traumatic tap from preexisting blood in the CSF.
51. Explain the importance of centrifuging red or yellow CSF.
52. State the length of time required for xanthochromia to appear after hemorrhage into the CSF.
53. Describe how to correct the WBC count in the CSF when RBCs are also present.
54. Define erythrophagocytosis and discuss its meaning.
55. State the three most common causes of CSF xanthochromia and describe how to distinguish them.
56. Enumerate the widely available laboratory tests on the CSF and give normal values for the constituents of the CSF routinely tested. Use Fig. 13-8 to remind you of the main headings and recite the tests under these headings. Also check Table 13-2 for values.

Learning Objectives for Chapter 13

57. Give the normal cell count in the CSF for young infants and mature Pts and state the only types of cells normally present.
58. State the normal value for the CSF glucose concentration and how it relates to the blood glucose level.
59. State the normal value for the CSF protein and describe, in principle, the importance of fractionating the immunoglobulins.
60. State how to correct the CSF protein value to compensate for blood in the CSF.
61. Describe the methods for cytologic analysis of CSF.
62. List some of the types of neoplastic cells that invade the CSF and state, in principle, how they are identified.
63. Describe, in principle, the methods for identifying the various common bacteria and viruses that cause meningitis and encephalitis.
64. Contrast the typical CSF profiles in encephalitis and meningitis (Table 13-2).
65. Describe the CSF profiles for multiple sclerosis and intrinsic neoplasms (Table 13-2).
66. Summarize the differences in the CSF pressure, cell count, and protein content from early infancy to maturity.
67. Explain why the vast array of laboratory tests available for the identification of microorganisms, abnormal cells, and other constituents places even more value on the clinical findings than ever before.

III. NEURORADIOLOGY

1. Enumerate, in principle, the anatomic features displayed by plain skull radiographs.
2. Discuss, in principle, the clinical indications for ordering plane skull radiographs.
3. Discuss, in principle, the indications for ordering plain spine radiographs.
4. Describe the structures visualized on CT scans not seen on plain films.
5. Describe some situations in which a CT is an acceptable substitute for MRI.
6. State the one major substance shown by CT that MRI does not visualize.
7. Cover only the text in the columns and rows of Table 13-4 and from the exposed headings recite the text for plain films, CT, and T1- and T2-weighted MRI.
8. State the procedure of choice to show intracranial calcification.
9. Name the contrast agents for angiography with CT and MRI.
10. Enumerate the major pathologic categories of CNS lesions disclosed by MRI (Fig. 13-11).
11. Explain which procedure, MRI or CT, is usually the procedure of choice to visualize most CNS lesions.
12. Recite the common indications for ordering an MRI scan.
13. State the additional information provided by an MRI scan enhanced with gadolinium.
14. State a special circumstance that would contraindicate an MRI scan because of physical danger to the Pt.
15. Describe what MRS displays in contrast to CT and MRI (Fig. 13-13).
16. Describe the use of ultrasound in neuroimaging and neurovascular imaging.
17. Describe the significance of decreased NAA on spectroscopy.
18. Describe the significance of increased Cho levels on spectroscopy.
19. Name some clinical applications for spectroscopy.
20. State some functions that radionuclide brain scans localize.

Learning Objectives for Chapter 13

21. Name the two major types of radionuclide scan in current use.
22. Describe several clinical applications of SPECT and PET.
23. Describe several different ways to visualize the arteries and veins of the CNS.
24. Distinguish between the difference in information obtained by Doppler sonography and radiographic imaging of vessels.
25. Describe some vascular lesions demonstrable by angiography (Fig. 13-12).
26. Describe the risks of invasive angiography by direct injection of contrast material into the vascular system.

14 Clinical and Laboratory Tests to Distinguish Conversion Disorder and Malingering from Organic Disease

Much will be gained if we succeed in transforming your hysterical misery into common unhappiness.

—**Sigmund Freud (1856–1939)**

I. THE GENERAL CLINICAL FEATURES OF CONVERSION DISORDER AND MALINGERING

A. Definition of conversion disorder

Conversion disorder (previously referred to as hysteria) means a temporary disorder of mental, voluntary motor, or sensory functions that mimics neurologic disease but is caused by unconscious determinants, not by organic lesions in the neuroanatomic sites that should produce the dysfunctions. Table 14-1 reviews some common dysfunctions in patients with conversion disorder.

B. Primary and secondary gain

Classic psychoanalytic theory holds that conversion disorders arise from unconscious mental mechanisms that relieve overwhelming anxiety by converting it into symptoms (Weintraub, 1995; Woolsey, 1976). The symptom provides **primary** and **secondary gains** for the Pt.

1. The **primary gain** consists of the relief of anxiety.
2. The **secondary gains** consist of manipulative control over the emotional responses, attention, and actions of other persons and relief from responsibilities. Apparently the gains make the symptom more acceptable to the Pt than the anxiety that the symptom relieves.

TABLE 14-1 · Symptoms and Signs of Conversion Disorder

A. Mental
   1. Pseudoepileptic seizures
   2. Amnestic and fugue states
B. Motor
   1. Paralysis (monoplegia, paraplegia, or hemiplegia)
   2. Hyperkinesia: tremors, flailing, and spasms
   3. Astasia-abasia
   4. Aphonia-dysphagia
   5. Hyperventilation, often with dizziness and syncope; weak, shallow respiration; or grunting, demonstrative respiration
   6. Blepharospasm, convergence spasm, pseudo–VIth nerve palsy, and ptosis
C. Sensory
   1. Anesthesia, paresthesia, hyperesthesia, or pain
   2. Dimness of vision, tunnel vision and spiral fields, blindness, double vision, and photophobia
   3. Deafness and dizziness
   4. Globus hystericus
   5. Multisystem complaints, especially gastrointestinal, genitourinary, and reproductive system/sexual/menstrual
   6. Urinary retention

3. Walker et al. (1989) suggested that operant conditioning, with its theory of reinforcement of behavior by reward, provides an alternative paradigm to psychoanalytic theory. They stated "Simply put, those behaviors that obtain reward are those that are expressed."

C. Distinction between conversion disorder, factitious disorder, and malingering

1. The *Diagnostic and Statistical Manual of Mental Disorders,* Fourth Edition. (DSM-IV) distinguishes between **conversion disorder factitious disorder,** and **malingering** for Pts who have symptoms and signs that are not caused by organic disease. In conversion disorder, the dysfunction and the purposes it serves seem to arise at a subconscious level, but the Pt experiences the illness as genuine. At the opposite pole stands the frank *malingerer* who consciously fakes an illness to achieve some tangible external goal, such as getting money in a lawsuit or avoiding criminal prosecution. The DMS-IV Text Revision (DSM-IV-TR) recognizes three main types of factitious disorders: (1) factitious disorders with predominantly psychological signs and symptoms, (2) factitious disorders with predominantly physical signs and symptoms, and (3) factitious disorders with combined psychological and physical signs and symptoms. Munchausen's syndrome (a chronic variant of factitious disorder with predominantly physical signs and symptoms) means the deliberate production of signs and symptoms to assume the role of a sick person. Often the Pt has had multiple surgical procedures that have failed to disclose an organic lesion or to affect a cure.
2. A large spectrum of symptoms and signs, such as non-epileptic seizures and many chronic pain syndromes, can occur as a conversion disorder in one Pt or as malingering in another. Rather than debating the question of the conscious or unconscious origin of the symptoms, the examiner's (Ex's) immediate operational task is to differentiate the nonorganic disorders of whatever origin from the known and diagnosable organic disorders. This is always the first dichotomy in diagnosis: Is the disorder nonorganic or organic? (Is there a lesion? See Table 15-3.) Fortunately, the same bedside techniques and laboratory tests serve to make this dichotomy irrespective of the particular DSM-IV diagnosis. To make a formal DSM-IV distinction between conversion reaction and malingering requires a decision about conscious simulation. To remain noncommittal, some clinicians choose simply to call these disorders *psychogenic, functional,* neurologically unexplained

or *nonorganic*. Careful selection of terms is important because of medicolegal considerations and because Pts have access to their own medical records. In the end, the Ex will need to make a DSM-IV diagnosis because the management of conversion disorder and malingering differ, but both types of Pt are entitled to an understanding, empathetic physicians (neurologists, psychiatrists, psychologists and general practitioners working in collaboration.

D. DSM-IV criteria for the diagnosis of conversion disorder

1. **Learn Table 14-2.**

TABLE 14-2 · Criteria for the Diagnosis of Conversion Disorder

1. Presence of symptoms and signs that imitate neurologic disease but do not match organic patterns of illness. The symptoms reflect the patient's mental image of the body and the way it functions rather than the wiring diagram and neurophysiology of the nervous system.
2. Absence of signs of organic illness. Symptoms abound, but signs can't be found.
3. History of preexisting psychiatric problems and of a precipitating or triggering incident.
4. Full remission of the symptom with time.

2. **The medical history in conversion disorder**
   a. Women, usually between 10 and 35 years of age, predominate at about 3:1. However, the quoted ratio may reflect a diagnostic bias. Malingering is more common, particularly in prisoners.
   b. The history discloses longstanding personality problems, with some immediate emotional stress that triggers the index event. For example, a woman, after getting engaged, may display neurologically unexplained paraplegia as an unconscious defense against the sexual performance or the duties implied by marriage. A history of other medically unexplained symptoms, predisposing emotional problems, and of the precipitating event is essential to the diagnosis of conversion disorder. Don't diagnose conversion disorder in a previously well-adjusted 60-year-old Pt who suddenly has neurologic symptoms. **Always assume that such a Pt has organic disease until proven otherwise.**
   c. During the interview or neurologic examination (NE), when the Ex focuses on the dysfunction, such as a tremor, it worsens. The dysfunction also worsens in the presence of family members or significant acquaintances. The symptom varies with the attention directed to it or with the presence of emotionally significant people. It is socially dependent. Remember, however, that emotional stress may similarly enhance organic tremors and involuntary movements.
3. **The diagnosis of conversion disorder rests on two pillars**
   a. **Pillar 1:** The negative pillar is the absence of neurologic signs that would have to be present if an organic lesion caused the disability.
   b. **Pillar 2:** The positive pillar is the history of overt psychiatric stress and the complete resolution of the symptoms with time as the psychiatric problems resolve.

E. Affective status in conversion disorder

1. No single affect or personality pattern accompanies conversion disorder (Woolsey, 1976). Some Pts appear blandly indifferent (*la belle indifférence*) to the disability by accepting it stoically or good-naturedly, as it were. However, the usefulness of this clinical sign is controversial (Stone et al., 2006) and not useful in distinguishing between conversion disorder and organic disease. Pts do not ask about or seem concerned about the cause or prognosis.

2. In contrast to the bland indifference of some Pts, others with neurologically unexplained symptoms, particularly sensory ones, such as pain, overreact histrionically, with much wailing or dramatic prostration. The art of diagnosis—the art—is to recognize the *disproportionate* underreaction or overreaction.
3. **Caveats for the history**
   a. In searching for psychiatric stressors, the naive Ex may overlook the **high achiever syndrome** or even misinterpret it as evidence against hysteria. Consider the Super-Kid or All-American Kid syndrome. The Pt, a straight-A student, runs cross country in the fall, plays varsity basketball in the winter, plays Little League baseball, swims competitively in the summers, and receives the yearly citizenship award at school. After school hours, the child goes to choir practice and baby-sits for the mother on weekends. The overscheduling denies the child a childhood. In desperation, the child becomes paraplegic. In such a Pt, the unremitting excellence of function, maintained at too high a cost in psychic energy, constitutes the psychiatric predisposition.
   b. Some Pts with multiple sclerosis, frontal lobe damage, anosognosia, abulia, or Anton's cortical blindness may seem blandly unconcerned about their disability and its implications.

II. PSYCHOGENIC DISORDERS OF MOTOR FUNCTION

A. Range of motor disorders

1. Somatoform disorders may cause paresis, paralysis, hypokinesia, or hyperkinesia. Handedness does not influence lateralization of the observed motor abnormalities, and unilateral motor and sensory symptoms are as common on either side of the body (Stone et al., 2002). The hyperkinesias usually take the form of tremor, spasms, or flailing about. The paralysis may affect cranial nerve muscles, causing aphonia or dysphagia, or it may affect the rest of the body in monoplegic, hemiplegic, or paraplegic distributions. Motor conversion disorders presenting as quadriplegia virtually never occurs.
2. Psychogenic impotence, a very common form of psychogenic dysfunction, does not qualify as conversion disorder, because it represents failure of autonomic function rather than volitional muscular activity.

B. Psychogenic oculomotor signs

1. **Some oculomotor manifestations:** Excessive blinking, squinting or blepharospasm, convergence spasm, pseudo–VI nerve palsy, and pseudoptosis.
2. **Convergence spasm:** The pupils constrict along with the forceful adduction of the eyes, indicating an overactive accommodation mechanism (Griffin et al., 1976). Review accommodation in Table 4-3.
3. **Pseudo-abducens nerve palsy:** The Pt, on attempting to look to one side, say the right, will move the eyes conjugately to, or a little past, the midline. Then the *ab*ducting, i.e, leading, eye deviates inward, as if the lateral rectus muscle had failed. The *ad*ducting, i.e., following, eye continues to progress to the right. Careful inspection will show that the Pt has learned to use convergence, as in volitionally looking cross-eyed. When the leading eye breaks from its abducting movement to the right, the pupils simultaneously constrict. Thus a volitional convergence stimulus has arrested the abduction of the eye, not weakness of the lateral rectus muscle (Troost and Troost, 1979). In organic VI nerve palsy, the failure of abduction does not cause pupilloconstriction.
4. **Pseudoptosis:** In organic ptosis, the Pt tends to lift the eyebrow up, using the action of the frontalis muscle. In pseudoptosis, the voluntary contraction of the orbicularis oculi causes the eyebrow to descend. The contraction of the orbicularis oculi muscle may be extreme enough to cause blepharospasm. The malingerer with pseudoptosis may also use mydriatic drops to dilate the pupil, further simulating a III nerve palsy (Keane, 1982).

5. **Caveats:** Blepharospasm more commonly occurs secondary to dystonia or to ocular inflammation with photophobia. When organic disease causes convergence spasm, the Pt usually has other midbrain and pretectal signs (Table 5-2). Tourette's syndrome may cause a variety of tics affecting the eyelids and causing excessive blinking.
6. Describe some associated findings or neighborhood signs if an organic lesion causes convergence spasm.

   ____

   See Table 5-2.

7. Describe the critical finding that distinguishes a pseudo-abducens palsy from an organic palsy.

   ____

   See frame II B 3.

C. Psychogenic dysfunctions of voice production, swallowing, and breathing

1. **Range of dysfunction:** Mutism or low voice volume, dysphagia, and respiratory dysrhythmias.
2. **Psychogenic mutism:** Pts with conversion muteness may exhibit complete mutism or speak with a low voice volume. Although aphonic, the Pt has normal vocal cord action during laryngoscopy or shows pure adductor palsy, but the Pt can produce a Valsalva maneuver or a normal strong cough, proving that the adductor muscles of the vocal cords can, in fact, act forcefully. The Pt has no palatal palsy, breathes and swallows normally, and may whisper with perfect articulation. The Pt may talk or phonate during sleep, thus establishing the integrity of the vocal apparatus.
3. **Spasmodic dysphonia:** When the Pt attempts to speak, the vocal cords go into spasm, causing a tight, hoarse, or strained voice (Aminoff et al., 1978).
4. **Psychogenic dysphagia:** The Pt chokes, or cannot swallow, but may have no accompanying signs of palatal, laryngeal, or pharyngeal dysfunction. The Pt swallows normally when asleep. The Pt may also experience **globus hystericus,** a distressing sensation of a lump lodged in the throat.
5. **Respiratory dysrhythmias:** Disorders include apnea, often in association with a Valsalva maneuver, hyperventilation, weak, shallow, or "asthenic" breathing in a Pt who avoids eye contact, or theatrical gagging, with guttural noises, stridor, rolling of the head and trunk and demonstrative, expressive eyes (Walker et al., 1989). Walker and colleagues (1989) likened the latter state of respiratory gymnastics to astasia and abasia: in both states, the Pt flirts with disaster but escapes. Hyperventilation may accompany or precede hysterical symptoms such as dizziness. Most Pts with psychogenic breathing disorders show no cyanosis and have a normal arterial O_2 but, if misdiagnosed, may be mistakenly intubated (Walker et al., 1989).
6. **Caveats:** Dystonia may cause spasmodic dysphonia. Early stages of several organic diseases—such as amyotrophic lateral sclerosis and myasthenia gravis—may cause dysphonia and dysphagia without other signs early in the course of the diseases. Always consider myasthenia gravis when the Pt has any unexplained weakness of bulbar muscles. Semirhythmic contractions of the abdominal wall and diaphragmatic flutter may be secondary to "belly dancer's" dyskinesia (Iliceto et al, 2004). Dyphagia lusoria may be associated with an aberrant right subclavian artery. A review of patients previously diagnosed with psychogenic dysphagia showed that a medical cause was found in two-thirds of cases (Ravich et al., 1990).

D. Psychogenic vomiting

In Pts with conversion disorder and malingering, the vomiting occurs mainly in the presence of emotionally significant people. Malingerers may simulate gastrointestinal bleeding by secretly adding blood to their vomitus or stool. The Pt with anorexia nervosa or bulimia vomits in the bathroom or in secret.

E. Psychogenic disturbances of station and gait

1. **General features of astasia-abasia:** Most common gait disorders are hemiparetic, paraparetic, ataxic, or trembling gait (Keane, 1989), and astasiaabasia. ***Astasia*** means the inability to stand, and ***abasia*** means the inability to walk. Taken together the two words imply total inability to stand and walk, but often with the Ex's suggestion the Pt may attempt to do so (Keane, 1989). Patients with atasia-abasia show wild gyrations when standing or walking. The Pt rarely falls, or falls into the Ex's arms (or a chair) without suffering bodily injury. The flamboyant gyrations without falling testify eloquently to the competency of the Pt's motor system and balance. When in bed or sitting, the Pt may show no disability or only minor disturbances of movement. On the *Romberg test*, the Pt will usually sway much more with the eyes closed. Review pages 410–411 for the methods of diverting the Pt into a normal performance on this test.
2. **Hemiparetic and hemiplegic gaits:** In psychogenic hemiplegia, the lower part of the face ipsilateral to the hemiplegia is not involved; the protruded tongue, if it deviates at all, deviates toward the normal side (Keane, 1986). Tongue deviation is uncommon in organic hemiplegia, but when it occurs the deviation is to the hemiplegic side. The arm and leg do not assume true hemiplegic postures when the Pt is at rest or when walking (Fig. 12-15; Keane, 1989). The leg of the organic hemiplegic turns outward when the Pt is recumbent. The abdominal, plantar, and muscle stretch reflexes are always normal. The hand is not preferentially affected as in organic hemiparesis.
3. **Dragging monoplegic gait:** The Pt walks with the good leg forward and the monoplegic limb dragging behind. The foot may be turned out or inverted or everted (Stone et al., 2002). Sudden buckling of the knee is also common.
4. **Psychogenic paraplegia:** Key differences on the NE are the presence of normal abdominal or cremasteric, muscle stretch, and plantar reflexes, normal muscle tone, and retention of bowel and bladder control in psychogenic paraplegia and their usual impairment in organic paraplegia (Baker and Silver, 1987).
    a. Sensory changes tend to be highly variable, may not match the motor level, and do not show the dissociated loss between anterolateral and dorsal columns or the sacral sparing that may characterize organic paraplegia (Table 14-3).

TABLE 14-3 · Differentiation of Psychogenic and Organic Paraplegia

	Nonorganic paraplegia	Organic paraplegia
Onset	Usually arises suddenly after stress in a person with a psychiatric predisposition	May evolve slowly or suddenly in a patient with a predisposing organic cause
Attitude to illness	May seem indifferent or histrionic	Appropriate concern
MSR	Present and normal	Absent in spinal shock or very brisk
Clonus	Absent or unsustained	Sustained
Muscle tone	Normal	Flaccid acutely, then spastic
Plantar response	Normal plantar flexion of great toe	Dorsiflexion of great toe unless spinal shock is present
Abdominal/cremasteric reflex	Present	Absent, depending on level
Umbilical migration	Absent	Upward migration if lesion affects T10 (Beevor's sign)
Sensory level	Extends horizontally around waist; variable; differs from motor level	Slants obliquely downward; constant border if lesion static
Inadvertent leg use	May move legs inadvertently for postural support, in sleep, or with Hoover's test	Does not move legs if the paraplegia is complete but may show flexor spasms
Sphincter control	Present	Lost
Anal wink reflex	Present	Lost in stage of spinal shock
MRI, SSEV, and cystometrogram	Normal but usually not needed	Abnormal

ABBREVIATIONS: MRI = magnetic resonance imaging; MSR = muscle stretch reflex; SSEP = somatosensory evoked potentials.

b. The T10 level of the spinal cord supplies the umbilical level of the abdomen (Fig. 2-10). With organic paraplegia from a T10 level lesion, the skeletal muscles of the lower two quadrants of the abdomen are paralyzed along with all other muscles distal to T10. The upper quadrant skin-muscle reflexes will be preserved but absent in the lower two quadrants. The Pt shows Beevor's sign when attempting to do a sit-up, i.e., the intact upper quadrant abdominal muscles cause the umbilicus to migrate *upward* because of no corresponding anchoring pull from the muscles of the paralyzed lower quadrants. This sign never occurs in psychogenic paraplegia.

6. **Caveats:** Recall that Pts with the rostral or caudal vermis syndromes may show little dysfunction when reclining but display dystaxia when walking, particularly when tandem walking. Camptocormia (bent spine), initially attributed to a psychogenic disorder, can have many causes including a variety of neuromuscular disorders, flexion dystonia of the trunk, extensor myopathy, and parkinsonism. Patients with involuntary movement syndromes, in particular dystonia musculorum deformans, frequently get diagnosed as having a psychogenic disorder in the early stages of their illness. Astasia abasia has also been related to normal pressure hydrocephalus. Status cataplecticus ("limp man syndrome" due to narcolepsy has been mistaken for a psychogenic disorder (Simon et al., 2004). See the gait essay at the end of Chapter 8.

F. Techniques and observations that separate psychogenic paresis or paralysis of trunk and limbs from organic paralysis

1. **Demeanor of the Pt:** The Pt's demeanor during testing of strength often provides a clue to psychogenic weakness. Usually the Pt with psychogenic paralysis makes a great show of effort to move the afflicted part, but to no avail. Thus, the Pt may grimace, grunt, or squirm, and show obvious strain, but the part does not move. It is a dramatic performance meant to communicate sincerity of effort, rather than a simple attempt to move the part, as in organic paralysis. The hysteric with partial paralysis usually moves the part very slowly. Often the Ex can see and feel that the putatively weak muscles in such a movement in fact contract very strongly. Thus, in grip testing, the Pt often co-contracts the flexors and extensors very strongly, demonstrating intact innervation, which the Ex can see and palpate. Because the Pt contracts all muscles isometrically, the Pt's fingers only encircle the Ex's fingers very lightly, not actually closing tightly on them. When the Ex tugs against a muscle to test strength, the Pt may offer considerable resistance and then yield suddenly, or may show a series of jactitating, cogwheel-like releases. Objective recording of strength by myometry shows different patterns of contractions in psychogenic weakness, normal individuals, and organically paralyzed Pts (van der Ploeg and Oosterhuis, 1991).
2. **Distribution of psychogenic paralysis:** Although the psychogenic paralysis may follow monoplegic, hemiplegic, or paraplegic distributions, it seldom affects individual muscles or groups of muscles innervated by one peripheral nerve or root. The limbs do not assume organic postures, as in organic hemiplegia, and the overall lack of signs, particularly the normal reflexes, establishes the psychogenic nature of the paralysis.
3. **Eliciting inadvertent or automatic movements (synkinesias) of the paralyzed parts in psychogenic motor disorders**

   a. **Sleep:** Several inadvertent or synkinetic movements establish the integrity of the putatively paralyzed part. The Pt with psychogenic monoplegia, hemiplegia, or paraplegia moves the parts in the normal manner during sleep. When dressing the Pt may inadvertently reach out with the affected part or use it automatically for postural support. This is a key principle: **The Ex finds some way to activate the putatively paralyzed muscles inadvertently or synkinetically.**

   b. **Monrad-Krohn's cough test for arm monoparesis (1922):** To identify psychogenic paralysis of the arm, the Ex stands behind the Pt and grasps the two latissimus dorsi muscles between the thumb and fingers of the right and left hands. The Ex asks the Pt to cough forcefully. Both latissimus dorsi muscles synkinetically contract strongly, thus establishing the integrity of the motor pathway through the brachial plexus.

c. **Double-crossed-arm pull test for psychogenic arm monoparesis**

   i. When required to use both sides simultaneously and unexpectedly, the psychogenic Pt will generally inadvertently contract the putatively weak side along with the normal side.

   ii. Start with the Pt upright and the forearms crossed and flexed (Fig. 14-1). If the Pt's arm is completely paralyzed, hold it in place.

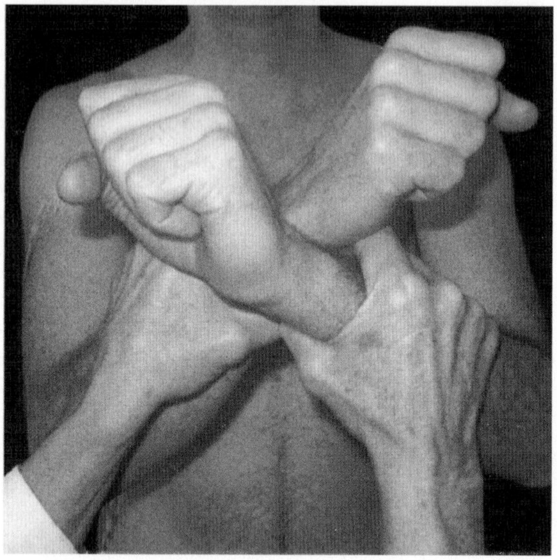

FIGURE 14-1. The double-crossed-arm pull test for psychogenic paresis of one arm. The examiner's hands grip the patient's forearms. See text for instructions.

   iii. While holding the Pt's forearms as shown in Fig. 14-1, say: "When I say *now,* try to pull back strongly away from me, and I'll hold you in place." Then say *now* after a brief pause. Usually the Pt braces the paretic and nonparetic arms when pulling back.

d. **Make-a-fist test for psychogenic wrist drop**

   i. To distinguish a psychogenic wrist drop from a radial nerve palsy, ask the Pt to extend the arm out straight. The putatively paralyzed wrist hangs limply (Fig. 14-2A).

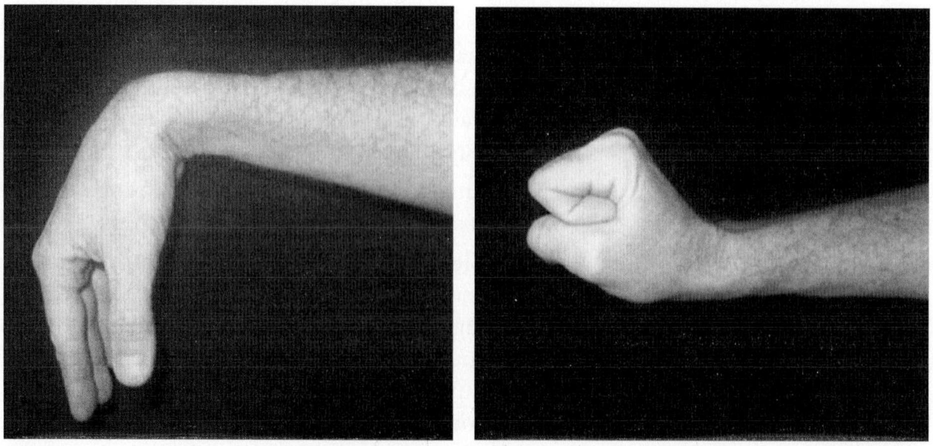

A B

FIGURE 14-2. Make-a-fist-test for psychogenic wrist drop. (A) With the forearm extended, the patient has an apparent wrist drop. (B) When the patient makes a fist, the wrist automatically dorsiflexes, proving that the extensor muscles are intact.

ii. Instruct the Pt to suddenly make a strong fist when you say *now*.

iii. If intact, the putatively paralyzed wrist extensors automatically cock the hand up into the "anatomic position" when the Pt makes a fist (Fig. 14-2B). Try this test yourself. In a true radial palsy, the wrist does not cock up.

iv. As a refinement of the test, ask the Pt to grip a screwdriver or rod strongly or to grip the rod strongly with both hands simultaneously.

e. **Reversed hands test for arm monoparesis**

i. To identify psychogenic hand paralysis, the Ex has the Pt reverse and invert the hands (Figs. 14-3A and 14-3B).

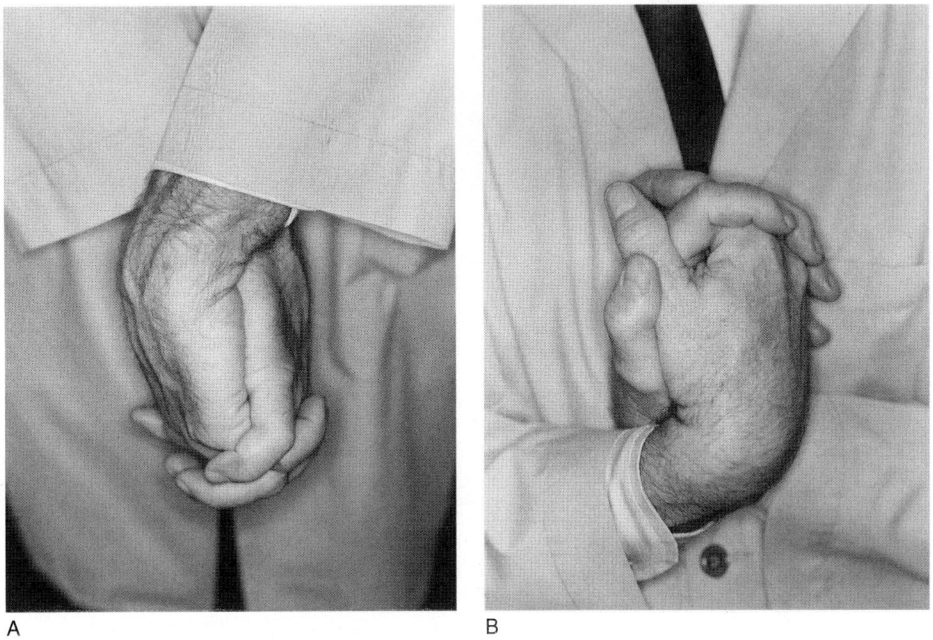

FIGURE 14-3. Inverted-hands test for psychogenic loss of sensation or motor function. (A) Clasp fingers as shown, with hands crossed and palms together. (B) Invert the hands. The final posture in B reverses right for left. See text for further instruction.

ii. Then ask the Pt to look at the fingers. The Ex then points to but does not touch a finger and asks the Pt to move that finger. Usually the Pt moves the finger of the hand opposite to the one pointed to by the Ex. Try this test on a partner. After a few trials, the subject learns to respond accurately. Thus, the test serves best during the first trials. The test also works for psychogenic anesthesia. With the Pt's eyes closed, the Ex actually touches the finger of one hand or the other. The Pt usually moves the finger of the putatively anesthetic hand.

f. **Backward displacement test for psychogenic foot drop**

i. To distinguish a psychogenic foot drop from a peroneal nerve palsy, ask the Pt to stand with the eyes closed.

ii. Place one hand flat on the Pt's sternum and suddenly displace the Pt backward, using the other hand on the Pt's back to prevent a fall.

iii. The Ex will see the dorsiflexor tendons of the feet spring into action as the Pt automatically reacts to the displacement.

g. **Hoover's test for psychogenic leg monoparesis**

i. With the Pt recumbent, stand at the foot of the examination table with one palm under each of the Pt's heels (Fig. 14-4A).

ii. Ask the Pt to press down with the putatively paretic leg. The heel will not press down on the Ex's palm.

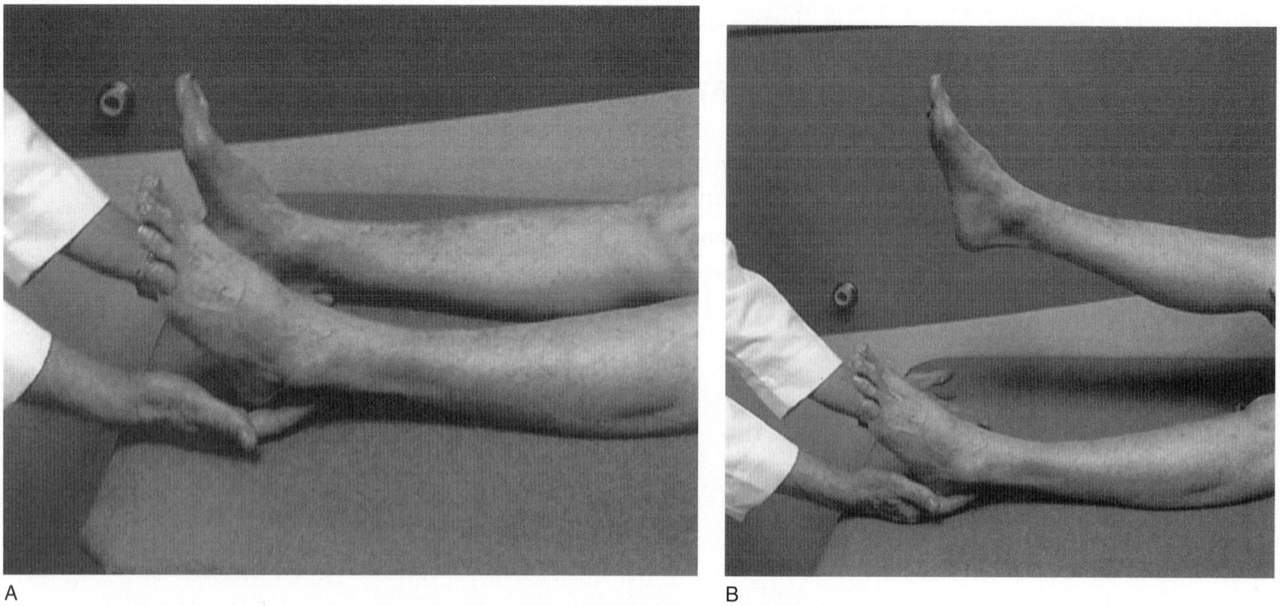

FIGURE 14-4. Hoover's leg-elevation test for psychogenic paralysis of one leg. The examiner places a hand under each of the patient's heels. Then the examiner asks the patient to forcefully raise the normal leg. The patient will inadvertently push down with the putatively paralyzed leg.

iii. Ask the Pt to lift the *normal* leg up briskly in one motion. The paretic leg will press down against the Ex's palm as an automatic, synkinetic counteraction that the Ex can feel and see (Fig. 14-4B; Stone et al., 2002).

iv. Ask the Pt to press down with both heels. Usually the Pt with psychogenic paralysis presses down with both heels, whereas the Pt with organic paralysis does not.

v. As a refinement of this test, place one hand under the paralyzed limb, press down on the knee of the sound limb, and instruct the Pt to lift it as strongly as possible. The putatively paralyzed limb will synkinetically press down.

h. **Raimiste's leg adduction-abduction synkinesis for psychogenic leg monoparesis**

i. The same principle of inadvertent synkinetic bracing of the putatively paralyzed part applies in testing adduction and abduction of the legs.

ii. With the Pt recumbent, place your hands on the Pt's knees and ask the Pt to squeeze the legs together strongly as you hold your hands in place, in opposition to the Pt's action (Fig. 14-5A).

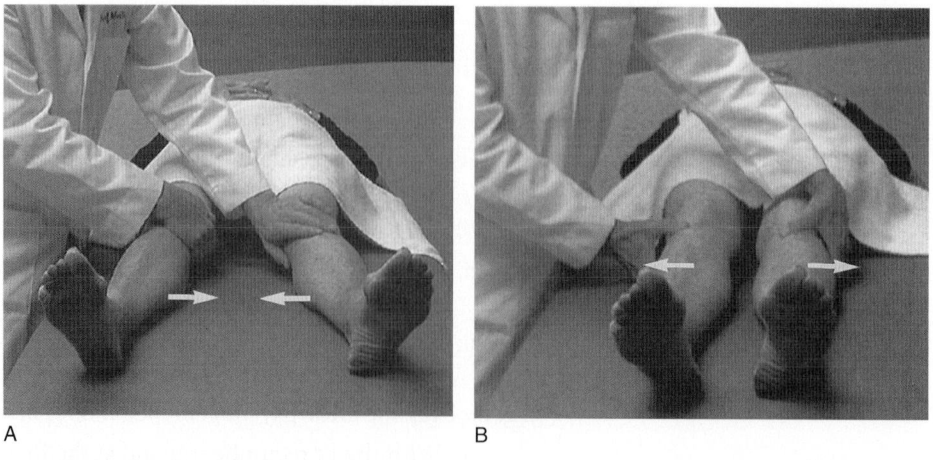

FIGURE 14-5. Raimiste's leg-adduction and -abduction test for psychogenic leg paresis. (A) The patient tries to *ad*duct, i.e., squeeze both legs strongly together (arrows) against the examiner's manual opposition. (B) The patient tries to *ab*duct, i.e., separate both legs strongly (arrows) against the examiner's manual opposition. In each case, the patient synkinetically braces the putatively paretic leg.

iii. The Pt usually braces the putatively paralyzed limb in automatic opposition to the action of the intact limb.

iv. Similarly, ask the Pt to press the legs apart strongly against your manual resistance. The putatively paralyzed limb usually will abduct in automatic opposition (Fig. 14-5B).

4. **Review of formal tests to produce synkinetic movements of putatively paralyzed muscles in Pts with psychogenic weakness**

a. Describe the Monrad-Krohn cough test for psychogenic brachial plexus/arm paralysis. ______________________________

See frame II F 3 b.

b. Name the muscle tested in the foregoing test ______________.

latissimus dorsi

c. Test for psychogenic arm monoparesis (double pull test). ______________________________

See frame II F 3 c.

d. Test for psychogenic wrist drop. ______________________________

See frame II F 3 d.

e. What major nerve, when interrupted, causes a wrist drop? ______________________________

Radial nerve.

f. Test for psychogenic foot drop. ______________________________

See frame II F 3 f.

g. What major nerve, when interrupted, causes a foot drop? ______________________________

Common peroneal nerve.

h. Test for psychogenic leg monoparesis (Hoover's test). ______________________________

See frame II F 3 g.

i. Describe how to do Raimiste's adduction-abduction test for psychogenic leg paralysis. ______________________________

See frame II F 3 h.

j. Try all of the foregoing tests on a companion.

5. Magnetic stimulation of the motor cortex can move the putatively paralyzed limb, thus proving that the pyramidal and peripheral pathways are intact (Pilai et al., 1991).

G. Psychogenic tremors

The tremor varies greatly in intensity and frequency and is present at rest, during a sustained posture, and during movement, in contrast to most organic tremors (Koller et al., 1989), midbrain or so-called rubral tremor excepted (Reza Samie et al., 1990). See Chapter 7 and Table 14-4.

TABLE 14-4 · Clinical Features of Psychogenic Tremor

1. Abrupt onset
2. Static course
3. Spontaneous remissions
4. Unclassifiable tremors (complex tremors)
5. Clinical inconsistencies (selective disabilities)
6. Changing tremor characteristics
7. Unresponsiveness to antitremor drugs
8. Tremor increases with attention
9. Tremor lessens with distractibility
10. Responsiveness to placebo
11. Absence of other neurologic signs
12. Remission with psychotherapy

SOURCE: Koller W, Lang A, Vetere-Overfield B, et al. Psychogenic tremors. *Neurology* 1989;39:1094–1099.

III. PSYCHOGENIC DISORDERS OF VISION

A. Range of symptoms

The visual symptoms consist of diminished vision or blindness, nonanatomic visual field defects, diplopia, and photophobia.

B. Psychogenic blindness

1. **Establishing the integrity of the visual pathways**
   a. The Pt retains pupillary light reactions, and the fundi appear normal.
   b. The Pt has no signs of cerebral lesions extensive enough to cause cortical blindness and no history compatible with such lesions.
   c. The organically blind Pt moves cautiously and slowly, rarely banging into objects. Psychogenically blind persons may bang into objects, as if to prove they can't see.
   d. The eyes of the psychogenically blind Pt may glance at a moving object that appears unexpectedly. Placing a mirror directly in front of the Pt and moving it may cause the Pt's eyes to pursue their reflection. The Pt may show optokinetic nystagmus (railroad nystagmus) when exposed to a rotating drum or moving stripes. However, Pts can inhibit optokinetic nystagmus. Its presence thus establishes the integrity of the retinogeniculo-calcarine pathway and the efferent optomotor pathway to the brainstem from the occipital cortex, but the absence of nystagmus does not prove that the Pt has a lesion.
   e. If the Pt has monocular psychogenic blindness, the swinging flashlight test will not demonstrate an afferent defect (Chapter 4, Section VI A 5).
   f. The Ex may induce the Pt to have double vision by applying canthal compression (Fig. 4-4), or the ophthalmologist can use prisms to prove that the putatively blind eye sees. Different colored lenses on each eye serve the same purpose (Liu et al., 2001).
   g. **Electrical tests:** The electroretinogram in patients with psychogenic disorders of vision remains normal, the electroencephalogram (EEG) shows a photic driving response, and visual evoked potential studies prove that impulses reach the visual cortex (Chapter 13).
2. **Caveats**
   a. Even evoked responses are not beyond manipulation, because the Pt's thoughts can change the pattern evoked (Bumgartner and Epstein, 1982; Tan et al., 1984).
   b. Acute retrobulbar neuritis can cause acute, complete blindness in an eye with a normal-appearing fundus before optic atrophy sets in. The diseased eye will show a diminished or absent direct pupillary light reflex, and the opposite pupil will fail to show a consensual reflex. The swinging flashlight test will show the afferent defect (Chapter 4, Section VI A 5).
   c. In Anton's syndrome, a bilateral, occipital lobe lesion causes bilateral cortical blindness, but the pupillary responses remain intact. Although obviously blind, the Pt confabulates vision, describing nonexistent scenes around him. The disorder qualifies as an anosognosia for blindness. During the diaschisis that may follow an acute, severe unilateral occipital lobe lesion, Anton's syndrome may occur temporarily. In these cases, magnetic resonance imaging will show the cerebral lesion.

C. Psychogenic visual field defects

The typical psychogenic visual field defect consists of constriction of the diameter of the field, thereby producing tunnel or tubular vision, as if the person were looking through a tunnel. In a closely allied phenomenon, the spiral visual field, the size of the field diminishes on successive trials. In tunnel vision, the visual field remains the same diameter for near and far objects (Fig. 14-6).

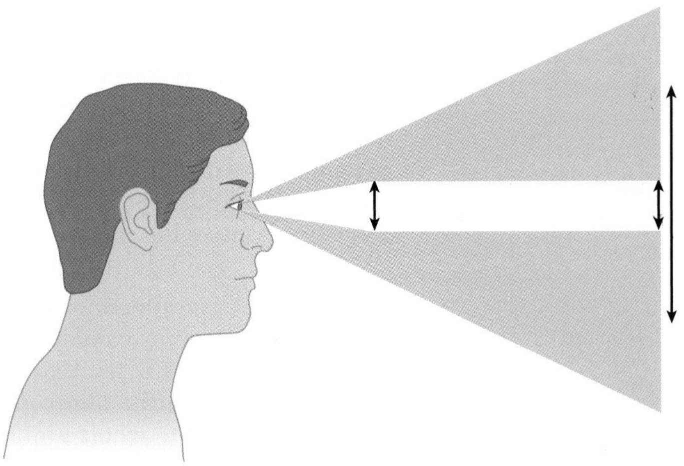

FIGURE 14-6. Illustration of tunnel vision in a patient with hysteria. The normal visual field expands. In tunnel vision the field remains the same size for targets at different distances.

D. Monocular diplopia

1. The spectrum of psychogenic ophthalmologic manifestations include monocular diplopia. The diplopia will not follow any of the laws of diplopia (Chapter 4), the corneal light reflections remain aligned, and the cover-uncover test remains normal.
2. **Caveat:** A dislocated lens; a fold, detachment, or elevation of the retina; or a hole in the iris may cause organic monocular diplopia, but the ocular examination and ophthalmoscopy easily differentiate these conditions.

E. Photophobia

Pain in the eyes on exposure to light may occur with hysteria or with organic illnesses, e.g., iritis. Careful slit-lamp examination and ophthalmologic investigation must rule out definable organic disease.

IV. PSYCHOGENIC DEAFNESS

A. Clinical and laboratory tests to establish the integrity of the auditory pathway

The psychogenically deaf Pt may turn when addressed unexpectedly from the side or may show a startle response to sudden sound when awake or asleep. The presence of a response indicates an intact auditory pathway, but absence of a response does not establish organic deafness. The tuning-fork tests of Weber and Rinne described in Chapter 9 may produce bizarre results. Audiologists have several methods of manipulating sound to recognize hysterical deafness, which, combined with the brainstem evoked response test (Chapter 13) showing evoked potentials recorded over the auditory cortex, document the integrity of the auditory pathways.

B. Caveat: acute viral illness, vascular occlusion, or pontine tegmental lesions can cause sudden deafness, with no other evidence of neurologic disease

V. PSCHOGENIC DISORDERS OF SOMATIC SENSATION

A. Range of disorders

Patients with psychogenic somatosensory disorders may complain of anesthesia, paresthesia, hyperesthesia, or pain in the body or extremities. The anesthesia usually affects all sensory modalities. If the Pt loses one modality, it usually affects touch or pain, not vibration or position sense.

B. Nonanatomic distribution of psychogenic sensory loss

1. Psychogenic sensory losses follow nonanatomic distributions and often have variable but very sharp borders from examination to examination. **Psychogenic sensory losses conform to the Pt's mental image of the body, not to the actual anatomic pattern of innervation by peripheral nerves, nerve roots, or central pathways** (Fig. 10-3). Chapter 10 explained how organic facial anesthesia from a V nerve lesion spares the angle of the mandible, which receives its sensory innervation from C2. See Figs. 10-2 and 14-7A.
2. In psychogenic anesthesia of an extremity, the loss usually includes the hand or foot and extends proximally to stop abruptly at a line transverse to the long axis of the limb, as if the extremity were amputated (seemingly a mental amputation). Often the transverse line crosses the wrist or elbow. In hysterical anesthesia of the whole arm, the loss often stops sharply at the shoulder joint, thus conforming to the Pt's mental image of an arm but not to the actual innervation by dermatomes, peripheral nerves, or central pathways. See Figs. 14-7C and 14-7D. In psychogenic lower extremity anesthesia, the proximal border often falls at the waist or the gluteal fold posteriorly or the inguinal line anteriorly (Figs. 14-7E and 14-7F). As the anesthesia improves, the border moves distally along the limb, stopping at successive transverse levels until it disappears.

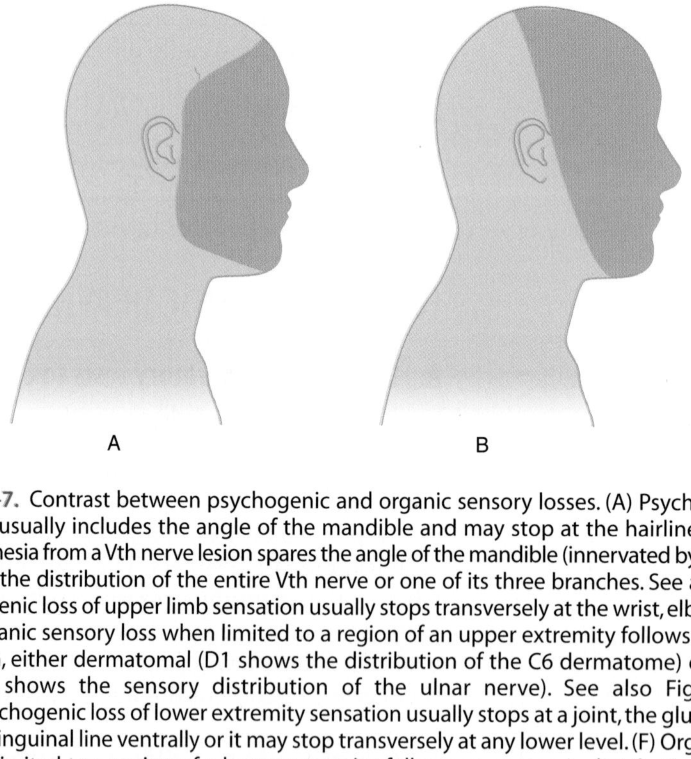

FIGURE 14-7. Contrast between psychogenic and organic sensory losses. (A) Psychogenic facial anesthesia usually includes the angle of the mandible and may stop at the hairline. (B) Organic facial anesthesia from a Vth nerve lesion spares the angle of the mandible (innervated by C2). The border follows the distribution of the entire Vth nerve or one of its three branches. See also Fig. 10-2. (C) Psychogenic loss of upper limb sensation usually stops transversely at the wrist, elbow, or shoulder. (D) Organic sensory loss when limited to a region of an upper extremity follows an anatomic distribution, either dermatomal (D1 shows the distribution of the C6 dermatome) or peripheral nerve (D2 shows the sensory distribution of the ulnar nerve). See also Figs. 2-10 and 2-11. (E) Psychogenic loss of lower extremity sensation usually stops at a joint, the gluteal fold dorsally, or the inguinal line ventrally or it may stop transversely at any lower level. (F) Organic sensory loss, when limited to a region of a lower extremity, follows an anatomic distribution, either dermatomal (F1 shows L5 dermatome) or peripheral nerve (F2 shows lateral femoral cutaneous nerve). See also Figs. 2-10 and 2-11.

3. In psychogenic paraplegia with a sensory level, the line circles the body horizontally; in organic paraplegia, the dermatomes slant downward in the abdomen; but this distinction is not absolute (Fig. 2-10 and Table 14-3). The abdominal reflexes and other reflexes below the level remain.

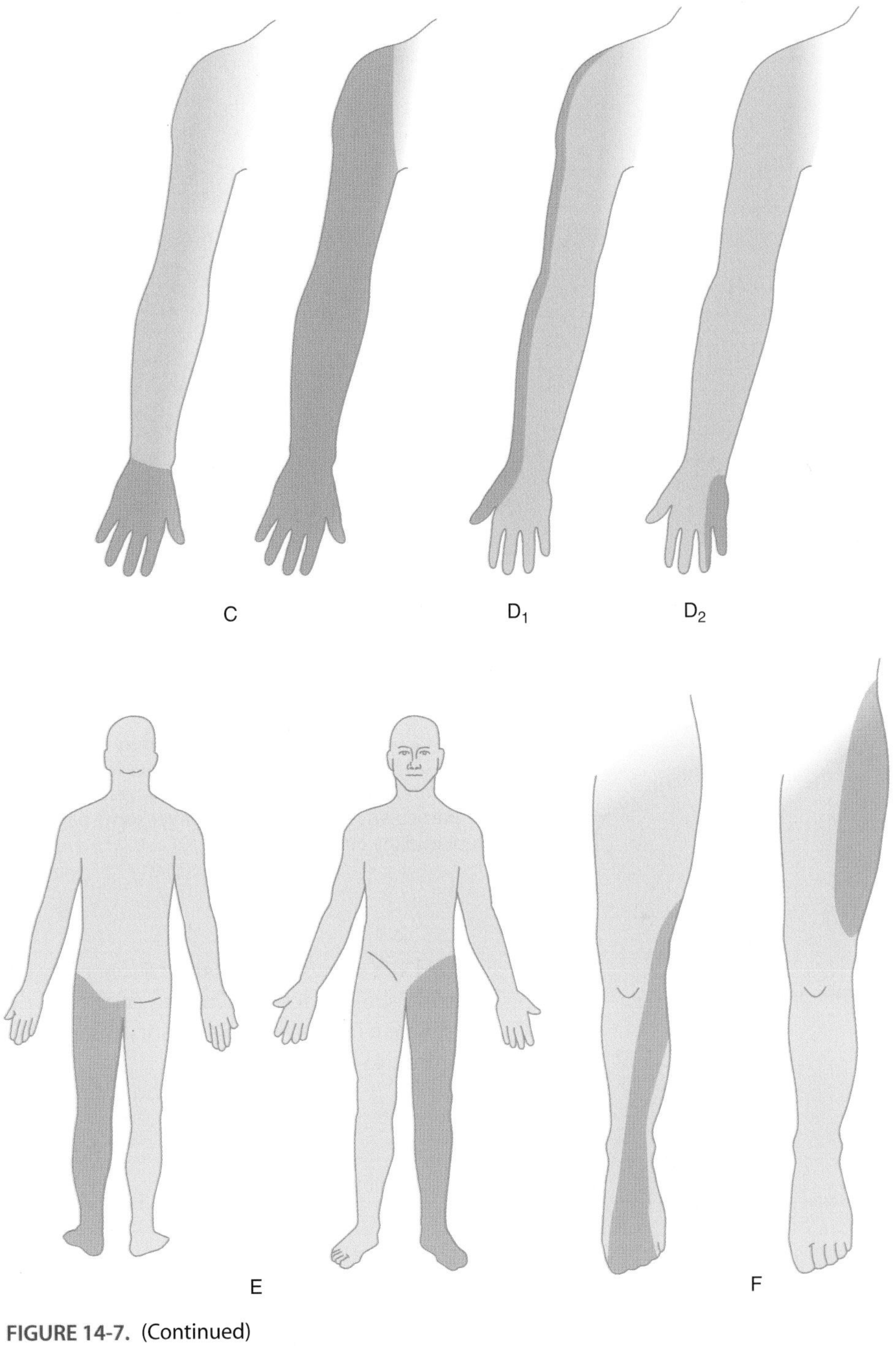

FIGURE 14-7. (Continued)

4. Some Pts show psychogenic hemianesthesia. The Pt not only loses all somatic sensation from one-half of the body but also may lose sight, hearing, taste, and smell on the affected side, an obvious anatomic impossibility. In psychogenic hemianesthesia, the sensory loss stops sharply at the midline and may run up the entire body and head as in the mental image of one-half of the body. The psychogenic Pt with hemisensory loss, for example, reports complete absence of vibratory sensation when a tuning fork, applied to the sternum or forehead, just reaches the midline. In fact, the vibration travels some distance through the bone, and its perception does not cut off sharply at the midline (Figs. 14-8A and 14-8B). Patients with organic hemisensory loss also may show a sharp cutoff. Thus, the finding is not pathognomonic of psychogenic disease (Stone et al., 2002).

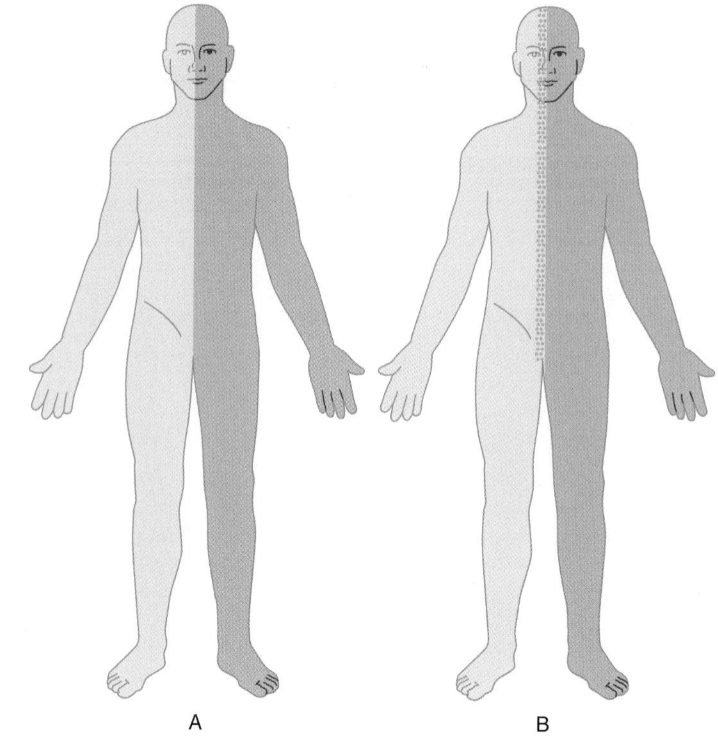

FIGURE 14-8. Some differences in the borders of psychogenic and organic sensory losses in hemianesthesia. (A) In psychogenic hemianesthesia, the sensory loss usually stops abruptly at the midline for all modalities. (B) In organic hemianesthesia, the sensory loss may fade gradually at the midline, particularly for vibration. However, some patients with organic hemisensory loss also have an abrupt midline cutoff.

5. Figure 14-9 shows the usual differences in the border zone of organic and psychogenic sensory losses. The site of the border between the anesthetic and the normal zone in psychogenic sensory disorders, although usually sharp, may change from time to time.

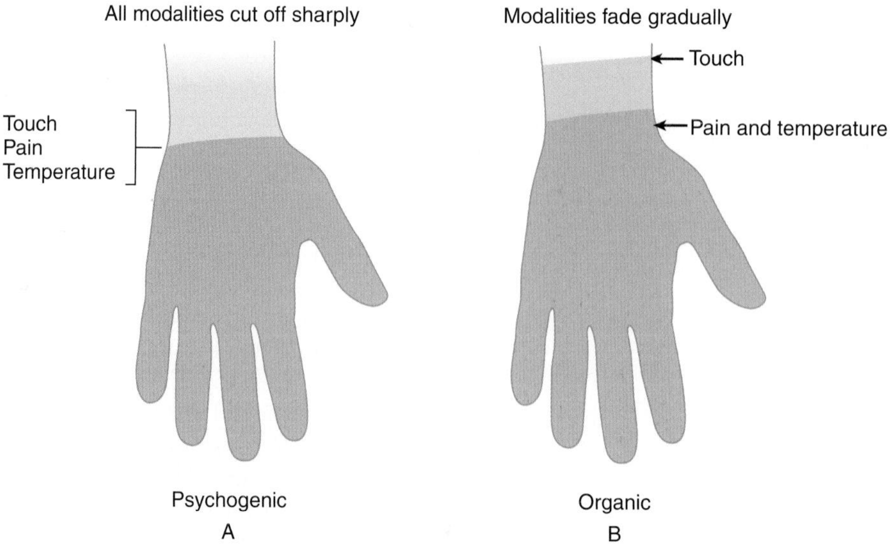

FIGURE 14-9. Contrast between psychogenic and organic stocking-glove sensory loss. (A) In psychogenic stocking-glove sensory loss, the proximal border stops sharply at a joint line or skin crevice for all modalities. (B) In organic stocking-glove sensory loss, the proximal border usually fades gradually and differs for the various modalities.

C. Inadvertent proof that a sensory deficit is nonorganic

1. **Normal motor function:** If the Pt has psychogenic anesthesia for all modalities, not anesthesia plus paralysis, the Pt may use the part completely normally, which is impossible without proprioception. This fact plus the *preservation* of stretch reflexes and *absence* of hypotonia, atrophy, and dystaxia prove that the Pt cannot have organic anesthesia. Complete sensory loss must produce areflexia, hypotonia, and sensory dystaxia. (Review Table 10-3 for the features of sensory dystaxia.) During sleep the Pt will withdraw the putatively anesthetic extremity from pain.
2. **Rhythmic responses:** In testing touch or pain responses, the Ex may elicit a rhythm of answering that inadvertently discloses the integrity of the sensation in the putatively anesthetic or analgesic area. Ordinarily, to maintain the Pt's attention, the Ex avoids such a rhythm in Pts with organic sensory deficits. Starting with areas of intact sensation, get the Pt to respond by saying *yes* when you apply the stimulus or *no* when you withhold it. Then, unexpectedly, out of rhythm, incorporate the anesthetic region in the testing. If the Pt says *no* each time just after the Ex unexpectedly touches the anesthetic zone, then at some level of consciousness, the Pt has perceived the stimulus.
3. **Pattern of exactly opposite responses:** In responding to position sense testing, the psychogenic Pt may give exactly opposite answers, saying, e.g., *down* each time for *up*. The fact that the Pt gives exactly the opposite response each time means that position sense has to be intact. Even with total absence of position sense, the Pt should guess the right answer about half of the time. Malingerers are more likely to produce this pattern.
4. **Histrionic underreaction or exaggerated overreaction:** Some Pts respond very slowly and deliberately to sensory tests. The Pt conveys the impression of trying very hard to feel the stimulus and report it correctly, i.e., a *pseudo*-cooperation. Other Pts give a studied response of feeling it "just a little bit," even after strong stimulation. In psychogenic analgesia, do not continue to apply increasingly strong pain stimuli to prove a point (or express frustration with a puzzling sensory examination). In contrast to these underreacting Pts, others overreact to sensory stimuli. The Ex learns to recognize the histrionic overreaction or studied underreaction as inadvertent evidence of the nonorganic nature of the sensory deficit.

D. Caveats

In deciding whether a sensory loss is psychogenic or not, review the Steps in the Analysis of a Sensory Complaint (Chapter 10, Section XI). Recall also that organic pain may be referred to or radiate beyond the confines of an anatomic territory; conversely, the Pt with organic loss may impose a "body scheme" pattern. Some Pts with organic disease have true hyperesthesia, sometimes of excruciating type, as in causalgia, or trigger zones where the slightest stimulus of a particular site elicits unbearable pain, as in trigeminal neuralgia. Some Pts with thalamic or parietal lesions will show hemisensory losses that imitate a midline psychogenic pattern (Stone et al., 2002; Yarnell et al., 1978). See Fig. 14-8.

VI. PSYCHOGENIC NONEPILEPTIC SEIZURES

A. Definition

Psychogenic nonepileptic seizures are episodes of altered motor, sensory, or mental function that resemble epileptic seizures but arise from psychological disturbances rather than from an abnormal hypersynchronous discharge of neurons (see the definition of epilepsy, page 306). The spells occur after some identifiable precipitating event. Most commonly, they occur in the presence of someone emotionally significant to the Pt, such as a parent or lover, or to avoid some unpleasant obligation. No single pathognomonic clinical feature separates true from pseudoepileptic seizures.

Pseudoepileptic seizures may manifest as pure unresponsiveness without motor activity—in other words, a swoon or staring spell (Geyer et al., 2000; Leis et al., 1992)—or with motor actions.

B. Motor manifestations of psychogenic seizures

1. The pseudoepileptic motor activities include bizarre patterns of flailing, thrashing, or quivering. In contrast, a true generalized motor seizure presents a stereotyped sequence of an aura, a cry, a fall, the tonus, the clonus, incontinence, and postictal confusion and somnolence. The clonic movements die gradually in a characteristic way. Pseudoseizure Pts show more random, out-of-phase movements, with the extremities on the two sides often doing different things. Epileptic movements are more often rhythmic, in-phase bilaterally symmetrical tonic-clonic jerks; however, myoclonic seizures may present as random jerks.
2. In addition to extremity movements, the Pts with psychogenic seizures make side-to-side rocking head and body movements, rarely seen in true epilepsy. The posturing and jerking vary in intensity during the seizure (Meierkord et al., 1991; Rowan and Gates, 1993). Epileptic Pts may injure themselves by falling or biting their tongues. Pseudoseizure Pts may do the same, although much less frequently.
3. Patients with epileptic or psychogenic seizure show pelvic thrusting. Pelvic thrusting is strongly associated only with the thrashing type of pseudo-seizure (Geyer et al., 2000).

C. Physiologic changes in psychogenic versus true seizures

1. Usually, in psychogenic seizures, the blood pressure, pulse rate, and pupillary size do not change materially, whereas in organic seizures they often change dramatically. Particularly with quiet staring spells of organic origin, the heart rate increases more than 30%, whereas in psychogenic seizures it does not (Opherk and Hirsch, 2002). True crying may occur in psychogenic seizures but excessively rarely in epileptic seizure (Lesser, 1996). However, laughter occurs in some epileptic seizures.
2. Serum prolactin, when measured at 10 to 20 minutes after a suspected ictal event, is elevated in approximately 90% of Pts who have just had a generalized tonic-clonic seizure and more than 50% of those who have had complex partial seizures.
3. Table 14-5 summarizes the differences between psychogenic and true seizures.
4. Two spells that, broadly considered, fall into the psychogenic category but are distinct clinically from the usual psychogenic seizure are breath-holding spells in infants and young children (page 527) and behavioral "tuning out" or staring spells. Normal babies, normal older persons, and especially learning disabled children frequently show spells consisting of an arrest of activity and a blank stare. You likely have noticed a tendency to sit and stare, to "blank out," at times, when events seem overwhelming or insolvable. The learning disabled child may show these spells repeatedly in the classroom or at home. The hallmark is that the observer can always terminate the spell abruptly by a stimulus such as touching the person or calling that person's name.

D. Caveats

1. **Range of true epileptic seizures:** Almost every conceivable neurologic symptom or sign has occurred in some Pt at some time as a true epileptic seizure. Epileptic seizures that arise in the frontal lobes may manifest by bicycle peddling motions, asymmetric tonic posturing (fencing position), often without loss of consciousness. Seizures arising in the supplementary motor area may also manifest as screaming, and even sexual activity (genital manipulation, pelvic thrusting). No matter how bizarre, the attack may be organic, including fugue states or confusional attacks (Ellis and Lee, 1978; Manford and Shorvon, 1992; Markand et al., 1978). **In many instances, even the most experienced neurologist observing an**

attack cannot distinguish psychogenic attacks from organic ones. Pseudoepileptic seizures occur in adolescents and children, but rarely before age 8 to 10 years. Although pseudoseizures can occur at night, they do so only when the Pt is already awake, but true epileptic seizures may occur during sleep (Lesser, 1996).

TABLE 14-5 · Differentiation of Psychogenic and Epileptic Seizures

	Psychogenic nonepileptic seizures	Epileptic seizures
Cause	Psychiatric predisposition always present; comorbid depression, sexual/physical abuse, anxiety, dissociative, and somatoform disorders; differentiate culture-bound syndromes	Hypersynchronous neuronal discharge based on anatomic or metabolic disease; specific triggers uncommon, but touch, sight, sound, or mental activities, e. g., calculation, may elicit a seizure
Onset	Onset often gradual, over minutes	Onset with brief aura or instantaneously
Location/ circumstances	Usually at home, in the presence of emotionally significant persons; do not occur while asleep	Occur anywhere, anytime, night or day, during sleep or wakefulness, and may follow a diurnal pattern
Induction of seizure	Often inducible by suggestion, or placebo challenge, i.e., IV saline, etc; patient may hyperventilate	Not induced by suggestion; hyperventilation may induce a seizure, especially petit mal
Vocalization/ Emotion	Vocalization may take the form of sobbing, yelling, or bizarre utterances	Overt, single outcry may initiate a generalized seizure, but formed words or sobbing are rare; laughter may occur (gelastic epilepsy)
Frequency	May be several per day	Except for petit mal and myoclonic seizures, other seizure types usually less than one per day
Motor activity	Variability from moment to moment; arrhythmic or out-of-phase movements on the two sides; rolling, side-to-side head or trunk movements; pelvic thrusting common with thrashing type of seizures; may be simply staring or akinetic	Usually follow a stereotyped pattern, depending on seizure type; staring spells often accompanied by twitch of face, blinking, or lip smacking; pure akinetic seizures are rare; pelvic thrusting uncommonly occurs
Duration	Often prolonged, >5 min, and may imitate status epilepticus; may come out of spell when addressed or stimulated	Usually <3 min but may have status epilepticus; addressing or stimulating the patient does not terminate the seizure
Incontinence	Very rare	Not uncommon
Autonomic changes	Do not occur	Increased pulse rate, sometimes cardiac dysrhythmias, pupillodilation, sweating, cyanosis, excessive salivation, and slobbering
Injury	Unusual; tongue biting very rare	Sometimes injury from falling or tongue biting
Postictal state	May remember events during episode; overt postictal confusion and somnolence unusual	Amnestic for time of seizure, except for some focal seizures; often postictal confusion or somnolence
Response to anticonvulsants	No response despite therapeutic levels and multiple drugs	Depending on seizure type and cause, patient usually responds to appropriate anticonvulsants
Objective laboratory signs	Video-EEG always normal; serum and CSF prolactin levels normal	Video-EEG always abnormal (if electrodes are properly situated); increased serum prolactin in the appropriate setting at 10-20 min after a suspected event

ABBREVIATIONS: CSF = cerebrospinal fluid; EEG = electroencephalogram.

2. **Triggering of seizures:** Hyperventilation can precipitate pseudoseizures and organic seizures, in particular petit mal. Rarely, thought processes such as calculation or playing games such as chess or cards may trigger true seizures (Goossens et al., 1990). The resolution requires combined video and EEG monitoring in a laboratory or ambulatory monitoring until the attacks can be recorded (Rowan and Gates, 1993).
   a. Normal records during an attack virtually exclude epilepsy, but the EEG, which depends on surface electrical activity, rarely may appear normal, even during some epileptic attacks.
   b. The most difficult problem is the combination of seizures and pseudo-seizures that occurs in about 10% of epileptics (Benbadis et al., 2001). Patients with unrecognized pseudoepileptic seizures erroneously sometimes get intubated and receive intravenous medication for status epilepticus (Leis et al., 1992).
3. **Rule out hypoglycemia:** Whenever a Pt exhibits any undiagnosed attack that alters consciousness or results in a frank seizure, always measure the blood glucose level and, if indicated, other blood constituents.

4. **Comorbid psychiatric disorders:** Psychiatric illnesses are expected in pseudoseizures (Bowman, 2000).

VII. FACTITIOUS FEVERS

Malingerers may produce false temperature readings by manipulating a thermometer. If a Pt has a puzzling fever or hypothermia of unknown origin, measure a fresh sample of urine with your own thermometer. The urine specimen will reflect the true body temperature, thus bypassing any manipulation the Pt manages with the thermometer (Murray et al., 1977). The Ex always has to consider doing a lumbar puncture and culturing the blood and urine in Pts with true fever of unknown origin.

VIII. THE AMNESIAS: PSYCHOGENIC (DISSOCIATIVE) AND ORGANIC

A. Psychogenic amnesia

1. Recognition of psychogenic amnesia rests on the psychiatric history and mental status examination rather than on bedside techniques such as those described for detecting other psychogenic signs and symptoms.
2. DSM-IV divides the psychogenic amnesias into *localized, selective, generalized,* and *systematized amnesias* and *fugue states*. Psychogenic amnesias often start suddenly and generally are selective or restricted. Organic dementias tend to be global rather than selective and are accompanied by other evidence of organic brain impairment.

B. Some special types of organic amnesia

1. Organic amnesia follows an overt disease that obviously affected the brain, such as head trauma, limbic encephalitis, (infectious, autoimmune, paraneoplastic) and substance abuse, or occurs in the context of a neuronal degenerative disease.
2. **Korsakoff's syndrome** (Korsakoff's psychosis, amnestic-confabulatory syndrome) occurs most commonly in the context of profound alcoholism and delirium tremens.
3. The **transient global amnesia (TGA) syndrome** involves middle-aged to elderly Pts, the opposite age range from psychogenic amnesia. The Pt becomes temporarily disoriented for person, place, and date, but has no loss of consciousness, and fully recovers within a few hours, leaving a memory gap regarding events during the episode. During the attack, there is inability to learn both verbal and nonverbal material. TGA may follow various precipitating events, such as emotional stress, contact with cold water, physical exercise, sexual intercourse, and a variety of medications and/or medical procedures. The pathogenesis is unknown but it occurs in mentally normal persons.
4. In the **pure amnestic syndrome** the Pt has retrograde and anterograde amnesia but retains a normal IQ. Damage to the medial quadrant of the temporal lobe causes it.

IX. PAIN, ESPECIALLY HEADACHE AND BACKACHE

A. Organic and psychogenic pain

1. Pain presents the most common and most difficult differential diagnosis of all, particularly separating psychogenic pain, malingering, depression, and organic disease.
2. Organic pain may affect facial expression resulting in grimacing and eyelid narrowing. It may increase the pulse rate, blood pressure, respiratory rate, and pupillary size and result in defensive postures to relive pain.

3. Pure organic pain syndromes without explicit interictal signs, such as migraine or trigeminal neuralgia, present in patterns recognizable by the history. Pain of visceral origin, such as gallbladder pain that is intermittent, causes no interictal signs. However, definable or diagnosable organic causes of the two most common pain disorders, headache and low backache, usually offer one or more objective signs that certify the diagnosis. Because every practitioner will have Pts with these two pain syndromes, I review next the objective findings that point toward the organic diagnosis or that mandate further study by imaging, electromyography, or cerebrospinal fluid examination. With no objective findings on the NE, the likelihood of organic disease or of a specific diagnosis by laboratory further studies becomes very small (Lewis et al., 2002), and the psychiatric investigation becomes paramount.

B. Signs of organic headaches associated with definable lesions

Use the following tests or procedures to screen Pts for organic causes of headache:

1. Palpate/percuss for pain over various sites on the head and neck:
   a. The entire scalp
   b. Sinuses and mastoid
   c. Exit sites of the ophthalmic and maxillary divisions of CrN V and the greater occipital nerve
   d. Temporal artery
   e. Masseters and neck muscles for tenderness or spasm
2. Test for consistent alteration of pain by posture and position, particularly straining, bending forward, and the Valsalva maneuver.
3. Test for nuchal rigidity or some other limitation of neck movement.
4. Listen for bruits over neck vessels or head and palpate neck for masses.
5. Inspect the ear drum for otitis.
6. Check fundi for absence of venous pulsation, papilledema and hypertensive exudates.

C. Signs of organic low back pain or sciatica

Patients with low backache or sciatica syndrome will generally show at least one of the following signs (review Chapter 10, Section VII A to I):

1. Resistance to movement or jarring
2. Characteristic antalgic gait
3. Tilt of the spine
4. Characteristic rising from a chair by bracing the arms to push up
5. Flat lumbar curve
6. Paravertebral muscle spasm
7. If the Pt has a radicular syndrome look for:
   a. Slight flexion of affected leg when standing and "soft" Achilles tendon
   b. Decreased or absent triceps sure muscle stretch reflex
   c. Atrophy of the calf on the side of radiating pain
   d. Weakness of the extensor hallucis longus and foot dorsiflexion
   e. Pain elicited by leg-raising tests

X. SOME FINAL CAVEATS ON THE DIAGNOSIS OF PSYCHOGENIC DISORDERS

A. Consider an organic illness with a psychogenic (functional) overlay

Organic pain may not follow standard textbook distributions. Some Pts with undiagnosed illnesses, in shopping from physician to physician, elaborate on or exaggerate their organic symptoms in desperation as they try to convince physicians of the reality of their illness. The many previous physicians will have asked the same questions over and over in the review of systems, inadvertently suggesting symptoms for the Pt to worry about or to imagine. Such Pts may be neither malingering nor frankly hysterical, but legitimately worried about their health. The Ex always has to consider that an organic disease underlies the seemingly psychogenic complaints (DePaulo and Folstein, 1978; Stone et al., 2002). See Table 14-6.

TABLE 14-6 · Organic Disorders with Bizarre or Subtle Neurologic Manifestations Often Mistaken for Psychogenic Illness

Early multiple sclerosis: fleeting sensory loss, retrobulbar neuritis, transient paraplegia
Porphyria: abdominal pain, peripheral neuropathy, seizures, and mental changes
Endocrinopathies: fatigue, weakness, nervousness, and tremors
Involuntary movement syndromes with bizarre gait disturbances, in particular dystonia with tortipelvis and camptocormia, early degenerative diseases such as spinocerebellar degenerations, certain channelopathies, and paroxysmal kinesigenic and non-kinesigenic dyskinesias.
Seizures with bizarre auras affecting vision, somatic sensation, and visceral auras with crawling sensations, abdominal auras of something like fluid running through the chest or abdomen, odd smells or odors, sexual feelings such as orgasm, forced thoughts, and forced laughter
Myasthenia gravis with transient cranial nerve dysfunction, fatigability, and weakness
Neuropathies, particularly carpal tunnel syndrome, causalgia (reflex sympathetic dystrophy), and autonomic neuropathies
Early Tourette's syndrome with multiple tics, throaty sounds, and urgent, obsessive personality patterns
Midline neoplasms or butterfly gliomas with personality changes preceding objective neurologic signs
Collagen-vascular disease with neuropathy, fleeting central nervous system symptoms, fatigue, and fever
Syringomyelia with dissociated pain and temperature loss
Foramen magnum or spinal level meningioma with spastic-ataxic gait

B. Remain patient

The diagnosis rests on the totality of the clinical evidence from the history and NE, not on any pathognomonic single finding or parlor trick that fools the Pt. During the history and examination, avoid the impression of trying to unmask or expose the Pt. Avoid confrontation and tricks, such as hypnosis or electric shocks, to "speed up" recovery. **Ridding the Pt of psychogenic symptoms does not rid the Pt of the psychogenic illness.** The symptom is not the problem—something else is.

C. Maintain professionalism to avoid diagnostic errors

Those puzzling and troublesome Pts whose illnesses consist of organic, psychogenic, and factitious factors often provoke anger. Neophyte physicians may refer to these Pts by inexcusable names such as "crocks," "gomers," or "gorks." Remember yet another aphorism: **If you deprecate the Pt, you have failed to understand the Pt's problem.** The psychogenic symptom is a way of communicating something that the Pt cannot face or verbalize, a distinct cry for help. Whatever the diagnostic label, whether an hysteric or malingerer, the Pt is distressed. Such Pts need a physician who remains receptive and potentially helpful, rather than dismissing the person as a cheat, a liar, or a fraud. Regard every event in the consulting room, whether an extensor plantar response or a factitious fever, neutrally as a clinical phenomenon. Reacting with hostility or overt disbelief will degrade the quality of your examination and greatly increase the possibility of an error in diagnosis or management. Avoid adversarial polarization with the Pt trying to prove the reality of an illness and you trying to disprove it. Retain the grace and humility to recognize the fallibility of your own judgments. Never dismiss the Pt with a belittling: "It's all in your head." At the end of the encounter, you can hint that the findings suggest a disorder that may end in recovery, but let the Pt retain the refuge of "patient-hood."

D. Avoid the patient's trap

The intimacy of the medical examination provides a prime opportunity for some Pts to indulge in pathologic manipulation. Such Pts may act seductively, try to exploit their illness for pity or favors, or consciously or subconsciously try to provoke hostility. If duped by these maneuvers, you lose any possibility of helping the Pt. For this and many other reasons, the medical model forbids the physician to succumb emotionally to the Pt, whether with love, pity, or hostility.

E. Beware of Munchausen's syndrome and Munchausen's syndrome by proxy

1. A practiced Pt with factitious disorder or Munchausen's syndrome can fool many of the tests described in this text, including falsifying a Babinski sign.
2. In Munchausen's syndrome by proxy, the parent or spouse acts as an enabler or frankly creates the illness of another family member. In children be wary of illness willfully perpetuated by a parent. Here are two of the worst cases in my experience. The first was a registered nurse whose son repeatedly presented at the emergency room with hypoglycemic seizures. Immunoassay of the child's blood showed porcine insulin. Sometime later the mother herself presented to an emergency room with hypoglycemia induced by self-administered insulin. In the second instance, a hospitalized child repeatedly had mysterious fevers caused by coliform bacteria septicemia. A video camera hidden in the hospital room showed the mother injecting feces into the child's intravenous tube. In view of the male propensity to batter children, we have to conclude that not all parents, mothers or fathers, love their children.

F. Following-up

A diagnostic feature of hysteria is the disappearance of the symptom with time. Schedule follow-up appointments to ensure that your proffered diagnosis was the correct diagnosis.

G. The patient may have some disease you hadn't thought of or even heard of

Never diagnose a psychogenic illness by exclusion because you cannot find another diagnosis. Call in a consultant who just may recognize the porphyria, smoldering collagen disease, occult carcinoma, parasitic infestation, chronic liver abscess, multiple sclerosis, or masked depression that you didn't even consider. Remember this:

There are more things in heaven and earth, Horatio, than are dreamt of in your philosophy.

—William Shakespeare (1564–1616), Hamlet

BIBLIOGRAPHY · Clinical and Laboratory Tests to Distinguish Conversion Disorder and Malingering from Organic Disease

Allanson J, Bass C, Wade DT. Characteristics of patients with severe disability and medically explained neurological symptoms: A pilot study. J Neurol Neursurg Psychiatry 2002; 73:307–309.

American Psychiatric Association. *Diagnostic and Statistical Manual of Mental Disorders,* Fourth ed. Washington, DC, American Psychiatric Association, 1994.

American Psychiatric Association. *Diagnostic and Statistical Manual of Mental Disorders,* Text Revision (DSM-IV-TR). Washington, DC, American Psychiatric Association, 2000.

Aminoff MJ, Dedo HH, Izdebski K. Clinical aspects of spasmodic dysphonia. *J Neurol Neurosurg Psychiatry* 1978;41:361–365.

Azher SN, Jankovic J. Camptocormia: Pathogenesis, classification, and response to therapy. Neurology 2005;65:355–369.

Baker JHE, Silver JR. Hysterical paraplegia. *J Neurol Neurosurg Psychiatry* 1987;50: 375–382.

Benbadis SR, Agrawal V, Tatum IV WO. How many patients with psychogenic nonepileptic seizures also have epilepsy? *Neurology* 2001;57:915–917.

Bowman ES. The differential diagnosis of epilepsy, pseudoseizures, dissociative identity disorder, and dissociative disorder not otherwise specified. *Bull Menninger Clin* 2000;64:164–180.

Bumgartner J, Epstein CM. Voluntary alteration of visual evoked potentials. *Ann Neurol* 1982;12:475–478.

Butler C, Zeman AZG. Neurological syndromes which can be mistaken for psychiatric conditions. *J Neurol Neurosurg Psychiatry* 2005;76:131–138.

DePaulo JR, Folstein MF. Psychiatric disturbances in neurological patients: detection, recognition, and hospital course. *Ann Neurol* 1978;4:225–228.

Ellis JM, Lee SI. Acute prolonged confusion in later life as an ictal state. *Epilepsia* 1978;19:119–128.

Geyer J, Payne TA, Drury I. The value of pelvic thrusting in the diagnosis of seizures and pseudoseizures. *Neurology* 2000;54:227–229.

Goossens LAZ, Andermann F, Andermann E, et al. Reflex seizures induced by calculation, card or board games, and spatial tasks: a review of 25 patients and delineation of the epileptic syndrome. *Neurology* 1990;40:1171–1176.

Griffin JF, Wray SH, Anderson DP. Misdiagnosis of spasm of the near reflex. *Neurology* 1976:26:1018–1020.

Iliceto G, Thompson PD, Day BL, et al. Diaphragmatic flutter, the moving umbilicus syndrome, and "belly dancer's" dyskinesia. Movement Disorders 2004;5(1):15–22.

Keane AM, Morris HH, Luders H, et al. Supplementary motor seizures mimicking pseudoseizures: some clinical differences. *Neurology* 1990;40:1404–1407.

Keane JR. Hysterical gait disorders. *Neurology* 1989;39:586–589.

Keane JR. Neuro-ophthalmic signs and symptoms of hysteria. *Neurology* 1982;32:757–762.

Keane JR. Wrong-way deviation of the tongue with hysterical hemiparesis. *Neurology* 1986;36:1406–1407.

Koller W, Lang A, Vetere-Overfield B, et al. Psychogenic tremors. *Neurology* 1989;39:1094–1099.

La France WC. Somatoform disorders. Sem Neurol 2009;29:234–246.

Leis AA, Ross MA, Summers AK. Psychogenic seizures: ictal characteristics and diagnostic pitfalls. *Neurology* 1992;42:95–99.

Lesser RP. Psychogenic seizures. *Neurology* 1996;46:1499–1506.

Lewis DW, Ashwal S, Dahl G, et al. Practice parameter: evaluation of children and adolescents with recurrent headaches: report of the Quality Standards Subcommittee of the American Academy of Neurology and the Practice Committee of the Child Neurology Society. *Neurology* 2002;59:490–498.

Manford M, Shorvon SD. Prolonged sensory or visceral symptoms: an under-diagnosed form of non-convulsive focal (simple partial) status epilepticus. *J Neurol Neurosurg Psychiatry* 1992;55:714–716.

Markand ON, Wheeler GL, Pollack SL. Complex partial status epilepticus. *Neurology* 1978;28:189–196.

Meierkord H, Will B, Fish D, et al. The clinical features and prognosis of pseudoseizures diagnosed using video-EEG telemetry. *Neurology* 1991;41:1643–1646.

Meyers JE, Volbrecht ME. A validation of multiple malingering detection methods in a large clinical sample. *Arch Clin Neuropsychol* 2003;18:261–276.

Monrad-Krohn GH. On the function of the latissimus dorsi muscle as a sign of functional dissociation in simulated and "functional" paralysis of the arm. *Acta Med Scand* 1922;56:9–11.

Murray HW, Tuazon CU, Guerrero IC, et al. Urinary temperature: a clue to early diagnosis of factitious fever. *N Engl J Med* 1977;296:23.

Opherk C, Hirsch LJ. Ictal heart rate differentiates epileptic from non-epileptic seizures. *Neurology* 2002;58:636–638.

Pilai JJ, Markind S, Streletz LJ, et al. Motor evoked potentials in psychogenic paralysis. *Neurology* 1991;42:935–936.

Ravich WJ, Wilson RS, Jones B, Donner MW. Psychogenic dysphagia and globus: reevaluation of 23 patients. *Dysphagia* 1990;4(4):244.

Reuber M, Mitchell AJ, Howlett SJ, et al. Functional symptoms in neurology: questions and answers. *J Neurol Neurosurg Psychiatry* 2005;76:307–314.

Reza Samie M, Selhorst JBG, Koller WC. Post-traumatic midbrain tremors. *Neurology* 1990;40:62–66.

Rowan AJ, Gates JR. *Non-Epileptic Seizures.* Stoneham, Butterworth-Heinemann, 1993.

Schrag A, Brown RJ, Trimble MR. Reliability of self-reported diagnoses in patients with neurologically unexplained symptoms. *J Neurol Neurosurg Psychiatry* 2004;75:608–611.

Simon DK, Nishino S, Scammell TE. Mistaking diagnosis of psychogenic gait disorders in a man with status cataplecticus ("Limp Man Syndrome"). *Mov Disorders* 2004;19(7): 838–840.

Stone J, Carson A, Sharpe M. Functional symptoms and signs in neurology: assessment and diagnosis. J Neurol Neurosurg Psychiatry 2005;76 (suppl 1):2–12.

Stone J, Sharpe M, Carson A, et al. Are functional motor and sensory rarely more frequent on the left? A systematic review. *J Neurol Neurosurg Psychiatry* 2002;73:548–558.

Stone J, Smyth R, Carson A, et al. La belle indifference in conversion symptoms and hysteria. *Br J Psychiatry* 2006;188:204–209.

Stone J, Zeman A, Sharpe M. Functional weakness and sensory disturbance. *J Neurol Neurosurg Psychiatry* 2002;73:241–245.

Tan CT, Murray NMF, Sawyers D, et al. Deliberate alteration of the visual evoked potential. *J Neurol Neurosurg Psychiatry* 1984;47:518–523.

Tong DC, Grossman M. What causes transient global amnesia? New insights from DWI. *Neurology* 2004;62(12):2154–2155.

Troost BT, Troost EG. Functional paralysis of horizontal gaze. *Neurology* 1979;29: 82–85.

van der Ploeg RJO, Oosterhuis HJGH. The "make/break test" as a diagnostic tool in functional weakness. *J Neurol Neurosurg Psychiatry* 1991;54:248–251.

Walker FO, Alessi AG, Digre KB, et al. Psychogenic respiratory distress. *Arch Neurol* 1989;46:196–200.

Weintraub MI. Malingering and conversion reactions. *Neurol Clin* 1995;13:229–450.

Woolsey RM. Hysteria: 1875–1975. *Dis Nerv Syst* 1976;37:379–386.

Yarnell P, Melamed E, Silverberg R. Global hemianesthesia: a parietal perceptual distortion suggesting non-organic illness. *J Neurol Neurosurg Psychiatry* 1978;41:843–846.

Learning Objectives for Chapter 14

I. THE GENERAL CLINICAL FEATURES OF CONVERSION DISORDER AND MALINGERING

1. Define conversion disorder.
2. Describe the *primary* and *secondary gains* in conversion disorder.
3. Describe the most important distinction between conversion disorder and malingering.
4. Distinguish between the usual goals of Pts with factitious disorders and the malingerer.
5. Discuss whether exacerbation of a symptom or sign by emotional stress establishes a psychogenic origin.
6. Name some organic neurologic conditions in which Pts may appear to be indifferent to their symptoms.

II. PSYCHOGENIC DISORDERS OF MOTOR FUNCTION

1. Describe some of the common psychogenic movement disorders of the eye and its associated muscles.
2. Describe the pseudo-VIth nerve palsy syndrome and state how to prove that the arrest of abduction is not due to a VIth nerve palsy.
3. Describe the difference in the action of the frontalis muscle, and the corresponding height of the eyebrow, in hysterical pseudoptosis and organic ptosis.
4. Describe some of the ways conversion disorder affects the oropharyngeal muscles and breathing.
5. Describe how to divert the Pt to elicit a more normal performance on the Romberg swaying test.
6. Imitate an organic hemiplegic gait (Fig.12-15).
7. Define *astasia-abasia* and explain how the condition proves that the Pt has a very competent motor system.
8. Describe the outstanding differences between psychogenic and organic paraplegia (Table 14-3).
9. Describe how the attempt to do a sit-up in a Pt with a T10 level lesion affects the location of the umbilicus.
10. Contrast the difference in the demeanor and amount of effort overtly displayed by Pts with psychogenic and organic illness when they try to move a paralyzed part.
11. State what observations, during grip testing, show that the functionally paralyzed Pt actually has intact forearm muscles.
12. Explain the value of observing a paralyzed Pt with conversion disorder during sleep.
13. Describe and demonstrate how to produce inadvertent or synkinetic movement of the putatively paralyzed parts in psychogenic paralysis: arm paralysis, wrist drop, foot drop, and leg paralysis (Figs. 14-1 to 14-5).
14. Describe a laboratory procedure that can prove that the pyramidal tract is intact.
15. Describe some major differences in psychogenic and organic tremors (Table 14-4).

III. PSYCHOGENIC DISORDERS OF VISION

1. List some psychogenic disorders of vision.
2. Describe some bedside methods of establishing the integrity of the retino-geniculo-calcarine pathway in psychogenic blindness.
3. Describe the results of the swinging flashlight test in monocular psychogenic blindness.

Learning Objectives for Chapter 14

4. Describe how to use the canthal compression test to establish vision in psychogenic monocular blindness.
5. Describe some laboratory tests that will establish the integrity of the visual pathways.
6. Name a lesion of sudden onset that may cause complete blindness in an eye without ophthalmoscopic changes early in the course.
7. Describe the differences in the NE that would distinguish psychogenic monocular blindness from retrobulbar neuritis.
8. Explain whether the presence of the pupillary light reflexes would exclude cortical blindness.
9. Describe the typical nonorganic visual field defects in Pts with conversion disorder (Fig. 14-6).
10. Name some organic causes for monocular diplopia.

IV. PSYCHOGENIC DEAFNESS

Describe some clinical and laboratory methods for establishing that a putatively deaf Pt has intact auditory pathways.

V. PSYCHOGENIC DISORDERS OF SOMATIC SENSATION

1. Describe the common kinds of functional somatic sensory disturbances (exclusive of special senses).
2. Explain this aphorism: Pts with conversion disorder lose sensation according to their mental image of the body rather than the anatomy and physiology of the nervous system. Give some examples of this principle (Figs. 14-7 to 14-9).
3. Describe how to use vibration sense to help distinguish organic from nonorganic hemianesthesia (Fig. 14-8).
4. Describe the difference in the stocking-glove distribution of psychogenic and organic sensory loss (Fig. 14-9).
5. Describe objective findings on the NE that prove that a Pt cannot have an organic basis for total anesthesia of a limb.
6. Describe how to use the inverted hands test to disclose nonorganic sensory loss (Fig. 14-3).
7. Describe some of the characteristic ways that functional Pts respond to sensory stimuli that may provide clues to the nonorganic nature of the disorder.
8. Explain the interpretation when the Pt gives exactly opposite answers to the up or down position of the digit when the Ex tests position sense.
9. Describe some of the demeanors or patterns of reaction of the Pt with conversion disorder to sensory testing that suggest nonorganic sensory loss.
10. List some organic sensory disorders that may be mistaken for hysteria.

VI. PSYCHOGENIC NONEPILEPTIC SEIZURES

1. Define psychogenic seizures.
2. Describe some circumstances that might elicit or trigger pseudoepileptic seizures.
3. Contrast the motor activities typically demonstrated in psychogenic seizures with a classic generalized motor seizure.
4. Explain why even an experienced observer has difficulty in distinguishing a psychogenic seizure from an epileptic seizure, even when viewing it in person.
5. Name the one most important procedure that will distinguish true from psychogenic seizures.

Learning Objectives for Chapter 14

6. Describe some objective autonomic signs of an epileptic seizure that are unlikely to occur in psychogenic seizures.
7. State which blood chemistry determinations the Ex should consider when observing any undiagnosed attack that alters consciousness, causes a frank loss of consciousness, or could be an epileptic seizure.
8. Summarize the major differences between psychogenic and true epileptic seizures (Table 14-5).

VII. FACTITIOUS FEVERS

Describe a simple, foolproof method of measuring the true body temperature without the Pt's having any knowledge of what you are doing.

VIII. THE AMNESIAS: PSYCHOGENIC (DISSOCIATIVE) AND ORGANIC

1. Describe major differences in the histories of Pts with psychogenic or organic amnesia.
2. State the usual illness that causes Korsakoff's amnesia.
3. Describe the transient global amnesia syndrome.

IX. PAIN, ESPECIALLY HEADACHE AND BACKACHE

1. Name some causes of intermittent pains of organic origin that lack signs in the interictal period.
2. Describe the physical examination necessary to search for organic causes of a headache.
3. Describe the physical examination necessary to search for organic causes of low backache.

X. SOME FINAL CAVEATS ON THE DIAGNOSIS OF PSYCHOGENIC DISORDERS

1. Discuss the concept of overlay and some reasons why organic pain may seem psychogenic or why the Pt might elaborate on it.
2. Discuss whether the physician should focus on early elimination of symptoms when the findings suggest a nonorganic illness.
3. Discuss the danger of the common practice of applying pejorative names to Pts with puzzling and troublesome neuropsychiatric syndromes.
4. Discuss why the medical model calls for the physician to respond neutrally to all events in the transaction between Pt and physician and to forgo judgment, moralizing, and emotional responses.
5 Explain how adherence to the medical model keeps the manipulative, seductive, or hostility-provoking Pt from gaining control over the physician.
6. Explain the meaning of *Munchausen's syndrome by proxy*.
7. Explain the importance of follow-up appointments in the management of psychogenic illnesses.
8. List several organic disorders that may present with puzzling symptoms that may suggest psychogenic illness (Table 14-6).

15 A Synopsis of the Neurologic Investigation and a Formulary of Neurodiagnosis

In clinical situations there are three principal factors that can legitimately influence the decision making process. These are:

1. *The scientific evidence*
2. *The practitioner's clinical experience*
3. *The practical situation, including the patient's wishes, other people's concerns, the patient's lifestyle and culture, the social environment, and realistic observations to the delivery of technically ideal interventions*

These can be thought of as a triangle of forces.

There are some problems with each of these factors as a primary guide to treatment. Consequently, they should remain metaphorically in a state of balance in the clinician's mind, so that he is able to establish treatment plans that are evidence based (but not mechanistic), patient centered and contextualized (but not irrational), and informed by experience (rather than by a faith in idiosyncratic ideas). Treatment frequently goes wrong because one or more of these factors have been neglected.

Rob Poole & Robert Hisso.
(Clinical Skills in Psychiatric Treatment. Cambridge University Press, 2008.)

I. THE ROUTINE SCREENING NEUROLOGIC EXAMINATION WHEN THE PATIENT HAS NO SYMPTOMS SUGGESTING NEUROLOGIC DISEASE

A. What is the minimum allowable neurologic examination

Every new patient (Pt) and every routine physical checkup requires the examiner (Ex) to complete a minimum screening neurologic examination (NE) of all body systems. To this requirement students often respond fretfully: "But it takes too long to do the

NE on everyone!" In fact, with sufficient practice, you can learn to do a basic screening NE in about 6 minutes in the mentally normal, cooperative Pt who has no neurologic symptoms. This statement presupposes a thorough history. The better the history, the briefer the examination required. The Ex need not and should not do every test on every Pt but should expand or trim the examination to fit the Pt's history. If a Pt presents only with a sore throat and has no neurologic symptoms whatsoever, the Ex squanders time in testing smell and taste, doing caloric irrigation, a detailed aphasia examination, and in tugging against every muscle. The expanded examination to explore neurologic symptoms often requires the time for these tasks. For a brand new Pt, we schedule a full hour to complete the history and physical examination, dictate notes, and arrange for laboratory tests or referrals. Recall that the history and clinical examination still constitute the most efficient methods known to establish the relationship between physician and the Pt that is optimum for detecting disease, and for planning a healthy lifestyle.

B. Format for the mandatory 6-minute neurologic examination for every patient

1. **Appraisal during the history:** During the history, the Ex appraises the Pt's mental status, notes the facial features, the eyes and ears, ocular movements, speech and swallowing and observes the posture, gait, and movement patterns.
2. **Examination of the head:** Inspect the head shape and palpate the head. Record the occipitofrontal circumference (OFC) of every infant.
3. **Visual system:** Test visual acuity (central fields), peripheral fields, do ophthalmoscopy, and test the pupillary reflexes.
4. **Do the 45-seconds motor examination of cranial nerves III, IV, V, VI, VII, IX, X, XI, and XII** (Table 6-8).
5. **Hearing:** Test by conversational voice and by finger rustling.
6. **Somatic motor examination**
   a. Undress the Pt, note the somatotype, and inspect for muscle atrophy, fasciculations, tremors, involuntary movements, and neurocutaneous stigmata.
   b. Test gait by free walking; toe, heel, and tandem walking, and deep knee bend.
   c. Test strength of abduction of arms, wrist dorsiflexion, grip, hip flexion, and foot dorsiflexion.
   d. Test cerebellar function by finger-to-nose and heel-to-knee tests, in addition to the gait.
   e. Elicit muscle stretch reflexes of biceps, quadriceps femoris, and triceps surae.
   f. Elicit plantar reflexes.
7. **Somatosensory examination**
   a. Test *superficial* sensation by light touch and temperature discrimination on the face, hands, and feet (Fig. 10-4).
   b. Test *deep* sensation by the directional scratch test (Chapter 10, Section VIII), position sense in fingers and toes, and vibration sense at the ankles.
   c. Test for astereognosis with coins or paper clips.

C. Recording the routine neurologic examination

When we read someone else's NE, we want to find out the mental status and whether the Pt can see, hear, talk, swallow, breathe, stand, walk, and feel normally. Surprisingly, many write-ups fail to include that information. Hurriedly scribbling that the "neuro exam is physiological" or "WNL" just won't do. When a Pt has neurologic findings, no forms or checkoff lists record the NE as well as a series of statements, best dictated and typed. If the Pt has no neurologic findings, you still may prefer to write out the screening NE, but a checkoff sheet can save time, and you may expand it as needed to record positive findings. See Table 15-1.

TABLE 15-1 · Recording the 6-Minute Screening Neurologic Examination for Patients without Neurologic Symptoms

Name:		#	Date:	Occupation:
Normal	Abnormal			
_____	_____	**1. Appearance and mental status:**_______old; race/ethnicity _____; male/female; affect:______________; oriented:__________ memory:__________		
_____	_____	**2. Head:** normocephalic, no bumps, tenderness, or depressions. OFC____		
_____	_____	**3. Visual system** a. Acuity and visual fields b. Pupils:_____ mm in size, react to light____; accom.____ c. EOM full. No nystagmus d. Fundi: describe/draw		
_____	_____	**4. Nonocular motor cranial nerves** a. Facial movements b. Tongue, jaw, and palate midline c. Word articulation d. Swallowing e. Breathing		
_____	_____	**5. Motor system** a. Gait/station: free walking; toe, heel, tandem; and deep knee bend b. Atrophy/fasciculations c. Tremor/involuntary movements d. Dystaxia/dysdiadochokinesia e. Strength: deltoids, grip, dorsiflexors hands and feet, and hip flexors f. Muscle tone/spasm		
_____	_____	**6. Sensory system** a. Hearing: voice, finger rustling b. Touch and temperature discrimination over the face, hands, and feet c. Directional scratch test, position, vibration, and coin recognition		
_____	_____	**7. Skin**		
_____	_____	**8. Dysmorphic features**		
		9. Case summary (no more than three lines):		
		10. Provisional diagnosis/differential diagnosis:		
		11. Recommendations:		
			Signature:__________________	

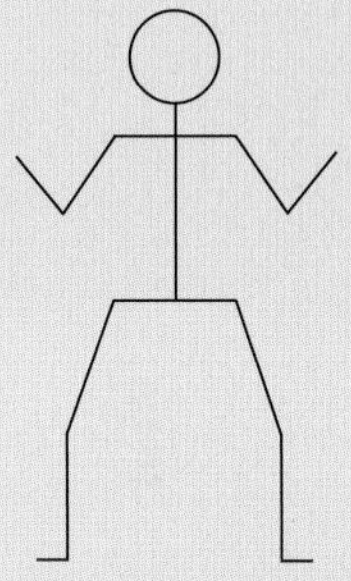

ABBREVIATIONS: accom. = accommodation; EOM = extraocular movements; OFC = occipitofrontal circumference.

II. THE CONCEPT OF "SOFT" NEUROLOGIC SIGNS

A. Definition

Many of the neurologic signs described thus far result from a lesion at a known site or that affect a known pathway. The presence of the sign essentially mandates the presence of a lesion. These "hard" signs contrast with "soft" signs that bear a statistical correlation with brain impairment but do not arise from specific, known central nervous system (CNS) lesions or even mandate a brain lesion. **A soft sign is any structural or functional deviation found more frequently in brain-impaired persons than in normal persons but that does not directly correlate with any particular type of brain lesion at any particular site, or interruption of any particular tract.** Table 15-2 lists several examples of soft signs.

TABLE 15-2 · Examples of "Soft" Signs of Brain Impairment

Dysmorphic soft signs	Neurologic soft signs
OFC <2 SD or >2 SD from the mean	Nystagmus
Skull asymmetry	Heterotropia
Hyper- and hypotelorism	Asymmetric facial movements
Unusual hair whorls	Dysarthria
Unusually fine or coarse hair	Dysprosody
Synophrys	Inability to wink eyes separately
Malformed ears	Saccadic smooth pursuit
Epicanthal folds	Measures of balance coordination, and steadiness
Cleft lip	Whole body clumsiness
Iris coloboma	Motor impersistence (inability to maintain a posture)
Iris heterochromia	Inability to hop on one foot
Micro- or macrostomia	Thumb-finger opposition: (Failure of successively touching of the thumb to the four fingers)
Broad or absent philtrum	Persistence of letter reversals
High arched palate	"Overflow" movements
Micrognathia	Excessive "piano-playing" movements of the outstretched fingers
Pectus excavatum	Choreiform twitches of the fingers when performing designated motor actions
Single palmar crease	Irregular alternating movements
Short, incurved little finger (clinodactyly)	Hypo- or hypertonia
Polydactyly	Poor comprehension of instructions for performing fine or gross motor tasks
Syndactyly	Right-left confusion
Abnormal toe lengths	
Dorsal midline defects: nevus, hair patch, dimple	

ABBREVIATIONS: OFC = occipitofrontal circumference; SD = standard deviation.

B. Implications of soft signs

Many soft signs are simply variations of normal or overlap in brain-impaired and normal populations. An example is the single palmar crease that regularly occurs in certain malformation syndromes with mental retardation, such as Down's syndrome, but also occurs in some neurologically normal persons. Other signs by themselves are hard signs of a neurologic lesion but not of brain impairment per se. A lateral rectus palsy necessitates a lesion but usually in the peripheral nervous system (PNS), not in the CNS. However, if we select a lateral rectus palsy as the independent variable, it will occur more frequently in brain-impaired persons than in normal persons. Hence, it is a hard sign of a neurologic lesion but a soft sign of a brain lesion. Dysmorphic soft signs suggest a prenatal teratogen or genetic cause for the brain impairment. Populations with an increased incidence of soft signs include children with mental retardation, learning disabilities, and behavioral disorders, and adult schizophrenics (Ardila, 1996; Dazzan and Murray 2002; Ismail et al., 2000; Tupper, 1986).

BIBLIOGRAPHY · The Concept of Soft Neurologic Signs

Ardila A. Correlation between scholastic performance and soft neurological signs in children. *Int Pediatr* 1996;11:284–287.

Dazzan P, Murray RM. Neurological soft signs in first-episode psychosis: a systematic review. *Br J Psychiatry* 2002;181:350–357.

Ismail B, Cantor Graae E, McNeil TF. Minor physical anomalies in schizophrenia: cognitive, neurological and other clinical correlates. *J Psychiatr Res* 2000;34:45–56.

Tupper DE, ed. *Soft Neurological Signs*. Orlando, Grune & Stratton, 1986.

III. THE CONCEPT OF "FALSE" LOCALIZING SIGNS

A. Definition

A false localizing sign is a true sign that occurs secondary to a lesion elsewhere in the CNS. The sign is not false, but it is distant from the actual site of the primary lesion (Larner, 2003).

B. Causes

1. False localizing signs are caused mainly by shifts of the brain that compress or displace structures distant from the lesion or that compress blood vessels that supply distant sites.
2. Obstructive hydrocephalus may cause compression of cranial nerve VI along the base of the skull, even with the primary lesion at the foramen magnum. Similarly, aqueductal enlargement in hydrocephalus may cause features of the pretectal (Sylvian aqueduct) syndrome, such as impaired upward gaze.
3. False localizing oculomotor disturbances may be associated with ruptured intracranial aneurysms.
4. Shifts of the brain from large unilateral lesions may compress the anterior cerebral artery under the falx or the posterior cerebral artery against the edge of the tentorium. See the section on brain herniations in Chapter 12.

BIBLIOGRAPHY · The Concept of "False" Localizing Signs

Larner AJ. False localizing signs. *J Neurol Neurosurg Psychiatry* 2003;74:416–418.

McKenna C, Fellus J, Barrett AM. False localizing signs in dramatic brain injury. *Brain Injury* 2009;23(7-8):597–601.

Suzuki J, Iwabuchi T. Ocular motor disturbances occurring as false localizing signs in ruptured intracranial aneurysms. *Acta Neurochirurgica* 1974;30(1-2):119–128.

IV. CLOSING THE NEUROLOGIC EXAMINATION WHEN THE PATIENT HAS SYMPTOMS OR SIGNS SUGGESTING NEUROLOGIC DISEASES

A. Hypothesis testing and reaching a provisional diagnosis

When the history suggests neurologic disease, the NE must include the critical tests for the integrity of neural structures that the lesion or disease could affect. The goal is to achieve the best provisional diagnosis. To reach a provisional diagnosis, the Ex poses and tests numerous diagnostic hypotheses during the history, physical examination, and, later, the laboratory work-up. The thinking process is one of posing if's: "If the Pt has such and such a disease or sign, then I should also find so and so. Very well, I will look for that next."

B. The concept of closure (cloture)

After the history, after the examination, and after the hypothesizing, the next event in the medical process is the **cloture.** *Cloture* is a technical term meaning, now that the arguments have been heard and the data presented, the time has come to pose the critical question(s) for decision and action. The provisional diagnosis and the differential diagnosis derived from it are the outcomes of the cloture, and the medical management is the action (Fig. 15-1).

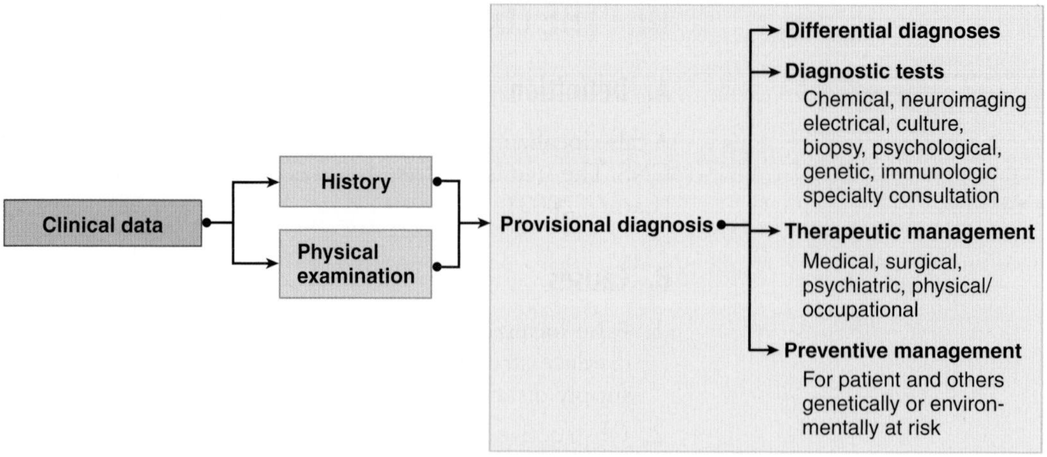

FIGURE 15-1. Summary of the operational steps for cloture. The clinical data lead to a provisional diagnosis. The provisional diagnosis is the critical link in the process because it determines the differential diagnoses, leads to the final diagnosis, and justifies all of the remaining steps in management.

C. The diagnostic catechism

The cloture requires six questions, three primary and the three derivative, that form the diagnostic catechism (Table 15-3).

TABLE 15-3 · The Diagnostic Catechism for Cloture

1. Is there a lesion or disease?
2. If so, where is the lesion or the disease?
3. What is the lesion or the disease (the provisional diagnosis)?
4. What is the optimum diagnostic management? What clinical or laboratory tests, if any, will confirm or reject the provisional diagnosis?
5. What is the optimum therapeutic management?
6. What is the optimum preventative management?

D. Is there a lesion (Table 15-3, question 1)?

The first dichotomy is whether the disorder is organic or psychogenic. That is the meaning of the first question, "Is there a lesion or a disease?" The Ex initially tries to discover neurologic signs that identify an anatomic lesion. Then the Ex considers organic disorders with biochemical lesions, such as some types of epilepsy or migraine, that exhibit no physical signs in the interictal examination. Next, the Ex considers emotional disorders with no lesion. The Ex must try to separate psychogenic from organic disorders because the provisional diagnosis thus achieved determines the extent and type of clinical and laboratory tests required to establish the final diagnosis. To answer *yes* to the question, "Is there a lesion?" the Ex hopes to find at least one sign. One firm sign may mean more than a multitude of symptoms. In answering the question, think through Fig. 15-2 to start generating the possibilities in your mind.

E. Where is the lesion or the disease (Table 15-3, question 2)?

If the clinical evidence suggests a lesion or disease, ask these questions:

1. Is the lesion or disease in the structure or the biochemistry of the Pt?
2. Is it at the level of gene, chromosome, or cell? Is it at the level of blending of cells into tissues or of tissues into organs, or of organs into systems, or of systems into

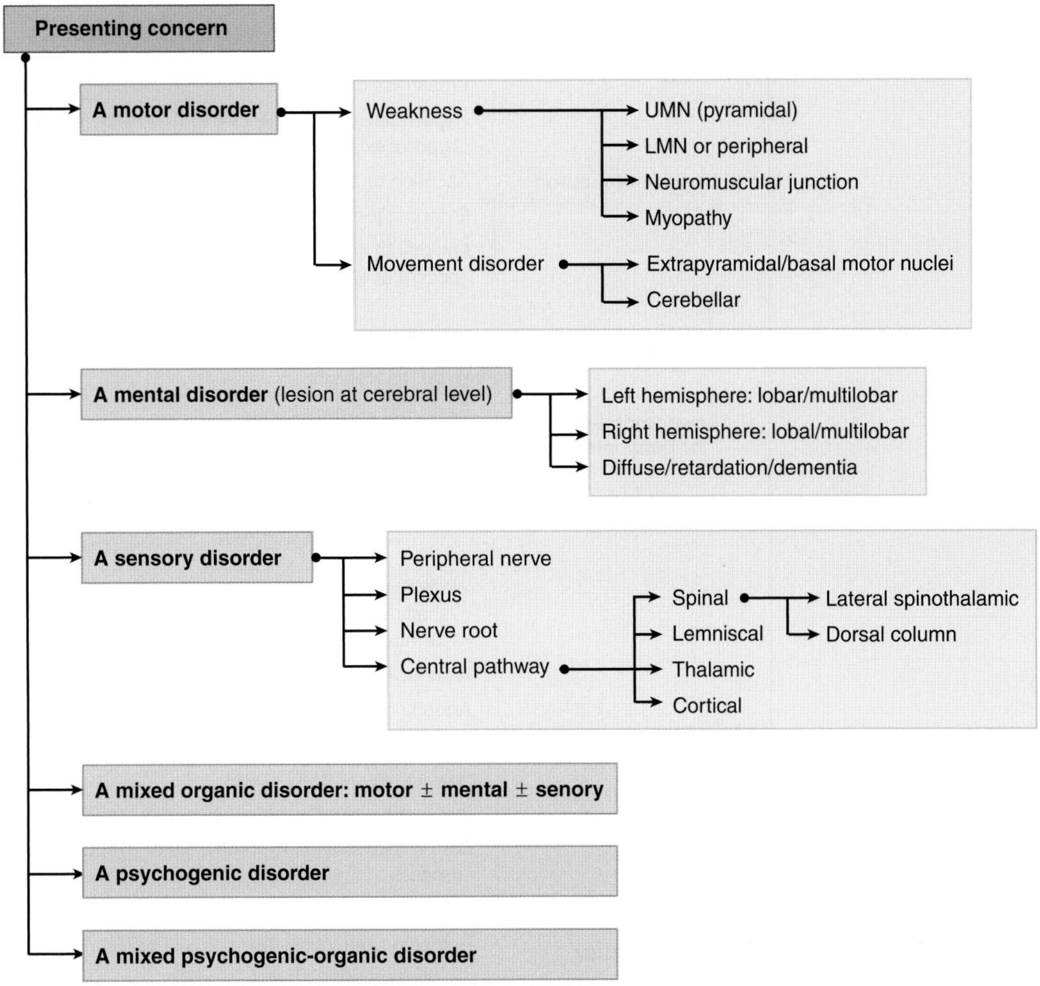

FIGURE 15-2. Preliminary possibilities when the patient's complaint and the neurologic examination suggest neurologic disease. Are the symptoms and signs motor, mental, or sensory? Are they organic or psychogenic, or some combination? LMN = lower motoneuron; UMN = upper motoneuron.

the general somatotype of the Pt? Do the findings constitute a diagnostic neuroanatomic, morphologic, biochemical, or genetic syndrome?

3. Can a decision be made as to the organ or organs, system or systems involved by the lesion? If it affects the nervous system, is the lesion:
   a. In the PNS or CNS?
   b. If the lesion involves the CNS, is it intra-axial or extra-axial?
   c. If intra-axial, is it *focal:* in the cerebrum, ventricular cavities or passageways, basal ganglia, brainstem, cerebellum, or spinal cord; or is it *multifocal* or *diffuse?*
   d. If the lesion could be extra-axial, is it:
      i. In a meningeal or bony covering?
      ii. In a meningeal space: epidural, subdural, or subarachnoid?
      iii. In a nerve root, plexus, peripheral nerve, neuromuscular junction, or muscle?
4. When the Pt's symptoms and signs suggest a neurologic disease, try to classify it as *motor, sensory, sensorimotor, headache,* or *organic mental syndrome.*
   a. If motor, think through Fig. 15-3 to locate the neuronal system affected; if an involuntary movement syndrome, see Fig. 15-4.
   b. If sensory, see Fig. 15-5.
   c. If a headache, see Fig. 15-6.
   d. If an organic mental syndrome, see Fig. 15-7.

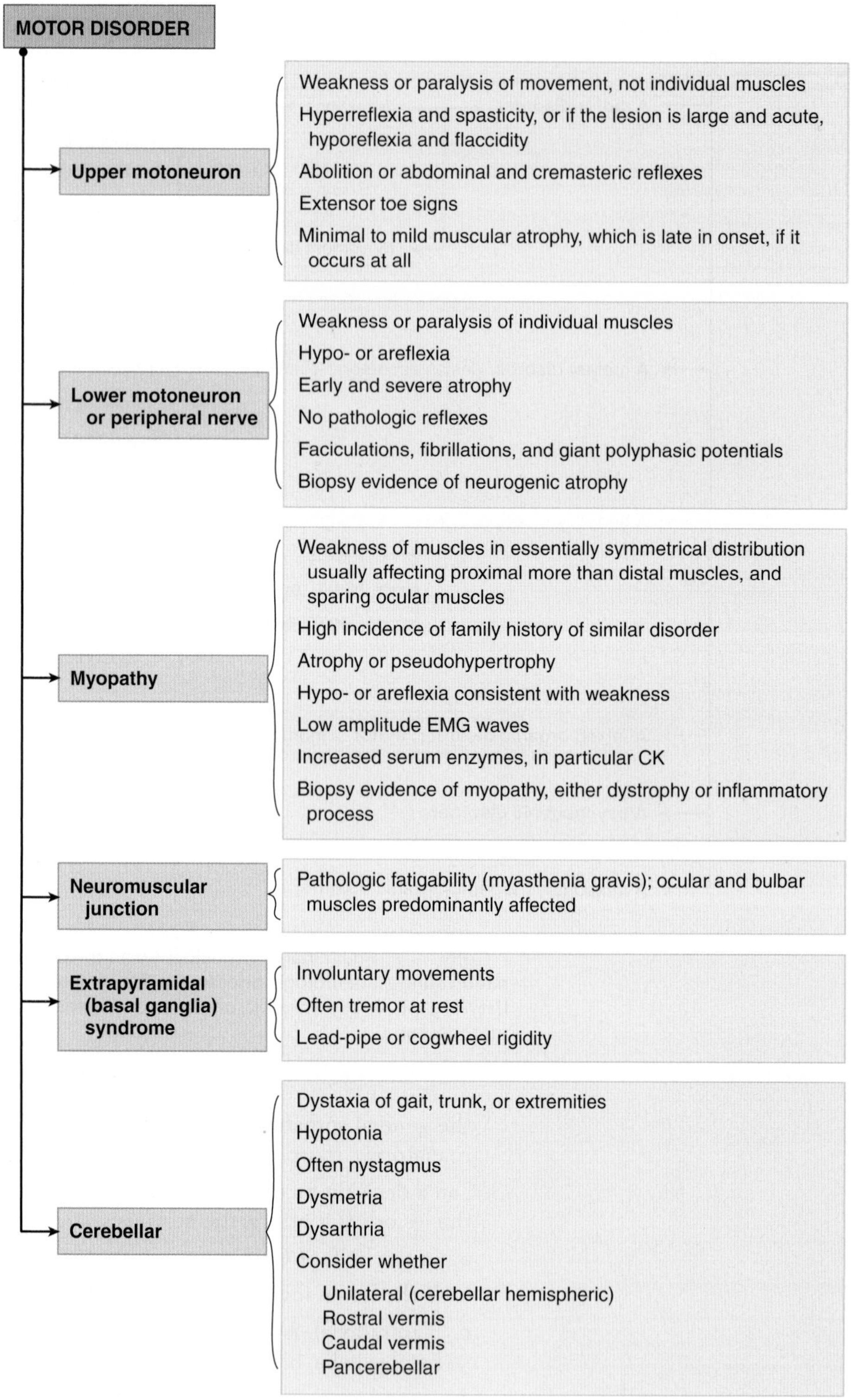
MOTOR DISORDER
Upper motoneuron
Weakness or paralysis of movement, not individual muscles
Hyperreflexia and spasticity, or if the lesion is large and acute, hyporeflexia and flaccidity
Abolition or abdominal and cremasteric reflexes
Extensor toe signs
Minimal to mild muscular atrophy, which is late in onset, if it occurs at all
Lower motoneuron or peripheral nerve
Weakness or paralysis of individual muscles
Hypo- or areflexia
Early and severe atrophy
No pathologic reflexes
Faciculations, fibrillations, and giant polyphasic potentials
Biopsy evidence of neurogenic atrophy
Myopathy
Weakness of muscles in essentially symmetrical distribution usually affecting proximal more than distal muscles, and sparing ocular muscles
High incidence of family history of similar disorder
Atrophy or pseudohypertrophy
Hypo- or areflexia consistent with weakness
Low amplitude EMG waves
Increased serum enzymes, in particular CK
Biopsy evidence of myopathy, either dystrophy or inflammatory process
Neuromuscular junction
Pathologic fatigability (myasthenia gravis); ocular and bulbar muscles predominantly affected
Extrapyramidal (basal ganglia) syndrome
Involuntary movements
Often tremor at rest
Lead-pipe or cogwheel rigidity
Cerebellar
Dystaxia of gait, trunk, or extremities
Hypotonia
Often nystagmus
Dysmetria
Dysarthria
Consider whether
Unilateral (cerebellar hemispheric)
Rostral vermis
Caudal vermis
Pancerebellar

FIGURE 15-3. Consider these loci as possible lesion sites if the patient has symptoms and signs suggesting an organic disorder of the motor system. CK = creatine kinase; EMG = electromyographic.

F. What is the lesion or the disease (Table 15-3, question 3)?

Having hypothesized the neuronal system, or systems, involved, and the lesion site, the Ex next has to hypothesize *what* the lesion is. For this purpose, systematically think through the entities shown in Fig. 15-8. Then state a provisional diagnosis according to the principle of parsimony: the simplest diagnosis that will explain the signs and symptoms.

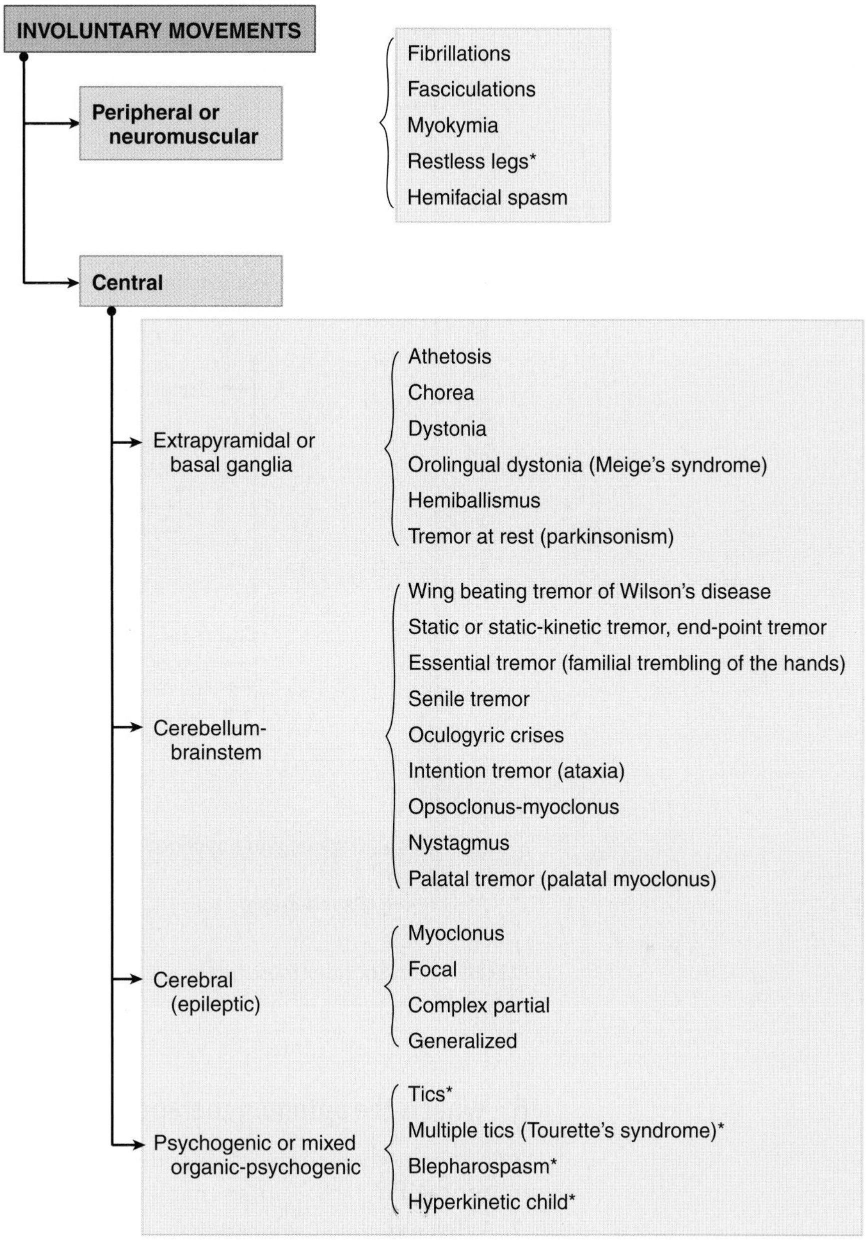

*Pathophysiology unclear disorder classified more or less arbitrarily

FIGURE 15-4. Consider these loci as possible lesion sites if the patient has an involuntary movement disorder.

G. What is the optimum diagnostic management (Table 15-3, question 4)?

What tests, clinical or laboratory, will confirm or reject the provisional diagnosis and establish the final diagnosis?

1. The explicitly stated provisional diagnosis provides the basis to generate a differential diagnosis list. The Ex selects any further clinical tests that will best affirm or deny the provisional diagnosis or point to another diagnosis. Having exhausted all clinical tests, the Ex selects laboratory tests according to these principles:
   a. Select the one or two *best* tests to support or reject the provisional diagnosis.
   b. Given tests of approximately equal clinical value, select the simplest, safest, and cheapest ones, but never curtail the investigation in the sole interest of "cost containment." Failure to diagnose a diagnosable disease is the costliest mistake of all.
   c. When faced with a hopeless or untreatable disorder, take all reasonable steps to exclude a treatable disorder.
2. To select the most appropriate laboratory tests, review the possible ones listed in Table 13-1.

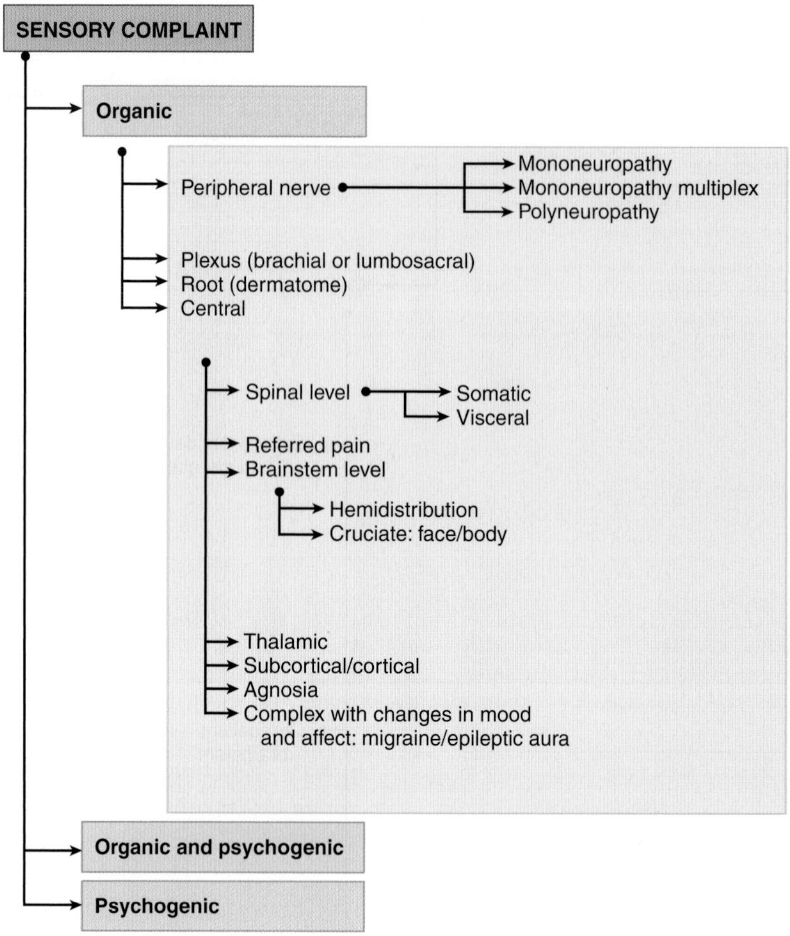

FIGURE 15-5. Consider these loci as possible lesion sites if the patient has a sensory complaint.

H. What is the optimum therapeutic management (Table 15-3, question 5)?

1. State the therapeutic goals and how to meet them. Just what can you hope to do for the Pt?
2. What emotional, educational, or socioeconomic perils does the Pt face because of the illness? What agencies—lay, rehabilitative, vocational, or governmental—might help?

I. What is the optimum preventative management (Table 15-3, question 6)?

1. Having identified the Pt's illness, the Ex has to identify other persons at risk. How can they be reached and offered prophylaxis? Consider for Pts with environmentally induced, contagious or infectious, or hereditary diseases.
2. Follow the Pt to ensure that your final diagnosis is indeed final and that the Pt's subsequent course continues to confirm its finality.

V. A PRÉCIS FOR SUCCESS IN THE NEUROLOGIC EXAMINATION

A. Attitudes for success in the neurologic examination

1. **Maintain professionalism:** Accept neutrally, as purely clinical phenomena, every behavior and every revelation made by the Pt. If you react emotionally to the Pt, you lose the objective judgment required to make correct clinical decisions.

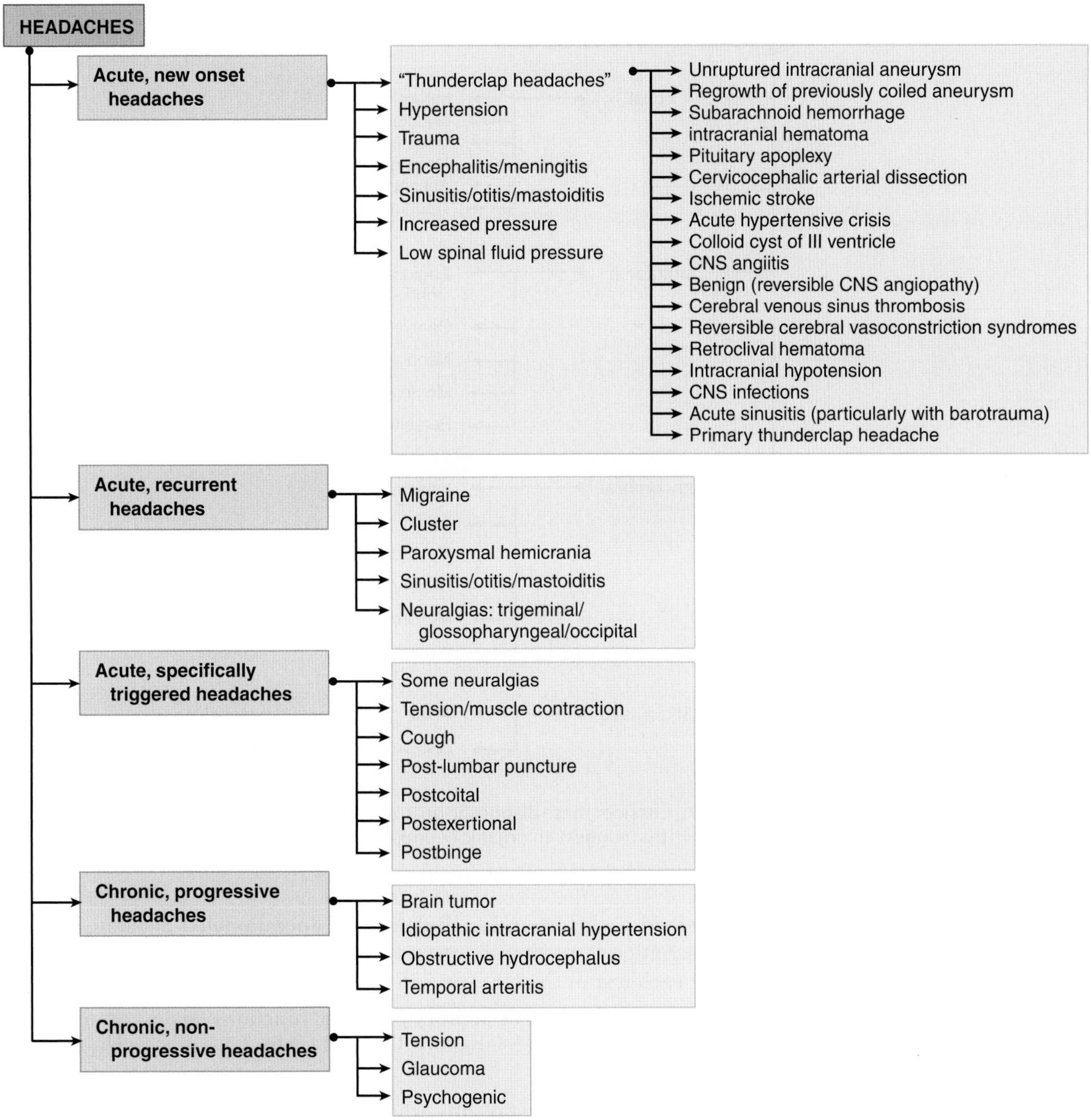

FIGURE 15-6. Consider these diagnostic possibilities if the patient has headaches. A-V = arteriovenous.

2. **Expect the abnormal:** By expecting every finding to be abnormal, you will do a much more vigilant examination than if you expect normality.
3. **Enjoy the NE:** Make the NE a game of friendly challenges to maintain the interest of both yourself and Pt in the outcome of each test. "Let's see how light a touch you can feel?" Or "How soft a sound you can hear." "Hold your hands out in front and let's see how still you can keep them." In testing strength, "Do your best, don't let me win," etc.

B. Overall principles for performance of the neurologic examination

1. **Do an organized NE:** A disorganized examination is the most common error of all. Correct it by laying out your instruments in order of use and proceeding rostrocaudally, doing the head and cranial nerve examination, motor examination, and sensory examination in order (see the Standard NE at the start of the text).
2. **Ensure the Pt's comfort and safety during each test.**

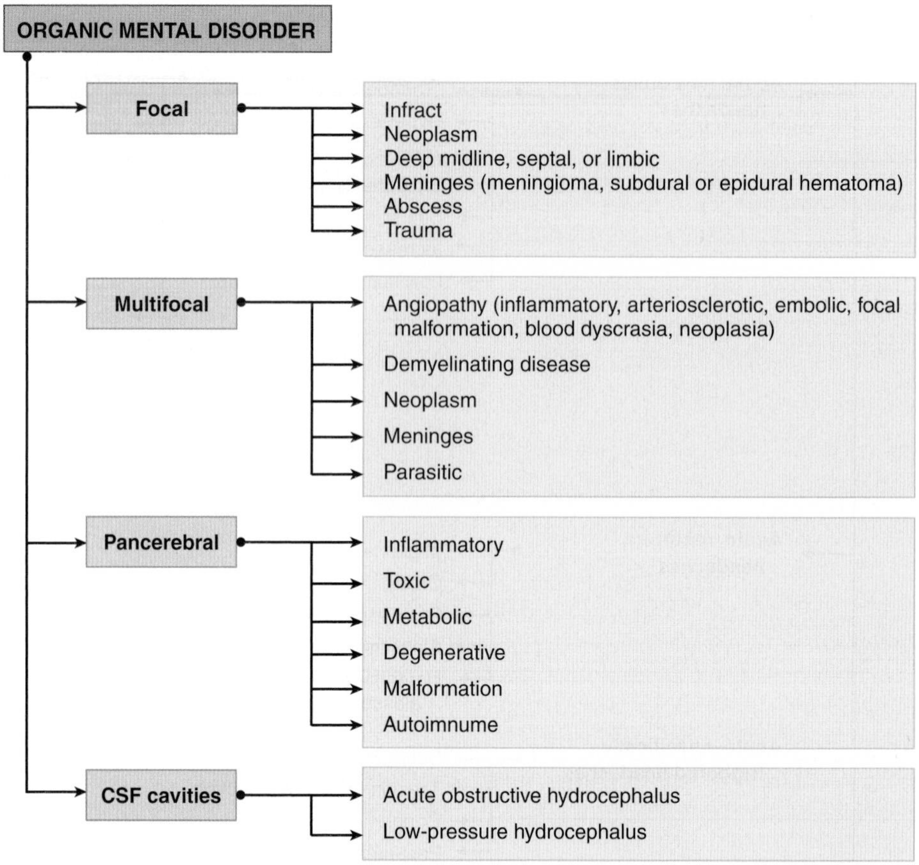

FIGURE 15-7. Consider these diagnostic possibilities if the patient has mental, emotional, or intellectual deficits that suggest an organic neurologic disorder.

3. **Understand each test and each definition operationally:** Separate observation and description from interpretation. If you understand the operation and the purpose of each test of the NE, you will interpret the findings correctly.
4. **Titrate, or match, the Pt's sensory or motor functions against yours, whenever possible:** Titrate or match visual fields, visual acuity, vibration and hearing thresholds, and strength.
5. **Quantify or scale the test results, whenever possible:** Measure circumferences of the head and extremities. Scale dysfunctions as minimal, mild, moderate, or severe, or enumerate on a scale from 0 to 4+.
6. **Think circuitry:** Visualize each neuroanatomic circuit as you test it. Unless you review circuitry daily, you forget it. If you find a neurologic abnormality, review the neighborhood signs that should accompany it by visualizing the conjunction of the circuits of the nervous system and test for these neighborhood signs. If you suspect a CNS lesion, actually draw a cross section of the CNS at the level of the suspected lesion and locate and label the clinically relevant nuclei and tracts. If you suspect a lesion of the PNS, draw the course of the relevant nerve.
7. **Consider whether any unusual finding is a normal variation that simply reflects the genetic background of the Pt:** Commonly, the Ex fails to call in and examine the entire family to decide about pseudopapilledema, the OFC, height of the arch of the foot, facial features, overall somatotype, etc.
8. **Consider whether any finding preexisted:** Ptosis, VI nerve palsy, anisocoria, hemiplegia, and atrophy. This precaution is especially important in examining the comatose Pt when a preexisting finding, such as anisocoria, may mislead you. Get old photographs or family videos.
9. **Extend the basic NE when required:** Reproduce triggering factors: hyperventilation, fatigability during exercise, dizziness on change of position, or trouble in swallowing. Have the Pt return when symptomatic and repeat the tests.

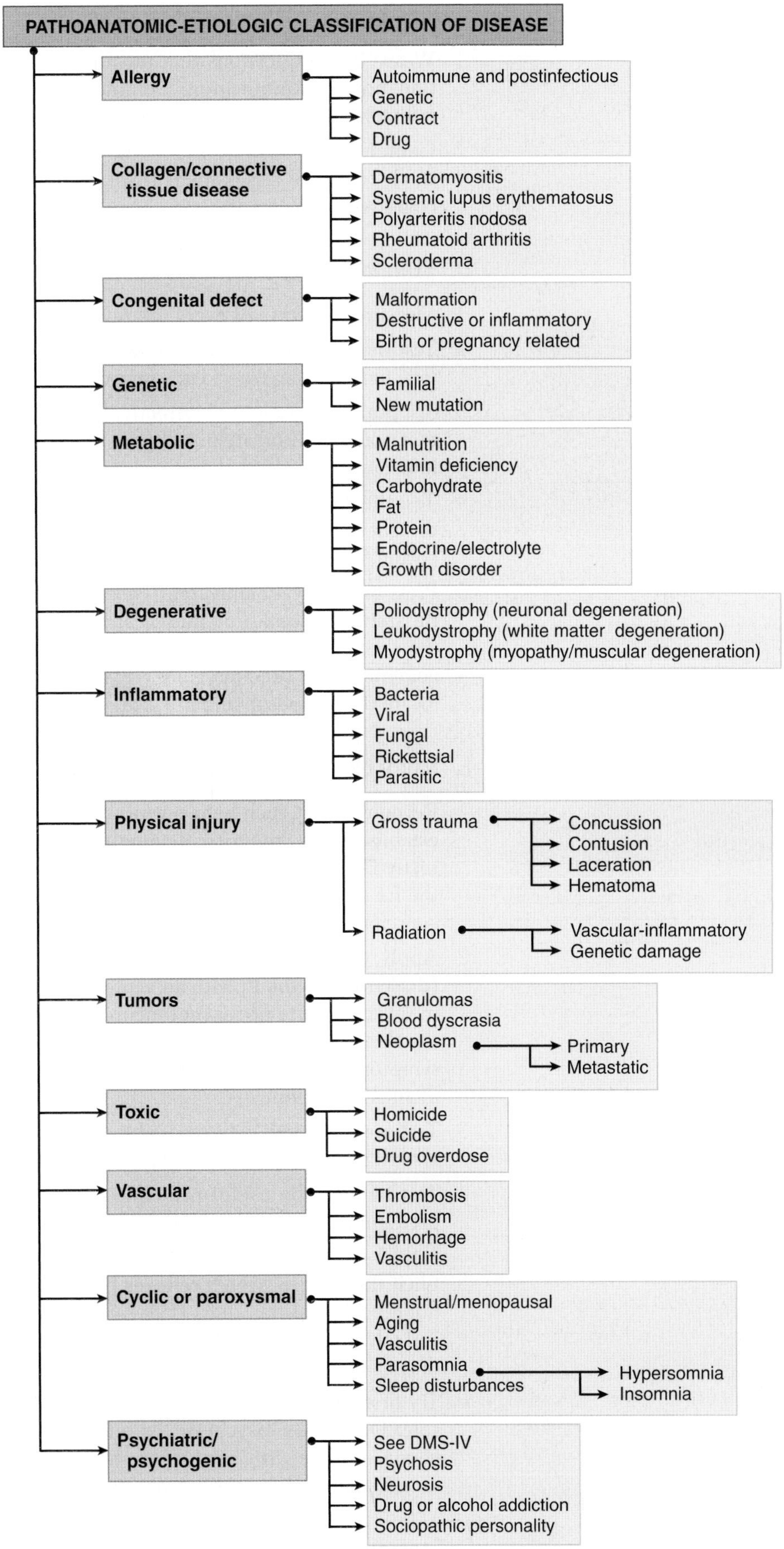

FIGURE 15-8. Brief pathoanatomic and etiologic classification of disease. Review this dendrogram systematically for each patient to generate the gamut of etiologic possibilities that may cause the clinical findings. The branching of the dendrogram vertically and to the right can be continued almost endlessly. DSM-IV = *Diagnostic and Statistical Manual,* 4th ed.

C. The mental status examination

1. **Weave in the questions that test the sensorium skillfully, as ordinary conversation, not as an inquisition:** Do not ask the *who, where, when,* and *what* questions in machine-gun style, except in an acute head injury.
2. **Complete the Mini-Mental-State Examination (MMSE) battery and the Montreal Cognitive Assessment (MoCA) test, if the history raises the question of cognitive impairment.**

D. Examination of the cranial nerves and head

1. **Measure the OFC of every infant.**
2. **Test the visual fields on the diagonals, not on the meridians:** Testing on the vertical or horizontal meridians may entirely miss a quadrantic defect (Fig. 3-13).
3. **Test pupilloconstriction correctly:** Darken the room, ask the Pt to fixate on a distant point to eliminate pupilloconstriction from accommodation, and flash a light into each eye separately from the side. Then do the swinging flashlight test.
4. **Test the corneal reflex from the side:** Bring the cotton wisp in from the side, out of sight of the Pt's vision, to avoid a visually induced blink response. Don't use the cotton tip of an applicator stick (no sticks around the eyes).
5. **Press on the zygomatic arch (cheekbone), not on the jaw, to test the strength of the sternocleidomastoid muscle and other rotators of the head:** Direct pressure on the cheekbone tests the head rotators without working through the lateral pterygoid muscles. If the pterygoids are weak, strong lateral pressure on the jaw may dislocate the temporomandibular joint, especially in elderly and edentulous Pts.

E. Motor examination

1. **Recognize that each behavior produced by the conscious or the unconscious Pt establishes the integrity of some neuroanatomic circuit:** By observing and correctly interpreting all spontaneous and elicited behaviors of the unconscious Pt, the Ex can test most of the sensory and motor circuits that can be tested in the conscious Pt.
2. **Apply the concept of deficit and release phenomena and of neural shock (diaschisis) to the Pt with an acute neurologic lesion:** Neural shock (depression) means that acute upper motoneuron lesions manifest only by deficit signs, not by the classic release signs as with chronic lesions. Because of neural shock, signs and symptoms temporarily extend beyond those expected by the actual anatomic size of an acute lesion.
3. **Test every Pt's gait, when possible.** Nothing tests the integrity of the Pt's nervous system so quickly (Chapter 8, Section VI), but Exs often fail to test it.
4. **Test strength by use of principles:** Review the length-strength law, the law of predominant strength of the antigravity muscles, and the law of matching the Pt and Ex muscle to muscle, particularly in testing finger strength (Fig. 7-3).
5. **Elicit the muscle stretch reflexes by a whiplash swing, not a peck.** Be a swinger, not a pecker, of hammers (Fig. 7-5). If no reflexes are elicited, try repositioning and relaxing the part, altering the pressure or tension on the tendon, and use Jendrassik's reinforcement.
6. **Try first to elicit the extensor toe sign from the lateral side of the foot, not the sole:** Demented, psychotic, or retarded Pts, the elderly and often the ticklish young, or those with painful peripheral neuropathies resist the discomfort of plantar stimulation but may tolerate pressure on the lateral side of the foot.

F. Sensory examination

1. **Establish good communication:** Inform the Pt of the nature of the stimulus and the response to make. "Which is the sharpest, number 1 or number 2?" "Is the toe up or down?" etc.

2. **Isolate the modality to be tested:** Conceal the test object from sight or perception by any modality other than the one being tested.
3. **Monitor the Pt's attention and reliability:** The Ex sometimes withholds a stimulus when the Pt expects it, and forewarns the Pt of that possibility.
4. **Test temperature discrimination rather than pain around the face and in children:** Test temperature discrimination by the tuning-fork and finger methods shown in Fig. 10-4. Pain and temperature sensations test the same pathways. In this time of acquired immunodeficiency syndrome, the fewer the pinpricks, the better. Testing temperature discrimination is far more comfortable for every Pt. Children will not accept pain testing, but children as young as 3 years will play the temperature game.

G. Closure (cloture) of the neurologic examination

1. **Write out the NE informatively or use a check list to state what you have actually tested and found to be negative or positive** (Table 15-1): At least your notes should enable the reader to find out about the Pt's mental state and whether the Pt can sit, stand, walk, talk, breathe, see, hear, and feel normally. I'd rather you simply state that than write out every negative finding, but some negatives are important as exclusionary evidence.
2. **Write a three-line summary:** If you have come to grips with the clinical problem, you can write it out in no more than three lines, no matter how complicated. **Your ability to summarize the findings is the best single test of your ability to function as a physician.** "This is a 64-year-old hypertensive African American salesman who had the acute onset of headache, unresponsiveness, eyes deviated to the left, flaccid right hemiplegia, and nuchal rigidity." From that summary, the probable diagnosis leaps out at you: left hypertensive putaminal hemorrhage probably extending into the ventricle and subarachnoid space.
3. **Always recite the diagnostic catechism** (Table 15-3): If tempted to make a nonorganic diagnosis, review the list of organic diseases commonly misdiagnosed (Table 14-6).
4. Review the pathoanatomic and etiologic classifications of disease to ensure that you have considered the gamut of possible causes for the clinical findings (Fig. 15-8).

VI. COMFORT: THE ULTIMATE OBJECTIVE OF EVERY CONTACT BETWEEN PATIENT AND PHYSICIAN

For hundreds, even thousands of years, physicians have understood the goals of the medical model and have expressed them in aphorisms. The two given here apparently arose in the Middle Ages, but their exact authorship is unknown. Here is the first:

> A painless examination
> A complete cure
> Leaving no blemish behind

And here is the other:

> The physician can only rarely cure,
> Can sometimes palliate,
> But can always give comfort.

At the end of every Pt-physician contact, the Pt should at least feel benefited and comforted, even when the physician cannot cure or even palliate. Comfort comes not from false optimism, pity, patronizing pap, or condescending platitudes, but from empathy and competence. Each Pt-physician contact remains incomplete, the ring remains open, and the physician remains but a technocrat, until the Pt feels this beneficence.

Learning Objectives for Chapter 15

I. THE ROUTINE SCREENING NEUROLOGICAL EXAMINATION WHEN THE PATIENT HAS NO SYMPTOMS SUGGESTING NEUROLOGIC DISEASE

1. List the parts of the Standard NE that you can electively omit for the screening examination.
2. Demonstrate the 45-seconds examination of the motor cranial nerves (Table 6-8).
3. Describe and demonstrate the screening examination for strength.
4. Demonstrate the directional scratch test that can be used as a substitute for more time-consuming dorsal column tests in the screening examination.
5. Describe what to include in your notes for a screening NE (Table 15-1).

II. THE CONCEPT OF "SOFT" NEUROLOGIC SIGNS

1. Define a soft sign.
2. List several examples of dysmorphic soft signs (Table 15-2).
3. Explain the etiologic implications of multiple dysmorphic soft signs.

III. THE CONCEPT OF "FALSE" LOCALIZING SIGNS

1. Define a false localizing sign.
2. Describe some causes of false localizing signs in the CNS.
3. Explain how hydrocephalus can cause false localizing signs.

IV. CLOSING THE NEUROLOGIC EXAMINATION WHEN THE PATIENT HAS SYMPTOMS OR SIGNS SUGGESTING NEUROLOGIC DISEASE

1. Discuss the importance of posing diagnostic hypotheses during the history and the examination.
2. Explain how the provisional diagnosis links the clinical input from the history and physical examination with the output or result for the Pt.
3. Define *cloture* as a technical term and explain its application to the encounter between Pt and Ex.
4. State the six questions of the diagnostic catechism (Table 15-3).
5. Explain the meaning of each of the six questions of the diagnostic catechism.
6. Describe how and why to use differential diagnostic dendrograms to analyze the Pt's presenting complaint (Figs. 15-2 through 15-8).
7. Enumerate the major pathoanatomic and etiologic categories of disease to consider in the differential diagnosis. (If you wish, make a dendrogram and extend it vertically and horizontally to the right; Fig. 15-8.)
8. State the principles involved in selecting laboratory tests.

V. A PRÉCIS FOR SUCCESS IN THE NEUROLOGIC EXAMINATION

1. Describe some techniques for making a friendly contest or game out of the NE that maintains the interest of the Ex and the Pt.
2. Describe some techniques for ensuring an orderly NE.
3. Describe the meaning of "think circuitry" in trying to localize a lesion from the symptoms and signs.
4. Explain how to use the *who, where, when,* and *what* questions in the mental status examination.
5. Describe the correct technique for examining the visual fields, pupilloconstriction, and the corneal reflex.

Learning Objectives for Chapter 15

6. Describe where to press with your hand to test the strength of the sternocleidomastoid muscle.
7. Explain the significance of any spontaneous or elicited movement observed in an unconscious Pt.
8. Discuss the concept of deficit and release phenomena in the interpretation of the clinical signs of acute and chronic CNS lesions.
9. Recite the main principles or laws for clinical testing of muscular strength.
10. Demonstrate the correct method of swinging a reflex hammer (Fig. 7-5).
11. Explain why in some Pts the Ex should begin testing the planter reflex by stimulating the lateral side rather than the sole of the foot.
12. Explain how to optimize the sensory examination.
13. Describe the most comfortable method of screening for interruption of the pain and temperature pathways.
14. Explain why a summary of no more than three lines of the clinical features of a Pt is essential to the cloture.
15. In a single word, state the physician's goal for every encounter with a Pt, even when unable to cure the Pt.

INDEX

NOTE: Page numbers followed by *f* and *t* indicate figures and tables.

C